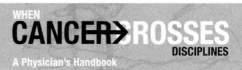

WHEN
CANCER➤CROSSES
DISCIPLINES
A Physician's Handbook

diagnosis

lifestyle modifications

surgery

chemotherapy

radiotherapy

genetics

endocrine

complementary therapies

medicine

Editors

Monica Robotin
Cancer Council NSW and University of Sydney, Australia

Ian Olver
Cancer Council Australia

Afaf Girgis
University of Newcastle, Australia

ICP

Imperial College Press

Published by

Imperial College Press
57 Shelton Street
Covent Garden
London WC2H 9HE

Distributed by

World Scientific Publishing Co. Pte. Ltd.
5 Toh Tuck Link, Singapore 596224
USA office: 27 Warren Street, Suite 401-402, Hackensack, NJ 07601
UK office: 57 Shelton Street, Covent Garden, London WC2H 9HE

British Library Cataloguing-in-Publication Data
A catalogue record for this book is available from the British Library.

WHEN CANCER CROSSES DISCIPLINES
A Physician's Handbook

ISBN-13 978-1-84816-364-5
ISBN-10 1-84816-364-9

Typeset by Stallion Press
Email: enquiries@stallionpress.com

Printed by FuIsland Offset Printing (S) Pte Ltd, Singapore

Contents

Contributors   xi

Foreword   xxv

SECTION I: CANCER PREVENTION

Cancer and the Epidemiologist

1.   Cancer and Tobacco: Its Effects on Individuals   1
     and Populations
     Bernard W. Stewart, Patricia F. Cotter
     and James F. Bishop

2.   Reviewing the Evidence on the Effectiveness   33
     of Smoking Cessation Interventions
     Nicholas Zwar

3.   Diet, Physical Activity and Cancer —   49
     The Epidemiological Evidence
     Erica L. James, Victoria M. Flood, Bruce Armstrong
     and Fiona Stacey

4.   Sun Exposure, Vitamin D and Cancer   79
     Bruce Armstrong and Anne Kricker

5. Oral Contraceptives, Hormone Replacement   111
    Therapy, and Cancers of the Female
    Reproductive System
    Karen Canfell and Emily Banks

6. Involuntary Exposures — Can Knowledge Keep   131
    Pace with Perceptions?
    Bernard W. Stewart

SECTION II: INTERDISCIPLINARY MANAGEMENT
ISSUES IN CANCER TREATMENT

IIa: Beyond Cancer Treatment

7. Diagnostic Dilemmas During and After   161
    Chemotherapy Treatment
    Ian N. Olver

8. Acute and Late Radiation Therapy Effects   179
    Sandro V. Porceddu, Jarad M. Martin,
    Brian O'Sullivan and Michael Fay

9. Oncological Emergencies: Diagnosis   201
    and Management
    Desmond Yip and Nicole Gorddard

10. Managing Cancer in Pregnancy   231
    Belinda E. Kiely and Kelly-Anne Phillips

11. Addressing the Nutritional Needs of Patients   267
    Undergoing Cancer Treatment — A Dietitian's View
    Judy Bauer, Jane Read and Kathy Chapman

12. Beyond Conventional Cancer Treatments: 285
    The Use of Complementary Therapies During
    Cancer Treatment: Implications for Clinicians
    Stephen J. Clarke, Andrew J. McLachlan,
    Darrin Brown, Stephen Carbonara and Rachel Kissane

13. What Matters to Patients and Carers   317
    Kendra J. Sundquist and Monica C. Robotin

IIb: Cancer and the Surgeon

14. Neurosurgical Involvement with Cancer Patients   343
    Mark A. J. Dexter and Juyong Cheong

15. Cancer and the Thoracic Surgeon   367
    Edmund Kassis and Stephen C. Yang

16. Cancer and the Oesophageal Surgeon   395
    Urs Zingg, Reginald V. Lord and David I. Watson

17. Abdominal Emergencies in Cancer Patients: 421
    Diagnosis and Management
    Brian Badgwell and Barry Feig

18. Peri-operative Management of Patients with GI   439
    Malignancy: The Interdisciplinary Approach
    Ross C. Smith

19. Management Challenges Following Rectal   465
    Cancer Treatment
    Margaret Schnitzler

20. Management of Nutritional Issues After Major   487
    Pancreatic Resections
    Nam Q. Nguyen, Neil D. Merrett and Andrew V. Biankin

21. Management Decisions in Primary and Secondary   507
    Liver Cancer
    Mark E. Brooke-Smith and Robert T. A. Padbury

22. Cancer and the Gynaecological Oncologist   547
    D. E. Marsden

23. Orthopedic Emergencies in Oncology   569
    Valerae O. Lewis and Jeffrey T. Luna

24. Recognition, Treatment and Management 603
of Post-cancer Treatment Lymphoedema
Neil Piller

25. Diagnostic and Management Challenges Following 627
Radical Prostatectomy
Manish I. Patel

26. Plastic and Reconstructive Surgery in Oncological 647
Surgery
Sean Nicklin and Mohammad Rahnavardi

27. Cancer and the ENT Surgeon 673
*Timothy P. Makeham, Julia Crawford, Mark Smith,
Meville Da Cruz and Carsten E. Palme*

IIc: Cancer and the Physician

28. Thyroid Cancer and the Endocrinologist 703
Nirusha Arnold and Howard C. Smith

29. The Effects of Cancer Therapy on Gonadal 729
Function and Fertility
Howard C. Smith

30. Cancer and Thrombosis 753
Jerry Koutts

31. Haematological Abnormalities in Cancer Patients 783
Philip J. Crispin and Ian W. Prosser

32. Managing the Patient with Chronic Viral Hepatitis 813
Receiving Chemotherapy
Venessa Pattullo and Jacob George

33. Management of Malignant Gastrointestinal Tract 833
Obstruction
Eric Y. T. Lee, Vu Kwan and Michael J. Bourke

34. Cancer and the Heart: The Good, the Bad   859
    and the Ugly
    Liza Thomas and David Richards

35. No-Man's Land: Between Paediatric and Adult   885
    Medical Oncology
    Lisa M. Orme, Susan Palmer and David Thomas

36. Cancer and the Geriatrician — Managing Cancer   907
    in Older People
    Robert J. Prowse

37. Cancer and the General Practitioner. The Role   917
    of the GP in Cancer Diagnosis and Treatment
    Moyez Jiwa

IId: Cancer and the Geneticist

38. Genetic Testing for Cancer Susceptibility: 931
    How and When?
    Judy Kirk

39. Management of Women at High Familial Risk   941
    of Breast and Ovarian Cancer
    Kathryn M. Field and Kelly-Anne Phillips

40. Management of High Genetic Risk Bowel Cancer   969
    Barbara Leggett

41. Hereditary Mutations and Cancer Management   981
    Alison H. Trainer and Robyn Ward

SECTION III: SURVIVING CANCER

IIIa: Survivorship Issues

42. Cancer and the Psycho-Oncologist. Psychosocial   1005
    Well-Being of Cancer Survivors
    Jane Turner, Katharine Hodgkinson and Allison Boyes

43. Understanding and Managing Changes in Survivor   1023
    Identity and Relationships
    Paul Y. Cheung and Ian H. Kerridge

44. Survivors of Childhood Cancer: Issues and   1047
    Challenges
    Carmen L. Wilson, Richard J. Cohn and Lesley J. Ashton

45. The Benefits of Nutrition and Physical Activity   1077
    for Cancer Survivors
    Kathy Chapman, Erica L. James, Jane Read
    and Judy Bauer

IIIb: Cancer, Palliative Care and End of Life Issues

46. Palliative and Supportive Care   1099
    Geoffrey Mitchell and David C. Currow

47. Cancer Care and General Practice Palliative Care   1121
    Paul Mercer

48. Spiritual and Existential Issues at the End of Life   1139
    Bruce Rumbold

Index   1161

Contributors

Bruce Armstrong
School of Public Health, University of Sydney
Sydney, NSW, Australia

Nirusha Arnold
Department of Diabetes and Endocrinology
Westmead Hospital, Sydney, NSW, Australia

Lesley J. Ashton
Children's Cancer Institute Australia for Medical Research
Randwick, Sydney, NSW, Australia

Brian Badgwell
University of Arkansas for Medical Sciences
Winthrop P. Rockefeller Cancer Institute, USA

Emily Banks
The 45 and Up Study
National Centre for Epidemiology and Population Health
The Australian National University
Canberra, ACT, Australia

Judy Bauer
The Wesley Hospital, Brisbane, Australia

Andrew V. Biankin
Department of Upper Gastrointestinal Surgery
Bankstown Hospital
Bankstown, NSW
Cancer Research Program, Garvan Institute of Medical Research
Sydney, NSW, Australia

James F. Bishop
The Cancer Institute NSW
Alexandria, NSW, Australia

Michael J. Bourke
Westmead Hospital, Sydney West Area Health Service
Westmead, NSW, Australia

Allison Boyes
Centre for Health Research and Psycho-oncology
Cancer Council NSW,
University of Newcastle
    and Hunter Medical Research Institute, NSW, Australia

Mark E. Brooke-Smith
Flinders Medical Centre/Royal Adelaide Hospital
Bedford Park, SA, Australia

Darrin Brown
Faculty of Pharmacy, University of Sydney
Centre for Education and Research on Ageing
Concord Hospital, NSW, Australia

Karen Canfell
Cancer Epidemiology Research Unit
Cancer Council NSW
Sydney, NSW, Australia

Stephen Carbonara
Faculty of Pharmacy, University of Sydney
Centre for Education and Research on Ageing
Concord Hospital, NSW, Australia

Kathy Chapman
Cancer Council NSW
Sydney, NSW, Australia

Juyong Cheong
Department of Neurosurgery
Westmead Hospital
Westmead, NSW, Australia

Paul Y. Cheung
Centre for Values, Ethics and the Law in Medicine
Faculty of Medicine
The University of Sydney, NSW, Australia

Stephen J. Clarke
Faculty of Medicine, University of Sydney
Cancer Pharmacology Research Group
Concord Hospital, NSW, Australia

Richard J. Cohn
Centre for Children's Cancer and Blood Disorders
Sydney Children's Hospital
Children's Cancer Institute Australia for Medical Research
Randwick, Sydney, NSW, Australia

Patricia F. Cotter
Cancer Prevention Division
The Cancer Institute NSW
Alexandria, NSW, Australia

Julia Crawford
Department of Otolaryngology Head Neck Surgery
University of Sydney, Westmead Hospital
Westmead, NSW, Australia

Phillip J. Crispin
Haematology Department, The Canberra Hospital
Australian National University Medical School
ACT, Australia

David C. Currow
Department of Palliative and Supportive Services
Flinders University, Adelaide, SA, Australia

Meville Da Cruz
Department of Otolaryngology Head Neck Surgery
University of Sydney, Westmead Hospital
Westmead, NSW, Australia

Mark A. J. Dexter
Department of Neurosurgery
Westmead Hospital
Westmead, NSW, Australia

Michael Fay
Department of Radiation Oncology
Royal Brisbane and Women's Hospital, Brisbane

Barry Feig
University of Texas M.D. Anderson Cancer Center
Houston, Texas, USA

Kathryn M. Field
Division of Hematology and Medical Oncology
Peter MacCallum Cancer Centre, VIC, Australia

Victoria M. Flood
Public Health Nutrition Group
Institute of Obesity, Nutrition and Exercise
University of Sydney, NSW, Australia

Department of Ophthalmology, University of Sydney
Centre for Vision Research, Westmead Millennium Institute
Westmead Hospital, NSW, Australia

Jacob George
Storr Liver Unit, Westmead Millennium Institute
University of Sydney, Westmead Hospital
Westmead, NSW, Australia

Nicole Gorddard
Medical Oncology, The Canberra Hospital
ANU Medical School
Australian National University, Australia

Katharine Hodgkinson
Department of Gynecological Cancer
Westmead Hospital
Westmead, NSW, Australia

Erica L. James
Centre for Health Research and Psycho-Oncology (CHeRP)
Cancer Council NSW
University of Newcastle
    and Hunter Medical Research Institute
NSW, Australia

Moyez Jiwa
Curtin Health Innovation Research Institute
Curtin University of Technology
Perth, WA, Australia

Edmund Kassis
The Department of Thoracic and Cardiovascular Surgery
The University of Texas M.D. Anderson Cancer Center
Houston, Texas, USA

Ian H. Kerridge
Centre for Values, Ethics and the Law in Medicine
Faculty of Medicine
The University of Sydney, Australia

Belinda E. Kiely
Division of Haematology and Medical Oncology
Peter MacCallum Cancer Centre
East Melbourne, VIC, Australia

Judy Kirk
Familial Cancer Service
Westmead Hospital
Westmead, NSW, Australia

Rachel Kissane
Faculty of Pharmacy, University of Sydney
Centre for Education and Research on Ageing
Concord Hospital, Sydney, NSW, Australia

Jerry Koutts
Institute of Clinical Pathology and Medical Research
Westmead Hospital, Westmead, NSW
Faculty of Medicine, University of Sydney, Australia

Anne Kricker
School of Public Health, University of Sydney
NSW, Australia

Vu Kwan
Department of Gastroenterology and Hepatology
Westmead Hospital, Sydney West Area Health Service
Westmead, NSW, Australia

Eric Y. T. Lee
Gastroenterology Department, St Michael's Hospital
Toronto, Ontario, Canada

Barbara Leggett
Royal Brisbane and Womens Hospital
Herston, Queensland, Australia

Valerae O. Lewis
Department of Orthopaedic Oncology
The University of Texas M. D. Anderson Cancer Center
Houston, Texas, USA

Reginald V. Lord
Department of Surgery
University of New South Wales
St. Vincent's Hospital
Darlinghurst, NSW, Australia

Jeffrey T. Luna
Department of Orthopaedic Oncology
The University of Texas M. D. Anderson Cancer Center
Houston, Texas, USA

Timothy P. Makeham
Department of Otolaryngology Head Neck Surgery
University of Sydney, Westmead Hospital
Westmead, NSW, Australia

D. E. Marsden
University of New South Wales
Gynaecological Cancer Centre
Royal Hospital for Women
Randwick, NSW, Australia

Jarad M. Martin
Radiation Oncology Queensland
St. Andrew's Cancer Care Centre
Department of Medicine, The University of Queensland
Faculty of Science, University of Southern Queensland
Australia

Andrew J. McLachlan
Faculty of Pharmacy, University of Sydney
Centre for Education and Research on Ageing
Concord Hospital, Sydney, NSW, Australia

Paul Mercer
Silky Oaks Medical Practice
Manly, Brisbane
Queensland, Australia

Neil D. Merrett
Department of Upper Gastrointestinal Surgery
Bankstown Hospital
Cancer Research Program, Garvan Institute of Medical Research
Darlinghurst, Sydney, NSW, Australia

Geoffrey Mitchell
Department of General Practice
The University of Queensland
Brisbane, QLD, Australia

Nam Q. Nguyen
Department of Gastroenterology, Bankstown Hospital
Cancer Research Program, Garvan Institute of Medical Research
Darlinghurst, Sydney, NSW, Australia

Sean Nicklin
Department of Plastic Surgery, Prince of Wales Hospital
High St., Randwick, NSW, Australia

Ian N. Olver
Cancer Council Australia
Surry Hills, Sydney, NSW, Australia

Lisa M. Orme
Children's Cancer Centre
The Royal Children's Hospital
onTrac@PeterMac: Victorian Adolescent
    and Young Adult Cancer Service
Peter McCallum Cancer Centre
Melbourne, Australia

Brian O'Sullivan
Department of Radiation Oncology
University of Toronto, Canada
Princess Margaret Hospital, Toronto, Canada

Robert T. A. Padbury
Division of Surgical and Specialty Services
Flinders Medical Centre
Bedford Park, SA, Australia

Carsten E. Palme
Department of Otolaryngology Head Neck Surgery
University of Sydney, Westmead Hospital
Westmead, NSW, Australia

Susan Palmer
onTrac@PeterMac: Victorian Adolescent
    and Young Adult Cancer Service
Peter McCallum Cancer Centre
Melbourne, VIC, Australia

Manish I. Patel
University of Sydney, Westmead Hospital
Westmead, NSW, Australia

Venessa Pattullo
Storr Liver Unit, Westmead Millennium Institute
University of Sydney, Westmead Hospital
Westmead, NSW, Australia

Kelly-Anne Phillips
Division of Hematology and Medical Oncology
Peter MacCallum Cancer Centre
East Melbourne, VIC, Australia

Neil Piller
Lymphoedema Assessment Clinic, Flinders Surgical Oncology
Department of Surgery, Flinders Medical Centre
Bedford Park, SA, Australia

Sandro V. Porceddu
Division of Cancer Services
Princess Alexandra Hospital
Brisbane, Australia

The University of Queensland
School of Medicine
Queensland, Australia

Ian W. Prosser
Australian National University Medical School
Haematology Department, The Canberra Hospital
Woden, ACT, Australia

Robert J. Prowse
Royal Adelaide Hospital
North Terrace
Adelaide, SA, Australia

Mohammad Rahnavardi
Department of Plastic Surgery, Prince of Wales Hospital
Randwick, NSW, Australia

Jane Read
Fresh Nutrition Solutions
Sydney, Australia

David Richards
Cardiology Department
University of New South Wales
Liverpool Hospital
Liverpool, NSW, Australia

Monica C. Robotin
Cancer Council NSW
School of Public Health
The University of Sydney
NSW, Sydney, Australia

Bruce Rumbold
Palliative Care Unit, School of Public Health
La Trobe University, VIC, Australia

Margaret Schnitzler
Royal North Shore Hospital
University of Sydney
St. Leonards, NSW, Australia

Howard C. Smith
Department of Diabetes and Endocrinology
Westmead Fertility Centre
Westmead Hospital, NSW, Australia

Mark Smith
Department of Otolaryngology Head Neck Surgery
University of Sydney, Westmead Hospital
Westmead, NSW, Australia

Ross C. Smith
University of Sydney
Royal North Shore Hospital
St. Leonards, NSW, Australia

Fiona Stacey
Centre for Health Research and Psycho-Oncology (CHeRP)
The Cancer Council NSW
University of Newcastle
    and Hunter Medical Research Institute, NSW, Australia

Bernard W. Stewart
Faculty of Medicine, University of New South Wales
Cancer Control Program, South Eastern Sydney
    and Illawarra Public Health Unit
Randwick, NSW, Australia

Kendra J. Sundquist
Cancer Council NSW
Sydney, NSW, Australia

David Thomas
onTrac@PeterMac: Victorian Adolescent
    and Young Adult Cancer Service
Peter McCallum Cancer Centre
Melbourne, Australia

Liza Thomas
Cardiology Department
University of New South Wales
Liverpool Hospital
Liverpool, NSW, Australia

Alison H. Trainer
Prince of Wales Clinical School
Faculty of Medicine
University of New South Wales
Sydney, Australia

Jane Turner
The School of Medicine
The University of Queensland
Brisbane, Australia

Robyn Ward
Prince of Wales Clinical School
Faculty of Medicine
University of New South Wales
Sydney, Australia

David I. Watson
Department of Surgery, Flinders University
Hepatobiliary and Oesophagogastric Surgical Unit
Flinders Medical Centre
Bedford Park, SA, Australia

Carmen L. Wilson
Children's Cancer Institute Australia for Medical Research
Randwick, NSW, Australia

Stephen C. Yang
The Division of Thoracic Surgery
Department of Surgery
Johns Hopkins Medical Institutions
Baltimore, Maryland, USA

Desmond Yip
Medical Oncology, The Canberra Hospital
ANU Medical School, ACT
Australian National University, Australia

Urs Zingg
Hepatobiliary and Oesophagogastric Surgical Unit
Flinders Medical Centre
Bedford Park, SA, Australia

Nicholas Zwar
School of Public Health and Community Medicine
University of New South Wales
Sydney, Australia

Foreword

....

Oncology: Beyond the Oncologist

Oncology is an increasingly complex field with constant improvements in surgery, radiation energy and computer-based treatment planning, and emerging molecular therapeutics. Furthermore, advances in diagnostic and functional imaging, molecular genetics and pathology, and minimally invasive procedures performed by an array of surgical and non-surgical specialists, have led to more robust and refined interdisciplinary cancer care. Just as importantly, improved adjunctive therapies and supportive measures during and after cancer treatment now mandate greater involvement of non-oncology specialists. In this century, no single oncologist can manage all patient needs through the spectrum of prevention, diagnosis, treatment, supportive care, and survivorship.

This reference is of great value to all practitioners who care for patients in need of cancer prevention, screening, therapy, and survivorship care. In addition to the perspectives provided by expert oncologists, a large component of the book illustrates the important contributions of non-oncology consultants in optimizing survival and enhancing quality of life. The text is therefore partitioned into appropriate sections so the reader can quickly find practical advice for particular oncologic problems and comorbidities frequently encountered in these patients.

Required Reading

In addition to the specific subspecialty topics covered in this book, there are several important chapters which cut across all disciplines: *Cancer and the Epidemiologist, Cancer and the Geneticist, Cancer and Complementary Medicine, Cancer and the Psycho-Oncologist,* and *Cancer and the Palliative Care Specialist* provide important information for all caregivers and reading them is encouraged. *Cancer and the Epidemiologist* reviews our current knowledge about smoking, smoking cessation, and cancer, diet and cancer risk, and emerging data about vitamin D and hormone replacement in cancer risk and prevention. These topics are among the most frequently raised by patients and loved ones before and after a cancer diagnosis.

Second, *Cancer and the Geneticist* provides a snapshot of current evidence about genetic mutations which increase the risk of certain cancers. Moreover, this chapter gives us a window into the future of personalized cancer care: genetic testing to identify those who may harbor a mutation, which will increasingly require specific screening efforts and interventions (medical and surgical) to minimize cancer risk. It also suggests what is coming: therapy specifically designed for a given genetic mutation as the concept of synthetic lethality becomes more broadly appreciated. These strategies will certainly be a larger part of oncology in the 21st century and beyond. Third, while not necessarily embraced by all clinicians, *Cancer and Complementary Medicine* is a "must read". Having either a dismissive or uninformed attitude about complementary or integrative medicine will not serve our patients well and obtaining a working knowledge of the principles and evidence-basis for this discipline is strongly recommended.

Cancer and the Psycho-Oncologist and *Cancer and the Palliative Care Physician* are also essential reading. The physical and psychosocial problems facing cancer patients and survivors can be daunting, and often not fully appreciated by treating physicians. Sensitivity to these tribulations is inherent to high-quality care and it is the duty of all physicians to minimize suffering. Acknowledgement and management of pain, grief, and loss and open discussions at the end of life are responsibilities that must be shared, not delegated, and doing so helps our patients and ourselves.

Cancer Care in the 21st Century: The Information Age Meets Team Oncology

Most importantly, as our understanding of the molecular basis of neoplasia accelerates and our appreciation for the total care needs of our cancer patients grows, modern cancer care must be transformed. The boom in information technology has facilitated much of the revolution in oncology and must also be part of the solution to deliver sophisticated, high-quality, interdisciplinary care in small community centers and larger academic ones. How this is accomplished, who is involved, and what professional attributes are necessary to deliver this care cannot be answered directly by this reference. However, as you read it, reflect on the environment in which you practice and how to best interact with a dynamic team of specialists, all of whom play an essential role in patient care. In larger centers, this may take the form of multidisciplinary, disease-specific clinics staffed by surgeons, medical oncologists, and radiotherapists, with ready access to experts in pathology, radiology, gastroenterology, pulmonary medicine, or supportive care. In other centers, regularly held multidisciplinary cancer conferences, which bring a number of subspecialists together in case-presentation format may be required, as a practical substitute for a multidisciplinary clinic. In many clinical settings, communications might have to be carried out electronically through secure web-based information systems and electronic mail. This is increasingly feasible as electronic medical records, web-based digital radiology files, and soon, digital photomicrographs, become widely available across the world; these innovations must be embraced and utilized by all.

Lastly, how physicians interact with each other and with patients in this new century will be a critical component of quality care and scrutinized by professional societies in the years to come. Interpersonal and communication skills are not just buzz words: consensus-building and consistent communication of information to patients is vital to the effectiveness of increasingly complex care plans. In this regard, physicians must assume different roles at various times during a course of treatment and longitudinal care: either as team leader, or team player. These roles may change at transition points of care, and as the team lead shifts, a clear understanding of who is in charge should always be conveyed to the patient.

In summary, this text is an exciting and refreshing edition which reflects the emergence of "team oncology". I hope it broadens and deepens your perspective on the future of oncology care and causes you to reflect on how your practice habits should change in this dynamic era.

Robert A. Wolff, M.D.
Professor, Department of Gastrointestinal Medical Oncology
Deputy Head, Clinical and Educational Affairs
Division of Cancer Medicine
University of Texas, M.D. Anderson Cancer Center, USA

1

Cancer and Tobacco: Its Effects on Individuals and Populations

Bernard W. Stewart,
Patricia F. Cotter and
James F. Bishop

Abstract

Tobacco smoking as the major cause of cancer is unrivalled and as western countries come to terms with its toll and smoking rates decline, the burden of tobacco-caused disease is far from reaching its peak in developing countries. Tobacco smoking causes cancer of the lung, as well as cancer of the oral cavity, naso-, oro- and hypopharynx, nasal cavity and paranasal sinuses, larynx, oesophagus, stomach, pancreas, liver, kidney (body and pelvis), ureter, urinary bladder, uterine cervix and bone marrow (myeloid leukaemia).

For lung cancer, incidence is almost precisely correlated with mortality and the only option currently available to markedly reduce the burden of lung cancer in the community is to reduce tobacco consumption.

For the cancer patient, continued smoking carries an increased risk of treatment complications or a second malignancy at the same or another site and the increased risk of a new primary cancer for many years after the original diagnosis. There is substantial medical evidence that continued smoking may reduce the effectiveness of treatment or worsen side effects of treatment.

The risk of death from smoking is substantial: about half of all cigarette smokers are eventually killed by their habit. Physicians and health professionals are in a unique position to capitalise on the teachable moment presented by the diagnosis of a smoking-caused disease and advise all smokers to quit. Unless these and other effective measures are implemented to prevent people from smoking and to help current users quit, tobacco will kill one billion people in the 21st century.

Keywords: Tobacco, environmental tobacco smoke, teachable moment, treatment effects.

1.   The Need to Eliminate Tobacco-Induced Cancer

Reference to tobacco occupies a singular position in any overview of cancer biology and clinical oncology. Theoretically, exogenous causative factors may be considered with reference to any tumour type and any such discussion has ramifications for prevention and the possibility of reducing the burden of incidence and mortality. Exogenous carcinogens include tobacco, alcoholic beverages, ultraviolet light and a range of occupational and environmental exposures.

In the classic appraisal made by Doll and Peto in 1981[1] regarding the causation of cancer in the USA, 30% of all cancer deaths were attributable to tobacco, with no other single agent of comparable standing with regards to cancer causation.[2] Lung cancer is the leading cause of cancer-related mortality worldwide, with almost 1.2 million deaths per year.[3] In delineating the role of tobacco smoking in lung cancer, many studies are directed to a heterologous grouping identified as non-small-cell lung cancer (NSCLC, comprising 80% of lung cancers), which includes adenocarcinoma, bronchioloalveolar, squamous, anaplastic and large-cell carcinomas.

1.1   *Causation proven*

The overwhelming body of epidemiological evidence indicates that the risk of lung and other cancers is determined by the duration of smoking, the amount of tobacco smoke inhaled (usually expressed in 'pack years') and the intensity of exposure, as indicated by the depth of inhalation. The carcinogenicity of tobacco smoke is clear both from such epidemiological studies and also from a huge spectrum of experimental data. The vital contribution of experimental studies has come through detailed analyses of the processes whereby the multiple carcinogens in tobacco smoke cause malignant transformation of respiratory and other epithelial tissue.

The particulate phase of tobacco smoke contains nicotine, nitrosamines, *N*-nitrosonornicotine, metals (cadmium, nickel and polonium-210), polycyclic aromatic hydrocarbons and carcinogenic aromatic amines (4-aminophenyl). The vapour phase contains carbon monoxide, carbon dioxide, benzene, ammonia, formaldehyde, hydrogen cyanide, and nitrosamines. Approximately 60 recognised carcinogens are present, along with toxic agents likely to induce tissue injury and consequent proliferative activity in respiratory epithelium.[4] Nicotine may contribute directly to carcinogenesis by stimulating cell proliferation and inhibiting apoptosis, thereby mediating promotion and progression of lung cancer.[5]

In the face of such a carcinogenic insult, which may continue over several decades, the lung is remarkably resistant to tumourigenesis. Only a minority of heavy smokers — 16% of men and 9.5% of women — develop lung cancer.

1.2   *Multiple target organs*

The most authoritative statements on the carcinogenicity of particular agents are evaluations made in the context of *IARC Monographs on the Evaluations of the Carcinogenic Risks to Humans*, edited by the International Agency for Research on Cancer, an arm of the World Health Organization (WHO). *IARC Monographs* on Tobacco Smoking and on Involuntary Smoking were published in 2004 and are the definitive publications in relation to a range of matters.[6] Tobacco smoking causes cancer of the lung, as well as cancer of the oral cavity, naso-, oro- and hypopharynx, nasal cavity and paranasal sinuses, larynx, oesophagus, stomach, pancreas, liver, kidney (body and pelvis), ureter, urinary bladder, uterine cervix and bone marrow (myeloid leukaemia). Available data indicate that tobacco smoking does not cause cancers of the female breast and endometrium.

The *IARC Monograph* on tobacco smoking provides comprehensive information in relation to each of the tumour types caused by smoking. Such details include the relationship of risk to exposure, the proportion of disease attributable to tobacco and the extent of reversibility of risk consequent upon smoking cessation. The causation of each of the tumour types known to be a consequence of tobacco smoking may be analysed with reference to the route of exposure to tobacco smoke or related metabolites, organic-specific metabolism of particular carcinogens and the cell biology of relevant tumours.

In respect of tobacco-induced lung cancer, the basics have been known for decades, though even in relation to lung cancer, new insights regarding tobacco continue to be revealed. The most important matter resolved in recent years concerns the carcinogenicity of so-called 'light' or 'mild' cigarettes. Cigarettes formulated to deliver less tar when subjected to 'smoking machine' analysis were marketed and advertised as presenting a lesser risk of ill-health than regular cigarettes. It is now established that smokers of light or mild cigarettes are essentially subject to the same risk of lung cancer as smokers of regular cigarettes.[7] The data indicate that smoking behaviour is dominated by the smoker's need to achieve a given intake of nicotine. Low or mild cigarettes provoke changes in smoking behaviour: more frequent inhalation, deeper inhalation and/or consumption of a greater number of cigarettes per day.[8] It is hypothesised that the usage of light or mild cigarettes accounts for an increasing proportion of adenocarcinoma by comparison with other histological types of non-small cell lung cancer.

Despite early implications, recent data suggest that women are no more susceptible than men to the carcinogenic effects of cigarette smoking to the lung.[9] Paradoxically, in the same study amongst those reporting having never smoked tobacco in any form, women had slightly higher rates of lung cancer than men. Lung cancer is a lethal disease and although some progress has been made in recent years, the five-year survival rate in developed countries remains less than 15%. For lung cancer, incidence is almost precisely correlated with mortality, which is not the situation for the other common cancers in developed countries: breast, colon and prostate cancer. As a consequence, the only option currently available to markedly reduce the burden of lung cancer in the community is to reduce tobacco consumption.

2.   The Genetics of Susceptibility

Knowledge of the genes mediating metabolism of tobacco smoke-derived carcinogens and those genes accounting for the repair of such damage was vigorously pursued. A specific stimulus for this research was the hypothesis that individual susceptibility to lung cancer may be revealed by genetic variation amongst such genes. Information concerning genetic determination of susceptibility to lung cancer independent of smoking behaviour and for suscepti-bility to nicotine addiction is available,[10] but will not be considered here. On the specific issue of genetic determination of susceptibil-ity to tobacco smoke carcinogenesis, there has been no consistent association between specific SNPs in XRCC1 and risk of lung cancer.

2.1   *Lung cancer is a different disease in smokers*

The characteristics of lung cancer in smokers, as distinct from lung cancer in never smokers, are sufficiently marked as to justify char-acterising these as two different tumour types with reference to both aetiology and clinical course.[11] A difference between the puta-tively distinct tumour types is most clearly indicated by mutation in epidermal growth factor receptor (EGFR). EGFR mutations are much more common in lung cancers afflicting people who have never smoked (45%), by comparison with those with tobacco-associated disease (7%).[12] This scenario is correlated with markedly increased responsiveness to the corresponding low molecular weight kinase inhibitors erlotinib and gefitinib. Patients likely to respond to these kinase inhibitors are those who are non-smokers, women and those of Asian ancestry; smokers with lung cancer show little response.[13] Lung cancers in smokers exhibit distinct patterns of TP53 and KRAS mutations, with KRAS mutations almost unknown in never smoker lung cancers. Indeed, it appears that EGRF and KRAS mutations are mutually exclusive.[14] Histologically, adenocarcinomas are considered to be less commonly attributable to tobacco smoking than squamous or large cell lung cancers. The distinction being drawn between apparently different lung tumour types affecting smokers and never smokers means that smoking status and history are not only relevant to public health, but to the clinical management of lung cancer. In a recent Japanese study, the 'never-smoking NSCLC' patient group exhibited significantly superior overall and cancer-specific survival than the 'smoking NSCLC' group.[15]

2.2 *Evidence of reversibility*

Elucidation of the molecular processes resulting in cancer causation by tobacco smoke has contributed directly to proving that the epidemiological association between smoking and lung cancer is causal. A decreased risk of cancer amongst former smokers indicates the degree to which carcinogenesis is reversible, which is consistent with both cellular and molecular data.[16,17]

Once direct exposure to tobacco smoke ceases, the tissue and molecular injury, which may otherwise contribute to cancer development, tends toward normal.[18] Accordingly, the aetiology of tobacco-induced lung cancer strongly favours smoking cessation as the most immediate, and effective, preventive measure. Both public health policy and primary health care are properly based on smoking cessation as a central tenet of cancer control.

3.   Prospects for Population-Based Screening

In developed countries, risk factors for lung cancer are clear. As summarised by Spitz and her colleagues, for never smokers they include regular exposure to environmental tobacco smoke and a family history of cancer in two or more first-degree relatives. For former smokers, risk factors are emphysema, no prior hay fever, dust exposure, and family history of cancer in two or more first-degree relatives. For current smokers, additional risk factors include asbestos exposure, and the family history variable involves one or more first-degree relatives with a smoking-related cancer.[19]

With criteria which clearly establish persons at high risk of lung cancer being evident over decades, and the clinical prospect of extremely poor survival once diagnosis is made, the context and benefits of population-based screening for lung cancer are immediately clear, and have been so for years.

In the 1950s autopsy studies showed that the lungs of heavy smokers were affected by multiple sites of preinvasive and early invasive cancer associated with the clinical disease leading to the patients' death. Protocols for lung cancer screening initially involved chest X-rays and sputum cytology and prior to 1980, evaluation of such procedures was undertaken in multiple studies. The results of these trials were uniformly negative, insofar as none showed any reduction in lung cancer mortality in the group subject to X-ray, with or without sputum cytology.[20] Chest X-ray was effective at identifying many additional small tumours in the lung that could be removed. However, that intervention did not reduce the likelihood that individuals would be diagnosed with new cases of advanced lung cancer or would die of lung cancer.

3.1 *Current status of computed tomography (CT) screening*

Current approaches to lung cancer screening are totally focused on CT because this technology is demonstrably more sensitive for the detection of very small nodules. That said, the titles of recent editorials — referring to 'are we ready?', 'spiraling into confusion' and 'yet another problem'[21–23] — clearly indicate that no basis has been established for the widespread introduction of CT screening for lung cancer. A central consideration is that the available data do not reveal a consistent reduction in lung cancer mortality as a consequence of CT-based screening. As might be anticipated from the earlier X-ray studies, many more patients with stage one disease are identified amongst those at risk as subjected to CT than amongst controls. Some insight into the challenge posed by data currently available is posed by Black and Baron,[21] who asked "How is it possible that two large studies published within six months of each other could lead to such dramatically different conclusions about the effectiveness of CT screening?" The best explanation for the paradox is the difference in the primary outcome measurements. One study,[24] concluding that asymptomatic individuals should not be screened, relied on mortality. The other,[25] which focused on survival, suggested that CT screening of high-risk individuals could prevent 80% of lung cancer deaths. Prolonged survival need not imply reduced mortality in the population.

There is direct evidence that, by comparison with chest X-ray and sputum cytology, spiral CT is a more effective screening methodology, and has the potential to detect disease more accurately. However, the potential for over diagnosis is also evident.[26] For lung cancer screening purposes, publications involving CT include 11 observational studies and six randomised trials.[20] Taking these data into account, Field and Duffy conclude that "we still do not have experimental evidence for or against the implementation of this screening modality". It may be, however, that lung cancer screening predicated on the detection of early stage lesions is an inherently flawed approach. The notion that for a period before advanced disease, lung cancer is localised and treatable may be wrong. Perhaps the early stage lesions currently detected in trials are not the precursors of advanced disease, which otherwise develops via a different pathway[27] and attempts are being made to characterise subsets of early disease in order to clarify this matter. A significant fraction of patients (30–40%) with stage one disease who undergo surgery die of recurrent disease. Such patients appear to be characterised by methylation of the promoter regions of four particular genes.[28]

3.2   *Genetic profiling of pre-malignant tissue*

Gene expression profiling has been extensively assessed in relation to clinical disease, specifically as a possible means to predict metastatic behaviour.[29] The same technology has been applied to bronchial epithelium at risk of tobacco smoke-induced malignant transformation. Spira and colleagues[30] analysed histologically normal large-airway cells obtained at bronchoscopy from smokers, to determine whether gene expression data might be used for biomarker purposes. They identified an 80-gene biomarker that distinguished smokers with and without lung cancer (80% sensitive, 84% specific). Combining cytopathology of lower airway cells with the biomarker suggested a means of assessing cancer-specific airway-wide responses to cigarette smoke, as a means of indicating individuals at highest risk. In a further study, the independence of the biomarker from other clinical risk factors was demonstrated, suggesting that use of a 'clincogenomic' model may expedite more invasive testing and definitive therapy for smokers with lung cancer and reduce invasive diagnostic procedures for individuals without lung cancer.[31]

4.   Chemoprevention

Granted the ready identification of persons at high risk for lung cancer (i.e. current and former smokers), chemoprevention has been, and continues to be, an immediately attractive and obvious consideration. Cancer chemoprevention is, in large part, predicated on epidemiological data indicating above average consumption of fresh fruit and vegetables as reducing cancer risk for multiple tumour types, and the efficacy of micronutrients in reducing, if not preventing, carcinogenesis in rodents.[32] However, attempts to prevent lung cancer by relatively short-term consumption of certain vitamins and antioxidants met with spectacular failures: a slightly increased incidence of lung cancer was recorded by comparison with relevant control groups in a trial context. In the case of a trial based in Finland, β-carotene-induced lung cancer elevation was most pronounced in men who smoked heaviest and drank the most.[33] In the US trial a similar effect was most pronounced in current (as opposed to former) smokers and in participants with the highest alcohol intake.[34] Better results might be obtained using different agents over a longer timeframe, and using biomarkers rather than cancer diagnosis as an end point.[35] For the moment, there appears to be few if any attempts to present chemoprevention as a credible response to the burden of tobacco-induced lung cancer.

5.   Passive Smoking

No level of exposure to environmental tobacco smoke may be regarded as safe. Apart from cancer, passive smoking can cause heart disease in non-smoking adults and increase the risk of sudden infant death syndrome, acute respiratory infections, middle-ear disease and exacerbation of asthma in children. This discussion of the hazard is limited to cancer causation.

As established in active smokers, tobacco smoke is carcinogenic, with the polycyclic hydrocarbons and nitrosamines therein exhibiting a genotoxic mechanism of action. On this basis, any level of exposure to such a biological toxin would be anticipated to present a carcinogenic risk. Accordingly, good public health practice would dictate that preventable exposure to any level of tobacco smoke should not occur. The present discussion of passive smoking (which is synonymous with exposure to environmental tobacco smoke, or to secondhand smoke) might therefore proceed directly to the implementation of practicable measures to prevent exposure. In practice, however, the social and economic considerations which surround tobacco smoking have dictated that specific research be conducted to establish that exposure to environmental tobacco smoke — investigated in its own right — does present a carcinogenic hazard to humans.

5.1. *Chemical composition*

Environmental tobacco smoke consists of a mixture of exhaled mainstream smoke and smoke emitted from the burning tip of the cigarette (or its equivalent in relation to other smoking techniques), called sidestream smoke, all diluted with ambient air. Environmental tobacco smoke consists of a particulate and a gaseous phase, and the chemical composition of mainstream and sidestream smoke have been extensively documented.[36] Carcinogens that occur in environmental tobacco smoke include benzene, 1,3-butadiene, benzo[a]pyrene, 4-(methyl-nitrosamino)-1-(3-pyridyl)-1-butanone and many others. Such compounds may mediate specific mutations of genes encoding for cell cycle and growth control, thereby leading to tumourigenesis. Moreover, epigenetic mechanisms, which could result in gene silencing without any effect on the coding sequence of the gene in question, may also be involved in malignant transformation occurring as a result of passive smoking.[37]

Cotinine, and its parent compound nicotine, are highly specific for exposure to secondhand smoke; cotinine is currently the most suitable biomarker for assessing recent exposure to environmental tobacco smoke.[38] Several studies have shown that concentrations of smoke-derived carcinogen adducts, including haemoglobin adducts of aromatic amines, are higher in adult involuntary smokers and in the children of smoking mothers than in individuals not exposed to secondhand smoke. Metabolites of the tobacco-specific carcinogen, 4-(methylnitrosamino)-1-(3-pyridyl)-1-butanone, have been found to be consistently elevated in passive smokers.[6,39]

Exposure to secondhand smoke may occur in many contexts, but has been most extensively investigated in relation to smoking by spouses at home, and in the workplace. Before various smoking restrictions were adopted, particularly high levels of environmental tobacco smoke were encountered by flight attendants and hospitality workers.

5.2 ETS and cancer causation

In its 2002 evaluation of 'Involuntary Smoking', the IARC noted more than 50 relevant studies concerning risk of lung cancer, concerning which there are a limited number of meta-analyses.[6] These show a statistically significant and consistent association between lung cancer risk in spouses of smokers and exposure to secondhand smoke from the smoking spouse. The excess risk is of the order of 20% for women and 30% for men, and the excess risk increases with increasing exposure. Lung cancer in never-smokers subject to passive smoking at work exhibits an increase in risk of 12–19%. The evidence is sufficient to conclude that involuntary smoking is a cause of lung cancer (IARC Group one carcinogen). Evidence in relation to other cancers, specifically including breast cancer and childhood cancer, is equivocal in relation to establishment of causation.

In the United States, exposure to secondhand smoke declined approximately 70% from the late 1980s through 2002.[40] Restrictions placed on smoking indoors in jurisdictions throughout the world have reduced exposure to environmental tobacco smoke. However, it is evident that not all options are equally effective in this regard. Within single buildings, the banning of smoking in particular areas or rooms is markedly ineffective so far as protecting non-smokers is concerned, with levels of smoke-related pollutants and particulates in such areas sometimes being comparable to those where smoking is allowed.[41] The US Surgeon General has concluded that protecting non-smokers from environmental tobacco smoke can only be accomplished by completely eliminating smoking in indoor places.

Measures to prevent involuntary exposure to secondhand smoke have been developed and adopted widely and recently, IARC assessed the evidence for effectiveness of such policies.[42] Where studied, smoke-free workplace policies consistently decrease exposure to secondhand smoke in high-exposure settings by 80–90%, and can lead to widespread decreases in exposure of up to 40%. Studies of workers affected by workplace smoking restrictions reveal individual decreased cigarette use of two to four cigarettes per day. The weight of evidence suggests that smoke-free work places do not result in increased smoking at home.

6.   Cancer Patients Who Smoke

6.1   *The effects of smoking on survival*

The diagnosis of cancer provides an incentive for many patients to make a serious attempt to quit smoking.[43] The diagnosis provides a 'teachable moment' for clinicians. Assisting smokers to quit may also have a favourable outcome on their long term prognosis.[44] In contrast, continued smoking carries an increased risk of treatment complications or a second malignancy at the same or another site and the increased risk of a new primary cancer for many years after the original diagnosis. There is substantial medical evidence that continued smoking may reduce the effectiveness of treatment or worsen side effects of treatment. This section focuses on the outcomes expected for those current and former smokers who have a cancer diagnosis and how their cancer prognosis is affected by their ability to quit.

Both current and former smokers may be expected to have an increased number and severity of tobacco-related co-morbid conditions that would adversely affect their general health status, symptom experience and quality of life.[44] The long term effects of smoking in cancer patients are uniformly negative, although risk will decline with time since cessation.[44] Independent of the aetiologic effects of tobacco carcinogens in relation to numerous tumour types, a growing literature also documents the direct and indirect adverse effects of smoking on oncologic treatment efficacy (short and long term outcomes), treatment-related toxicity and consequent morbidity, quality of life, recurrence of primary disease, second primary tumours and survival time.[43]

Specifically for NSCLC patients, smoking is both the cause of lung cancer and, when it continues following diagnosis, is also a cause of worse prognosis.[45,46] Smoking is an important independent predictor of poor lung cancer prognosis, increasing the hazard of dying by approximately one third compared to former or never smokers.[46,47] With regards to overall survival, the outcome is significantly more positive for former smokers (RR = 0.543), recent quitters (RR = 0.340) and non-smokers (RR = 0.447), when compared to current smokers.[46] This adverse effect on patients with lung cancer occurs relatively late in the course of management and may in part be due to the ongoing smoking that occurs after diagnosis.[47] The effect of smoking on survival has also been studied among breast cancer patients. A history of smoking increased mortality following diagnosis from causes other than breast cancer, but not mortality from breast cancer.[48,49] However, one study found conflicting associations between hormone receptor status and smoking, where women with oestrogen receptor (ER) and progesterone receptor (PR) positive tumours who were current smokers had an increased risk of breast cancer death, compared with never smokers.[49] Another study has suggested that the lower survival rate of smokers with breast cancer may be the result of an impairment of immunity or that smoking may promote the development of more aggressive, oestrogen-receptor negative tumours. Further, exposure to HRT before diagnosis was associated with an improved prognosis among smokers.[48]

6.2 Smoking as a risk factor for increased cancer stage at diagnosis

The effects of smoking on the spread of cancer have not been widely studied. However there is some evidence that smoking is associated with an increased stage at diagnosis and an adverse affect on metastatic behaviour.[50]

6.2.1 Increased secondary primary tumours

The information reported about second lung cancers in patients treated for NSCLC is quite different from that reported about patients treated for SCLC. Patients with NSCLC develop second primary cancers at a rate of approximately 1–2% per year. Patients successfully treated for SCLC develop second primary lung cancers at an average rate of approximately 6% per year, which increases from 2% to more than 10% per patient per year after ten years.[51] Cancer patients who smoke have a significantly increased risk of secondary primary tumours, with an elevated risk observed regardless of whether the initial malignancy is related to smoking or not.[44] For example, individuals treated with radiation therapy to the chest (e.g. for breast cancer) are at increased risk of secondary primary tumours of the lung if they smoke.[44] Smoking increases the risk of SCLC from six-fold to 15-fold in patients treated for Hodgkin disease and breast cancer. This suggests a multiplicative interaction between smoking and chest radiotherapy in patients treated for small-cell lung cancer, Hodgkin disease, and breast cancer.[51]

In patients with small-cell lung carcinoma who continue to smoke, the risk of a second lung cancer is approximately doubled overall.[52] In two studies of survivors of SCLC, the risk of a second cancer (mostly non-SCLC) was 3.5-fold to 4.4-fold higher than in the general population. In those who continued to smoke, the risk was far higher in those who also received chest irradiation (RR = 21.0) and alkylating agents (RR = 19.0).[52–54] This risk increased over time for SCLC survivors, with a cumulative incidence of 44% at 14 years.[55] In contrast, patients with a first primary tobacco-related cancer such as NSCLC also have a high risk of a second tobacco-related cancer, but their risk appears to remain more stable over time.[55]

6.3 Treatment

6.3.1 Surgery and wound healing

Smoking has major consequences for patients who undergo surgery and specifically in relation to the period immediately following surgery. Smoking affects tissue oxygenation, heart rate, airways clearance, immune response, and circulation. In addition, smokers on average also require higher doses of analgesia for pain relief.[56]

Respiratory complications in the post-operative period, such as some combination of pulmonary infections, atelectasis, bronchospasm, and the need for prolonged ventilation, as well as a higher post-operative mortality rate, are more common in smokers.[57] In addition, reconstructive survey may be compromised, as smoking substantially increases the risk of wound infection, flap necrosis, and fat necrosis, and these complications may also delay adjuvant chemotherapy and radiotherapy.[58] Smoking cessation for longer than three weeks before reconstructive head and neck surgery is beneficial for all smokers and reduces the incidence of impaired wound healing.[59]

The Faculty of Anaethesists of the Royal Australian College of Surgeons advises that smokers be counselled to stop smoking completely, or failing that, to abstain for at least six to eight weeks before surgery. Abstinence for the 12 hours immediately prior to surgery is particularly important, in order to achieve maximum tissue oxygenation.[60] The timing of cessation is relevant, as a reduction in peri-operative complications is not seen until a period of abstinence of five to eight weeks' duration. In general, smokers have a nearly six-fold increase in risk of a post-operative pulmonary complication.[61] In addition, several early studies have documented that smokers who decrease consumption but do not quit entirely, or quit but have been abstinent for less that two months, may have a higher rate of complications post-operatively.[62] Recently the issue of smoking cessation and peri-operative complications has been studied specifically in patients undergoing thoracotomy for primary or secondary lung tumours. In this study there was no evidence of a paradoxical increase in pulmonary complications among those who quit smoking within two months of undergoing surgery. However the types of complications differed between the recent quitter and ongoing smoker subgroups. All the complications in the ongoing smoker group were pneumonias; in the recent quitter subgroup fewer pneumonias occurred.[59,63] There is a strong incentive to advise patients to quit smoking immediately and capitalise on the 'teachable moment' that a cancer diagnosis provides.

6.3.2 *Radiation therapy and chemotherapy*

Smoking cigarettes during radiotherapy appears to prolong the period of reaction and may reduce the chance of cure.[64] Radiation therapy for head and neck cancer patients who continue to smoke has been associated with lower rates of complete response (45% in smokers vs. 74% in non-smokers) and a poorer two-year survival (39% in smokers vs. 66% in non-smokers).[65] In addition, among NSCLC patients diagnosed with early stage disease, current smokers have a poorer prognosis for survival after radiation therapy.[66] Similarly, in patients with advanced NSCLC, never smokers have an improved outcome over smokers when treated with chemotherapy.[67] This effect has also be demonstrated in lung cancer patients (both NSCLC and SCLC), where those with a cigarette burden of 40 or over pack years have a worse response to platinum-based chemotherapy, compared to those who have a cigarette burden of less than 40 pack years.[68]

Radiotherapy for breast cancer also significantly increases the risk of lung carcinoma more than ten years after exposure in women who smoked at the time of their breast cancer treatment. The increased risk is restricted to women who smoked at the time of radiotherapy and is not evident in non-smoking women. Squamous cell carcinoma of the lung appears to be the histopathologic subgroup most closely related to ionizing radiation.[69] Complications for patients receiving radiation therapy for cervical cancer are also more evident among patients who smoke, as they experience an increased incidence of gastro-intestinal complications.[70] Smokers present with higher risk grade prostate cancers[71] and smokers (both current and previous), treated with external beam radiotherapy for localised prostate cancer appear to be at a greater risk of developing metastatic disease.[72]

In addition, particular attention should be devoted to preventing patients from both smoking and taking antioxidant supplements during radiation therapy, as this combination appears to reduce the efficacy of radiation therapy.[73]

6.4 Drug interactions

Treatment-related weight loss and cachexia would be expected to be exacerbated by smoking, as smoking suppresses appetite and weight gain. In addition nicotine, via the induction of hepatic enzymes, increases metabolism of many pharmaceutical agents and potentially decreases their efficacy.[44] The effect of smoking on the pharmacology of many anti-cancer drugs is not well understood.

6.5 Inflammatory markers

Inflammation is associated with poor prognosis and decreased survival in many types of cancer, and higher levels of inflammatory markers have been seen in smokers.[74] These in turn may influence drug pharmacology and are implicated as prognostic markers.

6.6 Future directions/further research

Tobacco smoking is the largest single preventable cause of death and disease in Australia today. More than 50 years ago Doll and Bradford Hill in the UK and Wynder in the US reported that smoking and lung cancer appeared to be causally linked.[56] Since that time the health consequences of smoking have been widely studied and extensively reported, but in comparison the effects of smoking on cancer patients are relatively under-researched. Table 1 outlines some areas of potential future research.

Table 1. Recommendations for future research on smoking in cancer patients.

Area of research	Recommendation
Pharmacotherapy for nicotine dependence treatment	• Evaluate the efficacy of NRT (gum, patch, nasal spray, inhaler), non-nicotine medications (bupropion, clonidine, nortriptyline, and varenicline), and combination therapies (e.g. high-dose NRT, combined NRT and bupropion) in increasing tobacco abstinence rates in oncology patients.

(Continued)

Table 1. (*Continued*)

Area of research	Recommendation
	• Assess the efficacy of nicotine and non-nicotine medications in managing symptoms of nicotine withdrawal, craving, stress, and depression among cancer patients. • Assess the effect of nicotine in cigarettes and nicotine in NRT on cancer drugs/treatment.
Methodologic issues	• Obtain sample sizes needed to provide adequate statistical power for hypothesis testing. • Collect and report demographic and medical data including disease site, type, stage, and treatment. • Report on the timing of intervention relative to time of cancer diagnosis and treatment. • Include at least six-month outcomes to assess stability of treatment effects. • Assess tobacco use status using both seven-day point prevalence and continuous abstinence.
Prevention of disease recurrence	• Examine factors predictive of smoking relapse and relapse in cancer patients. • Evaluate relapse prevention strategies within nicotine dependence treatment interventions: cognitive-behavioural strategies, long-term use of pharmacotherapy, support mechanisms, and extended follow-up may increase abstinence maintenance.
Cancer treatment and quality of life	• Studies to determine the extent of interaction of radiation and chemotherapy agents in smokers compared to non-smokers. Further determine the type and extent of physical and psychological benefits experienced by cancer patients who stop smoking. This research is needed across cancer sites, as benefits may differ. • Clinical trials should routinely collect smoking status and include primary outcomes related to quality of life and oncology treatment. • Quality of life assessment may include global measures and site-specific measures.

Source: Adapted from Ref. 86.

7. Cancer Prevention — Reversal of Risk Upon Quitting

7.1 *The individual*

For much of the 20th century, smoking was regarded as a socially learned habit and as a personal choice, but it is now recognised that cigarette smoking is primarily a manifestation of nicotine addiction and that smokers individualise their level of nicotine intake. Although by the age of 20, 80% of cigarette smokers regret that they ever started, as a result of their addiction to nicotine, many will continue to smoke for a substantial proportion of their adult life.[75]

The risk of death from smoking is substantial: about half of all cigarette smokers are eventually killed by their habit.[76] Many are killed while they are still only in middle age (35–69 years of age), and could have anticipated living for another ten, 20, 30 or more years.[77] Those who continue to smoke lose on average about ten years of life, compared to non-smokers. Individuals who stop smoking at around 60, 50, 40, or 30 years gain respectively about three, six, nine, or ten years of life compared with those who continue to smoke.[76] Hence, those who stop smoking in early middle age (around the age of 40) avoid most of their risk of being killed by tobacco smoking.

The risk of dying from lung cancer for people who never smoke, is less than 1% (Fig. 1). However the risk of lung cancer is high for people who smoke all their lives, but this risk can be substantially modified if quitting occurs at any age.[77]

Sixteen percent of smokers will die from lung cancer by age 75 if they don't die from something else first. Smoking causes even more deaths from other diseases than from lung cancer; overall, half of all persistent smokers are killed by tobacco. For people who stop at age 50, the risk of dying of lung cancer is only about 6%.[77]

The main findings of Sir Richard Doll's study on smoking and death in British doctors are that the chances of a 35-year-old surviving to age 70 and beyond are 81% for non-smokers, compared to only 58% for smokers. A quarter of all the smokers were

Stopping smoking: avoiding lung cancer

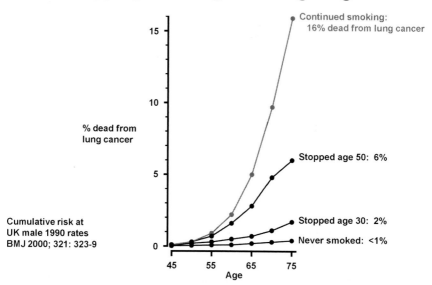

Figure 1. Risk of lung cancer with smoking cessation.[87]

killed by tobacco when they were aged 35 to 69 years, mainly from diseases such as lung cancer, coronary events and chronic lung disease. On average, the doctors who smoked died ten years earlier than non-smokers (Fig. 2). But it is not just a question of mortality: long-term smokers suffer more disease and disability before they die at younger ages. On average smokers suffer reduced quality of life for a greater number of years than non-smokers.[78]

The other main finding from Richard Doll's study was that stopping smoking was remarkably effective (Fig. 3). Even in early middle age (or at about age 40 years), those who stopped before they had incurable lung cancer or some other fatal disease avoided most of their risk of being killed by tobacco, and stopping before middle age was even more effective.

There are health benefits of quitting for all smokers, regardless of age, sex or length of time that they have been smoking.

Survival to age 70 and beyond: effect of smoking in male British doctors

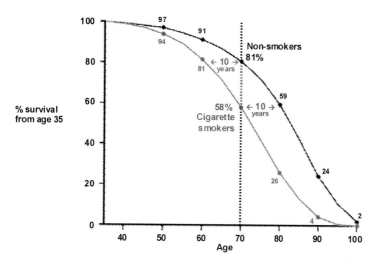

% survival from age 35

Non-smokers 81%

Cigarette smokers 58%

Age

Figure 2. Survival from age 35 years in British doctors.[88]

Effect of stopping smoking at about age 40

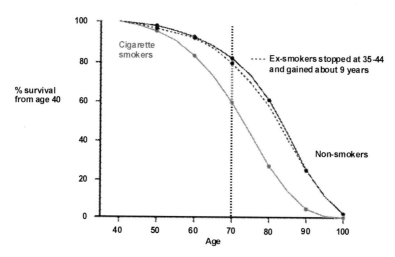

% survival from age 40

Cigarette smokers

Ex-smokers stopped at 35-44 and gained about 9 years

Non-smokers

Age

Figure 3. Effect of smoking cessation at age 40 years.

People who have already developed smoking-related health problems, like heart disease, can still benefit from quitting. For example, compared to continuing smokers, people who quit smoking after having a myocardial infarction reduce their chances of having another one by 50%. There are many benefits to quitting, with some even occurring within hours of stopping smoking.

7.2   Cancer patients

Some information about barriers to smoking cessation can be inferred from the characteristics of patients who continue to smoke following a cancer diagnosis (Table 2). Patients diagnosed with tobacco-related cancers typically report long histories of heavy tobacco use, indicating strong nicotine dependence.[79] Success in quitting smoking may also be challenged by the pressure for abrupt and immediate cessation following diagnosis. In addition, the cancer diagnosis is often confirmation of a smoker's worst fears and a reinforcement of their previous inability to quit leading to the fatalistic belief that it is too late to quit. The psychological distress of a cancer diagnosis is likely to lead heavily nicotine-dependent smokers to rely on smoking to regulate mood and cope with distress.[79]

Table 2.   Benefits and barriers to quitting.

Benefits	Barriers
Improved survival rate	High psychological distress
Fewer treatment complications	High nicotine dependence
Improved treatment efficacy	Abrupt cessation vs. 'commitment to abstinence'
Reduced risk of disease recurrence and second primary tumour	Low quitting self-efficacy
Improved mastery and control	Knowledge deficits
	Negative social support

Source: Ref. 79.

7.3   The population perspective

Around 30% of male cancer deaths are smoking-related, compared to around 13% of female cancer deaths; two in five of all deaths caused by smoking are from cancer.[80] Unlike many other areas of public health, there is little debate about the best way to mitigate the tobacco problem. The seven components of a comprehensive strategy were originally laid out in the landmark 1962 Smoking and Health Report of the Royal College of Physicians.[81] These components — public education, restriction of sales to minors, restriction of tobacco promotion, restricting smoking in public places, increasing tobacco tax/price, consumer information and production regulation, and cessation support services — are required to act synergistically to reduce smoking rates in a population.

It has been estimated that $2 has been saved on health care for each $1 spent on tobacco control programs to date.[82] The total economic benefits of tobacco control programs are estimated to exceed health-related and other expenditure by at least fifty to one.[83]

7.4   A global perspective

Tobacco is the largest cause of preventable death in the world, causing one in ten deaths worldwide. If current trends continue, it is projected that by 2030 tobacco will result in ten million deaths annually, of which 70% will have occurred in developing countries.[84]

The total number of smokers is increasing mainly due to expansion of the world's population; by 2030 there be at least another two billion people. Unless smoking prevalence rates decline dramatically, the absolute number of smokers will increase. The expected continuing decrease in male smoking prevalence also may be offset, in part, by a potentially dangerous increase in female smoking rates, especially in developing countries.[85]

One hundred million people died from tobacco use in the 20th century and unless effective measures are implemented to prevent people from smoking and to help current users quit, tobacco will kill one billion people in the 21st century.[85]

Acknowledgements

The authors wish to thank Usha Salagame for assistance with retrieving references and with formatting the reference list for publication.

Figures 1 to 3 of this chapter are obtained from "Deaths from Smoking" © 2006 International Union Against Cancer (UICC), available online at www.deathsfromsmoking.net. (Copyright waiver: Because this resource is intended to communicate the evidence that it summarises, any part of it may be reproduced for bona fide educational purposes without seeking copyright permission from the publisher or authors.)

References

1. R. Doll and R. Peto, The causes of cancer: Quantitative estimates of avoidable risks of cancer in the United States today, *J. Natl. Cancer Inst.* **66**: 1192–1308 (1981).
2. *World Cancer Report* (IARC Press, Lyon, 2003).
3. A. Jemal, R. Siegel, E. Ward, Y. Hao, J. Xu, T. Murray and M. J. Thun, Cancer statistics, 2008. *CA Cancer J. Clin.* **58**: 71–96 (2008).
4. S. S. Hecht, Cigarette smoking and lung cancer: Chemical mechanisms and approaches to prevention, *Lancet Oncol.* **3**: 461–469 (2002).
5. A. Catassi, D. Servent, L. Paleari, A. Cesario and P. Russo, Multiple roles of nicotine on cell proliferation and inhibition of apoptosis: Implications on lung carcinogenesis, *Mutat. Res.* **659**: 221–231 (2008).
6. IARC, *IARC Monographs on the Evaluation of Carcinogenic Risks to Humans. Volume 83. Tobacco Smoke and Involuntary Smoking* (International Agency for Research on Cancer, Lyon, 2004).
7. J. E. Harris, M. J. Thun, A. M. Mondul and E. E. Calle, Cigarette tar yields in relation to mortality from lung cancer in the cancer prevention study II prospective cohort, 1982–8, *Br. Med. J.* **328**: 72 (2004).
8. N. L. Benowitz, P. Jacob, III, J. T. Bernert, M. Wilson, L. Wang, F. Allen and D. Dempsey, Carcinogen exposure during short-term switching from regular to "light" cigarettes, *Cancer Epidemiol. Biomarkers Prev.* **14**: 1376–1383 (2005).
9. N. D. Freedman, M. F. Leitzmann, A. R. Hollenbeck, A. Schatzkin and C. C. Abnet, Cigarette smoking and subsequent risk of lung cancer in

men and women: Analysis of a prospective cohort study, *Lancet Oncol.* **9**: 649–656 (2008).

10. G. K. Alderton, Predisposing to behaviour?, *Nat. Rev. Cancer* **8**: 321 (2008).

11. S. Sun, J. H. Schiller and A. F. Gazdar, Lung cancer in never smokers — A different disease, *Nat. Rev. Cancer* **7**: 778–790 (2007).

12. J. Subramanian and R. Govindan, Molecular genetics of lung cancer in people who have never smoked, *Lancet Oncol.* **9**: 676–682 (2008).

13. S. V. Sharma, D. W. Bell, J. Settleman and D. A. Haber, Epidermal growth factor receptor mutations in lung cancer, *Nat. Rev. Cancer* **7**: 169–181 (2007).

14. I. Y. Tam, L. P. Chung, W. S. Suen, E. Wang, M. C. Wong, K. K. Ho, W. K. Lam, S. W. Chiu, L. Girard, J. D. Minna, A. F. Gazdar and M. P. Wong, Distinct epidermal growth factor receptor and KRAS mutation patterns in non-small cell lung cancer patients with different tobacco exposure and clinicopathologic features, *Clin. Cancer Res.* **12**: 1647–1653 (2006).

15. T. Yano, N. Miura, T. Takenaka, A. Haro, H. Okazaki, T. Ohba, H. Kouso, T. Kometani, F. Shoji and Y. Maehara, Never-smoking non-small cell lung cancer as a separate entity: Clinicopathologic features and survival, *Cancer* **113**: 1012–1018 (2008).

16. R. H. Breuer, A. Pasic, E. F. Smit, E. van Vliet, N. A. Vonk, E. J. Risse, P. E. Postmus and T. G. Sutedja, The natural course of preneoplastic lesions in bronchial epithelium, *Clin. Cancer Res.* **11**: 537–543 (2005).

17. Y. E. Miller, P. Blatchford, D. S. Hyun, R. L. Keith, T. C. Kennedy, H. Wolf, T. Byers, P. A. Bunn, Jr., M. T. Lewis, W. A. Franklin, F. R. Hirsch and J. Kittelson, Bronchial epithelial Ki-67 index is related to histology, smoking and gender, but not lung cancer or chronic obstructive pulmonary disease, *Cancer Epidemiol. Biomarkers Prev.* **16**: 2425–2431 (2007).

18. F. Veglia, S. Loft, G. Matullo, M. Peluso, A. Munnia, F. Perera, D. H. Phillips, D. Tang, H. Autrup, O. Raaschou-Nielsen, A. Tjonneland and P. Vineis, DNA adducts and cancer risk in prospective studies: A pooled analysis and a meta-analysis, *Carcinogenesis* **29**: 932–936 (2008).

19. M. R. Spitz, W. K. Hong, C. I. Amos, X. Wu, M. B. Schabath, Q. Dong, S. Shete and C. J. Etzel, A risk model for prediction of lung cancer, *J. Natl. Cancer Inst.* **99**: 715–726 (2007).

20. J. K. Field and S. W. Duffy, Lung cancer screening: The way forward, *Br. J. Cancer* **99**: 557–562 (2008).
21. W. C. Black and J. A. Baron, CT screening for lung cancer: Spiraling into confusion?, *J. Am. Med. Assoc.* **297**: 995–997 (2007).
22. S. G. Spiro, Screening for lung cancer: Yet another problem, *Thorax* **62**: 105–106 (2007).
23. J. Aisner, CT screening for lung cancer: Are we ready for wide-scale application? *Clin. Cancer Res.* **13**: 4951–4953 (2007).
24. P. B. Bach, J. R. Jett, U. Pastorino, M. S. Tockman, S. J. Swensen and C. B. Begg, Computed tomography screening and lung cancer outcomes, *J. Am. Med. Assoc.* **297**: 953–961 (2007).
25. C. I. Henschke, D. F. Yankelevitz, D. M. Libby, M. W. Pasmantier, J. P. Smith and O. S. Miettinen, Survival of patients with stage I lung cancer detected on CT screening, *N. Engl. J. Med.* **355**: 1763–1771 (2006).
26. Y. Toyoda, T. Nakayama, Y. Kusunoki, H. Iso and T. Suzuki, Sensitivity and specificity of lung cancer screening using chest low-dose computed tomography, *Br. J. Cancer* **98**: 1602–1607 (2008).
27. P. B. Bach, Is our natural-history model of lung cancer wrong?, *Lancet Oncol.* **9**: 693–697 (2008).
28. M. V. Brock, C. M. Hooker, E. Ota-Machida, Y. Han, M. Guo, S. Ames, S. Glockner, S. Piantadosi, E. Gabrielson, G. Pridham, K. Pelosky, S. A. Belinsky, S. C. Yang, S. B. Baylin and J. G. Herman, DNA methylation markers and early recurrence in stage I lung cancer, *N. Engl. J. Med.* **358**: 1118–1128 (2008).
29. P. Workman and P. Johnston, Genomicprofiling of cancer: What next?, *J. Clin. Oncol.* **23**: 7253–7256 (2005).
30. A. Spira, J. E. Beane, V. Shah, K. Steiling, G. Liu, F. Schembri, S. Gilman, Y. M. Dumas, P. Calner, P. Sebastiani, S. Sridhar, J. Beamis, C. Lamb, T. Anderson, N. Gerry, J. Keane, M. E. Lenburg and J. S. Brody, Airway epithelial gene expression in the diagnostic evaluation of smokers with suspect lung cancer, *Nat. Med.* **13**: 361–366 (2007).
31. J. Beane, P. Sebastiani, T. H. Whitfield, K. Steiling, Y. M. Dumas, M. E. Lenburg and A. Spira, A prediction model for lung cancer diagnosis that integrates genomic and clinical features, *Cancer Prev. Res.* **1**: 56–64 (2008).
32. B. W. Stewart, D. McGregor and P. Kleihues, *Principles of Chemoprevention* (IARC Scientific Publications, Lyon, 1996).
33. D. Albanes, O. P. Heinonen, P. R. Taylor, J. Virtamo, B. K. Edwards, M. Rautalahti, A. M. Hartman, J. Palmgren, L. S. Freedman,

J. Haapakoski, M. J. Barrett, P. Pietinen, N. Malila, E. Tala, K. Liippo, E. R. Salomaa, J. A. Tangrea, L. Teppo, F. B. Askin, E. Taskinen, Y. Erozan, P. Greenwald and J. K. Huttunen, Alpha-tocopherol and beta-carotene supplements and lung cancer incidence in the alpha-tocopherol, beta-carotene cancer prevention study: Effects of base-line characteristics and study compliance, *J. Natl. Cancer Inst.* **88**: 1560–1570 (1996).

34. G. S. Omenn, G. E. Goodman, M. D. Thornquist, J. Balmes, M. R. Cullen, A. Glass, J. P. Keogh, F. L. Meyskens, Jr., B. Valanis, J. H. Williams, Jr., S. Barnhart, M. G. Cherniack, C. A. Brodkin and S. Hammar, Risk factors for lung cancer and for intervention effects in CARET, the Beta-Carotene and Retinol Efficacy Trial, *J. Natl. Cancer Inst.* **88**: 1550–1559 (1996).

35. R. L. Keith and Y. E. Miller, Lung cancer: Genetics of risk and advances in chemoprevention, *Curr. Opin. Pulm. Med.* **11**: 265–271 (2005).

36. M. R. Law and A. K. Hackshaw, Environmental tobacco smoke, *Br. Med. Bull.* **52**: 22–34 (1996).

37. A. Besaratinia and G. P. Pfeifer, Second-hand smoke and human lung cancer, *Lancet Oncol.* **9**: 657–666 (2008).

38. S. Willers, G. Skarping, M. Dalene and S. Skerfving, Urinary cotinine in children and adults during and after semiexperimental exposure to evironmental tobacco smoke, *Arch. Environ. Health* **50**: 130–137 (1995).

39. M. Neri, D. Ugolini, S. Bonassi, A. Fucic, N. Holland, L. E. Knudsen, R. J. Sram, M. Ceppi, V. Bocchini and D. F. Merlo, Children's exposure to environmental pollutants and biomarkers of genetic damage. II. Results of a comprehensive literature search and meta-analysis, *Mutat. Res.* **612**: 14–39 (2006).

40. J. L. Pirkle, J. T. Bernert, S. P. Caudill, C. S. Sosnoff and T. F. Pechacek, Trends in the exposure of nonsmokers in the U.S. population to secondhand smoke: 1988–2002, *Environ. Health Perspect.* **114**: 853–858 (2006).

41. T. Cains, S. Cannata, R. Poulos, M. J. Ferson and B. W. Stewart, Designated "no smoking" areas provide from partial to no protection from environmental tobacco smoke, *Tob. Control* **13**: 17–22 (2004).

42. J. P. Pierce and M. E. Leon, Effectiveness of smoke-free policies, *Lancet Oncol.* **9**: 614–615 (2008).

43. E. R. Gritz, D. J. Vidrine and M. C. Fingeret, Smoking cessation a critical component of medical management in chronic disease populations, *Am. J. Prev. Med.* **33**(6S), 414–422 (2007).

44. E. R. Gritz, C. Dresler and L. Sarna, Smoking, the missing drug interaction in clinical trials: Ignoring the obvious, *Cancer Epidemiol. Biomarkers Prev.* **14**(10): 2287–2293 (2005).

45. A. Bryant and R. J. Cerfolio, Differences in epidemiology, histology, and survival between cigarette smokers and never-smokers who develop non-small cell lung cancer, *Chest* **132**(1): 185–192 (2007).

46. P. S. Nia, J. Weyler, C. Colpaert *et al.*, Prognostic value of smoking status in operated non-small cell lung cancer, *Lung Cancer* **47**: 351–359 (2005).

47. C. M. Tammemagi, C. Neslund-Dudas, M. Simoff *et al.*, Smoking and lung cancer survival. The role of comorbidity and treatment, *Chest* **125**(1): 27–37 (2004).

48. J. Manjer, I. Andersson, G. R. Berglund *et al.*, Survival of women with breast cancer in relation to smoking, *Eur. J. Surg.* **166**: 852–858 (2000).

49. M. D. Holmes, S. Murin, W. Y. Chen *et al.*, Smoking and survival after breast cancer diagnosis, *Int. J. Cancer* **120**: 2672–2677 (2007).

50. N. L. Kobrinsky, M. G. Klug, P. J. Hokanson *et al.*, Impact of smoking on cancer stage at diagnosis, *J. Clin. Oncol.* **21**(5): 907–913 (2003).

51. B. E. Johnson, Second lung cancers in patients after treatment for an initial lung cancer, *J. Natl. Cancer Inst.* **90**(18): 1335–1345 (1998).

52. M. A. Tucker, N. Murray, E. G. Shaw *et al.*, Second primary cancers related to smoking and treatment of small-cell lung cancer, *J. Natl. Cancer Inst.* **89**(23): 1782–1788 (1997).

53. G. E. Richardson, M. A. Tucker, D. J. Venzon *et al.*, Smoking cessation after successful treatment of small-cell lung cancer is associated with fewer smoking-related second primary cancers, *Ann. Intern. Med.* **119**(5): 383–390 (1993).

54. T. Kawaguchi, A. Matsumura, K. I. S. Ishikawa *et al.*, Second primary cancers in patients with stage iii non-small cell lung cancer successfully treated with chemo-radiotherapy, *Japan J. Clin. Oncol.* **36**(1): 7–11 (2006).

55. B. S. Glisson and W. K. Hong, Survival after treatment of small-cell lung cancer: An endless uphill battle, *J. Natl. Cancer Inst.* **89**(23): 1745–1747 (1997).

56. M. Winstanley, S. Woodward and N. Walker, *Tobacco in Australia: Facts and Issues*, 2nd ed. (Victorian Smoking and Health Program, Melbourne, 1995), p. 2.

57. S. Murin, Smoking cessation before lung resection, *Chest* **127**(6): 1873–1875 (2005).

58. M. J. Peters and L. Glantz, Should smokers be refused surgery? *Br. Med. J.* **334**: 20–21 (2007).

59. M. Kuri, M. Nakagawa, H. Tanaka *et al.*, Determination of the duration of preoperative smoking cessation to improve wound healing after head and neck surgery, *Anesthesiology* **102**: 892–896 (2005).

60. M. Winstanley, S. Woodward and N. Walker, *Tobacco in Australia: Facts and Issues*, 2nd ed. (Victorian Smoking and Health Program, Melbourne, 1995), p. 369.

61. L. G. Bluman, L. Mosca, N. Newman *et al.*, Preoperative smoking habits and postoperative pulmonary complications, *Chest* **113**(4): 883–889 (1998).

62. A. A. Vaporciyan, K. W. Merriman, F. Ece *et al.*, Incidence of major pulmonary morbidity after pneumonectomy: Association with timing of smoking cessation, *Ann. Thorac. Surg.* **73**: 420–426 (2002).

63. R. Barrera, W. Shi, D. Amar *et al.*, Smoking and timing of cessation: Impact on pulmonary complications after thoracotomy, *Chest* **127**(6): 1977–1983 (2005).

64. C. D. Rochers, S. Dische and M. I. Saunders, The problem of cigarette smoking in radiotherapy for cancer in the head and neck, *Clin. Oncol.* **4**: 214–216 (1992).

65. G. P. Browman, G. Wong, I. Hodson *et al.*, Influence of cigarette smoking on the efficacy of radiation therapy in head and neck cancer, *N. Engl. J. Med.* **328**(3): 159–163 (1993).

66. J. L. Fox, K. E. Rosenzweig and J. S. Ostroff, The effect of smoking status on survival following radiation therapy for non-small cell lung cancer, *Lung Cancer* **44**: 287–293 (2004).

67. A. S. Tsao, D. Liu, J. J. Lee *et al.*, Smoking affects treatment outcome in patients with advanced nonsmall cell lung cancer, *Cancer* **106**(11): 2428–2436 (2006).

68. R. Duarte, R. Luiz and M. Paschoal, The cigarette burden (measured by the number of pack-years smoked) negatively impacts the response rate to platinum-based chemotherapy in lung cancer, *Lung Cancer* **61**(2): 244–254.

69. M. Prochazka, P. Hall, G. Gagliardi *et al.*, Ionizing radiation and tobacco use increases the risk of a subsequent lung carcinoma in women with breast cancer: Case-only design, *J. Clin. Oncol.* **23**(30): 7467–7474 (2005).

70. P. J. Eifel, A. Jhingran, D. C. Bodurka *et al.*, Correlation of smoking history and other patient characteristics with major complications of pelvic radiation therapy for cervical cancer, *J. Clin. Oncol.* **20**(17): 3651–3657 (2002).

71. T. Pickles, M. Liu, E. Berthelet *et al.*, The effect of smoking on outcome following external radiation for localized prostate cancer, *J. Urol.* **171**: 1543–1546 (2004).

72. J. Pantarotto, S. Malone, S. Dahrouge *et al.*, Smoking is associated with worse outcomes in patients with prostate cancer treated by radical radiotherapy, *Br. J. Urol. Int.* **99**: 564–569 (2006).

73. F. Meyer, I. Bairati, A. Fortin *et al.*, Interaction between antioxidant vitamin supplementation and cigarette smoking during radiation therapy in relation to long-term effects on recurrence and mortality: A randomized trial among head and neck cancer patients, *Int. J. Cancer* **122**: 1679–1683 (2008).

74. D. Il'yasova, L. H. Colbert, T. B. Harris *et al.*, Circulating levels of inflammatory markers and cancer risk in the health aging and body composition cohort, *Cancer Epidemiol. Biomarkers Prev.* **14**(10): 2413–2418 (2005).

75. M. J. Jarvis, ABC of smoking cessation. Why people smoke, *Br. Med. J.* **328**: 277–279 (2004).

76. R. Doll, R. Peto, J. Boreham *et al.*, Mortality in relations to smoking: 50 years' observations on male British doctors, *Br. Med. J.* **328**: 1519 (2004).

77. International Union Against Cancer (UICC), Deaths from smoking, available at http://www.deathsfromsmoking.net/ (accessed 30 October 2008), Switzerland, Geneva, 2008.

78. H. Bronnum-Hansen and K. Juel, Abstention from smoking extends life and compresses morbidity: A population based study of health expectancy among smokers and never smokers in Denmark, *Tob. Control* **10**: 273–278 (2001).

79. C. M. McBride and J. S. Ostroff, Teachable moments for promoting smoking cessation: The context of cancer care and survivorship, *Cancer Control* **10**(4): 325–333 (2003).

80. B. Ridolfo and C. Stevenson, *The Quantification of Drug-Caused Mortality and Morbidity in Australia, 1998* (Australian Institute of Health and Welfare (AIHW), Canberra, 2001).

81. *Smoking and Health: A Report of the Royal College of Physicians on Smoking in Relation to Cancer of the Lung and Other Diseases* (Pitman Medical Publishing Co. Ltd, London, 1962).

82. D. J. Collins and H. M. Lapsley, *Counting the Cost: Estimates of the Social Costs of Drug Abuse in Australia in 1998–99. National Drug Strategy Monograph Series No. 49* (Commonwealth Department of Health and Ageing, Canberra, 2002).

83. Returns on investment in public health: An epidemiological and economic analysis (Department of Health and Ageing, 2003).

84. Curbing the epidemic: Governments and the economics of tobacco control, in *Development in Practice* (The World Bank, Washington D.C., 1999).

85. J. Mackay and M. Eriksen, *The Tobacco Atlas* (World Health Organization, Geneva, 2002).

86. L. Sanderson Cox, N. L. Africano, K. P. Tercyak *et al.*, Nicotine dependence treatment for patients with cancer, *Cancer* **98**(3): 632–644 (2003).

87. R. Peto, S. Darby, H. Deo, P. Silcocks, E. Whitley and R. Doll, Smoking, smoking cessation and lung cancer in the UK since 1950: Combination of national statistics with two case-control studies, *Br. Med. J.* **321**: 323–329 (2000).

88. The Clinical Trial Service Unit and Epidemiological Studies Unit at the University of Oxford, *Survival to Age 70 and Beyond: Effect of Smoking in Male British Doctors*, available at www.deathsfromsmoking.net.

2

Reviewing the Evidence on the Effectiveness of Smoking Cessation Interventions

Nicholas Zwar

Abstract

Smoking cessation is of great health benefit to cancer patients and the diagnosis of cancer presents an opportunity to encourage cessation. There is limited evidence on the efficacy of smoking cessation interventions in cancer patients. In the absence of specific studies, interventions that have been shown to be effective in the general population should be offered to patients with cancer. They include:

- health professional advice to quit;
- referral to telephone help lines;
- individual counselling, group counselling and computerised quit support; and
- smoking cessation pharmacotherapy.

Combining some form of counselling support with pharmacotherapy is a commonly used and evidence-based approach. The evidence on interventions specifically designed for patients with cancer suggests that more intensive interventions, offered over a number of sessions by a health professional such as a nurse or a peer counsellor, can be effective. Interventions are most effective when smoking cessation pharmacotherapy is also provided.

Keywords: Smoking cessation, cancer, pharmacotherapy, help lines.

1.   Introduction

Stopping smoking is frequently the single most important thing people can do to improve their health. This is true of cancer patients, as well as the general population. This chapter examines the evidence on the effectiveness of smoking cessation interventions, comprising interventions tested in the general population, as well as the much smaller literature of interventions tested in people with cancer. The rationale for considering both the broad and cancer specific literature is that in the absence of specific studies, it is reasonable to apply interventions found to be effective in the general population to special populations.[1]

2.   Effectiveness of Smoking Cessation Interventions in the General Population

Tobacco dependence can be viewed as a chronic disease that often requires repeated intervention and multiple attempts to quit.[2] Interventions that aim to assist quitting need to be seen in the context of public health approaches to discourage tobacco use and encourage cessation. These include restrictions on tobacco advertising and sale, taxation, restriction on smoking in public places and social marketing campaigns. The most common method of attempted cessation is unsupported quitting,[3] however only 3–5% of smokers who try to quit without treatment remain abstinent six to twelve months later.[4] A variety of approaches are available to support smoking cessation and the evidence on the effectiveness of major approaches is summarised below.

2.1   *Health professional advice*

There is evidence that advice from health professionals is effective in encouraging smoking cessation. A Cochrane review examined evidence from 41 trials, involving approximately 31,000 smokers.[5] The most common setting for advice was primary care. The pooled data from 17 trials revealed a small but significant increase in the odds of quitting at six months (relative risk 1.66, 95% confidence interval 1.42 to 1.92) of brief advice, compared to no advice (or usual care). Brief advice was defined as smoking cessation advice provided during a single consultation lasting less than 20 minutes plus up to one follow-up visit. This equates to an absolute difference in the cessation rate of about 2.5%, or one extra quitter for every 40 patients provided brief advice. In 11 trials where the intervention was more intensive, the estimated effect was higher (RR: 1.84, 95% CI: 1.60 to 2.13). Further evidence that spending more time has a greater effect comes from the meta-analysis for the US Clinical Practice Guideline.[1] In this meta-analysis, minimal duration counselling (up to three minutes) was found to result in an abstinence rate of 13.4% at six months (2.5% higher than controls); low intensity (3–10 minutes) in an abstinence rate of 16.0% (5% higher than controls); and higher intensity (more than 10 minutes) in an abstinence rate of 22.1% (11% higher than controls).

A Cochrane Review of randomised trials of smoking cessation interventions delivered by nurses and involving at least six months follow-up also show a benefit (RR: 1.28, 95% CI: 1.18 to 1.38).[6] The major effect of advice from health professionals is to motivate a quit attempt (3–5-fold increase). It is important to remember that combining brief advice with other effective interventions such as pharmacotherapy can considerably reduce the number needed to treat (NNT).

Most of the studies examining physician advice were conducted in community settings; however smoking cessation interventions delivered to hospitalised patients can also be effective. There is evidence that augmented in-hospital interventions for smoking cessation are more effective than usual care.[1,7] A Cochrane review concluded that at least one month of follow-up after discharge is needed to achieve an increase in abstinence at six months after the start of the intervention, compared to usual care.[7]

2.2 Telephone helplines

Telephone counselling provided through state-based or national services is available in many countries. There has been considerable research on quitline effectiveness in recent years and the U.S.

Treating Tobacco Use and Dependence 2008 Update conducted an meta-analysis of quitline intervention versus minimal or no contact or self-help materials.[2] In this analysis quitline interventions were defined as telephone counselling in which at least some of the contacts are initiated by the counselor to deliver tobacco use interventions, including call-back counselling. The meta-analysis of 11 studies found a robust effect of quitline counselling, with an odds ratio of 1.26 (95 CI: 1.4 to 1.8). The estimated abstinence rate with quitline counselling was 12.7% and 8.5% in the comparison group. A meta-analysis of six studies combining quitline counselling and medication also showed benefit over medications alone (OR: 1.3, 95% CI: 1.1–1.6).[2]

2.3 *Psychological methods*

Individual behavioural counselling involves individual face-to-face assistance from a trained counselor outside normal clinical care. The counsellor may work with the patient to increase motivation, identify high risk situations for relapse, develop problem solving skills, provide social support as part of treatment and help smokers obtain social support outside of treatment.[1,8] A Cochrane review identified 21 trials with over 7000 participants and concluded that individual behavioural counselling was more effective than control with an odds ratio for successful cessation of 1.56 (95% CI: 1.32–1.84).[8]

Group counselling, which focuses on skills training and providing mutual support can also be effective for assisting smoking cessation. The meta-analysis for the U.S. Clinical Practice guideline found an odds ratio of 1.3 (95% CI: 1.1–1.6) with an abstinence rate of 13.9% at six months follow-up.[1] Group programs do not suit all smokers, but are likely to be helpful for those who do find them appealing.[9] Self-help intervention such as pamphlets, booklets, audiotapes and videotapes were found to be of marginal benefit in the meta-analysis done for the U.S. Clinical Practice Guideline.[1] Computerised interventions are increasingly being used and the recent update of the U.S. Treating Tobacco Use and Dependence Guideline concluded that e-health tobacco interventions have generally yielded positive results.[2] A review of studies in adult smokers found that in seven of 15 studies there were significantly improved outcomes, compared to control groups.[10]

2.4   Alternative methods

2.4.1   Acupuncture

Acupuncture as an aid to smoking cessation has been the subject of a number of controlled studies and two meta-analyses have reviewed the results of controlled studies.[1,11] There was no significant difference between 'active' acupuncture or 'inactive' or sham acupuncture procedures. Positive expectations of the effect of acupuncture may therefore be the factor responsible for the benefit seen in uncontrolled studies, rather than the acupuncture itself.

2.4.2   Hypnosis

Hypnotherapy as an aid to smoking cessation has been the subject of a number of studies, including some controlled trials, a Cochrane Collaboration review of evidence in 1998 concluded that there was such heterogeneity between methods and results, that a meta-analysis was not feasible at that time.[12] The review concluded that hypnotherapy does not show a greater effect on six month quit rates than other interventions or no treatment.

2.5   Pharmacological agents

2.5.1   Nicotine replacement therapy

The aim of nicotine replacement therapy (NRT) is to replace some of the nicotine from cigarettes without the harmful constituents found in tobacco smoke. NRT reduces withdrawal symptoms associated with nicotine addiction, allowing the smoker to focus on the psychosocial aspects of quitting.[13] Meta-analyses of the evidence on the efficacy of NRT published by the Cochrane Library[14] and US Public Health Service[1] conclude that NRT is effective. The Cochrane review looked at 65 studies and found an overall odds ratio of 1.71 (95% CI: 1.60, 1.82), when comparing cessation rates at 12 months of various forms of NRT to placebo or no treatment.[14] The effect sizes (difference in abstinence rate between intervention and control groups) for different forms of NRT ranged from 5–12%, but no form of NRT (patch, gum, lozenge, microtab and inhaler) was significantly better than another. In the meta-analysis of 47 studies by Fiore, et al., the odds ratios ranged from 1.6–2.7 and effect sizes from 7–17% comparing various forms of NRT to placebo at six months follow-up.[1]

Highly dependent smokers (20 or more cigarettes per day) benefit more from 4 mg than 2 mg gum and there may be a small benefit of higher dose patches across the range of 15 to 42 mg in 16-hour or 24-hour patches.[14,15] Rapid onset and slower onset nicotine delivery systems have been combined in a number of studies, such as the transdermal patch for a steady background supply of nicotine, supplemented by gum for immediate relief of craving.[16,17] A meta-analysis of combination therapies showed that combination therapy almost doubles cessation rates at 12 months, compared to one form of therapy.[1] Pre-treatment NRT, where patients who are reluctant to quit using NRT in the standard way start using NRT while they reduce smoking and then progress to a quit attempt, has been shown to be of value.[18]

NRT can be used safely in people with stable cardiovascular disease but should be used with caution in people with recent myocardial infarction, unstable angina, severe arrhythmias and recent cerebrovascular accident. NRT should be considered when a pregnant woman is otherwise unable to quit, and when the likelihood and benefits of cessation outweigh the risks of NRT.[13] Intermittent dosage forms such as gum, lozenge, inhaler and microtab are preferred in pregnancy due to the possible risks to the foetus of continuous exposure to nicotine. Common adverse effects with NRT depend on the dosage form. For patch they include skin erythema and allergy and sleep disturbance; for gum, lozenge and microtab dyspepsia and nausea; and for inhaler mouth and throat irritation.[13]

2.5.2 Bupropion sustained release

Originally developed as an antidepressant, bupropion is a non-nicotine, oral therapy which reduces the urge to smoke and symptoms from nicotine withdrawal. Bupropion doubles the cessation rate compared to placebo: over 12 months. Data from two randomised, controlled trials showed 9% and 19% of smokers had not smoked for the 12 months following placebo and bupropion therapy, respectively.[19,20] Bupropion has been shown to be effective in a range of patient populations, including smokers with depression, cardiac disease and respiratory diseases including chronic obstructive pulmonary disease.[21] It has also been shown to improve short-term abstinence rates for people with schizophrenia.[22]

Bupropion is contraindicated in patients with a history of seizures, eating disorders and patients taking monoamine oxidase inhibitors. It should be used with caution in people taking medications that can lower seizure threshold, such as antidepressants and oral hypoglycaemic agents.[23,24] The most clinically important adverse effect is seizures (0.1% risk). Common adverse effects are insomnia, headache, dry mouth, nausea, dizziness and anxiety.[21,25]

2.5.3 *Varenicline*

Developed specifically for smoking cessation, varenicline acts by targeting the nicotine acetylcholine receptor in the reward centres in the brain. Varenicline binds with high affinity at the $\alpha 4\beta 2$ nicotinic acetylcholine receptor, where it acts as a partial agonist to alleviate symptoms of craving and withdrawal. At the same time, it blocks nicotine from binding to the $\alpha 4\beta 2$ receptor, thus reducing the intensity of the rewarding effects of smoking.[25] In two randomised double-blind clinical trials with identical study designs varenicline was compared to both bupropion and to placebo. All three groups received brief behavioural counselling. Varenicline produced a continuous abstinence rate from week 9 through to one year of 21.9% (compared to 8.4% in the placebo group [$p < 0.001$] and 16.1% in the bupropion group [$p = 0.057$]), and 23% (10.3% in the placebo group [$p < 0.001$] and 14.6% in bupropion group [$p = 0.004$]), respectively.[26,27] The abstinence rate for varenicline was significantly better than both bupropion and placebo in the long term. There has been one published open label study comparing varenicline to nicotine replacement therapy, which showed a benefit for varenicline. However this did not reach statistical significance for the primary outcome measure of continuous abstinence from weeks 9 through 52.[28]

Prolonged use of varenicline has also been shown to reduce relapse. In subjects who stopped smoking at the end of 12 weeks of treatment; an additional 12 weeks of treatment was more beneficial than placebo in maintaining abstinence to the end of treatment and to one year from the start of treatment, although the difference in continuous abstinence for weeks 13–52 between intervention and control groups was small.[29] The benefit only appears to be maintained for the period of use of varenicline.

Nausea is the most common adverse effect with varenicline and in these studies it was reported in almost 30% of smokers, although less than 3% discontinued treatment due to nausea.[27,28] Abnormal dreams were also more common in the varenicline group (13.1%) than either the bupropion (5.9%) or placebo groups (3.5%). The effectiveness and safety of varenicline has not been studied in patients with psychiatric conditions. Post-marketing, there have been reports of mood changes, depression, behaviour disturbance and suicidality possibly associated with varenicline[30] and prescribers have been advised to monitor patients for emergence of these problems.

2.5.4 *Nortriptyline*

The tricyclic antidepressant nortriptyline has been shown to approximately double cessation rates compared to placebo (OR = 2.1).[24,31] A recent systematic review shows that the use of nortriptyline for smoking cessation resulted in higher prolonged abstinence rates after at least six months, compared to placebo treatment.[32] The efficacy of nortriptyline does not appear to be affected by a past history of depression; it is, however, limited in its application by its potential for serious side effects including dry mouth, constipation, nausea, sedation and headaches, and a risk of arrhythmia in patients with cardiovascular disease.[25]

3. Effectiveness of Cessation Interventions in Cancer Patients

It has been suggested that the diagnosis of serious illness presents a 'teachable moment' for intervention on tobacco dependence,[1] and that many cancer survivors who smoke are motivated to quit.[33] Quit rates have been reported to be higher in patients with cancers related to smoking[34,35] and it has been suggested that raising awareness of the connection between the diagnosis and tobacco use may facilitate smoking cessation.[36] Despite this, there are a limited number of published studies which have empirically tested the effectiveness of smoking cessation interventions in cancer patients. In a review of the evidence on smoking cessation interventions designed specifically for cancer patients, Gritz, *et al.* identified only six studies.[36] All but one involved patients with smoking-related cancers. Intervention initiated in hospital by a nurse and followed up with telephone support after discharge increased short term abstinence from between 43–50% in the control group to 65–75% for the intervention group.[37,38] In lung cancer patients a pre-/post-evaluation of the same intervention model found abstinence in 40% of patients at six weeks,[39] while a controlled study of a brief version of the same intervention found only a small difference in abstinence from 21% in intervention group, compared to 14% in control group at six weeks follow-up.[40] In a study of brief advice from a surgeon or dentist in patients with head and neck squamous cell carcinoma, both intervention groups had high quit rates (70% continuous abstinence at one year), with no greater quit rate in the group that got a quit contract, tailored booklets and follow-up in addition to brief advice.[41] The only study identified in this review which did not focus on patients with smoking related cancers found no difference between unstructured brief advice, versus a structured programme delivered by a physician based on National Institutes of Health Guidelines.[42]

A more recent systematic review identified eight further relevant studies.[43] However the intervention resulted in significantly increased smoking cessation rates in cancer patients in only two of these studies. A randomised trial of a peer counselling program compared to self-help in adult survivors of childhood cancer by Emmons *et al.* found that the intervention group had a significantly higher quit rate at both the 8-month (16.8% v 8.5%, $p < .01$) and 12-month follow up points (15% v 9%, $p \leq .01$).[44] The intervention included six telephone calls from a trained childhood cancer survivor, involving motivational interviewing, tailored and targeted materials and free nicotine replacement therapy.

A randomised trial by Duffy, *et al.* allocated head and neck cancer patients who had smoked in the last six months and had co-morbid alcohol problem and/or depression to either a nurse-led cognitive behaviour therapy (CBT) program and pharmacotherapy with NRT and/or bupropion or to a control group, offered referral to smoking cessation, alcohol treatment and/or psychiatric evaluation.[45] At six months the quit rate in the intervention group was 47% versus 31% in the control group. An Australian randomised trial of a motivational interviewing approach to encouraging cessation in cancer patients was not included in either systematic review. At six months this study found no significant difference in biochemically confirmed quit rates between intervention (5%) and control (6%) groups.[46]

The review by de Moor, *et al.*[42] identified the following characteristics of effective interventions in cancer patients:

(1) attention to health risk behaviours that may impact smoking status and smoking cessation;
(2) designing intervention content around a theoretical framework;
(3) tailoring intervention content to survivor's stage of readiness to quit smoking;
(4) using "peers" to deliver intervention content;
(5) regular reinforcement of the importance of smoking cessation;
(6) a combination of nicotine replacement therapy or other pharmacotherapy and behavioural strategies for smoking cessation; and
(7) high intensity delivery over multiple sessions.

It should be noted that although the use of stage-based interventions was recommended in this review, there is currently a lack of evidence that such interventions are more effective;[47] furthermore, there is some evidence that, in the general population at least, unplanned quit attempts are as likely to be successful as planned attempts.[48]

The systematic review of de Moor[43] and colleagues notes the importance of higher intensity interventions with cancer survivors involving more contacts and longer follow-up. People with cancer who continue to smoke after diagnosis may be strongly addicted to tobacco. They may also be using smoking to cope with stress and therefore find it difficult to quit at the time of a health crisis. For both these reasons, high intensity interventions with multiple contacts may be needed to help people with cancer overcome tobacco dependence.

4.   Conclusion

A diagnosis of cancer can create a teachable moment, when cancer patients are motivated to quit. This is particularly the case where there is a link between the cancer and tobacco use. Explaining this link to patients may help to increase motivation to quit, but clinicians also need to be mindful of how in a stressful situation such as a health crisis, many tobacco users see smoking as a coping strategy.

In the absence of extensive empirical studies on the effect of smoking cessation interventions in cancer patients, interventions that have been shown to be effective in the general population should be offered. These include advice from a health professional such as a physician or nurse, individual or group counselling, telephone helplines and pharmacotherapy. There is increasing evidence that computerised support can also be effective. Combining some form of counselling support with pharmacotherapy is a commonly used and evidence-based approach.

The literature on interventions specifically designed for cancer patients is limited. However, the evidence suggests that more intensive interventions offered over a number of sessions by a health professional, such as a nurse or a peer counselor can be effective. Interventions are most effective when smoking cessation pharmacotherapy is also provided.

References

1. M. C. Fiore, B. W. Bailey, S. J. Cohen *et al.*, *Treating Tobbaco Use and Dependence*, Clinical Practice Guideline (U.S. Department of Health and Human Services, Public Health Service, 2000).
2. M. C. Fiore, C. R. Jaen. T. B. Baker *et al.*, *Treating Tobacco Use and Dependence: 2008 Update*, Clinical Practice Guideline (U.S.

Department of Health and Human Services, Public Health Service, 2008).

3. C. M. Doran, L. V., M. Robinson, H. Britt and R. P. Mattick, Smoking status of Australian general practice patients and their quit attempts, *Addict. Behav.* **31**: 758–766 (2006).

4. J. R. Hughes, J. Keely and S. Naud, Shape of the relapse curve and long-term abstinence among untreated smokers, *Addiction* **99**: 29–38 (2004).

5. L. F. Stead, G. Bergson and T. Lancaster, Physician advice for smoking cessation, *Cochrane Database Syst. Rev.* **2**: CD000165 (2008).

6. V. H. Rice and L. F. Stead, Nursing interventions for smoking cessation, *Cochrane Database Syst. Rev.* **1**: CD001188 (2008).

7. N. A. Rigotti, M. R. Munato and L. F. Stead, Interventions for smoking cessation in hospitalised patients, *Cochrane Database Syst. Rev.* **3**: CD001837 (2007).

8. T. Lancaster and L. F. Stead, Individual behavioural counselling for smoking cessation, *Cochrane Database Syst. Rev.* **2**: CD001292 (2005).

9. L. F. Stead and T. Lancaster, Group behaviour therapy programmes for smoking cessation, *Cochrane Database Syst. Rev.* **2**: CD001007 (2005).

10. S. T. Walters, J. A. Wright and R. Shegog, A review of computer and Internet-based interventions for smoking behavior, *Addict. Behav.* **31**: 264–277 (2006).

11. A. R. White, K. L. Resch and E. Ernst, A meta-analysis of acupuncture techniques for smoking cessation, *Tob. Control* **8**: 393–397 (1999).

12. N. C. Abbot, L. F. Stead, A. R. White and J. Barnes, Hypnotherapy for smoking cessation, *Cochrane Database Syst. Rev.* **2**: CD001008 (1998).

13. N. Zwar, R. Richmond, R. Borland, S. Stillman, M. Cunningham and J. Litt, *Smoking Cessation Guidelines for Australian General Practice* (Commonwealth Department of Health and Ageing, Canberra, 2004).

14. L. F. Stead, R. Perera, C. Bullen, D. Mant and T. Lancaster, Nicotine replacement therapy for smoking cessation, *Cochrane Database Syst. Rev.* **1**: CD000146 (2008).

15. J. Hughes, G. R. Lesmes, D. K. Hatsukami, R. Richmond *et al.*, Are higher doses of nicotine replacement more effective for smoking cessation? *Nicotine Tob. Res.* **1**: 169–174 (1999).

16. M. Kornitzer, M. Boutsen, M. Dramaix *et al.*, Combined use of nicotine patch and gum in smoking cessation: Placebo controlled trial, *Prevent. Med.* **24**: 41–47 (1995).

17. P. Puska, H. J. Korhonen, E. Vartianinen, E. L. Urjanheimo, G. Gustavsson and A. Westin, Combined use of nicotine patch and gum compared with gum alone in smoking cessation: A clinical trial in North Karelia, *Tob. Control* **4**: 231–235 (1995).

18. S. Shiffman and S. G. Fergusar, Nicotine patch therapy prior to quitting smoking: A meta-analysis, *Addiction* **103**: 557–563 (2008).

19. R. D. Hurt, D. P. Sacns, E. D. Glover, K. P. Offord, J. A. Johnston, L. C. Dale *et al.*, A comparison of sustained-release bupropion and placebo for smoking cessation, *N. Engl. J. Med.* **227**: 1195–1202 (1997).

20. D. E. Jorenby, S. J. Leischow, M. A. Nides, S. J. Rennard, J. A. Johnston, A. R. Hughes *et al.*, A controlled trial of sustained-release bupropion, a nicotine patch, or both for smoking cessation, *N. Engl. J. Med.* **340**: 685–691 (1999).

21. R. Richmond and N. Zwar, Therapeutic review of bupropion sustained release, *Aust. Drug Alcohol Rev.* **22**: 203–220 (2003).

22. A. E. Evins, C. Cather, T. Deckersbach, O. Freudenreich, M. A. Culhane, C. M. Olm-Shipman *et al.*, A double-blind placebo-controlled trial of bupropion sustained-release for smoking cessation in schizophrenia, *J. Clin. Psychopharmacol.* **25**: 218–225 (2005).

23. J. R. Hughes, L. F. Stead and T. Lancaster, Nortriptyline for smoking cessation: A review, *Nicotine Tob. Res.* **7**: 491–499 (2005).

24. J. R. Hughes, L. F. Stead and T. Lancaster, Antidepressants for smoking cessation, *Cochrane Database Syst. Rev.* **1**: CD000031 (2007).

25. N. Zwar, R. Richmond, R. Borland, M. Peters, S. Stillman, J. Litt, J. Bell and B. Caldwell, *Smoking Cessation Pharmacotherapy: An Update for Health Professionals* (Royal Australian College of General Practitioners, Melbourne, 2007).

26. D. Gonzales, S. I. Rennard, M. Nides, C. Oncken, S. Azoulay, C. B. Billing *et al.*, Varenicline, an α4β2 nicotinic acetylcholine receptor partial agonist, vs. sustained-release bupropion and placebo for smoking cessation, *J. Am. Med. Assoc.* **296**: 47–55 (2006).

27. D. E. Jorenby, J. T. Hays, N. A. Rigotti, S. Azoulay, E. J. Watsky, K. E. Williams *et al.*, Efficacy of varenicline, an α4β2 nicotinic acetylcholine receptor partial agonist, vs. placebo or sustained-release bupropion for smoking cessation, *J. Am. Med. Assoc.* **296**: 56–63 (2006).

28. H.-J. Aubin, A. Bobak, J. R. Britton, C. Oncken, C. B. Billing, J. Gong, K. E. Williams and K. R. Reeves, Varenicline versus transdermal

nicotine patch for smoking cessation: Results from a randomized open-label trial, *Thorax* **63**: 717–724 (2008).

29. S. Tonstad, P. Tønnesen, P. Hajek, K. E. Williams, C. B. Billing *et al.*, Effect of maintenance therapy with varenicline on smoking cessation, *J. Am. Med. Assoc.* **296**: 64–71 (2006).

30. K. Cahill, L. F. Stead and T. Lancaster, Nicotine receptor partial antagonists for smoking cessation, *Cochrane Database Syst. Rev.* **3**: CD006103 (2008).

31. J. R. Hughes, L. F. Stead and T. Lancaster, Nortriptyline for smoking cessation: A review, *Nicotine Tob. Res.* **7**: 491–499 (2005).

32. E. J. Wagena, P. Knipschild and M. P. Zeegers, Should nortriptyline be used as a first-line aid to help smokers quit? Results from a systematic review and meta-analysis, *Addiction* **100**: 317–326 (2005).

33. J. L. Ostroff, P. B. Jacobsen, A. B. Moadel *et al.*, Prevalence and predictors of continued tobacco use after treatment of patients with head and neck cancer, *Cancer* **75**: 569–576 (1995).

34. E. R. Gritz, C. R. Carr, D. Rapkin *et al.*, Predictors of long-term smoking cessation in head and neck cancer patients, *Cancer Epidemiol. Biomarkers Prev.* **2**: 261–270 (1993).

35. E. R. Gritz, R. Nisenbaum, R. E. Elashoff and E. C. Holmes, Smoking behavior following diagnosis in patients with stage 1 non-small cell cancer, *Cancer Causes Control* **2**: 105–112 (1991).

36. E. R. Gritz, M. C. Fingeret, D. J. Vidrine, A. B. Lasev, N. V. Mehta and G. P. Reece, Successes and failures of the teachable moment; smoking cessation in cancer patients, *Cancer* **1206**: 17–27 (2006).

37. A. E. Stanislaw and M. E. Wewers, A smoking cessation intervention with hospitalized surgical cancer patients: A pilot study, *Cancer Nurs.* **17**: 81–86 (1994).

38. M. E. Wewers, J. M. Bowen, A. E. Stanislaw and V. B. Desimone, A nurse delivered smoking cessation intervention among hospitalized postoperative patients — Influence of a smoking related diagnosis: A pilot study, *Heart Lung* **23**: 151–156 (1994).

39. M. E. Wewers, L. Jenkins and T. Mignery, A nurse-managed smoking cessation intervention during diagnostic testing for lung cancer, *Oncol. Nurs. Forum* **24**: 1419–1422 (1997).

40. B. Griebel, M. E. Wewers and C. A. Baker, The effectiveness of a nurse-managed minimal smoking cessation intervention among hospitalized patients with cancer, *Oncol. Nurs. Forum* **25**: 897–902 (1998).

41. E. R. Gritz, C. L. Carmack, C. de Moor *et al.*, First year after head and neck cancer: Quality of life, *J. Clin. Oncol.* **17**: 352–360 (1999).

42. R. A. Schnoll, B. Zhang, M. Rue *et al.*, Brief physician-initiated quit smoking strategies for clinical oncology settings: A trial coordinated by the Eastern Cooperative Oncology Group, *J. Clin. Oncol.* **21**: 355–365 (2003).

43. J. S. de Moor, K. Elder and M. Emmons, Smoking prevention and cessation interventions for cancer survivors, *Sem. Oncol. Nurs.* **24**: 180–192 (2008).

44. K. M. Emmons, E. Puleo, E. Park, E. R. Gritz, R. M. Butterfield, J. C. Weeks, A. Mertens and F. P. Li, Peer-delivered smoking cessation counseling for childhood cancer survivors increases rate of cessation: The partnership for health study, *J. Clin. Oncol.* **23**: 6515–6523 (2005).

45. S. A. Duffy, D. L. Ronis, M. Valenstein *et al.*, A tailored smoking, alcohol and depression intervention for head and neck cancer patients, *Cancer Epidemiol. Biomarkers Prev.* **15**: 2203–2208 (2006).

46. M. Wakefield, I. Olver, H. Whitford and E. Rosenfeld, Motivational interviewing as a smoking cessation intervention for patients with cancer: Randomized controlled trial, *Nurs. Res.* **53**(6): 396–405 (2004).

47. K. Cahill and N. Green, Stage-based interventions for smoking cessation, *Cochrane Database Syst. Rev.* **3**: CD004492 (2007).

48. R. West and T. Sohal, "Catastropic" pathways to smoking: Findings from a national survey, *Br. Med. J.* **332**: 458–460 (2006).

3

Diet, Physical Activity and Cancer — The Epidemiological Evidence

Erica L. James,
Victoria M. Flood,
Bruce Armstrong
and Fiona Stacey

Abstract

This review of the epidemiological evidence for diet and physical activity and the risk of cancer primarily summarises the recommendations of the World Cancer Research Fund (WCRF) and the American Institute of Cancer Research (AICR). Recommendations include the topics of: body fatness, plant foods, animal foods, alcoholic drinks, dietary supplements, and physical activity. For each of these recommendations we review the level of evidence used to determine the final recommendations, discuss potential limitations of dietary and physical activity measures, and review the study designs that underpin the existing evidence base. In addition, we briefly describe the biological mechanisms underlying the hypotheses around diet and physical activity and cancer and finally we describe more recent research published since the release of the WCRF/AICR recommendations.

There is "convincing" or "probable" evidence of the positive relationship between cancer and: body and abdominal fatness; alcohol; red and processed meats; and high-dose beta-carotene supplements. There is "convincing" or "probable" evidence of a protective effect of consumption of fruit and vegetables; calcium and selenium; and physical activity on cancer risk. Lifestyle modification has the potential to result in a substantial reduction in cancer incidence. If this potential is to be realised, policies and programmes that modify behavioural and environmental factors are required.

Keywords: Diet, nutrition, physical activity, BMI.

1. Introduction

Epidemiological interest in the relationship of cancer risk with diet was stimulated by ecological studies, which showed quite strong correlations of a population's apparent consumption of foods or nutrients with its risk of a range of cancers. Many of the large cohort studies have based their dietary measurements on food frequency questionnaires (FFQ), which generally do not provide good estimates of absolute food and nutrient intake, but may rank people well,[1] so risk is often assessed in terms of the highest category of intake (e.g. fifth quintile) compared to the lowest category of intake (first quintile). However, the correlations between dietary intakes in validation studies are rarely high (for example, FFQ data may be associated with a greater degree of measurement error, compared with dietary assessment which involves shorter memory recall or food records) and thus random error might cause estimates of the strength of associations of dietary variables with cancer risk to be substantially weaker than they really are.[2]

Most work on diet and cancer has been "reductionist" in its approach, both in humans and in experimental animals, where a particular food or nutrient has been studied in relation to its impact on tumour formation, or regression at a particular site of the body.[3] An approach that considers particular dietary components outside their whole dietary and, perhaps, lifestyle context, may be quite misleading. More recently, the effects of defined dietary patterns have been studied (such as a "prudent diet", compared with a

"Western diet")[4] — an approach that may provide, in the longer term, a better way to define diets that are associated with the lowest risk of cancer.

There have been few randomised intervention studies of diet and cancer and generally they have focussed on vitamin supplements, not dietary patterns. A major difficulty for intervention studies of diet is compliance with diet over a long period of time, as is required, due to the possibly long lag time for an influence on cancer to be seen.

The evidence base for a relationship between cancer and physical activity is also based on observational epidemiological studies and mechanistic studies exploring reasons why physical activity may protect against cancer (or why sedentary living may promote cancer). Large epidemiological studies carried out in the USA have shown that physical inactivity is associated with higher overall cancer incidence and mortality.[5-7] Mechanistic hypotheses why physical activity may protect against cancer include healthier levels of circulating hormones and the ability of the more active body to consume more food and nutrients without gaining weight.

The following section of this chapter discusses specific recommendations for diet and physical activity and reduction of cancer risk. It is based predominantly on the World Cancer Research Fund (WCRF)/American Institute of Cancer Research (AICR) report's recommendations, together with additional commentary on aspects of the literature and application of the recommendations. Where relevant, we have added more recent literature to that reviewed by WCRF/AICR. Two of the common sources of recent evidence are from two large prospective cohorts underway in Europe and the United States. The European Prospective Investigation into Cancer and Nutrition (EPIC) was designed to investigate the relationships between diet, nutritional status, lifestyle and environmental factors and the incidence of cancer and other chronic diseases. EPIC is a large study of diet and health, having recruited over half a million (520,000) people in ten European countries: Denmark, France, Germany, Greece, Italy, The Netherlands, Norway, Spain, Sweden and the United Kingdom. The National Institutes of Health (NIH)-AARP study cohort consists of 567,169 American Association of Retired Persons (AARP) members, including 340,148 men and 227,021 women, between the ages of 50 and 71 in 1995–96, who resided in California, Florida, Pennsylvania, New Jersey, North Carolina, Louisiana, and metropolitan Atlanta and Detroit. For sake of brevity, we have not dealt with the WCRF/AICR recommendations on foods and drinks that promote body fatness (the subject is adequately covered under body fatness); preservation, processing and preparation of food (there is insufficient evidence to make any recommendations) and breastfeeding (because of its limited relevance to adult behaviour).

2.   Recommendations

2.1   *Body fatness*

WCRF states "Be as lean as possible within the normal range of body weight". The normal range refers to ranges given by national governments or, the World Health Organization (WHO), as considered appropriate for different population groups. There is *convincing* evidence that greater body fatness increases the risk of cancers of the oesophagus, pancreas, colon and rectum (assessed together), breast (after the menopause), endometrium and kidney. There is *convincing* evidence that greater abdominal fatness increases the risk of colon and rectal cancers (assessed together).

Body fatness *probably* increases the risk for gallbladder cancer. Abdominal obesity *probably* increases the risk of pancreatic cancer, post-menopausal breast cancer and endometrial cancer. Greater body fatness *probably reduces* the risk of pre-menopausal breast cancer.

BMI (body mass index — weight divided by height squared), the commonly used measure, is not a perfect marker of body fatness. More precise techniques, such as underwater weighing, magnetic resonance imaging, computerised tomography, or dual energy X-ray absorptiometry are rare in large-scale epidemiological studies, due to their difficulty and expense. Abdominal fatness is usually measured either using the waist to hip ratio, or the waist circumference alone. There is a lack of consensus on how abdominal fatness is best measured, and measurement error is more likely than for some other anthropometric measures such as height and weight. The currently proposed maximum "cut-off" points for "healthy" waist circumferences (94 cm or 37 inches for men; 80 cm or 31.5 inches for women) and for "healthy" waist to hip ratios (1.0 for men; 0.8 for women) are based almost exclusively on studies of cardiovascular or type 2 diabetes risk in white populations in high-income countries.[8] It is not known whether they can be applied to other ethnic groups or outcomes. The relationship between waist circumference and the size of intra-abdominal fat stores (as opposed to subcutaneous abdominal fat stores) may vary between different ethnic groups.[9] As body fatness tends to increase with age in most populations, and is characteristically higher in women than in men, it is important that studies take into account both age and sex. Measurement of change in weight tends to be more precise than static measures such as weight or BMI.

Objective measures of height and weight, and therefore BMI, are reliable. However, many studies rely on self-reporting, which is liable to introduce bias. Although reported and actual weights are correlated, weight tends to be under-reported, especially by overweight and obese people.[10] BMIs calculated from self-reported data will therefore tend to be lower than those from more objective measures.

2.1.1 *Study designs*

The WCRF reviewed many studies, generally cohort and case-control studies, with a higher proportion of cohort studies reported in more recent epidemiological literature. The WCRF recommendations regarding *body fatness* were based on 161 different prospective cohort studies, across nine different cancer types. Of the 161 cohort studies, 117 reported an increased risk with higher levels of body fatness.

The WCRF recommendations regarding *abdominal fatness* were based on 19 separate prospective cohort studies, across four different cancer types. All 19 cohort studies reported an increased risk with higher levels of abdominal fatness.

2.1.2 *Recent literature*

Since the WCRF report, two meta-analyses[11,12] and a large cohort study[13] have provided further evidence for the relationship between total body fat and colorectal cancer. In addition, EPIC findings concluded that abdominal obesity is an equally strong risk factor for colon cancer in men and women, whereas body weight and BMI were associated with colon cancer risk in men, but not in women. These data suggest that fat distribution is a more important risk factor than body weight and BMI for colon cancer in women.[14]

Similarly, recent findings from cohort studies[15–17] have confirmed the previously described associations between overweight and obesity and increased risk of post-menopausal breast cancer. Furthermore, these data suggest that weight gain during adult life, specifically after menopause, increases the risk of breast cancer among post-menopausal women, while weight loss after menopause is associated with a decreased risk of breast cancer.[17]

Three large cohort studies published since WCRF[18–20] have provided further evidence of the relationship between total body fatness and risk of endometrial cancer. One found a six-fold increase in risk among very obese women (BMI > 40), compared to those of normal BMI (20–24), whereas those women with a BMI less than 20 had only half the risk.[20] In addition, BMI significantly modified the association between physical activity and endometrial cancer risk.[21]

Recent prospective findings have indicated that the risk of testicular cancer decreased modestly with increasing adult BMI and increased modestly with increasing adult height.[22] Similarly, for bladder cancer there was a modest, but graded positive association between BMI and risk of bladder cancer (and compared with normal weight, overweight was associated with 15% increase in risk, and obesity was related to an up to 28% increased risk).[23] The first relevant meta-analysis concluded that overweight and obesity are associated with increased risk of multiple myeloma. The association was similar among men and women and also among whites and blacks.[24]

2.1.3 *Mechanisms of carcinogenesis*

The age-specific pattern of association of breast cancer with BMI, is largely explained by its relationship with endogenous sex hormone levels.[25] The inflammatory state associated with obesity may promote cancer.[25,26] In contrast, energy restriction delays the onset of many age-related diseases, including cancer.

In the case of **gallbladder cancer**, body fatness probably increases the risk of cancer directly and indirectly through the formation of gallstones. Excess body weight (particularly abdominal fatness) exacerbates insulin resistance, which leads to the pancreas producing more insulin. Hyperinsulinaemia increases the risk of **colorectal and endometrial** cancer, and possibly **pancreatic and kidney** cancer.[26] Increased circulating leptin levels are associated with an increased risk of **colorectal and prostate** cancer. [27,28]

2.2   *Plant foods*

WCRF recommends to eat mostly foods of plant origin. The direct evidence that cereals (grains), roots, tubers, or plantains affect the risk of any cancer remains unimpressive. However, foods containing dietary fibre *probably* protect against colorectal cancer. Dietary fibre is mostly found in cereals, roots and tubers, and also in vegetables, fruits, and pulses (legumes). All of these are highest in dietary fibre when in whole or minimally processed forms. Foods high in dietary fibre may also have a protective effect indirectly because they are relatively low in energy density.

Non-starchy vegetables *probably* protect against cancers of the mouth, pharynx, and larynx, and those of the oesophagus and stomach. Fruits in general *probably* protect against cancers of the mouth, pharynx, and larynx, and those of the oesophagus, lung, and stomach. Allium vegetables (such as onions, garlic, and leeks) *probably* protect against stomach cancer. Garlic (an allium vegetable, commonly classed as a herb) *probably* protects against colorectal cancer.

In the WCRF report, the terms "vegetables" and "fruits" were used according to their culinary definition. Some studies have included pulses as vegetables whereas others have classified these as a separate entity or not at all. Smokers consume fewer vegetables and fruits than non-smokers.[29,30] Fat intake inversely correlates with vegetable and, particularly, fruit intake in the

USA.[31] Recent studies of the effects of fruits and vegetables in cancers thought to be caused by smoking have controlled for the effect of smoking.

Studies using self-reporting tend to over-report vegetable and fruit consumption.[32] Where an effect exists, results from such studies are liable to underestimate the extent to which vegetables and fruits modify the risk of cancer.

2.2.1 *Study designs*

The evidence was too limited in amount, consistency, or quality to draw any conclusions regarding cereals (grains) or roots and cancer risk. However, for foods containing dietary fibre an association was apparent from many, though not all, cohort studies and risk of colorectal cancer. The Harvard pooled analysis from 13 prospective cohort studies (725,628 participants, followed up for six to 20 years, 8081 colorectal cancer cases) concluded there was a significant inverse association in the age-adjusted model (0.84, 95% CI 0.77–0.92).[33] However, the association was attenuated and no longer statistically significant after adjusting for other risk factors (0.94, 95% CI 0.86–1.03). The pooled analysis therefore found that, after accounting for other dietary risk factors, high dietary fibre intake was not associated with a reduced risk of colorectal cancer.

The WCRF recommendations regarding *non-starchy vegetables* were based on 52 separate prospective cohort studies, across five different cancer types. Of the 52 cohort studies, 40 reported a decreased risk with higher levels of consumption of non-starchy vegetables. The WCRF recommendations regarding *allium vegetables* were based on four different prospective cohort studies, across two different cancer types. Of the four cohorts, all reported a decreased risk with higher levels of consumption of allium vegetables.

The WCRF recommendations regarding *fruit* were based on 64 different prospective cohort studies, across seven different cancer types. Of the 64 cohorts, 50 reported a decreased risk with higher levels of fruit consumption.

2.2.2   Recent literature

Recently published data from large cohorts supports the probable relationship between fruit and vegetable consumption and decreased risk of esophageal and lung cancer.[34,35]

2.2.3   Mechanisms of carcinogenesis

Vegetables could plausibly protect against cancer by way of glucosinolates. Certain hydrolysis products of glucosinolates, including indoles and isothiocyanates, have shown anti-carcinogenic properties in laboratory experiments and in diets in live experiments in animals.[36] The human genotype of glutathione S-transferase has been shown to have an important role in the metabolism of these phytochemicals and may be able to modify their anti-cancer properties.[37,38]

Colorectal cancer

Fibre exerts several effects in the gastrointestinal tract but the precise mechanisms for its probable protective role are not under-stood. Fibre dilutes faecal contents, decreases transit time, and increases stool weight.[39] Fermentation products, especially short-chain fatty acids, are produced by the gut flora from a wide range of dietary carbohydrates that reach the colon. Short-chain fatty acids, particularly butyrate, can induce apoptosis and cell cycle arrest, and promote differentiation. Fibre intake is also strongly correlated with intake of folate.

2.3   Animal foods

WCRF recommends to limit intake of red meat and avoid processed meat. The evidence that red meats and processed meats are a cause of colorectal cancer is *convincing*. Cantonese-style salted fish is a *probable* cause of nasopharyngeal cancer. This finding does not apply to any other type of fish product.

As yet, there is no agreed definition for "processed meat". Some studies count minced meat, or ham, bacon, and sausages as processed meats; others do not. Some research has found people who consume large amounts of meat and processed meats tend to consume less poultry, fish and vegetables and *vice versa*[40] though this is not consistently the case in all sub-populations, for example in an older Australian population, people who consumed higher quantities of lean red meat also consumed higher quantities of fish and vegetables.[41] So an apparent effect of meat and processed meat could possibly be due, at least in part, to low intakes of these other foods.

2.3.1 *Study designs*

The WCRF recommendations regarding *red meat* were based on 25 different prospective cohort studies, across five different cancer types. Of the 25 cohorts, 24 reported an increased risk with higher levels of consumption of red meat. There were more cohorts investigating colorectal cancer than the other cancer types. For red meat and colorectal cancer, there were 16 cohort studies and meta-analysis of seven studies resulted in a summary effect estimate of 1.43 (95% CI 1.05–1.94) per times/week.[40]

The WCRF recommendations regarding *processed meats* were based on 31 different prospective cohort studies, across five different cancer types. Of the 31 cohorts, 26 reported an increased risk with higher levels of consumption of processed meat. There were more cohorts investigating colorectal cancer than the other cancer types. For processed meat and colorectal cancer, there were 14 cohort studies and meta-analysis of five of these studies resulted in a summary effect estimate of 1.21 (95% CI 1.04–1.42) per 50 g/day.[40]

The WCRF conclusion that Cantonese-style salted fish is probably a cause of nasopharyngeal cancer is based on one cohort study[42] and 21 case-control studies.

2.3.2 *Recent literature*

Recent research from the EPIC cohort classifying whole diet has supported the WCRF conclusion regarding meat consumption and colorectal cancer.[43] However, a population-based prospective cohort study in Japan found no significant associations between meat consumption and the risk of colorectal cancer.[44] In this study, no specific meat type showed a dose-response relationship to the risk of colorectal cancer, but intake of chicken showed a significant positive dose-response relationship to the risk of colon cancer (P-trend = 0.03).[44]

Two cohorts and one meta-analysis published since the WCRF report provide contradictory evidence regarding the role of fish being protective or otherwise on colorectal cancer.[45-47]

Whilst the WCRF report concluded limited evidence for the relationship between red meat consumption and endometrial cancer, a recent meta-analysis of 16 case control studies concluded that meat consumption, in particular red meat consumption, increases endometrial cancer risk.[48]

The WCRF report also concluded there was limited evidence for the relationship between processed meat consumption and stomach cancer. A recent meta-analysis of ten cohorts and 19 case-control studies supports a positive relationship between processed meat consumption and risk of stomach cancer.[49] Overall, an increase in processed meat consumption of 30 g/day was associated with statistically significant 15% and 38% increased risks of stomach cancer in cohort studies and case-control studies, respectively. Among the individual processed meat items, findings were most consistent for bacon consumption. Summary results indicate that there was a statistically significant 37% higher risk of stomach cancer among those in the highest relative to the lowest category of bacon consumption.[49]

2.3.3 *Mechanisms of carcinogenesis*

Red meat can be relatively high in animal fats and can be energy dense and thus contribute to body fatness (see Section 2.1). Red meat consumption, particularly of processed meats, may increase the generation of carcinogenic N-nitroso compounds by stomach and gut bacteria. Some red meats are also cooked at high temperatures, resulting in the production of carcinogenic heterocyclic amines and polycyclic aromatic hydrocarbons.[40] Haem promotes the formation of N-nitroso compounds and also contains iron. Free iron can lead to production of free radicals and iron overload activates oxidative responsive transcription factors, pro-inflammatory cytokines, and iron-induced hypoxia signalling.[50,51]

2.4 *Alcohol*

WCRF recommends to limit alcoholic drinks. If alcoholic drinks are consumed, limit consumption to no more than two drinks a day for men and one drink a day for women. The evidence that alcoholic drinks are a cause of cancers of the mouth, pharynx and larynx, oesophagus, colorectum (men), and breast is *convincing*. Alcoholic drinks are *probably* a cause of liver cancer, and of colorectal cancer in women.

At high levels of consumption, the effects of alcohol are heavily confounded by other behaviours, such as smoking tobacco. Self-reporting consumption of alcoholic drinks is liable to underestimate consumption, sometimes grossly, because alcohol is known to be unhealthy and undesirable, and is sometimes drunk secretly. Heavy drinkers usually underestimate their consumption, as do drinkers of illegal or unregulated alcoholic drinks. In recent years, the strength and serving size of some alcoholic drinks have increased. For example, in the UK, wine is commonly served in 250 ml glasses as opposed to the standard 125 or 175 ml glass. In addition, alcohol content of drinks varies widely. Studies that measure consumption in terms of number of drinks may be referring to very different amounts of alcohol.

2.4.1 *Study designs*

The WCRF recommendations were based on 58 different prospective cohort studies, across six different cancer sites (treating mouth, pharynx and larynx as one). Of the 58 cohort studies, 47 reported an increased risk with higher levels of alcohol consumption. Meta-analysis on total alcoholic drinks from two cohorts concluded a summary effect estimate of 1.24 (95% CI 1.18–1.30) per drink/week for mouth, pharynx and larynx cancers.[40] For colorectal cancer, meta-analysis of six cohort studies provided a summary effect estimate of 1.01 (95% CI 0.95–1.08) per drink/week (for men RR = 1.09 (95% CI 1.02–1.15); for women RR = 1.00 (95% CI 0.89–1.40).[40] In the case of breast cancer, meta-analysis of three cohort studies resulted in a summary effect estimate of 1.07 (95% CI 0.89–1.29) per five times/week.[40]

2.4.2 Recent literature

Longitudinal research conducted in Japan and published since the WCRF report has strengthened the evidence that alcohol is associated with a high risk of oral cancers.[52] Cohort data from Singapore, adjusted for smoking, concluded that alcohol consumption was not a risk factor for nasopharyngeal cancer.[53]

The WCRF conclusion that there is convincing evidence for the association between alcohol consumption and colorectal cancer in men is given further support by findings from a recent meta-analysis[54] and EPIC.[55] Interestingly, unlike the WCRF findings that concluded there was only *probable* evidence for women, the EPIC cohort concluded the relationship was maintained after adjustment for a series of relevant dietary and lifestyle confounding factors and was not heterogeneous by gender or anatomical sub-site.[55]

The convincing evidence that alcohol consumption increases risk of breast cancer has additional weight by recent studies including from the EPIC cohort[56] and a Danish cohort that concluded the risk is minor for moderate levels of weekly alcohol intake, but increases for each extra drink consumed.[57] Weekend consumption and binge drinking seem to be related to an additionally increased risk of breast cancer.[57]

2.4.3 Mechanisms of carcinogenesis

Evidence suggests that reactive metabolites of alcohol, such as acetaldehyde, may be carcinogenic. The association between alcohol intake and colorectal cancer risk may be modified by acetaldehyde dehydrogenase and alcohol dehydrogenase genetic status[58,59] and intestinal bacteria, which have high alcohol dehydrogenase activity, can produce levels of acetaldehyde in colorectal tissue up to 1000-fold higher than that in blood.[40] The effects of alcohol may also be mediated through the production of prostaglandins, lipid peroxidation, and the generation of free-radical oxygen species. Alcohol also acts as a solvent, enhancing penetration of carcinogens into cells.[2] For mouth, pharynx and larynx cancers, tobacco may induce specific mutations in DNA that are less efficiently repaired in the presence of alcohol. Alcohol has been demonstrated to alter retinoid status in rodent studies and, as a result, cellular growth, cellular differentiation, and apoptosis are adversely altered. For all these pathways, genetic polymorphisms might also influence risk.[60,61] Alcohol interferes with oestrogen pathways in multiple ways, which may be important to its association with breast cancer. Regular, high levels of alcohol consumption cause liver damage, which may have a tumour promoting effect through associated liver cell proliferation. Heavy consumers of alcohol may have diets deficient in essential nutrients, making tissue susceptible to carcinogenesis.[40] Alcohol may also induce folate deficiency by other means and disrupt one-carbon metabolism.

2.5   *Dietary supplements*

WCRF recommends meeting nutritional needs through diet alone and that dietary supplements are not recommended for cancer prevention. The evidence that high-dose beta-carotene supplements are a cause of lung cancer in tobacco smokers is *convincing*. Calcium *probably* protects against colorectal cancer. At specific doses, selenium *probably* protects against prostate cancer.

Randomised controlled trials (RCTs) using nutrient supplements provide strong evidence. But the evidence can only be taken to apply to supplements at the doses and in the form given, under the specific experimental conditions. Importantly, inferences are also limited by the length of follow-up after supplementation began; thus often only relatively short term outcomes are reported. The doses used in trials are often pharmacological, in which case they cannot be taken as directly relevant to the nutrients as contained in foods and diets.

2.5.1   *Study designs*

The WCRF conclusion that *beta-carotene* is related to an increased risk of lung cancer is based on five RCTs and one cohort. Four of the five RCTs reported increased risk with *beta-carotene* intervention and meta-analysis of three trials gave a summary effect estimate of 1.10 (95% CI 0.89–1.36) for *beta-carotene* supplementation versus none.[40] The WCRF recommendation regarding *beta-carotene* and prostate cancer having no effect is based on three RCTs and two cohorts. All failed to demonstrate a protective effect. The WCRF recommendation regarding *beta-carotene* and skin cancer having no effect is based on three RCTs and three cohorts; none of which demonstrated a positive effect.

The basis on which the WCRF recommendations are made about the following selected nutrients are:

(i) There is limited evidence for **alpha-tocopherol** and prostate cancer based on one RCT of male smokers which showed a statistically significant decreased risk effect estimate of 0.66 (95% CI 0.52–0.86).[62,63]

(ii) **Calcium** is probably protective of colorectal cancer based on seven cohorts; six of the seven cohorts demonstrated a decreased risk for *calcium* supplementation.

(iii) **Selenium** is probably protective of prostate cancer based on one RCT and two cohorts. All showed a decreased risk with *selenium* supplementation and this is supported by dietary *selenium* data.[40] The WCRF recommendation that there is limited evidence that *selenium* is protective of lung cancer is based on one RCT which showed a non-significant decreased risk with an effect estimate of 0.74 (95% CI 0.44–1.24).[64] The WCRF recommendation that there is limited evidence that *selenium* is protective of skin cancer is based on one RCT and one cohort study. The RCT suggested an increased risk with supplementation (1.18; 95% CI 0.49–2.85) which was not present for the cohort study.[65,66] The WCRF recommendation that there is limited evidence that specific doses of *selenium* are protective of colorectal cancer is based on one RCT and one cohort study. Evidence from the trial and dietary *selenium* data are supportive of an effect but this did not occur in the cohort study.

2.5.2   *Recent literature*

Recent findings from the EPIC cohort observed no difference in plasma concentrations of carotenoids and overall risk of prostate cancer.[67]

A recent systematic review concluded that antioxidant intake may be protective against oesophageal cancer[68] however a large RCT observed no overall effect of long-term alpha-tocopherol and/or beta-carotene supplementation on the incidence of, or mortality from, oral/pharyngeal, oesophageal, and laryngeal cancers.[69] The beta-carotene supplement, however, may have had some benefit against early-stage laryngeal cancers.[69] Similarly, a recent RCT found no convincing evidence that antioxidant supplements prevent gastrointestinal cancers, in fact, antioxidant supplements seem to increase overall mortality.[70] A recent meta-analysis supports the relationship between beta-carotene and lung cancer.[71]

Large cohort data from China supports the probable protective effect of calcium on colorectal cancer in women.[72] Similarly, RCT data from USA also supports the protective effect of calcium on all-cause cancer amongst women[73] and results indicate contrasting effects of calcium and vitamin D by concurrent oestrogen therapy on colorectal cancer risk.[74] In terms of prostate cancer and calcium, recent studies indicate mixed results with one cohort[75] and a large RCT[76] indicating increased risk, whilst a separate large cohort demonstrated no increased risk[77] and a meta-analysis of observational studies concluded no increased risk existed with dairy product use.[78]

A recent Cochrane review concluded that the potential cancer preventive effect of selenium should be tested in adequately conducted randomised trials.[70] Reid *et al.* suggests a threshold effect of selenium with the 200-mcg/day selenium treatment demonstrating decreased total cancer incidence by a statistically significant 25%; however, 400-mcg/day of selenium had no effect on total cancer incidence.[79] For prostate cancer specifically, a recent North and Central American RCT concluded selenium or vitamin E, alone or in combination, did not prevent prostate cancer.[80]

2.5.3 *Mechanisms of carcinogenesis*

Phytochemicals

Various phytochemicals have been shown to have antioxidant, anti-carcinogenic, anti-inflammatory, immunomodulatory, and anti-microbial effects in laboratory experiments.

Selenium

Dietary selenium deficiency causes a lack of selenoprotein expression. A number of selenoproteins have important anti-inflammatory and antioxidant properties.[81,82] These enzymes are rapidly degraded during selenium deprivation. Selenoproteins appear to reach their maximal levels relatively easily at normal dietary selenium intake and not to increase with selenium supplementation. It is, however, plausible that supraphysiological amounts of selenium might affect programmed cell death, DNA repair, carcinogen metabolism, immune system, and anti-angiogenic effects.[83] For prostate cancer specifically, selenoproteins are involved in testosterone production, which is an important regulator of normal and abnormal prostate growth.[40]

Beta-carotene and lung cancer

A protective association present at dietary intake amounts of carotenoids may be lost or reversed by pharmacological supplementation and the higher levels that this may supply. In one animal study, low-dose beta-carotene protected against smoking-induced changes in p53, while high doses promoted these changes.[84] It is also possible that the protective associations seen in observational studies are not due to the specific agent used in supplement studies, but rather to other carotenoids present in diet[85] or to other associated dietary or health-related behaviours.

Calcium and colorectal cancer

Intracellular calcium is a pervasive second messenger acting on many cellular functions, including cell growth. It has direct growth-restraining and differentiation- and apoptosis-inducing actions on normal and colorectal tumour cells.[86]

2.6   *Physical activity*

WCRF recommends to be physically active as part of everyday life. The evidence that physical activity protects against colon cancer is *convincing*. Physical activity *probably* protects against post-menopausal breast cancer and cancer of the endometrium. Taken together, the evidence suggests that all types and degrees of physical activity are or may be protective, excluding extreme levels of activity: the evidence for any specific type or degree of physical activity is limited. The evidence is consistent with the message that the more physically active people are the better.

Large studies of physical activity are mainly undertaken in high-income countries. Such studies tend to pay most attention to voluntary recreational activity and may therefore have limited relevance to populations in lower-income countries. In these countries, overall activity levels may be higher and physical activity is mostly of the type classed as occupational, household, or transport.

There is currently no generally agreed classification of different levels of overall physical activity, with quantified degrees of activity corresponding to terms such as "active" and "sedentary". Physical activity is rarely measured precisely.

2.6.1 *Study designs*

The WCRF recommendations were based on 86 different prospective cohort studies, across six different cancer types. Of the cohort studies, 25 investigated total physical activity, 22 occupational physical activity and 38 recreational physical activity. Of the 86 cohort studies, 56 reported a decreased risk with higher levels of physical activity. There were more cohorts investigating colorectal cancer than the other cancer types and many of the cohorts investigating breast cancer did not specify menopausal status.

2.6.2 *Recent literature*

Colorectal

There have been a further six large cohort studies published since the WCRF report[87–92] all of which reinforce the WCRF findings of convincing evidence for the protective effect of physical activity on colorectal cancer. Some of these more recent cohorts provide evidence of the efficacy of walking and additional evidence for the protective effect for women specifically.

Breast

Of five recently published large cohorts,[93–97] one emphasised the protective effect of strenuous recreational physical activity as opposed to moderate activity on risk of breast cancer.[93] For those that investigated post-menopausal breast cancer, all supported the protective effects of vigorous physical activity with differing conclusions regarding the underlying mechanisms and impact of receptor status.[94,96,97] In a large American cohort of pre-menopausal women, those who had engaged in at least 39 MET-h/wk of total activity on average from ages 12 years onward had a 23% lower risk of pre-menopausal breast cancer than the least active women.[95] This activity level translates to about 3.25 hour/week of running or 13 hour/week of walking. This is an important addition to the evidence base given the WCRF conclusion that there was limited evidence for the protective effect of physical activity on pre-menopausal breast cancer.

Endometrial

A recent review adds weight to the existing evidence of a probable protective effect of physical activity on endometrial cancer by concluding that most of the studies reviewed observed an inverse association between physical activity and endometrial cancer risk, with an average risk reduction of around 30%.[98] Four other recent large cohorts provided mixed findings with regard to the impact of exercise intensity with one indicating a protective effect from light and moderate levels of physical activity,[21] whilst another concluding there was a need for vigorous physical activity.[99]

2.6.3 *Mechanisms of carcinogenesis*

Fat oxidation is an important physiological consequence of physical activity. Regular exercise increases fat oxidation in both healthy and obese people, a mechanism that is thought to occur as a result of improved insulin sensitivity,[100] although it may be attenuated in obese people. Evidence has shown that physical activity could influence appetite control by: increasing the sensitivity of satiety signals; altering food choice or macronutrient preference; and modifying the pleasure response to food. People can also tolerate substantial negative energy balance during sustained physical activity, thus resulting in weight loss. Eventually, food intake will increase to compensate for the exercise-induced energy loss, but the degree of compensation may vary greatly between individuals.[101,102] Specific effects of exercise against colon cancer may include effects on endogenous steroid hormone metabolism, and reduced gut transit time.[26,103] Specific effects for breast and endometrial cancer include effects on endogenous steroid hormone metabolism and a reduction in levels of circulating oestrogens and androgens.[40,104]

3.   Conclusion

There is "convincing" or "probable" evidence of the positive relationship between cancer and: body and abdominal fatness; alcohol; red and processed meats; and high-dose beta-carotene supplements. There is "convincing" or "probable" evidence of a protective effect of consumption of fruit and vegetables; calcium and selenium; and physical activity on cancer risk.

More than one in every three of the seven million deaths from cancer worldwide is caused by nine potentially modifiable risk factors (including fruit and vegetable consumption, physical inactivity, high BMI and alcohol consumption).[105] In Australia, the possible cancer burden due to diet and sedentary behaviour based on the most recent authoritative estimates indicate high body mass (3.9%), physical inactivity (5.6%), alcohol (3.1%) and low consumption of fruit and vegetables (2.0%) contribute a total of 13.7% of the total attributable cancer burden in DALYs.[106] Parkin and colleagues estimate that 31.5% of colorectal cancers in men and 18.4% in women could be prevented if reasonable targets with respect to diet (reduced consumption of red meat, increased fruit and vegetables), exercise (30 minutes, five days a week), alcohol consumption (no more than three standard drinks a day for men, two standard drinks for women) and weight control were achieved.[107] These predictions suggest that realistic lifestyle modifications can result in a substantial reduction in cases of this major cancer. These findings reinforce the importance of policies and programmes that modify behavioural and environmental factors to reduce the burden of cancers.

Acknowledgements

Our thanks to Sarah Duncan and Shari Bonnette for assistance with referencing.

References

1. R. S. Gibson, *Principals of Nutritional Assessment*, 2nd edn. (Oxford University Press, New York, 2005).
2. S. Bingham, A. Welch, A. McTaggart, A. Mulligan, S. Runswick, R. Luben, S. Oakes, K.-T. Khaw, N. Wareham and N. Day, Nutritional methods in the European Prospective Investigation of Cancer in Norfolk, *Public Health Nutr.* **4**: 847–858 (2001).
3. M. S. Donaldson, Nutrition and cancer: A review of the evidence for an anti-cancer diet, *Nutr. J.* **3**: 1–21 (2004).
4. M. L. Slattery, K. M. Boucher, B. J. Caan, J. D. Potter and K.-N. Ma, Eating patterns and risk of colon cancer, *Am. J. Epidemiol.* **148**: 4–16 (1998).
5. D. Albanes and A. Blair, Physical activity and risk of cancer in the NHANES I population, *Am. J. Public Health* **79**: 744–750 (1989).
6. S. N. Blair, H. W. Kohl 3rd, R. S. Paffenbarger Jr., D. G. Clark, K. H. Cooper and L. W. Gibbons, Physical fitness and all-cause mortality. A prospective study of healthy men and women, *J. Am. Med. Assoc.* **262**: 2395–2401 (1989).
7. R. S. Paffenbarger Jr., R. T. Hyde and A. L. Wing, Physical activity and incidence of cancer in diverse populations: A preliminary report, *Am. J. Clin. Nutr.* **45**: 312–317 (1987).
8. M. B. Snijder, R. M. van Dam, M. Visser and J. C. Seidell, What aspects of body fat are particularly hazardous and how do we measure them?, *Int. J. Epidemiol.* **35**: 83–92 (2006).
9. A. Misra, J. S. Wasir and N. K. Vikram, Waist circumference criteria for the diagnosis of abdominal obesity are not applicable uniformly to all populations and ethnic groups, *Nutrition* **21**: 969–976 (2005).
10. V. M. Flood, K. L. Webb, R. Lazarus and G. Pang, Use of self-report to monitor overweight and obesity in populations: Some issues for consideration, *Aust. N. Z. J. Public Health* **24**: 96–99 (2000).
11. Z. Dai, Y. C. Xu and L. Niu, Obesity and colorectal cancer risk: A meta-analysis of cohort studies, *J. Gastroenterol.* **13**: 4199–4206 (2007).

12. A. A. Moghaddam, M. Woodward and R. Huxley, Obesity and risk of colorectal cancer: A meta-analysis of 31 studies with 70,000 events, *Cancer Epidemiol. Biomarkers Prev.* **16**: 2533–2547 (2007).

13. K. F. Adams, M. F. Leitzmann, D. Albanes, V. Kipnis, T. Mouw, A. Hollenbeck and A. Schatzkin, Body mass and colorectal cancer risk in the NIH-AARP cohort, *Am. J. Epidemiol.* **166**: 36–45 (2007).

14. T. Pischon, P. H. Lahmann, H. Boeing, C. M. Friedenreich *et al.* Body size and risk of colon and rectal cancer in the European Prospective Investigation into Cancer and Nutrition (EPIC), *J. Natl. Cancer Inst.* **98**: 920–931 (2006).

15. J. Ahn, A. Schatzkin, J. V. Lacey Jr., D. Albanes, R. Ballard-Barbush, K. F. Adams, V. Kipnis, T. Mouw, A. F. Hollenbeck and M. F. Leitzmann, Adiposity, adult weight change, and post-menopausal breast cancer risk, *Arch. Intern. Med.* **167**: 2091–2102 (2007).

16. S. Borgquist, K. Jirstrom, L. Anagnostaki, J. Manjer and G. Landberg, Anthropometric factors in relation to different tumor biological subgroups of postmenopausal breast cancer, *Int. J. Cancer* **124**: 402–411 (2009).

17. A. H. Eliassen, G. A. Colditz, B. Rosner, W. Willett and S. E. Hankinson, Adult weight change and risk of postmenopausal breast cancer, *J. Am. Med. Assoc.* **296**: 193–201 (2006).

18. S. Chang, J. V. Lacey Jr., L. A. Brinton, P. Hartge, K. Adams, T. Mouw, L. Carroll, A. Hollenbeck, A. Schatzkin and M. F. Leitzmann, Lifetime weight history and endometrial cancer risk by type of menopausal hormone use in the NIH-AARP diet and health study, *Cancer Epidemiol. Biomarkers Prev.* **16**: 723–730 (2007).

19. C. M. Friedenreich, A. E. Cust, P. H. Lahmann, K. Steindorf, M.-C. Boutron-Ruault *et al.*, Anthropometric factors and risk of endometrial cancer: The European Prospective Investigation into Cancer and Nutrition, *Cancer Causes Control* **18**: 399–413 (2007).

20. K. Lindemann, M. Ellstrom-Engh and A. Eskild, Body mass, diabetes and smoking, and endometrial cancer risk: A follow-up study, *Br. J. Cancer* **98**: 1582–1585 (2008).

21. A. V. Patel, H. S. Feigelson, J. T. Talbot, M. L. McCullough, C. Rodriguez, R. C. Patel, M. J. Thun and E. E. Calle, The role of body weight in the relationship between physical activity and endometrial cancer: Results from a large cohort of US women, *Int. J. Cancer* **123**: 1877–1882 (2008).

22. T. Bjorge, S. Tretli, A. K. Lie and A. Engeland, The impact of height and body mass index on the risk of testicular cancer in 600,000 Norwegian men, *Cancer Causes Control* **17**: 983–987 (2006).

23. C. Koebnick, D. S. Michaud, S. C. Moore, Y. Park, A. Hollenbeck, R. Ballard-Barbush, A. Schatzkin and M. F. Leitzmann, Body mass index, physical activity and bladder cancer in a large prospective study, *Cancer Epidemiol. Biomarkers Prev.* **17**: 1214–1221 (2008).

24. S. C. Larsson and A. Wolk, Body mass index and risk of multiple myeloma: A meta-analysis, *Int. J. Cancer* **121**: 2512–2516 (2007).

25. Cancer Council New South Wales, *Overweight, Obesity and Cancer Prevention*, Position Statement (Cancer Council New South Wales, Sydney, 2008).

26. E. E. Calle and R. Kaaks, Overweight, obesity and cancer: Epidemiological evidence and proposed mechanisms, *Nat. Rev. Cancer* **4**: 579–591 (2004).

27. S. Chang, S. D. Hursting, J. H. Contois, S. S. Strom, Y. Yamamura and R. J. Babaian, Leptin and prostate cancer, *Prostate* **46**: 62–67 (2001).

28. P. Stattin, A. Lukanova, C. Biessy, S. Soderberg, R. Palmqvist and R. Kaaks, Obesity and colon cancer: Does leptin provide a link?, *Int. J. Cancer* **109**: 149–152 (2004).

29. J. B. McPhillips, C. B. Eaton, K. M. Gans, C. A. Derby, T. M. Lasater, J. L. McKenney and R. A. Carleton, Dietary differences in smokers and nonsmokers from two southeastern New England communities, *J. Am. Diet. Assoc.* **94**: 287–292 (1994).

30. A. Morabia and E. L. Wynder, Dietary habits of smokers, people who never smoked, and exsmokers, *Am. J. Clin. Nutr.* **52**: 933–937 (1990).

31. G. Ursin, R. G. Ziegler, A. F. Subar, B. I. Graubard, R. W. Haile and R. Hoover, Dietary patterns associated with a low-fat diet in the National Health Examination Follow-up Study: Identification of potential confounders for epidemiologic analyses, *Am. J. Epidemiol.* **137**: 916–927 (1993).

32. W. Willett, *Nutritional Epidemiology*, 2nd ed. (Oxford University Press, New York, 1998).

33. Y. Park, D. J. Hunter, D. Spiegelman, L. Bergkvist, F. Berrino, P. A. van den Brandt *et al.*, Dietary fiber intake and risk of colorectal cancer: A pooled analysis of prospective cohort studies, *J. Am. Med. Assoc.* **294**: 2849–2857 (2005).

34. N. D. Freedman, Y. Park, A. F. Subar, A. Hollenbeck, M. F. Leitzmann, A. Schatzkin and C. C. Abnet, Fruit and vegetable intake and

espohageal cancer in a large prospective cohort study, *Int. J. Cancer* **121**: 2753–2760 (2007).

35. J. Linseisen, S. Rohrmann, A. B. Miller, H. B. Bueno-de-Mesquita, F. L. Buchner *et al.*, Fruit and vegetable consumption and lung cancer risk: Updated information from the European Prospective Investigation into Cancer and Nutrition (EPIC), *Int. J. Cancer* **121**: 1103–1114 (2007).

36. C. W. Boone, G. J. Kelloff and W. E. Malone, Identification of candidate cancer chemopreventive agents and their evaluation in animal models and human clinical trials: A review, *Cancer Res.* **50**: 2–9 (1990).

37. P. Brennan, C. C. Hsu, N. Moullan, N. Szeszenia-Dabrowska, J. Lissowska, D. Zaridze, P. Rudnai, E. Fabianova, D. Mates, V. Bencko, L. Foretova, V. Janout, F. Gemignani, A. Chabrier, J. Hall, R. J. Hung and P. Boffeta and F. Canzian, Effect of cruciferous vegetables on lung cancer in patients stratified by genetic status: A mendelian randomisation approach, *Lancet* **366**: 1558–1560 (2005).

38. Cancer Council New South Wales, *Fruit, Vegetables and Cancer Prevention,* Position Statement (Cancer Council New South Wales, Sydney, 2007).

39. J. H. Cummings, Dietary fibre and large bowel cancer, *Proc. Nutr. Soc.* **40**: 7–14 (1981).

40. World Cancer Research Fund/American Institute for Cancer Research, *Food, Nutrition, Physical Activity, and the Prevention of Cancer: A Global Perspective* (AICR, Washington DC, 2007).

41. V. M. Flood, K. L. Webb, G. Burlutski, E. Rochtchina, W. Smith and P. Mitchell, Healthy ageing: 10 year trends in food and nutrient intakes among older Australians, *Asia Pac. J. Clin. Nutr.* **15**(Suppl. 3): S102 (2006).

42. X. Zou, J. Li, J. Li *et al.*, The preliminary results of epidemiology investigation in the role of Epstein-Barr Virus and salty fish in nasopharyngeal carcinoma in Sihu area, Guangdong province, *China Carcinoma* **3**: 23–25 (1994).

43. E. Keese, F. Clavel-Chapelon and M.-C. Boutron-Ruault, Dietary patterns and risk of colorectal tumors: A cohort of French women of the National Education System (E3N), *Am. J. Epidemiol.* **164**: 1085–1093 (2006).

44. Y. Sato, N. Nakaya, S. Kuriyama, Y. Nishino, Y. Tsubono and I. Tsuji, Meat consumption and risk of colorectal cancer in Japan: The Miyagi Cohort Study, *Eur. J. Cancer Prev.* **15**: 211–218 (2006).

45. D. Engeset, V. Anderson, A. Hjartaker and E. Lund, Consumption of fish and risk of colon cancer in the Norwegian Women and Cancer (NOWAC) study, *Br. J. Nutr.* **98**: 576–582 (2007).
46. A. Geelen, J. M. Schouten, C. Kamphuis, B. E. Stam, J. Burema, J. M. S. Renkema, E. Bakker, P. van't Veer and E. Kampman, Fish consumption, n-3 fatty acids and colorectal cancer: A meta-analysis of prospective cohort studies, *Am. J. Epidemiol.* **166**: 1116–1125 (2007).
47. M. N. Hall, J. E. Chavarro, I. Lee, W. Willett and J. Ma, A 22-year prospective study of fish, n-3 fatty acid intake and colorectal cancer risk in men, *Cancer Epidemiol. Biomarkers Prev.* **17**: 1136–1143 (2008).
48. E. V. Bandera, L. H. Kushi, D. F. Moore, D. M. Gifkins and M. L. McCullough, Consumption of animal foods and endometrial cancer risk: A systematic literature review and meta-analysis, *Cancer Causes Control* **18**: 967–988 (2007).
49. S. C. Larsson, N. Orsini and A. Wolk, Processed meat consumption and stomach cancer risk: A meta-analysis, *J. Natl. Cancer Inst.* **98**: 1078–1087 (2006).
50. X. Huang, Iron overload and its association with cancer risk in humans: Evidence for iron as a carcinogenic metal, *Mutat. Res.* **533**: 153–171 (2003).
51. Cancer Council New South Wales, *Meat and Cancer Prevention*, Position Statement (Cancer Council New South Wales, Sydney, 2007).
52. R. Ide, Y. Fujino, Y. Hoshiyama, K. Sakata, A. Tamakoshi and T. Yoshimura, Cigarette smoking, alcohol drinking, and oral and pharyngeal cancer mortality in Japan, *Oral Dis.* **14**: 314–319 (2008).
53. J. T. Friborg, J. Yuan, R. Wang, W. Koh, H. Lee and M. C. Yu, A prospective study of tobacco and alcohol use as risk factors for pharyngeal carcinomas in Singapore Chinese, *Cancer* **109**: 1183–1191 (2007).
54. A. Moskal, T. Norat, P. Ferrari and E. Riboli, Alcohol intake and colorectal cancer risk: A dose–response meta-analysis of published cohort studies, *Int. J. Cancer* **120**: 664–671 (2006).
55. P. Ferrari, M. Jenab, T. Norat, A. Moskal, N. Slimani, A. Olsen *et al.*, Lifetime and baseline alcohol intake and risk of colon and rectal cancers in the European Prospective Investigation into Cancer and Nutrition (EPIC), *Int. J. Cancer* **121**: 2065–2072 (2007).
56. A. Tjonneland, J. Christensen, A. Olsen, C. Stripp, B. L. Thomsen *et al.*, Alcohol intake and breast cancer risk: The European

Prospective Investigation into Cancer and Nutrition (EPIC), *Cancer Causes Control* **18**: 361–373 (2007).

57. L. S. Morch, D. Johansen, L. C. Thygesen, A. Tjonneland, E. Lokkegaard, C. Stahlberg and M. Gronbaek, Alcohol drinking, consumption patterns and breast cancer among Danish nurses: A cohort study, *Eur. J. Public Health* **17**: 624–629 (2007).

58. M. Murata, M. Tagawa, S. Watanabe, H. Kimura, T. Takeshita and K. Morimoto, Genotype difference of aldehyde dehydrogenase 2 gene in alcohol drinkers influences the incidence of Japanese colorectal cancer patients, *Cancer Sci.* **90**: 711–719 (1999).

59. E. W. Tiemersma, P. A. Wark, M. C. Ocke, A. Bunschoten, M. H. Otten, F. J. Kok and E. Kampman, Alcohol consumption, alcohol dehydrogenase 3 polymorphism, and colorectal adenomas, *Cancer Epidemiol. Biomarkers Prev.* **12**: 419–425 (2003).

60. R. G. Dumitrescu and P. G. Shields, The etiology of alcohol-induced breast cancer, *Alcohol* **35**: 213–225 (2005).

61. Cancer Council New South Wales, *Alcohol and Cancer Prevention*, Position Statement (Cancer Council New South Wales, Sydney, 2008).

62. J. Virtamo, P. Pietinen, J. K. Huttunen, P. Korhonen, N. Malila, M. J. Virtanen, D. Albanes, P. R. Taylor and P. Albert, Incidence of cancer and mortality following alpha-tocopherol and beta-carotene supplementation, *J. Am. Med. Assoc.* **290**: 476–485 (2003).

63. O. P. Heinonen, D. Albanes, J. Virtamo, P. R. Taylor, J. K. Huttunen, A. M. Hartman, J. Haapakoski, N. Malila, M. Rautalahti, S. Ripatti, H. Maenpaa, L. Teerenhovi, L. Koss, M. Virolainen and B. K. Edwards, Prostate cancer and supplementation with alpha-tocopherol and beta-carotene: Incidence and mortality in a controlled trial, *J. Natl. Cancer Inst.* **90**: 440–446 (1998).

64. M. E. Reid, A. J. Duffield-Lillico, L. Garland, B. W. Turnbull, L. C. Clark and J. R. Marshall, Selenium supplementation and lung cancer incidence: An update of the Nutritional Prevention of Cancer Trial, *Cancer Epidemiol. Biomarkers Prev.* **11**: 1285–1291 (2002).

65. L. C. Clark, G. F. Combs, Jr., B. W. Turnbull, E. H. Slate, D. K. Chalker, J. Chow, L. S. Davis, R. A. Glover, G. F. Graham, E. G. Gross, A. Krongrad, J. L. Lesher, K. Park, B. B. Sanders, C. L. Smith and J. R. Taylor, Effects of selenium supplementation for cancer prevention in patients with carcinoma of the skin: A randomized controlled trial. Nutritional Prevention of Cancer Study Group, *J. Am. Med. Assoc.* **276**: 1957–1963 (1996).

66. S. A. McNaughton, G. C. Marks, P. Gaffney, G. Williams and A. C. Green, Antioxidants and basal cell carcinoma of the skin: A nested case-control study, *Cancer Causes Control* **16**: 609–618 (2005).

67. T. J. Key, P. N. Appleby, N. E. Allen, R. C. Travis, A. W. Roddam *et al.*, Plasma cartenoids, retinol, and tocopherols and the risk of prostate cancer in the European Prospective Investigation into Cancer and Nutrition Study, *Am. J. Clin. Nutr.* **86**: 672–681 (2007).

68. A. Kubo and D. A. Corley, Meta-analysis of antioxidant intake and the risk of esophageal and gastric cardia adenocarcinoma, *Am. J. Gastroenterol.* **102**: 2323–2330 (2007).

69. M. E. Wright, J. Virtamo, A. M. Hartman, P. Pietinen, B. K. Edwards, P. R. Taylor, J. K. Huttunen and D. Albanes, Effects of alpha-tocopherol and beta-carotene supplementation on upper aerodigestive tract cancers in a large, randomized controlled trial, *Cancer* **109**: 891–898 (2007).

70. G. Bjelakovic, D. Nikolova, R. Simonetti and C. Gluud, Antioxidant supplements for preventing gastrointestinal cancers, *Cochrane Datab. Syst. Rev.* **3**: CD004183 (2008).

71. T. Tanvetyanon and G. Bepler, Beta-carotene in multivitamins and the possible risk of lung cancer among smokers versus former smokers: A meta-analysis and evaluation of national brands *Cancer* **113**: 150–157 (2008).

72. A. Shin, H. Li, X.-O. Shu, G. Yang, Y.-T. Gao and W. Zheng, Dietary intake of calcium, fiber and other micronutrients in relation to colorectal cancer risk: Results from the Shanghai Women's Health Study, *Int. J. Cancer* **119**: 2938–2942 (2006).

73. J. Lappe, D. Travers-Gustafson, K. Davies, R. Recker and R. Heaney, Vitamin D and calcium supplementation reduces cancer risk: Results of a randomized trial, *Am. J. Clin. Nutr.* **85**: 1586–1591 (2007).

74. E. Ding, S. Mehta, W. Fawzi and E. Giovanucci, Interaction of estrogen therapy with calcium and vitamin D supplementation on colorectal cancer risk: Reanalysis of Women's Health Initiative randomized trial, *Int. J. Cancer* **122**: 1690–1694 (2008).

75. H. G. Skinner and G. G. Schwartz, Serum calcium and incident and fatal prostate cancer in the National Health and Nutrition Examination Survey, *Cancer Epidemiol. Biomarkers Prev.* **17**: 2302–2305 (2008).

76. P. N. Mitrou, D. Albanes, S. J. Weinstein, P. Pietinen, P. R. Taylor, J. Virtamo and M. F. Leitzmann, A prospective study of dietary

calcium, dairy products and prostate cancer risk (Finland), *Int. J. Cancer* **120**: 2466–2473 (2007).

77. K. A. Koh, H. D. Sesso, R. S. Paffenbarger Jr. and I.-M. Lee, Dairy products, calcium and prostate cancer risk, *Br. J. Cancer* **95**: 1582–1585 (2006).

78. M. Huncharek, J. Muscat and B. Kupelnick, Dairy products, dietary calcium and vitamin D intake as risk factors for prostate cancer: A meta-analysis of 26,769 cases from 45 observational studies, *Nutr. Cancer* **60**: 421–441 (2008).

79. M. Reid, A. Duffield-Lillico, E. Slate, N. Natarajan, B. Turnbull, E. Jacobs, G. F. Combs Jr., D. S. Alberts, L. C. Clark and J. R. Marshall, The nutritional prevention of cancer: 400 mcg per day selenium treatment, *Nutr. Cancer* **60**: 155–163 (2008).

80. S. M. Lippman, E. A. Klein, P. J. Goodman, M. S. Lucia, I. M. Thompson *et al.*, Effect of selenium and vitamin E on risk of prostate cancer and other cancers: The Selenium and Vitamin E Cancer Prevention Trial (SELECT), *J. Am. Med. Assoc.* **301**: 39–51 (2009).

81. H. E. Ganther, Selenium metabolism, selenoproteins and mechanisms of cancer prevention: Complexities with thioredoxin reductase, *Carcinogenesis* **20**: 1657–1666 (1999).

82. Cancer Council New South Wales, *Selenium and Cancer*, Position Statement (Cancer Council New South Wales, Sydney, 2006).

83. G. F. Combs Jr., Status of selenium in prostate cancer prevention, *Br. J. Cancer* **91**: 195–199 (2004).

84. C. Lui, R. M. Russell and X. D. Wang, Low dose [beta]-carotene supplementation of ferrets attenuates smoke-induced lung phosphorylation of JNK, p38 MAPK, and p53 proteins, *J. Nutr.* **134**: 2705–2710 (2004).

85. G. E. Goodman, S. Schaffer, G. S. Omenn, C. Chen and I. King, The association between lung and prostate cancer risk, and serum micronutrients: Results and lessons learned from {beta}-carotene and retinol efficacy trial, *Cancer Epidemiol. Biomarkers Prev.* **12**: 518–526 (2003).

86. S. A. Lamprecht and M. Lipkin, Cellular mechanisms of calcium and vitamin D in the inhibition of colorectal carcinogenesis, *Ann. N. Y. Acad. Sci.* **952**: 73–87 (2001).

87. B. A. Calton, J. V. Lacey Jr., A. Schatzkin, C. Schairer, L. H. Colbert, D. Albanes and M. F. Leitzmann, Physical activity and the risk of colon cancer among women: A prospective cohort study (United States), *Int. J. Cancer* **119**: 385–391 (2006).

88. C. Friedenreich, T. Norat, K. Steindorf, M.-C. Boutron-Ruault, T. Pischon *et al.*, Physical activity and risk of colon and rectal cancers: The European Prospective Investigation into Cancer and Nutrition, *Cancer Epidemiol. Biomarkers Prev.* **15**: 2398–2407 (2006).

89. R. A. Howard, D. M. Freedman, Y. Park, A. Hollenbeck, A. Schatzkin and M. F. Leitzmann, Physical activity, sedentary behavior and the risk of colon and rectal cancer in the NIH-AARP diet and health study, *Cancer Causes Control* **19**: 939–953 (2008).

90. P. Schnohr, M. Gronbaek, L. Petersen, H. O. Hein and T. I. A. Sorensen, Physical activity in leisure-time and risk of cancer: 14-year follow-up of 28,000 Danish men and women, *Scand. J. Public Health* **33**: 244–249 (2005).

91. H. Takahashi, S. Kuriyama, Y. Tsubono, N. Nakaya, K. Fujita, Y. Nishino, D. Shibuya and I. Tsuji, Time spent walking and risk of colorectal cancer in Japan: The Miyagi Cohort Study, *Eur. J. Cancer Prev.* **16**: 403–409 (2007).

92. K. Y. Wolin, I.-M. Lee, G. A. Colditz, R. J. Glynn, C. S. Fuchs and E. Giovannucci, Leisure-time physical activity patterns and risk of colon cancer in women, *Int. J. Cancer* **121**:2776–2781 (2007).

93. C. M. Dallal, J. Sullivan-Halley, R. K. Ross, Y. Wang, D. Deapen *et al.*, Long-term recreational physical activity and risk of invasive and *in situ* breast cancer, *Arch. Intern. Med.* **167**: 408–415 (2007).

94. M. F. Leitzmann, S. C. Moore, T. M. Peters, J. V. Lacey Jr., A. Schatzkin, C. Schairer, L. A. Brinton and D. Albanes, Prospective study of physical activity and risk of postmenopausal breast cancer, *Breast Cancer Res.* **10**: R92 (2008).

95. S. S. Maruti, W. Willett, D. Feskanich, B. Rosner and G. A. Colditz, A prospective study of age-specific physical activity and premenopausal breast cancer, *J. Natl. Cancer Inst.* **100**: 728–737 (2008).

96. T. M. Peters, A. Schatzkin, G. L. Gierach, S. C. Moore, J. V. Lacey Jr., N. Wareham, U. Ekeland, A. Hollenbeck and M. F. Leitzmann, Physical activity and postmenopausal breast cancer risk in the NIH-AARP diet and health study, *Cancer Epidemiol. Biomarkers Prev.* **18**: 289–296 (2009).

97. B. Tehard, C. M. Friedenreich, J.-M. Oppert and F. Clavel-Chapelon, Effect of physical activity on women at increased risk of breast cancer: Results from the E3N cohort study, *Cancer Epidemiol. Biomarkers Prev.* **15**: 57–64 (2006).

98. A. E. Cust, B. K. Armstrong, C. M. Friedenreich, N. Slimani and A. Bauman, Physical activity and endometrial cancer risk: A review of the current evidence, biologic mechanisms and the quality of physical activity assessment methods, *Cancer Causes Control* **18**: 243–258 (2007).

99. G. L. Gierach, S. Chang, L. A. Brinton, J. V. Lacey Jr., A. Hollenbeck, A. Schatzkin and M. F. Leitzmann, Physical activity, sedentary behavior and endometrial cancer risk in the NIH-AARP diet and health study, *Int. J. Cancer* **124**: 2139–2147 (2009).

100. J. Achten and A. E. Jeukendrup, Optimizing fat oxidation through exercise and diet, *Nutrition* **20**: 716–727 (2004).

101. J. E. Blundell, R. J. Stubbs, D. A. Hughes, S. Whybrow and N. A. King, Cross talk between physical activity and appetite control: Does physical activity stimulate appetite?, *Proc. Nutr. Soc.* **62**: 651–661 (2003).

102. Cancer Council New South Wales, *Physical Activity and Cancer Prevention*, Position Statement (Cancer Council New South Wales, Sydney, 2009).

103. M. H. Lewin, N. Bailey, T. Bandaletova, R. Bowman, A. J. Cross, J. Pollock, D. E. G. Shuker and S. A. Bingham, Red meat enhances the colonic formation of the DNA adduct O6-carboxymethyl guanine: Implications for colorectal cancer risk, *Cancer Res.* **66**: 1859–1865 (2006).

104. H. Vainio and F. Bianchini (eds.), *IARC Handbooks of Cancer Prevention: Weight Control and Physical Activity* (IARC Press, Washington DC, 2002).

105. G. Danaei, S. Van der Hoorn, A. D. Lopez, C. J. L. Murray, M. Ezzati, and the Comparative Risk Assessment Collaborating group (Cancers), Causes of cancer in the world: Comparative risk assessment of nine behavioural and environmental risk factors, *Lancet* **366**: 1784–1793 (2005).

106. S. Begg, T. Vos, B. Barker, C. Stevenson, L. Stanley and A. Lopez, *The Burden of Disease and Injury in Australia 2003* (Australian Institute of Health and Welfare, Canberra, 2007).

107. D. M. Parkin, A.-H. Olsen and P. Sasieni, The potential for prevention of colorectal cancer in the UK, *Eur. J. Cancer Prev.* **18**: 179–190 (2009).

4

Sun Exposure, Vitamin D and Cancer

**Bruce Armstrong
and Anne Kricker**

Abstract

Exposure to sunlight is the main source of Vitamin D. The first evidence that Vitamin D might protect against cancer came from ecological studies showing, mainly in the USA, that the rates of a range of cancers were lower where ambient solar radiation was higher. Prompted by these findings and evidence of Vitamin D's anti-carcinogenic effects in basic biological studies, a number of epidemiological studies have investigated the possible inverse associations of sun exposure and Vitamin D with cancer. While a number of different types of cancer have been studied, the strongest available evidence suggests that high serum Vitamin D levels protect against colorectal cancer and that sun exposure probably protects against non-Hodgkin lymphoma. While it is plausible that a protective effect of sun exposure against cancer would be mediated through production of Vitamin D, there is currently little direct evidence of it. Present evidence does not justify giving or taking Vitamin D to prevent cancer. It is sufficient, however, to justify randomised controlled trials of doses of 1000 IU to 2000 IU of Vitamin D a day to see if it will prevent cancer. Known harmful effects of Vitamin D do not occur at these levels of intake.

Keywords: Cancer aetiology, sun exposure, ultraviolet rays, blood vitamin D, dietary vitamin D.

1. Introduction

Vitamin D is essential to healthy life. Its best known function is maintenance of calcium homeostasis, which it does primarily by promoting intestinal absorption of calcium and phosphorous, decreasing their clearance by the kidneys and promoting bone mineralisation.[1] There is increasing evidence, however, that it has other physiological functions, some of which may protect against, or improve the outcome of cancer.[2] In this chapter, we will use the term Vitamin D to refer to the chemical forms of Vitamin D that are physiologically active or able to be activated and use the names of individual Vitamin D compounds when it is relevant to a clear understanding.

Vitamin D$_3$ (cholecalciferol) is produced in skin exposed to sunlight by photo-isomerisation of 7-dehydrocholesterol, which is present in sufficient quantities to allow production of all the Vitamin D required. The short wavelength, ultraviolet (UV) B radiation required for this chemical change covers the same spectrum of UV radiation as that which is most active in causing skin cancer. Vitamin D$_3$ is not physiologically active; to become so, it is first changed to 25-hydroxy cholecalciferol (25OH Vitamin D) in the liver and then to 1,25-dihydroxy cholecalciferol (1,25diOH Vitamin D) in the kidneys or, locally, in many other tissues of the body. 25OH Vitamin D is the form of Vitamin D in highest concentration in blood, and is used to evaluate sufficiency in Vitamin D. The very low concentrations of 1,25diOH Vitamin D in blood derive mainly from that produced in the kidneys; these concentrations are very tightly regulated by parathyroid hormone, as it regulates blood calcium concentrations.

Vitamin D is also present in food, mainly fish liver, fish oils, fatty fish and egg yolks.[1] Some countries require fortification of some foods with Vitamin D, mostly milk or milk products, cereal, margarine and infant formula. Exposure to sunlight is the main source of Vitamin D for human populations except at high latitudes, where the level of UV B radiation in sunlight is low, and in people who eat large amounts of fatty fish.

The basic biological evidence for anti-carcinogenic effects of Vitamin D is quite strong.[3] Vitamin D plays a role in controlling cell proliferation and differentiation and can activate apoptotic pathways and inhibit angiogenesis, effects that could lead to suppression of carcinogenesis or, perhaps, cancer itself. Many cancers express the Vitamin D receptor and the 1α hydroxylase required to convert circulating 25OH Vitamin D to 1,25diOH Vitamin D. Thus they have the potential to be affected by circulating Vitamin D.[3]

In this chapter, we will summarise evidence that suggests that populations with higher exposure to solar UV B radiation have lower cancer mortality, and possibly incidence rates and evidence from observational studies that a person's sun exposure might reduce their risk of some cancers. We will also review evidence that Vitamin D protects against cancer and, to a limited extent, that it mediates the possible beneficial effects of sun exposure against cancer.

2. Ambient Solar Radiation and Cancer Incidence and Mortality

Ecological studies, mainly from the USA, provide evidence that mortality rates for some cancers are lower in areas where ambient levels of solar radiation are higher.[4-6] By ecological study, we mean a study in which the units of study are populations, not individual people, and the exposure of people in those populations, in this case to solar radiation, is inferred from measurements in the whole of each population or its environment. Such studies are generally considered capable only of generating hypotheses about causation, or providing some credibility for a hypothesis derived from another source, but not of providing direct support for a causal relationship. Essentially, this is because they permit inferences only at the group level, not at the individual level, and because it is not possible to effectively disentangle the relationship of an ecological measure of exposure with population risk of a disease from the effect of some other factor that is correlated with the exposure and is causally related to the disease.[7]

Apperly first reported a negative correlation of mortality from all cancers in 1934–38 with an index of solar radiation across states of the USA.[4] He noted that it was evident that men and women at higher latitudes in New Hampshire, Vermont, and Massachusetts had greater risks of dying from cancer than those of similar ages who lived in southern states like Texas, Georgia and Alabama.[4] He suggested that "the relative immunity to cancer is a direct effect of sunlight".

After a gap of almost 40 years, the relationship between mortality from colon cancer and sunlight was examined by Garland and Garland,[5] again showing a negative correlation. A recent systematic review has tabulated 14 reports of ecological studies of the association of solar radiation with mortality from or incidence of cancer.[8] Seven studies originated in the USA, one each in England and Wales, the former USSR and Japan, and four across multiple countries. With a few inconsistent exceptions, mortality from, or incidence of cancer tended to fall, as ambient solar radiation increased. The measures of ambient solar UV used varied from simple latitude to model-based estimates or direct measurements of solar UV B irradiance. The cancers studied included cancers of the salivary glands, oesophagus, stomach, colon, rectum, liver, pancreas, nasal cavity and sinuses, larynx, lung, breast, kidney, bladder, cervix, body of uterus, ovary, prostate, thyroid, and brain, and non-Hodgkin lymphoma, multiple myeloma and other neoplasms of lymphoid and histiocytic tissues (see also Grant[9] for several cancers not tabulated by van der Rhee et al.[8]). Only mortality rates were used, except in three studies examining incidence rates of non-Hodgkin lymphoma. The meta-analysis did not include an additional contemporary analysis that found inverse associations of ambient UV B radiation across European countries with mortality from cancers of the breast, body of uterus, ovary, prostate and kidney, and multiple myeloma and non-Hodgkin lymphoma (NHL), but not from colon cancer.[10] Giovanucci[11] noted that it was remarkable to have so consistent a pattern of inverse relationships as observed for solar radiation across a wide range of different kinds of cancer with diverse risk factors.

These inverse associations are consistent with the possibility that Vitamin D protects against cancer occurrence or death, if it is assumed that mean blood Vitamin D concentrations in populations vary directly with ambient solar irradiance and inversely with latitude. A comprehensive review of published studies of blood Vitamin D in different populations suggests that this is not necessarily true.[1] While studies in the United Kingdom, France and Argentina have shown clear latitude gradients in the expected direction, weaker latitude gradients have been reported for the

USA and Australia. In a systematic review of continental European studies at single locations, latitude was only a weak predictor of mean blood 25OH Vitamin D concentrations.[1] There was, however, a strong interaction between latitude and age in predicting population mean Vitamin D. In people 18–65 years of age, levels fell with increasing latitude by an average of just 3.4 nmol/l between 35° and 70° North. In people more than 65 years of age, mean blood Vitamin D increased by an average of 23.1 nmol/l over the same latitude range. The measurements included in this systematic review were done by many different methods on variously representative samples of the population and probably with widely varying quality. Clearly, however, it cannot be assumed at present that there is necessarily a simple inverse relationship between blood Vitamin D concentration and latitude, or a direct relationship between it and ambient solar irradiance.

3. Individual Sun Exposure, Vitamin D and Cancer Occurrence

3.1 *Colorectal cancer*

3.1.1 *Sun exposure*

Freedman *et al.*[12] conducted a death certificate based case-control study of cancers of the colon, breast, ovary and prostate based on death certificates from 24 states of the USA for 1985 to 1995. Cases were people whose deaths were due to one of the index cancers and controls were people who had died of other conditions, excluding cancer and a few others conditions possibly associated with sun exposure. The relative risk (RR, estimated in case control studies from the odds ratio) for colon cancer death with high residential sunlight exposure (based on state of residence at birth and at death) was somewhat reduced (RR 0.73, 95% confidence interval (CI) 0.71–0.74), with a trend from a smaller reduction with medium exposure (RR 0.90). There was also a small reduction in RR with occupational sun exposure in non-farming outdoor jobs (0.90, 95% CI 0.86–0.94) but not in farming (1.04). While the study design allowed some control for possible confounding of these associations with physical activity (occupational only), which is a known cause of colon cancer, and socioeconomic status (based on occupation), possible confounding with other risk factors, such as dietary red meat and body fatness (see Chapter 3), was not controlled for. It is important to note that the main measure of sun exposure in this study, ambient solar radiation in the state of residence, was ecological, not individual. However, the fact that there were individual measures of and adjustment for two possible confounding variables allows for some control of confounding.

In a large, population-based case control study of colon cancer in three US states, 1993 cases and 2410 controls were asked about the number of hours they spent outdoors each week in each season two years before entry to the study. There was no appreciable association between sun exposure and colon cancer risk.[13]

A number of studies have investigated the occurrence of colorectal cancer following skin cancer on the basis that, since sun exposure is an established cause of skin cancer, risk of colorectal cancer (and perhaps other cancers) should be less in people who have had a previous skin cancer than those who have not. Large studies based on population-based cancer registries, however, have given conflicting results and, on balance, appear to show a small increase, rather than a decrease, in the risk of colorectal cancer following skin cancer.[1] An IARC Working Group on Vitamin D concluded:[1] "The incidence of second cancers in individuals is elevated by several known and unknown mechanisms, including common aetiological factors and predispositions, and influenced by possible biases in the ascertainment of second cancers... The net direction of these influences will mostly be in the direction of elevated occurrence of second cancers, against which a possible effect of sunlight and Vitamin D ... could be difficult to detect". Thus, while these studies also provide evidence related to some other cancers reviewed below, they will not be discussed further here.

3.1.2 Vitamin D

The IARC Working Group on Vitamin D has recently published meta-analyses of published data on the associations of blood 25OH Vitamin D with colorectal, breast and prostate cancers.[1] It included nine studies published between 1989 and 2008, 5330 cases and 20,394 controls. The summary relative risk for the highest exposure category relative to the lowest was 0.56 (95% CI 0.43–0.74) (Table 1)

Table 1. Results of meta-analyses of published data on the association of blood 25OH vitamin D concentrations and risk of occurrence of colorectal, breast and prostate cancers.[1]

Cancer	No. of studies	Countries[a]	Study designs	Cases	Controls	RR, 95% CI
Colorectal	9	USA 5, EU 1, Finland 1, Japan 1, Turkey 1	Case control 1, nested case control 7, cohort 1	5330	20,384[b]	0.56, 0.42–0.74
Breast	5	USA 3, UK 1, Germany 1	Case control 2, nested case control 2, cohort 1	3307	20,091[b]	0.46, 0.21–1.03
Prostate	7	USA 7, Finland 1	Nested case control 6, cohort 1	1909	19,281[b]	0.83, 0.61–1.12

[a]Numbers refer to the numbers of studies from each country and number of studies with each design, respectively.
[b]Includes 16,818 unaffected subjects in the cohort study.

and the pooled relative risk per ng/ml increase in serum Vitamin D was estimated at 0.983 (95% CI 0.976–0.990) or 1.7% (95% CI 2.3%–10%) reduction in risk per ng/ml increase in Vitamin D. There was significant heterogeneity in relative risks across the nine studies: $p = 0.02$. Sensitivity analyses by characteristics of studies (case control compared with nested case control or cohort, adjustment for body fatness (by BMI) or not, publication year and upper vitamin D concentration for the reference category) and of subjects (gender and age) showed no important effects on the pooled relative risk. Only three of the studies had adjusted for alcohol intake, BMI and physical activity and two had adjusted for meat intake.

The IARC Working Group[1] also reviewed studies of the association between estimated dietary intake of Vitamin D and colorectal cancer. The RR for the highest intake category was below unity for five of seven case control studies and for eight of 12 cohort studies. IARC concluded there was limited evidence that high intakes of foods containing Vitamin D protect against colorectal cancer. In one of the case control studies reviewed,[13] dietary Vitamin D was not associated with colorectal cancer risk, but Vitamin D supplements were: RR 0.6 (95% CI 0.4–0.9). A very recent Japanese case control study found no association between dietary Vitamin D and colorectal cancer;[14] another, however, did: 0.63 (0.36–1.08), p for trend 0.02, adjusted for residence, sex, age, job, parental history of colorectal cancer, smoking, alcohol drinking, body mass index, leisure-time physical activity, and intakes of energy, vegetable, fruit, and red meat.[15]

While dietary Vitamin D is usually a minority contributor to total Vitamin D availability, it has generally been shown to be positively associated with blood Vitamin D levels. However, the fact that dietary Vitamin D is measured with considerable error will militate against finding a true association, if there is one, between it and cancer occurrence.

Two randomised controlled trials have examined the effect of Vitamin D supplementation on the risk of colorectal cancer. The first, a pilot study for a planned larger study recruited subjects from participants age 65–85 in the British Doctors Study and people registered with a single UK general practice; 1345 received 100,000 IU of Vitamin D orally every four months (average of ~800 IU daily) for five years and 1341 received a matching placebo.[16] The primary endpoint was fractures; total cancer mortality and colorectal cancer mortality were measured as secondary endpoints. The intervention reduced the fracture rate, RR 0.78 (95% CI 0.61–0.99). The RRs for death from cancer and colorectal cancer were, respectively, 0.86 (95% CI 0.61–1.20) and 0.62 (95% CI 0.24–1.60). Thus while a protective effect against all cancers, and colorectal cancer specifically, is a possibility, the evidence for it in this study is weak.

In a US Women's Health Initiative trial, 36,282 post-menopausal women received 500 mg of elemental calcium and 200 IU of Vitamin D_3 twice daily (18,176 women), or a matching placebo (18,106), for an average of 7.0 years, with hip fracture the primary endpoint.[17] There were 168 cases of invasive colorectal cancer — a designated secondary endpoint — in those who received the intervention and 154 in those who received the placebo, RR 1.08 (95% CI 0.86–1.34). There was nothing to suggest a protective effect of the intervention. However, a case control study (317 cases and 317 matched controls) nested within the cohort found a trend towards increasing RRs for colorectal cancer with decreasing baseline serum Vitamin D (RR 2.53 95% CI 1.49–4.32 for serum Vitamin D <31.0 nmol/litre). Various arguments have been advanced to explain this "negative" result, of which an insufficient dose of Vitamin D is probably the most plausible. It is argued that substantially higher doses might be needed to obtain the full benefits of Vitamin D.[18] Another perspective is offered by the clear association of baseline serum Vitamin D with colorectal cancer risk: the presence of this effect in the absence of any effect of the intervention, suggests that a low serum Vitamin D might indicate people who are going to develop cancer, but does not itself influence cancer risk.[1]

3.2 *Breast cancer*

3.2.1 *Sun exposure*

Five studies have examined the association between measures of sun exposure and breast cancer risk, with conflicting results (Table 2). The first, a case-control study nested within the US Nurses Health Study, assessed sun exposure from location of residence.[19] While the RRs were greater in women residing at entry to the study in each of three more northerly regions relative to the South, they were only a little above unity (RRs 1.03–1.13). Results restricted to women who had lived in one region the whole of their lives were little different, except in California, RR 1.35 (95% CI 1.02–1.78), where solar irradiance is high in much of the state. In the two other studies that used residence to estimate sun exposure,[12,20] reduced relative risks (0.73 or 0.74) were observed with residence in a high solar radiation environment at different times of life, although in only one did the 95% confidence interval exclude unity.

In four studies that had sun exposure measures specific to individuals (Table 2), the results showed stronger evidence of protective effects of sun exposure. In the death certificate-based case control study of Freedman *et al.*,[12] a non-farming outdoor occupation at the time of death was associated with an 18% lower risk of breast cancer; for farming the reduction was just 8%. In one cohort study (based on the first National Health and Nutrition Survey population) and two population-based case control studies, in which participants were interviewed, four out of five self-reported measures of sun exposure from two of the studies[20,21] were moderately strongly associated with lower risks of breast cancer (RRs 0.61–0.66). In the remaining study,

Table 2. Results of studies of the association of measures of individual sun exposure with breast cancer occurrence: Relative risks for highest exposed category with reference to lowest, except as otherwise specified.

Author, year and population	Study design and subject numbers	Sun exposure measure	Relative risk, 95% CI	Covariates included in analysis
Laden 1997 USA	Nested case control study Controls 455 Cases 3603	Residential location with reference to the South		Age, age at menarche, parity, age at first birth, oral contraceptive use, menopause, hormone replacement therapy, family history, benign breast disease, body fatness
		California	1.13, 0.99–1.29	
		Northeast	1.05, 0.94–1.17	
		Midwest	1.03, 0.91–1.17	
John 1999 USA	Population-based cohort study Cohort 5009 Cases 190	High solar radiance in state of birth	0.73, 0.49–1.09	Age, education, age at menarche, age at menopause, body fatness, alcohol, physical activity
		High solar radiance in state of longest residence	0.73, 0.50–1.08	
		High recreational sun exposure	0.66, 0.44–0.99	
		High occupational sun exposure	0.64, 0.41–0.98	

(Continued)

Table 2. *(Continued)*

Author, year and population	Study design and subject numbers	Sun exposure measure	Relative risk, 95% CI	Covariates included in analysis
Freedman 2002 USA	Death certificate-based case-control study Controls 70,081 Cases 130,261	High residential sunlight exposure	0.74, 0.72–0.76	Age, race, occupational physical activity, socioeconomic status (based on occupation)
		Outdoor occupation — non-farmer	0.82, 0.70–0.97	
		Outdoor occupation — farmer	0.92, 0.77–1.10	
John 2007 San Francisco Bay Area, USA	Population-based case control study Controls 2523 Cases 1788	High lifetime outdoor activity[a]	0.92, 0.77–1.10	Age, ethnicity, education, family history, number of full term pregnancies, height and other variables[b]
		High sun exposure index[a]	1.04, 0.87–1.26	
Knight 2007 Ontario, Canada	Population-based case control study Controls 1135 Cases 972	High outdoor activity at ages 10 to 19	0.65, 0.50–0.85	Age, ethnicity, family history, ever breast-fed, age at menarche, age first birth
		Outdoor job >1 year at ages 10 to 19	0.61, 0.46–0.80	
		High outdoor activity at ages 20 to 29	0.65, 0.50–0.85	

[a]Summary relative risks across three categories of constitutive pigmentation and localised and advanced breast cancer calculated using a simple fixed-effects meta-analysis; there was little heterogeneity in individual relative risks contributing to the summaries. The sun exposure index was based on the difference in skin reflectance between skin usually protected from and skin usually exposed to the sun when outdoors.
[b]Additional covariates were included in models for women with light and medium constitutive pigmentation.

high lifetime outdoor activity and a high sun exposure index (based on a comparison of measured reflectance of usually exposed and usually unexposed skin) were only weakly associated with breast cancer, and in opposing directions.

3.2.2 Vitamin D

The IARC Working Group[1] meta-analysis estimated the pooled relative risk for breast cancer across five studies, 3307 cases and 20,091 controls, to be 0.46 (95% CI 0.21–1.03) for the highest relative to the lowest category of blood Vitamin D (Table 1). There was highly significant heterogeneity in relative risks among the studies ($p < 0.001$), which was more a consequence of variation in the observed level of apparent protection against breast cancer in four of the studies, than to the distribution of individual study relative risks above and below the null. Three of the five studies had adjusted for body fatness, alcohol intake and hormone therapy.

Among the studies of dietary Vitamin D and breast cancer reviewed by the IARC Working Group[1] one of two case-control studies and two of three cohort studies reported reduced RRs in the highest intake category. In two cohort studies, this decrease was largely or solely observed in pre-menopausal women.

Invasive breast cancer was a secondary outcome in the Women's Health Initiative randomised controlled trial of calcium and Vitamin D referred to above (Sec. 3.1.2). There were 528 cases in women who received calcium and Vitamin D and 546 in women who received placebo; the RR was 0.96 (95% CI 0.85–1.09). Breast cancer was also the subject of a nested case control study of baseline serum Vitamin D (1067 cases and 1067 matched controls); RR for breast cancer was weakly increased, 1.22 (95% CI 0.89–1.67), in those with serum 25OH Vitamin D <32.4 nmol/l.

3.3 Prostate cancer

3.3.1 Sun exposure

The first direct evidence of a protective effect of sun exposure against the occurrence of prostate cancer, and perhaps any cancer, came from a case-control study of 422 prostate cancer patients and

290 controls patients who had benign prostatic hypertrophy.[22,23] In it, sun exposure was measured with a validated questionnaire used in the South Wales skin cancer study. The RR for prostate cancer in those with highest lifetime sun exposure was 0.32 (95% CI 0.20–0.51) (Table 3). High exposure categories of other sun-related variables, sunbathing, regular foreign holidays and childhood sunburn, were similarly associated with a lower risk of prostate cancer.

Three subsequent studies have also shown some evidence of a protective effect of residence in a high solar radiation environment against prostate cancer[12,24,25] (Table 3), but not of an outdoor occupation or, in one study, self-reported recreational sun exposure, or physician assessed sun exposure, or actinic skin damage.[26] One study, which included only cases of primary advanced prostate cancer, reported an appreciably reduced prostate cancer risk, with high values of a sun exposure index (based on a comparison of measured reflectance of usually exposed and usually unexposed skin) OR = 0.51 (95% CI 0.33–0.80)[25] (Table 3).

3.3.2 *Vitamin D*

The IARC Working Group meta-analysis estimated the pooled relative risk for prostate cancer across seven studies of men, 1909 cases and 19,281 controls, to be 0.83 (95% CI 0.61–1.12) for the highest relative to the lowest category of blood Vitamin D (Table 1).[1] There was some heterogeneity in relative risks among the studies ($p = 0.032$); five studies had RRs close to the null, three below and two above; the other two had low RRs. Four studies had adjusted for body fatness and one for several dietary variables also.

Three studies have examined the association between estimated dietary intake of Vitamin D and prostate cancer; in none was there evidence of a possible protective effect.[27–29]

3.4 *Non-Hodgkin lymphoma*

3.4.1 *Sun exposure*

While a range of early, mainly ecological studies, suggested that sun exposure might increase risk of non-Hodgkin lymphoma (NHL),[30] studies of individual sun exposure appear to suggest that

Table 3. Results of studies of the association of measures of individual sun exposure with prostate cancer occurrence. Relative risks for highest exposed category with reference to lowest, except as otherwise specified.

Author, year and population	Study design and subject numbers	Sun exposure measure	Relative risk, 95% CI	Covariates included in analysis
Luscombe 2001 and Bodiwala 2003[a] England	Hospital-based case control study Controls 290[b] Cases 422	Low lifetime sun exposure	0.32, 0.20–0.51	Age[d]
		History of childhood sunburn	0.29, 0.17–0.48	
		Sunbathing score[c]	0.81, 0.77–0.86	
		History of regular foreign holidays	0.48, 0.34–0.68	
Freedman 2002 24 US states	Death certificate-based case control study Controls 83,421 Cases 97,873	High solar radiation in state of birth and death	0.90, 0.87–0.93	Age, race, occupational physical activity, socioeconomic status (based on occupation)
		Outdoor occupation — non-farmer	1.00, 0.96–1.05	
		Outdoor occupation — farmer	1.16, 1.11–1.22	

(*Continued*)

Table 3. (Continued)

Author, year and population	Study design and subject numbers	Sun exposure measure	Relative risk, 95% CI	Covariates included in analysis
John 2004 and John 2007 USA	Population-based cohort study Cohort 3367 Cases 161	High solar radiation in state of birth	0.49, 0.27–0.90	Age[e]
		High solar radiation in state of longest residence	0.80, 0.44–1.49	
John 2005 San Francisco Bay	Population-based case control study in men 40–79 yrs Controls 455 Cases 450[f]	High solar radiation in state of birth	1.01, 0.73–1.39	Age and family history of prostate cancer
		High lifetime hours per week spent outdoors	0.95, 0.62–1.45	
		High sun exposure index[g]	0.51, 0.33–0.80	
		High lifetime hours per week in outdoor jobs	0.73, 0.48–1.11	

[a]These two papers report results from two phases of one study; their results have been combined by a simple fixed effects meta-analysis.
[b]Controls were men with benign prostatic hypertrophy.
[c]Relative risk per unit increase in score.
[d]Confounding with vasectomy status, diet and occupation were also assessed without effect on the results.
[e]Sun exposure in state of birth and state of longest residence each adjusted for the other.
[f]Cases were men with primary *advanced* prostate cancer.
[g]Based on the difference in skin reflectance between skin usually protected from and skin usually exposed to the sun when outdoors.

recreational sun exposure decreases its risk. A pooled analysis of original data from 8243 cases and 9697 controls in ten member studies of the InterLymph Consortium was published early in 2008.[31] The results from eight studies in which similar exposure variables could be defined are summarised in Fig. 1. For a composite measure of total sun exposure (recreational + non-recreational exposure) in these studies, the RR fell weakly with increasing sun exposure to 0.87 (95% CI 0.71–1.05) in the fourth quarter of exposure. There was

(a) Total sun exposure

	Q 1 Cases/controls	Q 4 Cases/controls	OR[1] (95% CI)
NSW	227/165	153/165	0.65 (0.47-0.90)
BC	160/150	137/147	0.87 (0.61-1.22)
NCI-SEER	136/103	132/107	0.73 (0.49-1.09)
Connecticut	121/165	155/166	1.32 (0.95-1.84)
Nebraska	107/152	93/126	0.99 (0.66-1.47)
Mayo	66/96	32/95	0.45 (0.26-0.78)
Epilymph 2[2]	221/332	239/331	0.99 (0.75-1.29)
UK	176/274	146/227	0.99 (0.74-1.33)
Pooled OR[3]	1214/1437	1087/1364	0.87 (0.71-1.05)

(b) Recreational sun exposure

	Q 1 Cases/controls	Q 4 Cases/controls	OR[1] (95% CI)
NSW	238/176	120/160	0.48 (0.34-0.67)
BC	170/139	136/150	0.69 (0.49-0.98)
NCI-SEER	156/106	107/94	0.54 (0.36-0.82)
Connecticut	118/178	136/175	1.22 (0.87-1.71)
SCALE	792/657	599/689	0.72 (0.62-0.85)
Epilymph 1	97/150	94/150	1.01 (0.69-1.48)
Epilymph 2[2]	235/323	245/349	0.92 (0.71-1.19)
UK	236/288	147/252	0.70 (0.53-0.92)
Pooled OR[3]	2042/2017	1584/2019	0.76 (0.63-0.91)

[1] Odds ratio (OR) for highest exposure quarter (Q 4) with reference to baseline (Q 1); adjusted for covariates including age, sex, ethnicity, regional centres, skin colour and sun sensitivity.
[2] adjusted for questionnaire type.
[3] pooled OR adjusted for study centre.

Figure 1. Results of pooled analysis of original data from ten case control studies on sun exposure and risk of non-Hodgkin lymphoma — Relative risks for highest quarters of total (a) and recreational sun exposure (b) with reference to lowest quarters. Abbreviations and acronyms in first column refer to study centres. Reproduced with permission from Kricker *et al.* (2008).[31]

a steeper downtrend for recreational exposure to an RR of 0.76 (95% CI 0.63–0.91; p for trend 0.005) in the fourth quarter, but no appreciable downtrend for non-recreational exposure. Limited control of potential confounding was possible in this analysis: all results were adjusted for ethnic origin, pigmentary characteristics and sun sensitivity, and available data on socioeconomic status, tobacco and alcohol intake in individual studies did not suggest they confounded the association of NHL with recreational sun exposure. Data were not available, however, on physical activity, obesity and diet, which might be confounding factors. The authors argued that the effect of recreational exposure, which was strongest for exposure in the ten years before diagnosis, is consistent with Vitamin D production as a mechanism by which sun exposure might protect against NHL. Net production of Vitamin D in the skin is greatest during the period immediately after exposure begins and therefore might be better predicted by exposure received more intermittently than more continuously.[32]

3.4.2 *Vitamin D*

Lim *et al*.[33] nested a case control study of lymphoid neoplasms within the Alpha-Tocopherol Beta-Carotene Cancer Prevention Study cohort of Finnish male smokers; serum Vitamin D was measured for 270 cases and 538 controls matched by birth year and month of blood draw. Overall, there was little association between serum Vitamin D and NHL risk, the RRs for the second and third tertiles relative to the first were 0.75 (95% CI 0.50–1.14) and 0.82 (95% CI 0.53–1.26), respectively. However, on the grounds that the apparent protection of sun exposure against NHL was greatest for sun exposure in the ten years before diagnosis,[31] the authors examined the association of serum Vitamin D with NHL for measurements made <7 and ≥7 years before diagnosis, which divided subjects into two groups of similar size. There was a trend towards lower risk of NHL with increasing serum Vitamin D measured <7 years before diagnosis, second tertile RR 0.60 (95% CI 0.33, 1.10) and third tertile 0.43 (95% CI 0.23, 0.83; p for trend <0.01). The RRs in this study were adjusted only for age and month of blood collection. Separately, however, the authors established that physical activity, obesity and smoking did not confound the association of serum Vitamin D with NHL.

Three case-control studies have reported on associations of dietary Vitamin D intake and NHL. In two (one including Vitamin D supplements) there was no direct evidence that dietary Vitamin D was protective against NHL.[34,35] In one of these, however, there was a quite strong inverse association between fatty fish intake, which is a rich source of vitamin D, and NHL.[34] The RRs for the second and third tertiles of intake respectively were 0.8 (95% CI 0.6–1.2) and 0.5 (95% CI 0.3–0.9; p for trend 0.02). The third, a small hospital-based case control study from southern Italy,[36] reported an inverse association of dietary Vitamin D intake with NHL risk: RRs for second and third tertiles of intake respectively were 0.8 (95% CI 0.5–1.2) and 0.6 (95% CI 0.4–0.9; $p < 0.05$). These results were adjusted for gender, age, centre, education, place of birth, hepatitis C virus infection, and total energy intake.

3.5   Other cancers

3.5.1   Oesphageal and gastric cancers

A case-cohort study was nested within a cohort of 29,584 people in Linxian County, China.[37] Serum 25OH Vitamin D was measured for 545 oesophageal (all squamous cell cancers), 353 gastric cardia, and 81 gastric noncardia cancer patients and 1105 other subjects sampled from the cohort. The RRs, adjusted for age, sex, smoking and alcohol, were 1.06 (95% CI 1.01–1.13) for oesophageal cancer, 1.03 (95% CI 0.96–1.10) for gastric cardia cancer and 0.98 (95% CI 0.86–1.12) for gastric non-cardia cancers per 15 nmol/l increase in serum Vitamin D. Addition of any of body fatness and serum selenium, cholesterol, retinol and α-tocopherol did not change the results.

In an analysis based on the male US Health Professionals Follow-Up Study, an estimation model for plasma 25OH Vitamin D concentrations was created in a sample of 1095 men for whom these concentrations had been measured.[38] This model contained factors for race, area of residence, leisure-time physical activity, body mass index, dietary Vitamin D, supplementary Vitamin D and season of blood draw. Model estimates of plasma 25OH Vitamin D were then made for all 47,800 men in the cohort and used to study the relationship of estimated Vitamin D concentration with cancer incidence (4286 cases) and cancer mortality (2025 deaths). The RRs

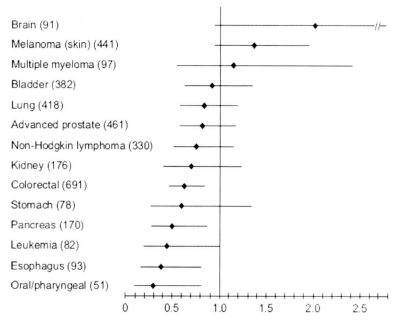

Figure 2. Multivariable relative risks and 95% confidence intervals for an increment of 25 nmol/l in predicted plasma 25OH vitamin D level for individual cancers in the Health Professionals Follow-up Study (1986 to 2000). Numbers in parentheses are numbers of cases. Co-variables included in the Cox proportional hazards model were age, height, smoking history, and intakes of total calories, alcohol, red meat, calcium, retinol, and total fruits and vegetables. Reproduced with permission from Giovannucci *et al.* (2006) and Oxford University Press.[38]

for individual cancers in the report of this study are shown in Fig. 2. The RR for oesophageal cancer was about 0.4 (95% CI 0.1–0.8) and that for stomach cancer 0.6 (95% CI 0.3–1.4).

3.5.2 *Pancreatic cancer*

In a nested case-control study with 184 cases of pancreatic cancer and 368 matched controls from the Prostate, Lung, Colorectal, and Ovarian Screening Trial cohort, serum 25OH Vitamin D was not appreciably associated with cancer risk.[39] The RR for the fifth quintile of Vitamin D was 1.45 (95% CI 0.66–3.15), adjusted for age, race, sex, and date of blood draw, body fatness and smoking; RRs for all other quintiles were close to unity. This result is in marked contrast to that obtained by the same investigators in an analysis of data from the Alpha-Tocopherol Beta-Carotene Cancer Prevention Study cohort of Finnish male smokers, in which the corresponding RR was 2.92 (95% CI 1.56–5.48).[39] The RR from the male US Health Professionals Follow-Up Study (Fig. 2) was about 0.5 (95% CI 0.3–0.9).[38]

3.5.3 Lung cancer

Serum Vitamin D concentrations were measured in a Finnish cohort of 6937 people from whom blood was collected in 1978 to 1980.[40] During a maximum of 24 years of follow-up, 122 lung cancers were identified. The RR for lung cancer was 0.72 (85% CI 0.43–1.19) for the highest relative to the lowest tertile of serum Vitamin D.

3.5.4 Skin cancers

Probably all skin cancers are caused by sun exposure; consequently all of them are probably positively associated with vitamin D produced by sun exposure. This probability is illustrated by the result for melanoma in the analysis of the male US Health Professionals Follow-Up Study referred to in Section 3.5.1 — a RR for melanoma of about 1.4 (95% CI 0.9–2.0) per 25 nmol/l (Fig. 2).[38] It is one of only three cancers reported in this study for which risk was higher with higher levels of vitamin D.

In spite of the difficulty in determining whether Vitamin D from sun exposure might protect against skin cancer, there is evidence that skin keratinocytes produce 1,25diOH Vitamin D and increasing basic biological evidence that it is active in physiological pathways in the skin that may protect against skin cancer.[41]

Two US, clinic-based case-control studies have examined the association of estimated dietary intake of Vitamin D with melanoma.[42,43] In one, there was weak evidence of a trend towards lower risk of melanoma with higher intake of Vitamin D, RR 0.6 (95% CI 0.4–1.0) for the highest intake quintile.[43] Any trend in the other was in the opposite direction, RR for highest quintile 1.8 (95% CI 0.9–3.5).

3.5.5 Ovarian cancer

In the death certificate-based case-control study referred to in Sec. 3.1.1, mortality from ovarian cancer was inversely associated with high residential ambient solar radiation, OR 0.84 (95% CI 0.81–0.88) for the highest category.[12] It was not associated with outdoor work.

A case control study of 224 cases and 603 controls nested in three large US cohort studies of women found no overall association of blood Vitamin D with ovarian cancer, RR 0.83 (95% CI 0.49–1.39) adjusted for ever use of post-menopausal hormones, body fatness, parity, lactose intake, duration of oral contraceptive use and season of blood draw.[44]

3.5.6 Other lymphomas and leukaemia

Three case control studies have reported on the association between sun exposure and Hodgkin lymphoma. In one, RR fell with increasing frequency of sunbathing and sunburn;[45] in another it fell with increasing sunny vacations, but not other recreational exposure or occupational exposure;[46] and in the third there was little indication of a falling risk with increasing time spent outdoors.[47] In one case control study, there was a weak trend towards a falling risk of multiple myeloma with increasing time spent outdoors.[47]

In the male US Health Professionals Follow Up Study analysis with estimated serum Vitamin D concentrations, the RR for multiple myeloma was about 1.2 (95% CI 0.6–2.4) per 25 nmol/l increase in serum Vitamin D and that for leukaemia of all kinds was 0.4 (95% CI 0.2–1.0).[38]

A moderate sized US case control study found a weak inverse association between estimated dietary Vitamin D and multiple myeloma, a lymphoid neoplasm closely related to NHL.[48] The RR for the highest Vitamin D intake category was 0.5 (95% CI 0.3–1.0).

3.5.7 All cancers

Three studies have examined the association of blood Vitamin D concentration with incidence of or mortality from all cancers together. Using model-estimated serum Vitamin D concentrations in the male US Health Professionals Follow-Up Study (see Sec. 3.5.1), the RR for occurrence of any cancer was 0.83 (95% CI 0.74–0.92) and for death from any cancer it was 0.71 (95% CI 0.60–0.83) per 25 nmol/l increase in serum Vitamin D level.[38] In an analysis of the relationship of serum 25OH Vitamin D with cancer mortality, based on 536 cancer deaths identified on follow-up of participants of the third US National Health and Nutrition Survey, the RR for death from cancer in the highest category of serum Vitamin D ($\geq$120 nmol/l) was 1.49 (95% CI 0.85–2.64).[49] A cohort of 3299 patients referred for coronary angiography, who also had their serum 25OH Vitamin D concentrations measured, was followed up for a median time of 7.75 years and 95 deaths from cancer ascertained.[50] The RRs for the second, third and fourth quartiles of serum Vitamin D were 0.87 (95% CI 0.50–1.52), 0.73 (95% CI 0.40–1.32) and 0.45 (95% CI 0.22–0.93) respectively, adjusted for age, sex, body fatness, smoking, serum retinol, physical activity, alcohol, and diabetes mellitus.

The incidence of all cancers except skin cancers was examined as a secondary endpoint in a randomised controlled trial in 1180 women >55 years of age randomised to taking 1400 mg or 1500 mg of calcium alone, calcium with 1100 IU of Vitamin D, or placebo, with fracture as the primary endpoint.[51] Women were treated and followed up for four years, during which time 50 were diagnosed with cancer. The RR of cancer in women receiving calcium alone was reported as 0.53 (95% CI 0.27–1.03) and that for calcium and Vitamin D 0.40 (95% CI 0.20–0.82). Thus while calcium appeared to reduce cancer incidence, there was little evidence of benefit from addition of Vitamin D. The authors, however, hypothesised that no benefit of Vitamin D would have been likely in the first year of treatment and repeated the analysis on the follow-up experience of the second to fourth years. The RR for calcium only changed a little, 0.59 (95% CI 0.29–1.21), while that for calcium and Vitamin D fell to 0.23 (95% CI 0.09–0.60). The authors concluded "that improving Vitamin D nutritional status substantially reduced all-cancer risk in post-menopausal women". This conclusion is not valid, given that it is based on what was probably an a *posteriori* decision to exclude the first year of follow-up from the analysis.

4. Does Vitamin D Mediate Apparently Protective Effects of Sun Exposure Against Cancer?

In principle, this question could be answered it two ways. First, Vitamin D mediation of a protective effect of sun exposure might be demonstrated by measuring both sun exposure and blood Vitamin D concentration in a case control or cohort study of a cancer (preferably the latter, because of the prospective nature of both measurements) and determining whether a protective effect of sun exposure could be substantially attenuated by adjustment for Vitamin D concentration. Second, it might be demonstrated by seeing, in a case control or cohort study, whether genetic variants that impair the action of available Vitamin D modify the effect of sun exposure on risk of the cancer. For example, presence of one or two copies of an activity impairing variant in the Vitamin D receptor gene might attenuate or eliminate a protective effect of sun exposure that is seen in the absence of the variant.

We know of no examples of the first of these possible approaches. There are, however, a few examples of the second in studies of sun exposure, Vitamin D receptor variants and cancers of the breast[52] and prostate,[25] and NHL.[53] While they suggest that Vitamin D does mediate apparent effects of sun exposure on prostate cancer and NHL, they are by no means persuasive and will require much larger numbers of subjects, probably gained through pooling data from a number of studies,[54] to provide the statistical power needed to be convincing.

5. Conclusions

We have summarised in Table 4 the epidemiological evidence presented above for possible protective effects of sun exposure and Vitamin D against cancer. We have not included in it any mention of ecological studies, which initiated this line of research; not because they were unimportant but because, having provided the initial hypothesis, they contribute little of value to making decisions about cause and effect. In addition to an account of the volume of evidence relevant to each of the major types of cancer for which there is some evidence, we have also roughly indicated in Table 4

Table 4. Summary of the epidemiological evidence for protective effects of sun exposure and vitamin D against cancer: The evidence summarised includes observational studies in individuals and randomised controlled trials but not ecological studies.

Cancer type	Number of studies				Evaluation
	Sun exposure	Blood vitamin D	Dietary vitamin D	RCT with vitamin D	
Oesophagus and stomach					Inadequate
Number of studies	0	2	0	0	
Protective effect	0	1	0	0	
Colorectal					Sufficient
Number of studies	2	9	21	2	
Protective effect	1	7	14	1[a]	
Pancreas					Inadequate
Number of studies	0	3	0	0	
Protective effect	0	1	0	0	
Lung					Inadequate
Number of studies	0	1	0	0	
Protective effect	0	0	0	0	
Melanoma of skin					Inadequate
Number of studies	NA	NA	1	0	
Protective effect			1	0	

(Continued)

Table 4. (Continued).

Cancer type	Number of studies				Evaluation
	Sun exposure	Blood vitamin D	Dietary vitamin D	RCT with vitamin D	
Breast					Inadequate
Number of studies	5	5	5	2	
Protective effect	3	4	3	0	
Ovary					Inadequate
Number of studies	1	1	0	0	
Protective effect	1	0	0	0	
Prostate					Inadequate
Number of studies	4	7	3	0	
Protective effect	3	2	0	0	
Non-Hodgkin lymphoma					Limited
Number of studies	10	1	3	0	
Protective effect	6	1	1	0	
Other lymphomas and leukaemia					Inadequate
Number of studies	3	1	1	0	
Protective effect	2	0	1	0	
All cancers					Inadequate
Number of studies	0	3	0	1	
Protective effect	0	2	0	0	

[a]While there is clear evidence of a protective effect in this one study, the confidence interval is wide, RR 0.62 (95% CI 0.24–1.60), and is wholly consistent with the null result of the other trial, RR 1.08 (95% CI 0.86–1.34).

the weight of evidence in support of a protective effect of sun exposure and/or Vitamin D and our evaluation of the strength of the evidence's support for causation. In doing the latter, we have followed IARC's guidance for evaluating evidence of causation from epidemiological studies (http://monographs.iarc.fr/ENG/Preamble/CurrentPreamble.pdf).

We conclude that the evidence for a causal relationship between sun exposure or Vitamin D and all except two of the cancer types listed is *inadequate*. By "inadequate", IARC means: "The available studies are of insufficient quality, consistency or statistical power to permit a conclusion regarding the presence or absence of a causal association between exposure and cancer". The exceptions are colorectal cancer, for which we think the evidence for a causal relationship is *sufficient*, "That is, a positive relationship has been observed between the exposure and cancer in studies in which chance, bias and confounding could be ruled out with reasonable confidence"; and NHL for which we think the evidence is *limited*, that is "a causal interpretation is considered … to be credible, but chance, bias or confounding could not be ruled out with reasonable confidence".

For NHL, the judgement for limited evidence is probably not controversial. It is based on the association between recreational sun exposure and NHL in a pooled analysis of all relevant studies.[31] Recreational exposure was pinpointed in the first such study to be published,[55] it has been confirmed as associated with NHL in four subsequent studies (Fig. 1), and the association is statistically significant in the pooled analysis ($p = 0.005$). It was strongest for exposure in the past ten years and, in the only study of NHL that included it, serum Vitamin D measured within seven years of diagnosis was also inversely associated with NHL risk.[33] On the negative side, all the studies of individual sun exposure are case-control studies and they had generally poor control subject participation rates. Thus we cannot rule out the possibility that control subjects who chose to participate had higher recreational sun exposure than those who refused. That adjustment for socioeconomic status did not weaken the association is, perhaps, against this explanation but we do not think it can be ruled out entirely. It was also not possible to adequately control in the pooled analysis, for possible confounding of recreational sun exposure with physical activity, diet and energy balance, which might plausibly be associated with NHL.

The judgement for sufficient evidence for colorectal cancer is based on the IARC meta-analysis of serum Vitamin D and colorectal cancer and its low relative risk and narrow 95% confidence interval, 0.56 (95% CI 0.43–0.74) (Table 1) rule out chance as more than a remotely possible explanation for the association. Eight of the nine studies in the meta-analysis were based on cohort studies, which eliminates selection bias; blood Vitamin D is an objective measure, which largely rules out information bias; and differential completeness of follow-up according to blood Vitamin D concentration seems improbable and should be eliminated in nested case control study designs, which were used for analysis of most of the cohorts. Confounding of serum Vitamin D with age, sex, and ethnicity were dealt with by all studies and three, including the two largest, also controlled for alcohol, body fatness and physical activity, which are known risk factors for colorectal cancer and are associated with serum Vitamin D. The IARC Working Group on Vitamin D[1] has argued that poor health status may itself be a cause of lower serum Vitamin D levels, for a range of reasons. However, people who agree to join cohort studies are generally healthy and it would have been rarely the case that someone already ill with colorectal cancer would have joined. Thus we think that confounding as an explanation for the association is implausible.

In considering the significance of the judgement that there is sufficient evidence that serum Vitamin D is causally associated with colorectal cancer, it is important to appreciate that IARC's approach to evaluation of evidence was developed in the context of preventing hazard, not proposing a public health intervention. We would argue that the "sufficient evidence" should not be taken as justifying routine, or even exceptional, use of Vitamin D as a way to prevent cancer. It would, however, justify the conduct of a randomised controlled trial in healthy people, to see whether or not supplementary Vitamin D in an appropriate dose can prevent cancer. While concerns about toxicity might be cited, there is persuasive evidence that Vitamin D is not toxic at the doses of 1000 IU to 2000 IU a day that might be proposed.[18,56]

References

1. IARC Working Group on Vitamin D, *Vitamin D and Cancer*, IARC Working Group Reports, International Agency for Research on Cancer, Lyon (2008). Ref Type: Serial (Book, Monograph).
2. D. D. Bikle, Vitamin D receptor, UVR, and skin cancer: A potential protective mechanism, *J. Invest Dermatol.* **128**: 2357–2361 (2008).
3. K. K. Deeb, D. L. Trump and C. S. Johnson, Vitamin D signalling pathways in cancer: Potential for anticancer therapeutics, *Nat. Rev. Cancer* **7**: 684–700 (2007).
4. F. L. Apperly, The relation of solar radiation to cancer mortality in North America, *Cancer Res.* **1**: 191–195 (1941).
5. C. F. Garland and F. C. Garland Do sunlight and vitamin D reduce the likelihood of colon cancer? *Int. J. Epidemiol.* **9**: 227–231 (1980).
6. F. C. Garland, C. F. Garland, E. D. Gorham *et al.*, Geographic variation in breast cancer mortality in the United States: A hypothesis involving exposure to solar radiation, *Prev. Med.* **19**: 614–622 (1990).
7. P. Waltz and G. Chodick, Assessment of ecological regression in the study of colon, breast, ovary, non-Hodgkin's lymphoma, or prostate cancer and residential UV, *Eur. J. Cancer Prev.* **17**: 279–286 (2008).
8. H. J. van der Rhee, E. de Vries and J. W. Coebergh, Does sunlight prevent cancer? A systematic review, *Eur. J. Cancer* **42**: 2222–2232 (2006).
9. W. B. Grant, An estimate of premature cancer mortality in the U.S. due to inadequate doses of solar ultraviolet-B radiation, *Cancer* **94**: 1867–1875 (2002).
10. W. B. Grant, Ecologic studies of solar UV-B radiation and cancer mortality rates, *Recent Results Cancer Res.* **164**: 371–377 (2003).
11. E. Giovannucci, The epidemiology of vitamin D and cancer incidence and mortality: A review (United States), *Cancer Causes Control* **16**: 83–95 (2005).
12. D. M. Freedman, M. Dosemeci and K. McGlynn, Sunlight and mortality from breast, ovarian, colon, prostate, and non-melanoma skin cancer: A composite death certificate based case-control study, *Occup. Environ. Med.* **59**: 257–262 (2002).
13. E. Kampman, M. L. Slattery, B. Caan *et al.*, Calcium, vitamin D, sunshine exposure, dairy products and colon cancer risk (United States), *Cancer Causes Control* **11**: 459–466 (2000).

14. J. Ishihara, M. Inoue, M. Iwasaki *et al.*, Dietary calcium, vitamin D, and the risk of colorectal cancer, *Am. J. Clin. Nutr.* **88**: 1576–1583 (2008).

15. T. Mizoue, Y. Kimura, K. Toyomura *et al.*, Calcium, dairy foods, vitamin D, and colorectal cancer risk: The fukuoka colorectal cancer study, *Cancer Epidemiol. Biomarkers Prev.* **17**: 2800–2807 (2008).

16. D. P. Trivedi, R. Doll and K. T. Khaw, Effect of four monthly oral vitamin D-3 (cholecalciferol) supplementation on fractures and mortality in men and women living in the community: Randomised double blind controlled trial, *Br. Med. J.* **326**: 469–472 (2003).

17. J. Wactawski-Wende, J. M. Kotchen, G. L. Anderson *et al.*, Calcium plus vitamin D supplementation and the risk of colorectal cancer, *N. Engl. J. Med.* **354**: 684–696 (2006).

18. R. Vieth, H. Bischoff-Ferrari, B. J. Boucher *et al.*, The urgent need to recommend an intake of vitamin D that is effective, *Am. J. Clin. Nutr.* **85**: 649–650 (2007).

19. F. Laden, D. Spiegelman, L. M. Neas *et al.*, Geographic variation in breast cancer incidence rates in a cohort of U.S. women, *J. Natl. Cancer Inst.* **89**: 1373–1378 (1997).

20. E. M. John, G. G. Schwartz, D. M. Dreon *et al.*, Vitamin D and breast cancer risk: The NHANES I Epidemiologic follow-up study, 1971–1975 to 1992. National Health and Nutrition Examination Survey, *Cancer Epidemiol. Biomarkers Prev.* **8**: 399–406 (1999).

21. J. A. Knight, M. Lesosky, H. Barnett *et al.*, Vitamin D and reduced risk of breast cancer: A population-based case-control study, *Cancer Epidemiol. Biomarkers Prev.* **16**: 422–429 (2007).

22. C. J. Luscombe, A. A. Fryer, M. E. French *et al.*, Exposure to ultraviolet radiation: Association with susceptibility and age at presentation with prostate cancer, *Lancet* **358**: 641–642 (2001).

23. D. Bodiwala, C. J. Luscombe, S. Liu *et al.*, Prostate cancer risk and exposure to ultraviolet radiation: Further support for the protective effect of sunlight, *Cancer Lett.* **192**: 145–149 (2003).

24. E. M. John, D. M. Dreon, J. Koo *et al.*, Residential sunlight exposure is associated with a decreased risk of prostate cancer, *J. Steroid Biochem. Mol. Biol.* **89–90**: 549–552 (2004).

25. E. M. John, G. G. Schwartz, J. Koo *et al.*, Sun exposure, vitamin D receptor gene polymorphisms, and risk of advanced prostate cancer, *Cancer Res.* **65**: 5470–5479 (2005).

26. E. M. John, J. Koo and G. G. Schwartz, Sun exposure and prostate cancer risk: Evidence for a protective effect of early-life exposure, *Cancer Epidemiol. Biomarkers Prev.* **16**: 1283–1286 (2007).

27. A. R. Kristal, J. H. Cohen, P. Qu *et al.*, Associations of energy, fat, calcium, and vitamin D with prostate cancer risk, *Cancer Epidemiol. Biomarkers Prev.* **11**: 719–725 (2002).

28. M. Tseng, R. A. Breslow, B. I. Graubard *et al.*, Dairy, calcium, and vitamin D intakes and prostate cancer risk in the National Health and Nutrition Examination Epidemiologic Follow-up Study cohort, *Am. J. Clin. Nutr.* **81**: 1147–1154 (2005).

29. S. Y. Park, S. P. Murphy, L. R. Wilkens *et al.*, Calcium, Vitamin D, and dairy product intake and prostate cancer risk: The Multiethnic Cohort Study, *Am. J. Epidemiol.* **166**: 1259–1269 (2007).

30. B. K. Armstrong and A. Kricker, Sun exposure and non-Hodgkin lymphoma, *Cancer Epidemiol. Biomarkers Prev.* **16**: 396–400 (2007).

31. A. Kricker, B. K. Armstrong, A. M. Hughes *et al.*, Personal sun exposure and risk of non Hodgkin lymphoma: A pooled analysis from the Interlymph Consortium, *Int. J. Cancer* **122**: 144–154 (2008).

32. A. R. Webb, B. R. DeCosta and M. F. Holick, Sunlight regulates the cutaneous production of vitamin D3 by causing its photodegradation, *J. Clin. Endocrinol. Metab.* **68**: 882–887 (1989).

33. U. Lim, D. M. Freedman, B. W. Hollis *et al.*, A prospective investigation of serum 25-hydroxyvitamin D and risk of lymphoid cancers, *Int. J. Cancer* **124**: 979–986 (2009).

34. E. T. Chang, K. M. Balter, A. Torrang *et al.*, Nutrient intake and risk of non-Hodgkin's lymphoma, *Am. J. Epidemiol.* **164**: 1222–1232 (2006).

35. P. Hartge, U. Lim, D. M. Freedman *et al.*, Ultraviolet radiation, dietary vitamin D and risk of non-Hodgkin lymphoma (United States), *Cancer Causes Control* **17**: 1045–1052 (2006).

36. J. Polesel, R. Talamini, M. Montella *et al.*, Linoleic acid, vitamin D and other nutrient intakes in the risk of non-Hodgkin lymphoma: An Italian case-control study, *Ann. Oncol.* **17**: 713–718 (2006).

37. W. Chen, S. M. Dawsey, Y. L. Qiao *et al.*, Prospective study of serum 25(OH)-vitamin D concentration and risk of oesophageal and gastric cancers, *Br. J. Cancer* **97**: 123–128 (2007).

38. E. Giovannucci, Y. Liu, E. B. Rimm *et al.*, Prospective study of predictors of vitamin D status and cancer incidence and mortality in men, *J. Natl. Cancer Inst.* **98**: 451–459 (2006).

39. R. Z. Stolzenberg-Solomon, R. B. Hayes, R. L. Horst *et al.*, Serum vitamin D and risk of pancreatic cancer in the prostate, lung, colorectal, and ovarian screening trial, *Cancer Res.* **69**: 1439–1447 (2009).

40. A. Kilkkinen, P. Knekt, M. Heliovaara *et al.*, Vitamin D status and the risk of lung cancer: A cohort study in Finland, *Cancer Epidemiol. Biomarkers Prev.* **17**: 3274–3278 (2008).

41. R. Gupta, K. M. Dixon, S. S. Deo *et al.*, Photoprotection by 1,25 dihydroxyvitamin D3 is associated with an increase in p53 and a decrease in nitric oxide products, *J. Invest. Dermatol.* **127**: 707–715 (2007).

42. M. A. Weinstock, M. J. Stampfer, R. A. Lew *et al.*, Case-control study of melanoma and dietary vitamin D: Implications for advocacy of sun protection and sunscreen use, *J. Invest. Dermatol.* **98**: 809–811 (1992).

43. A. E. Millen, M. A. Tucker, P. Hartge *et al.*, Diet and melanoma in a case-control study, *Cancer Epidemiol. Biomarkers Prev.* **13**: 1042–1051 (2004).

44. S. S. Tworoger, I. M. Lee, J. E. Buring *et al.*, Plasma 25-hydroxyvitamin D and 1,25-dihydroxyvitamin D and risk of incident ovarian cancer, *Cancer Epidemiol. Biomarkers Prev.* **16**: 783–788 (2007).

45. K. E. Smedby, H. Hjalgrim, M. Melbye *et al.*, Ultraviolet radiation exposure and risk of malignant lymphomas, *J. Natl. Cancer Inst.* **97**: 199–209 (2005).

46. T. Weihkopf, N. Becker, A. Nieters *et al.*, Sun exposure and malignant lymphoma: A population-based case-control study in Germany, *Int. J. Cancer* **120**: 2445–2451 (2007).

47. L. Grandin, L. Orsi, X. Troussard *et al.*, UV radiation exposure, skin type and lymphoid malignancies: Results of a French case-control study, *Cancer Causes Control* **19**: 305–315 (2008).

48. H. D. Hosgood, III, D. Baris, S. H. Zahm *et al.*, Diet and risk of multiple myeloma in Connecticut women, *Cancer Causes Control* **18**: 1065–1076 (2007).

49. D. M. Freedman, A. C. Looker, S. C. Chang *et al.*, Prospective study of serum vitamin D and cancer mortality in the United States, *J. Natl. Cancer Inst.* **99**: 1594–1602 (2007).

50. S. Pilz, H. Dobnig, B. Winklhofer-Roob *et al.*, Low serum levels of 25-hydroxyvitamin D predict fatal cancer in patients referred to coronary angiography, *Cancer Epidemiol. Biomarkers Prev.* **17**: 1228–1233 (2008).

51. J. M. Lappe, D. Travers-Gustafson, K. M. Davies *et al.*, Vitamin D and calcium supplementation reduces cancer risk: Results of a randomized trial, *Am. J. Clin. Nutr.* **85**: 1586–1591 (2007).

52. E. M. John, G. G. Schwartz, J. Koo *et al.*, Sun exposure, vitamin D receptor gene polymorphisms, and breast cancer risk in a multiethnic population, *Am. J. Epidemiol.* **166**: 1409–1419 (2007).
53. M. P. Purdue, P. Hartge, S. Davis *et al.*, Sun exposure, vitamin D receptor gene polymorphisms and risk of non-Hodgkin lymphoma, *Cancer Causes Control* **18**: 989–999 (2007).
54. P. Boffetta, B. Armstrong, M. Linet *et al.*, Consortia in cancer epidemiology: Lessons from InterLymph, *Cancer Epidemiol. Biomarkers Prev.* **16**: 197–199 (2007).
55. A. M. Hughes, B. K. Armstrong, C. M. Vajdic *et al.*, Sun exposure may protect against non-Hodgkin lymphoma: A case-control study, *Int. J. Cancer* **112**: 865–871 (2004).
56. R. P. Heaney, Vitamin D: Criteria for safety and efficacy, *Nutr. Rev.* **66**: S178–S181 (2008).

5

Oral Contraceptives, Hormone Replacement Therapy, and Cancers of the Female Reproductive System

Karen Canfell and
Emily Banks

Abstract

In developed countries, approximately 1.5 million women are diagnosed with cancer every year and almost half of these are cancers of the female reproductive organs. Oestrogens and progestogens, prescribed as oral contraceptives and hormone replacement therapy (HRT), are among the most commonly used medications worldwide. Oral contraceptives increase breast cancer risk while being used, although this excess risk diminishes following cessation of use. Oral contraceptives also increase the risk of cervical cancer, but they result in a long lasting reduction in the risk of ovarian and endometrial cancers. The combination of these risks means that, overall, use of combined oral contraceptives results in a net reduction in the lifetime risk of breast, ovarian and endometrial cancers. Use of oestrogen-only HRT increases the risk of breast, endometrial and ovarian cancer. Compared to oestrogen-only HRT, use of combined oestrogen-progestogen HRT results in a greater increase in breast cancer risk, a similar elevation in the risk of ovarian cancer, and a decreased or null effect on the risk of endometrial cancer. There is limited evidence available on the association between use of HRT and cervical cancer risk. Overall, the use of oestrogen-only or combined HRT results in a net increase in the risk of cancer of the breast, ovary and endometrium. Therefore, oral contraceptives and HRT have differing effects on the risk of developing reproductive system cancers. The net effect of oral contraceptives is likely to be protective in developed countries, whereas the net effect of combined HRT is to elevate the risk of reproductive system cancers.

Keywords: Oestrogen, progestogen, hormone replacement therapy, HRT, oral contraceptives, breast cancer, ovarian cancer, endometrial cancer.

1.   Introduction

In developed countries, approximately 1.5 million women are diagnosed with cancer every year, with almost half of these cancers involving the female reproductive organs, including cancers of the breast, ovary, uterine corpus or cervix.[1] Oestrogens and progestogens, prescribed as oral contraceptives and hormone replacement therapy (HRT), are among the most commonly used medications worldwide. Around 100 million women, or approximately 10% of women of reproductive age, are estimated to be currently using combined oral contraceptives and around 300 million women are estimated to have used oral contraceptives at some stage in their lives.[2] HRT is used predominantly in industrialised countries — in the mid-to-late 1990s an estimated 20 million women were using HRT in developed countries.[1] Major findings on the adverse effects of HRT were published in 2002 and 2003[3,4] and this was followed by substantial declines in the numbers of women using HRT. The numbers of prescriptions fell by more than 50% in the US between 2001 and 2004[5] and these declines were mirrored in other industrialized countries.[6-8]

Oral contraceptives and HRT have differing effects on the risk of developing cancer at various reproductive system sites. Because of this, and because of differences in levels of background risk at the age when these agents are used, the overall net effect of oral contraceptives on reproductive system cancers differs to that of HRT — while use of combined oral contraceptives results in a net decrease in the lifetime risk of cancer of the breast, ovary or endometrium, use of HRT results in an average net increase in the lifetime risks of these cancers. The International Agency for Research on Cancer (IARC), the cancer research arm of the World Health Organization, classifies oestrogen-only HRT and combined oestrogen-progestogen HRT as Group 1 carcinogens, concluding that there is sufficient evidence to indicate that they are carcinogenic to humans.[2,9]

This chapter will summarise the evidence for the relationship between use of oral contraceptives and use of HRT, and risk of cancer at various reproductive system sites.

2.   Oral Contraceptives

During reproductive years, oestradiol and progesterone levels are generally high and show large variations over the course of each menstrual cycle — normal oestradiol levels vary from 100 to 1700 pmol/L over the cycle.[10] Combined oral contraceptives contain both oestrogens and progestogens and suppress the production of endogenous oestradiol and progesterone. Although it is difficult to make direct quantitative comparisons, the hormonal stimulation received by the breast tissue of women taking combined oral contraceptives may not differ substantially from that in non-users.[11] Combined oral contraceptives also lead to the suppression of ovulation and atrophic effects on the endometrium. Progestogen-only oral contraceptives are used less commonly than combined oral contraceptives and lead to variable levels of suppression of ovulation and of hormone levels.

2.1   *Oral contraceptives and breast cancer*

The summary of worldwide evidence shows that oral contraceptives increase the risk of breast cancer. A recent IARC evaluation found that there is sufficient evidence to conclude that combined oral contraceptives lead to an increased risk of cancer of the breast in current and recent users.[2] A pooled analysis of data from over 50,000 women with breast cancer and 100,000 controls, conducted by the Collaborative Group for Hormonal Factors in Breast Cancer published in 1996, found that women currently using oral contraceptives have a 24% (95% CI: 15–33%) higher risk of breast cancer, compared to women who have never used oral contraceptives.[12] No significant trend in breast cancer risk is observed with increasing duration of use. The risk gradually diminishes following cessation of use and returns to the level of a woman who has never used oral contraceptives within around ten years after ceasing use.[12] The additional breast cancers observed in users of combined oral contraceptives are mainly localised to the breast.[12]

The evidence regarding the relationship between progestogen-only oral contraceptives and breast cancer is extremely limited — the combined worldwide studies include data on fewer than 800 women with breast cancer exposed to progestogen-only oral contraceptives.[12,13] These data show that the relative risk of breast cancer among women who had used progestogen-only oral contraceptives in the previous five years was 1.17 (SD 0.09; $p = 0.06$), compared to women who had never used oral contraceptives, with no significant increase in risk among women who had ceased used ten or more years earlier (relative risk 0.94; SD 0.1).[12] Although the data are not definitive, these findings are broadly comparable to those observed for combined oral contraceptives.

The background risk of breast cancer among women of reproductive age is relatively low, but increases with age. Since the use of oral contraceptives increases the risk of breast cancer while they are being used and for around ten years afterwards, it follows that the older women are when they use oral contraceptives, the greater the number of excess breast cancers resulting from use.

2.2   Oral contraceptives and ovarian cancer

Women who have used combined oral contraceptives have a reduced risk of ovarian cancer, compared to women who have never used oral contraceptives. Importantly, this protection is long-lasting. The 2008 pooled analysis of the Collaborative Group on Epidemiological Studies of Ovarian Cancer investigated risk in 23,257 women with ovarian cancer and 87,303 controls, and found that the reduction in risk persisted for more than 30 years after combined oral contraceptive use had ceased, though this reduction became, somewhat attenuated over time.[14] The proportional risk reductions per five years of use of combined oral contraceptives were 29% (95% CI: 23–34%) for use that had ceased within the last ten years, 19% (95% CI: 14–24%) for use ceasing ten to 19 years previously, and 15% (95% CI: 9–21%) for use ceasing 20 to 29 years previously. The average duration of use for women included in the analysis was four to five years. It was found that the reduction in risk of ovarian cancer was greater with longer durations of use — the reduction in risk for women who had used oral contraceptives for 15 or more years was 0.42 (95% CI: 0.36–0.49), compared to never-users.[14] This effect did not vary according to the calendar period when oral contraceptives were used, suggesting that the high dose preparations used in earlier years had similar effects to later lower dose formulations.[14] It has been estimated that use of oral contraceptives reduced the number of ovarian cancer cases by around 9% in the 1990s and 13% in the first decade of the 21st century, compared to the numbers expected in the absence of oral contraceptives.[14]

2.3 *Oral contraceptives and endometrial cancer*

The risk of endometrial cancer is reduced in women who have used oral contraceptives and this reduction in risk is greater with increasing duration of use.[2] Although the results are yet to be summarised in a pooled analysis, case-control and cohort studies show a general reduction in endometrial cancer of the order of 40 to 90% among women who have ever used combined oral contraceptives, compared to never-users. Data from several case-control studies suggest that the protective effect persists for at least ten to 20 years.[2] No summary information on the effect of dose, type or time since last use is available at present.

2.4 *Oral contraceptives and cervical cancer*

The primary cause of cervical cancer is known to be infection with oncogenic types of the human papillomavirus (HPV), but use of oral contraceptives appears to act as a co-factor in progression from HPV infection to cervical cancer. A number of studies conducted in the 1990s suggested that the use of oral contraceptives increases the risk of developing high grade pre-neoplastic disease, or invasive cervical cancer. However, confounding between use of oral contraceptives and sexual behavioural variables (which might influence the risk of HPV acquisition) was a concern in the interpretation of the early studies. In addition, the magnitude of the effect of oral contraceptives was uncertain and not always statistically significant.[15] The effects of oral contraceptives have now been clarified through several important pooled analyses. The first of these involved a meta-analysis of data pooled from eight case-control studies conducted by IARC.[16] In women infected with an oncogenic type of HPV, the risk of disease did not increase if oral contraceptives had been used for less than five years, but for users of more than five years duration the relative risk was 2.82 (95% CI: 1.46–5.42), and for users of more than ten years duration the relative risk was 4.03 (95% CI: 2.09–8.02), compared with HPV positive never-users. A later analysis of the pooled worldwide data on more than 16,500 cervical cancers by the International Collaboration for the Epidemiological Studies of Cervical Cancer found that the relative risks for current users of oral contraceptives were 1.90 (95% CI: 1.69–2.13) for users of five or more years duration.[17] After ceasing use, the risks declined to baseline levels after ten years. The use of oral contraceptives appears to be associated with an elevation in risk for adenocarcinoma, of a similar magnitude as that for squamous cell cancers.[17–20]

It does not appear that the use of oral contraceptives increases the risk of HPV acquisition or persistence. In the IARC study,[16] rates of HPV infection were examined amongst controls (i.e. participants with no evidence of cervical disease), and it was found that oral contraceptive users were not more likely to be infected with HPV DNA. This result was confirmed by another case-control study,[15] by a subsequently published systematic review of the literature[21] and by the findings of the pooled analysis of worldwide data.[17] These results, in conjunction with the overall increase in risk of cervical cancer associated with use of oral contraceptives, suggest that they have an impact on the progression of existing HPV infections, rather than acting to increase the probability of acquiring an HPV infection or increasing its persistence.

3.   Hormone Replacement Therapy

Hormone replacement therapy (HRT) preparations vary in the combination of steroids, the route of administration (oral, transdermal or topical), the dose schedule, and local or systemic effects.[22,23] HRT is prescribed as oestrogen-only therapy or combined therapy with oestrogen and progestogen. After menopause, endogenous oestradiol levels fall, such that oestradiol levels are around 70–200 pmol/L in post-menopausal women[10] and endogenous progesterone production ceases. Use of HRT substantially increases the level of oestradiol in post-menopausal women and, in the case of combined oestrogen-progestogen HRT, results in exposure to significant levels of progestogens. This is likely to stimulate the development of cancers that are sensitive to these hormones, including cancers of the female reproductive system. Figure 1 shows the age-specific mortality rates for female reproductive cancers in developed countries, on a log scale, and demonstrates the inflection (levelling off) of cancer rates occurring around the time of menopause for cancers of the breast, ovary and endometrium. When age is taken into account, this translates into

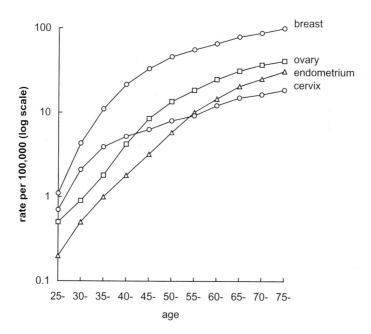

Figure 1. Mortailty rates by age for female reproductive cancers in developed countries (1990).

a reduction in risk of these cancers in post-menopausal, compared to pre-menopausal, women and is in keeping with the observed increase in the risk of these cancers seen with exposure to exogenous oestrogens and progestogens.

HRT is highly effective in the treatment of hot flushes, night sweats and vaginal dryness related to menopause.[24] Women using HRT must balance relief of these symptoms against the increased risk of serious disease attributable to the use of HRT, including stroke and venous thrombosis, in addition to the effect on the risk of developing reproductive system cancers.[2] The effect of HRT on other non-life threatening conditions, such as increased risk of incontinence[25] and gallbladder disease[26,27] and reduced peripheral fractures[28] should also be considered. The US Food and Drug Administration,[29] the UK Medicines and Healthcare Products Regulatory Agency,[30] and the Australian Therapeutic Goods Administration[31] have formulated broadly similar recommendations for HRT use, which may be generally summarised as follows:

- HRT should be used for the short term treatment of menopausal symptoms (hot flushes, night sweats, vaginal dryness) only;
- women considering the use of HRT should be informed of its risks and benefits;
- HRT should not be used for the prevention of disease, or in general as first-line treatment for osteoporosis; and
- HRT should be used for as short a period of time as possible and the need for continuing use should be reviewed six-monthly[31] or annually.[30]

3.1   *HRT and breast cancer*

Evidence from a large body of research shows that exposure to higher levels of oestrogen increases the risk of breast cancer. This evidence includes findings of reduced breast cancer risk with oophorectomy,[32,33] natural menopause,[12] use of oestrogen antagonists such as tamoxifen,[34,35] and low endogenous oestradiol levels.[33] The increased risk of breast cancer with increasing obesity in post-menopausal women can be explained by their elevated oestradiol levels, compared with post-menopausal women of healthy weight.[36] The findings regarding HRT and breast cancer are consistent with the overall picture of the relationship between hormones and breast cancer. Progestogens (also termed progestins) also increase the risk of breast cancer and exposure to combined oestrogens and progestogens increases the risk of breast cancer to a greater extent than exposure to oestrogen alone. Exactly how oestrogens and progestogens increase breast cancer risk is unknown. Oestrogens increase the mitotic rate of cells in the breast,[11] increasing the risk of mutation and acting as a neoplastic promoter.[37]

The most recent independent quantitative review of the effect of HRT on serious disease is the UK Public Assessment Report (UK Medicines and Healthcare product Regulatory Authority).[30] This review, supplemented by data from other large scale studies, shows that current users of HRT are at an increased risk of developing breast cancer, and that breast cancer risk is elevated with the use of all HRT types, but is much greater in users of combined oestrogen-progestogen than in users of oestrogen-only HRT.[30] The relative risk of breast cancer increases with increasing duration of use.[4,12,30] However, the increase in breast cancer risk wears off within a few years of ceasing use of HRT.[4,12] The risk of death from breast cancer is also elevated in women who are currently using HRT.[4,38] Use of HRT by women with a previous diagnosis of breast cancer increases the risk of recurrence.[38] Screening mammography is less effective in women currently using HRT, with increased false positive screens and a greater chance that breast cancers will be missed at screening.[39,40]

The relative risk of breast cancer (i.e. the percentage increase in risk) associated with HRT use does not vary significantly according to a woman's age. However, the background absolute risk of breast cancer does vary by age and this difference in background rate means that the same duration of use of HRT at an older age will result in a greater number of cases of breast cancer and other serious disease than use at a younger age. The largest relative risks in current users of HRT compared to non-users are observed for lobular, mixed ductal-lobular and tubular breast cancers.[41]

Apart from the difference between oestrogen-progestogen and oestrogen-only HRT, the risk of breast cancer relating to current use of different chemical formulations and doses of systemic HRT has not been shown to differ significantly.[4] The only factor found to significantly modify the effect of HRT on the risk of breast cancer is body size.[30,42] HRT results in a larger increase in the risk of breast cancer in women who have a lower, compared to a higher body mass index. Consistent with this is the finding that the effect of HRT on breast cancer is greater in Europe than in North America (where average BMI levels are higher).[30]

In the European context, five years use of oestrogen-only HRT results in a 20% (95% CI: 10–40%) increase in breast cancer risk, or two additional breast cancers per 1000 users aged 50–59, and three additional breast cancers per 1000 users aged 60–69.[42] Five years use of combined oestrogen-progestogen HRT results in a 60% (95% CI: 50–70%) increase in breast cancer, or six additional breast cancers per 1000 users aged 50–59, and nine additional breast cancers per 1000 users aged 60–69.[42] To provide context for these absolute and relative risks, in the European setting, ten in 1000 women aged 50–59 and 15 women aged 60–69 would be expected to develop breast cancer over a five-year period.[42] One additional unit of alcohol per day increases breast cancer risk by 7%[43] and an extra unit of Body Mass Index (equivalent to a weight gain of around 2.6 kg for a woman of average height) is associated with a 4% increase in post-menopausal breast cancer risk.[44] Hence, five years of oestrogen-only use is equivalent to around two to three additional alcoholic drinks per day or 13 kg weight gain for a woman of average height. Five years of oestrogen-progestogen HRT is the equivalent of around eight extra drinks per day, or a 39 kg weight gain. Having a mother or a sister with breast cancer is associated with a 65% increase in breast cancer risk for women aged 50 and over,[45] which is equivalent to five years of combined oestrogen-progestogen therapy.[42]

3.2 HRT and ovarian cancer

Cohort and case-control studies indicate the risk of ovarian cancer is moderately elevated in current users of HRT. However, no summary analysis of the world-wide data is available at the current time. The Million Women Study followed 948,576 post-menopausal women without previous cancer or bilateral oophorectomy and found that the relative risk of ovarian cancer in current users of HRT was 1.20 (95% CI: 1.09–1.32), compared to non-users.[46] The relative risk of dying of ovarian cancer in current versus never users was 1.23 (95% CI: 1.09–1.38). Among current users, risk increased gradually with increasing duration of use, such that current users with more than ten years of use had a relative risk of 1.31 (95% CI: 1.12–1.53) compared to non-users. No significant differences in effect were identified according to type of HRT (oestrogen-only versus oestrogen-progestogen), mode of administration or hormonal constituents. Among past users, no significant elevation in risk was seen, with a relative risk of 0.98 (95% CI: 0.88–1.11) for incident ovarian cancer and a relative risk of 0.97 (95% CI: 0.84–1.11) for ovarian cancer mortality.[46]

3.3   HRT and endometrial cancer

It has long been established that women using oestrogen-only HRT are at an increased risk of endometrial cancer, and this risk increases with duration of use.[9] As a consequence, many women with an intact uterus are prescribed combined oestrogen and progestogen HRT. Although the limited information available suggested that combined HRT did reduce the risk of endometrial cancer compared with oestrogen-only HRT,[2] until recently there was little data available to quantify the magnitude of the effect. In 2005, the UK Million Women Study reported results for a total of 716,738 postmenopausal women in the UK without previous hysterectomy.[47] It was found that use of continuous combined preparations was associated with a reduced risk of endometrial cancer, with a relative risk of 0.71 (95% CI: 0.56–0.90), compared with never users. However the use of cyclic combined preparations was not associated with any change in risk compared to never users, with a relative risk of 1.05 (95% CI: 0.91–1.22). In contrast, oestrogen-only HRT was associated with an elevated risk of 1.45 (95% CI: 1.02–2.06). These associations were modified according to body mass index, such that the beneficial effects of combined HRT were greater in obese women, and the adverse effects of oestrogen-only HRT were greatest in non-obese women.[47]

Although combined HRT is associated with a protective effect for endometrial cancer, particularly in the case of obese women and when continuous preparations were used, this benefit is outweighed by the adverse effects of combined HRT on the risk of breast cancer. When cancers of the endometrium and breast are considered together, there is a greater increase in total incidence with combined HRT, than with oestrogen-only HRT.[47]

3.4 HRT and cervical cancer

A number of studies have examined the possibility that the use of HRT influences the acquisition or persistence of HPV infection. As noted earlier, there is no evidence for such an effect with oral contraceptive use, which suggests that a link between HPV infection and use of HRT is unlikely, and this is borne out by the available data.[2] It is difficult to reliably assess the association between the use of HRT and the risk of high grade pre-neoplastic disease, or of invasive cervical cancer. It has been demonstrated that users of HRT can be more likely to have opportunistic cervical screening assessments when they visit a general practitioner for prescription or adjustment of their hormonal medication than women who do not use HRT.[48] If the confounding effect of screening cannot be fully taken into account, HRT may appear to be associated with a protective effect for invasive cervical cancer, because pre-neoplastic disease in HRT users may tend to be identified and treated at an earlier stage. On the other hand, if the end point for assessment is related to the development of pre-neoplastic lesions, these are likely to be identified more consistently in women screened more frequently, thus leading to an apparent increase in risk in HRT users.

Two randomised, placebo-controlled trials of combined HRT therapy have reported on the risk of abnormal cervical smears in HRT users — the Heart and Estrogen/Progestin Replacement Study (HERS) and the Women's Health Initiative (WHI). The HERS study examined the incidence of abnormal smears over a two-year follow-up period in 2561 post-menopausal women with normal cytology upon entry into the study.[49] Participants in the study were randomised to combined HRT therapy or to placebo. After one year, the incidence of abnormal smears was 3.0% across the study cohort, and after the second year of follow-up an additional 1.4% had abnormal smears. The relative risk of any cytological abnormality in HRT users versus placebo was 1.36 (95% CI: 0.93–1.99), but this effect appeared to be wholly explained by an increase in low grade equivocal smears in HRT users, with a relative risk of 1.58 (95% CI: 0.99–2.52). The relative risk for more severe cytological changes was found to be unity, 1.02 (95% CI: 0.53–1.95). Importantly, women in the HERS study were followed for a further two years after assessing abnormal smear rates, in order to obtain a final diagnosis. The results suggested that HRT impacts the rate of equivocal low grade smear abnormalities, without affecting the rate of underlying pre-neoplastic disease.

The WHI Study involved 16,608 post-menopausal non-hysterectomised women randomised to combined HRT or placebo, and followed up with Pap smears at least every three years for an average of 5.6 years.[50] Women in the HRT group had a significantly higher incidence of abnormal cervical smears ($p < 0.001$). A total of 646 (8.1%) abnormal smears were observed in the HRT group and 452 (5.9%) abnormal smears were observed in the placebo group. However, the number of high grade pre-neoplastic abnormalities was similar in the two groups, with most of the increased incidence in the HRT group related to equivocal and low grade smears.

A small number of observational studies have attempted to directly assess the risk of developing invasive cervical cancer in HRT users. One study involved long term follow-up of a cohort of more than 22,000 Swedish women and examined the incidence and mortality of a number of cancers in relation to use of oestrogen-only HRT. A slightly non-significantly decreased risk of invasive cervical cancer was identified in HRT users after an average follow-up of 6.7 years, with a relative risk of 0.8 (95% CI: 0.5–1.2), compared to the background population, but a relative risk of 0.9 was observed after correction for differences in hysterectomy rates between the cohort and the background population.[51] After an average of 13 years of follow-up of the cohort, the risk of incident invasive cervical cancer in HRT users remained lower that that in the background population (but not-significantly so), with a relative risk of 0.8 (95% CI: 0.6–1.1) after correcting for differences in hysterectomy rates.[52] A significant, apparently protective effect of HRT use on cervical cancer mortality was observed, with a relative risk of 0.3 (95% CI: 0.2–0.6) observed in HRT users. This pattern of a non-significant impact on cancer incidence, but a significant impact on mortality, is suggestive of a screening effect, leading to differential diagnosis patterns in HRT users and non-users. Similar results were obtained from a British study which examined rates of invasive cervical cancer in a cohort of more than 4500 women who had received an average of 67 months of HRT, with 43% of the participants using combined HRT.[53] Two cases of invasive cervical cancer were observed among the cohort. This was associated with a non-significant reduction in risk in HRT users, with a relative risk of 0.5 (95% CI: 0.1–1.7) for the development of carcinoma *in situ* or invasive cervical cancer, compared to expected rates in the general population of women after correcting for hysterectomy. Another case-control study of oestrogen-only HRT, performed in Italy, identified a similar (but significant) reduction in the relative risk of invasive cervical cancer of 0.5 (95% CI: 0.3–0.8) in HRT users, with a decreasing risk for increased duration of HRT use, and a decreasing risk for women who started using HRT before age 50 years.[54] This study used hospital-based controls, although women admitted for gynaecological, hormonal or neoplastic disease, or women with a hysterectomy were excluded from the control group. In this study, only adjustment for the lifetime number of cervical smears was performed.

In summary, there is no evidence for any difference in HPV prevalence in users and non-users of HRT, as would be expected from the analogy with the results for users of oral contraceptives. This suggests that if HRT has any effect, it operates as a co-factor in HPV progression, rather than by increasing the probability of viral infection, or by increasing the duration of initial infection. The results from randomised trials show that the use of HRT increases the incidence of equivocal cytological smears, but there is no evidence to show that HRT increases the risk of high grade pre-neoplastic abnormalities; and it is not known whether the increase in equivocal cytology reflects an increase in the rate of actual underlying pre-neoplastic abnormalities.[55] The effect of HRT on invasive cervical cancer is also not clear, because of concerns over residual confounding, due to differential screening effects in users and non-users of HRT.

4.   Conclusions

Oral contraceptives increase the risk of breast cancer while being used, although this excess risk diminishes following cessation of use. Oral contraceptives also increase the risk of cervical cancer;

but they result in a long lasting reduction in the risk of ovarian and endometrial cancers. The combination of these risks means that, overall, use of combined oral contraceptives results in a reduction in the lifetime risk of cancers of the breast, ovary and endometrium.

Use of oestrogen-only HRT increases the risk of breast, endometrial and ovarian cancers. Use of combined oestrogen and progestogen HRT results in a greater increase in the risk of breast cancer, a similar elevation in risk of ovarian cancer, and a decreased or null effect on the risk of endometrial cancer. There is limited evidence available on the association between use of HRT and risk of cervical cancer. Overall, use of both oestrogen-only combined oestrogen-progestogen HRT results in a net increase in the risk of cancers of the breast, ovary and endometrium. Therefore, regulatory bodies in several jurisdictions recommend that HRT should be used for the short term treatment of menopausal symptoms (hot flushes, night sweats, vaginal dryness) only and not be used for the prevention of any chronic disease, or as first line treatment for osteoporosis. Women considering use of HRT should be informed of its risks and benefits; HRT should be used for as short a period of time as possible and the need for continuing use should be reviewed regularly.

References

1. V. Beral, E. Banks, G. Reeves and P. Appleby, Use of HRT and the subsequent risk of cancer, *J. Epidemiol. Biostat.* **4**(3): 191–210 (1999).
2. International Agency for Research on Cancer, *IARC Monographs on the Evaluation of Carcinogenic Risk to Humans: Combined Estrogen-Progestogen Contraceptives and Combined Estrogen-Progestogen Menopausal Therapy*, Vol. 91 (IARC, Lyon, France, 2007).
3. Writing Group for the Women's Health Initiative Investigators, Risks and benefits of estrogen plus progestin in healthy postmenopausal women: Principal results from the Women's Health Initiative randomized controlled trial, *J. Am. Med. Assoc.* **288**(3): 321–333 (2002).
4. Million Women Study Collaborators, Breast cancer and hormone-replacement therapy in the Million Women Study, *Lancet* **362**(9382): 419–427 (2003).
5. P. M. Ravdin, K. A. Cronin, N. Howlader, C. D. Berg, R. T. Chlebowski, E. J. Feuer *et al.*, The decrease in breast-cancer incidence in 2003 in the United States, *N. Engl. J. Med.* **356**(16): 1670–1674 (2007).

6. K. Canfell, E. Banks, A. M. Moa and V. Beral, Decrease in breast cancer incidence following a rapid fall in use of hormone replacement therapy in Australia, *Med. J. Aust.* **188**(11): 641–644 (2008).

7. K. Canfell, E. Banks, M. Clements, Y. J. Kang, A. Moa, B. Armstrong *et al.*, Sustained lower rates of HRT prescribing and breast cancer incidence in Australia since 2003, *Breast Cancer Res. Treat.*, February 15 [E pub ahead of print] (2009).

8. M. Kumle, Declining breast cancer incidence and decreased HRT use, *Lancet* **372**(9639): 608–610 (2008).

9. IARC, *IARC Monographs on the Evaluation of Carcinogenic Risks to Humans. Hormonal Contraception and Post-Menopausal Hormonal Therapy*, Vol. 72 (IARC, Lyon, France, 1999).

10. The Royal College of Pathologists of Australasia, *Manual of Use and Interpretation of Pathology Tests*, RCPA (1990).

11. T. J. Key, P. K. Verkasalo and E. Banks, Epidemiology of breast cancer, *Lancet Oncol.* **2**(3): 133–140 (2001).

12. Collaborative Group on Hormonal Factors in Breast Cancer, Breast cancer and hormonal contraceptives: Collaborative reanalysis of individual data on 53,297 women with breast cancer and 100,239 women without breast cancer from 54 epidemiological studies, *Lancet* **347**(9017): 1713–1727 (1996).

13. Collaborative Group on Hormonal Factors in Breast Cancer, Breast cancer and hormonal contraceptives: Further results, *Contraception* **54**(Suppl. 3): 1S–106S (1996).

14. Collaborative Group on Epidemiological Studies of Ovarian Cancer, V. Beral, R. Doll, C. Hermon, R. Peto and G. Reeves, Ovarian cancer and oral contraceptives: Collaborative reanalysis of data from 45 epidemiological studies including 23,257 women with ovarian cancer and 87,303 controls, *Lancet* **371**(9609): 303–314 (2008).

15. J. M. Deacon, C. D. Evans, R. Yule, M. Desai, W. Binns, C. Taylor *et al.*, Sexual behaviour and smoking as determinants of cervical HPV infection and of CIN3 among those infected: A case-control study nested within the Manchester cohort, *Br. J. Cancer* **83**(11): 1565–1572 (2000).

16. V. Moreno, F. X. Bosch, N. Munoz, C. J. Meijer, K. V. Shah, J. M. Walboomers *et al.*, Effect of oral contraceptives on risk of cervical cancer in women with human papillomavirus infection: The IARC multicentric case-control study, *Lancet* **359**(9312): 1085–1092 (2002).

17. International Collaboration of Epidemiological Studies of Cervical Cancer, P. Appleby, V. Beral, A. Berrington de González, D. Colin, S. Franceschi, A. Goodhill *et al.*, Cervical cancer and hormonal contraceptives: Collaborative reanalysis of individual data for 16,573 women with cervical cancer and 35,509 women without cervical cancer from 24 epidemiological studies, *Lancet* **370**(9599): 1609–1621 (2007).

18. A. Berrington de González, P. Jha, J. Peto, J. Green and C. Hermon, Oral contraceptives and cervical cancer, *Lancet* **360**(9330): 410 (2002).

19. J. Green, A. Berrington de González, S. Sweetland, V. Beral, C. Chilvers, B. Crossley *et al.*, Risk factors for adenocarcinoma and squamous cell carcinoma of the cervix in women aged 20–44 years: The UK National Case-Control Study of Cervical Cancer, *Br. J. Cancer* **89**(11): 2078–2086 (2003).

20. A. Berrington de González, S. Sweetland and J. Green, Comparison of risk factors for squamous cell and adenocarcinomas of the cervix: A meta-analysis, *Br. J. Cancer* **90**(9): 1787–1791 (2004).

21. J. Green, A. Berrington de González, J. S. Smith, S. Franceschi, P. Appleby, M. Plummer *et al.*, Human papillomavirus infection and use of oral contraceptives, *Br. J. Cancer* **88**(11): 1713–1720 (2003).

22. M. L. Gilliam, Local and systemic options for hormone replacement therapy, *Int. J. Fertil. Womens Med.* **46**(4): 222–227 (2001).

23. G. A. Greendale, N. P. Lee and E. R. Arriola, The menopause, *Lancet* **353**: 571–580 (1999).

24. A. MacLennan, J. Broadbent, S. Lester and V. Moore, Oral oestrogen and combined oestrogen/progestagen therapy versus placebo for hot flushes, *Cochrane Database Syst. Rev.* **4**: CD002978 (2004).

25. S. Hendrix, B. Cochrane, I. Nygaard *et al.*, Effects of estrogen with and without progestin on urinary incontinence, *J. Am. Med. Assoc.* **293**: 935–948.

26. J. A. Simon, D. Hunninghake, S. K. Agarwel *et al.*, Effect of estrogen plus progestin on risk for biliary tract surgery in postmenopausal women with coronary artery disease, *Ann. Intern. Med.* **135**: 493–501 (2001).

27. B. Liu, V. Beral, A. Balkwill *et al.*, Gallbladder disease and use of transdermal versus oral hormone replacement therapy in postmenopausal women: prospective cohort study, *Br. Med. J.* **337**: a386 (2008).

28. J. A. Cauley, J. Robbins, Z. Chen *et al.*, Effects of estrogen plus progestin on risk of fracture and bone mineral density: The Women's Health Initiative Randomised Trial, *J. Am. Med. Assoc.* **290**: 1729–1738 (2003).

29. United States Department of Health and Human Services Food and Drug Administration, *Guidance for Industry Noncontraceptive Estrogen Drug Products for the Treatment of Vasomotor Symptoms and Vulvar and Vaginal Atrophy Symptoms — Recommended Prescribing Information for Health Care Providers and Patient Labeling*, Draft guidelines. Revision 4, 2005, http://www.fda.gov/cder/guidance/6932dft.pdf (accessed July 2008).

30. Medicines and Healthcare Products Regulatory Agency, UK Public Assessment Report, *Hormone-Replacement Therapy: Safety Update* (MHRA, London, 2007), http://www.mhra.gov.uk/home/groups/plp/documents/websiteresources/con2032228.pdf (accessed July 2008).

31. Australian Drug Evaluation Committee, *ADEC Summary Statement on HRT*, Canberra, Australia (Australian Government Department of Health and Ageing, Therapeutic Goods Administration, 2004), http://www.tga.gov.au/docs/html/hrtadec3.htm (accessed July 2008).

32. M. J. Clarke, Ovarian ablation in breast cancer, 1896 to 1998: Milestones along hierarchy of evidence from case report to Cochrane review, *Br. Med. J.* **317**(7167): 1246–1248 (1998).

33. T. J. Key and P. K. Verkasalo, Endogenous hormones and the aetiology of breast cancer, *Breast Cancer Res.* **1**(1): 18–21 (1999).

34. A. Thomsen and J. M. Kolesar, Chemoprevention of breast cancer, *Am. J. Health Syst. Pharm.* **65**(23): 2221–2228 (2008).

35. A. Howell, The endocrine prevention of breast cancer, *Best Pract. Res. Clin. Endocrinol. Metab.* **22**(4): 615–623 (2008).

36. Endogenous Hormones Breast Cancer Collaborative Group, Body mass index, serum sex hormones, and breast cancer risk in post-menopausal women, *J. Natl. Cancer Inst.* **95**(16): 1218–1226 (2003).

37. G. A. Colditz, Decline in breast cancer incidence due to removal of promoter: Combination estrogen plus progestin, *Breast Cancer Res.* **9**: 108 (2007) [erratum *Breast Cancer Res.* **9**: 401 (2007)].

38. E. Banks, V. Beral and G. Reeves, For the Million Women Study Collaborators, Published results on breast cancer and hormone replacement therapy in the Million Women Study are correct, *Climacteric* **7**: 415–416 (2004).

39. L. Holmberg and H. Anderson, HABITS (hormonal replacement therapy after breast cancer — Is it safe?), a randomised comparison: Trial stopped, *Lancet* **363**: 453–455 (2004).

40. E. Banks, G. Reeves, V. Beral *et al.*, How personal characteristics of individual women influence the sensitivity and specificity of mammography in the Million Women Study: Cohort study, *Br. Med. J.* **329**: 477 (2004).

41. G. K. Reeves, V. Beral, J. Green, T. Gathani and D. Bull, Hormonal therapy for menopause and breast-cancer risk by histological type: A cohort study and meta-analysis, *Lancet Oncol.* **7**(11): 910–918 (2006).

42. E. Banks, K. Canfell and G. Reeves, HRT and breast cancer: Recent findings in the context of the evidence to date, *Womens Health (Lond. Engl.)* **4**(5): 427–431 (2008).

43. Collaborative Group on Hormonal Factors in Breast Cancer, Alcohol, tobacco and breast cancer: Collaborative reanalysis of individual data from 53 epidemiological studies, including 58515 women with breast cancer and 95067 women without the disease, *Br. J. Cancer* **87**: 1234–1245 (2002).

44. G. Reeves, K. Pirie, V. Beral, J. Green and E. Spencer, For the Million Women Study Collaborators, Cancer incidence and mortality in relation to body mass index in the Million Women Study: Cohort study, *Br. Med. J.* **335**: 1134–1139 (2007).

45. Collaborative Group on Hormonal Factors in Breast Cancer, Familial breast cancer: Collaborative reanalysis of individual data from 52 epidemiological studies including 58,209 women with breast cancer and 101,986 women without the disease, *Lancet* **358**: 1389–1399 (2001).

46. V. Beral, D. Bull, J. Green and G. Reeves, Ovarian cancer and hormone replacement therapy in the Million Women Study, *Lancet* **369**(9574): 1703–1710.

47. V. Beral, D. Bull and G. Reeves, Endometrial cancer and hormone-replacement therapy in the Million Women Study, *Lancet* **365**(9470): 1543–1551 (2005).

48. C. Finley, E. W. Gregg, L. J. Solomon and E. Gay, Disparities in hormone replacement therapy use by socioeconomic status in a primary care population, *J. Commun. Health* **26**(1): 39–50.

49. G. F. Sawaya, D. Grady, K. Kerlikowske, J. L. Valleur, V. M. Barnabei, K. Bass *et al.*, The positive predictive value of cervical smears in previously screened postmenopausal women: The Heart and Estrogen/progestin Replacement Study (HERS), *Ann. Intern. Med.* **133**(12): 942–950.

50. G. L. Anderson, H. L. Judd, A. M. Kaunitz, D. H. Barad, S. A. Beresford, M. Pettinger *et al.*, Effects of estrogen plus progestin on gynecologic

cancers and associated diagnostic procedures: The Women's Health Initiative randomized trial, *J. Am. Med. Assoc.* **290**(13): 1739–1748 (2003).

51. H. O. Adami, I. Persson, R. Hoover, C. Schairer and L. Bergkvist, Risk of cancer in women receiving hormone replacement therapy, *Int. J. Cancer* **44**(5): 833–839 (1989).

52. I. Persson, J. Yuen, L. Bergkvist and C. Schairer, Cancer incidence and mortality in women receiving estrogen and estrogen-progestin replacement therapy — Long-term follow-up of a Swedish cohort, *Int. J. Cancer* **67**(3): 327–332 (1996).

53. K. Hunt, M. Vessey, K. McPherson and M. Coleman, Long-term surveillance of mortality and cancer incidence in women receiving hormone replacement therapy, *Br. J. Obstet. Gynaecol.* **94**(7): 620–635 (1987).

54. F. Parazzini, C. La Vecchia, E. Negri, S. Franceschi, S. Moroni, L. Chatenoud *et al.*, Case-control study of oestrogen replacement therapy and risk of cervical cancer, *Br. Med. J.* **315**(7100): 85–88 (1997).

55. K. Canfell, V. Beral and A. R. McLean, *Use of Hormone Replacement Therapy as a Potential Co-factor in the Neoplastic Progression of HPV-Related Cervical Disease*, Thesis (Life and Environmental Sciences Division, University of Oxford, 2004).

6

Involuntary Exposures — Can Knowledge Keep Pace with Perceptions?

Bernard W. Stewart

Abstract

Cancer in humans may be caused by exposure to carcinogens which occurs against the will of the individuals affected. Such cancers can be distinguished from those caused by tobacco smoking, alcohol drinking and deliberate sun exposure, together with malignancies for which diet, obesity, exercise, reproductive history, sexual behaviour and the like are risk factors, all often described as cancers associated with lifestyle. Involuntary exposure to carcinogens is best characterised in the workplace. Most of the substances known to be carcinogenic for humans have been identified following epidemiological study of particular workers. Occupational cancer may be prevented by regulation, once carcinogens or hazardous environments have been recognised, despite unacceptable delays in the case of asbestos specifically. Wider pollution of the environment is generally attributable to industrial practice, though arsenic contamination of water supplies in some locations also occurs naturally. Atmospheric pollution causes lung cancer, with worst exposures now involving developing countries. Local pollution by asbestos, polycyclic aromatic hydrocarbons, or heavy metals may cause cancer amongst residents, but clear proof of causation in relation to pesticides, solvents and industrial waste in such situations is difficult. Media attention to cancer allegedly associated with a variety of consumer products (apart from tobacco and alcohol) raises anxiety and expectations. Specific actions have been taken in some circumstances, but expectations regarding absolute safety can never be met. Cancer clusters are also extensively reported. Corresponding investigations serve to address neighbourhood concerns, but have not revealed modes of cancer causation which would have otherwise remained unknown. Overall, involuntary exposures account for a small proportion of cancer cases, but such cancers are preventable and the community demands no less.

Keywords: Environmental carcinogen, occupational cancer, pollution, consumer products, cancer cluster.

1. Cancers That Should be Prevented

Earlier chapters in this section address certain risk factors for cancer that have been investigated both in relation to cancer aetiology and also in relation to cancer prevention. In all cases, correct appreciation of the impact of relevant risk factors depends primarily on an understanding of epidemiological data. Appreciation of the extent to which preventive measures might be adopted and could be effective also involves epidemiological assessment, as well as input from a range of non-clinical professionals, extending from laboratory scientists through to experts in both behaviour and communication. Unlike the earlier chapters, which deal with risks arising as a consequence of lifestyle choices (tobacco usage, alcohol consumption, diet, exercise, sexual behaviour, etc.), risks discussed here arise independently of conscious choice, and are generated contrary to the wishes of those affected.

Present understanding is that involuntary exposures account for a minor fraction of the cancer burden. An assessment of cancer causes in Europe in 2008[1] identified tobacco smoking and consumption of alcoholic beverages as the major risk factors, accounting for 27% and 11% respectively of cancer in men, the corresponding figures for women being 6% and 5%. Other lifestyle-related risk factors, such as excess weight, relative lack of physical activity, infection and sunlight, variously account for between 1% and 5% of malignant disease, with the exception of reduced physical activity in men being responsible for <1% of cancer. By comparison, occupational exposure (3% of cancer in men, and <1% of cancer in women) and environmental exposure (<1% for both sexes) were seen to account for a small proportion of the total cancer burden.

Involuntary exposure to carcinogens specifically includes hazardous circumstances which occur in the workplace, and in the wider environment due to pollution of air, water and soil. The term also includes exposures consequent upon using a variety of consumer products. Cancer clusters are invariably reported to health authorities with the suspicion that involuntary exposures are responsible. Across this spectrum of circumstances, the community requires that action be taken to prevent cancer causation; carcinogenesis is simply unacceptable.

When a patient with cancer seeks to know the cause of his or her malignancy, almost invariably, the focus is on exposures to which that individual has been subjected in circumstances beyond his or her control. Provision of adequate information then becomes an aspect of clinical care, requiring the oncologist to address non-clinical disciplines. As will become clear, information that may be responsibly conveyed varies markedly across the spectrum of involuntary exposures. At one extreme, occupational cancer is explicable and should be prevented; at the other, cancer clusters provide no insight regarding causation, but do represent a burden of care that may be alleviated if relevant data are correctly understood. Community perceptions, however, do not vary according to the circumstances of exposure and risk. These perceptions generally involve a clear-cut understanding of cause and effect, untrammeled by limited evidence and alternative explanations. This may lead to dissatisfaction with health authorities and inadequate attention to other scenarios that provide an opportunity for risk reduction or cancer prevention.

2. Occupational Cancer: Prevention is Achievable

Occupational cancer has been, and is, the primary context in which cancer can be correctly perceived as a preventable environmental disease.[2] Most of the chemicals currently recognised as being capable of causing cancer in humans were revealed as occupational carcinogens (the next-largest such category being iatrogenic carcinogens). Occupational cancer most commonly involves lung or skin cancer; a distribution of disease which clearly implicates particular routes of exposure.[3] However, study of cancer in the workplace has revealed a more complex situation than might be understood from the scenario of being occupationally exposed to potent carcinogenic substances. Increased incidence of cancer is readily evident in certain occupations, although specific agents that might account for such an outcome have not been identified.

The total burden of occupational cancer is not clear, the matter being most famously addressed by Doll and Peto in relation to their estimates of attributable risk of cancer in the United States was published in 1981.[4] They estimated the proportion of cancers caused by occupational factors to be 4%, and more than 25 years later, it is unclear whether that estimate was accurate. That the matter is unclear is readily apparent, since a whole conference was devoted to this question.[5] Much more recently, it has been suggested that in Australia, 10.8% of cancer (excluding non-melanoma skin cancer) in males and 2.2% of cancer cases in females are caused by occupational exposures.[6] In contrast, comparable figures for a typical European country are suggested to be 3% in males and <1% in females.[1] Means to determine the accuracy of such estimates are not clear. However, granted that, for example, the proportion of cancer attributable to tobacco is not subject to contention or widely differing estimates, it is problematic that the medico-scientific community cannot provide a definitive determination in relation to what is an ostensibly simple question. In any event, there seems little doubt that occupational exposure accounts for a minor fraction of all cancer worldwide,[7] and the burden of occupational cancer is assuredly greater in developing countries.[8] However, while the burden of occupational cancer is difficult to quantify, this does not detract from the priority that should be accorded to its prevention. Prevention of cancer consequent upon lifestyle choices must focus on individual behaviour, and adoption of regulatory measures only plays a supportive role. In contrast, occupational cancer is recognised as being wholly preventable by regulation.[9]

2.1   *Carcinogens identified*

In the first instance, cancer occurs in workers who produce, handle or encounter carcinogens in the workplace. Asbestos fibres caused, and continue to account for emerging cases of mesothelioma, as well as lung cancer and exposure to vinyl chloride resulted in polymerisation workers developing angiosarcoma of the liver.[10]

Reference to asbestos or vinyl chloride as examples of occupational carcinogens may convey the impression that such carcinogens, or indeed carcinogens generally, may be definitively specified as a single category. This is not the case: all authorities categorising agents in relation to causation of cancer in humans use a range of categories or Groups in the case of International Agency for Research on Cancer (IARC — an arm of World Health Organization). IARC allocate agents for which there is some evidence of carcinogenicity, according to whether the available data definitively establish that the agent causes cancer in humans (Group 1), probably (Group 2A) or possibly (Group 2B) causes cancer in humans, or that evidence is not adequate to infer carcinogenicity (Group 3). Categorisation occurs in the context of *IARC Monographs on the Evaluation of Carcinogenic Risks to Humans*, of which approximately 100 volumes have been published since 1972.[11]

The *IARC Monograph* evaluations may serve as a database for the purposes of listing occupational carcinogens. The exercise is not simple. In *IARC Monographs*, information summarised under *Production and Use* (Sec. 1.2) and *Occurrence* (Sec. 1.3) may be used to identify those agents categorised Group 1, Group 2A and Group 2B which have been encountered in the workplace.[12] Such information, however, does not necessarily identify those agents which are encountered by specific individuals, or those agents which are best targeted at the present time in relation to regulations calculated to prevent occupational cancer. Inevitably, epidemiological evidence concerning occupational cancer is predicated on specific past practice. Some work practices resulting in identification of occupational cancer may have been discontinued long ago, and a limited number of agents, such as 2-naphthylamine, are no longer used. Otherwise, current manufacturing or industrial processes may be modified so that past exposures no longer occur.

The understanding that *past* rather than current practice is reflected in today's burden of occupationally-induced cancer is most starkly, and tragically, illustrated by asbestos. Addressing 'The European mesothelioma epidemic' in 1999, Peto and colleagues[13] determined that death from mesothelioma would progressively increase in Western European countries, including Great Britain until at least 2020. After that date, current restrictions on use of asbestos could be reasonably expected to account for a decline. Regulatory control of occupational exposure to asbestos was initially focused on those involved in mining and milling asbestos, insulation workers, dockside workers and demolition workers. Determining the full scope of exposure is ongoing, with particular occupations such as automobile workers clearly implicated.[14] This scenario can be generalised to many carcinogens: job descriptions of those exposed may extend well beyond the workforce primarily engaged in handling the agent in question.

Chemicals proven to cause cancer (IARC Group 1) in those occupationally exposed cover a broad scope of substances (Table 1).

Table 1. Non-radioactive substances established as causing cancer in humans (IARC Group 1) and which are encountered in an occupational context.

4-Aminobiphenyl	Methylenebis(chloroaniline) (MOCA)
Asbestos	Mineral oils, untreated and mildly
Benzene	treated
Benzidine	Mustard gas
Benzo[*a*]pyrene	2-Naphthylamine
Beryllium	Nickel compounds
Bis(chloromethyl)ether	Shale-oils
1,3-Butadiene	Silica
Cadmium	Soots
Chromium[VI]	Strong-inorganic-acid mists containing
Coal-tar pitches	sulphuric acid
Coal-tars	Talc containing asbestiform fibres
Dyes metabolised to benzidine	2,3,7,8-Tetrachlorodibenzo-*para*-dioxin
Erionite	*ortho*-Toluidine
Ethylene oxide	Vinyl chloride
Formaldehyde	Wood dust
Gallium arsenide	

An additional number of specific substances are strongly implicated in the causation of cancer in the workplace as indicated by their IARC Group 2A categorisation. These include (but are not limited to) acrylonitrile, 1,3-butadiene, chlorinated toluenes, such as trichlorobenzene, ethylene dibromide, polychlorinated biphenyls, and trichloroethylene. Such substances are implicated by epidemiological investigations and cause cancer in experimental animals, though not necessarily at the same anatomical site as appears relevant to humans.[15] A much more numerous category of agents are those encountered in the course of particular industrial processes, but for which evidence of carcinogenicity is restricted to results in experimental animals. Typically, but not by definition, such agents are IARC Group 2B — possibly cause cancer in humans.[12]

2.2   Hazardous workplaces and occupations

The burden of occupational cancer cannot be fully addressed by reference to the carcinogenicity of specific substances. Account must also be taken of circumstances in which increased risk of cancer in the workplace is evident, although the corresponding specific causal agents are, at best, implicated, and at worst, unknown. This matter has been included in the *IARC Monograph* program by a series of evaluations involving particular 'exposures'. Group 1 exposures — that is, those situations in which increased incidence of cancer has been demonstrated unequivocally — include:

- aluminium production;
- boot and shoe manufacture and repair;
- chimney sweeping;
- coal gasification, coal-tar distillation and coke production;
- furniture and cabinet making;
- hematite mining;
- iron and steel founding;
- isopropyl alcohol manufacture;
- magenta production;
- painting; and
- rubber production.

Group 2A exposures, which indicates strongly suggestive, but not definitive evidence include petroleum refining, production of glass and pressed ware, work as a hairdresser or barber and work applying insecticides. In the absence of specific preventive measures, it is reasonable to presume that the corresponding occupational risks remain current. Thus, work as a painter continues to involve exposure to a range of organic solvents, chemical dyes and other materials. Apart from benzene, organic solvents generally have not been definitively established as carcinogenic for humans.[16] However, it is established that painters, as an occupational category, are at increased risk of lung cancer. Comparable evidence is less definitive in relation to those spraying or applying insecticides (apart from arsenical insecticides). There are many work situation in which it has proved difficult to single out the particular agents mediating carcinogenesis, despite evidence of increased risk of cancer associated with particular job descriptions.[17,18]

Though a primary consideration, it does not follow with certainty that increased risk of cancer in an occupational setting is attributable to a particular class of chemicals, or even to chemicals at all. Increased risk of lymphoma has been strongly associated with agricultural work in US studies. Data from Scandinavia clearly implicate chlorophenoxy compounds, but findings in relation to these specific agents, or in relation to unspecified agricultural chemicals, have been equivocal.[19,20] More generally, there are job categories associated with excess risk of one or more tumour types, which are not readily related to particular chemical exposures. Thus chemists or chemical workers are variously reported to be at increased risk for brain, breast, cervix, genitourinary, large intestine, lung, haematopoietic, ovary, skin or testis tumours, while there are also at least seven studies which fail to record any increased risk.[21] Such data implicate differences in work situations, despite a common job description. Possibly increased risk of breast cancer among teachers and nurses has been recorded in some studies, but such an outcome has not been consistently observed.[22,23] Work as a teacher or nurse does not involve industrial-level chemical exposures, but any consistent findings of increased risk would warrant scrutiny of particular duties.[24]

2.3 *Achieving prevention*

Means to prevent occupational cancer, in those situations where specific carcinogenic agents have been identified, are little short of self-evident. Exposure to workplace carcinogens mandates consideration of the following options:

- replace known carcinogens with non-carcinogens having identical or at least comparable chemical properties;
- modify production processes, such that hazardous compounds are not present;
- adopt closed systems to prevent workplace (and environmental) contamination; and
- alter relevant work practices.

Lastly, and only if other options prove impractical, workers should be equipped with personal protective equipment to reduce or eliminate the extent of their exposure. The extent to which any of these measures have been adopted, and are effective, varies markedly with the situation being addressed. Measures to prevent occupational cancer are usually mandated by regulation. The history of relevant legislation in UK has been reviewed by Alderson,[10] and by Bingham and Reid[25] in relation to practice in USA. Consequently, regulations are in place, particularly in developed countries, to prevent occupational exposure to recognised carcinogens. In general, the agents that are subject to regulation are determined by national statutory authorities, and corresponding regulation may also involve state or provincial levels of government.

Currently, there is widespread discussion of a proposed international ban on asbestos.[26] Such circumstances may well have to take account of differences between chrysotile (white asbestos) and the more bio-persistent needle-like amphiboles, including crocidolite (blue asbestos). At present there are extensive limitations, if not unequivocal bans, on the use of asbestos in many countries.

Replacement of carcinogenic agents may occur in the absence of unequivocal proof that cancer has arisen because of current practice. Short of bans, regulations may provide for maximal workplace concentrations of specific substances, including benzene and vinyl chloride. Thus the *IARC Monograph* on 1,3-butadiene includes eight-hour time-weighted average exposure levels for butadiene in various plants and production facilities, together with statutory exposure limits and guidelines, as are in force in 18 countries.[27]

Workers potentially exposed to carcinogens may be subject to surveillance procedures to assess their individual situations.[9] Personal monitors may be worn. Biological monitoring involves the measurement of particular chemicals or their metabolites in tissues or fluids, such as urine or blood.[28] Finally, in limited circumstances, clinical examination may be adopted in a screening context as a means of providing for earliest possible intervention in the event of cancer development.[9]

2.4 *The task is ongoing*

With regard to current studies, some newly investigated circumstances do not reveal increased risk. Thus in a study of bauxite miners, who are potentially exposed to silica (Group 1, IARC), there was little evidence of increased cancer incidence of mortality.[29] In terms of potential case numbers, transport workers exposed to engine emissions[30] may exemplify modern workers at risk of occupational cancer.

Occupational cancer is brought to the community's attention either in relation to the award of damages, or as background to the wider distribution of a carcinogen otherwise confined to the workplace. Expectations of a safe workplace are enshrined in legislation and regulatory machinery is available to address potentially carcinogenic exposures in the course of employment. The decades required from the time at which asbestos was demonstrated to be cause occupational cancer through to when the material was effectively banned, are a tragic testimony to inadequate urgency and the influence of vested interests. The brief outline of preventive measures (Sec. 2.3) is evidence of progress, but it is argued that the rate of progress is not adequate.[31]

3. Environmental Cancer: Prevention is Evolving

The phrase 'environmental cancer' is ambiguous, if not contentious.[32] Though arguably being relevant to the aetiology of all non-heritable malignant disease,[33] the term is usually identified with the disease attributable to pollution.[34] Taking a slightly broader perspective, the term 'environmental cancer' will be used here to mean non-heritable cancer which is not attributable to voluntary exposures or 'lifestyle choices'. The distinction between voluntary exposures and the impact of pollution may involve a degree of semantics: tobacco smoke is a voluntary exposure so far as the active smoker is concerned, but is an environmental pollutant for persons encountering 'second-hand smoke'.

By comparison with the workplace, demonstrating causation of cancer by environmental pollution and determining the proportion of malignant disease attributable to such exposure is inherently difficult. There are relatively few specific examples (Table 2). Of course, such a scenario does not necessarily indicate that cancer causation has not occurred. On the contrary, evidence of carcinogenicity for the agents involved clearly implicates the possibility of causation if exposure is known to occur.[35]

Prevention of environmental cancer generally involves reducing pollution.[2] Air may be polluted with polycyclic aromatic hydrocarbons, benzene or other carcinogens arising from industrial emissions, engine exhaust, tobacco smoke or other sources. Similarly, water may be polluted with arsenic, present in the soil due to mining or industrial waste. In many instances, action to reduce exposure to particular agents is justified, even if cancer causation under pre-existing circumstances cannot be shown. Overall, therefore, knowledge about environmental cancer offers clear opportunities to reduce the burden of malignant disease.

3.1 *General pollution*

3.1.1 *Air*

When unqualified, the term 'air pollution' is generally understood to indicate outdoor air pollution. Multiple studies have established

Table 2. Examples of environmental cancer.

Situation	Persons exposed	Carcinogen	Principal route(s) of exposure	Target organ (or tumour type)
Proven risk (involving exposure to recognised carcinogen in circumstance subject to epidemiological study)				
Residing near point sources of recognised carcinogens causing extreme local pollution	Relevant local populations	Asbestos Coke oven and iron foundry emissions Arsenic, cadmium and nickel compounds	Inhalation in all cases	Lung and other sites depending on pollutant
Passive smoking	Children and adults in smoker household; persons exposed as a consequence of smoking in the workplace and other environments	Tobacco smoke passively inhaled	Inhalation	Lung; some evidence regarding larynx and other sites

(Continued)

Table 2. (Continued)

Situation	Persons exposed	Carcinogen	Principal route(s) of exposure	Target organ (or tumour type)
Drinking water contamination from industrial sources of arsenic	Surrounding communities	Arsenic compounds	Ingestion	Urinary bladder and others
Residential exposure to radon	Occupants of particular houses	Radon	Inhalation and irradiation (Yes: studies involving home exposure indicate causality)	Lung

Likely risk (involving evidence of exposure to recognised or probable carcinogens)

Local atmospheric pollution from point sources of industrial emissions	Residents of particular local communities	Multiple, often unspecified, from petrochemical, steel and other industry	Inhalation	Lung
General atmospheric pollution (excluding tobacco smoke)	Whole population	Pollutants include — diesel exhaust — gasoline exhaust — sulphur dioxide	Inhalation	Lung

(Continued)

Table 2. (Continued)

Situation	Persons exposed	Carcinogen	Principal route(s) of exposure	Target organ (or tumour type)
Living near a properly-operating nuclear facility	Local community	Ionising radiation	Irradiation	Leukaemia, breast, thyroid
Asbestos in drinking water	Particular communities	Asbestos	Ingestion	Colo-rectum and possibly other sites

increased risk of lung cancer attributable to air pollution, with relative risks from cohort and case control studies typically being 1.3–1.7.[34] The data are consistent with fine particles ($PM_{2.5}$) being the most relevant indicator of atmospheric pollution. On this basis, the proportion of lung cancer in Europe attributable to air pollution is 10.7%, corresponding to 27,000 cases annually with three quarters of these being in men.[36] Characterisation of individual substances as accounting for cancer or health risks consequent upon air pollution is challenging. A study in Houston, Texas examined 179 candidate substances of which 12 were deemed to present a definite health risk, nine were considered probably responsible and 24 were deemed to present possible risks.[37] For lung cancer specifically, outdoor air pollutants of greatest concern are polycyclic hydrocarbons, acetaldehyde, and 1,3-butadiene.[38]

In the 1990s, Eastern Europe provided some of the highest recorded levels of air pollution. More recently, air pollution in cities in developing countries such as China and India has been implicated as contributing to the burden of lung cancer.[39] All such studies are complicated by the extent to which active smoking accounts for the burden of lung cancer.[40]

Indoor air pollution specifically includes environmental tobacco smoke, for which over 50 epidemiological studies are available. The data typically indicate relative risks for lung cancer of 1.22 in women and 1.36 in men as a consequence of spousal smoking, the respective figures being 1.15 and 1.28 as a consequence of workplace exposure.[41] More generally, substances responsible for indoor pollution in developed countries include chloroform, formaldehyde and naphthalene.[38] However, the burden of cancer attributable to indoor air pollution is greatest in developing countries, where the problem largely centres on ventilation (or lack of it) for various types of cooking.[42]

3.1.2 *Water*

The most important carcinogenic water pollutant is arsenic. There is unequivocal evidence for causation of urinary bladder, lung and skin cancer by arsenic in drinking water. Any potential confounding effect of smoking in relation to lung cancer has been excluded in studies from Taiwan and Chile.[43]

The possibility that chlorination of water may result in carcinogenic by-products is under active investigation.[44] That consideration acknowledged, it must be stated that the benefits of disinfection of water by chemical methods, are irrefutable. Any major change to this practice would need to be evaluated fully, not only with regard to the need to maintain microbiological safety, but also with regard to the possible long-term adverse effects of alternatives to chlorination.

As many as 500 chlorination by-products have been identified, including trihalomethanes and halogenated acids and aldehydes, some of which are carcinogenic to experimental animals. Only a small fraction of the chlorination by-products that have been identified in drinking water have been tested for carcinogenicity. None of the disinfectant by-products can be considered individually as the plausible causes for cancers observed in human studies.[45]

Drinking chlorinated water has been reported to be associated with the development of some cancer. Evaluating chlorinated drinking water as a carcinogenic hazard in 1991,[46] IARC noted that available studies showed moderately consistent correlation between consumption of chlorinated water and cancers of the stomach, colon, rectum, urinary bladder and lung, with the most consistent findings concerning cancer of the urinary bladder. Nonetheless, it was found that there was inadequate evidence for the carcinogenicity of chlorinated drinking water (IARC Group 3). When the potency of the chlorination by-products that have been tested for carcinogenicity is viewed in the context of their concentrations in drinking water, these are at least three orders of magnitude too low to account for the risk implied.

3.2   Localised pollution

3.2.1   Spatial aggregation studies

In many instances, spatial analysis of cancer aggregation has suggested hypotheses concerning causation, exemplified by the association between bladder cancer and US counties with chemical industry.[47] More recent studies have focused on the association of agricultural chemicals with childhood cancer[48] or breast cancer, the latter being studied both in the US[49,50] and the UK.[51] Understanding that broad classes of pesticides may be characterised as xenoestrogens[52] underpins a broad spectrum of investigation concerning possible causation of breast cancer by pesticides. It may be indicative of the limitation of power of epidemiological investigations generally that the causative implications of the various scenarios mentioned have not been established.

Once particular spatial aggregations of cancer are demonstrated, secondary studies to elucidate causes may be initiated. Perhaps the most extensive study of environmental influences on risk of such cancer has involved investigation of the relatively increased incidence of breast cancer among residents of Long Island.[50] More than ten projects were designed to establish the possible causes. Primary focus involved organochloride pesticides, because laboratory animals exposed to these agents develop mammary tumours. However, there was no association between breast cancer risk and breast tissue levels of DDT, PCBs and related compounds. Generally, there was no evidence that environmental exposures were responsible for the increased risk of disease.[49] A possible relationship between pesticide usage and childhood cancer has yet to be excluded.[48]

3.2.2 Point sources

A conspicuous subset of situations involving the impact of environmental carcinogens are those in which the exposure concerned is confined to a specific geographical location. Foremost in this category are cancers consequent upon the explosion of nuclear bombs in Nagasaki and Hiroshima.[53] Nagasaki and Hiroshima have principally involved causation of leukaemia and breast cancer; failure of the nuclear reactor at Chernobyl in the Ukraine caused increased incidence of thyroid cancer.[54]

The immediate chemical counterparts to the scenarios involving extreme exposure to ionizing radiation include Seveso in Italy, where an industrial accident resulted in massive community exposure to 2,3,7,8-tetrachlorodibenzo-p-dioxin (TCDD, also referred to as 'dioxin') to the extent that chloracne was observed. The health of those exposed has been extensively monitored. The most recent report documents follow-up of 276,108 exposed persons, divided between zones corresponding to very high (A), high (B) and low (R) exposure. Results confirmed previous findings of excesses of lymphatic and hematopoietic tissue neoplasms, with a rate ratio of 2.23 (six deaths) in zone A and of 1.59 (28 deaths) in zone B. There were no soft-tissue sarcomas and no excess of breast or gynaecological cancer.[55]

Localised pollution by certain carcinogens emanating from industrial sites at which the material is used or generated as a by-product is associated with increased incidence of cancer in the local community. Obviously, confidence in a causal relationship is vastly increased if the tumour type evident in the community is known to be caused by the agent in question, usually by dint of increased risk of disease amongst the relevant workforce. Increased incidence of mesothelioma in a community located near to an asbestos mining or milling site[56] is a clear example. Cause-effect is readily established, since 90% of mesothelioma cases amongst men may be shown to involve exposure to asbestos. Increased risk of lung cancer is evident in communities surrounding iron founding and metal smelting.[57] The atmospheric pollutants are known to include polycyclic aromatic hydrocarbons, as well as compounds of chromium and nickel which cause lung cancer in smelter workers. In relation to water pollution, mention has been made of industrial sources of arsenic in groundwater (see Sec. 3.1.2).

For many other point sources of pollution, causation of increased cancer in the local community appears a reasonable likelihood, but is difficult to demonstrate.[58] The most extensively investigated point sources of potential or demonstrable carcinogen exposure have been toxic waste dumps, particularly in US.[59] Such sources of pollution have rarely, if ever, been demonstrated to be associated with increased risk of malignant disease. Environmental sources of TCDD are known to include incinerators, but efforts to demonstrate increased incidence of cancer attributable to incinerator emissions have proved elusive.[60] In UK, in communities around vinyl chloride polymerisation plants, no evidence could be found of angiosarcoma cases attributable to environmental, as distinct from occupational, exposure.[61]

3.3 *Keeping pace with community expectations*

Community dissatisfaction is probably underpinned by naïve perceptions of cause and effect in relation to cancer aetiology. Dissatisfaction might also be expressed by the medico-scientific community because knowledge does not evolve as might be anticipated. Consider the causation of breast cancer by industrial chemicals. Mechanisms by which xenoestrogens could cause breast cancer are evident[62] and, more generally, over 200 substances have been identified as causing mammary tumours in rodents.[63] Yet no industrial pollutant has been definitively identified as causing human breast cancer. The available data do not allow specification of related measures to reduce pollution as being known to reduce the burden of breast cancer. Hopefully, measures predicated on reducing exposure to toxins generally will have such an effect. Community expectations may be met in this fashion.

4. Consumer Products: Prevention in Specific Instances

4.1 *Diverse findings*

Historically, food additives were listed by Doll and Peto in 1981[4] as accounting for up to 1% of cancer in the United States. Since that time, additional positive evidence of this particular risk has not been forthcoming. There are almost no studies which purport to directly assess the carcinogenic risk of food additives generally, and the matter is rarely reviewed. Amongst additives, colouring agents are probably the most intensively investigated, but no particular agents or class of compound has emerged as being of greatest concern. It has long been recognised that nitrite, added to meat and some other foods as a preservative, may contribute to the formation of nitroso compounds. Dietary exposure to nitrate and nitrite is complex, and the use of nitrite as a preservative is subject to regulation.[64] Apart from this, at least in developed countries, there is no evidence of dietary contamination by potent carcinogens, specifically as a consequence of the use of permitted colouring, preservative or flavouring agents. Artificial sweeteners have long been subject to inquiry, but available evidence suggests an absence of risk.[65] Likewise, consumption of coffee is more often reported in relation to reduced risk of cancer than in any other context.[66] Definitive evidence in relation to the possible contamination of deep-fried food by acrylamide is yet to become available, but changes have been made to relevant food processing to reduce, or eliminate, this contaminant.

Hair dyes and pesticides exemplify the principle that those employed to manufacture or apply products which the broader community may encounter as consumers are exposed to higher concentrations of the respective agents than those who use them in a consumer context. Thus risk of cancer consequent upon work as a hairdresser was recently re-evaluated by IARC and confirmed as Group 2A (probably carcinogenic for humans) while personal use of hair colourants is Group 3, the category of 'cannot be evaluated as to its carcinogenicity' indicating that data which are available fail to establish that the agent possibly causes cancer in humans. Aromatic diamines shown to cause cancer in experimental animals were phased out as components in semi-permanent hair dyes in the 1980s.[67] Similarly, though it has not been possible to indicate unequivocally which agents account for risk, pesticide applicators are subject to increased risk of some cancers; no such generalisation can be made concerning people living in houses that have been sprayed.

The precautionary principle[68] is central to consumer protection from environmental carcinogens, particularly if a relevant exposure is demonstrated unequivocally. At perhaps the most unequivocal end of the spectrum, the flame retardant tris (2,3-dibromopropyl) phospate was found to be carcinogenic in rats and mice, and could be recovered from urine when it was used as a flame retardant for children's sleepwear. Such use of the compound was banned under many jurisdictions. At the other extreme, evidence that mobile (cell) phones cause cancer is far from definitive, inference of a hazard being most readily made from the association between electromagnetic fields from overhead powerlines and risk of childhood leukaemia.[69] Requirements to shield phone users and recommendations concerning usage of these phones have been widely adopted.

4.2 *Community expectations*

The community expects consumer products to be 'safe', a characterisation which whatever its ramifications, certainly includes the assurance that any inherent risk of cancer causation has been excluded. Obviously, consumer products in this context do not include smoking materials and alcoholic beverages. For everything else, and in relation to cancer specifically, the most important consideration is not some agreement between the community and those in authority as to what constitutes 'safe'. The most important consideration is that, in contrast to occupational and environmental cancer, various classes of consumer products subject to investigation have not proven to be hazardous to those who purchase and use them. As indicated in Sec. 4.1 above, there is no recognised burden of cancer attributable to consumer products so defined. To that extent, the community's expectations have been met.

5. Cancer Clusters: Prevention Impossible

Clusters of infectious disease have long provided insight regarding causation, and monitoring outbreaks of food poisoning or other infectious disease continues to be a vital and effective aspect of public health. Cancer clusters are markedly different from infectious disease clusters.

Cancer clusters are defined by a perceived greater-than-expected incidences of cancer involving a particular geographical region, which is reported to health authorities.[70] A very small proportion of cancer clusters are documented in the peer-reviewed medico-scientific literature.[71] Typically, cancer clusters are reported to authorities with reference to specific individual instances of disease, with case numbers involving less than 15 persons. Though it is intuitively appealing to view cluster reports as the opportunity to reveal otherwise unknown carcinogens, or the impact of known carcinogens in a novel exposure context, such circumstances have rarely been reported.

Cancer cluster investigations may be distinguished from various aspects of cancer epidemiology. Only in commentaries on cancer clusters are vinyl chloride, asbestos and/or diethyl stilboestrol identified as substances whose carcinogenicity was established due to the occurrence of clusters, and their investigation.[72] Discovery of carcinogenicity for these agents did not involve cluster reports; the relevant publications were case reports, there being no contemporary perception of increased incidence of cancer by the community or group at risk. Spatial aggregations of cancer are revealed in the context of systematic monitoring of the variation of cancer incidence according to county or local government area.[73] Areas exhibiting higher than national or other relevant average incidence are not cancer clusters as defined above (see Sec. 3.2.1). Once reports of cancer clusters are distinguished from case reports and those involving spatial aggregation,[74] it is evident that cluster investigations have never revealed a previously unknown carcinogen.

Cancer clusters cause community concern and anxiety. Most are investigated with reference to whether greater-than-expected incidence of cancer has occurred.[75] Generally, this procedure is flawed as a result of the populations being defined *a posteriori*, an incongruity often explained by reference to 'the Texas sharpshooter'.[76] Nonetheless, estimates of the degree to which clusters of cancer cases exceed what is expected underpin cluster investigation procedures. Explanations for cancer clusters are also considered in the context of cluster investigations. For the benefit of those at apparent risk, such investigations are usefully extended beyond exposure to agents which might account for the cluster, to include all agents which cause concern to those affected.[77] A specific goal of cancer cluster investigations is to provide assurances to those perceived to be at risk to the effect that circumstances causing cancer are not known to occur or to persist in a particular environment.

When it comes to community expectations, there is clear evidence via the media that cluster investigations have not lived up to the hope that was vested in the reporting process. In respect of every cluster, the hope is that a novel or unexpected carcinogenic influence might be revealed, with obvious benefits to the local group experiencing anxiety and people in similar circumstances elsewhere. In this regard, the community has it wrong. Exempting major disasters such as Hiroshima or Seveso, which immediately attract investigation, there is no recorded instance of a cluster investigation which resulted in the discovery of novel causation. In short, in relation to cancer clusters, community expectations are not being met because the expectations are misplaced.

6. Conclusion

Cancer is properly described as an environmental disease when the term 'environmental' is understood to include all non-heritable risk factors. The burden of disease attributable to risk factors arising from lifestyle choices is large by comparison to that arising from involuntary exposures: those exposures that people encounter either in the workplace, in the home or further afield and over which they have no direct control. These exposures, however, may variously account for cancer that is preventable. The community is entitled to demand continuing vigilance in relation to cancer causation by involuntary exposures, and, when appropriate, effective action to reduce or eliminate risk.

References

1. J. M. Martin-Moreno, I. Soerjomataram and G. Magnusson, Cancer causes and prevention: A condensed appraisal in Europe in 2008, *Eur. J. Cancer* **44**: 1390–1403 (2008).
2. *World Cancer Report* (IARC Press, Lyon, 2003).
3. P. Boffetta and M. Kogevinas, Occupational cancer in Europe, *Environ. Health Perspect.* **107**(Suppl. 2): 227 (1999).
4. R. Doll and R. Peto, The causes of cancer: Quantitative estimates of avoidable risks of cancer in the United States today, *J. Natl. Cancer Inst.* **66**: 1192–1308 (1981).
5. *Quantification of Occupational Cancer, Banbury Report 9* (Cold Spring Harbor Laboratory Press, Cold Spring Harbor, 1981).
6. L. Fritschi and T. Driscoll, Cancer due to occupation in Australia, *Aust. N. Z. J. Public Health* **30**: 213–219 (2006).
7. G. Danaei, H. S. Vander, A. D. Lopez, C. J. Murray and M. Ezzati, Causes of cancer in the world: Comparative risk assessment of nine behavioural and environmental risk factors, *Lancet* **366**: 1784–1793 (2005).

8. *Occupational Cancers in Developing Countries, IARC Scientific Publications No. 129* (International Agency for Research on Cancer, Lyon, 1994).

9. AFOM Working Party on Occupational Cancer, *Occupational Cancer. A Guide to Prevention, Assessment and Investigation* (The Australasian Faculty of Occupational Medicine, Sydney, 2003).

10. M. Alderson, *Occupational Cancer* (Butterworths, London, 1986).

11. IARC, *IARC Monographs on the Evaluation of Carcinogenic Risks to Humans*, International Agency for Research on Cancer. Available at monographs.iarc.fr/ (accessed August 2008).

12. J. Siemiatycki, L. Richardson, K. Straif, B. Latreille, R. Lakhani, S. Campbell, M. C. Rousseau and P. Boffetta, Listing occupational carcinogens, *Environ. Health Perspect.* **112**: 1447–1459 (2004).

13. J. Peto, A. Decarli, C. La Vecchia, F. Levi and E. Negri, The European mesothelioma epidemic, *Br. J. Cancer* **79**: 666–672 (1999).

14. O. Wong, Malignant mesothelioma and asbestos exposure among auto mechanics: Appraisal of scientific evidence, *Regul. Toxicol. Pharmacol.* **34**: 170–177 (2001).

15. Y. Yoshida, M. Tatematsu, K. Takaba, S. Iwasaki and N. Ito, Target organ specificity of cell proliferation induced by various carcinogens, *Toxicol. Pathol.* **21**: 436–442 (1993).

16. E. Lynge, A. Anttila and K. Hemminki, Organic solvents and cancer, *Cancer Causes Control* **8**: 406–419 (1997).

17. M. C. Alavanja, M. Dosemeci, C. Samanic, J. Lubin, C. F. Lynch, C. Knott, J. Barker, J. A. Hoppin, D. P. Sandler, J. Coble, K. Thomas and A. Blair, Pesticides and lung cancer risk in the agricultural health study cohort, *Am. J. Epidemiol.* **160**: 876–885 (2004).

18. J. Dich, S. H. Zahm, A. Hanberg and H. O. Adami, Pesticides and cancer, *Cancer Causes Control* **8**: 420–443 (1997).

19. N. Pearce and D. McLean, Agricultural exposures and non-Hodgkin's lymphoma, *Scand. J. Work Environ. Health* **31**(Suppl. 1): 18–25 (2005).

20. J. C. Schroeder, A. F. Olshan, R. Baric, G. A. Dent, C. R. Weinberg, B. Yount, J. R. Cerhan, C. F. Lynch, L. M. Schuman, P. E. Tolbert, N. Rothman, K. P. Cantor and A. Blair, Agricultural risk factors for t(14;18) subtypes of non-Hodgkin's lymphoma, *Epidemiology* **12**: 701–709 (2001).

21. R. R. Monson, Occupation. In: *Cancer Epidemiology and Prevention*, eds. D. Schottenfeld and J. F. Fraumeni (Oxford University Press, New York, 1996), pp. 373–405.

22. S. A. Petralia, J. E. Vena, J. L. Freudenheim, A. Michalek, M. S. Goldberg, A. Blair, J. Brasure and S. Graham, Risk of premenopausal breast cancer and patterns of established breast cancer risk factors among teachers and nurses, *Am. J. Ind. Med.* **35**: 137–141 (1999).

23. E. E. Calle, T. K. Murphy, C. Rodriguez, M. J. Thun and C. W. Heath Jr., Occupation and breast cancer mortality in a prospective cohort of US women, *Am. J. Epidemiol* **148**: 191–197 (1998).

24. H. K. Gunnarsdottir, T. Aspelund, T. Karlsson and V. Rafnsson, Occupational risk factors for breast cancer among nurses, *Int. J. Occup. Environ. Health* **3**: 254–258 (1997).

25. E. Bingham and J. Reid, Prevention and regulation approaches to carcinogens. In: *Molecular Carcinogenesis and the Molecular biology of Human Cancer*, eds. D. Warshawsky and J. R. Landolph (Taylor & Francis, Boca Raton, 2006), pp. 547–558.

26. M. Camus, A ban on asbestos must be based on a comparative risk assessment, *Can. Med. Assoc. J.* **164**: 491–494 (2001).

27. IARC, 1,3-Butadiene. In: *IARC Monographs on the Evaluation of Carcinogenic Risks to Humans, Vol. 71, Re-evaluation of some Organic Chemicals, Hydrazine and Hydrogen Peroxide* (International Agency for Research on Cancer, Lyon, 1999), pp. 109–225.

28. D. Cavallo, C. L. Ursini, B. Perniconi, A. D. Francesco, M. Giglio, F. M. Rubino, A. Marinaccio and S. Iavicoli, Evaluation of genotoxic effects induced by exposure to antineoplastic drugs in lymphocytes and exfoliated buccal cells of oncology nurses and pharmacy employees, *Mutat. Res.* **587**: 45–51 (2005).

29. L. Fritschi, J. L. Hoving, M. R. Sim, A. Del Monaco, E. MacFarlane, D. McKenzie, G. Benke and N. de Klerk, All cause mortality and incidence of cancer in workers in bauxite mines and alumina refineries, *Int. J. Cancer* **123**: 882–887 (2008).

30. F. Laden, J. E. Hart, A. Eschenroeder, T. J. Smith and E. Garshick, Historical estimation of diesel exhaust exposure in a cohort study of U.S. railroad workers and lung cancer, *Cancer Causes Control* **17**: 911–919 (2006).

31. R. O'Neill, S. Pickvance and A. Watterson, Burying the evidence: How Great Britain is prolonging the occupational cancer epidemic, *Int. J. Occup. Environ. Health* **13**: 428–436 (2007).

32. P. Boffetta, J. K. McLaughlin, C. La Vecchia, P. Autier and P. Boyle, 'Environment' in cancer causation and etiological fraction: Limitations and ambiguities, *Carcinogenesis* **28**: 913–915 (2007).

33. G. N. Wogan, S. S. Hecht, J. S. Felton, A. H. Conney and L. A. Loeb, Environmental and chemical carcinogenesis, *Semin. Cancer Biol.* **14**: 473–486 (2004).

34. P. Boffetta, Human cancer from environmental pollutants: The epidemiological evidence, *Mutat. Res.* **608**: 157–162 (2006).

35. D. Belpomme, P. Irigaray, L. Hardell, R. Clapp, L. Montagnier, S. Epstein and A. J. Sasco, The multitude and diversity of environmental carcinogens, *Environ. Res.* **105**: 414–429 (2007).

36. P. Vineis, G. Hoek, M. Krzyzanowski, F. Vigna-Taglianti, F. Veglia, L. Airoldi, H. Autrup, A. Dunning, S. Garte, P. Hainaut, C. Malaveille *et al.*, Air pollution and risk of lung cancer in a prospective study in Europe, *Int. J. Cancer* **119**: 169–174 (2006).

37. K. Sexton, S. H. Linder, D. Marko, H. Bethel and P. J. Lupo, Comparative assessment of air pollution-related health risks in Houston, *Environ. Health Perspect.* **115**: 1388–1393 (2007).

38. M. M. Loh, J. I. Levy, J. D. Spengler, E. A. Houseman and D. H. Bennett, Ranking cancer risks of organic hazardous air pollutants in the United States, *Environ. Health Perspect.* **115**: 1160–1168 (2007).

39. H. Ishikawa, Y. Tian, F. Piao, Z. Duan, Y. Zhang, M. Ma, H. Li, H. Yamamoto, Y. Matsumoto, S. Sakai, J. Cui, T. Yamauchi and K. Yokoyama, Genotoxic damage in female residents exposed to environmental air pollution in Shenyang city, China, *Cancer Lett.* **240**: 29–35 (2006).

40. F. Chen, P. Cole and W. F. Bina, Time trend and geographic patterns of lung adenocarcinoma in the United States, 1973–2002, *Cancer Epidemiol. Biomarkers Prev.* **16**: 2724–2729 (2007).

41. IARC, *IARC Monographs on the Evaluation of Carcinogenic Risks to Humans, Vol. 83. Tobacco Smoke and Involuntary Smoking* (International Agency for Research on Cancer, Lyon, 2004).

42. N. Bruce, R. Perez-Padilla and R. Albalak, Indoor air pollution in developing countries: A major environmental and public health challenge, *Bull. World Health Organ.* **78**: 1078–1092 (2000).

43. S. Tapio and B. Grosche, Arsenic in the aetiology of cancer, *Mutat. Res.* **612**: 215–246 (2006).

44. C. M. Villanueva, K. P. Cantor, J. O. Grimalt, N. Malats, D. Silverman, A. Tardon, R. Garcia-Closas, C. Serra, A. Carrato, G. Castano-Vinyals, R. Marcos, N. Rothman, F. X. Real, M. Dosemeci and M. Kogevinas, Bladder cancer and exposure to water disinfection by-products

through ingestion, bathing, showering, and swimming in pools, *Am. J. Epidemiol.* **165**: 148–156 (2007).

45. IARC, *IARC Monographs on the Evaluation of Carcinogenic Risks to Humans, Vol. 84. Some Drinking-Water Disinfectants and Contaminants, Including Arsenic* (International Agency for Research on Cancer, Lyon, 2004).

46. IARC, Chlorinated drinking water. In: *IARC Monographs on the Evaluation of Carcinogenic Risks to Humans*, Vol. 52 (International Agency for Research on Cancer, Lyon, 2008), pp. 45–141.

47. R. Hoover and J. F. Fraumeni Jr., Cancer mortality in U.S. counties with chemical industries, *Environ. Res.* **9**: 196–207 (1975).

48. S. E. Carozza, B. Li, K. Elgethun and R. Whitworth, Risk of childhood cancers associated with residence in agriculturally intense areas in the United States, *Environ. Health Perspect.* **116**: 559–565 (2008).

49. D. M. Winn, The Long Island Breast Cancer Study Project, *Nature Rev. Cancer* **5**: 986–994 (2005).

50. M. D. Gammon, A. I. Neugut, R. M. Santella, S. L. Teitelbaum, J. A. Britton *et al.*, The Long Island Breast Cancer Study Project: Description of a multi-institutional collaboration to identify environmental risk factors for breast cancer, *Breast Cancer Res. Treat.* **74**: 235–254 (2002).

51. K. Muir, S. Rattanamongkolgul, M. Smallman-Raynor, M. Thomas, S. Downer and C. Jenkinson, Breast cancer incidence and its possible spatial association with pesticide application in two counties of England, *Public Health* **118**: 513–520 (2004).

52. S. Safe and S. Papineni, The role of xenoestrogenic compounds in the development of breast cancer, *Trends Pharmacol. Sci.* **27**: 447–454 (2006).

53. D. A. Pierce and M. Vaeth, The shape of the cancer mortality dose-response curve for the A-bomb survivors, *Radiat. Res.* **126**: 36–42 (1991).

54. P. Jacob, T. I. Bogdanova, E. Buglova, M. Chepurniy, Y. Demidchik, Y. Gavrilin, J. Kenigsberg, R. Meckbach, C. Schotola, S. Shinkarev, M. D. Tronko, A. Ulanovsky, S. Vavilov and L. Walsh, Thyroid cancer risk in areas of Ukraine and Belarus affected by the Chernobyl accident, *Radiat. Res.* **165**: 1–8 (2006).

55. D. Consonni, A. C. Pesatori, C. Zocchetti, R. Sindaco, L. C. D'Oro, M. Rubagotti and P. A. Bertazzi, Mortality in a population exposed

to dioxin after the Seveso, Italy, accident in 1976: 25 years of follow-up, *Am. J. Epidemiol.* **167**: 847–858 (2008).

56. A. Reid, J. Heyworth, N. H. de Klerk and B. Musk, Cancer incidence among women and girls environmentally and occupationally exposed to blue asbestos at Wittenoom, Western Australia, *Int. J. Cancer* **122**: 2337–2344 (2008).

57. V. E. Archer, Air pollution and fatal lung disease in three Utah counties, *Arch. Environ. Health* **45**: 325–334 (1990).

58. A. Kibble and R. Harrison, Point sources of air pollution, *Occup. Med. (Lond.)* **55**: 425–431 (2005).

59. M. Vrijheid, Health effects of residence near hazardous waste landfill sites: A review of the epidemiologic literature, *Environ. Health Perspect.* **108**(Suppl. 1): 101–112 (2000).

60. R. J. Roberts and M. Chen, Waste incineration — How big is the health risk? A quantitative method to allow comparison with other health risks, *J. Public Health* **28**: 261–266 (2006).

61. P. Elliott and I. Kleinschmidt, Angiosarcoma of the liver in Great Britain in proximity to vinyl chloride sites, *Occup. Environ. Med.* **54**: 14–18 (1997).

62. L. S. Birnbaum and S. E. Fenton, Cancer and developmental exposure to endocrine disruptors, *Environ. Health Perspect.* **111**: 389–394 (2003).

63. R. A. Rudel, K. R. Attfield, J. N. Schifano and J. G. Brody, Chemicals causing mammary gland tumors in animals signal new directions for epidemiology, chemicals testing, and risk assessment for breast cancer prevention, *Cancer* **109**: 2635–2666 (2007).

64. Y. Grosse, R. Baan, K. Straif, B. Secretan, F. El Ghissassi and V. Cogliano, Carcinogenicity of nitrate, nitrite, and cyanobacterial peptide toxins, *Lancet Oncol.* **7**: 628–629 (2006).

65. S. Gallus, L. Scotti, E. Negri, R. Talamini, S. Franceschi, M. Montella, A. Giacosa, L. Dal Maso and C. La Vecchia, Artificial sweeteners and cancer risk in a network of case-control studies, *Ann. Oncol.* **18**(1): 40–44 (2006).

66. S. C. Larsson, E. Giovannucci and A. Wolk, Coffee consumption and stomach cancer risk in a cohort of Swedish women, *Int. J. Cancer* **119**: 2186–2189 (2006).

67. H. M. Bolt and K. Golka, The debate on carcinogenicity of permanent hair dyes: New insights, *Crit. Rev. Toxicol.* **37**: 521–536 (2007).

68. P. Grandjean, Implications of the precautionary principle for primary prevention and research, *Annu. Rev. Public Health* **25**: 199–223 (2004).

69. G. Draper, T. Vincent, M. E. Kroll and J. Swanson, Childhood cancer in relation to distance from high voltage power lines in England and Wales: A case-control study, *Br. Med. J.* **330**: 1290 (2005).
70. Centers for Disease Control and Prevention, Guidelines for investigating clusters of health events, *Morbidity and Mortality Weekly Report* **39**: 1–23 (1990).
71. C. W. Trumbo, Public requests for cancer cluster investigations: A survey of state health departments, *Am. J. Public Health* **90**: 1300–1302 (2000).
72. M. J. Thun and T. Sinks, Understanding cancer clusters, *CA Cancer J. Clin.* **54**: 273–280 (2004).
73. M. Kulldorff, E. J. Feuer, B. A. Miller and L. S. Freedman, Breast cancer clusters in the Northeast United States: A geographic analysis, *Am. J. Epidemiol.* **146**: 161–170 (1997).
74. A. D. Langmuir, Formal discussion of epidemiology of cancer: Spatial-temporal aggregation, *Cancer Res.* **25**: 1384–1386 (1965).
75. B. S. Kingsley, K. L. Schmeichel and C. H. Rubin, An update on cancer cluster activities at the Centers for Disease Control and Prevention, *Environ. Health Perspect.* **115**: 165–171 (2007).
76. K. J. Rothman, A sobering start for the cluster busters' conference, *Am. J. Epidemiol.* **132**: S6–13 (1990).
77. B. W. Stewart, "There will be no more!": The legacy of the Toowong breast cancer cluster, *Med. J. Aust.* **187**: 178–180 (2007).

7

Diagnostic Dilemmas During and After Chemotherapy Treatment

Ian N. Olver

Abstract

The symptoms of cancer or its recurrence must be distinguished from the early and late side effects of anti-cancer treatment, other drugs, or unrelated concomitant illnesses. Symptoms of cancer may be directly due to the effects of the primary tumour or its metastases on surrounding tissue, or the manifestations of paraneoplastic syndromes, which are distant effects often mediated by hormones or cytokines, but not directly due to the local effect of tumour. Systemic symptoms of cancer include weight loss, fatigue, pruritus and fever and sweats, which must be distinguished from unrelated illnesses. Organ-specific cancers cause symptoms either due to the mass effect, such as tumour blockage of hollow passages like the airways, gastrointestinal tract or urogenital tract, or cause organ dysfunction, as may occur in the liver or lungs. Pain may occur with nerve compression, blockage of hollow organs, or the stretching of organ capsules, as occurs in the liver.

The side effects of chemotherapy are part of the differential diagnosis of symptoms which could mimic those of conditions unrelated to the cancer. Examples include emesis, infection, anaemia, or cumulative organ toxicities. Some toxicities manifest themselves very late after the treatment, such as second cancers and sterility.

Keywords: Cancer, chemotherapy, symptoms, side effects, paraneoplastic syndrome.

1. Introduction

This chapter could have been subtitled, "Patients with cancer can develop acute appendicitis too". With all of the emphasis on the local and generalised symptoms of a patient's cancer or its recurrence and the acute and late effects of the treatments, unrelated illnesses as a cause of symptoms can be overlooked. Patients can acquire acute illnesses, such as influenza, to which they may be prone when it appears in a community, or indeed they may develop acute appendicitis. They may have other common chronic conditions, such as heart disease or endocrine diseases and in addition are often prescribed multiple drugs, which may have side effects or interact with each other.

Case 1

A patient with small cell lung cancer with painful liver metastases is mid-cycle after his fourth cycle of chemotherapy. He develops drowsiness, confusion, is nauseated and complains of abdominal pains and constipation and is dehydrated, which he experiences as a dry mouth.

What is the differential diagnosis? He could have progressive disease despite the chemotherapy and have developed cerebral metastases, which would explain the confusion. Alternatively he may have become febrile when he was neutropenic at mid-cycle as a side effect of chemotherapy, which could explain the drowsiness, confusion and dehydration. If he was taking opiate analgesia for the pain from his liver metastases, the drowsiness, confusion and dry mouth can be explained as side effects of that medication. However, the case was written with a symptom complex that was a "full hand" for hypercalcaemia. How could this be explained? The man may have progressive disease and have developed bone metastases, which could result in hypercalcaemia. If the underlying cancer was a non-small cell lung cancer, hypercalcaemia could be a paraneoplastic manifestation, but this is one of the paraneoplastic effects not seen with small cell lung cancer. Therefore, he could have hyperparathyroidism as a concomitant illness and consulting an endocrinologist may be helpful.

The case illustrates the importance of knowing about the likely symptoms of the cancer and the acute and late side effects of treatment, which become part of the differential diagnosis of a new symptom. If they can be excluded, then other conditions unrelated to cancer can be considered. However, this is complicated by the fact that some of the symptoms of cancer are paraneoplastic syndromes, which are symptoms due to the presence of cancer, but are not caused by the local pressure of the cancer or its metastases. Instead they are due to hormones secreted by the tumour, or an immune response to the tumour, and are diagnoses of exclusion.[1]

Late effects describe problems which occur months or years after diagnosis and will depend on the site and extent of the primary cancer and the intensity and nature of the initial treatment.[2] Although often focussing upon physical symptoms, late effects do include psychosocial problems, and in a broad sense, economic, insurance and employment issues after surviving cancer as well.

2. The Symptoms of Cancer or Its Recurrence After Therapy

When making a differential diagnosis from presenting symptoms, the main characteristic of a cancer related symptom is persistence. For example, respiratory infections causing cough and dyspnoea will resolve over time, but if the same symptoms are due to an underlying cancer, they will persist and worsen over weeks or months. Back pain due to an injury will wax and wane, but if due to bone metastases will progressively worsen and may be exacerbated by other causes of pain if the tumour presses on surrounding nerves. Persistence will be a feature of either the presentation of a primary cancer, or relapse after treatment, and cancer will probably be the first of the differential diagnosis of a new symptom which needs to be excluded.

The symptoms of cancer can be general, including the paraneoplastic syndromes, or localised and organ-specific. It is important to note that cancers can present without symptoms and simply be detected on scans performed for other reasons. This will occur if the tumour exerts no pressure on a hollow viscous, or arises deep in the parenchyma of an organ like the liver, well away from stretching the nerve-rich capsule and causing pain.

2.1 *General and paraneoplastic symptoms*

The most common general symptoms are weight loss, fatigue and sweats and fevers. Paraneoplastic manifestations can be associated with any organ system, and are commonly of hormonal, neurological, haematological, renal, or dermatological nature, or occur in supportive tissues as in hypertrophic pulmonary osteoarthropathy.[3–7] Endocrinologic paraneoplastic symptoms, for example, can mimic Cushing's syndrome, hyperparathyroidism, or a syndrome of inappropriate anti-diuretic hormone secretion and need to be distinguished from them.[8]

2.2 *Weight loss*

Weight loss in cancer is not simply due to starvation, because of decreased appetite or gastrointestinal obstruction. Cancer cachexia is due to the tumour itself and mediated by cytokines such as tumour necrosis factor alpha (TNFα) and inflammatory mediators causing weight loss, particularly loss of lean body mass.[9] This paraneoplastic syndrome is a diagnosis of exclusion after other causes, including infectious diseases and eating disorders have been excluded.

2.3 *Fatigue*

Fatigue is a very common symptom of cancer and has many causes.[10] Patients describe fatigue as encompassing decreased energy levels, tiredness and the need to sleep during the day and even weakness. It can be associated with anaemia or depression or lost sleep at night, often due to other symptoms of cancer such as poorly controlled pain. As well as medication directed at associated conditions, exercise is helpful in abrogating this symptom.[11]

2.4 Fever and sweats

Fever associated with cancer can be due to infections, drug reactions, blood transfusions, hormonal changes, or graft versus host disease after bone marrow or stem cell transplantation. As a diagnosis of exclusion, the tumour can cause unexplained fever. Fever and sweats are symptoms most commonly identified with Hodgkin's disease and non-Hodgkins lymphomas, as so-called B symptoms are associated with a poorer prognosis. Often the pattern is of a swinging fever, peaking in the late afternoon. Symptomatically, a tumour-related fever can be relieved with non-steroidal anti-inflammatory drugs. Likewise sweating can be related to the cancer, chemotherapy, menopause or other unrelated sweating disorders.[12]

2.5 Pruritus

Pruritus is a symptom associated with cancers such as Hodgkin's disease and lymphomas and precedes other symptoms by several months. The underlying cause is unknown, but may be related to the release of cytokines.[13]

3. Local Symptoms of Cancer in Specific Organs

Many cancers present or relapse as lumps. The critical differential of a lump is whether it is benign or malignant. One characteristic of a malignant lump is its consistency, ranging from the rubbery feel of a lymphoma to the rock hard feel of a squamous cell cancer. It may be of irregular shape, but the main feature of cancers is their changing nature and size, due to growth. The major differential diagnosis when a lymph node is involved is infection, but the persistence, or the lack of response to antibiotics in the case of suspected bacterial infections, is the trigger for further investigation; often the definitive test is a biopsy. The accompanying symptoms may be helpful. However symptoms such as fever or bruising could occur both with haematological malignancies and with infections. Cancer is a differential diagnosis of fever of unknown origin, particularly a relapsing fever.

Inflammatory breast cancer may present as a diffuse redness rather than a lump, in which case a differential diagnosis of mastitis maybe considered.[14] The local lump, however, may be a manifestation of secondary spread, rather than the tumour's primary site, so knowing the pattern of spread of a cancer is important. Breast cancer, for example, most commonly spreads to the liver, lungs, bones and brain, so recurrence after treatment may be diagnosed due to symptoms in one of those organs.

Lung cancer can present with symptoms including cough, dyspnoea, wheeze or stridor, haemoptysis, chest pain, superior vena caval obstruction or Horner's syndrome from a Pancoast tumour.[15] These symptoms are quite non-specific, so only on investigation will the differential between cancer, infection and chronic lung disease become apparent.

Bowel cancer often presents as an altered bowel habit with alternating constipation or diarrhoea, which may be spurious diarrhoea in the case of impending bowel obstruction. Anaemia may be the presenting symptom of a cancer in the ascending colon, while lesions in the descending colon more often present with obstruction.[16] Symptoms include griping pain, abdominal swelling and vomiting, or rectal bleeding. Many of these symptoms could also occur with conditions ranging from irritable bowel syndrome to inflammatory bowel disease, or even as was alluded to at the beginning, acute appendicitis.

Upper gastrointestinal cancers commonly present with dysphagia. The differential diagnosis of dysphagia starts with a history of whether the symptom is worse upon the ingestion of solids or liquids, to distinguish obstructive from neuromuscular causes. Indigestion or early satiety are common symptoms of gastric cancer, but also of peptic ulcer disease.[17]

Overlapping with the bowel symptoms can be the presentation of gynaecologic malignancies, with abdominal bloating and discomfort, or ascites heralding ovarian cancer, which can otherwise be asymptomatic.[18] There may be more specific gynecological symptoms, such as vaginal bleeding, particularly with uterine and cervical cancer. Again, as the differential diagnosis includes many benign conditions, from pregnancy to fibroids, gynecological expertise may be required.

Urologic cancer can present with haematuria.[19] An abdominal mass or abdominal discomfort may alert the clinician to a kidney cancer, or this may be found incidentally on a scan for another reason or an abdominal examination. A painless lump is the usual presentation of testicular cancer, but if painful, orchitis or torsion become differential diagnoses. With prostate cancer, obstruction to urine flow is common, but this does not distinguish it from the more common benign prostatic hyperplasia. Moreover it can present with symptoms only from its secondaries, which will most likely cause bone pain or a fracture, which will need to be distinguished from traumatic or rheumatological causes of these symptoms.

Brain tumours classically present with a headache, typically worse in the morning and improving over the day, as opposed to the pattern of tension headaches, which worsen as the day progresses.[20] More specific symptoms include seizures and neurological symptoms, such as visual disturbances, limb or facial weakness, altered sensations, a balance disorder, memory disturbance (typically short term memory loss), receptive and expressive dysphasia, or altered consciousness. However, many of these symptoms could occur with a range of epileptic conditions, strokes of even cyclically, presenting as migraine headaches.

Finally, a symptom may be organ-specific, with pain arising from the involvement of specific organs. However some organs (e.g. the liver) only have pain receptors in their capsule, which react specifically to being stretched, so even a large tumour may not cause pain. A cancer can block a tube or hollow organ, often causing griping pain, or could press on adjacent structures like nerves, where pain may only occur with movement.

4. The Side Effects of Chemotherapy

The acute and late side effects of chemotherapy must be considered in the differential diagnosis of symptoms occurring during and after treatment. They can be classified by whether they occur hours or days after the chemotherapy, or are delayed by months or years (Table 1). Late effects, in this context, usually refer to toxicities which occur at least six months after therapy, where they are part of a differential diagnosis that includes tumour recurrence or progression, or symptoms of an unrelated illness. For the purpose of

Table 1. Toxicities of chemotherapy.

Immediate (hours–days)	Early (days–weeks)	Delayed (weeks–months)	Late (months–years)
Extravasation	Myelosuppression	Cardiotoxicity	Second cancer
Emesis	Mucositis	Pulmonary fibrosis	Encephalopathy
Hypersensitivity	Alopecia	Periph. neuropathy	Sterility
Tumour lysis	Cystitis	Hepatotoxicity	Teratogenicity
		Nephrotoxicity	

this discussion, I will consider those side effects which pose issues in the differential diagnoses of symptoms.

4.1 Acute side effects

4.1.1 Hypersensitivity

Some chemotherapy drugs are associated with hypersensitivity reactions. Flushing, bronchospasm and hypotension can occur. For example hypersensitivity was seen in the initial clinical trials of paclitaxel, where it was thought to be due to the vehicle, cremophore EL, used in its formulation.[21] Hypersensitivity reactions can be prevented by premedicating with steroids and antihistamines; they have been reported with cisplatin, carboplatin, oxaliplatin, paclitaxel, liposomal doxorubicin, doxorubicin, rituximab, bleomycin and procarbazine. Immunological sensitisation with L-asparaginase occurs in a third of treated patients.[22] However, some individuals can be allergic to other substances in the medical environment such as latex, or other supportive drugs, like antibiotics. Even food allergies may be a relevant differential diagnosis, if patients are being fed when they need to stay for several hours to have their chemotherapy.

4.1.2 Extravasation

It is not uncommon that chemotherapy drugs may irritate the vein they are infused into, or cause a flare reaction in the skin overlying it. This must be distinguished from the situation where a vesicant drug leaks into the tissues around the intravenous cannula. For drugs such as doxorubicin, an initial mild erythema and swelling around where the cannula is inserted may progress to deep ulceration and tissue destruction within a few days. Formerly it was recommended that plastic surgeons be consulted to debride the area immediately, but now antidotes such as DMSO, applied liberally to the site, will prevent the progression to ulceration.[23] For most drugs, the initial treatment after stopping the drug should be to apply ice (possibly with the exception of vinca alkaloid drugs, where heat may be better) and then see if a more specific treatment is recommended.

4.1.3 Emesis

Nausea and vomiting are common side effects associated with the administration of cytotoxic chemotherapy. With drugs that are highly likely to cause emesis, such as cisplatin or combinations such as doxorubicin and cyclophosphamide, prophylactic antiemetics are administered. There are three phases of emesis associated with chemotherapy. Acute post-chemotherapy emesis occurs within the first 24 hours, delayed emesis may persist for a week, and anticipatory emesis is a learned response which can occur in subsequent cycles of chemotherapy, if emesis was problematic in the previous cycle. Antiemetic regimens incorporating two classes of drugs: the 5 hydroxytryptamine 3 inhibitors (5HT3) and the neurokinin 1 inhibitors (NK1) with corticosteroids represent great progress in controlling emesis.[24]

However, emesis is also a common symptom of an underlying cancer or its recurrence. Patients with cerebral or liver metastases, or those who have tumours causing bowel obstruction, may present with emesis. Other drugs, particularly opiate analgesia, also have to be recognised as a potential source of a patient's emesis. The differential diagnosis should be broadened, to consider organ failure such as renal or hepatic failure, which will also cause emesis. A variety of endocrine diseases, from diabetes to hypercalcaemia, as illustrated in the case above, must also be considered.

4.1.4 Bone marrow suppression

Most cytotoxic drugs cause myelosuppression. Characteristically the nadir counts occur between days 10 and 14 and recovery between days 21 and 28, or longer with stem cell toxicity as it occurs with nitrosoureas. Neutropenia is the most important risk factor for infection. Patients presenting with febrile neutropenia should be commenced on broad spectrum antibiotics after cultures of blood, urine and other potential sources of infection, such as sputum, secretions from wounds, peri anal lesions or sites of stomatitis have been taken. Originally, gram negative organisms, such as Pseudomonas, dictated antibiotic policy, but more recently gram positive organisms are becoming more problematic. Staphylococci can colonise venous access devices. In patients who remain febrile, resistant staphylococci or fungi should be considered and antibiotics added accordingly. Prophylactic use of granulocyte colony stimulating factors (G-CSF) in patients having curative chemotherapy who develop febrile neutropenia may enable maintenance of dose intensity in subsequent courses.[25]

The main differential diagnosis is tumour-related fever. Characteristically this is a cyclical fever which peaks in the afternoon. It may occur more often when there are liver metastases and responds symptomatically to non-steroidal anti-inflammatory drugs. The biological targeted therapies such as the monoclonal antibodies rituximab and trastuzumab cause fever as a side effect, often temporally associated with receiving a dose.

Thrombocytopenia is usually transient, but platelet transfusions may be required if bleeding or bruising occurs, or to prevent spontaneous haemorrhage. The main differential diagnosis of this side effect is bone marrow infiltration by cancer, which can often be seen as a leucoerythoblastic blood film.

Anaemia can occur as a cumulative toxicity with drugs such as cisplatin. Blood transfusions are usually advised when the patient becomes symptomatic with weakness and exertional dyspnoea.[26]

Case 2

A man with cancer of unknown primary and presenting initially with weight loss, is being treated with a broad spectrum chemotherapy regimen including cisplatin.He begins to feel lethargic, is breathless on exertion, looks pale and is found to have a low haemoglobin. What is the differential diagnosis?

Anaemia could be simply treatment-related, after serial doses of cisplatin, or secondary to bleeding accompanying extreme thrombocytopenia. The tumour could cause anaemia by bone marrow infiltration, but an occult primary in the ascending colon could be the cause of slow blood loss and an iron deficiency pattern. If weight loss is partly caused by nutritional deficiency, folate deficiency may contribute to anaemia. Finally, as a diagnosis of exclusion, is the tumour-related paraneoplastic anaemia of chronic disease?

5.   Late Effects of Chemotherapy

5.1   *Organ toxicities*

Chemotherapy affecting various organs is usually a cumulative toxicity which takes months to manifest itself. The anthracyclines, doxorubicin and daunorubicin are commonly associated with cardiotoxicity. Acutely, a myocarditis/pericarditis syndrome can occur, causing arrhythmias. The chronic effect is a dose dependent cardiomyopathy. This occurs at cumulative doses over $450 \, mg/m^2$ of doxorubicin, where a drop in ejection fraction can be seen, with subsequent congestive cardiac failure. Trastuzumab has also been associated with cardiotoxicity. Some recovery, with improvement of the ejection fraction occurs over many months following cessation of the chemotherapy. 5-Fluorouracil and related drugs can cause coronary artery spasm, giving very similar chest pain to angina. High dose cyclophosphamide can rarely cause haemorrhagic myocarditis. Rituximab has been associated with cardiac arrhythmias. Cardiologists are often called to manage these toxicities, which can have more dramatic impact if they occur on the background of pre-existing cardiac disease.[27,28]

Pulmonary toxicity, commencing as an acute pneumonitis and progressing to fibrosis, can present as dyspnoea with a dry cough, malaise and fever. Pulmonary function tests show a restrictive defect, with a reduced diffusing capacity. The drug most commonly causing this complication is bleomycin. This is a cumulative toxicity, particularly with doses of bleomycin over 360 mg and in patients over 60 years, or those receiving concomitant radiation or oxygen therapy and in those with renal impairment. Other drugs exhibiting pulmonary toxicity include the alkylating agents, busulphan, carmustine, cyclophosphamide, chlorambucil, melphalan, the antimetabolites methotrexate and cytosine arabinoside, and procarbazine. Stopping the drug may prevent severe damage and corticosteroids can help with symptom control.[29] The differential diagnosis can include pulmonary metasases, or pulmonary infections acquired in the community, or when neutropenic, or reactivation of pre-existing infections such as tuberculosis, when immunosuppressed on chemotherapy.

Cumulative peripheral neuropathy occurs with the vinca alkaloids, particularly vincristine. A glove and stocking sensorimotor neuropathy can occur, but an autonomic neuropathy, with constipation and paralytic ileus is also described. Only some improvement occurs with withdrawal of the drug. Cisplatin, oxaliplatin, etoposide, hexamethylmelamine and paclitaxel are also associated with neuropathy, which is usually a cumulative toxicity. Peripheral neuropathy can occur as a paraneoplastic syndrome. The tumour can also directly impinge on nerves and nerve roots, but this most often causes unilateral signs. Other common co-morbid illnesses have to be considered, such as diabetes or chronic alcoholism and non-cytotoxic drugs that can cause neuropathy. There is slow recovery at the conclusion of chemotherapy.[30]

Encephalopathy is often due to high concentrations of a drug in the CNS. Methotrexate can cause motor dysfunction and cranial nerve palsies, particularly when given intrathecally, but also when delivered with cranial irradiation. 5-Fluorouracil can cause somnolence, cerebellar ataxia and an upper motor neurone syndrome. Ataxia and disorientation is a feature of high dose Cytosine arabinoside. Ifosfamide can also cause cerebellar dysfunction, coma and seizures. The great concern when such symptoms occur is that cerebral metastases have developed. This can often be excluded by a CT or MRI scan, but meningeal disease can be more difficult to diagnose. Other drugs such as opiates, corticosteroids or psychotropic drugs can cause disordered mental states.[31] Opportunistic CNS infection such as toxoplasmosis can be difficult to diagnose until specifically considered. Then, of course, patients with cancer may develop psychiatric illnesses which may be a diagnosis of exclusion in this situation.

Cytotoxic drugs can be toxic to the liver. Some drugs, such as anthracyclines, which are metabolised by the liver, will require dosage reduction in the presence of liver dysfunction. Methotrexate causes acute and chronic liver toxicity. High dose Ara-C can cause enzyme elevations. Bleomycin has caused hyperbilirubinaemia, while dacarbazine can cause severe hepatic necrosis. These causes of liver impairment must be distinguished from underlying liver diseases, or liver involvement with cancer.[32]

Cisplatin is the most common cytotoxic agent to cause kidney damage. It causes proximal tubular damage, which can be limited by vigorous pre-hydration with saline. Methotrexate is excreted by the kidneys and can cause damage by precipitating in the renal tubules. This can be prevented by hydration and alkalinisation of the urine. Methyl-CCNU causes progressive renal tubular atrophy, while mitomycin C can cause microangiopathic changes in the renal vessels, and high cumulative doses of streptozotocin cause proteinuria. Agents such as bisphosphonates can also cause renal dysfunction. Underlying kidney disease must be considered, but any problem due to the underlying cancer is more likely to manifest itself as ureteric obstruction, which may need to be relieved by stents or urostomies.[33]

Other tissues can be affected by chemotherapy. For example regimens containing corticosteroids can lead to late bone effects, such as avascular necrosis.[34] Steroid administration may also result in cataracts. As both bone and joint problems and cataracts can occur with aging, the cause may be difficult to discern.

5.2 Second cancers

Perhaps the most unfortunate of the late effects of chemotherapy are second cancers which occur several years after treatment, usually when a complete remission has occurred after treating the first cancer. These second cancers are often related to the use of alkylating agents, the duration of chemotherapy and the use of chemotherapy in patients over forty years of age. The most common second malignancy is acute leukaemia. Chromosomal abnormalities, such as on chromosomes 7 or 5 occur with the development of the leukaemia and these secondary leukaemias have a worse prognosis than similar primary leukaemias. Non-Hodgkin's lymphomas or solid tumours can occur as second malignancies. Examples are bladder cancers developing after treatment with cyclophosphamide, gastrointestinal or skin cancers after chlorambucil, or sarcomas after combined chemotherapy and radiotherapy. The most obvious differential diagnosis is recurrence of the initial cancer.[35]

5.3   *Reproductive function*

Sterility is a late effect of chemotherapy, however with some cancers such as germ cell tumours, fertility may be impaired prior to chemotherapy. Chemotherapy can affect both germ cell production and endocrine function. In males germinal aplasia results in elevated follicle stimulating hormone (FSH). In females an early menopause with the associated acute changes of vasomotor symptoms, musculoskeletal complaints, urinary incontinence and sexual difficulties, such as dyspareunia occur, with the late effects of osteoporosis and lipid changes and an increase in cardiovascular disease risk. These may be exacerbated if anti-cancer hormonal therapy is employed. The major agents responsible are chlorambucil, cyclophosphamide, nitrogen mustard, busulphan, procarbazine and nitrosoureas, while doxorubicin, vinblastine, cytosine arabinoside and cisplatin are probable candidates. In 50% of the patients with testicular cancer, sperm counts may recover in 2–3 years, but 75% have compromised sperm counts prior to chemotherapy. In females, follicular maturation is arrested and patients can become menopausal, particularly if older than 40 years. Attempts to suppress gonadal function with hormones to protect fertility have variable results.[36] In pregnancies following chemotherapy there is no strong evidence of an excess risk of cancer in the baby.

Impotence can occur in relation to chemotherapy. During the treatment, side effects and fatigue are physical problems, but other issues may be related to loss of body image, be it surgical removal of a breast or testicle, or hair loss from chemotherapy. Endocrine dysfunction secondary to cancer and its treatment may require assessment by an endocrinologist and appropriate hormone replacement instituted. As a late effect, many barriers to a satisfying sex life may be psychological, rather that just physical, and if recognised, may be managed with appropriate support and counselling.[37]

Pregnancy is contraindicated during cancer therapy because most chemotherapy drugs are teratogenic.[38] The greatest problems occur in the first trimester. Some drugs such as alkylating agents are more teratogenic than others.

6.   Conclusions

It is important to think beyond the cancer and the treatment in considering the differential diagnosis of new symptoms. Although cancer or its recurrence must be excluded and the therapy has a myriad of immediate, cumulative and late effects, unrelated concomitant conditions may require referral to other specialists to assist with their management.

References

1. E. J. Dropcho, Principles of paraneoplastic syndromes, *Ann. N. Y. Acad. Sci.* **841**: 246–261 (1998).
2. A. H. Partridge and E. P. Winer, Long-term complications of adjuvant chemotherapy for early stage breast cancer, *Breast Dis.* **21**: 55–64 (2004).
3. F. Graus and J. Dalmau, Praneoplastic neurological syndromes: Diagnosis and treatment, *Curr. Opin. Neurol.* **20**: 732–737 (2007).
4. H. Straszewski, Hematologic paraneoplastic syndromes, *Semin. Oncol.* **24**: 329–333 (1997).
5. J. K. Maesaka, S. K. Mittal and S. Fishbane, Paraneoplastic syndromes of the kidney, *Semin. Oncol.* **24**: 373–381 (1997).
6. C. A. Pipkin and P. A. Lio, Cutaneous manifestations of internal malignancies: An overview, *Dermatol. Clin.* **26**: 1–15 (2008).
7. K. Mito, R. Maruyama, Y. Uenishi, K. Arita, H. Kawano, K. Kashima and M. Nasu, Hypertrophic pulmonary osteoarthropathy associated with non-small cell lung cancer demonstrated growth hormone-releasing hormone by immunohistochemical analysis, *Intern. Med.* **40**: 532–535 (2001).
8. B. A. DeLellis and L. Xia, Paraneoplastic endocrine syndromes: A review, *Endocr. Pathol.* **14**: 303–317 (2003).
9. S. Acharyya, K. J. Ladner, L. L. Nelsen, J. Damrauer, P. J. Reiser, S. Swoap and D. C. Guttridge, Cancer cachexia is regulated by selective targeting of skeletal muscle gene products, *J. Clin. Invest.* **114**: 370–378 (2004).

10. G. Prue, J. Rankin, J. Allen, J. Gracey and F. Cramp, Cancer related fatigue: A critical appraisal, *Eur. J. Cancer* **42**: 846–863 (2006).

11. N. Humpel and D. C. Iverson, Review and critique of the quality of exercise recommendations for cancer patients and survivors, *Support. Care Cancer* **13**: 493–502 (2005).

12. D. S. Zhukovsky, Fever and sweats in the patient with advanced cancer, *Heamatol. Oncol. Clin. North Am.* **16**: 579–588 (2002).

13. P. G. Gobbi, C. Cavalli, A. Gendarini, A. Crema, G. Ricevuti, M. Federico, U. Prisco and E. Ascari, Reevaluation of prognostic significance of symptoms in Hodgkin's disease, *Cancer* **56**: 2874–2880 (1985).

14. S. E. Singletary and M. Cristofanilli, Defining the clinical diagnosis of inflammatory breast cancer, *Semin. Oncol.* **35**: 7–10 (2008).

15. J. R. Molina, P. Yang, S. D. Cassivi, S. E. Schild and A. A. Adjei, Non-small cell lung cancer: Epidemiology, risk factors, treatment and survivorship, *Mayo Clin. Proc.* **83**: 584–594 (2008).

16. M. S. Cappell, Pathophysiology, clinical presentation, and management of colon cancer, *Gastroenterol. Clin. North Am.* **37**: 1–24 (2008).

17. J. F. Gibbs, A. Rajput, K. S. Chadha, W. G. Douglas, H. Hill, C. Nwogu, H. R. Nava and M. S. Sabel, The changing profile of oesophageal cancer presentation and its implications for diagnosis, *J. Natl. Med. Assoc.* **99**: 620–626 (2007).

18. L. H. Smith, Early detection of ovarian cancer: A review of the evidence, *Expert Rev. Anticancer Ther.* **6**: 1045–1052 (2006).

19. E. K. Johnson, S. Daignault, Y. Zhang and C. T. Lee, Patterns of haematuria referral to urologists: Does a gender disparity exist? *Urology* **72**: 498–502 (2008).

20. S. R. Chandana, S. Movva, M. Arora and T. Singh, Primary brain tumours in adults, *Am. Fam. Physician* **77**: 1423–1430 (2008).

21. R. B. Weiss, R. C. Donehower, P. H. Wiernik, T. Ohnuma, R. J. Gralla, D. L. Trump, J. R. Baker Jr., D. A. Van Echo, D. D. Von Hoff and B. Leyland-Jones, Hypersensitivity reactions form taxol, *J. Clin. Oncol.* **8**: 1263–1268 (1990).

22. G. M. Shepherd, Hypersensitivity reactions to chemotherapeutic drugs, *Clin. Rev. Allergy Immunol.* **24**: 253–262 (2003).

23. I. N. Olver, J. Aisner, A. Hament, L. Buchanan, J. K. Bishop and R. S. Kaplan, A prospective study of topical dimethyl sulphoxide (DMSO) for treating anthracycline extavasations, *J. Clin. Oncol.* **6**: 1732–1735 (1988).

24. I. N. Olver, Prevention of chemotherapy-induced nausea and vomiting: Focus on fosaprepitant, *Ther. Clin. Risk Manage.* **4**: 501–506 (2008).

25. M. E. Falagas, K. Z. Vardakas and G. Saonis, Decreasing the incidence and impact of infections in neutropenic patients: Evidence form meta-analyses of randomised controlled trials, *Curr. Med. Res. Opin.* **24**: 215–235 (2008).

26. S. E. Kurtin, A time for hope: Promising advances in the management of anaemia, neutropenia, thrombocytopenia and mucositis, *J. Support. Oncol.* **4**(Suppl. 2): 85–88 (2007).

27. R. L. Jones, C. Swanton and M. S. Ewer, Anthracycline cardiotoxicity, *Expert Opin. Drug Saf.* **5**: 791–809 (2006).

28. R. L. Jones and M. S. Ewer, Cardiac and cardiovascular toxicity of nonanthracycline anticancer drugs, *Expert Rev. Anticancer Ther.* **6**: 1249–1269 (2006).

29. B. Vahid and P. E. Marik, Pulmonary complications of novel antineoplastic agents for solid tumours, *Chest* **133**: 528–538 (2008).

30. A. J. Windebank and W. Grisold, Chemotherapy-induced neuropathy, *J. Periph. Nerv. Syst.* **13**: 27–46 (2008).

31. J. Hildebrand, Neurological complications of cancer chemotherapy, *Curr. Opin. Oncol.* **18**: 321–324 (2006).

32. P. D. King and M. C. Perry, Hepatotoxcity of chemotherapy, *Oncologist* **6**: 162–176 (2001).

33. M. Darmon, M. Ciroldi, G. Thiery, B. Schlemmer and E. Azoulay, Clinical revew: Specific aspects of acute renal failure in cancer patients, *Crit. Care* **10**: 211 (doi:10.1186/cc4907) (2006).

34. H. Gogas and D. Fennelly, Avascular necrosis following extensive chemotherapy and dexamethasone treatment in a patient with advanced ovarian cancer: Case report and review of the literature, *Gynecol. Oncol.* **63**: 379–381 (1996).

35. L. B. Travis, C. S. Rabkin, L. M. Brown, J. M. Allan, B. P. Alter, C. B. Ambrosone, C. B. Begg, N. Caporaso, S. Channock, A. DeMichele, W. D. Figg, M. K. Gospodarowicz, E. J. Hall, M. Hisada, P. Inskip, R. Kleinerman, J. B. Little, D. Malkin, A. G. Ng, K. Offit, C. H. Pui, L. L. Robison, N. Rothman, P. G. Shields, L. Strong, T. Taniguchi, M. A. Tucker and M. H. Greene, Cancer survivorship — Genetic susceptibility and second primary cancers: Research strategies and recommendations, *J. Natl. Cancer Inst.* **98**: 15–25 (2006).

36. B. Koczwara, Addressing fertility needs of breast cancer patients: Oncology perspective, *Expert Rev. Anticancer Ther.* **8**: 1323–1330 (2008).
37. M. E. Galbraith and F. Crighton, Alterations of sexual function in men with cancer, *Semin. Oncol. Nurs.* **24**: 102–114 (2008).
38. D. Meirow and E. Schiff, Appraisal of chemotherapy effects on reproductive outcome according to animal studies and clinical data, *J. Natl. Cancer Inst. Monogr.* **34**: 21–25 (2005).

8

Acute and Late Radiation Therapy Effects

Sandro V. Porceddu,
Jarad M. Martin,
Brian O'Sullivan
and Michael Fay

Abstract

Radiation therapy (RT) is associated with acute and late effects of normal tissues. Acute effects are often expressed during or immediately after RT and are transient, while late effects may be expressed months to years after completion of treatment and are often irreversible and may be progressive. In addition, radiation effects may clinically appear as other conditions, not related to the cancer or its treatment.

This chapter describes the RT effects associated with commonly treated malignancies, the differential diagnosis and methods to treat or limit the adverse sequelae of radiation treatment.

Keywords: Radiation therapy, acute and late effects, normal tissues.

1. Introduction

Radiation Therapy (RT) is the use of ionising radiation to treat malignancies and related diseases. RT is used as either the primary (curative), pre-operative, post-operative or palliative treatment in a wide range of cancers.[1]

Whether a RT effect is expressed early or late relates to the rate of cell turnover for a particular tissue or organ. In general, **acute effects** are expressed soon after the commencement or shortly after completion of RT. **Late effects** are expressed well after the RT has been completed, ranging from three months to years.[1,2]

The majority of cancers receiving RT are treated with external beam radiotherapy (EBRT) delivered by a linear accelerator. RT fields are tailored to deliver a high dose to the tumour, while minimising dose to the surrounding normal tissues.

The use of computerised planning software allows design of conformal fields known either as three-dimensional conformal radiotherapy or intensity modulated radiotherapy (IMRT).

Brachytherapy may be used either alone, or in combination with EBRT. This is the use of radioactive sources such as seeds or needles (e.g. Iridium-192, Iodine-125) which are either implanted in tissue or inserted intra-cavitary, and deliver a very high dose at the interface, with a rapid dose fall-off, minimising dose to surrounding tissues beyond the area of interest.

Despite the use of highly conformal treatments, the majority of patients receiving RT will experience some degree of acute and/or late radiation effects.

It is not possible to discuss all possible RT effects, however, this chapter will detail acute and late RT effects experienced for commonly treated cancers, and some side effects which are less common, but important to recognise and address early.

RT effects can mimic other non-treatment related conditions and therefore it is important to be able to differentiate these. For example RT skin reaction may mimic cellulitis and therefore be treated inappropriately with antibiotics. RT to the pelvis may result in dysuria which may mimic a urinary tract infection. Conversely symptoms such as cough, shortness of breath and changes on the chest X-ray may be mistaken for radiation pneumonitis when in fact may represent lymphangitis carcinomatosis. Throughout this chapter various radiation effects and their differentiation diagnosis and how they may be distinguished will be discussed.

2. Acute and Late Radiation Effects of Normal Tissue

2.1 *Acute radiation effects*

The majority of normal tissue RT effects are a result of direct cell killing. The main targets that lead to expression of acute RT effects are the stem cells (which give rise to progenitor cells) and the progenitor cells (which differentiate into mature cells). Depletion of the stem cells and progenitor cells leads to tissues becoming denuded, as the normal cell loss is not matched with proliferation of new cells.[1]

Some side effects, such as fatigability, somnolence, nausea and vomiting are more likely to be mediated by radiation-induced release of cytokines and can mimic flu-like illness.

Tissues that express early or acute RT effects are those that are turning over rapidly, such as the mucosa of the alimentary tract and skin and they tend to be transient and recover after a few weeks following RT.

2.2 *Subacute effects*

Transient RT effects may be seen between six weeks to three months following treatment and are often reversible. Examples of subacute effects include somnolence following RT to the brain, **L'hermitte's syndrome** (shooting pains down the spine occurring on head flexion) after spinal irradiation, and pneumonitis following irradiation to the chest. The precise pathophysiology underlying these effects remains uncertain, in particular those affecting neurological tissues, since these structures are not examined pathologically, due to the reversible nature of the condition.

2.3 *Late RT effects*

Late RT effects are those seen months to years following a course of RT and, unlike acute effects, late effects tend to be irreversible. Common examples of late reacting tissues include the brain, the spinal cord and the heart.

The process of late effects is not yet fully understood. For many years, similar to acute effects, direct cell kill of "target cells" leading to a functional deficient has been considered the main cause of late effects. The latency of expression of these effects is thought to be due to the slow turnover of the "target cells". In addition, damage to the microvasculature that supplies these tissues, and loss of supporting tissue such as oligodendrocytes resulting in demyelination, have also been considered to play a part in augmenting this process.[1] It has now been recognised that severe acute RT effects may result in greater late effects, known as **consequential effects**, related to inadequate recovery of the depleted stem cell population.

In recent times there has been a paradigm shift in the understanding of the cause of late effects. From radiobiological and molecular research, it would appear that ionising radiation causes early activation of cytokine cascades, which leads to fibrogenesis and excessive extracellular matrix and collagen deposition. This results in the development of excessive fibrosis in addition to cell depletion and microvascular compromise.[3]

2.4   *Factors affecting acute and late RT effects*

2.4.1 *Radiotherapy dose and fractionation*

The unit of absorbed dose is known as Gray (Gy). Conventional RT is the use of 1.8–2.0Gy daily treatment, five days per week.

Delivering a total dose of RT using a series of smaller doses, fractionated RT, facilitates sparing of normal tissues, by allowing repair of sublethal DNA damage between treatments and repopulation of normal cells.[1] The presence of tumour hypoxia is an important adverse determinant of treatment outcome with RT. Fractionation allows re-oxygenation and re-assortment of tumour cells into a more radiosensitive phase of the cell cycle.[1]

Acute reacting tissues are sensitive to total dose and overall treatment time. The **severity** of the acute reaction is dependent on the **rate** of accumulation of dose (overall time), while **healing time** is more reliant on the **total dose**.

Late reacting tissues have different radiobiological characteristics and are more sensitive to the total dose and **dose/fraction**.

For the same total dose, if the treatment is delivered using larger doses/fraction compared with conventionally fractionated RT, an increase in severity of late effects may be seen. Tolerance doses for various organs have been described that predict the 5% probability of a severe late RT effect occurring with conventionally fractionated RT at 5 years ($TD_{5/5}$).[3,4]

2.4.2 Altered fractionation

Various fractionation schedules are used to exploit different radiological characteristics of the tumour or normal tissues.[1]

These include hyperfractionated, accelerated, accelerated-hyperfractionated and hypofractionated RT.

2.4.3 Concurrent chemotherapy/radioprotectants

Concurrent chemotherapy is commonly used with RT in a range of malignancies, because of the proven benefits in outcome in a number of studies. However this is associated with an increase in acute RT effects and potentially late effects.

A number of radioprotectants have been developed, such as amifostine, but further evaluation is required to assess safety and efficacy. Palifermin is another agent that is undergoing assessment in reducing RT induced mucositis.

Immunosuppressants, such as methotrexate used for rheumatoid arthritis have radiosensitising properties and ceasing these agents prior to RT is required.

2.4.4 Pre-existing conditions

There are also genetically transmitted DNA repair deficiencies which can result in increased RT sensitivity, such as ataxia-telangiectasia, and connective tissue diseases such as scleroderma.[5]

2.5 Acute/Late grading scoring system

Over the years multiple scoring systems have been devised. The currently used scoring system is Common Terminology Criteria Adverse Events (CTCAE) v3.0.[6]

This system and others generally score toxicity from absent/ none through to severe. In the current CTCAE v3.0, toxicity is scored in five grades: Grade 0 — absent or none, Grade 1 — mild, Grade 2 — moderate, Grade 3 — severe, Grade 4 — life-threatening, and Grade 5 — death.[7]

3. Common Clinical Scenarios

3.1 *Head and neck radiotherapy*

RT side effects associated with head and neck treatment are common and can be severe. It is important to manage these symptoms early, to prevent detrimental treatment delays. **Cessation of smoking** is important, as this will negate the benefits of RT and also appears to be a significant contributing factor to the development of osteoradionecrosis (ORN).

Acute effects

The common acute side effects include

- dermatitis;
- mucositis;
- odynophagia;
- dysphagia;
- salivary changes;
- hoarseness;
- loss of taste;
- hair loss; and
- weight loss.

RT dermatitis is usually seen in the first 1–2 weeks and may be mistaken for cellulitis. Patients should avoid direct sunlight and chemical irritants, such as perfumed creams or alcohol-based lotions. Appropriate skin care products used to moisten the skin are available. When moist desquamation/skin breakdown occur, gel-based products are used to protect and promote wound healing.

Mucositis begins with erythema then patchy ulcerations, usually in weeks 2–3, followed by confluent ulcerations by weeks 4–6.

The white patches can sometimes be mistaken for oral candidiasis (these tend to appear more as white plaques).

Mouth care begins at the beginning of RT. This involves attention to oral hygiene, with the use of mouthwashes (usually salt/bicarbonate based), nystatin to prevent oral candidiasis, brushing teeth with a soft tooth brush, use of topical agents such as lignocaine mouthwash and systemic analgesics which include paracetamol syrup or narcotic medications. In addition patients should avoid spicy or abrasive foods that may cause trauma.

A number of agents have been studied or are undergoing clinical trials to evaluate their role in reducing mucositis. These include

- sucralfate;
- amifostine;
- granulocyte-macrophage colony-stimulating factor;
- zinc; and
- palifermin.

Many of these agents require additional evaluation for safety and efficacy. There is a theoretical concern that some of these agents, such as amifostine and palifermin may either protect the tumour (amifostine) or stimulate tumour growth (palifermin).

Dysphagia (difficulty swallowing) and **odynophagia** (painful swallowing) occur due to the resulting mucositis and pain, thickening of saliva and oedema of the mucosa and soft tissues of the neck. This can lead to nutritional disturbances and weight loss. All patients require nutritional assessment prior to the commencement of and during treatment. Nutritional problems can be exacerbated by nausea or vomiting related to low dose brain-stem irradiation, or more commonly as a consequence of the taste dysfunction and the influence of thickened mucoid saliva associated with radiotherapy to this region.

Late effects

Late side effects include

- xerostomia;
- dental complications;

- osteoradionecrosis (ORN);
- trismus;
- swallowing dysfunction;
- hoarseness;
- fibrosis to pharynx and soft tissues of the neck;
- thyroid disorder; and
- carotid stenosis.

Neurological complications, such as brachial plexopathy, injury to optic structures, myelopathy or brainstem myelopathy are rare with modern RT techniques and will not be discussed further in this section.

Xerostomia is a common long-term sequel of head and neck RT. Conformal treatments such as IMRT can spare the parotids and minimise long-term xerostomia.

Salt/bicarbonate mouthwashes can help with breaking up the tenacious thick sputum and keeping the mouth clean.

Products that can help include;

- **Artificial salivary products** provide temporary relief.
- **Sialagogues**, such as pineapple, sugarless gum or **pilocarpine** (shown to reduce oral dryness in randomised trials). However, pilocarpine use has not been widely adopted, due to associated parasympathomimetic stimulation.
- **Amifostine** reduces the rate of xerostomia with RT alone, but benefit with chemo-RT is uncertain. It is not available in all countries, is expensive and is administered as a daily intravenous dose.[8]

Dental problems following RT are common, due to reduced production and alteration of the chemical composition of normal saliva, which in turn is associated with a change in the microbial flora.

All patients should have a pre-treatment dental evaluation and commence fluoride prophylaxis, preferably using **fluoride mouth trays** in patients with teeth.

Osteoradionecrosis (ORN) is a complication seen in approximately 5–10% of people who receive head and neck RT, which may be either asymptomatic or symptomatic. Patients who continue to smoke and have pre-existing conditions which impair blood supply, such as a connective tissue disease or diabetes, or who require teeth extraction post-therapy are at higher risk. Following RT, pre-extraction **hyperbaric oxygen (HBO)** may be useful in preventing its development in patients requiring dental extraction within high-dose RT fields.[9]

Recurrent tumour and osteomyelitis should be excluded in the presence of suspected ORN.

For **minor ORN** consisting of bone exposure management involves improving nutrition and oral hygiene, cessation of smoking, optimising diabetic control, minimising trauma caused by dentures and a trial of oral antibiotics such as penicillin or clindamycin. In some cases if healing is slow some minor debridement of the bone and a graft repair over the exposed area may be helpful.

For **major ORN**, characterised by radiologic changes, pain and/or fracture, the principles described above are applied, but patients may require major surgery with reconstructive surgical flaps, analgesia and intravenous antibiotics. The value of HBO in established ORN is not fully resolved and costly.

Trismus, due to fibrosis of the muscles of mastication, leads to reduced ability to open the mouth and inability to chew adequately. Early recognition and referral to a speech pathologist is essential. Muscle relaxants, such as benzodiazepines, are used as a last resort in severe cases.

Long term **swallowing problems,** mainly dysphagia, are common sequelae and can lead to nutritional problems and aspiration.

Factors leading to swallowing problems include lack of saliva, mucosal and soft tissue oedema of the pharynx, fibrosis of soft tissues and neck muscles and pharyngeal stenosis. Symptoms can range from *mild*, requiring alteration in diet and pharyngeal muscle strengthening to *moderate*, requiring swallowing retraining to *severe*, requiring pharyngeal dilatation or permanent enteral feeding.

Asymptomatic biochemical **hypothyroidism** may occur, but clinical hypothyroidism is rare.

3.2   *Lung radiotherapy*

Acute effects

RT can initiate a cascade of inflammatory mediators in the lung. In a small percentage of patients this is clinically evident as a syndrome of **radiation pneumonitis,** with cough and progressive dyspnoea. Progressive scarring of the lung can result and occasionally even respiratory failure. Respiratory infection can present in a very similar manner and antibiotics should usually be instituted in the first instance. The radiologic imaging will tend to show opacities matching the RT fields with pneumonitis, rather than following anatomical (e.g. lobar) boundaries. The risk factors are not entirely clear, but the volume of lung receiving a high RT dose appears important. Some patients are intrinsically more sensitive to lung RT — such as patients with Systemic Lupus Erythematosus (SLE).

Toxicity is higher where the RT is given twice a day, with concurrent chemotherapy and to larger volumes (such as primary and involved mediastinal nodes).

Lung function tests are usually measured both to assess suitability to tolerate RT and to estimate its consequences. Medication for intercurrent respiratory disease, such as chronic obstructive airways disease, should be optimised.

Fatigue is almost universal; starting early in treatment and lasting four to six weeks after completion of the course.

Oesophagitis can occur if the high dose volume includes a significant length of oesophagus. Topical anaesthetics (e.g. Xylocaine viscous) and analgesics may help. Nutritional support and insertion of a feeding tube are occasionally required.

Pain can occur from swelling of the tumour or pleural irritation.

Lower respiratory tract infection can arise from obstruction of part of the lung by tumour. Patients can become extremely unwell, requiring parenteral antibiotics and occasionally surgery.

Subacute effects

Radiation pneumonitis can appear up to six months following treatment and oral corticosteroids can be helpful in this case. Asymptomatic radiologic changes are much more common and would not usually be an indication for treatment. **Lymphangitis carcinomatosis** may mimic radiation pneumonitis.

Late effects

The long-term consequence of lung inflammation is pulmonary fibrosis. The clinical effect depends on the volume of lung affected and the pre-existing degree of pulmonary compromise. Pre-treatment lung function tests can give some indication of the risk, but are not particularly sensitive.

Oesophageal strictures or fistulae are rare developments with modern treatment. They usually require endoscopic dilatation or bronchial stent placement in the case of fistulae.

3.3   *Breast RT and cardiac toxicity*

3.3.1   *Breast cancer RT*

RT for breast cancer (BC) is commonly delivered as adjuvant treatment following definitive breast conserving surgery. The three cornerstones of breast RT are eradication of remaining cancer cells, maintenance of a cosmetically acceptable breast, and minimisation of cardiac toxicity.

A conventional course of RT will generally last between 5–6 weeks, with treatment five times per week, directed at the entire breast. Partial breast RT (PBRT) is now an active area of research, as it is recognised that the primary site is at greatest risk of recurrence, rather than sites on the breast located away from the original tumour. This approach has the advantage of potentially reducing toxicity, and because of the reduced RT fields required, such treatment can be delivered in less than one week. Although still being validated in phase 3 clinical trials, it is likely that such an approach will become more common for selected patients within the next five years.

Acute effects

Skin erythema is a very common side effect. While no topical preparation can prevent it, moisturisers will palliate the burning sensation. This will occasionally progress to moist desquamation, most commonly in the inframammory fold, especially in women with larger breasts. Keeping the region dry and using a non-underwired bra may help, but usually non-adhesive wound care incorporating surgical gels are required for pain control and to prevent ongoing excoriation. Reassurance is required that although such problems tend to worsen in the 10–14 days following the completion of RT, they would have usually resolved 4–6 weeks after the last treatment. It is important to communicate this to the patient and to primary carers, as the appearance can mimic severe **cellulitis**. Both the natural history and clearly demarcated borders corresponding to the RT treatment fields should aid in the differential diagnosis.

Subacute effects

In the longer term **breast lymphoedema** can develop following the axillary surgery and breast RT. The discomfort of a hot, swollen, heavy breast tends to deteriorate during the day and improve at night, as recumbency can aid postural lymphatic drainage. Referral to a physiotherapist is helpful, to teach breast massage away from the affected axillary lymphatics.

Late effects

Lymphodema of the arm can develop following RT to the axilla and supraclavicular regions. This is part of the reason axillary RT is now infrequently performed following axillary dissection, as the combination of surgery and RT have a multiplicative effect on the risk of arm lymphoedema.

Teleangiectasia may evolve years after the RT, and in the early stages may alarm some women, who may fear that they are suffering from disease recurrence.

More severe contractures of the breast with increasing **fibrosis** are rare in the modern era, and probably more a reflection of an idiosyncratic radiosensitivity, although a complicated post-operative course may contribute. In extreme situations, a mastectomy and reconstruction may be required.

The only intervention that has been shown to modify the natural history of breast RT toxicity is the use of **IMRT**. A randomized trial showed a 17% reduction in the rate of moist desquamation in the acute setting, and a separate trial showed improved late cosmesis due to better dose uniformity.[10,11] Such techniques are now receiving wide acceptance, on the basis of this evidence.

3.3.2 *Cardiac toxicity*

The **Early Breast Cancer Trialists Collaborative Group** meta-analysis showed that although adjuvant RT reduced the risk of a subsequent BC related death, it provided no additional advantage for overall survival.[12] This was because of excess cardiac mortality. Further work has identified a higher risk of cardiac morbidity and mortality for women with tumours on the left side compared to the right, and that such differences take at least ten years to become apparent.[13] Functional imaging and angiographic studies have shown higher than expected instances of atherosclerotic plaques in the left anterior descending (LAD) coronary artery in women who have had their left breast irradiated.[14]

It is important to engage in primary cardiovascular (CV) risk minimisation with women having RT for BC. Smoking cessation, and discussions regarding hypertension, lipid and glycaemic control are all important. There is some suggestion that with modern RT delivery techniques the risk of CV toxicity will be reduced, although the long natural history of this process requires that all avenues for risk reduction be used. The use of IMRT may allow reduced radiation dose to be delivered to the LAD and PBRT may also hold similar potential.

3.4 *Prostate radiotherapy and rectal toxicity*

Prior to commencing RT for prostate cancer (PC), a number of technical factors will determine the likelihood of side effects. Key amongst these is the dose of RT prescribed. Although six randomised trials have shown improvements in surrogate endpoints, such as prostatic specific antigen (PSA) relapse, with the use of increased doses, this comes at the price of a higher risk of late effects. This has prompted the implementation of two key preventative technologies:

- **Image Guided Radiotherapy (IGRT)**: Since the prostate moves in an unpredictable fashion, some form of soft tissue imaging prior to treatment each day is required to ensure accurate treatment delivery. This translates into not only less inadvertent dose to neighbouring structures such as the rectum, but higher doses being delivered to the targeted prostate.

- **IMRT**: The use of dynamic RT fields helps to mould the radiation dose to the shape of the prostate. This reduces the proportion of the rectum being treated to high doses; there is some evidence to suggest that this reduces the risk of severe late reaction from 1–2% down to around 0.1%.[15]

Acute effects

Acute toxicities tend to accumulate towards the second half of the treatment course, and tend to persist for around two weeks following the completion of treatment, before improving back towards baseline in the 3–4 subsequent weeks. Hence the strategy is to prophylactically mitigate against the risk of severe toxicity, differentiate from alternative pathologies and palliate symptoms through to resolution.

Men who suffer from excessive obstructive urinary symptoms prior to starting RT are at higher risk of severe acute **urinary toxicity** during treatment. Such men may benefit from a bladder neck incision, or trans-urethral resection of the prostate 2–3 months prior to starting treatment. It is rare to see significant urinary irritation in the first weeks of treatment, and hence the potential of a **urinary tract infection** needs to be considered in this instance.

RT can cause either **irritative** or **obstructive symptoms**, both of which are managed differently. In both symptom clusters the man can have symptoms of urinary frequency and increased nocturia.

- **Irritative** symptoms tend to be dominated by dysuria and excessive urgency. This is thought to be caused by inflammatory changes in the urothelium, exposing the underlying bladder and urethra to the relatively acidic urine. The cornerstone of management here is urinary alkalinisation (e.g. cranberry juice, Ural), reduction of irritants (especially caffeine), with occasional recourse to anti-inflammatory medication.
- **Obstructive symptoms** include the classic cluster of hesitancy, poor stream and terminal dribbling. Consideration of

alpha-blockade is required in the first instance. It is rare (<1%) for men to require catheterisation for such side effects.

Perianal toxicity, including haemorrhoidal type irritation respond to hygienic manoeuvres (e.g. salt water baths), and topical analgesic/steroidal preparations.

Diarrhoea can be managed with a low fibre diet, escalating to the use of anti-motility agents. Excessive mucous, frequency and bleeding refractory to the above may indicate a more severe **radiation proctitis.** In this instance steroid administration may be required, usually per rectum (e.g. colifoam enema), but occasionally administered orally. The advent of IGRT has reduced the incidence of such toxicity.[15]

Late effects

It is controversial whether the target for RT damage regarding **erectile dysfunction** (ED) is the penile bulb, pudendal artery, or periprostatic nerves. In any instance, the best predictor of function following RT is erectile function at baseline. There is some circumstantial evidence that prophylactic use of a phosphodiesterase inhibitor (PDEI), such as sildenafil may decrease the development of ED. The use of such drugs can certainly be helpful to manage ED once it occurs, although other methods, such as penile prostaglandin injections, penile implants or vacuum pumps can also be helpful.

Around 20% of men will have significant chronic **urinary toxicity** from baseline levels, usually relating to urinary urgency and frequency. Since the prostatic urethra runs directly through the RT target volume, despite the development of IGRT or IMRT, sparing of this structure from radiation dose is difficult. Such problems can respond to alpha blockade or detrusor stabilisation medication.

Radiation cystitis is always a diagnosis of exclusion made on cystoscopy, so any haematuria occurring following RT needs full work-up, including urinary cytology and urological examination. This toxicity can be very difficult to manage, although encouraging results are reported with **HBO.**

Moderate long term **rectal toxicity** such as change in bowel habit, frequency or increased mucous discharge can be managed with dietary manipulation, usually via increased soluble fibre. **Severe radiation proctitis (RP)** leading to ongoing bleeding can mimic a plethora of bowel pathologies, and mandates endoscopic evaluation to exclude a metachronous process. RP is a clinical diagnosis made by visualising teleangiectasia on the anterior rectal wall, just posterior to the position of the prostate, in the absence of other pathologies. The endoscopist needs to be made aware of this differential diagnosis, because biopsy is both unnecessary and potentially dangerous. This is because the irradiated region does not heal well after trauma, and has the potential to ulcerate and even develop into a fistula. Currently the best results for managing this problem seem to be from laser photocoagulation.[16]

3.5   *Central nervous system (CNS)*

There are a number of RT effects on the central nervous system, ranging from mild fatigue to radionecrosis. The **volume** irradiated and **anatomical site** within the brain can play an important part on acute and late RT effects.[17]

There is marked heterogeneity amongst the volume of brain irradiated for different indications. Whole brain RT may be prescribed for brain metastases, where a small dose is given to the whole intracranial volume. In treatment of high grade gliomas, a much larger dose is given to part of the brain. Stereotactic radiosurgery is a highly focussed form of RT given to a very small volume of the brain. Doses given are much higher — typically 18 to 24Gy as a single fraction.

Prior to treatment the following assessments may be relevant:

- **Ophthalmologic assessment** in any radical treatment where the eye may receive a significant dose of RT.
- Baseline **pituitary gland** function. Panhypopituitarism can result — often with a latency of many years.
- **Neurocognitive assessment** is increasingly felt to be of value, especially in protocols involving paediatric patients and clinical research trials.

Acute effects

Fatigue is an almost universal complaint. It usually begins in the first or second week and continues for up to six weeks after RT. There is no specific treatment.

Alopecia occurs over the RT field entry and exit point. With whole brain RT, there is total alopecia. Hair usually grows back, unless the scalp has received a large dose (>60Gy).

Nausea and vomiting respond well to 5-hydroxytryptamine-3 receptor antagonists (e.g. ondansetron) or dexamethasone. Acute hydrocephalus should be considered if there is any alteration in the level of consciousness and an urgent CT or MRI scan of the brain should be performed.

Mild confusion is not uncommon, especially in older patients and may require increased nursing supervision.

Seizures can occasionally result when the lesion is close to the motor strip and there is marked oedema. Dexamethasone can assist in decreasing oedema. Patients should be strongly advised not to drive while undergoing treatment.

Subacute effects

Somnolence syndrome is an uncommon symptom cluster usually seen in children, of tiredness, irritability and loss of appetite. It is associated with demyelination and is self-limiting.

Late effects

Late neurocognitive changes are much more common at the extremes of age (in younger than three years and adults over 70 years). Care should be taken when ascribing these changes to RT if they were not present at baseline. Similarly, in the era of combined modality treatment, defining the contribution of each modality to toxicity can be very difficult. Disease recurrence should not be overlooked as a cause of progressive symptoms.

The **optic chiasm** doses are restricted to 54Gy, or blindness can result in up to 1–5% of cases. This requires identification of the chiasm on the planning CT (or usually fused diagnostic CT and MRI) and avoidance of dose to this volume. Unilateral blindness can (rarely) be caused by excessive dose to the retina. A small dose to the lens can cause **cataracts** (around 6–10Gy).

Pituitary gland function should be checked routinely after treatment if the pituitary was irradiated. Cortisol is of prime importance, but thyroid function, gonadotrophins and growth hormone should not be forgotten. The development of biochemical abnormalities may appear many years after treatment.[18]

Second tumours are not uncommon after brain RT, particularly after the successful treatment of tumours such as medulloblastoma in children. Meningioma is the most commonly diagnosed tumour following brain RT.

Radiation necrosis is often difficult to differentiate from tumour recurrence. Symptoms can vary from mild headache to seizures, paralysis and coma. Modalities which can help separate the two entities are magnetic resonance spectroscopy (MRS) and positron emission tomography (PET). Surgery may sometimes be required, where the necrotic brain is causing mass effect. HBO has been advocated in the past with little evidence of benefit. Steroids can be of benefit in decreasing oedema.

4. Less Common, but Important Clinical Scenarios

4.1 *Effects on fertility*

Total body irradiation in children leads to less than 2% of them becoming biological parents.[19,20] In adults the sperm count may be reduced by as little as 0.1Gy. A biologically equivalent dose of 6–8Gy to the germinal stem cells may lead to sterility for years.[1] The testicular Leydig cells are significantly more radioresistant and testosterone production may remain adequate with up to 12Gy.[20]

Permanent infertility may be caused by:

- depletion of germinal stem cells;
- damage to testicular testosterone production; or
- secondary endocrine dysfunction.

RT to the para-aortic nodes is unlikely to cause a significant scattered dose to the testes. However, in the case of RT to the pelvis, the dose can be reduced from 1.5–3.0Gy to 0.5–0.8Gy, by shielding or displacing the gonads.

Oocytes are sensitive to 0.12Gy, and 4Gy is considered the lethal dose to ovaries in 50% of patients. Ovarian failure occurs through loss of ovarian follicle production, which in turn leads to loss of endocrine function. RT to other glands in the hypothalamic-pituitary axis may also affect fertility.[1,19,20] There is no evidence for radioactive iodine treatment causing infertility, miscarriage or congenital complications, however, it is prudent for women to avoid pregnancy for one year.

4.2   *Interventions for fertility preservation*

- sperm banking;
- embryonic cryopreservation, and
- gonadal shielding and oophoropexy to move ovaries out of the radiation field.

Investigational techniques such as cryopreservation of ovarian or testicular tissue and hormonal manipulation are not widespread at present.[19,20]

4.3   *Radiation-induced malignancy*

This is one of the most feared complications of RT treatment and is the factor limiting its use in benign conditions. Much of the data comes from treatment of benign conditions or tumours cured with RT (such as Hodgkin Disease).[21-23] The other population studied are the atomic bomb survivors, but it is unclear how well this can be generalised to the population treated with medical radiation.[24]

Ionising radiation can induce a cancer in any tissue irradiated. The mechanism is thought to be incomplete or disrupted DNA repair following RT. There is usually a long latency, a median of seven years, from the time of irradiation to developing a cancer.

The type of cancer resulting can be as varied as the tissue irradiated. It should be noted that chemotherapy can influence this risk (as was seen with MOPP chemotherapy used in Hodgkin Disease).

Age at irradiation is especially important.[23] For example irradiation of the breast bud has a higher likelihood of inducing a breast cancer than RT in an older woman.

Treatment of radiation-induced malignancies is particularly difficult. The patient will often have been treated to RT tolerance doses, leaving little room for re-treatment.

Despite this, the risk of an induced malignancy is small (around 1–2% at ten years) and needs to be weighted against the potential benefits of RT.

4.4   *Radiation recall reactions*

Some drugs (especially chemotherapeutics) can cause a recurrence of the radiotherapy reaction in the irradiated tissue.[25] Skin rash is most commonly noted and occurs within eight days of application of the promoting stimulus. Some drugs (such as gemcitabine) seem to be particularly prone to result in this reaction.

5.   Summary of Key Points

- Acute effects are seen during and shortly after RT and are transient.
- Late effects are seen months to years following RT.
- RT effects on tissues are influenced by the total dose, dose per fraction, rate of delivery, concurrent chemotherapy, use of certain medications and pre-existing conditions.
- Acute and late radiation effects may mimic other non-cancer or treatment-related conditions.
- A number of strategies can reduce the acute and late RT effects, which include the use of certain radioprotectants and modern conformal RT techniques, such as IMRT.
- RT may cause infertility and cancer and therefore the benefits of RT need to be weighed by the potential long-term sequelae of treatment.

Acknowledgements

The authors wish to acknowledge the assistance of Jacki Doughton in the preparation of this manuscript.

References

1. E. J. Hall and A. J. Giaccia, *Radiobiology for the Radiologist*, 6th ed. (Lippincott Williams and Wilkins, 2005).
2. P. Rubin, L. Constine and J. Williams, Late effects of cancer treatment: Radiation and drug toxicity. In: *Principles and Practice of Radiation Oncology*, 3rd ed., eds. C. Perez and L. Brady (Lippincott-Raven Publishers, Philadelphia, 1998), pp. 155–211.
3. B. Emami, J. Lyman, A. Brown *et al.*, Tolerance of normal tissue to therapeutic irradiation, *Int. J. Radiat. Oncol. Biol. Phys.* **21**(1): 109–122 (1991).
4. M. T. Milano, L. S. Constine and P. Okunieff, Normal tissue tolerance dose metrics for radiation therapy of major organs, *Semin. Radiat. Oncol.* **17**(2): 131–140 (2007).
5. T. Holscher, S. M. Bentzen and M. Baumann, Influence of connective tissue diseases on the expression of radiation side effects: A systematic review, *Radiother. Oncol.* **78**(2): 123–130 (2006).
6. A. Trotti, A. D. Colevas, A. Setser *et al.*, CTCAE v3.0: Development of a comprehensive grading system for the adverse effects of cancer treatment, *Semin. Radiat. Oncol.* **13**(3): 176–181 (2003).
7. A. Trotti, Toxicity in head and neck cancer: A review of trends and issues. *Int. J. Radiat. Oncol. Biol. Phys.* **47**(1): 1–12 (2000).
8. D. M. Brizel, T. H. Wasserman, M. Henke *et al.*, Phase III randomized trial of amifostine as a radioprotector in head and neck cancer, *J. Clin. Oncol.* **18**(19): 3339–3345 (2000).
9. M. H. Bennett, J. Feldmeier, N. Hampson, R. Smee and C. Milross, Hyperbaric oxygen therapy for late radiation tissue injury, *Cochrane Database Syst. Rev.* 2005(3): CD005005.
10. E. Donovan, N. Bleakley, E. Denholm *et al.*, Randomised trial of standard 2D radiotherapy (RT) versus intensity modulated radiotherapy (IMRT) in patients prescribed breast radiotherapy, *Radiother. Oncol.* **82**(3): 254–264 (2007).
11. J. P. Pignol, I. Olivotto, E. Rakovitch *et al.*, A multicenter randomized trial of breast intensity-modulated radiation therapy to reduce acute radiation dermatitis, *J. Clin. Oncol.* **26**(13): 2085–2092 (2008).
12. M. Clarke, R. Collins, S. Darby *et al.*, Effects of radiotherapy and of differences in the extent of surgery for early breast cancer on local recurrence and 15-year survival: An overview of the randomised trials, *Lancet* **366**(9503): 2087–2106 (2005).

13. S. H. Giordano, Y. F. Kuo, J. L. Freeman, T. A. Buchholz, G. N. Hortobagyi and J. S. Goodwin, Risk of cardiac death after adjuvant radiotherapy for breast cancer, *J. Natl. Cancer Inst.* **97**(6): 419–424 (2005).

14. C. R. Correa, H. I. Litt, W. T. Hwang, V. A. Ferrari, L. J. Solin and E. E. Harris, Coronary artery findings after left-sided compared with right-sided radiation treatment for early-stage breast cancer, *J. Clin. Oncol.* **25**(21): 3031–3037 (2007).

15. P. A. Kupelian, T. R. Willoughby, C. A. Reddy, E. A. Klein and A. Mahadevan, Impact of image guidance on outcomes after external beam radiotherapy for localized prostate cancer, *Int. J. Radiat. Oncol. Biol. Phys.* **70**(4): 1146–1150 (2008).

16. K. Leiper and A. I. Morris, Treatment of radiation proctitis, *Clin. Oncol. (R. Coll. Radiol.)* **19**(9): 724–729 (2007).

17. P. E. Valk and W. P. Dillon, Radiation injury of the brain, *Am. J. Neuroradiol.* **12**(1): 45–62 (1991).

18. M. Brada, B. Rajan, D. Traish *et al.*, The long-term efficacy of conservative surgery and radiotherapy in the control of pituitary adenomas, *Clin. Endocrinol.* **38**(6): 571–578 (1993).

19. S. J. Lee, L. R. Schover, A. H. Partridge *et al.*, American Society of Clinical Oncology recommendations on fertility preservation in cancer patients, *J. Clin. Oncol.* **24**(18): 2917–2931 (2006).

20. R. Grundy, R. G. Gosden, M. Hewitt *et al.*, Fertility preservation for children treated for cancer (1): Scientific advances and research dilemmas, *Arch. Dis. Child.* **84**(4): 355–359 (2001).

21. J. Franklin, A. Pluetschow, M. Paus *et al.*, Second malignancy risk associated with treatment of Hodgkin's lymphoma: Meta-analysis of the randomised trials, *Ann. Oncol.* **17**(12): 1749–1760 (2006).

22. R. S. Lavey, N. L. Eby and L. R. Prosnitz, Impact on second malignancy risk of the combined use of radiation and chemotherapy for lymphomas, *Cancer* **66**(1): 80–88 (1990).

23. A. J. Swerdlow, J. A. Barber, G. V. Hudson *et al.*, Risk of second malignancy after Hodgkin's disease in a collaborative British cohort: The relation to age at treatment, *J. Clin. Oncol.* **18**(3): 498–509 (2000).

24. D. L. Preston, E. Ron, S. Tokuoka *et al.*, Solid cancer incidence in atomic bomb survivors: 1958–1998, *Radiat. Res.* **168**(1): 1–64 (2007).

25. M. Caloglu, V. Yurut-Caloglu, R. Cosar-Alas, M. Saynak, H. Karagol and C. Uzal, An ambiguous phenomenon of radiation and drugs: Recall reactions, *Onkologie* **30**(4): 209–214 (2007).

9

Oncological Emergencies: Diagnosis and Management

Desmond Yip
and Nicole Gorddard

Abstract

Patients with cancer may develop oncological emergencies affecting a range of organ systems, due to either the progression of their disease, or as a complication of their treatment. Recognition of common oncological emergencies is important, in order to institute appropriate acute management and to involve the appropriate subspecialties early. This chapter will discuss a number of common oncological emergencies and cover presentation, investigations and management. Further detailed discussion may be found in the subspecialty chapters.

Keywords: Hypercalcaemia, hyponatraemia, tumour lysis syndrome, raised intracranial pressure, spinal cord compression, SVC obstruction, massive haemoptysis, pericardial effusion, malignant bowel obstruction, febrile neutropenia.

1. Metabolic Emergencies

1.1 *Hypercalcaemia*

1.1.1 *Presentation*

The symptoms of hypercalcaemia may be non-specific and difficult to distinguish from symptoms that may otherwise be attributed to the underlying cancer and the treatments for it such as chemotherapy or analgesics. These symptoms include lethargy, confusion, mental dullness, nausea, thirst, constipation, anorexia and worsening bone pains. In extreme cases patients may be delirious or comatose. Clinically patients are often dehydrated, but the severity of symptoms does not always correlate with the serum calcium level. It is important to have a high index of suspicion for malignant hypercalcaemia and to order a serum calcium level corrected for albumin level.

1.1.2 *Causes*

The commonest cause of hypercalcaemia in the community is primary hyperparathyroidism and this may still be a cause of hypercalcaemia in a cancer patient. It is worthwhile looking back on previous biochemistry profiles, to see if a patient has had an elevated calcium level in the past, predating the present illness or diagnosis of malignancy. A serum PTH (parathyroid hormone) level may be useful to determine whether hypercalcaemia is due to primary hyperparathyroidism (it may be normal or high in the face of hypercalcaemia).

Common tumours that are associated with malignant hypercalcaemia are:

- breast cancer;
- non-small cell lung cancer;
- squamous cell cancers;
- myeloma;
- renal cell cancers;
- bladder cancer; and
- cervical cancer.

There are three main mechanisms of hypercalcaemia in malignancy:

1. Humoral hypercalcaemia of malignancy, due to production of PRTrP (parathyroid related peptide), which leads to increased bone resorption and inhibition of renal excretion of calcium.
2. Cytokine release by tumour, stimulating loss of calcium from bone (occurring more commonly in myeloma, breast cancer and NSCLC).
3. Elevated serum calcitriol (occurring in lymphomas and seminoma).

It is important to note that the presence of bone metastases is not a prerequisite for malignant hypercalcaemia to occur.

1.1.3 *Management*

Rehydration with normal saline is an important first step to treating malignant hypercalcaemia. This expands the intravascular volume, to bring the calcium down by dilution and also increases renal excretion. Judicious use of loop diuretics for the management of fluid overload in patients who have been rehydrated can be considered. Thiazides should be avoided, as they can increase calcium resorption. However, saline forced diuresis is not recommended, now that potent bisphosphonates are available, due to the risk of fluid overload, electrolyte imbalance and the requirement for close haemodynamic and biochemical monitoring. Phosphate levels may be low and replacement should be carried out.

Intravenous bisphosphonates (zoledronic acid, pamidronate and bondronate sodium) are the mainstay of treatment of malignant hypercalcaemia and can be given early in the course of management. These act on the osteoclasts to inhibit their function and have a maximum effect within 2–4 days. Care is required to adjust the dose in renal impairment according to manufacturers' guidelines.

In emergent cases of malignant hypercalcaemia, it may be desirable to lower serum calcium quickly and there is a role for parenteral administration of calcitonin in this setting, along with the above measures.

For calcitriol-mediated hypercalcaemia, such as in lymphomas and myeloma, corticosteroids can be quite effective in reducing the calcium level. They are safe in renal failure, although care needs to be taken in patients at risk of tumour lysis.

1.2 Hyponatraemia

1.2.1 Presentation

Patients may be asymptomatic or have non-specific symptoms of lethargy, dizziness and altered mental state. In severe cases patients may be stuporose, confused or experience seizures.

1.2.2 Causes

Hyponatraemia in a patient with cancer may have many possible causes and it is important to have a systematic approach in attempting to find the cause, rather than acting hastily and administering normal saline. Serum osmolality should be checked to exclude factitious causes such as hyperlipidaemia or hyperglycaemia. The next important step relies on clinical examination to determine the patient's fluid status:

1. Hypovolaemic: Patient is volume depleted or dehydrated. Causes in this situation could be due to fluid loss from vomiting, diarrhoea, poor oral intake, third space losses or diuretic therapy.
2. Hypervolaemic: These are the oedema states that include cardiac failure, cirrhosis (including haepatic failure) and nephrotic syndrome or renal failure where low effective blood volume leads to ADH release, producing hyponatraemia.
3. Euvolaemic: This is mainly seen in the setting of SIADH (Syndrome of Inappropriate Antidiuretic Hormone). This can be due to ectopic secretion of ADH by tumours such as small cell lung cancer and head and neck cancers. Intracerebral or intrathoracic lesions can also be associated with SIADH. Chemotherapy drugs such as cisplatin, vincristine, cyclophosphamide and ifosfamide may produce SIADH, as well as supportive care medications such as opiates, carbamazepine,

tricyclic antidepressants and selective serotonin reuptake inhibitors (SSRIs). Hypothyroidism and Addison's disease can also cause euvolaemic hyponatraemia.

1.2.3 Investigations

A useful investigation to determine the cause of hyponatraemia is measuring urinary sodium and osmolality. However this is only interpretable if patients are not on diuretic therapy. A urinary sodium of less than 20 mmol/L is indicative of an appropriate response to hyponatraemia and would be consistent with an appropriate ADH response, as seen in either hypovolaemic or hypervolaemic states. In the presence of euvolaemic state, normal renal and hepatic function, a urinary sodium of over 20 mmol/L is diagnostic of SIADH. The urine is also concentrated with an osmolality of >300 mOsm.

1.2.4 Management

The goal of treatment is to restore the sodium level to normal and achieve or maintain normovolaemia.

1. Hypovolaemic state. Hydration with normal saline. If patient has an elevated creatinine, the fractional excretion of sodium index can help to determine whether the renal impairment is prerenal (<1%), or due to acute tubular necrosis (>2%).
2. Hypervolaemic state. The underlying cause of the oedema state should be treated. For example hepatic impairment may be treated with supportive measures, such as protein restriction, lactulose and treatment of the cancer, if this is causing liver dysfunction. Cardiac failure may be managed by fluid restriction, vasodilators, pressor agents and ACE inhibitors.
3. Euvolaemic state (SIADH). Drugs that are associated with SIADH should be withdrawn and the patient fluid restricted (to a total daily fluid intake of 800–1200 ml, depending on severity). Consideration should be given to treatment of the underlying malignancy. In patients who do not respond to fluid restriction demeclocycline if available may be used to produce a nephrogenic diabetes insipidus to offload water. Oral urea (which has an osmotic diuretic effect) and loop diuretics may be used to

augment excretion of electrolyte — free water in the urine. Normal isotonic saline is not suitable, as it causes net water retention, thereby worsening the hyponatraemia. In cases of severely symptomatic hyponatraemia, hypertonic saline 3% can be used, with care not to increase the serum sodium each day by more that 10 mmol. Serum electrolytes will need to be monitored every 6–8 hours initially for patients receiving hypertonic saline, to ensure sodium is not corrected too fast. Rapid correction of the sodium may precipitate central pontine myelinolyis that can lead to pseudobulbar palsy and spastic quadriparesis. Selective vasopressin 2 receptor antagonists (known as vaptans) have been undergoing clinical development. Conivaptan and mozavaptan are available commercially in some countries and have a role in treatment of SIADH.[1]

1.3   *Tumour lysis syndrome*

Tumour lysis syndrome is usually seen in patients with rapidly proliferating bulky tumours which are treatment sensitive (predominantly haematological malignancies). The syndrome arises from rapid tumour lysis with release of intracellular breakdown products into the circulation that can lead to multisystem complications.

1.3.1 *Presentation*

Signs of tumour lysis after initiation of antitumour therapy include weakness, paralytic ileus and oliguria. Associated electrolyte disturbances are: hyperkalaemia, hyperuricaemia, hyperphosphataemia and hypocalcaemia. Oliguric renal failure may occur, as well as cardiac arrest due to the metabolic complications. Tumour lysis may also be an initial presentation of rapidly progressive cancers even before any treatment has taken place and may also be precipitated by the use of corticosteroids alone.

1.3.2 *Prevention*

Patients at risk of this complication should be admitted to hospital and precautions initiated to prevent tumour lysis. This includes intravenous hydration to maintain urine output of 2.5L–3L per day, urinary alkalinisation (to keep urinary pH ≥ 7) and commencement of the xanthine oxidase inhibitor allopurinol. Rasburicase (recombinant urate oxidase) given intravenously may be used in paediatric patients or in patients who are unable to tolerate allopurinol.[2] It has a rapid onset of action. It is however contraindicated in patients with glucose-6-phosphate dehydrogenase deficiency and is expensive.

Tumours which may be prone to tumour lysis include the following:

- small cell lung cancer;
- germ cell tumours;
- high grade lymphoma (eg Burkitt's);
- neuroblastoma;
- acute lymphocytic leukaemia; and
- chronic myeloid leukaemia.

Risk factors for tumour lysis include:

- high tumour proliferation rate;
- chemosensitivity;
- pre-existing renal impairment;
- high LDH level; and
- high serum uric acid.

1.3.3 Treatment

Treatment of tumour lysis is aimed at managing the metabolic abnormalities and preventing end organ damage. Hyperkalaemia should be managed with insulin/dextrose infusion and resonium. If ECG changes are present, calcium gluconate should be given intravenously, to protect the heart. Hypocalcaemia should be treated with calcium replacement. Allopurinol or rasburicase may be used to treat the hyperuricaemia. Maintaining hydration, adequate urine output and alkalinisation of the urine is necessary to prevent precipitation of the uric acid in the renal tubules, leading to renal failure. In severe cases of tumour lysis, renal dialysis may be required, especially if there is progressive hyperkalaemia.

2. Neurological Emergencies

2.1 *Raised intracranial pressure*

2.1.1 *Presentation*

Occasionally patients with primary CNS neoplasms or brain metastases will present with altered level of consciousness and significant neurological deficits associated with raised intracranial pressure. Raised intracranial pressure can result from the tumour growing within the rigid confines of the cranium, in addition to peri-tumoral oedema. Vasogenic oedema surrounds many brain tumours and contributes significantly to tumour-related morbidity and symptoms. The oedema results from disruption of the blood-brain barrier, which allows protein-rich fluid to accumulate in the extracellular space. Raised intracranial pressure may result in global brain symptoms including headache (classically worse in the mornings), altered mental state and drowsiness or even coma. It may result in the herniation syndromes, which can lead to respiratory arrest and death. Herniation of the uncus of the temporal lobe through the tentorium cerebelli can occur, as can cerebellar herniation through the foramen magnum.

2.1.2 *Physical examination*

Focal neurological signs, such as pupillary dilatation and ptosis (due to compression of the oculomotor cranial nerve) may occur in uncal herniation. Papilloedema may also indicate raised intracranial pressure. Coma, rising blood pressure and bradycardia are late signs of increased intracranial pressure.

2.1.3 *Investigations*

Urgent CT scan with intravenous contrast should be performed. Findings may be contrast enhancing lesions with significant surrounding vasogenic oedema. Sulcal effacement and midline shift may occur, due to mass effect and raised intracranial pressure. Effacement of the ventricles or hydrocephalus with a midline tumour and CSF obstruction may also be seen. Lumbar puncture should be avoided in the setting of raised intracranial pressure, because of the possibility of precipitating herniation.

The patient should be examined to exclude infection, narcotic toxicity or other causes of altered mental state. Full blood count and serum electrolyte panel should be performed, and urinalysis and chest X-ray may help exclude infection. Occasionally EEG may be helpful if status epilepticus needs to be excluded.

2.1.4 Causes

A rapidly growing glioblastoma multiforme may occasionally present with raised intracranial pressure, but more commonly this occurs late in the disease course, when the tumour has become refractory to treatment. Acute bleeding into a brain tumour may precipitate raised intracranial pressure, and occasionally dramatic increase in the amount of vasogenic oedema may occur associated with hyponatraemia and hypoosmolar syndromes. Rarely a patient commenced on oral temozolomide for glioblastoma multiforme may experience this syndrome, possibly caused by rapid tumour breakdown associated with necrosis, inflammation and increasing oedema.[3] Raised intracranial pressure has also been noted to complicate recurrent/refractory seizures.

2.1.5 *Management*

Synthetic glucocorticoids, such as dexamethasone are effective in reducing peritumoral oedema and hence intracranial pressure, and have an effect within 6–8 hours. Patients with mild symptoms and signs may be commenced on oral corticosteroids, usually 4–8 mg dexamethasone twice daily. Patients with severe symptoms and signs, such as obtundation or coma and signs of herniation need immediate intravenous glucocorticoid. Generally a loading dose of 10 mg dexamethasone is administered, followed by 4mg qid (or 8 mg bd). For patients already on chronic steroid therapy at the time of deterioration, a larger dose of dexamethasone may be required — and up to 100 mg total daily dose may be used. In some patients who have become comatose or have signs of herniation, osmotic diuretics, e.g. mannitol may also be used when a more acute effect is required (within minutes). The usual dose is 1g/kg, which may repeated at

0.25–0.5 g/kg every 6–8 hours as needed. Serum osmolality and sodium may increase and need to be monitored in this setting. Mannitol should be used with caution if there is renal insufficiency.[4] Rapid decrease in blood pressure should be avoided if there is significant hypertension, to maintain adequate cerebral perfusion pressure, and patients should be nursed with the bedhead elevated.

Urgent radiotherapy or surgery should be considered, depending on the clinical situation and previous treatment. Surgical resection when the patient is clinically stable may be considered for patients who have single or low volume resectable brain lesions; stereotactic radiosurgery may be another option. Any other systemic disease should be under reasonable control to contemplate surgical resection. Whole brain radiotherapy is an appropriate option for patients with multiple brain metastases.

2.2 Spinal cord compression

Malignant spinal cord compression is an oncological emergency that requires prompt recognition, investigation and intervention, to prevent severe morbidity arising from a patient developing permanent paralysis. Early contact with the radiation oncology and neurosurgical teams should be made whilst a patient is being worked up.

2.2.1 Presentation

The most common symptom of cord compression is back pain. The pain may be localised to the affected vertebra(e) or radicular pain from nerve compression. Weakness of the legs is the next most common symptom and patients may complain of a heaviness or strange sensation in the legs, with difficulty in walking. Sensory loss may occur usually after development of weakness. Autonomic involvement, such as bowel and bladder disturbances occur late and predict a poor prognosis for recovery.

2.2.2 Physical examination

Physical examination will usually detect weakness of the lower limbs in an upper motor neurone pattern. Reflexes will be brisk but may be difficult to elicit if patients have pre-existing peripheral neuropathy. Plantar reflexes will be upgoing. A sensory level corresponding to the level of compression may be present and cauda equina involvement can produce a saddle distribution of sensory loss.

2.2.3 Investigations

Magnetic resonance imaging (MRI) is the most sensitive modality for diagnosing spinal cord compression. The imaging protocol should incorporate the entire spine, as multiple levels of compression (some asymptomatic), may be present in up to half of patients. In institutions where MRI is not available, or where MRI is contraindicated due to cardiac pacemakers or metallic implants, a CT myelogram is an alternative examination.

2.2.4 Causes

Cord compression can occur through a vertebral metastasis eroding into the vertebral space, a paravertebral mass entering the epidural space though the intervertebral foramina, or direct metastasis into the epidural space. Damage to the cord is sustained by axonal damage and demyelination from pressure effect and also by vascular compromise.

The most common primary tumour types responsible for malignant spinal cord compression are:

- breast cancer;
- lung cancer;
- prostate cancer;
- lymphoma;
- renal cancer; and
- myeloma.

2.2.5 Management

Corticosteroids should be commenced promptly where there is a high clinical suspicion of malignant spinal cord compression, to reduce oedema around the cord. Steroids may relieve pain, but narcotic analgesics may be required to control it. The dosage of steroids is still controversial. A moderate dose of dexamethasone 10 mg, followed by 4 mg qid is reasonable if patients have stable neurological deficits, or are still able to walk. In rapidly progressive spinal cord compression and in patients who are unable to walk, high dose dexamethasone (100 mg loading and 96mg per day) may be considered, as a dose response has been demonstrated in animal models. Radiotherapy should be commenced urgently after diagnosis of malignant spinal cord compression for the best chance of neurological recovery.

A randomised trial has compared radical surgery plus postoperative radiotherapy to radiotherapy alone.[5] It was found that surgery conferred an advantage in the retention of ability to walk, recovery of walking ability and improved survival. This study excluded certain radiosensitive tumours, such as lymphoma, leukaemia, multiple myeloma and germ cell tumours. Entry criteria for this study were:

- true displacement of spinal cord;
- one area of compression;
- paraplegic for less than 48 hours;
- acceptable surgical risk; and
- expected survival of at least three months.

The factors above should be used to assess patients for consideration of urgent neurosurgical decompression. Surgery should be also be considered in the following situations:[6]

- unknown primary tumour (to obtain histopathology to make diagnosis);
- relapse after radiotherapy;
- progression on radiotherapy; or
- unstable spine or pathological fracture with retropulsion.

3. Febrile Neutropenia

Febrile neutropenia is an oncologic emergency, because of the potential for overwhelming bacterial sepsis in these patients who are relatively immunosuppressed due to recent chemotherapy. Neutropenic patients also have an increased incidence of viral infections especially human herpes viruses. Invasive fungal infection can occur, usually following a longer period of absolute neutropenia (generally ≥10 days). The incidence of febrile neutropenia correlates with increasing duration of neutropenia, as well as the degree of absolute neutropenia. The neutrophil nadir will often occur 7–10 days after administration of chemotherapy. The duration of neutropenia is generally short (≤5 days) following standard chemotherapy for solid tumours. More prolonged neutropenia is expected with high dose or myeloablative chemotherapy often used for haematologic malignancy.

3.1 *Presentation*

Clinical signs of infection may be very subtle, due to the lack of neutrophils and hence poor inflammatory response e.g. tenderness may be the only sign of infection, and poorly circumscribed mild erythema may indicate a significant soft tissue infection. Positive culture results are usually significant, even in the absence of inflammatory cells (which have been suppressed by recent treatment). Occasionally neutropenic patients will not mount a fever, especially if they have been on recent steroid medication. Neutropenic patients who are systemically unwell (e.g. hypotensive, hypothermic or confused), may also have underlying sepsis and should be treated empirically. Patients who have been on chronic steroid medication may have suppression of their pituitary-adrenal axis and have an inadequate stress response to sepsis. They generally require appropriate corticosteroid coverage in addition to antibiotics.

A generally accepted definition of febrile neutropenia is a single temperature of 38.3°C, or at least 38°C sustained for an hour, with an absolute neutrophil count of <500 μL^{-1}, or <1000 μL^{-1} and expected to fall further.

If a patient presents with a fever in the setting of recent chemotherapy, they should be assumed neutropenic until proven otherwise.

3.2 *Physical examination*

Thorough examination includes initially ensuring the patient is haemodynamically stable. Patients who are hypoxic or hypotensive are more likely to develop septic shock/multiple organ dysfunction and may require intensive care. The intensive care team should be involved early in the care of these patients.

Meticulous examination of the chest, cardiovascular system and abdomen to exclude infection is important. Central venous catheter infection predisposes patients to right sided endocarditis; fundi should also be examined to exclude Roth's spots, and nails examined for splinter haemorrhages. The central venous catheter insertion site should be carefully examined for any redness, tenderness or fluctuance, which may be suggestive of infection. The oropharyngeal mucosa and skin are examined for any signs of gingivitis, ulceration, skin lesions or rash. Breaks in the integrity of the skin and mucosa may be a portal of entry for infection. Peri-anal inspection and palpation are performed, to look for any signs of peri-anal sepsis, such as an anal tear or fissure, perianal tenderness, swelling or fluctuance. Digital rectal examination is best avoided in patients who may be neutropenic, as it may induce transient bacteraemia. Sinuses should be palpated for tenderness.

3.3   Investigations

An urgent full blood count should be sent off, as well as biochemistry, to include serum creatinine, electrolytes and liver function. Two sets of blood cultures should be collected for bacteria and fungi. If the patient has a central venous catheter *in situ*, blood cultures should be sent from a peripheral site, as well as a set of cultures drawn through the central catheter lumen/s. This may help determine whether the catheter itself is the source of sepsis. Urinalysis and culture should be performed, as well as a chest X-ray if there are any respiratory symptoms or signs. Bacterial and viral throat culture should be requested if there is erythema or ulceration of the oropharynx. Any sputum should be sent for culture and skin lesions swabbed.

Imaging with ultrasound or CT scanning are helpful if an abscess, e.g. buttock/perineal abscess, are clinically suspected. Surgical consultation is important, if patients have evidence of an abscess which is likely to require surgical drainage. It should be noted that in cases of extreme neutropenia pus formation may not occur due to the lack of neutrophils and an abscess may not become evident until white cell recovery starts to occur.

3.4   *Management*

Both gram positive and gram negative infections are relatively common as the source of neutropenic fever. Bacterial transmigration may occur through the gut mucosa damaged due to recent chemotherapy. This probably accounts for many of the gram negative/coliform infections. Gram positive organisms are increasing in incidence, and account for the majority of bloodstream infections.[7-9] This may be partly due to increased use of central venous catheters/line sepsis, as well as some use of quinolones for prophylaxis of febrile neutropenia. Gram negative bacilli remain the most common cause of infections other than bacteraemia.[9] Incidence of polymicrobial infection is also significant, so even if there is a source of infection clinically, initial broad spectrum antibiotics are indicated rather than a more targeted approach for high risk patients. Antibiotics may then be tailored when culture results are available. Only 30–40% of patients will have a positive culture result, however, and it is likely that some of these patients do not have invasive infection, but transient bacteraemia. Occasionally the fever will be non-infectious in nature, e.g. tumour fever or a drug reaction.

3.4.1   *Initial management*

Initial treatment for febrile neutropenia usually includes broad spectrum intravenous antibiotics and hospitalisation. Intravenous fluid and oxygen support may also be required. Oral antibiotics have also been proven effective in patients with low risk febrile neutropenia, which will be discussed later. There are several choices for initial empiric therapy for patients with febrile neutropenia. The optimal regimen is not clear, and in addition effectiveness of antibiotics may vary among institutions according to local infection patterns, prevalent bacteria and antibiotic susceptibilities. This should be taken into account when an empiric regimen is selected for a particular institution.

Options for the empiric treatment of febrile neutropenia:

Monotherapy:

- 4th generation cephalosporins, e.g. ceftazidime, cefepime; or
- carbapenem (imipenem/meropenem).

Dual Therapy:

- extended spectrum penicillin, e.g. ticarcillin/clavulanate or piperacillin/tazobactam + aminoglycoside, e.g. gentamicin;
- 4th generation cephalosporin, e.g. ceftazidime or cefepime + aminoglycoside; or
- extended spectrum penicillin or cephalosporin + quinolone (ciprofloxacin).

These regimens all include broad spectrum gram negative coverage. *Esherichia coli*, *Klebsiella* and *Pseudomonas* species are common bacterial isolates in febrile neutropenia, and are well covered by all of these empiric regimens. Gram positive coverage is incomplete, but many gram positive infections are more indolent (but not *Staphylococcus aureus*). More specific gram positive coverage with the addition of vancomycin is not routinely justified and does not improve outcomes. Patients who present septic with hypotension may be infected with a resistant *Staphylococcus aureus* however, and should receive vancomycin as part of initial treatment. In addition to patients who are haemodynamically unstable, patients with suspected intravenous line infection, those with severe mucositis, and with a history of methicillin resistant staphylococcal infection or penicillin resistant streptococcal infection should also receive empiric vancomycin. Quinolones, or vancomycin and aztreonam are treatment options for patients with B-lactam allergy.

3.4.2 *Antibiotic treatment duration*

Patients with febrile neutropenia will generally require 7–14 days of antibiotic treatment. The shorter course of antibiotics may be appropriate in clinically well patients who have evidence of neutrophil recovery. It is desirable to have evidence of neutrophil recovery (>500 cells/μL^{-1}) for 48 hours before cessation of antibiotics. Some clinicians will stop antibiotic therapy in low risk patients who are culture negative once they have been afebrile for 48 hours, with neutrophil recovery. Antibiotics may be altered according to culture results to provide more specific cover. It is preferable to avoid frequent antibiotic changes in the first 72 hours, for patients who are clinically stable and without good clinical indication, e.g. positive culture results.

3.4.3 Monitoring response to treatment

Patients should be carefully examined daily, to detect developing clinical signs of infection. As neutrophils recover, signs of infection may become more evident, and pulmonary infiltrates may appear on chest X-ray. Vital signs should be regularly monitored as occasionally sudden clinical deterioration will occur. Blood tests should be performed at least every three days,[10] to evaluate for bone marrow recovery as well as to monitor organ function and antibiotic levels as appropriate. Systemic inflammatory markers (CRP and ESR) may be measured to monitor response to treatment. Levels of procalcitonin, C-reactive protein, serum amyloid A, and interleukins have been shown to be predictive of invasive infection and bacteraemia, and prognostic for infectious complications.[11,12] Their routine use is not recommended however, and monitoring clinical parameters is more important.

3.4.4 Management of persistent febrile neutropenia

If fever persists, patients should be carefully re-examined for a source of infection, and further sets of blood cultures sent. Imaging, e.g. CT scans, may be appropriate to exclude an infectious collection, especially if there is focal discomfort, and patients should have serial chest X-rays, to ensure there is no infiltrate developing. High resolution chest CT may be useful to exclude pulmonary disease. If there are pulmonary infiltrates, bronchoscopy with washings and biopsy should be considered.

Any indwelling device which may be a nidus for infection should be reviewed, e.g. biliary or ureteric stents may need changing, or central venous catheters may need to be removed. If there is a suspicion of central venous catheter infection, antibiotics should be given directly through the central catheter, and sometimes the catheter will be salvaged. However, if there is a history of rigors and hypotension when the catheter is used (septic flush), the catheter should not be accessed and needs to be removed. Septic emboli, periport or catheter tunnel infection, persistent fever and ongoing bacteraemia are further indications for catheter removal.[8]

Vancomycin may be added at any stage if gram positive cocci are detected on culture, whilst awaiting bacterial identification and sensitivities.[7-9] Vancomycin is often empirically added if there is ongoing fever and neutropenia after 3 days with no obvious source, although this approach is somewhat controversial.[13]

Antifungal treatment is generally added if patients remain febrile and neutropenic after five days, usually with amphotericin B. The newer antifungal agents voriconazole or caspofungin are also effective in this setting.[7,8,13] In patients with persistent fever and neutropenia, opportunistic infections e.g. with atypical mycobacteria should be considered. *Pneumocystis jiroveci* (*carinii*) pneumonia may occur in patients on chronic steroid therapy and this requires treatment with cotrimoxazole or pentamidine if sulphur allergic.

Antiviral medication is generally only used when viral infection is evident clinically or with laboratory confirmation.[8]

3.4.5 *Management of neutropenia with septicaemic shock*

Febrile neutropenia is a morbid and sometimes fatal condition hence the need for prompt treatment. Complication rates including death occur in 10–40% of febrile neutropenic patients in unselected series of patients. Chemotherapy-induced febrile neutropenia is a form of treatment toxicity which is reversible and generally should be managed aggressively. Patients who develop multiple organ dysfunction or respiratory failure may require admission to intensive care, inotrope support and short-term mechanical ventilation. Many of these patients will fully recover with appropriate treatment.

3.4.6 *Management of low risk neutropenia*

It is now clear that patients with febrile neutropenia are a heterogeneous group of patients, and a subset of patients at low risk of complications (≤5%) and death (≤2%) can be identified. These patients may not require such intensive or prolonged treatment, and have been successfully managed with broad-spectrum oral antibiotics as inpatients.[11,14]

There are different definitions of low risk febrile neutropenia. Generally they are younger, fitter patients, who have developed febrile neutropenia as an outpatient, and whose tumour is responding to treatment. Patients with solid tumours and a short duration of neutropenia are generally at lower risk of complications than patients who have received myeloablative therapy. Absence of hypotension, hypoxia and renal failure are important. They should not have underlying chronic obstructive pulmonary disease, evidence of pneumonia, or venous catheter infection. The Multinational Association for Supportive Care in Cancer (MASCC) risk-index score is an accepted and validated tool for assessing febrile neutropenic patients at low risk of complications.[10,15] In this model, patients who score at least 21 are at low risk of complications and death (see Table 1).

Low risk febrile neutropenic patients may potentially be managed with broad spectrum oral antibiotics and an early discharge plan if they are clinically stable and without evidence of bacteraemia or catheter associated infection.

Oral amoxicillin/clavulanate and ciprofloxacin are effective treatment for low risk febrile neutropenia and have been shown to

Table 1.   Scoring system (MASCC risk-index score).

Characteristic	Weight
Burden of illness: no or mild symptoms	5
No hypotension	5
No chronic obstructive pulmonary disease	4
Solid tumour or no previous fungal infection	4
No dehydration	3
Burden of illness: moderate symptoms	3
Outpatient status	3
Age <60 years	2

Note: Points attributed to the variable "burden of illness" are not cumulative. The maximum theoretical score is therefore 26.

be as effective as initial intravenous antibiotics for low-risk patients when managed on an inpatient basis.[11,14] One approach may be to commence low risk febrile neutropenic patients on oral antibiotics at the time of hospital admission, with a view to early discharge after 24–48 hours of observation if the patients are clinically stable and culture results are available and satisfactory.[16,17] Whether these patients can be managed entirely as outpatients from diagnosis is more contentious and is the subject of ongoing research. This approach is not generally recommended and should be limited to centres with expertise in managing such patients as well as excellent outpatient support.

3.4.7 Use of colony stimulating factors

White blood cell colony stimulating factors (G-CSF or GM-CSF) are known to shorten the duration of neutropenia associated with chemotherapy. They are used prophylactically to reduce the incidence of febrile neutropenia for chemotherapy regimens known to carry a substantial risk ($\geq20\%$) of developing febrile neutropenia. Their role in established febrile neutropenia is not clear, however. Colony stimulating factors are not generally recommended in the routine treatment of febrile neutropenia, as they have not been shown to reduce mortality.[8,18,19] They have been shown to shorten the duration of hospitalisation slightly, but whether this is cost effective, or clinically significant is unclear.

While not recommended for routine treatment of established febrile neutropenia, they may play a role in the management of high-risk patients, e.g. patients who are hypotensive, or requiring intensive care, those with pneumonia, or expected to have a prolonged duration of absolute neutropenia.[18,19] Daily filgrastim or lenograstim may be used in this situation, often until the neutrophil count is >5000 μL^{-1} for two consecutive days.

Patients who have experienced febrile neutropenia with chemotherapy are at increased risk of recurrent infection if their treatment continues without modification. Consideration should be given to use of white blood cell colony stimulating factors if not already in usage, or dosage reduction.

4. Superior Vena Caval Obstruction

Superior vena caval obstruction is often not considered as a true medical emergency. There is often sufficient time to perform appropriate investigations to determine a histological diagnosis in patients presenting with this as an initial manifestation of malignancy, in order to guide treatment.

4.1 *Presentation*

SVC obstruction can present with symptoms of dyspnoea, facial fullness, cough and headache. Symptoms may come on gradually or acutely.

4.2 *Physical examination*

Facial and upper trunk or arm swelling is common, with plethora of these areas. The jugular veins may be distended, as well as collateral veins on the chest wall, indicating subacute onset. Conjunctival injection and chemosis can be present. The patient should be examined for cervical lymphadenopathy.

4.3 *Investigation*

CT imaging of the chest with intravenous contrast should be performed to confirm a diagnosis of SVC obstruction. It will provide information as to the level of the obstruction and provide information as to its cause. In primary presentations, pathological diagnosis needs to be made by sputum cytology, bronchoscopy or fine needle biopsy of any accessible lesions, such as lymph nodes or intrathoracic masses. Tumour marker levels may give a clue as to the primary tumour.

4.4 *Causes*

SVC obstruction occurs due to extrinsic compression of the vessel by intrathoracic tumours or lymph nodes. Common tumours that are responsible for SVC obstruction include:

- small cell lung cancer;
- non small cell cancer;

- lymphoma;
- breast carcinoma
- germ cell tumour; or
- thymic carcinomas.

SVC obstruction may also occur due to thrombosis of the vessel.

4.5   Management

Elevation of the head and steroids may be used to provide some relief of symptoms. In chemotherapy-sensitive tumours, such as small cell lung cancer, germ cell tumour and lymphomas, rapid relief of obstruction may be obtained by initiating systemic therapy. Radiotherapy is another option, especially in less chemotherapy sensitive tumours. Insertion of a percutaneous venal caval stent should be considered in patients who are very symptomatic or distressed from SVC obstruction, especially if they are still being worked up for a diagnosis. This procedure usually provides rapid relief of symptoms. If the cause of obstruction is thrombosis, anticoagulation should be initiated, along with removal of any venous catheter.[20]

5.   Massive Haemoptysis

Massive haemoptysis is often defined as haemoptysis >300 mL/24 hours, or haemoptysis requiring intubation. It is a life-threatening condition, with a significant mortality rate (10–30%). Bronchogenic carcinoma or pulmonary metastases may cause massive haemoptysis. Bronchiectasis, pulmonary infections or infarction are other common causes of significant haemoptysis.

5.1   Investigations

The source of bleeding needs to be ascertained. Chest imaging with chest X-ray or CT scan should be performed. Fiberoptic bron-choscopy is a more accurate method of determining the site of pulmonary haemorrhage and may also be used for therapeutic effect.

5.2 Management

Patients with massive haemoptysis should be managed in an intensive care setting and may require intubation. A double lumen endotracheal tube may be required in some emergent situations, to maintain the airway and isolate the bleeding lung. Respiratory, interventional radiology and often thoracic surgical consultation are important. Good intravenous access needs to be secured and patients generally require intravenous fluid support and blood transfusion. Underlying coagulopathy or thrombocytopenia should be excluded as exacerbating factors, and anticoagulant or antiplatelet medications ceased.

Instillation of adrenaline may be helpful and cold saline lavage or balloon tamponade are also sometimes employed. Endoscopic laser treatment may also be used in centres with expertise in this procedure.

Bronchial artery embolisation using polyvinyl alcohol particles and/or gelfoam is a radiologic intervention which is minimally invasive and effective, and is gaining popularity. Surgical resection of the bleeding site with lobectomy or pneumonectomy is now generally reserved for bleeding not amenable or responsive to bronchial artery embolisation.[21–23]

6. Pericardial Tamponade

6.1 Presentation

Accumulation of the pericardial effusion may be slow, with insidious onset of symptoms that may be non-specific. Dyspnoea, cough, fatigue and chest pain or chest heaviness are common presenting symptoms, oedema may also be seen. A large (or rapidly developing) pericardial effusion may restrict filling of the heart causing pericardial tamponade. Untreated pericardial tamponade may result in cardiac failure and cardiac arrest. Dyspnoea and orthopnoea are common symptoms of pericardial tamponade.

6.2 Physical examination

Findings on examination may include tachycardia, raised jugular venous pressure, presence of pulsus paradoxus, narrowed pulse pressure, hypotension and muffled or distant heart sounds. Patients may also have signs of low cardiac output, e.g. peripheral vasoconstriction, poor capillary refill, or diaphoresis. It is important to distinguish pericardial tamponade from cardiac failure, due to their management options.

6.3   Investigations

The ECG is generally of low voltage in pericardial tamponade. Chest X-ray will classically show an enlarged cardiac silhouette, with a globular water-bottle appearance.

Echocardiography is the most important diagnostic test if cardiac tamponade is suspected clinically. This should confirm the presence of significant effusion in the pericardial sac; right atrial and right ventricular collapse are the most common echocardiographic findings. CT and MRI may be helpful to evaluate the pericardial and pleural space, e.g. the presence of loculations.

6.4   Causes

Malignant pericardial effusion may occur in advanced malignancy, due to direct tumour invasion of the pericardium or from lymphatic or haematogenous spread. It is most often seen in lung cancer, breast cancer and lymphoma/leukaemias. Occasionally idiopathic pericardial effusion will occur, or it will result from treatment, e.g. mediastinal radiation. It is often accompanied by malignant pleural effusion. Only rarely will a malignant pericardial effusion be the initial presentation of an extracardiac malignancy.

6.5   Management

Patients who have asymptomatic or minimally symptomatic pericardial effusion may be managed conservatively. More aggressive antineoplastic therapy may be effective. Patients who have evidence of pericardial tamponade however, require urgent treatment, unless this is medically inappropriate.

Pericardiocentesis usually provides immediate relief of symptoms and improved haemodynamics. Cytology should be requested, as cytology-positive malignant pericardial effusion carries a worse prognosis, with a median survival of only a few months.

The recurrence rate is high after simple pericardiocentesis, and for most patients a more definitive surgical or medical treatment should be considered. Subxiphoid or transthoracic pericardiostomy (pericardial window) may be the preferred treatment, with partial pericardiectomy reserved for patients with a more favourable overall prognosis (life expectancy >1 year). Prolonged pericardial catheter drainage, sometimes with the injection of sclerosing agents has also been used, but seems to have a higher complication and recurrence rate than formal pericardiostomy.[24,25]

7. Malignant Bowel Obstruction

Bowel obstruction as a complication is a common scenario in intra-abdominal tumours and may be responsible for great morbidity. Management often requires multidisciplinary input.

7.1 Presentation

Symptoms include nausea, vomiting, constipation, abdominal distension and pain.

7.2 Physical examination

This will give important clues as to the possible causes of the obstruction and also the level of obstruction. Absent bowel sounds can indicate ileus, whereas tinkling bowel sounds would be consistent with obstruction. Hernial orifices need to be checked for bowel incarceration and a rectal examination performed, to exclude low faecal impaction. Fluid status should be determined as patients are often dehydrated. Clinical evidence of shock or peritonism should alert the clinician to the possibility of a perforated viscus.

7.3 Investigations

Full blood count and electrolytes should be performed. Plain abdominal X-ray can confirm bowel obstruction, with the presence of fluid levels in dilated loops of bowel. Air under the diaphragm would indicate the presence of visceral perforation. The film may show faecal loading or impaction. A small bowel series or CT scan with oral contrast may locate a transition point indicating the level or levels of obstruction in the bowel.

7.4 Causes

Cancer can cause bowel obstruction in three ways: luminal obstruction, extrinsic compression of the bowel or neurological involvement of the mesenteric plexus, affecting bowel motility. It should never be assumed that the obstruction is solely due to cancer. Electrolyte disturbances leading to ileus, constipation producing faecal impaction, incarcerated hernias and post-operative or radiation-induced adhesions or strictures can be responsible for the presentation and may be readily reversible.

7.5 Management

The patient should be rehydrated with intravenous fluids and the electrolytes corrected. A nasogastric tube on drainage or suction may provide good palliation if there is vomiting or significant gaseous distension of the bowel. Enemas or suppositories can be used to treat constipation. Early surgical consultation should be initiated if there is evidence of localised mechanical obstruction in patients who are considered appropriate for surgery. If definitive surgery is not possible, surgical consultation may still be worthwhile. Some patients will receive good palliative relief from a defunctioning stoma to bypass a malignant obstruction, or a venting gastrostomy to prevent refractory nausea and vomiting if the former is not feasible.

8. Conclusion

Clinical deterioration in a cancer patient may result from complications of the cancer itself and/or its treatment, and may cause a complex array of clinical syndromes. Careful clinical evaluation and selected investigations are crucial to determine the cause of decline. Pressure or obstructive syndromes (e.g. spinal cord compression, malignant bowel obstruction, raised intracranial pressure) are fairly common complications of malignancy, as are metabolic emergencies and febrile neutropenia. These complications are often reversible with appropriate treatment, and optimal treatment may require a multidisciplinary approach. Especially in the pressure-related syndromes, systemic treatment of the malignancy and surrounding oedema is likely to be helpful, but the incorporation of surgery or radiotherapy may significantly improve local tumour control, and provide a more prompt response to treatment. Interventional radiologists are increasingly part of the multidisciplinary team managing cancer, e.g. for stenting vessels, and bronchial artery embolisation. Even in advanced incurable malignancy active treatment of complications may provide substantial palliative benefit to maintain quality of life in the time remaining and should be considered.

References

1. G. Decaux, V2-antagonists for the treatment of hyponatraemia, *Nephrol. Dial. Transplant.* **22**: 1853–1855 (2007).
2. B. T. Yim, R. P. Sims-McCallum and P. H. Chong, Rasburicase for the treatment and prevention of hyperuricemia, *Ann. Pharmacother.* **37**: 1047–1054 (2003).
3. M. A. Rosenthal, D. L. Ashley and L. Cher, Temozolomide-induced flare in high-grade gliomas: A new clinical entity, *Intern. Med. J.* **32**: 346–348 (2002).
4. P. Y. Wen, D. Schiff, S. Kesari, J. Drappatz, D. C. Gigas and L. Doherty, Medical management of patients with brain tumors, *J. Neurooncol.* **80**: 313–332 (2006).
5. R. A. Patchell, P. A. Tibbs, W. F. Regine, R. Payne, S. Saris, R. J. Kryscio, M. Mohiuddin and B. Young, Direct decompressive surgical resection in the treatment of spinal cord compression caused by metastatic cancer: A randomised trial, *Lancet* **366**: 643–648 (2005).
6. J. S. Cole and R. A. Patchell, Metastatic epidural spinal cord compression, *Lancet Neurol.* **7**: 459–466 (2008).
7. A. M. Bal and I. M. Gould, Empirical antimicrobial treatment for chemotherapy-induced febrile neutropenia, *Int. J. Antimicrob. Agents* **29**: 501–509 (2007).
8. W. T. Hughes, D. Armstrong, G. P. Bodey, E. J. Bow, A. E. Brown, T. Calandra, R. Feld, P. A. Pizzo, K. V. Rolston, J. L. Shenep and

L. S. Young, 2002 guidelines for the use of antimicrobial agents in neutropenic patients with cancer, *Clin. Infect. Dis.* **34**: 730–751 (2002).

9. K. V. Rolston, Challenges in the treatment of infections caused by gram-positive and gram-negative bacteria in patients with cancer and neutropenia, *Clin. Infect. Dis.* **40**(Suppl. 4): 246–252 (2005).

10. J. Klastersky, M. Paesmans, E. B. Rubenstein, M. Boyer, L. Elting, R. Feld, J. Gallagher, J. Herrstedt, B. Rapoport, K. Rolston and J. Talcott, The Multinational Association for Supportive Care in Cancer risk index: A multinational scoring system for identifying low-risk febrile neutropenic cancer patients, *J. Clin. Oncol.* **18**: 3038–3051 (2000).

11. A. Freifeld, D. Marchigiani, T. Walsh, S. Chanock, L. Lewis, J. Hiemenz, S. Hiemenz, J. E. Hicks, V. Gill, S. M. Steinberg and P. A. Pizzo, A double-blind comparison of empirical oral and intravenous antibiotic therapy for low-risk febrile patients with neutropenia during cancer chemotherapy, *N. Engl. J. Med.* **341**: 305–311 (1999).

12. A. Uys, B. L. Rapoport, H. Fickl, P. W. Meyer and R. Anderson, Prediction of outcome in cancer patients with febrile neutropenia: Comparison of the Multinational Association of Supportive Care in Cancer risk-index score with procalcitonin, C-reactive protein, serum amyloid A, and interleukins-1beta, -6, -8 and -10, *Eur. J. Cancer Care* **16**: 475–483 (2007).

13. C. Viscoli and E. Castagnola, Planned progressive antimicrobial therapy in neutropenic patients, *Br. J. Haematol.* **102**: 879–888 (1998).

14. W. V. Kern, A. Cometta, R. De Bock, J. Langenaeken, M. Paesmans and H. Gaya, Oral versus intravenous empirical antimicrobial therapy for fever in patients with granulocytopenia who are receiving cancer chemotherapy. International Antimicrobial Therapy Cooperative Group of the European Organization for Research and Treatment of Cancer, *N. Engl. J. Med.* **341**: 312–318 (1999).

15. A. Uys, B. L. Rapoport and R. Anderson, Febrile neutropenia: A prospective study to validate the Multinational Association of Supportive Care of Cancer (MASCC) risk-index score, *Support. Care Cancer* **12**: 555–560 (2004).

16. C. Girmenia, E. Russo, I. Carmosino, M. Breccia, F. Dragoni, R. Latagliata, S. Mecarocci, S. G. Morano, C. Stefanizzi and G. Alimena, Early hospital discharge with oral antimicrobial therapy in patients with hematologic malignancies and low-risk febrile neutropenia, *Ann. Hematol.* **86**: 263–270 (2007).

17. H. E. Innes, D. B. Smith, S. M. O'Reilly, P. I. Clark, V. Kelly and E. Marshall, Oral antibiotics with early hospital discharge compared with in-patient intravenous antibiotics for low-risk febrile neutropenia in patients with cancer: A prospective randomised controlled single centre study, *Br. J. Cancer* **89**: 43–49 (2003).

18. O. A. Clark, G. H. Lyman, A. A. Castro, L. G. Clark and B. Djulbegovic, Colony-stimulating factors for chemotherapy-induced febrile neutropenia: A meta-analysis of randomized controlled trials, *J. Clin. Oncol.* **23**: 4198–4214 (2005).

19. T. J. Smith, J. Khatcheressian, G. H. Lyman, H. Ozer, J. O. Armitage, L. Balducci, C. L. Bennett, S. B. Cantor, J. Crawford, S. J. Cross, G. Demetri, C. E. Desch, P. A. Pizzo, C. A. Schiffer, L. Schwartzberg, M. R. Somerfield, G. Somlo, J. C. Wade, J. L. Wade, R. J. Winn, A. J. Wozniak and A. C. Wolff, 2006 update of recommendations for the use of white blood cell growth factors: An evidence-based clinical practice guideline, *J. Clin. Oncol.* **24**: 3187–3205 (2006).

20. L. D. Wilson, F. C. Detterbeck and J. Yahalom. Clinical practice. Superior vena cava syndrome with malignant causes, *N. Engl. J. Med.* **356**: 1862–1869 (2007).

21. M. Fartoukh, A. Khalil, L. Louis, M. F. Carette, B. Bazelly, J. Cadranel, C. Mayaud and A. Parrot, An integrated approach to diagnosis and management of severe haemoptysis in patients admitted to the intensive care unit: A case series from a referral centre. *Respir. Res.* **8**: 11 (2007).

22. T. W. Lee, S. Wan, D. K. Choy, M. Chan, A. Arifi and A. P. Yim, Management of massive hemoptysis: A single institution experience, *Ann. Thorac. Cardiovasc. Surg.* **6**: 232–235 (2000).

23. T. H. Ong and P. Eng, Massive hemoptysis requiring intensive care, *Intensive Care Med.* **29**: 317–320 (2003).

24. C. A. Cullinane, I. B. Paz, D. Smith, N. Carter and F. W. Grannis Jr., Prognostic factors in the surgical management of pericardial effusion in the patient with concurrent malignancy, *Chest* **125**: 1328–1334 (2004).

25. R. J. Laham, D. J. Cohen, R. E. Kuntz, D. S. Baim, B. H. Lorell and M. Simons, Pericardial effusion in patients with cancer: Outcome with contemporary management strategies, *Heart* **75**: 67–71 (1996).

10

Managing Cancer in Pregnancy

Belinda E. Kiely
and Kelly-Anne Phillips

Abstract

Cancer is diagnosed in about 1 in 1000 pregnant women. The incidence is predicted to rise, as women increasingly delay their pregnancies until later in life. The most frequent cancers diagnosed in pregnancy are cervical, breast, leukaemia, Hodgkin lymphoma, malignant melanoma and thyroid. The optimal management of cancer in pregnancy requires a multidisciplinary team approach, with involvement of the medical oncologist, obstetrician, neonatologist, surgeon, radiation oncologist, allied health staff, general practitioner, nursing staff, pathologist, radiologist and pharmacist. Treatment should be carefully tailored to the specific circumstances of each case. The health and welfare of both the mother and the foetus must be considered, but these parties may have conflicting interests, particularly regarding the use of chemotherapy. Depending on the type of cancer and the stage at diagnosis, delaying chemotherapy until after delivery is not always an option and chemotherapy is often delivered during pregnancy. There is a paucity of prospective studies regarding diagnosis and treatment of cancer in pregnancy; however, there are numerous reports of the safe use of chemotherapy during the second and third trimesters. This chapter focuses on managing breast cancer and lymphoma during pregnancy.

Keywords: Pregnancy, cancer, chemotherapy, foetus.

1.   Overview

The occurrence of cancer in pregnant women is rare, with cancer complicating approximately 1 in 1000 pregnancies.[1,2] The most common female cancers are also those most frequently seen during the reproductive age of a woman. Cervical cancer, breast cancer, leukaemia, Hodgkin lymphoma, malignant melanoma and thyroid are the most frequently diagnosed gestational malignancies (Table 1).[1,3] Between 0.07% and 0.1% of all malignant tumours are diagnosed during pregnancy.[4] Because the risk of most cancers increases with age, the incidence of pregnancy-related cancers is predicted to rise, as women increasingly delay pregnancy into the later reproductive years. There are no strict guidelines for the management of cancer in pregnancy, but case series and reports provide information to guide treatment in a way that maximises the benefit to the mother, but minimises harm to the foetus and newborn. It is not always possible to delay cancer treatment until after delivery and treatment such as chemotherapy is often delivered during pregnancy. This chapter focuses on breast cancer and lymphoma because these are the cancers most likely to require chemotherapy during pregnancy and are therefore most likely to create dilemmas in management for oncologists.

Table 1.   Distribution of cancer in pregnancy.

Site	Proportion of cancers in pregnant women (%)
Cervix	26
Breast	26
Leukaemia	15
Lymphoma	10
Melanoma	8
Thyroid	4
Miscellaneous	11

Table modified and reproduced with permission from Pavlidis.[4]

2. Principles of Managing Cancer in Pregnancy

2.1 *Safety of chemotherapy in pregnancy*

Before starting any chemotherapy, an ultrasound of the foetus should be performed, to ensure the foetus appears normal and to confirm gestational age. Evaluation of foetal growth should be performed before every subsequent cycle of chemotherapy.

The risk of foetal malformation or death is dependent upon the stage of foetal development, the agent utilised, and the foetal dose of that agent. The first trimester is the most critical period for chemotherapeutic drug exposure, as implantation (weeks 1 to 2 after conception) and embryogenesis (weeks 3 to 8 after conception) proceed.[1] Cytotoxic chemotherapy during the first trimester should be avoided, due to its high potential for teratogenicity during organogenesis.[1,5] There are data supporting the safe administration of some chemotherapy agents during the second and third trimesters. Case series have reported a 10–20% rate of congenital malformations when chemotherapy is delivered in the first trimester, compared with a to 1–3% rate of malformations for second and third trimester exposure.[6] The rate of congenital malformations in the general population not exposed to chemotherapy is 2–3%.[7]

The major manifestations of first trimester chemotherapy exposure are spontaneous abortions during implantation and major morphological abnormalities during embryogenesis. Structures such as the limbs and palate have limited periods of vulnerability during embryogenesis, while others, such as the gonads and the central nervous system continue to develop and may be affected throughout all phases of embryogenesis, foetal development, and growth.[1,8] Despite this, the greatest risks of harm, and especially the risks of major malformation are over by the completion of the first trimester.

Foetal adverse effects following exposure to chemotherapy during the second and third trimesters are more subtle. The most common complications from individual case series include low birth weight, pre-term delivery, transient infant leucopaenia, transient tachypnoea of the newborn and intrauterine growth restriction.[6,8,9] Other potential toxic effects include a stillborn foetus, impaired functional development, diminished neurologic and/or intellectual function, diminished learning capability, decreased gonadal and reproductive function, mutagenesis of germ-line tissue, and carcinogenesis.[10] The quantitative data on these risks is limited.

2.2 Categorising risk of drugs in pregnancy

Drugs in pregnancy have been assigned a risk level (A, B, C, D or X) according to definitions provided by the Australian Drug Evaluation Committee (ADEC) (Table 2).[11] Most chemotherapeutic agents fall into the C or D categories. These drugs can be given in pregnancy, when the potential benefit justifies the potential risk to the foetus.

2.3 Breast feeding and cancer drugs

No chemotherapy drugs are proven safe during breast feeding. Many cytotoxic drugs, especially the alkylating agents, are excreted in breast milk. Neonatal neutropaenia has been reported in an infant breastfed during maternal treatment with cyclophosphamide.[12] Breast feeding is therefore contraindicated if chemotherapy is to continue post-partum. Women receiving tamoxifen should also be advised not to breastfeed.

2.4 Long term implications of chemotherapy for the child

The major *theoretical* long term concerns for children whose mothers received chemotherapy during pregnancy include physical development, neurodevelopment, heart function, secondary malignancies and infertility. Reviewing the data available, there does not appear to be a significant risk of these long term effects, especially following second and third trimester exposures.

A large study with a median follow up of 18.7 years reported on 84 children who were born to mothers who received chemotherapy during pregnancy for haematological malignancies.[13] The children were examined for physical health, growth, development, and haematological, cytogenetic, neurological, psychological, and

Table 2. Explanation of drug risk categories.

ADEC category	Explanation
A	Drugs which have been taken by a large number of pregnant women without any proven increase in the frequency of malformations or other direct or indirect harmful effects on the foetus having been observed.
B	Drugs which have been taken by a limited number of pregnant women without an increase in the frequency of malformation or other direct or indirect harmful effects on the human foetus having been observed. Human data are lacking or inadequate. Sub-categorisation is based on available animal data: B1 — no evidence of harm in animals B2 — limited animal data but no evidence of harm B3 — evidence of harm in animals.
C	Drugs which have caused, or may be suspected of causing, harmful effects on the human foetus or neonate without causing malformations. These effects may be reversible.
D	Drugs which have caused, are suspected to have caused or may be expected to cause, an increased incidence of human foetal malformations or irreversible damage. These drugs may also have adverse pharmacological effects.
X	Drugs which have such a high risk of causing permanent damage to the foetus that they should not be used in pregnancy or when there is a possibility of pregnancy.

ADEC — Australian Drug Evaluation Committee. Copyright Commonwealth of Australia, reproduced by permission.[11]

learning disorders. The occurrence of cancer was also considered. The children's ages ranged from 6 to 29 years at the time of assessment. Overall, the children demonstrated normal birth weight and normal learning and educational performance. There were no congenital, neurological, or psychological abnormalities and no reports of malignancies. Twelve second generation children were also assessed and displayed normal development.

The data regarding late effects of chemotherapy on children's neurodevelopment are limited. The majority of available reports have focused on immediate maternal and foetal pregnancy outcomes, not considering later neurodevelopment as a primary end point. The general impression based on the available data is that chemotherapy does not have a major impact on later neurodevelopment. A review of 111 children born to mothers treated with chemotherapy during pregnancy and followed up for 1 to 19 years reported all had normal late neurodevelopment, based on formal developmental and cognitive tests.[14]

2.5   *Pharmacokinetics and drug dosing in pregnancy*

The pharmacokinetics of chemotherapeutic agents in pregnancy has not been extensively studied.

Transfer of drugs across the placenta is favoured by high lipid solubility, low molecular weight and loose binding to plasma proteins. The placenta may itself help protect the foetus from chemotherapy. The gene encoding the multidrug resistant P-glycoprotein is over-expressed in the endometrium during pregnancy, which may offer, some toxicologic protection of the foetus from agents such as doxorubicin, vinblastine, vincristine and the taxanes.[15]

Pregnancy results in a 50% increase in plasma volume, as well as increased hepatic and renal clearance. These physiological changes might decrease active drug concentrations, compared with non-pregnant women of the same weight. Pregnancy can also diminish gastric motility, which may alter the absorption of orally administered drugs. Plasma albumin decreases in pregnancy, resulting in an increase in the amount of unbound active drug. However, the high levels of oestrogen during pregnancy cause an increase in other plasma proteins that likely counterbalance this effect. The third space potential of the amniotic fluid must also be considered when prescribing chemotherapy in pregnancy, particularly for drugs such as methotrexate.[16]

Whether any of these factors either compromise cure rates by reducing the effective drug concentrations, or results in excess toxicity is unclear, and it is difficult to predict if and how doses should be modified. Until further studies are undertaken, it is recommended that the standard weight-based chemotherapy doses used for non-pregnant patients are used for pregnant patients.[16–18]

2.6   Use of anti-emetics in pregnancy

Metoclopramide is a category A drug and is considered safe in all trimesters. Prochlorperazine (Stemetil) is in category C. There is evidence of harmful effects in animals, but inadequate evidence of the safety in human pregnancy. Stemetil has however been widely used during pregnancy for many years without apparent ill consequence and is generally considered safe. High doses during late pregnancy should be avoided, because such dosing has caused jaundice, hyper-reflexia, hyporeflexia or prolonged extrapyramidal disturbances in the child.[19]

5HT3 antagonists are category B1 drugs. They have not been associated with foetal malformations and have been safely used during all trimesters of pregnancy.[20] Corticosteroids are category A drugs and considered safe in all trimesters. First trimester exposure has been associated with cleft palate and skeletal malformations in animal experiments, but these findings are not considered relevant to humans.[19]

Aprepitant is categorised B1 and animal experiments have revealed it crosses the placenta. Reproductive studies performed in rats and rabbits at doses up to 1.5 times the systemic exposure at the adult human dose have revealed no evidence of harm to the foetus.[19] There are no well controlled studies in human pregnancy; however, in the limited number of pregnant women who have taken the drug, there has been no increase in the observed rate of foetal malformation or harm.[19] Because animal reproduction studies are not always predictive of human response, this drug should be used during pregnancy only if clearly indicated.

2.7   Use of growth factors in pregnancy

Granulocyte colony-stimulating factor (G-CSF) and erythropoietin have been used safely in pregnant patients.[21,22] Growth factors should be used as per standard chemotherapy protocols.

2.8   *Timing of delivery*

The recommended time for delivery is approximately three weeks after the last cycle of chemotherapy, to minimise the risk of maternal and foetal neutropaenia and subsequent infection as well as haemorrhage.[1,17,18] Chemotherapy should not be given after the 35th week of gestation, to reduce the risk of neutropaenia at the time of delivery.[1,23] Labour can be induced, or caesarean section performed when the maturation of the foetus is deemed sufficient. If possible, delivery should be timed for 34 or more weeks of gestation, at which time the morbidity of prematurity is relatively low.[18] If chemotherapy is to continue post-partum, the first dose should be given allowing time to recover from delivery and to minimise the risk of infection.

2.9   *Radiation therapy*

The use of radiation therapy is generally avoided during all trimesters of pregnancy, because of the risk to the foetus of teratogenicity and the potential induction of childhood malignancies and haematological disorders.[24,25] The amount of radiation to which the foetus is exposed depends upon the stage of pregnancy when therapeutic radiation is administered. The first trimester is the most crucial period for foetal harm. Foetal malformations have been associated with doses of 0.1Gy or more during the first trimester.[26] Later in pregnancy the foetus is more developed and therefore less sensitive to radiation. However, later in pregnancy the increasing uterine fundal height increases the foetal exposure from internal radiation scatter. Even with appropriate shielding, the closer the foetus is to the diaphragm, the greater the possible whole body foetal dose when the mother receives radiation above the diaphragm. As an example, the administration of 50Gy external beam irradiation to the breast could result in a first trimester foetal dose of 0.04 to 0.15Gy, or a third trimester dose as high as 2Gy.[27–29]

Although there are several case reports of normal infants born after their mothers had been irradiated, including one exposed in the first trimester,[29–31] irradiation is generally avoided in pregnant women, because absence of risk to the foetus cannot be guaranteed.[17,32]

2.10   *Metastases to the foetus*

Dissemination of tumour cells to the foetus is extremely rare. In the published literature, melanoma, leukaemia, lymphoma and one case of hepatocellular carcinoma have resulted in foetal metastases.[27] There are no reported cases of metastatic disease in the foetus from breast cancer, but there are four reported cases of placental metastasis from breast cancer, and one of these exhibited invasion of the chorionic villi.[2]

3.   Breast Cancer

3.1   *Epidemiology of breast cancer in pregnancy*

Gestational breast cancer is traditionally defined as breast cancer diagnosed during pregnancy, or in the first 12 months post-partum.[33-35] According to a Western Australian population based study, it accounts for 6.25% of breast cancers in women younger than 45 years.[33] Two-thirds are diagnosed post-partum and one-third are diagnosed during pregnancy.[33] The median age at diagnosis is 34 years.[33] Other case series report a similar median maternal age of 33 to 34 years.[22,36-38]

Breast cancer is the second most frequent cancer observed during pregnancy, estimated to affect 1 in 1500 to 1 in 4000 pregnancies.[33,39]

Pregnancy itself may transiently increase an individual woman's risk of developing breast cancer, despite its long-term protective effect on the development of the disease. This was illustrated by three population-based series in which pregnancy was followed by a period of increased breast cancer risk lasting three to ten years, which subsequently declined.[40-42]

3.2   *Diagnosis of breast cancer in pregnancy*

The diagnosis of pregnancy associated breast cancer is often delayed due to the difficulty of palpating a small lump in a breast that is engorged due to pregnancy and lactation.

Most women present with a painless lump, 90% of which are detected by self examination[4] and breast examination should therefore be performed at the first antenatal visit and all suspicious lesions biopsied. Core biopsy of a suspicious lesion can be safely performed in pregnancy and is the most reliable method of diagnosis of invasive carcinoma.[43] Cytology from fine needle aspiration biopsy lacks accuracy in pregnancy and lactation and its main value is to confirm suspected galactocoeles, or as therapy for symptomatic cysts.[43,44]

Breast imaging in pregnancy and lactation is extremely difficult and often leads to false diagnoses.[43] The increased breast density seen in pre-menopausal women, as well as the physiologic changes seen within the breast during pregnancy (increased water content, higher density, and loss of contrasting fat) make breast imaging difficult to interpret.

Ultrasound may be employed to confirm a tumour in the case of clinical suspicion. It can differentiate between solid and cystic lesions in 97% of cases.[6] Ultrasound does not expose the woman and foetus to radiation and has been reported to be more sensitive than mammography in detecting cancerous changes in the breasts of pregnant women.[45]

Mammography is not always essential in the diagnosis and management of gestational breast cancer, but if required, there is minimal risk to the foetus with modern techniques and use of abdominal shielding. A dose of 200–400mGy is delivered by standard bilateral mammography.[17] This results in less than 0.5µGy exposure to the embryo/foetus, well below the level of 100mGy that increases the risk of foetal malformation by 1%.[46]

The efficacy and safety of breast MRI has not been evaluated in gestational breast cancer and it is currently not recommended. There are concerns over the safety of gadolinium, which has been shown to cross the placenta and causes foetal abnormalities in rats.[17] Positioning the pregnant patient on her stomach for the MRI could also prove difficult.

3.3 *Pathology of breast cancer in pregnancy*

The predominant histology is invasive ductal carcinoma, with 80–100% of patients presenting with this histology.[22,36,38,47] Most tumours are high grade and hormone receptor negative,[36,37,47] similar to breast cancers in non-pregnant young women, suggesting that age at diagnosis, rather than the pregnant state, determines the biologic features of the tumour.[37,48] However, some series have reported a higher frequency of oestrogen receptor (ER) negative tumours in pregnant patients, compared to age matched controls,[47,49] suggesting the pregnancy may have some influence on the pathology. Lymphovascular invasion and lymph node involvement (56–67%) are commonly seen.[23,37] Some series report higher rates of inflammatory tumours in pregnant patients than in non-pregnant controls.[47] Case control studies have revealed Her2/neu status is positive in 28–58% of patients.[37,49,50] Based upon conflicting data from these case control studies, it remains unclear if Her2/neu receptor status differs compared to age matched controls.

3.4   *Staging of breast cancer in pregnancy*

Pregnant women tend to present with more advanced disease than non-pregnant women. This is at least partially explained by the frequently delayed diagnosis. One review showed that a pregnant woman has a 2.5-fold higher risk of presenting with disseminated breast cancer than a non-pregnant woman, and a significantly lower chance of being diagnosed with stage I disease.[23]

CT scans and bone scans are not recommended during pregnancy.[17,18,51] Chest X-rays with abdominal shielding and abdominal ultrasound are considered safe.[4,17,51,52] Non-contrast MRI is preferred for detection of bone and brain metastases if clinically indicated, although contrast agents such as gadolinium are best avoided.[17,51,52]

3.5   *Treatment of breast cancer in pregnancy*

Treatment should conform as closely as possible to standardised protocols for non-pregnant patients. If a woman is diagnosed with breast cancer in the first trimester, then the risks of delaying treatment until the second trimester and the potential need for an abortion should be discussed. Termination of pregnancy does not improve survival for breast cancer and is not routinely recommended.[5,23,53] The decision to continue or terminate the pregnancy should be individualised and made by a fully informed woman in conjunction with her physician.

Factors which should be considered in women with gestational breast cancer considering termination include:

- the possible risk of foetal toxicity or complications from breast cancer treatment during pregnancy;
- the woman's prognosis and ability to care for her offspring; and
- the effect of breast cancer treatment on the woman's future fertility.

3.6 Surgical treatment of breast cancer in pregnancy

Breast surgery can be safely performed during all trimesters of pregnancy, with minimal risk to the developing foetus.[36,54,55] Modified radical mastectomy with axillary lymph node dissection is the treatment of choice for operable disease, to avoid the need for radiation therapy and potential second surgery. Breast conserving surgery with axillary lymph node dissection can still be a safe option, but the potential risk of incomplete excision and the need for a second surgery must be explained. It is best considered in the second and third trimesters, to allow initiation of radiation therapy after delivery without a significant delay. The majority of women in published reports have been managed with mastectomy.[33]

Sentinel lymph node biopsy has not been systematically evaluated in pregnant patients and is not recommended. The potential efficacy and safety should be discussed with clinically node negative pregnant patients. The theoretical risk to the developing foetus of radiation delivered by the radioactive technetium must be considered. A few studies have sought to quantify the radiation absorbed dose to the foetus.[56–58] They have all concluded the radiation absorbed is negligible (< 0.014mGy) and lymphoscintigrophy and sentinel node biopsy can be performed safely during pregnancy. In addition to safety issues, it is not clear whether lymphatic pathways are altered in the breasts of pregnant women, making identification of the sentinel node more difficult. Further evaluation is required before formal recommendations can be made.

3.7 Systemic therapy for breast cancer in pregnancy

3.7.1 Timing of adjuvant chemotherapy

The improvement in maternal survival accruing from chemotherapy administered earlier (during pregnancy) rather than later (after delivery) has not been quantified. In early stage gestational breast cancer, there are no controlled data defining the extent to which a delay in the initiation of adjuvant chemotherapy impairs maternal survival outcomes. Retrospective studies in non-pregnant women have indicated relapse free survival and overall survival may be compromised if adjuvant chemotherapy is commenced more than 12 weeks after definitive surgery.[59,60] One retrospective review of premenopausal non-pregnant patients indicated that those with ER negative tumours had improved disease free survival when chemotherapy was commenced within 21 days of surgery.[61] Because most gestational breast cancers are ER negative, there may be a similar benefit in gestational breast cancer, however further studies are required.

Deferring adjuvant chemotherapy until the post-partum period remains a valid option for selected patients, such as hormone receptor positive, node negative patients presenting within the third trimester. For higher risk patients chemotherapy should be commenced within 12 weeks of surgery.

In advanced disease, a delay in initiating chemotherapy may impair progression free survival and lead to worsening symptoms depending on the sites and extent of metastatic disease.

3.7.2 Chemotherapy drugs used in breast cancer in pregnancy

There is considerable data addressing the use of anthracyclines in pregnant women, but very limited information exists on other agents such as taxanes and trastuzumab. The long term implications of exposure to these newer agents are not known and the safest option is to avoid use in pregnancy. The most commonly used regimen in pregnant women with breast cancer has been doxorubicin plus cyclophosphamide (AC) or 5-fluorouracil (5-FU), doxorubicin and cyclophosphamide (FAC). There is no data on the safety during pregnancy of dose-dense anthracycline containing regimens with or without taxanes. Dose dense regimens are therefore not recommended. The only consistent adverse effect in all of the case studies of antenatal chemotherapy in women with breast cancer is an increased risk of pre-term delivery. A summary of the common breast cancer drugs and the recommendations for use in pregnancy is given in Table 3.

Table 3. Breast cancer therapies and recommendations in pregnancy.

Drug	Class	Evidence	Summary
Anthracyclines (Doxorubicin)	D	Multiple case reports of safe use in 2nd and 3rd trimesters Long term follow-up	Appears safe in 2nd and 3rd trimesters
Cyclophosphamide	D	Case reports of safe use combined with anthracycline and 5-fluorouracil	Appears safe in 2nd and 3rd trimesters
5-Fluorouracil	D	Case reports of safe use combined with anthracycline and cyclophosphamide	Appears safe in 2nd and 3rd trimesters
Taxanes	D	Limited case reports in humans — no malformations	Insufficient evidence to assess safety
Trastuzumab	B2	Limited case reports in humans — risk of oligohydramnios — no malformations	Insufficient evidence to assess safety
Lapatinib	C	One human case report to date	Insufficient evidence to assess safety
Methotrexate	D	Risk of malformations and abortion	Avoid in all trimesters
Gemcitabine	D	No human reports	Insufficient evidence to assess safety
Vinorelbine	D	Limited case reports in humans — no malformations	Insufficient evidence to assess safety
Tamoxifen	B3	Risk of malformations	Avoid in all trimesters

Anthracycline-based regimens

Several case series report on the use of anthracyclines during pregnancy (Table 4). The largest of these series reports on embryo-foetal outcomes in 160 patients (34 with breast cancer) exposed to anthracyclines in all three trimesters of pregnancy.[62] The authors concluded that the risk of toxicity was low, especially after the first trimester and using doses of doxorubicin below 70mg/m² per cycle. Doxorubicin and daunorubicin were the most frequently administered anthracyclines and 90% received combination chemotherapy with at least one other agent. Of 15 foetal deaths, 6 were associated with maternal death, 13 were in patients with acute leukaemia and 11 had received daunorubicin. There were 5 malformations reported, 3 following first trimester chemotherapy exposure and two following second trimester exposure. The risk of severe foetal toxicity was increased 30-fold when the dose per cycle of doxorubicin exceeded 70mg/m² per cycle. The duration of exposure to anthracyclines was not associated with the occurrence of severe foetal toxicity.

Foetal cardiac toxicity must also be considered when administering anthracyclines during pregnancy. The available data is limited but suggest the risk of late cardiac toxicity is minimal. One study of 81 children over five years of age whose mothers were treated with cytotoxic drugs, including anthracyclines, during pregnancy showed no clinical or echocardiogram evidence of myocardial damage.[63] In another study foetal echocardiograms were performed every 2 weeks in a pregnant patient receiving doxorubicin and cyclophosphamide from 24 weeks gestation.[64] Unexposed foetuses were monitored as controls. With follow up to 2 years, no significant difference in systolic function was recorded between exposed and unexposed foetuses. In contrast to these reports, there are a few case reports of neonatal cardiac toxicity following in utero exposure to anthracyclines, mainly idarubicin and daunorubicin.[62,65–67] Because of these reports, doxorubicin is preferred over idarubicin or epirubicin for use in pregnancy.[1]

Taxanes

There are several case reports on taxane use during pregnancy, but there is little information on the long-term effects of foetal

Table 4. Use of anthracyclines during pregnancy.

References	Berry et al.[36]	Giacalone et al.[38]	Germann et al.[62]	Ring et al.[22]	Hahn et al.[121]
No. of pts.	24	14	160	16	57
Chemotherapy	FAC	FEC, EC, FAC, VEM	Multiple anthracycline regimens	AC and EC	FAC
Cancer	Breast	Breast	Mixed — 80 acute leukaemia, — 34 breast	Breast	Breast
Timing of chemotherapy	2nd and 3rd trimesters	All 3 trimesters	All 3 trimesters	2nd and 3rd trimesters	2nd and 3rd trimesters
Median gest. age at cycle 1	22 weeks	26 weeks (mean)	NR	20 weeks	23 weeks
Median cycles during pregnancy	4	2	NR	4	4
Median gest. age at delivery	38.0 weeks	34.7 weeks (mean)	NR	37 weeks	37 weeks
Foetal malformations	Nil	Nil	5 (3%) — 3 after 1st trimester exposure — 2 after 2nd trimester exposure	Nil	3 (5%) — Down syndrome — clubfoot — bilateral ureteral reflux

(Continued)

Table 4. (Continued)

References	Berry et al.[36]	Giacalone et al.[38]	Germann et al.[62]	Ring et al.[22]	Hahn et al.[121]
Foetal deaths	Nil	3 (21%) — 2 after 1st trimester exposure — 1 after 2nd trimester exposure	19 (12%) — 6 with maternal death — 13 mothers with acute leukaemia — 4 SA	Nil	Nil
Neonatal complications	— 2 (8%) resp. distress — 1 (4%) leucopaenia	— 1 (7%) resp. distress — 1 (7%) leucopaenia — 1 death D8	— 3 (2%) cardiac toxicity — 7 (4%) leucopaenia	— 1 IUGR — 2 resp. distress	— 10% resp. distress — 1 sub-arachnoid haemorrhage
Follow-up of offspring	Healthy at median 54 months	Healthy at median 19 months	NR	NR	Healthy at 2–157 months

A — Doxorubicin; C — cyclophosphamide; D — day; E — epirubicin; F — 5-fluorouracil; gest. — gestational; M — methotrexate; NR — not reported; resp. — respiratory; SA — spontaneous abortion; V — vinorelbine.

exposure. Because of the lack of long term data, international guidelines currently recommend avoiding taxanes.[17]

Taxanes have a low molecular weight and are highly lipophilic, so they would be expected to cross the placenta. However transplacental transfer is reduced by placental P-glycoprotein and the high protein binding of taxanes.

Case reports suggest the short-term safety of taxanes. Docetaxel was reported in six cases to have been used safely during the second and third trimesters of pregnancy with no adverse outcomes in the infant.[68–72] Docetaxel was administered as a single agent in only one case.[70]

There are nine reports documenting the use of paclitaxel during the second and third trimesters of pregnancy — four cases in breast cancer[73–76] and five cases in ovarian cancer. Paclitaxel was used as a single agent in only two cases. No malformation was reported and normal development was observed after a median follow up of 16 months. One report assessed the pharmacokinetics of paclitaxel at 34 and 36 weeks gestation.[77] The maximal plasma concentration and area under the curve were decreased compared with non-pregnant patients and the clearance, half life and volume of distribution were within range for non-pregnant women. The effect of these changes on patient outcomes has not been reported.

Vinorelbine

There are at least six cases reporting the safe use of vinorelbine during the second and third trimesters of pregnancy, five of these were for breast cancer treatment.[68,78–80] In five of these reports vinorelbine was given in combination with other agents (5-fluorouracil, cisplatin or trastuzumab). No malformations were reported and offspring seemed healthy with a median follow-up of 23 months.

Gemcitabine

Studies in animals have shown teratogenicity and embryotoxicity. No information on humans is available. Gemcitabine is currently not recommended in pregnancy on the basis of insufficient evidence.[19]

Trastuzumab

Trastuzumab has been assigned a category B2 pregnancy risk on the basis of trials in monkeys, which documented placental transfer of trastuzumab, but no apparent foetal harm.[81] Information on foetal outcome is currently limited to a number of case reports with differing outcomes.

Her2 is expressed in embryo-foetal tissue but its role in foetal development is unknown. In murine studies, deletion of the Her2 gene was fatal to embryos at early gestation, due to cardiac and neural dysfunction.[82] This suggests a possible role in cardiac and neural development.

Oligohydramnios and anhydramnios has been observed in four case reports and reversible foetal renal failure was associated with one of these cases.[72,75,82,83] Cardiac function in the foetus was monitored in one case with no reported problems. One infant died of multiple organ failure 21 weeks after delivery.[82] Three other case reports describe delivery of healthy infants following exposure in all three trimesters of pregnancy.[80,84,85] One of these children has been observed for five years and has normal growth and development. There have been no reports of foetal malformations following trastuzumab administration.

Evidence is currently insufficient to provide any recommendations, but in light of the case reports, delaying trastuzumab until after delivery is the safest option. Any pregnancies that are exposed to trastuzumab during the second trimester should be closely followed with particular attention to amniotic fluid volume and foetal renal function.

Lapatinib

Because there is very little experience of lapatinib use in pregnant women, the safest option is to avoid its use during pregnancy. Animal studies have found no treatment related malformations but minor skeletal variations and an increase in post-implantation losses have been observed.[19] One human case report describes 11 weeks of exposure to lapatinib in the first and second trimesters.[86] The pregnancy was uncomplicated and resulted in the delivery of a healthy baby. The child was developmentally normal at 18 months of age.

Methotrexate

Despite case reports of the safe use of CMF (cyclophosphamide, methotrexate, 5-fluorouracil) during pregnancy,[22,38] the abortifacient effect and teratogenic potential of methotrexate have led to the recommendation that it should be avoided in all trimesters.[18,19] Malformations similar to those in the aminopterin syndrome (cranial dysostosis, hypertelorism, wide nasal bridge, micrognanthia and ear anomalies) have been reported following exposure to doses greater than 10mg per week in the first trimester.[19,87] Increased methotrexate toxicity can result from delayed elimination of the drug from the amniotic fluid, which acts as a sequestered space.[18]

3.7.3 Endocrine therapy and breast cancer in pregnancy

Tamoxifen is not recommended during pregnancy.[17] There are reports of neonatal defects including ambiguous genitalia and craniofacial defects.[88] If indicated, endocrine therapy should be commenced after delivery. There are no reports of women with pregnancy associated breast cancer receiving aromatase inhibitors, although teratogenic effects have been described in animal models.[89] Long acting gonadotrophin releasing hormone agonists (GnRHa) are not advised during pregnancy, but were not associated with teratogenicity in a case series of 5 patients administered long acting GnRHa in early pregnancy.[90]

3.8 Radiation therapy for breast cancer in pregnancy

A standard 50Gy course of radiotherapy to the breast exposes the foetus to between 0.04Gy and 2Gy, depending on the gestational stage.[91] Although the risks are small, in order to minimise the risk of harm, the general recommendation is to postpone radiotherapy until after delivery.[17]

Delaying radiotherapy is usually feasible in these women, because their young age and high frequency of poor pathological prognostic factors mean that adjuvant chemotherapy is often indicated and radiotherapy is given after completion of surgery and chemotherapy. Studies in non-pregnant women have demonstrated radiation therapy should commence within six months of surgery in those receiving chemotherapy,[92,93] and within eight weeks of surgery in those not receiving chemotherapy.[94] Longer delays may compromise local control. In pregnant women, the decision to undergo breast conserving surgery followed by radiation therapy should be undertaken with these time frames in mind.

3.9 *Prognosis of breast cancer in pregnancy*

The relationship between pregnancy and the outcome of breast cancer remains controversial. Some studies have shown poorer prognosis in patients in whom breast cancer is diagnosed during pregnancy compared to age and stage matched controls,[33,47,95–97] while others have found no effect.[27,98–100]

The studies demonstrating gestational breast cancer has a worse prognosis than non-gestational breast cancer have not been able to explain why. It may be partly explained by the delay in diagnosis commonly seen in pregnancy. There is also the possibility that the pregnancy itself, and the associated hormonal milieu, influence the biologic behaviour of the breast cancer, resulting in a more aggressive phenotype.

One retrospective multi-centre study compared 154 patients with pregnancy-associated breast cancer to a control group of 308 non-pregnant breast cancer patients.[47] There was a significantly higher proportion of inflammatory breast cancer (26% v 9.1%; $p < 0.00001$), larger tumours and negative receptor status in the pregnancy group. The pregnancy group had a significantly worse five-year recurrence-free survival (69% v 81%; $p = 0.01$) and five-year overall survival (61% v 75%; $p = 0.001$) than the non-pregnancy group. Even when inflammatory breast cancers were excluded, the outcomes remained significantly worse in the pregnant women. Of interest, outcome was also significantly poorer after chemotherapy for patients in the pregnant group than in the non pregnant group. Multivariate analysis demonstrated that pregnancy was an independent and significant prognostic factor for overall survival.

A more recent Australian study reported an overall five-year survival for pregnancy associated breast cancer of 72.8%.[33]

This was still inferior to the five-year survival of 75–85% reported for all young Australian women diagnosed with breast cancer at the time.[101]

4. Lymphoma

Lymphoma is one of the most frequent malignancies diagnosed during pregnancy.[1,3,4] Hodgkin lymphoma has an early age peak from the teens through to 30 years old and is consequently the most common type of lymphoma diagnosed during pregnancy.[102] The incidence of Hodgkin lymphoma ranges from 1 in 1000 to 1 in 6000 pregnancies.[103,104] The mean age at diagnosis for Non-Hodgkin Lymphoma (NHL) is 42 and it is much less commonly diagnosed during pregnancy.

4.1 *Diagnosis of lymphoma in pregnancy*

Most women present with asymptomatic lymphadenopathy with or without B symptoms. Lymph node biopsy under local or general anaesthesia should be performed to confirm the diagnosis and is considered safe in all trimesters of pregnancy.[105,106]

4.2 *Staging of lymphoma in pregnancy*

Staging should be limited and based on history, physical examination, blood tests, bone marrow biopsies and CXR with abdominal shielding. Abdominal and pelvic CT should be avoided during pregnancy to minimise foetal radiation exposure.[105] However, abdominal ultrasound and/or MRI can be useful alternatives to CT. PET scans are not recommended during pregnancy, as (18)FDG can cross the placenta and may expose the foetus to higher radiation than CT.[107,108]

4.3 *Treatment of lymphoma in pregnancy*

The decision to treat or closely monitor the pregnant woman with lymphoma must be individualised. Therapy can sometimes be delayed until at least the second trimester to decrease the risk of foetal harm. This must however be balanced against the potential for maternal harm from treatment delay.

Chemotherapy has been safely administered to pregnant women with lymphoma; however the supporting data are limited and based on case reports. One series evaluated 84 children, aged 6 to 29 yrs, born to mothers with haematological malignancies who received chemotherapy including anthracyclines during pregnancy (see Sec. 2.4).[13] Twenty-nine women were treated for Non-Hodgkin lymphoma and twenty-six were treated for Hodgkin lymphoma. The authors concluded that full dose chemotherapy can be safely administered to pregnant women with aggressive haematological malignancies. This study is reassuring, but more reports are necessary to further evaluate the safety of chemotherapy during pregnancy.

4.3.1 Treatment of Hodgkin lymphoma in pregnancy

The nodular sclerosing histological subtype of Hodgkin lymphoma is the most prevalent in pregnant women, similar to non-pregnant women younger than 40 years.[105] Outside pregnancy, most patients with Hodgkin lymphoma are treated with combination chemotherapy and the most common chemotherapy regimen used is ABVD (doxorubicin, bleomycin, vinblastine, dacarbazine).

Patients with early stage disease diagnosed during the first trimester can generally be closely observed without treatment until the second trimester.[105] Radiotherapy with shielding can be considered for stage 1 disease with isolated involvement of neck or axillary lymph nodes if symptom control is necessary. The risk to the foetus is considered minimal in this setting, but absence of harm cannot be guaranteed.[32] Women presenting with advanced or bulky disease in the first trimester will usually require prompt treatment with an appropriate chemotherapy protocol such as ABVD. Because a delay in therapy may adversely affect survival and because chemotherapy in the first trimester can be teratogenic, pregnancy termination should be considered and discussed with the woman presenting with advanced disease in the first trimester.

Data based on case reports suggest patients presenting with Hodgkin lymphoma in the second or third trimesters can be treated with ABVD chemotherapy, similarly to non-pregnant women, without affecting foetal outcome.[1,13,109–111] There are no reports regarding foetal pulmonary damage or neurotoxicity associated with treatment with bleomycin or vinca-alkaloids, respectively.

There are also case reports describing the safe use of MOPP (mechlorethamine, vincristine, procarbazine and prednisone) after the first trimester,[13,112] however there is better data supporting the use of ABVD. Because MOPP or MOPP variants are rarely used to treat Hodgkin lymphoma in the current era, in non-pregnant women, it should be possible to avoid using MOPP in pregnancy.

There are no reports on treatment of pregnant patients with BEACOPP or escalated BEACOPP (bleomycin, etoposide, doxorubicin, cyclophosphamide, vincristine, procarbazine, and prednisone) and therefore these regimens are not recommended during pregnancy.[105]

The prognosis of Hodgkin lymphoma is believed to be unaffected by pregnancy. Relapse and mortality rates in pregnancy are similar to rates in age and stage matched non-pregnant women. A case-control study of 48 women with pregnancy associated Hodgkin lymphoma reported a 20-year survival rate similar to that of matched controls.[109] Two larger, but much older patient series reported similar outcomes for pregnant and non pregnant women.[113,114] It is difficult to know if the outcomes would still be similar today with current chemotherapy and radiotherapy regimens.

4.3.2 Treatment of non-Hodgkin lymphoma

Non-Hodgkin lymphoma (NHL) often has an aggressive histology in pregnancy. Diffuse large B-cell and peripheral T cell lymphomas are the most common in this context.[115]

Indolent NHL

This group, which includes follicular lymphoma, small lymphocytic lymphoma and chronic lymphocytic leukaemia, is extremely rare during pregnancy.[105] Indolent NHL is generally considered an incurable malignancy and even in non-pregnant patients, treatment is frequently delayed until the patient is symptomatic.[105] Therefore, during pregnancy, administration of chemotherapy during the first trimester is usually avoidable. Safe administration of rituximab during the first trimester has been reported[116,117] and could be considered if treatment during the first trimester is indicated.[105]

During the second and third trimesters, chemotherapy with CVP (cyclophosphamide, vincristine and prednisone) and CHOP (cyclophosphamide, doxorubicin, vincristine and prednisone) with or without rituximab can be considered. Existing data suggest that CHOP may be administered during the second and third trimesters without adverse foetal outcomes.[13,110,118] One case series reports on 18 pregnant women who received CHOP for Non-Hodgkin lymphoma. No congenital malformations were noted and all pregnancies were successfully delivered at 35 to 40 weeks.[119]

There are no reports regarding treatment with fludarabine during pregnancy and its use should therefore be avoided if possible.[105]

Aggressive NHL

This group represents the majority of NHL cases diagnosed during pregnancy. It includes diffuse large B-cell lymphoma, mantle cell lymphoma, mature T-cell neoplasms and NK-cell neoplasms. Most of these women require prompt treatment with intensive combination chemotherapy in order to produce the best outcomes. The few case reports that have described the administration of CHOP during the first trimester for the treatment of NHL have reported no increase in the risk of severe foetal malformation.[1,13,115] One first trimester exposure to CHOP did however result in transient complete foetal B cell depletion.[120] Therapeutic abortion should be strongly considered when aggressive NHL is diagnosed during the first trimester. The limited existing data suggest the combination of CHOP with rituximab may be considered safe during the second and third trimesters.[105]

Very aggressive NHL

This group includes Burkitt's lymphoma and precursor lymphoblastic leukaemia/lymphoma. Treatment should be initiated immediately after diagnosis, even during the first trimester, due to the aggressive course and poor prognosis of these lymphomas if untreated. Many chemotherapy regimens for very aggressive lymphoma include high dose methotrexate, which is teratogenic in the first trimester, and can cause severe foetal myelosupression during the second and third trimesters.[13] Whether conventional chemotherapy including high dose methotrexate can be safely administered during the second and third trimesters has not been determined and pregnancy termination should be strongly considered.

5. Conclusion

Although the occurrence of cancer in pregnancy is rare, the management of cancer in pregnancy is complex and requires a multidisciplinary team approach with involvement of the woman in decision making at all stages. Pregnancy termination is not always necessary. Depending on the characteristics of the cancer and the stage of the pregnancy, treatment may be delivered during pregnancy without demonstrable harm to the foetus, or deferred to the post-partum period without compromising the health of the mother. Although data concerning the long term risks of chemotherapy are limited, data concerning the short term safety of chemotherapy administered during the second and third trimesters are reassuring. To minimise foetal harm, radiation therapy and endocrine therapy are best delayed until after delivery. Management coordinated by a multidisciplinary team will ensure the best possible outcome for both mother and infant.

Acknowledgements

We would like express our sincere gratitude to Associate Professor Max Wolf from the Department of Haematology and Medical Oncology at Peter MacCallum Cancer Centre for critically reviewing the section on lymphoma.

References

1. E. Cardonick and A. Iacobucci, Use of chemotherapy during human pregnancy, *Lancet Oncol.* **5**: 283–291 (2004).
2. J. F. Potter and M. Schoeneman, Metastasis of maternal cancer to the placenta and fetus, *Cancer* **25**: 380–388 (1970).

3. T. E. Buekers and T. A. Lallas, Chemotherapy in pregnancy, *Obstet. Gynecol. Clin. North. Am.* **25**: 323–329 (1998).

4. N. A. Pavlidis, Coexistence of pregnancy and malignancy, *Oncologist* **7**: 279–287 (2002).

5. P. Eedarapalli and S. Jain, Breast cancer in pregnancy, *J. Obstet. Gynaecol.* **26**: 1–4 (2006).

6. J. C. Woo, T. Yu and T. C. Hurd, Breast cancer in pregnancy: A literature review, *Arch. Surg.* **138**: 91–98; discussion 99 (2003).

7. H. Kalter and J. Warkany, Congenital malformations (second of two parts), *N. Engl. J. Med.* **308**: 491–497 (1983).

8. A. Ring, Breast cancer and pregnancy, *Breast* **16**(Suppl. 2): S155–S158 (2007).

9. D. Zemlickis, M. Lishner, P. Degendorfer *et al.*, Fetal outcome after *in utero* exposure to cancer chemotherapy, *Arch. Intern. Med.* **152**: 573–576 (1992).

10. J. E. Garber, Long-term follow-up of children exposed *in utero* to antineoplastic agents, *Semin. Oncol.* **16**: 437–444 (1989).

11. Medicines in Pregnancy Working Party of the Australian Drug Evaluation Committee, Prescribing medicines in pregnancy. In: *An Australian Categorisation of Risk of Drug Use in Pregnancy*, 4th ed. (Commonwealth of Australia, Canberra, 1999), http://www.tga.gov.au/docs/html/medpreg.htm.

12. J. I. Durodola, Administration of cyclophosphamide during late pregnancy and early lactation: A case report, *J. Natl. Med. Assoc.* **71**: 165–166 (1979).

13. A. Aviles and N. Neri, Hematological malignancies and pregnancy: A final report of 84 children who received chemotherapy *in utero*. *Clin. Lymphoma* **2**: 173–177 (2001).

14. I. Nulman, D. Laslo, S. Fried *et al.*, Neurodevelopment of children exposed *in utero* to treatment of maternal malignancy, *Br. J. Cancer* **85**: 1611–1618 (2001).

15. R. J. Arceci, J. M. Croop, S. B. Horwitz *et al.*, The gene encoding multidrug resistance is induced and expressed at high levels during pregnancy in the secretory epithelium of the uterus, *Proc. Natl. Acad. Sci. USA* **85**: 4350–4354 (1988).

16. J. Stevenson, B. Giantonio, R. L. Boyd *et al.*, Adjuvant chemotherapy for breast cancer in pregnancy: Can recommendations be made with confidence. *Semin. Oncol.* **24**: xxv–xxxvi; discussion xxxvi, xxxix (1997).

17. S. Loibl, G. von Minckwitz, K. Gwyn *et al.*, Breast carcinoma during pregnancy. International recommendations from an expert meeting, *Cancer* **106**: 237–246 (2006).
18. A. Psyrri and B. Burtness, Pregnancy-associated breast cancer, *Cancer J.* **11**: 83–95 (2005).
19. *MIMS Online*, Managing editor: E. Donohoo, Copyright MIMS Australia Pty Ltd 2003, Health Communication Network Ltd (ACN 068 458 575): St Leonards NSW 2065. Viewed 7 July 2008, http://www.mims.com.au.
20. D. G. Tincello and M. J. Johnstone, Treatment of hyperemesis gravidarum with the 5-HT3 antagonist ondansetron (Zofran), *Postgrad. Med. J.* **72**: 688–689 (1996).
21. R. K. Freeman, S. J. Yaffe and G. G. Briggs, *Drugs in Pregnancy and Lactation: A Reference Guide to Fetal and Neonatal Risk* (Lippincott Williams & Wilkins, Philadelphia, 1998).
22. A. E. Ring, I. E. Smith, A. Jones *et al.*, Chemotherapy for breast cancer during pregnancy: An 18-year experience from five London teaching hospitals, *J. Clin. Oncol.* **23**: 4192–4197 (2005).
23. D. Zemlickis, M. Lishner, P. Degendorfer *et al.*, Maternal and fetal outcome after breast cancer in pregnancy, *Am. J. Obstet. Gynecol.* **166**: 781–787 (1992).
24. J. F. Greskovich Jr. and R. M. Macklis, Radiation therapy in pregnancy: Risk calculation and risk minimization, *Semin. Oncol.* **27**: 633–645 (2000).
25. H. B. Kal and H. Struikmans, Radiotherapy during pregnancy: Fact and fiction, *Lancet Oncol.* **6**: 328–333 (2005).
26. M. Otake and W. J. Schull, A review of forty-five years study of Hiroshima and Nagasaki atomic bomb survivors. Radiation cataract, *J. Radiat. Res. (Tokyo)* **32**(Suppl.): 283–293 (1991).
27. J. A. Petrek, Breast cancer during pregnancy, *Cancer* **74**: 518–527 (1994).
28. M. L. Gemignani, J. A. Petrek and P. I. Borgen, Breast cancer and pregnancy, *Surg. Clin. North Am.* **79**: 1157–1169 (1999).
29. C. Antypas, P. Sandilos, J. Kouvaris *et al.*, Fetal dose evaluation during breast cancer radiotherapy, *Int. J. Radiat. Oncol. Biol. Phys.* **40**: 995–999 (1998).
30. S. L. Ngu, P. Duval and C. Collins, Foetal radiation dose in radiotherapy for breast cancer, *Australas. Radiol.* **36**: 321–322 (1992).

31. P. H. Van der Giessen, Measurement of the peripheral dose for the tangential breast treatment technique with Co-60 gamma radiation and high energy X-rays, *Radiother. Oncol.* **42**: 257–264 (1997).

32. E. Fenig, M. Mishaeli, Y. Kalish *et al.*, Pregnancy and radiation, *Cancer Treat. Rev.* **27**: 1–7 (2001).

33. A. D. Ives, C. M. Saunders and J. B. Semmens, The Western Australian gestational breast cancer project: A population-based study of the incidence, management and outcomes, *Breast* **14**: 276–282 (2005).

34. A. Molckovsky and Y. Madarnas, Breast cancer in pregnancy: A literature review, *Breast Cancer Res. Treat.* **108**: 333–338 (2007).

35. R. F. Pommier and S. A. Fields, Breast cancer in pregnancy — A diagnostic and therapeutic challenge, *West. J. Med.* **163**: 70–71 (1995).

36. D. L. Berry, R. L. Theriault, F. A. Holmes *et al.*, Management of breast cancer during pregnancy using a standardized protocol, *J. Clin. Oncol.* **17**: 855–861 (1999).

37. L. P. Middleton, M. Amin, K. Gwyn *et al.*, Breast carcinoma in pregnant women: Assessment of clinicopathologic and immunohistochemical features, *Cancer* **98**: 1055–1060 (2003).

38. P. L. Giacalone, F. Laffargue and P. Benos, Chemotherapy for breast carcinoma during pregnancy: A French national survey, *Cancer* **86**: 2266–2272 (1999).

39. J. T. Parente, M. Amsel, R. Lerner *et al.*, Breast cancer associated with pregnancy, *Obstet. Gynecol.* **71**: 861–864 (1988).

40. J. Wohlfahrt, P. K. Andersen, H. T. Mouridsen *et al.*, Risk of late-stage breast cancer after a childbirth, *Am. J. Epidemiol.* **153**: 1079–1084 (2001).

41. M. Lambe, C. Hsieh, D. Trichopoulos *et al.*, Transient increase in the risk of breast cancer after giving birth, *N. Engl. J. Med.* **331**: 5–9 (1994).

42. G. Albrektsen, I. Heuch and G. Kvale, The short- and long-term effect of a pregnancy on breast cancer risk: A prospective study of 802,457 parous Norwegian women, *Br. J. Cancer* **72**: 480–484 (1995).

43. K. Bock, P. Hadji, A. Ramaswamy *et al.*, Rationale for a diagnostic chain in gestational breast tumor diagnosis, *Arch. Gynecol. Obstet.* **273**: 337–345 (2006).

44. D. B. Novotny, S. J. Maygarden, R. W. Shermer *et al.*, Fine needle aspiration of benign and malignant breast masses associated with pregnancy, *Acta Cytol.* **35**: 676–686 (1991).

45. T. Ishida, T. Yokoe, F. Kasumi *et al.*, Clinicopathologic characteristics and prognosis of breast cancer patients associated with pregnancy and lactation: Analysis of case-control study in Japan, *Jpn. J. Cancer Res.* **83**: 1143–1149 (1992).

46. M. Mazonakis, H. Varveris, J. Damilakis *et al.*, Radiation dose to conceptus resulting from tangential breast irradiation, *Int. J. Radiat. Oncol. Biol. Phys.* **55**: 386–391 (2003).

47. P. Bonnier, S. Romain, J. M. Dilhuydy *et al.*, Influence of pregnancy on the outcome of breast cancer: A case-control study. Societe Francaise de Senologie et de Pathologie Mammaire Study Group, *Int. J. Cancer* **72**: 720–727 (1997).

48. S. Shousha, Breast carcinoma presenting during or shortly after pregnancy and lactation, *Arch. Pathol. Lab. Med.* **124**: 1053–1060 (2000).

49. S. Aziz, S. Pervez, S. Khan *et al.*, Case control study of novel prognostic markers and disease outcome in pregnancy/lactation-associated breast carcinoma, *Pathol. Res. Pract.* **199**: 15–21 (2003).

50. R. M. Elledge, D. R. Ciocca, G. Langone *et al.*, Estrogen receptor, progesterone receptor, and HER-2/neu protein in breast cancers from pregnant patients, *Cancer* **71**: 2499–2506 (1993).

51. A. E. Ring, I. E. Smith and P. A. Ellis, Breast cancer and pregnancy, *Ann. Oncol.* **16**: 1855–1860 (2005).

52. A. H. Nicklas and M. E. Baker, Imaging strategies in the pregnant cancer patient, *Semin. Oncol.* **27**: 623–632 (2000).

53. R. M. King, J. S. Welch, J. K. Martin Jr. *et al.*, Carcinoma of the breast associated with pregnancy, *Surg. Gynecol. Obstet.* **160**: 228–232 (1985).

54. R. I. Mazze and B. Kallen, Reproductive outcome after anesthesia and operation during pregnancy: A registry study of 5405 cases, *Am. J. Obstet. Gynecol.* **161**: 1178–1185 (1989).

55. P. G. Duncan, W. D. Pope, M. M. Cohen *et al.*, Fetal risk of anesthesia and surgery during pregnancy, *Anesthesiology* **64**: 790–794 (1986).

56. N. Pandit-Taskar, L. T. Dauer, L. Montgomery *et al.*, Organ and fetal absorbed dose estimates from 99mTc-sulfur colloid lymphoscintigraphy and sentinel node localization in breast cancer patients, *J. Nucl. Med.* **47**: 1202–1208 (2006).

57. O. Gentilini, M. Cremonesi, G. Trifiro *et al.*, Safety of sentinel node biopsy in pregnant patients with breast cancer, *Ann. Oncol.* **15**: 1348–1351 (2004).

58. A. Keleher, R. Wendt 3rd, E. Delpassand *et al.*, The safety of lymphatic mapping in pregnant breast cancer patients using Tc-99m sulfur colloid, *Breast J.* **10**: 492–495 (2004).

59. C. Lohrisch, C. Paltiel, K. Gelmon *et al.*, Impact on survival of time from definitive surgery to initiation of adjuvant chemotherapy for early-stage breast cancer, *J. Clin. Oncol.* **24**: 4888–4894 (2006).

60. S. Cold, M. During, M. Ewertz *et al.*, Does timing of adjuvant chemotherapy influence the prognosis after early breast cancer? Results of the Danish Breast Cancer Cooperative Group (DBCG), *Br. J. Cancer* **93**: 627–632 (2005).

61. M. Colleoni, M. Bonetti, A. S. Coates *et al.*, Early start of adjuvant chemotherapy may improve treatment outcome for premenopausal breast cancer patients with tumors not expressing estrogen receptors. The International Breast Cancer Study Group, *J. Clin. Oncol.* **18**: 584–590 (2000).

62. N. Germann, F. Goffinet and F. Goldwasser, Anthracyclines during pregnancy: Embryo-fetal outcome in 160 patients, *Ann. Oncol.* **15**: 146–150 (2004).

63. A. Aviles, N. Neri and M. J. Nambo, Long-term evaluation of cardiac function in children who received anthracyclines during pregnancy, *Ann. Oncol.* **17**: 286–288 (2006).

64. M. Meyer-Wittkopf, H. Barth, G. Emons *et al.*, Fetal cardiac effects of doxorubicin therapy for carcinoma of the breast during pregnancy: Case report and review of the literature, *Ultrasound Obstet. Gynecol.* **18**: 62–66 (2001).

65. E. E. Reynoso and F. Huerta, Acute leukemia and pregnancy — Fatal fetal outcome after exposure to idarubicin during the second trimester, *Acta Oncol.* **33**: 709–710 (1994).

66. B. L. Siu, M. R. Alonzo, T. A. Vargo *et al.*, Transient dilated cardiomyopathy in a newborn exposed to idarubicin and all-trans-retinoic acid (ATRA) early in the second trimester of pregnancy, *Int. J. Gynecol. Cancer* **12**: 399–402 (2002).

67. C. Achtari and P. Hohlfeld, Cardiotoxic transplacental effect of idarubicin administered during the second trimester of pregnancy, *Am. J. Obstet. Gynecol.* **183**: 511–512 (2000).

68. M. De Santis, A. Lucchese, S. De Carolis *et al.*, Metastatic breast cancer in pregnancy: First case of chemotherapy with docetaxel, *Eur. J. Cancer Care (Engl.)* **9**: 235–237 (2000).

69. Y. Nieto, M. Santisteban, J. M. Aramendia *et al.*, Docetaxel administered during pregnancy for inflammatory breast carcinoma, *Clin. Breast Cancer* **6**: 533–534 (2006).

70. M. C. Gainford and M. Clemons, Breast cancer in pregnancy: Are taxanes safe? *Clin. Oncol. (R. Coll. Radiol.)* **18**: 159 (2006).

71. V. Potluri, D. Lewis and G. V. Burton, Chemotherapy with taxanes in breast cancer during pregnancy: Case report and review of the literature, *Clin. Breast Cancer* **7**: 167–170 (2006).

72. R. Sekar and P. R. Stone, Trastuzumab use for metastatic breast cancer in pregnancy, *Obstet. Gynecol.* **110**: 507–510 (2007).

73. A. Gadducci, S. Cosio, A. Fanucchi *et al.*, Chemotherapy with epirubicin and paclitaxel for breast cancer during pregnancy: Case report and review of the literature, *Anticancer Res.* **23**: 5225–5229 (2003).

74. A. M. Gonzalez-Angulo, R. S. Walters, R. J. Carpenter Jr. *et al.*, Paclitaxel chemotherapy in a pregnant patient with bilateral breast cancer, *Clin. Breast Cancer* **5**: 317–319 (2004).

75. A. A. Bader, D. Schlembach, K. F. Tamussino *et al.*, Anhydramnios associated with administration of trastuzumab and paclitaxel for metastatic breast cancer during pregnancy, *Lancet Oncol.* **8**: 79–81 (2007).

76. J. L. Lycette, C. L. Dul, M. Munar *et al.*, Effect of pregnancy on the pharmacokinetics of paclitaxel: A case report, *Clin. Breast Cancer* **7**: 342–344 (2006).

77. V. J. Wiebe and P. E. Sipila, Pharmacology of antineoplastic agents in pregnancy, *Crit. Rev. Oncol. Hematol.* **16**: 75–112 (1994).

78. C. Cuvier, M. Espie, J. M. Extra *et al.*, Vinorelbine in pregnancy, *Eur. J. Cancer* **33**: 168–169 (1997).

79. P. A. Janne, D. Rodriguez-Thompson, D. R. Metcalf *et al.*, Chemotherapy for a patient with advanced non-small-cell lung cancer during pregnancy: A case report and a review of chemotherapy treatment during pregnancy, *Oncology* **61**: 175–183 (2001).

80. M. A. Fanale, A. R. Uyei, R. L. Theriault *et al.*, Treatment of metastatic breast cancer with trastuzumab and vinorelbine during pregnancy, *Clin. Breast Cancer* **6**: 354–356 (2005).

81. K. K. Leslie, Chemotherapy and pregnancy, *Clin. Obstet. Gynecol.* **45**: 153–164 (2002).

82. I. D. Witzel, V. Muller, E. Harps *et al.*, Trastuzumab in pregnancy associated with poor fetal outcome, *Ann. Oncol.* **19**: 191–192 (2008).

83. W. J. Watson, Herceptin (trastuzumab) therapy during pregnancy: Association with reversible anhydramnios, *Obstet. Gynecol.* **105**: 642–643 (2005).

84. A. M. Waterston and J. Graham, Effect of adjuvant trastuzumab on pregnancy, *J. Clin. Oncol.* **24**: 321–322 (2006).

85. S. Pant, M. B. Landon, M. Blumenfeld *et al.*, Treatment of breast cancer with trastuzumab during pregnancy, *J. Clin. Oncol.* **26**: 1567–1569 (2008).

86. H. Kelly, M. Graham, E. Humes *et al.*, Delivery of a healthy baby after first-trimester maternal exposure to lapatinib, *Clin. Breast Cancer* **7**: 339–341 (2006).

87. M. Feldkamp and J. C. Carey, Clinical teratology counseling and consultation case report: Low dose methotrexate exposure in the early weeks of pregnancy, *Teratology* **47**: 533–539 (1993).

88. L. Barthelmes and C. A. Gateley, Tamoxifen and pregnancy, *Breast* **13**: 446–451 (2004).

89. G. M. Tiboni, Aromatase inhibitors and teratogenesis, *Fertil. Steril.* **81**: 1158–1159; author reply 1159 (2004).

90. O. Taskin, R. Gokdeniz, R. Atmaca *et al.*, Normal pregnancy outcome after inadvertent exposure to long-acting gonadotrophin-releasing hormone agonist in early pregnancy, *Hum. Reprod.* **14**: 1368–1371 (1999).

91. J. Petrek, Breast cancer and pregnancy, *J. Natl. Cancer Inst. Monogr.* **16**: 113–121 (1994).

92. T. I. Yock, A. G. Taghian, L. A. Kachnic *et al.*, The effect of delaying radiation therapy for systemic chemotherapy on local-regional control in breast cancer, *Breast Cancer Res. Treat.* **84**: 161–171 (2004).

93. J. M. Metz, D. J. Schultz, K. Fox *et al.*, Analysis of outcomes for high-risk breast cancer based on interval from surgery to postmastectomy radiation therapy, *Cancer J.* **6**: 324–330 (2000).

94. M. G. Ruo Redda, R. Verna, A. Guarneri *et al.*, Timing of radiotherapy in breast cancer conserving treatment, *Cancer Treat. Rev.* **28**: 5–10 (2002).

95. R. M. Clark and T. Chua, Breast cancer and pregnancy: The ultimate challenge, *Clin. Oncol. (R. Coll. Radiol.)* **1**: 11–18 (1989).

96. R. M. Clark and J. Reid, Carcinoma of the breast in pregnancy and lactation, *Int. J. Radiat. Oncol. Biol. Phys.* **4**: 693–698 (1978).

97. V. F. Guinee, H. Olsson, T. Moller *et al.*, Effect of pregnancy on prognosis for young women with breast cancer, *Lancet* **343**: 1587–1589 (1994).

98. J. A. Petrek, R. Dukoff and A. Rogatko, Prognosis of pregnancy-associated breast cancer, *Cancer* **67**: 869–872 (1991).

99. P. Nugent and T. X. O'Connell, Breast cancer and pregnancy, *Arch. Surg.* **120**: 1221–1224 (1985).

100. G. Ribeiro, D. A. Jones and M. Jones, Carcinoma of the breast associated with pregnancy, *Br. J. Surg.* **73**: 607–609 (1986).

101. Australian Institute Health Welfare, *Cancer Survival in Australia 2001 — Part 1 — National Summary Statistics* (Canberra, 2001).

102. A. B. Gelb, M. van de Rijn, R. A. Warnke *et al.*, Pregnancy-associated lymphomas. A clinicopathologic study, *Cancer* **78**: 304–310 (1996).

103. H. L. Riva, P. S. Andreson and J. W. O'Grady, Pregnancy and Hodgkin's disease; a report of eight cases, *Am. J. Obstet. Gynecol.* **66**: 866–870 (1953).

104. H. L. Stewart Jr. and R. W. Monto, Hodgkin's disease and pregnancy, *Am. J. Obstet. Gynecol.* **63**: 570–578 (1952).

105. D. Pereg, G. Koren and M. Lishner, The treatment of Hodgkin's and non-Hodgkin's lymphoma in pregnancy, *Haematologica* **92**: 1230–1237 (2007).

106. B. Weisz, D. Meirow, E. Schiff *et al.*, Impact and treatment of cancer during pregnancy, *Expert Rev. Anticancer Ther.* **4**: 889–902 (2004).

107. H. Benveniste, J. S. Fowler, W. D. Rooney *et al.*, Maternal-fetal *in vivo* imaging: A combined PET and MRI study, *J. Nucl. Med.* **44**: 1522–1530 (2003).

108. R. J. Hicks, D. Binns and M. G. Stabin, Pattern of uptake and excretion of (18)F-FDG in the lactating breast, *J. Nucl. Med.* **42**: 1238–1242 (2001).

109. M. Lishner, D. Zemlickis, P. Degendorfer *et al.*, Maternal and foetal outcome following Hodgkin's disease in pregnancy, *Br. J. Cancer* **65**: 114–117 (1992).

110. J. Zuazu, A. Julia, J. Sierra *et al.*, Pregnancy outcome in hematologic malignancies, *Cancer* **67**: 703–709 (1991).

111. C. Jacobs, S. S. Donaldson, S. A. Rosenberg *et al.*, Management of the pregnant patient with Hodgkin's disease, *Ann. Intern. Med.* **95**: 669–675 (1981).

112. B. Weisz, E. Schiff and M. Lishner, Cancer in pregnancy: Maternal and fetal implications, *Hum. Reprod. Update* **7**: 384–393 (2001).

113. T. J. Myles, Hodgkin's disease and pregnancy, *J. Obstet. Gynaecol. Br. Emp.* **62**: 884–891 (1955).

114. R. M. Barry, H. D. Diamond and L. F. Craver, Influence of pregnancy on the course of Hodgkin's disease, *Am. J. Obstet. Gynecol.* **84**: 445–454 (1962).

115. M. Lishner, D. Zemlickis, S. B. Sutcliffe *et al.*, Non-Hodgkin's lymphoma and pregnancy, *Leuk. Lymphoma* **14**: 411–413 (1994).

116. E. Kimby, A. Sverrisdottir and G. Elinder, Safety of rituximab therapy during the first trimester of pregnancy: A case history, *Eur. J. Haematol.* **72**: 292–295 (2004).

117. M. Ojeda-Uribe, C. Gilliot, G. Jung *et al.*, Administration of rituximab during the first trimester of pregnancy without consequences for the newborn, *J. Perinatol.* **26**: 252–255 (2006).

118. R. M. Peres, M. T. Sanseverino, J. L. Guimaraes *et al.*, Assessment of fetal risk associated with exposure to cancer chemotherapy during pregnancy: A multicenter study, *Braz. J. Med. Biol. Res.* **34**: 1551–1559 (2001).

119. A. Aviles, J. C. Diaz-Maqueo, A. Talavera *et al.*, Growth and development of children of mothers treated with chemotherapy during pregnancy: Current status of 43 children, *Am. J. Hematol.* **36**: 243–248 (1991).

120. B. Friedrichs, M. Tiemann, H. Salwender *et al.*, The effects of rituximab treatment during pregnancy on a neonate, *Haematologica* **91**: 1426–1427 (2006).

121. K. M. Hahn, P. H. Johnson, N. Gordon *et al.*, Treatment of pregnant breast cancer patients and outcomes of children exposed to chemotherapy *in utero*, *Cancer* **107**: 1219–1226 (2006).

11

Addressing the Nutritional Needs of Patients Undergoing Cancer Treatment — A Dietitian's View

Judy Bauer,
Jane Read
and Kathy Chapman

Abstract

Significant nutritional issues facing people with cancer undergoing treatment include weight loss, treatment-related side effects and the presence of nutritional impact symptoms. Appropriate nutritional care is an essential component of a comprehensive cancer care service and all members of the multidisciplinary team should play a proactive role in addressing the nutritional needs of patients. Key aspects include the identification of malnutrition by nutritional screening and assessment, setting of appropriate goals, nutritional intervention (determining the nutritional prescription and implementation of the nutritional care plan), evaluation and monitoring. The success of nutritional care in improving patient outcomes is dependent upon the intensity of the care provided and positive clinical outcomes, such as improvements in dietary intake, maintenance of nutritional status and improvement in quality of life have been demonstrated in recent randomised controlled studies.

Keywords: Nutrition, nutritional assessment, dietary intake, malnutrition, dietary counselling.

1.   Introduction

Comprehensive nutritional care of patients undergoing cancer treatment involves collaboration by all members of the multidisciplinary team, to ensure coordinated care along agreed nutrition goals and priorities. All team members need to recognise nutrition-related issues and be able to recommend and implement effective strategies that will lead to positive patient outcomes. Nutrition is an aspect of their daily lives in which many people with cancer and their carers feel they can play an active role and they may actively seek nutrition information from a variety of sources. It is important that patients' nutritional needs and concerns are identified and addressed as they arise, as an increasing number of patients with cancer use complementary or alternative diets and supplements that often have little or no evidence base or benefit.[1]

2.   Causes of Weight Loss in Cancer Patients

Although the majority of people with cancer experience weight loss as their disease progresses, the causes of weight loss are multifactorial and may be related to the types of treatment they undergo (i.e. surgery, chemotherapy or radiotherapy), mechanical gastro-intestinal obstruction, cachexia, or a combination of these factors. For example, surgery can lead to malabsorption, radiation treatment can be associated with nausea, pain, diarrhoea and mucositis, and chemotherapy with nausea, vomiting, diarrhoea and mucositis. Symptoms such as loss of appetite, nausea, vomiting, dysphagia, taste changes, early satiety, pain and bowel changes such as diarrhoea and/or constipation all can affect patients' ability to consume an adequate oral intake. Common side effects of cancer and its treatment that may preclude patients from meeting their nutritional requirements are listed in Table 1. Weight loss may also be due to mechanical obstruction caused by the cancer itself, such as obstruction of the oesophagus causing swallowing problems and reduced oral intake.

Cancer cachexia is a complex syndrome, characterised by a progressive loss of lean tissue, metabolic abnormalities, anorexia

Table 1. Symptoms which may affect the nutritional status of patients with cancer.

Constipation	Mouth ulcers and oral infection
Dyspepsia	Mucositis
Diarrhoea	Nausea
Depression	Oral candidiasis
Dysguesia	Pain
Dysphagia	Vomiting
Fatigue	Weakness
Loss of appetite	Xerostomia
Malabsorption	

and fatigue. A consensus conference in 2006 proposed the diagnostic criteria for cachexia as weight loss of at least 5% over 12 months or less in the presence of underlying illness, together with three of the following criteria: decreased muscle strength, fatigue, anorexia, low fat-free body mass index, or abnormal biochemistry (increased inflammatory markers; anaemia; low serum albumin).[2] Cachexia has been implicated in the deaths of 30 to 50% of all cancer patients, as many die from wasting associated with this condition.[3] The consequences of progressive weight loss and subsequent development of malnutrition include an increased risk of complications, decreased response to and tolerance of treatment, a lower quality of life, higher health-care costs and reduced survival.[4-6]

The old misconception that malnutrition associated with cancer is inevitable and unresponsive to treatment has been challenged by a body of high quality evidence supporting the positive role medical nutritional therapy can play in patients undergoing cancer treatment.[7,8] Nutritional care is being recognised as an essential component of cancer treatment and access to an accredited practicing dietitian should be an integral part of a comprehensive cancer care service.[9]

3.   Evidence Based Nutrition Guidelines

Evidence based practice guidelines for the nutritional management of cancer cachexia[7] and nutritional management of radiation therapy[8] have been published and are endorsed by the Dietitians Association of Australia. In today's information-rich environment, these guidelines can assist clinicians to access and utilise the best available evidence regarding the nutritional care of patients with cancer. The guidelines highlight the key aspects of the nutritional care process, which includes nutrition screening and assessment, establishing the goals of treatment, implementation of the nutritional care (nutrition prescription and counselling) and monitoring and evaluation.[10]

3.1 *Identifying malnutrition — Nutrition screening and assessment*

It is important that systems are in place to identify and prioritise patients in the most nutritional need and a screening program can expeditiously identify people who are malnourished or at risk of malnutrition, so that nutritional intervention can commence in a timely manner. Although a number of reliable and valid nutritional screening tools have been published, the Malnutrition Screening Tool (MST) has been validated to quickly identify nutritional risk in patients with cancer.[11,12] It consists of two questions related to recent weight loss and appetite and can be completed by patients, carers, clinic staff or clinicians in minimal time (Table 2).

Table 2. Malnutrition screening tool[©].[11]

Have you lost weight recently without trying?	
If no	0
If unsure	2
If yes, how much weight (kg) have you lost?	
0.5–5.0	1
> 5.0–10.0	2
> 10.0–15.0	3
> 15.0	4
Unsure	2
Have you been eating poorly because of a decreased appetite?	
No	0
Yes	1
If score 0 or 1 — Not at risk of malnutrition	
score ≥ 2 — At risk of malnutrition	

Nutritional screening should occur at the time of diagnosis and at regular intervals throughout treatment, so that nutrition-related issues can be addressed as they occur.

All people with cancer would benefit from individualised medical nutritional therapy, provided by an accredited practicing dietitian. As this may not be possible in all situations, the Oncology Nutrition Action Flowchart© has been developed to assist clinicians to guide nutrition care for people with cancer following nutritional screening (Fig. 1). For patients at low risk of malnutrition, provision of written information about nutritional issues in cancer from a credible source and rescreening at regular intervals throughout treatment is recommended. For patients at high nutritional risk, a variety of intervention strategies are available, which include advice regarding increasing protein and energy intake, using high protein and energy liquid supplements (either home-made or commercial) and consultation with an accredited practicing dietitian. The Oncology Nutrition Action Flowchart© can be used by the multidisciplinary team to guide and commence nutrition care as soon as nutrition-related issues are identified. This is particularly useful if there is delayed or limited access to an accredited practicing dietitian.

Nutritional assessment can be used to determine the nutritional status of patients at the time of diagnosis and for monitoring at regular intervals during cancer treatment. The scored Patient-Generated Subjective Global Assessment (PG-SGA) is a valid and reliable method of nutritional assessment specifically developed for use in cancer patients.[13–18] It consists of a comprehensive medical history (which documents changes in weight and dietary intake, the presence of nutritional impact symptoms persisting for longer than two weeks and an assessment of functional capacity) and a physical examination (looking for evidence of loss of subcutaneous fat, muscle wasting, oedema or ascites). These are combined into a global assessment of nutrition (as well or moderately well nourished, suspected of being malnourished or severely malnourished) and a score is calculated. A comprehensive nutritional assessment may not be realistic to implement for all patients in the absence of an accredited practicing dietitian. In these situations, the Oncology Nutrition Action Flowchart© can be used to guide nutritional care following screening.

What is your oncology patient's malnutrition risk?

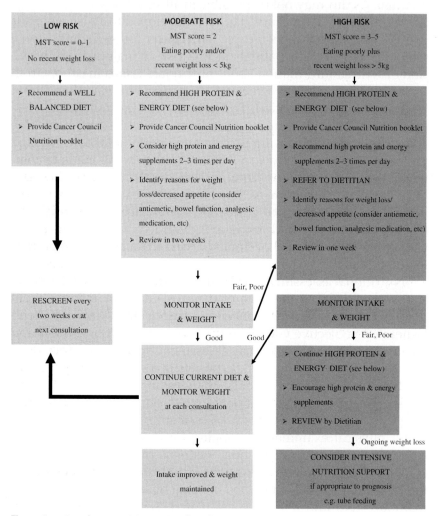

Figure 1. Oncology nutrition action flowchart.

HIGH ENERGY & PROTEIN DIET

- Try serving 6 smaller meals/snacks per day
- Include 3–4 extra serving of energy and protein-rich foods or drinks daily
  - Extra serves of eggs, meat, baked beans, cheese
  - Milk or soy-based drinks e.g. milkshakes, smoothies
  - Extra desserts e.g. ice cream, custard, cakes, biscuits
  - Dried fruit, nuts, chocolate, chips
- Fortify foods by adding milk powder, cream, butter, cheese
- For more nourishing diet ideas or advice regarding suitable commercial supplements contact your dietitian

Developed by the Cancer Cachexia Steering Committee, based on the Malnutrition Action Flowchart (©Merrilyn Banks, APD) *2006*

Figure 1. *(Continued)*

3.2 *Nutritional treatment goals*

The goals and priorities of nutritional care should be determined by the multidisciplinary team in conjunction with the patient. When discussing nutritional goals and intervention options with patients and carers, it is important to present realistic potential outcomes, which will be dependent on the patient's diagnosis and prognosis. There is a distinction between intensive nutritional care when an achievable outcome is viable and coercing patients to undergo intensive nutritional care when palliative support is more appropriate. Patients should be given clear messages of the likely benefits of nutrition care.[9] Traditionally, weight gain has been a goal of nutritional intervention, but in light of recent studies demonstrating that patients with cancer who stabilised their weight had increased survival and improved quality of life compared to those who continued to lose weight,[19–21] weight maintenance is now considered a suitable goal of nutrition care. The main goals of medical nutrition therapy are to:

- maintain weight and preserve lean body mass;
- minimise nutrition-related side effects and complications; and
- maximise quality of life.[22]

3.3 *Nutritional intervention*

There are two key aspects of the nutritional intervention — the nutritional prescription, and implementation of the nutritional care plan. The nutritional intervention plan may change as new issues are identified or the patient's condition changes.

3.3.1 *Nutritional prescription*

The type of cancer, disease stage and treatment modality may affect nutritional requirements. The energy expenditure of patients with cancer has been shown to vary greatly from hypo- to hypermetabolic.[23] Dietary intake is often reduced as a result of nutritional impact symptoms such as taste alterations, poor appetite and fatigue. An energy intake in excess of 120 kJ/kg/day and protein intake in excess of 1.4 g/kg/day are needed for weight maintenance in patients with cancer.[20,24] Any existing dietary modifications, such as lipid lowering or weight reduction should be reviewed during cancer treatment and in general, the prescription of a high protein and energy dense diet is recommended.

The prescription of pharmacological doses of eicosapentaenoic acid (EPA), an omega-3 polyunsaturated fat, is a recent novel nutritional intervention in patients with cancer cachexia. Early animal and human studies indicated that EPA supplementation reduces the production of pro-inflammatory cytokines (interleukin-6, interleukin-1 and tumour necrosis factor) and increases the cell death rate in cultured cancer cell lines.[25-28] A recent Cochrane review found insufficient data to establish whether supplementation with EPA (either in the form of capsules or high protein and energy enriched EPA supplements) is superior to placebo in patients with cancer cachexia.[29] Although improved outcomes (dietary intake, body composition, performance status, quality of life) have been demonstrated with high protein and energy EPA-enriched supplements in open studies, these results have not been confirmed in randomised trials. Issues such as adherence with the prescription,[30] duration of the intervention,[31] appropriateness of study endpoints,[32] advanced stage of cancer and the type of treatment (supportive care/chemotherapy/mixed therapy) are all important to consider when evaluating these trials. Further well-designed studies addressing these methodological issues are required, to determine whether there is a clinical benefit of EPA in patients with cancer.[7,29] A promising approach is multimodal therapy, which combines nutrition with a pharmacological intervention that addresses both the reduction in dietary intake and changes in metabolism that occurs in cancer.[33,34]

3.3.2 *Implementation of nutritional care*

This involves counselling the patient and/or carers to achieve the recommended dietary intake and facilitates the optimal control of nutritional impact symptoms, co-ordination of care and ongoing planning. Individualised nutritional counselling by a dietitian has been shown to increase intake, attenuate weight loss and improve quality of life and performance status in patients with cancer.[24,35–38] Appropriate nutritional advice may be provided by all members of the multidisciplinary health care team, and a consistent message, with reinforcement from multiple team members, may increase dietary intake and adherence. Patients should be encouraged to regard nutritional care as one of the key elements of their cancer treatment. Simple strategies, such as eating small frequent meals and snacks, replacing low energy fluids such as tea and coffee with high protein and energy drinks, enjoying favourite foods frequently and relaxing other dietary restrictions can be of assistance in increasing dietary intake.

Table 3 describes some helpful nutritional strategies to assist patients cope with the symptoms of cancer and its treatment. Patients need to be provided with sufficient information regarding the possible side effects and dietary changes that may be required during their treatment. Studies have shown that patients who receive proactive nutrition counselling and are prepared for the dietary changes necessary during their treatment achieve better outcomes such as weight maintenance, nutritional status and quality of life.[7–9] Patient education is essential to manage food aversions and help patients explore strategies to cope with the side effects of treatment. Optimal control of symptoms such as nausea and vomiting, pain, constipation, diarrhoea and mucosal toxicity is necessary for achieving dietary intake goals. Appropriate medications are important for symptom management and should be regularly reviewed by the medical team.

Patients unable to meet their nutritional requirements with food alone, despite adequate nutritional counselling, may benefit from oral nutritional supplements. These are especially useful for

Table 3. Common cancer- or treatment-related symptoms and some suggested strategies to alleviate them.

Symptom	Nutritional management
Anorexia	• Small high-protein and high-energy meals every 1–2 hours. • Add extra kilojoules and protein where possible to food (e.g. butter, skim milk powder, honey). • If ingesting solids is a problem, consume liquid supplements, soups, milk shakes and smoothies. • Snacks should be high in kilojoules and protein. • Prepare and store small portions of foods, so no preparation is required. • Try new foods. Patients should experiment with recipes, flavourings, spices, types, and consistencies of food.
Dysguesia (change in taste)	• Use plastic utensils if taste is metallic. • Rinse mouth thoroughly with water before eating. • Try citrus fruits, to flavour foods and drinks. • Zinc supplements may help improve the return of taste.
Dry mouth	• Use moist foods with extra sauces, gravies, butter, or margarine. • Suck on hard lollies or chew gum. • Clean teeth (including dentures) and rinse mouth at least four times per day (after each meal and before bedtime). • Keep water handy at all times, to moisten the mouth. • Avoid mouth rinses containing alcohol. • Drink fruit nectar instead of juice. • Commercial products are available as saliva substitutes.
Mouth sores	• Modify consistency of food (puree or mince the foods). • Add gravy, sauces to soften food. • Avoid rough, crunchy food, and cut food into small pieces. • Avoid spicy, salty food or highly acidic foods. • Use a straw to drink liquids. • Avoid very hot and very cold foods. Have them at room temperature. • Consider liquid nutritional supplements.
Nausea	• Eat small meals several times a day, and don't have long periods without food. • Minimize unpleasant sensory stimulants (cooking odours).

(Continued)

Table 3. *(Continued)*

Symptom	Nutritional management
	• Avoid foods likely to cause nausea (greasy, spicy, strong flavours). • Eat bland, light foods. • Sip fluids throughout the day. • Rinse mouth before and after eating.
Constipation	• Ensure adequate fluids. • Ensure adequate fibre.
Diarrhoea	• Ensure adequate fluids and fibre. • Consider pro-biotics if diarrhoea has been induced by antibiotics. • Limit vegetables which are gas-forming (cruciferous vegetables).

patients who experience dysphagia. Commercial high protein and energy supplements can provide patients with vital nutrients needed for cell regeneration and assist in meeting their energy and nutrient needs when intake of solid food becomes inadequate. New supplements should ideally be introduced when the patient has no major symptoms. For example, it is best to introduce them in between chemotherapy cycles, so patients do not develop food aversions. Various types of supplements are available, ranging in nutrient density, composition and flavour (milk, soy or fruit flavour based). It is important for patients to trial different types and flavours, in order to find a variety that best suits their needs, which may also change during treatment. Supplements may be used as between meal snacks or as full meal replacements, and should be provided with regular ongoing nutritional counselling. Although there is a wide range of commercially available high protein and energy liquid supplements, home-made drinks such as smoothies and milkshakes may be more cost effective and are well tolerated. Prognosis, economic circumstances and patient preferences need to be considered when recommending high protein and energy supplements. Some patients may be concerned that drinking nutrient-dense supplements between meals may reduce their meal intake. Studies in patients with cancer have shown that consumption of high protein and energy supplements increase overall dietary intake, without negatively impacting on spontaneous food intake.[24,37] Patients may experience acute enteritis due to high doses of chemotherapy, or radiotherapy to the pelvis. Others may have impaired gastrointestinal function due to the disease process or a bowel resection. Elemental oral supplements which are peptide-based or made up of single amino acids and sugars allow better absorption in these patients. A dietitian will be able to provide individualised advice for patients and tailor a specialised meal plan to meet their requirements.

If patients undergoing treatment for cancer are unable to meet their nutritional needs due to mechanical obstruction or treatment-related side effects, enteral nutritional support needs to be considered. The route of enteral feeding will depend on factors such as length of treatment, duration of ongoing symptoms and patient preference. Nasogastric or nasojejunal feeding are generally used in the short term and a percutaneous endoscopic gastrostomy (PEG) for longer term support. A wide variety of commercially available enteral formulae can provide patients with their complete nutritional needs. The selection of the appropriate formulae will depend upon the patients' nutrient requirements, gut function, cost and convenience. Patients receiving treatment for head and neck cancer may benefit from the placement of a prophylactic PEG prior to the commencement of treatment. This has been shown to reduce weight loss, treatment interruptions and hospitalisations.[8]

Parenteral nutritional support may be required for some patients with cancer who do not have a functional gastrointestinal tract, if oral intake is not tolerated due to severe nausea, vomiting and diarrhoea, or for those with significant mucositis, when placing a PEG or nasogatric tube may be unsafe. Patients receiving a bone marrow transplant may fall into this category. Key factors to consider prior to initiating parenteral nutrition include patient's prognosis, treatment, nutritional status, gastrointestinal function and the levels of monitoring and specialised care required.

Nutritional counselling is effective both during active treatment (chemotherapy and radiotherapy) and while receiving supportive care. The frequency of counselling is an important aspect of implementation of the nutrition care plan, having been shown to impact on patient adherence and outcomes. Recent studies in patients receiving radiation therapy or with cancer cachexia have demonstrated effective clinical outcomes with weekly to fortnightly nutrition intervention.[24,30,35,39] Several randomised clinical trials have demonstrated that appropriate nutritional care can help to overcome nutritional impact symptoms and assist patients to maintain weight and quality of life.[35,36] However if the weight loss is due to cachexia, the success of nutritional intervention may be more limited, due to the complex pathogenesis of the condition.[40] Nevertheless, medical nutrition therapy can still achieve positive outcomes, such as a decrease in the severity of symptoms, improvement in dietary intake and quality of life in patients with cancer.[9] For many patients with cancer and their carers, these patient focused outcomes are extremely important, especially for those with poor prognoses.[9]

3.3.3 *Monitoring and evaluation of nutritional care*

The final stage of the nutritional care process is the monitoring and evaluation of nutritional care, to ensure that the plan is responsive to the patients' needs. Multidisciplinary team meetings are the ideal forum to allow for interdisciplinary discussion and decision making regarding the nutrition care plan.

4. Summary and Conclusions

Appropriate nutritional care is an essential component of cancer treatment. All members of the multidisciplinary team should play a proactive role in identifying and managing nutrition issues faced by patients undergoing cancer treatment. Key aspects of the nutritional care process include identification of malnutrition by nutritional screening and assessment, setting of appropriate goals, intervention (prescription and implementation), evaluation and monitoring. Positive clinical outcomes, such as improvement in quality of life have been demonstrated with intensive nutrition care in recent randomised controlled studies. Further research is required to determine the optimal medical nutrition therapy for cancer patients and in particular for optimising the management of cancer cachexia.

References

1. C. L. Rock, V. A. Newman, M. L. Neuhouser, J. Major and M. J. Barnett, Antioxidant supplement use in cancer survivors and the general population, *J. Nutr.* **134**: 3194S–3195S (2004).
2. W. J. Evans, J. E. Morley, J. Argiles, C. Bales, V. Baracos *et al.*, Cachexia: A new definition, *Clin. Nutr.* **27**: 793–799 (2008).
3. M. R. Palomares, J. W. Sayre, K. C. Shekar, L. M. Lillington and R. Chlebowski, Gender influence of weight-loss pattern and survival of nonsmall cell lung carcinoma patients, *Cancer* **78**: 2119–2126 (1996).
4. M. Grant and L. Rivera, Impact of dietary counselling on quality of life in head and neck patients undergoing radiation therapy, *Qual. Life Res.* **3**: 77–78 (1994).
5. F. D. Ottery, Definition of standardized nutritional assessment and interventional pathways in oncology, *Nutrition* **12**(Suppl. 1): S15–19 (1996).
6. G. Nitenberg and B. Raynard, Nutritional support of the cancer patient: issues and dilemmas, *Crit. Rev. Oncol. Hematol.* **34**: 137–168 (2000).
7. J. D. Bauer, S. Ash, W. Davidson, J. M. Hill, T. Brown, E. Isenring and M. Reeves, Evidence based practice guidelines for nutritional management of cancer cachexia, *Nutr. Diet* **63**: S5–32 (2006).
8. E. Isenring, J. M. Hill, W. Davidson, T. Brown, L. Baumgartner, K. Kaegi, M. Reeves, S. Ash, S. Thomas, N. McPhee and J. D. Bauer, Evidence based practice guidelines for the nutritional management of patients receiving radiation therapy, *Nutr. Diet* **65**: S1–S20 (2008).
9. S. Capra, J. Bauer, W. Davidson and S. Ash, Nutritional therapy for cancer induced weight loss, *Nutr. Clin. Pract.* **17**: 210–213 (2002).
10. N. Hakel-Smith and N. M. Lewis, A standardized nutrition care process and language are essential components of conceptual model to guide and document nutrition care and patient outcomes, *J. Am. Diet Assoc.* **104**: 1878–1884 (2004).
11. M. Ferguson, J. Bauer, M. Banks and S. Capra, Development of a valid and reliable malnutrition screening tool for adult acute hospital patients, *Nutrition* **15**: 458–464 (1999).
12. M. L. Ferguson, J. Bauer, B. Gallagher, S. Capra, D. R. Christie and B. R. Mason, Validation of a malnutrition screening tool for patients receiving radiotherapy, *Australas. Radiol.* **43**: 325–327 (1999).
13. F. D. Ottery, Patient-generated subjective global assessment. In: *The Clinical Guide to Oncology Nutrition*, eds. P. D. McCallum and

C. G. Polisena (The American Dietetic Association, Chicago, 2000), pp. 11–23.

14. C. Persson, P.-O. Sjoden and B. Glimelius, The Swedish version of the patient-generated subjective global assessment of nutritional status: Gastrointestinal vs. urological cancers, *Clin. Nutr.* **18**: 71–77 (1999).

15. F. Ottery, F. Bender and S. Kasenic, The design and implementation of a model of nutritional oncology clinic, *Oncol. Issues Suppl.* **17**: 3–8 (2002).

16. J. Bauer, S. Capra and M. Ferguson, Use of the scored patient — Generated subjective global assessment as a nutrition assessment tool in patients with cancer, *Eur. J. Clin. Nutr.* **56**: 779–785 (2002).

17. E. Isenring, J. Bauer and S. Capra, The scored patient-generated subjective global assessment (PG-SGA) and its association with quality of life in ambulatory patients receiving radiotherapy, *Eur. J. Clin. Nutr.* **57**(2): 305–309 (2003).

18. J. A. Read, N. Crockett, D. H. Volker, P. MacLennan, S. T. B. Choy, P. Beale and S. J. Clarke, Nutritional assessment in cancer: Comparing the Mini-Nutritional Assessment (MNA) to the Scored Patient Generated Subjective Global Assessment (PGSGA), *Nutr. Cancer* **53**: 51–56 (2005).

19. H. J. Andreyev, A. R. Norman, J. Oates and D. Cunningham, Why do patients with weight loss have a worse outcome when undergoing chemotherapy for gastrointestinal malignancies? *Eur. J. Cancer* **34**: 503–509 (1998).

20. W. Davidson, S. Ash, S. Capra and J. Bauer, Weight stabilisation is associated with improved survival duration and quality of life in unresectable pancreatic cancer, *Clin. Nutr.* **23**: 239–247 (2004).

21. P. J. Ross, S. Ashley, A. Norton *et al.*, Do patients with weight loss have a worse outcome when undergoing chemotherapy for lung cancers? *Br. J. Cancer* **90**: 1905–1911 (2004).

22. M. Shike, Nutrition therapy for the cancer patient, *Hematol. Oncol. Clin. North Am.* **10**: 221–234 (1996).

23. M. M. Reeves, Estimating patients' energy requirements: cancer as a case study, PhD thesis, Queensland University of Technology, 2004.

24. J. Bauer and S. Capra, Intensive nutrition intervention improves outcomes in patients with cancer cachexia receiving chemotherapy — A pilot study, *Support. Care Cancer* **13**: 270–274 (2005).

25. S. Endres, R. Ghorgani, V. E. Kelly *et al.*, The effect of dietary supplementation with n-3 polyunsaturated fatty acids or the synthesis of

interleukin-1 and tumor necrosis factor by mononuclear cells, *New Engl. J. Med.* **320**: 265 (1989).

26. S. J. Wigmore, J. A. Ross, J. S. Falconer, C. E. Plester, M. J. Tisdale, D. C. Carter and K. C. Fearon, The effect of polyunsaturated fatty acids on the progress of cachexia in patients with pancreatic cancer, *Nutrition* **12** (Suppl. 1): S27–30 (1996).

27. M. J. Tisdale and S. A. Beck, Inhibition of tumour-induced lipolysis *in vitro* and cachexia and tumour growth *in vivo* by eicosapentaenoic acid, *Biochem. Pharmacol.* **41**: 103–107 (1991).

28. G. E. Caughey, E. Mantzioris, R. A. Gibson, L. G. Cleland and M. J. James, The effect on human tumor necrosis factor α and interleukin 1B production of diets enriched in n-3 fatty acids from vegetable oil or fish oil, *Am. J. Clin. Nutr.* **63**: 116–122 (1996).

29. A. Dewey, C. Baughan, T. Dean, B. Higgins and I. Johnson, Eicosapentaenoic acid (EPA, an omega-3 fatty acid from fish oils) for the treatment of cancer cachexia, *Cochrane Database Syst. Rev.* **24**(1): CD004597 (2007).

30. K. Fearon, M. von Meyenfeldt, A. Moses, R. van Geenan, A. Roy, D. Gouma, A. Giacosa, A. Van Gossum, J. Bauer, M. Barber, N. Aaronson, A. Voss and M. Tisdale, The effect of a protein and energy dense, n-3 fatty acid enriched oral supplement on loss of weight and lean tissue in cancer cachexia: A randomised double blind trial, *Gut* **52**: 1479–1486 (2003).

31. E. Bruera, F. Strasser, J. L. Palmer, J. Willey, K. Calder, G. Amyotte and V. Baracos, Effect of fish oil on appetite and other symptoms in patients with advanced cancer and anorexia/cachexia: A double-blind, placebo-controlled study, *J. Clin. Oncol.* **21**: 129–134 (2003).

32. A. Jatoi, K. Rowland, C. L. Loprinzi, J. A. Sloan, S. R. Dakhil, N. MacDonald, B. Gagnon, P. J. Novotny, J. A. Mailliard, T. I. Bushey, S. Nair and B. Christensen, North Central Cancer Treatment Group. An eicosapentaenoic acid supplement versus megestrol acetate versus both for patients with cancer-associated wasting: A North Central Cancer Treatment Group and National Cancer Institute of Canada collaborative effort, *J. Clin. Oncol.* **22**: 2469–2476 (2004).

33. G. Mantovani, A. Macciò, C. Madeddu, G. Gramignano, R. Serpe, E. Massa, M. Dessi, F. M. Tanca, E. Sanna, L. Deiana, F. Panzone, P. Contu and C. Floris, Randomized phase III clinical trial of five different arms of treatment for patients with cancer cachexia: interim results, *Nutrition* **24**: 305–313 (2008).

34. K. C. Fearon, Cancer cachexia: Developing multimodal therapy for a multidimensional problem, *Eur. J. Cancer* **44**: 1124–1132 (2008).

35. E. Isenring, S. Capra and J. Bauer, Nutrition intervention is beneficial in oncology outpatients receiving radiotherapy to the gastrointestinal, head or neck area, *Br. J. Cancer* **91**: 447–452 (2004).

36. P. Ravasco, I. Monteiro-Grillo, P. M. Vidal and M. E. Camilo, Dietary counseling improves patient outcomes: a prospective, randomized, controlled trial in colorectal cancer patients undergoing radiotherapy, *J. Clin. Oncol.* **23**(7): 1431–1438 (2005).

37. D. McCarthy and D. Weihofen, The effect of nutritional supplements on food intake in patients undergoing radiotherapy, *Oncol. Nurs. Forum* **26**: 897–900 (1999).

38. L. Ovesen, L. Allingstrup, J. Hannibal, E. L. Mortensen and O. P. Hansen, Effect of dietary counseling on food intake, body weight, response rate, survival, and quality of life in cancer patients undergoing chemotherapy: A prospective, randomized study, *J. Clin. Oncol.* **11**: 2043–2049 (1993).

39. A. W. G. Moses, C. Slater, T. Preston, M. D. Barber and K. C. H. Fearon, Reduced total energy expenditure and physical activity in cachectic patients with pancreatic cancer can be modulated by an energy and protein dense oral supplement enriched with n-3 fatty acids, *Br. J. Cancer* **90**: 996–1002 (2004).

40. M. J. Tisdale, The 'cancer cachectic factor', *Support. Care Cancer* **11**: 73–78 (2003).

12

Beyond Conventional Cancer Treatments: The Use of Complementary Therapies During Cancer Treatment: Implications for Clinicians

Stephen J. Clarke,
Andrew J. McLachlan,
Darrin Brown,
Stephen Carbonara
and Rachel Kissane

Abstract

An increasing proportion of patients suffering from cancer use complementary and alternative medicines (CAM). This use is frequently undertaken in addition to their prescribed treatments, often without their physician's knowledge. For many types of CAM, this concomitant use of treatments is without risk. However, for systemically administered CAM, such as herbal medicines, there are significant risks of adverse drug interactions between herbal medicines and anti-cancer agents, which may result in either increased drug toxicity or therapeutic failure. This review demonstrates the paucity of high quality randomised controlled data that are available to guide cancer clinicians in regard to potential adverse interactions between standard treatments and commonly used herbal medicines. It shows that certain combinations of herbal medicines and chemotherapy carry significant risks and are contraindicated. For instance, *in vivo* studies have shown that concomitant use of St John's Wort with cancer chemotherapy agents that are CYP3A4 substrates has the potential to cause therapeutic failure. *In vitro* and *in vivo* studies show that caution is warranted when considering concomitant Asian ginseng or fenugreek with CYP3A4 substrates and guarana with CYP1A2 substrates. A potential for pharmacodynamic interactions between herbal medicines and anti-cancer agents also exists. Patients with oestrogen receptor positive breast cancers should be advised to avoid administration of phyto-oestrogen containing herbal preparations. Currently there is a lack of conclusive information regarding interactions between feverfew, ginger, garlic, gingko, chamomile, milk thistle, grape seed, black cohosh, celery, devil's claw or cranberry when concomitantly taken with anti-cancer agents. Physicians should be proactive in ascertaining herbal medicine use in all their patients receiving cancer chemotherapy, in order to advise them appropriately.

Keywords: Chinese herbs, medical oncology, drug herb interactions.

1. Introduction

Complementary and Alternative Medicine (CAM) includes a diverse group of treatments that range from music therapy, exercise and massage to more invasive treatments such as acupuncture, nutritional therapies and herbal medicines. The last 15 years have seen a significant increase in the use of CAM. In 1990, a survey performed in the United States estimated that 34% of the respondents used at least one form of complementary therapy in the previous 12 months.[1] This figure had increased to 42% by 1997.[2] The popularity of CAM use has been mirrored in Australia.[3] In 2004, a South Australian survey reported 52% of respondents had used at least one non-medically prescribed CAM in the previous year. More than 57% of respondents reported using CAM without their health practitioner's knowledge and 50% took conventional medicines on the same day, creating the potential for drug-CAM interactions.[3]

Patients with cancer are also increasingly frequently using CAM. In 1998, a systematic review of the literature revealed a mean CAM use in 31% among cancer patients.[4] A number of recent studies have suggested that this figure may now exceed 80%, although there is variability in use depending on tumour type and ethnic group studied, CAM use being more common in breast cancer patients and individuals from Asian backgrounds.[5,6]

A recent systematic review attempted to identify the principal reasons cancer patients are using CAM. Although there was a wide range of responses, the most frequent were a perceived beneficial response (38%), wanting "control" (17%), CAM as a "last resort" (10%) and "finding hope" (10%).[7]

Not surprisingly therefore, CAM is big business. In the US alone, it has been estimated that cancer patients spend over $30 billion in out of pocket expenses on CAM, even though there are few data to indicate the cost effectiveness of CAM.[8] This increased use by patients with cancer and expense of CAM has highlighted issues in regard to the safety and efficacy of these treatments. This is particularly the case for systemically administered CAM, including herbal medicines, where there is the potential for clinically significant interactions with conventional anti-cancer treatment. Consequently, in this chapter we decided to restrict our discussions on CAM to systemically administered herbal medicines, in order to highlight the potential for herb-drug interactions with anti-cancer agents, to educate clinicians about these commonly used medicines and highlight the dearth of high quality data that are available.

2. Herb-Drug Interactions

The focus of this discussion is limited to more commonly used herbal medicines[9] and those mentioned in recent literature as causing or having the potential to cause herb-drug interactions with conventional anti-cancer medicines.[10–12] The anti-cancer agents investigated included those in common use and belonging to a variety of drug classes, including cytotoxic, hormonal and molecular targeted therapies. However, data on herb-drug interactions from *in vivo* trials, especially with regard to cancer chemotherapy agents, are extremely limited. This means that some of the concepts regarding potential drug interactions with anti-cancer drugs have had to be extrapolated from interactions with drugs from other therapeutic classes that have similar routes of metabolism.

Herb-drug interactions occur via several broad mechanisms, including pharmaceutical, pharmacokinetic (PK) and pharmacodynamic (PD) interactions (Table 1). Pharmacokinetic interactions can result when common pathways of absorption, metabolism, distribution or elimination exist between the constituents of herbal medicines and anti-cancer agents. These interactions most commonly involve intestinal and hepatic metabolising enzymes (cytochrome P450, or "CYP" enzymes) and drug transporters such as P-glycoprotein (P-gp), breast cancer resistance protein (BCRP) and multi-drug resistance proteins (MRPs) found not only in resistant tumour cells, but also in healthy tissue including the gut epithelium, liver and central nervous system.[13] Because most anti-cancer agents have a very narrow therapeutic index, any interaction affecting the clearance of parent or metabolites has considerable potential to result in toxicity or sub-therapeutic levels. Two of the most important CYP enzymes for metabolism of xenobiotics in humans are CYP3A4 and CYP2D6 (see Table 1). Substrates for CYP3A4 include many of the commonly used anti-cancer drugs such as exemestane, tamoxifen, letrozole, docetaxel, paclitaxel, vincristine, irinotecan, gefitinib and imatinib, among many.[12] Also, cyclophosphamide is a pro-drug, which is activated by CYP enzymes, including CYP3A4; however, it is also inactivated by CYP3A4 to the dechloroethyl metabolite. Toremifene, vinorelbine and vinblastine are also metabolised by CYP3A4, but are converted to active metabolites. Substrates for the drug transporter, P-gp, include many of the naturally derived anti-cancer drugs including the taxanes, vinca alkaloids, epipodophyllotoxins and anthracyclines. Pharmacodynamic interactions may occur when a herbal compound acts in an additive, synergistic or antagonistic fashion with an anti-cancer agent.

It is worth noting that disease states themselves can change the PK or PD of a drug and extrapolating data from healthy volunteers to patients with cancer is not always possible. For example, CYP

Table 1. Level of caution required for the concomitant use of selected anti-cancer agents with herbal medicines. The coloured classification system was derived by the authors based upon their critical, clinical evaluation of available literature. "Extreme" caution denotes high potential for adverse reactions confirmed from *in vivo* studies, concomitant use should be avoided; "Moderate" caution, denotes medium potential for adverse reactions (*in vitro* studies indicates possible interaction), concomitant use should only be administered under strict, clinical supervision; "Low" caution denotes little potential for adverse reactions, *in vivo* and *in vitro* studies indicate little potential for interactions concomitant use may be considered; "Unknown" caution denotes a lack of available clinical evidence to make an appropriate recommendation.

Level of caution required for concomitant use:
- Unknown (white)
- Low (light grey)
- Moderate (dark grey)
- Extreme (black)

Herb \ Agent	Aminoglutethimide	Bleomycin	Busulfan	Capecitabine	Carboplatin	Chlorambucil	Cisplatin	Cladribine	Cyclophosphamide	Cytarabine	Docetaxel	Doxorubicin	Epirubicin	Etoposide	Exemestane	Fluorouracil	Fotemustine	Gefitinib	Gemcitabine	Goserelin	Idarubicin	Ifosfamide	Imatinib	Irinotecan	Letrozole	Leuprorelin	Melphalan	Mercaptopurine	Methotrexate	Mitoxantron	Octreotide	Oxaliplatin	Paclitaxel	Pemetrexed	Prednisolone/Raltitrexed	Tamoxifen	Temozolamide	Teniposide	Thioguanine	Thiotepa	Topotecan	Toremifene	Vinblastine	Vincristine	Vinorelbine
Black Cohosh																																													
Celery																																													
Chamomile																																													
Chaste berry																									Moderate											Moderate									
Cranberry																																													
Devil's Claw																																													
Dong Quai																									Moderate																				
Echinacea									Extreme		Extreme		Moderate	Extreme	Extreme	Extreme							Extreme	Extreme	Extreme											Extreme						Extreme	Extreme	
Fenugreek										Moderate	Moderate	Moderate																																	
Feverfew																																													
Garlic																																													
Ginger																																													
Gingko																																													
Ginseng (Asian)									Extreme		Extreme	Extreme		Extreme			Moderate					Extreme											Extreme			Extreme							Extreme	Extreme	
Grape seed																																													
Green Tea																																													
Guarana											Low											Low																							
Horseradish																																													
Liquorice																									Moderate										Moderate										
Milk Thistle																																													
Passionflower																																													
Pau'Darco																																													
Red Clover	Extreme											Extreme							Extreme						Extreme											Extreme							Extreme		
Saw Palmetto																																													
Soy beans																									Moderate																				
St John's Wort									Extreme		Extreme	Moderate		Extreme			Extreme					Extreme	Extreme										Extreme			Extreme		Low					Extreme	Extreme	Extreme
Valerian																																													
Wild Yam																									Moderate											Moderate									

3A-mediated drug metabolism may be impaired in patients with a cancer related acute phase response and patients with advanced cancer often show marked variability in drug response.[14] While it may be seen as important to investigate herb-drug interactions in people with cancer, this is fraught with numerous clinical, ethical and logistical challenges. Furthermore, issues related to the study design and the nature of the herbal medicine product (including the dose, herbal extract and product quality) used in these studies can impact on the generalisability of such studies to the broader cancer patient population. For these reasons evidence of herb-drug interactions with anticancer therapies is based on a theoretical interaction potential extrapolated for *in vitro* or *in vivo* studies. It is not difficult to see how clinically significant interactions can occur when cytotoxic drugs with narrow therapeutic margins are then affected by inherent changes in metabolism, as well as changes in metabolism caused by herbal medicines or other conventional (pharmaceutical) medicines.

Although the potential for herb-drug interactions remains theoretical for many anti-cancer agents, the consequences are potentially significant in terms of disease outcome and morbidity and any theoretical interaction should be regarded as clinically relevant.

The following section reviews some of the more commonly ingested herbal medicines and discusses the evidence to support the potential for significant herb-drug interactions.

2.1   *Asian ginseng (Panax ginseng)*

Several different types of ginseng are used in herbal medicine products (Asian, Siberian, American and Japanese ginseng varieties), although Asian Ginseng is the most commonly used. Ginseng is widely used in an attempt to enhance the natural immune system, assist in recovery and reduce fatigue.[15] This herb is also purported to improve physical performance, strength and increase stamina, although rigorous data from controlled trials are lacking.

The main constituents of Asian ginseng include saponin glycosides; i.e. ginsenosides (also known as panaxosides), antioxidants, volatile oils, fatty acids, vitamins and polysaccharides.

The ginsenosides are believed to be responsible for Asian ginseng's effects.[15]

The effects of Asian ginseng on drug efficacy/drug metabolism *in vitro* and *in vivo* have not yet been fully elucidated and available data have been contradictory. Several *in vitro* studies have shown its constituents to have no significant effect on cytochrome P450 enzyme activity, however, one study performed using human liver microsomes suggested a crude ginseng extract had moderate inhibitory effects on CYP 1A1, 1A2, 1B1, 2D6, 2C19, 2C9, 2E1 and 3A4.[16] Further *in vitro* studies have shown high concentrations of ginsenosides (>200 mg/L) to have a moderate inhibitory effect on P-gp activity.[16]

Several reports of drug interactions between ginseng products and conventional medicines including monoamine oxidase inhibitors (MAOIs), warfarin, antidiabetic therapies, CNS drugs (including tranylcypromine and isocarboxazid), nifedipine and digoxin, have been described in the literature.[17,18] There have been no reports of any interaction between Asian ginseng and anti-cancer agents. However, in view of the interaction with these other compounds, caution may still be warranted with the administration of Asian ginseng together with anti-cancer agents that are CYP3A4 substrates.

2.2 *Black cohosh (Cimicifuga racemosa)*

Black cohosh is promoted for use in the treatment of menopausal symptoms and menstrual conditions, although its efficacy has yet to be conclusively substantiated in clinical trials. It may be misconceived as having estrogenic properties due to its effect in menopausal herbal medicine products, such as Remifemin®. However, black cohosh's effect may be due to more of a dopaminergic, rather than an oestrogenic profile,[19] or the result of constituents which have selective oestrogen receptor modulator (SERM) activity.[20] Therefore, the theoretical caution in regard to administration of black cohosh in patients with oestrogen-dependent tumours may be unfounded.

Whilst there have been no direct *in vivo* studies, an *in vitro* study suggests that black cohosh may also influence the efficacy of selected chemotherapeutic agents used in the treatment of breast cancer.[21] Results showed that black cohosh enhanced the sensitivity of mouse mammary cancer cells to doxorubicin and docetaxel, but reduced sensitivity to cisplatin. Whilst the mechanisms of interaction and clinical relevance of this study are not yet clear, caution may be warranted in cancer patients receiving black cohosh in conjunction with chemotherapy. An *in vivo* study in rats also investigated the use of black cohosh and tamoxifen on implanted endometrial adenocarcinoma cells and showed that black cohosh did not enhance or reduce the inductive effect of tamoxifen on tumour growth, but may have reduced the metastasizing potential of the tumour potentiated by tamoxifen.[22]

A number of randomised studies have failed to show benefit for black cohosh compared to placebo in the treatment of hot flushes[23] or vasomotor symptoms of menopause, which are common problems for women undergoing chemotherapy.[24]

A clinical trial has shown that black cohosh may have an inhibitory effect on CYP2D6 activity, but no significant effect on the activities of CYP3A4, CYP1A2 and CYP2E1, in healthy volunteers.[25] Caution may be warranted therefore in patients receiving anticancer agents metabolised by CYP2D6. A further study, again in healthy volunteers, has shown that black cohosh has no effect on the drug disposition of digoxin, which may be indicative of a lack of effect of the herb on the activity of P-gp.[26] There have also been reports of black cohosh inducing acute hepatotoxicity, leading in some instances to hepatic failure necessitating liver transplantation.[27]

In summary, evidence regarding the potential interaction between black cohosh and anti-cancer agents is limited, but caution is still appropriate for its use in this context.

2.3   *Celery (Apium graveolens)*

Celery has been traditionally used for the treatment of arthritic conditions and gout, as well as urinary tract infections. Celery extracts have also been shown to have a chemopreventive effect in pre-clinical models.[28,29] A pre-clinical study in mice pre-treated with celery and parsley juices also showed potentiation of the effects of pentobarbital, however statistical significance was only observed in parsley co-treated animals.[30] The likelihood of celery producing adverse interactions with anti-cancer agents is low, however, further investigation is warranted.

2.4 Chamomile (Matricaria recutita)

Chamomile is used topically for its anti-inflammatory effects and to treat skin disorders. It is also ingested orally for use as a mild sedative. Chamomile mouthwash may be of use in the prevention or treatment of mucositis induced by radiation and chemotherapy in patients, and a number of clinical trials have been carried out, albeit with conflicting results.[31,32] In terms of the potential for adverse drug interactions, a pre-clinical study found that the activity of CYP1A2 in rat liver microsomes treated with chamomile tea was significantly decreased by 24% ($p < 0.05$), however no significant changes were observed in the activities of CYP2D, CYP2E and CYP3A sub-families.[33] This finding suggests that there is limited potential for interactions between chamomile and anti-cancer agents when ingested systemically; however, more data will be needed to produce a more conclusive finding.

2.5 Echinacea (Echinacea purpurea)

Echinacea is traditionally used as an immunostimulant, antibacterial and antiviral, and is commonly used in cough and cold preparations in an attempt to alleviate symptoms.[34] Echinacea consists of a range of constituents including caffeic acid conjugates (caftaric acid, cichoric acid and echinacoside), alkylamides, glycoproteins and polysaccharides.[35,36]

In vivo evidence regarding the effect of echinacea on the activity of CYP enzymes has been conflicting. One clinical study showed that echinacea inhibits CYP1A2 activity and induces CYP3A activity, but had no effect on the activities of CYP2C9 or CYP2D6,[37] however, another study observed no effect on CYP3A4, CYP2D6, CYP1A2 or CYP2E1 activity.[38] It is likely that the effects of echinacea on CYP enzyme activity may be dependent on the preparation and/or dosage of echinacea used, which could explain these apparently conflicting results. Thus, caution is still warranted with the use of anti-cancer agents that are metabolised by CYP3A4 as they may interact with co-administered echinacea products.

2.6 Fenugreek (Trigonella foenum graecum)

The German Commission E has approved the internal use of fenugreek as an appetite stimulant and topically as a poultice to treat local inflammation. Although no herb-drug interactions have been reported for fenugreek, it has several constituents that could theoretically cause interactions with some medicines. It has been suggested that the coumarin content could theoretically potentiate the anticoagulant effect of warfarin. However a clinical study in patients with coronary artery disease receiving 5 g of fenugreek powder for three months found no significant effect on blood coagulation parameters although *in vitro* investigations showed inhibition of platelet aggregation.[39]

Fenugreek also contains several flavonoids, including quercetin, which has been implicated in CYP3A4 inhibition. One study demonstrated that quercetin increased the bioavailability of verapamil in rabbits *in vivo*, suggesting CYP3A4 inhibition as a possible mechanism.[40] Another trial showed that the AUC of cyclosporine (a CYP3A4 substrate) was increased when it was co-administered with quercetin to healthy volunteers ($n = 8$), the highest increase occurring when participants received quercetin for three days prior to commencement of cyclosporine.[41] An animal study also demonstrated that quercetin can increase the bioavailability of orally administered paclitaxel.[42] Increases in AUC and Cmax were observed when paclitaxel was administered with quercetin, possibly as a result of intestinal P-gp and CYP3A4 inhibition. Previous *in vitro* studies also demonstrated an inhibitory effect of quercetin on P-gp.[43] However, information regarding plasma concentrations and bioavailability of quercetin following oral administration of recommended doses of fenugreek is largely unknown. Thus, there is the potential for interaction between fenugreek and anti-cancer agents as a result of the quercetin content and caution is warranted in co-administering fenugreek together with anti-cancer agents that are CYP3A4 substrates and/or substrates for P-gp.

2.7 Feverfew (Tanacetum parthenium)

Feverfew is commonly used for migraine prophylaxis or treatment, although supporting randomised trial data are lacking.[44]

Parthenolide is thought to be the constituent responsible for feverfew's therapeutic effect.[45] There have been no reports of interactions with conventional medicines. Thus, it is probably safe to use feverfew with anti-cancer agents and recent reports even suggest an apoptotic effect in cancer cell lines, which might provide possible additional therapeutic benefit.[46]

2.8   Garlic (Allium sativum)

Garlic has traditionally been reported to have expectorant, diaphoretic, disinfectant, diuretic, antimicrobial, antihypertensive, lipid-lowering, fibrinolytic, antiplatelet and cancer protective properties. A number of systematic reviews have provided evidence for its efficacy in the treatment of hypertension, and hypercholesterolaemia.[47,48] A further systematic review has indicated a potential protective effect of high levels of raw or cooked garlic against colorectal and stomach cancers, although the evidence for this indication is of varying quality.[49]

An *in vitro* study found that garlic extracts may have an inhibitory effect on CYP 2C9*1, 2C9*2, 2C19, 2D6, 3A4, 3A5 and 3A7 and P-gp activity.[50] However, garlic extracts have been shown to not alter the disposition of co-administered medications primarily dependent on the CYP2D6 or CYP3A4 pathway of metabolism in healthy volunteers.[51]

A number of clinical studies investigating the potential interaction between garlic and the HIV protease inhibitor, saquinavir, have shown that garlic reduced drug bioavailability in healthy volunteers.[52,53] Whilst the mechanism of this interaction is not clear, the results indicate a possible inductive effect on CYP enzyme or P-gp activity and suggest that caution may be warranted with concomitant use of garlic and anti-cancer drugs metabolised by these mechanisms.

These studies highlight the unreliability of *in vitro-in vivo* correlations, and in the absence of confirmatory clinical studies, combined with the relative lack of involvement of the CYP2C class of isoenzymes in anti-cancer agent metabolism (except tamoxifen)[54] potential herb-drug interactions appear unlikely.

2.9   Ginger (Zingiber officinale)

Ginger is used for its antiemetic and antispasmodic effects, often in pregnancy.[55] Its main constituents include starch, lipids, volatile oils, monoterpenes, amino acids and proteins. *In vitro* studies have demonstrated its antiplatelet activity, its inhibitory effects on COX-2 and its glucose lowering effects through enhanced insulin sensitivity.[56–58] Ginger may cause potential pharmacodynamic interactions with anti-inflammatory or antidiabetic medicines, although there is no *in vivo* evidence to support this. Although the *in vitro* evidence suggests that ginger may cause an increased risk of bleeding with anti-platelet agents or anticoagulants, a recent study reported there were no interactions with warfarin at recommended doses and suggests that ginger has no effect on CYP2C9 activity *in vivo*.[59]

From the available clinical evidence it would appear that ginger is a relatively safe herbal medicine and should not produce adverse interactions with anti-cancer agents.

2.10   Ginkgo (Ginkgo biloba)

Ginkgo extracts are used mainly as enhancers of peripheral circulation in the treatment of cerebrovascular disorders, memory loss, Alzheimer's disease, multi-infarct dementia and free radical damage.[60] The majority of these studies have been conducted using the standardised EGb 761 extract of *ginkgo biloba*. Ginkgo consists of ginkgo flavonol glycosides: quercetin, kaempferol and isorhamnetin. Ginkgo extracts also contain biflavones including bilobetin, ginkgetin, and isoginkgetin as well as ginkgolides.[59,61]

As with garlic, clinical studies have shown that ginkgo extracts at recommended doses are unlikely to significantly alter the disposition of co-administered medications primarily dependent on the CYP2D6, CYP3A4,[61] CYP1A2 or CYP2E1 mediated pathways of elimination.[62]

Clinical studies have also shown that *ginkgo biloba* does not affect the drug disposition of digoxin, indicating there should be minimal potential for induction or inhibition of P-gp activity. Therefore clinically significant interactions with anti-cancer agents that are substrates for P-gp are unlikely.[63]

2.11   Grape seed (Vitis vinifera)

Grape seed extract is known for its potent antioxidant activity, as well as purported antibacterial, anti-inflammatory and anti-allergic properties. Grape seed extract at a concentration of 600 mg/mL has been shown to significantly increase the expression of CYP3A4 mRNA.[64] However as suggested by Sparreboom *et al.*,[11] it is unlikely that these levels can be reached in humans following the intake of commercial grape seed preparations.[11]

2.12   Green tea (Camellia sinensis)

The principal active constituents of green tea are catechins. Catechins have purported antioxidant, anti-carcinogenic and anti-atherogenic properties. In studies conducted in rodents, catechins have produced increases in the metabolism of substrates of CYP1A, 1A2, 2B and glutathione-S transferase, although decaffeinated extracts did not show these increases, implicating caffeine as the causative factor.[65] *In vitro* studies of individual purified catechins have shown inhibition of numerous CYPs including 1A1, 1A2, 2A6, 2C19, 2E1 and 3A4.[66] *In vitro* cell line assays have also shown that catechins decrease P-gp activity and are able to decrease the efflux of doxorubicin, a theoretical interaction which may increase the efficacy of doxorubicin although no *in vivo* studies have been performed to confirm this interaction.[67]

No evidence for *in vivo* herb-drug interactions between catechins and anti-cancer agents has been published. A pharmacokinetic study performed in healthy volunteers given green tea extracts showed no changes in the pharmacokinetics of dextromethorphan and alprazolam, indicating that decaffeinated green tea has no effect on the activity of CYP2D6 and CYP3A4, the major metabolising enzymes for these medicines respectively.[68]

There has been a single case report of a possible interaction between green tea and warfarin.[69]

Since *in vivo* drug interaction studies between green tea and anti-cancer agents have not been performed, caution should be observed before patients concomitantly ingest significant quantities of green tea whilst receiving chemotherapy.

2.13 Guarana (Paullinia cupana)

No *in vivo* drug interaction studies examining the effect of guarana or its extracts have been reported. Caffeine,[70] the main constituent of guarana, is a CYP1A2 substrate and the potential exists for competitive inhibition with other CYP1A2 substrates including the chemotherapeutic agents cyclophosphamide and ifosfamide. Patients undergoing chemotherapy with these medicines should be advised to avoid ingesting extreme quantities of caffeine-containing beverages.

2.14 Liquorice (Glycyrrhiza uralensis)

Liquorice root is used for its anti-inflammatory, anti-ulcer and anti-arthritic actions. The active components are glycyrrhizin and its more potent metabolite glycyrrhetinic acid.[71] Glycyrrhizin and glycyrrhetinic acid are inhibitors of cortisol metabolism.[72] Fluid retention, hypokalaemia, hypertension and aggravation of congestive heart disease are known adverse effects of long term or high dose use of liquorice root due to accumulation of mineralocorticoids.[73] Since glucocorticoids with significant mineralocorticoid effects (mainly dexamethasone and prednisone) are commonly used in chemotherapy and antiemetic protocols, cancer patients should be cautioned against administration of liquorice root to reduce the risk of excessive mineralocorticoid side effects.

No *in vivo* studies examining the effect that liquorice root or its extracts may have on anti-cancer treatment have been published. The major flavonoid component of liquorice, glabridin has been shown *in vitro* to irreversibly inhibit CYP3A4 and 2B6, possibly through destruction of the heme moiety by a reactive metabolite of glabridin.[74] In studies conducted in rodents, significantly different effects are seen on total CYP protein and mRNA depending on dosage regimens. Whilst single doses of liquorice extracts or purified glycyrrhizin had no effect, repeated dosing significantly induced CYP3A4 production in rats and mice, and CYP1A2 production in rats alone.[75] The implications for patients receiving cancer chemotherapy remain to be established.

2.15 Milk Thistle (Silybum marianum)

Milk Thistle is commonly used for its hepatoprotective properties and silymarin, a mixture of closely related flavonoids, is the principal constituent believed to be responsible for this effect.[76] Although clinical evidence to support the efficacy of this herb remains elusive, milk thistle continues to be one of the most commonly promoted and used herbal medicines.[77,78]

A number of *in vitro* studies have been carried out investigating the combination of milk thistle constituents and selected chemotherapeutic drugs. Results indicate that silybin may synergistically enhance the inhibition of ovarian cancer cell growth in combination with cisplatin and doxorubicin;[79] however, the clinical relevance of this observed positive effect is unclear and there is a lack of information regarding the potential toxic consequences of this combination *in vivo*.

Evidence regarding the effect of milk thistle on CYP enzymes *in vitro* is conflicting. One study investigated the effect of several silymarin flavonolignans, i.e. silybin, silydianin, silycristin, and dehydrosilybin (the oxidised product of silybin) on CYP3A4, 2D6 and 2E1 in human liver microsomes. The authors concluded that the activity of the human CYP enzymes was largely unaffected by flavonolignans in the silymarin complex at pharmacologically effective concentrations and, as a result, no drug interactions should be expected.[80] Other studies have demonstrated that milk thistle decreases CYP3A4 activity and inhibits P-gp cellular efflux *in vitro*.[81,82]

In vivo evidence from clinical studies has shown that recommended doses of a milk thistle preparation had no effect on the activity of CYP3A4, CYP2D6, CYP1A2 or CYP2E1 in healthy volunteers.[38] Furthermore, a recent randomised controlled clinical trial in 16 healthy volunteers investigated the combination of milk thistle with indinavir, a CYP3A4 substrate used in the treatment of HIV.[83] No significant difference was seen in the AUC for indinavir when milk thistle was added to the drug regimen indicating that it does not inhibit CYP3A4 *in vivo*. The findings of this latest study support results from earlier studies that indicated milk thistle had no inhibitory or inductive effects on P-gp or CYP3A4.[84,85]

Lack of an effect of milk thistle on the activity of P-gp seen has been further supported by a recent study in which the combination of milk thistle and digoxin in healthy volunteers was investigated.[26] There was no apparent effect of milk thistle on the disposition of digoxin, indicating a lack of effect of the herb on P-gp activity.

The balance of available evidence suggests milk thistle can be safely combined with cancer chemotherapy agents that are CYP 3A- or P-gp substrates, but close monitoring of changes in drug effects is appropriate.

2.16 *St Johns Wort (Hypericum perforatum)*

St. Johns Wort (SJW) is commonly used for the treatment of mild to moderate depression as well as other psychiatric disorders such as seasonal affective disorder and mild anxiety.[86] Although its overall mechanism of action is unclear, hyperforin is believed to be the constituent responsible for its antidepressant effect. Several *in vitro* studies have indicated hyperforin acts by inhibiting the re-uptake of neurotransmitters such as serotonin, noradrenaline and possibly dopamine.[87] Despite these findings, SJW herbal medicine products with minimal amounts of hyperforin present have been demonstrated to have some efficacy as an anti-depressant suggesting other constituents may also have a role.

SJW has been shown to be a potent modulator of several cytochrome P450 enzymes. Its constituents have both inductive and inhibitory effects. *In vitro* studies have shown that extracts of SJW significantly inhibit the activity of CYP1A2, 2D6, 2C9, 2C19 and 3A4. *In vivo* studies have shown SJW derivatives produce significant induction of hepatic and intestinal CYP3A4 if administered for longer than a two-week period while having no inductive effect on cytochromes P450 2C9 or 2D6[88] and a possible inductive effect on CYP1A2.[89] In the clinical setting the predominant effect of co-administration of SJW is indication of metabolism with the associated risk of lack of efficacy due to sub-therapeutic concentrations.

Hyperforin, a major constituents of SJW, is believed to be responsible for inducing intestinal expression of the MDR1 P-glycoprotein (P-gp), enhancing its drug efflux function.[90,91] Two studies have directly investigated clinically significant interactions between SJW and anti-cancer agents. The first of these examined the effect of SJW on the metabolism of irinotecan, a pro-drug of SN-38 and a known CYP3A4 substrate.[92] A 42% decrease in the area under the curve (AUC) was observed for the combination of irinotecan and SJW compared to irinotecan alone. The second study investigated the effect of SJW on imatinib and found that the clearance of imatinib increased by 43% when co-administered with SJW.[93] CYP3A4 is the major enzyme responsible for the metabolism of imatinib with CYPs 1A2, 2D6, 2C9 and 2C19 contributing to a lesser extent. These studies clearly indicate the potential for clinically significant interactions between SJW and anti-cancer agents.

The likelihood of SJW affecting chemotherapy agents that are substrates for CYP3A-enzymes has been supported by evidence from other trials demonstrating clinically significant interactions between SJW and conventional medicines.[94] Several case reports suggest SJW is responsible for interactions with cyclosporine with one case resulting in acute heart transplant rejection.[95] Two possible mechanisms of interaction between SJW and cyclosporine include induction of intestinal and hepatic CYP3A4 as well as induced expression of intestinal P-gp drug transporters.

SJW has also been shown to interact with fexofenadine, which is not metabolised by CYP enzymes but is a measure of MDR1 function providing further evidence as to the involvement of SJW in multiple induction mechanisms.[96] Thus, concomitant treatment with SJW and other anti-cancer agents that are CYP3A4 substrates or substrates for the P-gp drug transport system may affect the outcomes of cancer chemotherapy.

2.17 Saw palmetto (Serenoa repens)

Saw Palmetto is primarily used for treating prostatic conditions such as benign prostatic hypertrophy (BPH) because of its anti-androgenic properties and a systematic review supports the positive effects of saw palmetto on symptoms of BPH.[97] Although the exact mechanism of action is unknown, studies have shown that it acts as a mild inhibitor of 5-alpha-reductase, the enzyme responsible for the conversion of testosterone to the more active form, dihydrotestosterone (DHT).[98]

Its role in relieving symptoms of BPH also arises from its inhibition of cyclo-oxygenase and lipoxygenase pathways, thereby preventing the synthesis of prostaglandins and leukotrienes involved in inflammation.[99] This action has been implicated in a case report in which a patient suffered intraoperative haemorrhaging following the use of a saw palmetto extract.[100] There have been no reported interactions between saw palmetto and conventional medicines including anti-cancer agents.

An *in vitro* study found a potent inhibitory effect of saw palmetto on CYP3A4, 2D6 and 2C9,[101] however, *in vivo* pharmacokinetic studies have demonstrated that Saw Palmetto had no significant effect on cytochrome P450 isoenzymes, including CYP1A2 and CYP2E1 or CYP2D6 or CYP3A4 in healthy volunteers.[38,102]

In light of its anti-androgenic properties and until interaction studies prove otherwise, it would be advisable to avoid use of saw palmetto in cancer patients that are receiving hormonal therapy, due to the risk of possible additive pharmacodynamic effects.

2.18   *Valerian (Valeriana officinalis)*

Valerian is purported to be useful as an antispasmodic, an anxiolytic and an anti-depressant, but it is most often used to treat insomnia. It has a complex composition and contains three major sesquiterpenes — valerianic acid, valeranone, and kessyl glycol and monterpenes (primarily borneol). *In vitro* studies suggest that valerian inhibits CYP3A4 and P-gp.[103,104] However, *in vivo* studies indicate that valerian does not interact with CYPs 1A2, 2E1, 2D6 or 3A4/5 metabolism pathways at recommended doses.[25,105] While there may be some rationale against the concomitant use of barbiturates or other sedatives with valerian, there is no *in vivo* evidence of any interactions between it and anti-cancer agents or other conventional medicines.

2.19   *Other frequently used CAM*

2.19.1 *Evening primrose oil*

Evening primrose oil contains high levels of γ-linolenic acid (GLA), which exhibits anti-inflammatory, anti-proliferative and anti-thrombotic properties.[106] Evening primrose oil or GLA has been shown to be useful in the treatment of atopic eczema,[107] diabetic neuropathy,[108] and mastalgia.[109] There have also been a number of trials to investigate the use of evening primrose oil or GLA, in improving survival rates and outcomes of patients with primary liver cancer,[110] but without demonstrable survival advantage.

A more recent clinical study investigated the combined treatment of a high dose oral GLA supplement with tamoxifen in women with locally advanced or metastatic breast cancer compared to tamoxifen alone.[111] Results indicate that GLA supplementation significantly enhanced the efficacy of tamoxifen, resulting in more rapid response to treatment compared to patients receiving tamoxifen only. There were no adverse effects reported.

Overall, evening primrose oil and/or its constituent γ-linolenic acid have shown positive effects in the treatment of some cancers. However, evidence is limited and there have been no direct clinical studies to assess the potential risk of a negative interaction. Therefore, caution is warranted and patients receiving chemotherapy must be carefully monitored in the event of commencing supplementation.

2.19.2 Herbal medicines containing phyto-oestrogens

Many women with breast cancer self-medicate with complementary medicines to alleviate menopausal-like symptoms produced by their anti-cancer treatments.[112] *In vitro* studies have been performed investigating the proliferative effects of herbal substances and purified extracts that are marketed for menopausal symptom relief using MCF-7 cultured breast cancer cells. Products containing soy, red clover, dong quai and ginseng have all been shown to produce increases in MCF-7 cell proliferation in the absence of oestrogen.[113] A similar *in vitro* assay recently published investigating purified genistein, daidzein and resveratrol, all phyto-oestrogens also showed increases in the proliferation of MCF-7 cells.[114] Research conducted in athymic mice with implanted MCF-7 cells showed that dietary genistein was able to negate the anti-oestrogenic effects of concurrent tamoxifen.[115] These proliferative effects have not been shown *in vivo* however, since it is unlikely that any such study would be attempted. Therefore it would be prudent to advise women with oestrogen receptor positive breast cancers and who are undergoing treatment with anti-oestrogens to avoid self-medication with any herbs containing phyto-oestrogens.

2.20　*Other herbs*

2.20.1 *Devil's claw (Harpagophytum procumbens)*

Devil's Claw is used for the treatment of musculoskeletal conditions and shown to be effective in arthritic and chronic back pain.[116] It has been associated with an increased risk of bleeding in a patient receiving warfarin,[117] however, this interaction has not been confirmed and no further studies on potential drug interactions with devil's claw have been carried out.

2.20.2 *Cranberry (Vaccinium macrocarpon)*

Cranberry is primarily used in the prevention of urinary tract infections with some evidence of a beneficial effect.[118] Clinical studies have demonstrated that cranberry enhances the affect of warfarin.[119] The exact mechanism of this interaction has yet to be characterised and it remains unclear whether either cranberry will cause any significant interactions with anti-cancer agents, however, further investigations are required.

3.　　Conclusion

The increasing use of herbal medicines and complementary therapies amongst cancer patients has led to concerns about the appropriate concomitant use of pharmaceutical and herbal medicines. The data we have examined highlight the validity of concerns about potential adverse interactions between CAM and conventional anti-cancer treatments. However, there are enormous gaps in our knowledge because of the lack of well conducted clinical and pharmacokinetic studies of CAM and conventional treatments in cancer patients. It is imperative that these gaps be filled to ensure that cancer patients receive the safest and most effective therapies.

References

1. D. M. Eisenberg, R. C. Kessler, C. Foster, F. E. Norlock, D. R. Calkins and T. L. Delbanco, Unconventional medicine in the United States. Prevalence, costs, and patterns of use, *N. Engl. J. Med.* **328**(4): 246–252 (1993).
2. D. M. Eisenberg, R. B. Davis, S. L. Ettner, S. Appel, S. Wilkey, M. Van Rompay and R. C. Kessler, Trends in alternative medicine use in the United States, 1990–1997: Results of a follow-up national survey, *J. Am. Med. Assoc.* **280**(18): 1569–1575 (1998).
3. A. H. MacLennan, S. P. Myers and A. W. Taylor, The continuing use of complementary and alternative medicine in South Australia: Costs and beliefs in 2004, *Med. J. Aust.* **184**(1): 27–31 (2006).
4. E. Ernst and B. R. Cassileth, The prevalence of complementary/ alternative medicine in cancer: A systematic review, *Cancer* **83**(4): 777–782 (1998).
5. M. A. Richardson, T. Sanders, J. L. Palmer, A. Greisinger and S. E. Singletary, Complementary/alternative medicine use in a comprehensive cancer center and the implications for oncology, *J. Clin. Oncol.* **18**(13): 2505–2514 (2000).
6. H. S. Boon, F. Olatunde and S. M. Zick, Trends in complementary/ alternative medicine use by breast cancer survivors: Comparing survey data from 1998 and 2005, *BMC Womens Health* **7**: 4 (2007).
7. M. J. Verhoef, L. G. Balneaves, H. S. Boon and A. Vroegindewey, Reasons for and characteristics associated with complementary and alternative medicine use among adult cancer patients: A systematic review, *Integr. Cancer Ther.* **4**(4): 274–286 (2005).
8. P. M. Herman, B. M. Craig and O. Caspi, Is complementary and alternative medicine (CAM) cost-effective? A systematic review, *BMC Complement. Altern. Med.* **5**: 11 (2005).
9. M. Blumenthal, Herbal sales down 7% in mainstream market, *Herbal Gram* **66**: (2005).
10. D. Pal and A. K. Mitra, MDR- and CYP3A4-mediated drug-herbal interactions, *Life Sci.* **78**(18): 2131–2145 (2006).
11. A. Sparreboom, M. C. Cox, M. R. Acharya and W. D. Figg, Herbal remedies in the United States: Potential adverse interactions with anticancer agents, *J. Clin. Oncol.* **22**(12): 2489–2503 (2004).
12. I. Meijerman, J. H. Beijnen and J. H. Schellens, Herb-drug interactions in oncology: Focus on mechanisms of induction, *Oncologist* **11**(7): 742–752 (2006).

13. J. H. Beijnen and J. H. Schellens, Drug interactions in oncology, *Lancet Oncol.* **5**(8): 489–496 (2004).
14. L. P. Rivory, K. A. Slaviero and S. J. Clarke, Hepatic cytochrome P450 3A drug metabolism is reduced in cancer patients who have an acute-phase response, *Br. J. Cancer* **87**(3): 277–280 (2002).
15. Y. Z. Xiang, H. C. Shang, X. M. Gao and B. L. Zhang, A comparison of the ancient use of ginseng in traditional Chinese medicine with modern pharmacological experiments and clinical trials, *Phytother. Res.* **22**(7): 851–858 (2008).
16. B. C. Foster, J. T. Arnason and C. J. Briggs, Natural health products and drug disposition, *Ann. Rev. Pharmacol. Toxicol.* **45**: 203–226 (2005).
17. R. Bressler, Herb-drug interactions: Interactions between ginseng and prescription medications, *Geriatrics* **60**(8): 16–17 (2005).
18. K. Janetzky and A. P. Morreale, Probable interaction between warfarin and ginseng, *Am. J. Health Syst. Pharm.* **54**(6): 692–693 (1997).
19. G. B. Mahady, Is black cohosh estrogenic? *Nutr. Rev.* **61**(5 Pt 1): 183–186 (2003).
20. D. Seidlova–Wuttke, O. Hesse, H. Jarry, V. Christoffel, B. Spengler, T. Becker and W. Wuttke, Evidence for selective estrogen receptor modulator activity in a black cohosh (*Cimicifuga racemosa*) extract: Comparison with estradiol-17beta. *Eur. J. Endocrinol.* **149**(4): 351–362 (2003).
21. S. Rockwell, Y. Liu and S. A. Higgins, Alteration of the effects of cancer therapy agents on breast cancer cells by the herbal medicine black cohosh, *Breast Cancer Res. Treat.* **90**(3): 233–239 (2005).
22. T. Nisslein and J. Freudenstein, Concomitant administration of an isopropanolic extract of black cohosh and tamoxifen in the *in vivo* tumor model of implanted RUCA-I rat endometrial adenocarcinoma cells, *Toxicol. Lett.* **150**(3): 271–275 (2004).
23. B. A. Pockaj, J. G. Gallagher, C. L. Loprinzi, P. J. Stella, D. L. Barton, J. A. Sloan, B. I. Lavasseur, R. M. Rao, T. R. Fitch, K. M. Rowland, P. J. Novotny, P. J. Flynn, E. Richelson and A. H. Fauq, Phase III double-blind, randomized, placebo-controlled crossover trial of black cohosh in the management of hot flashes: NCCTG Trial N01CC1, *J. Clin. Oncol.* **24**(18): 2836–2841 (2006).
24. K. M. Newton, S. D. Reed, A. Z. LaCroix, L. C. Grothaus, K. Ehrlich and J. Guiltinan, Treatment of vasomotor symptoms of menopause with black cohosh, multibotanicals, soy, hormone therapy, or placebo: A randomized trial, *Ann. Intern. Med.* **145**(12): 869–879 (2006).

25. B. J. Gurley, S. F. Gardner, M. A. Hubbard, D. K. Williams, W. B. Gentry, I. A. Khan and A. Shah, *In vivo* effects of goldenseal, kava kava, black cohosh, and valerian on human cytochrome P450 1A2, 2D6, 2E1, and 3A4/5 phenotypes, *Clin. Pharmacol. Ther.* **77**(5): 415–426 (2005).

26. B. J. Gurley, G. W. Barone, D. K. Williams, J. Carrier, P. Breen, C. R. Yates, P. F. Song, M. A. Hubbard, Y. Tong and S. Cheboyina, Effect of milk thistle (*Silybum marianum*) and black cohosh (*Cimicifuga racemosa*) supplementation on digoxin pharmacokinetics in humans, *Drug Metab. Dispos.* **34**(1): 69–74 (2006).

27. E. C. Chow, M. Teo, J. A. Ring and J. W. Chen, Liver failure associated with the use of black cohosh for menopausal symptoms, *Med. J. Aust.* **188**(7): 420–422 (2008).

28. S. Sultana, S. Ahmed, T. Jahangir and S. Sharma, Inhibitory effect of celery seeds extract on chemically induced hepatocarcinogenesis: Modulation of cell proliferation, metabolism and altered hepatic foci development, *Cancer Lett.* **221**(1): 11–20 (2005).

29. G. Q. Zheng, P. M. Kenney, J. Zhang and L. K. Lam, Chemoprevention of benzo[a]pyrene-induced forestomach cancer in mice by natural phthalides from celery seed oil, *Nutr. Cancer* **19**(1): 77–86 (1993).

30. V. Jakovljevic, A. Raskovic, M. Popovic and J. Sabo, The effect of celery and parsley juices on pharmacodynamic activity of drugs involving cytochrome P450 in their metabolism, *Eur. J. Drug Metab. Pharmacokinet.* **27**(3): 153–156 (2002).

31. W. Carl and L. S. Emrich, Management of oral mucositis during local radiation and systemic chemotherapy: A study of 98 patients, *J. Prosthet. Dent.* **66**(3): 361–369 (1991).

32. P. Fidler, C. L. Loprinzi, J. R. O'Fallon, J. M. Leitch, J. K. Lee, D. L. Hayes, P. Novotny, D. Clemens–Schutjer, J. Bartel and J. C. Michalak, Prospective evaluation of a chamomile mouthwash for prevention of 5-FU-induced oral mucositis, *Cancer* **77**(3): 522–525 (1996).

33. P. P. Maliakal and S. Wanwimolruk, Effect of herbal teas on hepatic drug metabolizing enzymes in rats, *J. Pharm. Pharmacol.* **53**(10): 1323–1329 (2001).

34. R. Schoop, P. Klein, A. Suter and S. L. Johnston, Echinacea in the prevention of induced rhinovirus colds: A meta-analysis, *Clin. Ther.* **28**(2): 174–183 (2006).

35. A. Matthias, R. S. Addison, K. G. Penman, R. G. Dickinson, K. M. Bone and R. P. Lehmann, Echinacea alkamide disposition and

pharmacokinetics in humans after tablet ingestion, *Life Sci.* **77**(16): 2018–2029 (2005).

36. A. Matthias, E. M. Gillam, K. G. Penman, N. J. Matovic, K. M. Bone, J. J. De Voss and R. P. Lehmann, Cytochrome P450 enzyme-mediated degradation of Echinacea alkylamides in human liver microsomes, *Chem. Biol. Interact.* **155**(1–2): 62–70 (2005).

37. J. C. Gorski, S. M. Huang, A. Pinto, M. A. Hamman, J. K. Hilligoss, N. A. Zaheer, M. Desai, M. Miller and S. D. Hall, The effect of echinacea (Echinacea purpurea root) on cytochrome P450 activity *in vivo*, *Clin. Pharmacol. Ther.* **75**(1): 89–100 (2004).

38. B. J. Gurley, S. F. Gardner, M. A. Hubbard, D. K. Williams, W. B. Gentry, J. Carrier, I. A. Khan, D. J. Edwards and A. Shah, *In vivo* assessment of botanical supplementation on human cytochrome P450 phenotypes: *Citrus aurantium, Echinacea purpurea*, milk thistle, and saw palmetto, *Clin. Pharmacol. Ther.* **76**(5): 428–440 (2004).

39. A. Bordia, S. K. Verma and K. C. Srivastava, Effect of ginger (*Zingiber officinale* Rosc.) and fenugreek (*Trigonella foenumgraecum* L.) on blood lipids, blood sugar and platelet aggregation in patients with coronary artery disease, *Prostaglandins Leukot. Essent. Fatty Acids* **56**(5): 379–384 (1997).

40. J. S. Choi and H. K. Han, The effect of quercetin on the pharmacokinetics of verapamil and its major metabolite, norverapamil, in rabbits, *J. Pharm. Pharmacol.* **56**(12): 1537–1542 (2004).

41. J. S. Choi, B. C. Choi and K. E. Choi, Effect of quercetin on the pharmacokinetics of oral cyclosporine, *Am. J. Health Syst. Pharm.* **61**(22): 2406–2409 (2004).

42. J. S. Choi, B. W. Jo and Y. C. Kim, Enhanced paclitaxel bioavailability after oral administration of paclitaxel or prodrug to rats pretreated with quercetin, *Eur. J. Pharm. Biopharm.* **57**(2): 313–318 (2004).

43. G. Scambia, F. O. Ranelletti, P. B. Panici, R. De Vincenzo, G. Bonanno, G. Ferrandina, M. Piantelli, S. Bussa, C. Rumi, M. Cianfriglia *et al.*, Quercetin potentiates the effect of adriamycin in a multidrug-resistant MCF-7 human breast-cancer cell line: P-glycoprotein as a possible target, *Cancer Chemother. Pharmacol.* **34**(6): 459–464 (1994).

44. V. Pfaffenrath, H. C. Diener, M. Fischer, M. Friede and H. H. Henneicke-von Zepelin, The efficacy and safety of *Tanacetum parthenium* (feverfew) in migraine prophylaxis — A double-blind, multicentre, randomized placebo-controlled dose-response study, *Cephalalgia* **22**(7): 523–532 (2002).

45. C. Tassorelli, R. Greco, P. Morazzoni, A. Riva, G. Sandrini and G. Nappi, Parthenolide is the component of tanacetum parthenium that inhibits nitroglycerin-induced Fos activation: Studies in an animal model of migraine, *Cephalalgia* **25**(8): 612–621 (2005).
46. S. Zhang, C. N. Ong and H. M. Shen, Involvement of proapoptotic Bcl-2 family members in parthenolide-induced mitochondrial dysfunction and apoptosis, *Cancer Lett.* **211**(2): 175–188 (2004).
47. C. A. Silagy and H. A. Neil, A meta-analysis of the effect of garlic on blood pressure, *J. Hypertens.* **12**(4): 463–468 (1994).
48. C. Stevinson, M. H. Pittler and E. Ernst, Garlic for treating hypercholesterolemia. A meta-analysis of randomized clinical trials, *Ann. Intern. Med.* **133**(6): 420–429 (2000).
49. A. T. Fleischauer and L. Arab, Garlic and cancer: A critical review of the epidemiologic literature, *J. Nutr.* **131**(3s): 1032S–1040S (2001).
50. B. C. Foster, M. S. Foster, S. Vandenhoek, A. Krantis, J. W. Budzinski, J. T. Arnason, K. D. Gallicano and S. Choudri, An *in vitro* evaluation of human cytochrome P450 3A4 and P-glycoprotein inhibition by garlic, *J. Pharm. Pharm. Sci.* **4**(2): 176–184 (2001).
51. J. S. Markowitz, C. L. Devane, K. D. Chavin, R. M. Taylor, Y. Ruan and J. L. Donovan, Effects of garlic (*Allium sativum* L.) supplementation on cytochrome P450 2D6 and 3A4 activity in healthy volunteers, *Clin. Pharmacol. Ther.* **74**(2): 170–177 (2003).
52. E. Sussman, Garlic supplements can impede HIV medication, *AIDS* **16**(9): N5 (2002).
53. S. C. Piscitelli, A. H. Burstein, N. Welden, K. D. Gallicano and J. Falloon, The effect of garlic supplements on the pharmacokinetics of saquinavir, *Clin. Infect Dis.* **34**(2): 234–238 (2002).
54. Z. Desta, B. A. Ward, N. V. Soukhova and D. A. Flockhart, Comprehensive evaluation of tamoxifen sequential biotransformation by the human cytochrome P450 system *in vitro*: Prominent roles for CYP3A and CYP2D6, *J. Pharmacol. Exp. Ther.* **310**(3): 1062–1075 (2004).
55. F. Borrelli, R. Capasso, G. Aviello, M. H. Pittler and A. A. Izzo, Effectiveness and safety of ginger in the treatment of pregnancy-induced nausea and vomiting, *Obstet. Gynecol.* **105**(4): 849–856 (2005).
56. E. Tjendraputra, V. H. Tran, D. Liu–Brennan, B. D. Roufogalis and C. C. Duke, Effect of ginger constituents and synthetic analogues on cyclooxygenase-2 enzyme in intact cells, *Bioorg. Chem.* **29**(3): 156–163 (2001).

57. K. Sekiya, A. Ohtani and S. Kusano, Enhancement of insulin sensitivity in adipocytes by ginger, *Biofactors* **22**(1–4): 153–156 (2004).

58. E. Nurtjahja-Tjendraputra, A. J. Ammit, B. D. Roufogalis, V. H. Tran and C. C. Duke, Effective anti-platelet and COX-1 enzyme inhibitors from pungent constituents of ginger, *Thromb. Res.* **111**(4–5): 259–265 (2003).

59. X. Jiang, K. M. Williams, W. S. Liauw, A. J. Ammit, B. D. Roufogalis, C. C. Duke, R. O. Day and A. J. McLachlan, Effect of ginkgo and ginger on the pharmacokinetics and pharmacodynamics of warfarin in healthy subjects, *Br. J. Clin. Pharmacol.* **59**(4): 425–432 (2005).

60. D. J. McKenna, K. Jones and K. Hughes, Efficacy, safety, and use of ginkgo biloba in clinical and preclinical applications, *Altern. Ther. Health Med.* **7**(5): 70–86, 88–90 (2001).

61. J. S. Markowitz, J. L. Donovan, C. Lindsay DeVane, L. Sipkes and K. D. Chavin, Multiple-dose administration of Ginkgo biloba did not affect cytochrome P-450 2D6 or 3A4 activity in normal volunteers, *J. Clin. Psychopharmacol.* **23**(6): 576–581 (2003).

62. B. J. Gurley, S. F. Gardner, M. A. Hubbard, D. K. Williams, W. B. Gentry, Y. Cui and C. Y. Ang, Cytochrome P450 phenotypic ratios for predicting herb-drug interactions in humans, *Clin. Pharmacol. Ther.* **72**(3): 276–287 (2002).

63. V. F. Mauro, L. S. Mauro, J. F. Kleshinski, S. A. Khuder, Y. Wang and P. W. Erhardt, Impact of ginkgo biloba on the pharmacokinetics of digoxin, *Am. J. Ther.* **10**(4): 247–251 (2003).

64. J. L. Raucy, Regulation of CYP3A4 expression in human hepatocytes by pharmaceuticals and natural products, *Drug Metab. Dispos.* **31**(5): 533–539 (2003).

65. P. P. Maliakal, P. F. Coville and S. Wanwimolruk, Tea consumption modulates hepatic drug metabolizing enzymes in Wistar rats, *J. Pharm. Pharmacol.* **53**(4): 569–577 (2001).

66. S. Muto, K. Fujita, Y. Yamazaki and T. Kamataki, Inhibition by green tea catechins of metabolic activation of procarcinogens by human cytochrome P450, *Mutat. Res.* **479**(1–2): 197–206 (2001).

67. Y. Sadzuka, T. Sugiyama and T. Sonobe, Efficacies of tea components on doxorubicin induced antitumor activity and reversal of multidrug resistance, *Toxicol. Lett.* **114**(1–3): 155–162 (2000).

68. J. L. Donovan, K. D. Chavin, C. L. Devane, R. M. Taylor, J. S. Wang, Y. Ruan and J. S. Markowitz, Green tea (*Camellia sinensis*) extract does not alter cytochrome p450 3A4 or 2D6 activity in healthy volunteers, *Drug Metab. Dispos.* **32**(9): 906–908 (2004).

69. J. R. Taylor and V. M. Wilt, Probable antagonism of warfarin by green tea, *Ann. Pharmacother.* **33**(4): 426–428 (1999).

70. D. K. Bempong and P. J. Houghton, Dissolution and absorption of caffeine from guarana, *J. Pharm. Pharmacol.* **44**(9): 769–771 (1992).

71. A. Fugh-Berman and E. Ernst, Herb-drug interactions: Review and assessment of report reliability, *Br. J. Clin. Pharmacol.* **52**(5): 587–595 (2001).

72. P. Ferrari, A. Sansonnens, B. Dick and F. J. Frey, *In vivo* 11beta-HSD-2 activity: Variability, salt-sensitivity, and effect of licorice, *Hypertension* **38**(6): 1330–1336 (2001).

73. P. D. Coxeter, A. J. McLachlan, C. C. Duke and B. D. Roufogalis, Herb-drug interactions: An evidence based approach, *Curr. Med. Chem.* **11**(11): 1513–1525 (2004).

74. U. M. Kent, M. Aviram, M. Rosenblat and P. F. Hollenberg, The licorice root derived isoflavan glabridin inhibits the activities of human cytochrome P450S 3A4, 2B6, and 2C9, *Drug Metab. Dispos.* **30**(6): 709–715 (2002).

75. M. Paolini, J. Barillari, M. Broccoli, L. Pozzetti, P. Perocco and G. Cantelli-Forti, Effect of liquorice and glycyrrhizin on rat liver carcinogen metabolizing enzymes, *Cancer Lett.* **145**(1–2): 35–42 (1999).

76. B. P. Jacobs, C. Dennehy, G. Ramirez, J. Sapp and V. A. Lawrence, Milk thistle for the treatment of liver disease: A systematic review and meta-analysis, *Am. J. Med.* **113**(6): 506–515 (2002).

77. A. Rambaldi, B. P. Jacobs, G. Iaquinto and C. Gluud, Milk thistle for alcoholic and/or hepatitis B or C virus liver diseases, *Cochrane Database Syst. Rev.* (2): CD003620 (2005).

78. J. H. Hoofnagle, Milk thistle and chronic liver disease, *Hepatology* **42**(1): 4 (2005).

79. G. Scambia, R. De Vincenzo, F. O. Ranelletti, P. B. Panici, G. Ferrandina, G. D'Agostino, A. Fattorossi, E. Bombardelli and S. Mancuso, Antiproliferative effect of silybin on gynaecological malignancies: Synergism with cisplatin and doxorubicin, *Eur. J. Cancer* **32A**(5): 877–882 (1996).

80. R. Zuber, M. Modriansky, Z. Dvorak, P. Rohovsky, J. Ulrichova, V. Simanek and P. Anzenbacher, Effect of silybin and its congeners on human liver microsomal cytochrome P450 activities, *Phytother. Res.* **16**(7): 632–638 (2002).

81. R. Venkataramanan, V. Ramachandran, B. J. Komoroski, S. Zhang, P. L. Schiff and S. C. Strom, Milk thistle, a herbal supplement,

decreases the activity of CYP3A4 and uridine diphosphoglucurono-syl transferase in human hepatocyte cultures, *Drug Metab. Dispos.* **28**(11): 1270–1273 (2000).

82. S. Zhang and M. E. Morris, Effects of the flavonoids biochanin A, morin, phloretin, and silymarin on P-glycoprotein-mediated transport, *J. Pharmacol. Exp. Ther.* **304**(3): 1258–1267 (2003).

83. E. Mills, K. Wilson, M. Clarke, B. Foster, S. Walker, B. Rachlis, N. DeGroot, V. M. Montori, W. Gold, E. Phillips, S. Myers and K. Gallicano, Milk thistle and indinavir: A randomized controlled pharmacokinetics study and meta-analysis, *Eur. J. Clin. Pharmacol.* **61**(1): 1–7 (2005).

84. R. DiCenzo, M. Shelton, K. Jordan, C. Koval, A. Forrest, R. Reichman and G. Morse, Coadministration of milk thistle and indinavir in healthy subjects, *Pharmacotherapy* **23**(7): 866–870 (2003).

85. S. C. Piscitelli, E. Formentini, A. H. Burstein, R. Alfaro, S. Jagannatha and J. Falloon, Effect of milk thistle on the pharmacokinetics of indinavir in healthy volunteers, *Pharmacotherapy* **22**(5): 551–556 (2002).

86. J. Barnes, L. A. Anderson and J. D. Phillipson, St John's wort (*Hypericum perforatum* L.): A review of its chemistry, pharmacology and clinical properties, *J. Pharm. Pharmacol.* **53**(5): 583–600 (2001).

87. A. Singer, M. Wonnemann and W. E. Muller, Hyperforin, a major antidepressant constituent of St. John's Wort, inhibits serotonin uptake by elevating free intracellular Na+1, *J. Pharmacol. Exp. Ther.* **290**(3): 1363–1368 (1999).

88. Y. Chen, S. S. Ferguson, M. Negishi and J. A. Goldstein, Induction of human CYP2C9 by rifampicin, hyperforin, and phenobarbital is mediated by the pregnane X receptor, *J. Pharmacol. Exp. Ther.* **308**(2): 495–501 (2004).

89. M. Wenk, L. Todesco and S. Krahenbuhl, Effect of St John's wort on the activities of CYP1A2, CYP3A4, CYP2D6, N-acetyltransferase 2, and xanthine oxidase in healthy males and females, *Br. J. Clin. Pharmacol.* **57**(4): 495–499 (2004).

90. M. Hennessy, D. Kelleher, J. P. Spiers, M. Barry, P. Kavanagh, D. Back, F. Mulcahy and J. Feely, St Johns wort increases expression of P-glycoprotein: Implications for drug interactions, *Br. J. Clin. Pharmacol.* **53**(1): 75–82 (2002).

91. D. Durr, B. Stieger, G. A. Kullak–Ublick, K. M. Rentsch, H. C. Steinert, P. J. Meier and K. Fattinger, St John's Wort induces intestinal

P-glycoprotein/MDR1 and intestinal and hepatic CYP3A4, *Clin. Pharmacol. Ther.* **68**(6): 598–604 (2000).

92. R. H. Mathijssen, J. Verweij, P. de Bruijn, W. J. Loos and A. Sparreboom, Effects of St. John's wort on irinotecan metabolism, *J. Natl. Cancer Inst.* **94**(16): 1247–1249 (2002).

93. R. F. Frye, S. M. Fitzgerald, T. F. Lagattuta, M. W. Hruska and M. J. Egorin, Effect of St John's wort on imatinib mesylate pharmacokinetics, *Clin. Pharmacol. Ther.* **76**(4): 323–329 (2004).

94. E. Mills, V. M. Montori, P. Wu, K. Gallicano, M. Clarke and G. Guyatt, Interaction of St John's wort with conventional drugs: Systematic review of clinical trials, *Br. Med. J.* **329**(7456): 27–30 (2004).

95. F. Ruschitzka, P. J. Meier, M. Turina, T. F. Luscher and G. Noll, Acute heart transplant rejection due to St. John's wort, *Lancet* **355**(9203): 548–549 (2000).

96. G. K. Dresser, U. I. Schwarz, G. R. Wilkinson and R. B. Kim, Coordinate induction of both cytochrome P4503A and MDR1 by St John's wort in healthy subjects, *Clin. Pharmacol. Ther.* **73**(1): 41–50 (2003).

97. T. Wilt, A. Ishani and R. Mac Donald, *Serenoa repens* for benign prostatic hyperplasia, *Cochrane Database Syst. Rev.* (3): CD001423 (2002).

98. L. S. Marks, D. L. Hess, F. J. Dorey, M. Luz Macairan, P. B. Cruz Santos and V. E. Tyler, Tissue effects of saw palmetto and finasteride: Use of biopsy cores for *in situ* quantification of prostatic androgens, *Urology* **57**(5): 999–1005 (2001).

99. W. H. Goldmann, A. L. Sharma, S. J. Currier, P. D. Johnston, A. Rana and C. P. Sharma, Saw palmetto berry extract inhibits cell growth and Cox-2 expression in prostatic cancer cells, *Cell Biol. Int.* **25**(11): 1117–1124 (2001).

100. P. Cheema, O. El-Mefty and A. R. Jazieh, Intraoperative haemorrhage associated with the use of extract of Saw Palmetto herb: A case report and review of literature, *J. Intern. Med.* **250**(2): 167–169 (2001).

101. S. H. Yale and I. Glurich, Analysis of the inhibitory potential of *Ginkgo biloba, Echinacea purpurea*, and *Serenoa repens* on the metabolic activity of cytochrome P450 3A4, 2D6, and 2C9, *J. Altern. Complement. Med.* **11**(3): 433–439 (2005).

102. J. S. Markowitz, J. L. Donovan, C. L. Devane, R. M. Taylor, Y. Ruan, J. S. Wang and K. D. Chavin, Multiple doses of saw palmetto (*Serenoa repens*) did not alter cytochrome P450 2D6 and 3A4 activity in normal volunteers, *Clin. Pharmacol. Ther.* **74**(6): 536–542 (2003).

103. J. Strandell, A. Neil and G. Carlin, An approach to the *in vitro* evaluation of potential for cytochrome P450 enzyme inhibition from herbals and other natural remedies, *Phytomedicine* **11**(2–3): 98–104 (2004).

104. T. Lefebvre, B. C. Foster, C. E. Drouin, A. Krantis, J. F. Livesey and S. A. Jordan, *In vitro* activity of commercial valerian root extracts against human cytochrome P450 3A4, *J. Pharm. Pharm. Sci.* **7**(2): 265–273 (2004).

105. J. L. Donovan, C. L. DeVane, K. D. Chavin, J. S. Wang, B. B. Gibson, H. A. Gefroh and J. S. Markowitz, Multiple night-time doses of valerian (*Valeriana officinalis*) had minimal effects on CYP3A4 activity and no effect on CYP2D6 activity in healthy volunteers, *Drug Metab. Dispos.* **32**(12): 1333–1336 (2004).

106. U. N. Das, Can essential fatty acids reduce the burden of disease(s)? *Lipids Health Dis.* **7**: 9 (2008).

107. N. L. Morse and P. M. Clough, A meta-analysis of randomized, placebo-controlled clinical trials of Efamol evening primrose oil in atopic eczema. Where do we go from here in light of more recent discoveries? *Curr. Pharm. Biotechnol.* **7**(6): 503–524 (2006).

108. K. M. Halat and C. E. Dennehy, Botanicals and dietary supplements in diabetic peripheral neuropathy, *J. Am. Board. Fam. Pract.* **16**(1): 47–57 (2003).

109. J. Blommers, E. S. de Lange-De Klerk, D. J. Kuik, P. D. Bezemer and S. Meijer, Evening primrose oil and fish oil for severe chronic mastalgia: A randomized, double-blind, controlled trial, *Am. J. Obstet. Gynecol.* **187**(5): 1389–1394 (2002).

110. C. F. van der Merwe, J. Booyens, H. F. Joubert and C. A. van der Merwe, The effect of gamma-linolenic acid, an *in vitro* cytostatic substance contained in evening primrose oil, on primary liver cancer. A double-blind placebo controlled trial, *Prostaglandins Leukot. Essent. Fatty Acids* **40**(3): 199–202 (1990).

111. F. S. Kenny, S. E. Pinder, I. O. Ellis, J. M. Gee, R. I. Nicholson, R. P. Bryce and J. F. Robertson, Gamma linolenic acid with tamoxifen as primary therapy in breast cancer, *Int. J. Cancer* **85**(5): 643–648 (2000).

112. A. E. Lethaby, J. Brown, J. Marjoribanks, F. Kronenberg, H. Roberts and J. Eden, Phytoestrogens for vasomotor menopausal symptoms, *Cochrane Database Syst. Rev.* (4), CD001395 (2007).

113. C. Bodinet and J. Freudenstein, Influence of marketed herbal menopause preparations on MCF-7 cell proliferation, *Menopause* **11**(3): 281–289 (2004).

114. D. M. Harris, E. Besselink, S. M. Henning, V. L. Go and D. Heber, Phytoestrogens induce differential estrogen receptor alpha- or beta-mediated responses in transfected breast cancer cells, *Exp. Biol. Med.* (*Maywood*) **230**(8): 558–568 (2005).

115. Y. H. Ju, D. R. Doerge, K. F. Allred, C. D. Allred and W. G. Helferich, Dietary genistein negates the inhibitory effect of tamoxifen on growth of estrogen-dependent human breast cancer (MCF-7) cells implanted in athymic mice, *Cancer Res.* **62**(9): 2474–2477 (2002).

116. J. J. Gagnier, S. Chrubasik and E. Manheimer, Harpgophytum procumbens for osteoarthritis and low back pain: A systematic review, *BMC Complement. Altern. Med.* **4**: 13 (2004).

117. A. Fugh-Berman, Herb-drug interactions, *Lancet* **355**(9198): 134–138 (2000).

118. R. G. Jepson and J. C. Craig, Cranberries for preventing urinary tract infections, *Cochrane Database Syst. Rev.* (1): CD001321 (2008).

119. M. I. Mohammed Abdul, X. Jiang, K. M. Williams, R. O. Day, B. D. Roufogalis, W. S. Liauw, H. Xu and A. J. McLachlan, Pharmacodynamic interaction of warfarin with cranberry but not with garlic in healthy subjects, *Br. J. Pharmacol.* **154**(8): 1691–1700 (2008).

13

What Matters to Patients and Carers

Kendra J. Sundquist and
Monica C. Robotin

Abstract

The changes in health care and health care practices over the last decades have seen increased information sharing between health care professionals and patients, and encouragement for patients to participate in their medical care. The growth of internet technology and its increasing accessibility has shaped the health information seeking behaviours of people living in developed countries. Major cross-cultural and socioeconomic differences exist worldwide in regard to accessing information about cancer, and influence the way patients, carers and clinicians manage communication in the clinical setting.

People with cancer will continue to request more information in order to better understand their cancer and treatment options available. To enable them to participate as they wish in clinical decision-making, they require access to culturally appropriate health information that is trustworthy, timely and tailored to their level of literacy and understanding. Becoming more knowledgeable about CAM (Complementary or Alternative Medicine) can benefit patients in making informed treatment decisions and assist health care providers in advising against dangerous treatments, or those that may interact with standard anti-cancer therapies.

Keywords: Cancer, shared decision making, health seeking behaviours, Internet, communication, health information.

1.   Introduction

Cancer patients have many unmet needs,[1,2] which also include the need for information and psychological support.[2] Lack of sufficient information may be associated with increased uncertainty, anxiety, distress and dissatisfaction,[1] while cancer-relevant communication has been shown to play a key role in the reduction of the burden imposed by cancer on patients and carers.[3–5] For example, information seeking has been shown to be associated with more effective coping, stress reduction, improved understanding of the disease process, and more social support.[6] The context influences doctors' support of shared decision-making in cancer care.

Patients and carers seek honest and accurate information, provided with empathy and understanding[7] and clinician estimates of prognosis have been shown to have a profound impact on decisions about treatment, including life-sustaining treatment.

Access to reliable and appropriate information promotes understanding and increases psychological wellbeing. Patients, carers, families and friends need to be able to access reliable information and appropriate emotional and psychological support and a meta-analysis of 37 published outcome studies showed that such support improves the wellbeing of people with cancer.[8]

Two thirds of people with cancer experience long term psychological distress and approximately 30% experience clinically significant anxiety, while depression prevalence rates range from 20–35%.[9] Informal cancer carers also experience high rates of anxiety and depression, with 20–30% of all carers believed to be at high risk for psychiatric morbidity.[10] As many as 84% of cancer carers had above normal levels of psychological distress,[11] and over 50% showed clinical levels of depression, which is three times higher than the level found in community samples of people of the same age.[12]

Another study found that carers reported higher levels of cancer-related distress than either people with cancer, or survivors.[13] Women carers generally report higher rates of depression and anxiety, lower life satisfaction and quality of life ratings, when compared to men carers.[10,11,14]

While there has been a recent "explosion" of available cancer-related information through various media, including television coverage, print coverage, and the internet, the complexity of cancer-related information spanning prevention, early detection, treatment, recovery, and end-of-life issues challenges the public to remain abreast of the rapidly evolving scientific and clinical understanding of the disease.

The US National Cancer Institute (NCI) conducted the first Health Information National Trends Survey (HINTS) in 2003 and repeated it in 2005.[15] In the first survey, nearly 6500 Americans were contacted via telephone random digit-dialling. Most respondents were white (75.9%), aged 40 or older and 63% were female. Analyses of the HINTS 2003 data suggest significant differences in knowledge levels on preventable causes of cancer between socioeconomic groups, which may help explain some of the disparities reported in the literature. It is evident that high income and high education are associated with increased awareness about causes of major cancers such as lung and skin, and allows people to successfully minimize disease risks. Use of the Internet to obtain health information about topics other than cancer increased from the 2003 to the 2005 survey, with younger or more educated people more likely to use the Internet to seek health information.[15] Women were more likely to search for cancer information from all sources than men, and people aged 50 to 64 most frequently searched for cancer-specific information.[15]

2.   Who Seeks Health Information

Medical and social commentary suggests a shift in health care and health care practices over the last decade. Primarily, there has been a move towards information sharing between health care professionals and patients, with patients encouraged to participate in their medical care. The increasing availability of health information has been conducive to patients making more informed decisions.

Patients may possess different attitudes towards health and their own health care: whilst most patients seek out information about their disease (health seekers), others do not.

In general, health seekers have a health-conscious orientation towards issues of health and engage in positive health behaviours.[16] Amongst this group, differences have been noted in regards to using information to inform decisions and how actively they participate in health care decision making. Typologies of patient preferences, for example a desire for information and involvement in medical care and decisions, have emerged in recent years. They differ primarily in the number of categories delineated. Three such typologies are outlined in Table 1.

Czaja *et al.* stated that patients who **do not seek information** tend to be older, male; have lower levels of education and social support, be less familiar with the medical system, report less stress at diagnosis and express a preference for non-involvement in health care and less need for information and communication (they are termed 'passive patients').[17] **Seek and defer** patients have higher education levels, report intermediate levels of stress at diagnosis and social support, have a stronger preference for involvement in health care and tend to discuss information with health care professionals. The **seek and decide** patients are characterised by higher education levels and levels of reported stress at diagnosis, have good social support and familiarity with the medical system, report feeling comfortable asking questions, seek other sources of information, discuss their findings with health care professionals and actively participate in decision making.[17]

Overall, Maibach *et al.* concluded that the way patients valued, understood and accessed health information varied; the authors defined their categories along comparable demographics.[18] **Independent actives** tended to be younger, female, had higher education levels, and visited health care professionals more often. They sought information from a variety of sources and placed a high value on health. The **independent passives** were the youngest group. They were more likely to be male and Caucasian and less likely to seek out information. **Doctor-dependent actives** were the oldest group, had the lowest levels of education, lower income levels and reported more chronic conditions. They tended to seek out information regarding their conditions, although this was restricted to information from their health care provider. The **doctor-dependent passives** tended to report low levels of

Table 1. Typologies of information seeking and engagement in health care decisions.

Author(s)	Categories		
Bylund, Sabee, Imes & Aldridge–Sanford, 2007[95]	**Physician reliant** — Seek out information but defer to doctors for decision making	**Self reliant** — Seek out information and view doctor as an advisor. They are actively involved in health care decisions	
Czaja, Manfredi & Price, 2003[17]	**Non-seekers** — Do not seek information and are not involved in decision making	**Seek and Defer** — Seek out information and desire to be informed about their conditions. However, they do not participate in making decisions	**Seek and Decide** — Seek out information and use this to inform decisions. They are actively involved in health care decisions
Maibach, Weber, Massett, Hancock & Price, 2006[18]	**Doctor-dependent passives** — Do not seek out information and are not involved in decision making	**Independent passives** — Do not seek out information but make decisions independent of doctors	**Doctor-dependent actives** — Seek out information but defer to doctors for decision making	**Independent actives** — Seek out information and are actively engaged in decision making

education, were more likely to be male and visited their health care professional often. They were less likely to seek out health information.[18] Patients with an active outlook were more likely than those with a passive orientation to read for information, while passives tended to watch more television.

Such typologies suggest effective ways in which health information could be targeted to communicate with these varying groups, by targeting information at the appropriate educational level and in settings which are appropriate to each sub-group.[18] Doctor-dependent passives tend to visit health care professionals regularly and have low levels literacy, but would benefit most from doctor-initiated communication. For those classified as independent passives, barriers primarily relate to attitudes and beliefs about health. As they tend to be younger, have few chronic problems and rarely seek out information, mass media campaigns may be the most suitable means of imparting health information for this group.

3.   Trends in Seeking Health Information

In the US it is estimated that 80% of online adults search for health information,[19] and The National Cancer Institute reports that 53% of their sample (2003) accessed information specifically related to cancer.[15] By 2005, this figure had increased to 61.5%. Participation in online support groups also increased from 4% in 2003 to 4.4% in 2005.

The Health Information National Trends Survey (HINTS) data portray a significant shift in the ways in which patients consume health and medical information, with more patients looking for information online before talking with their treating doctors. While the level of use of the Internet as a source for cancer-specific information remained relatively unchanged from 2003 to 2005, the number of people using the Internet to communicate with their healthcare provider, or their provider's office, either by emailing questions or setting up appointments through a website, increased from 7% in 2003 to 10% in 2005.[15]

While information on the use and effectiveness of various channels of information remains scarce, studies suggest that people use multiple sources, including healthcare professionals, other patients, family or friends, information sessions, telephone helpline, the printed media, and in recent times, the internet.[18–23] Generally the most influential and the most preferred sources of information are health care professionals.[20–23]

Information seeking varies with age across a range of sources: NCI data found that over 80% of participants indicated they would seek information from health care providers and the internet first.[15] Older people were nearly ten times more likely to prefer a visit to a health care professional to seek information, compared to using the internet. However, across all age groups, the number of people who first went to the internet for information exceeded those who first went to a health care professional.

Active channels, such as the internet, books, helplines and narratives are preferred by those who have a health oriented outlook, as they are willing to look for health information and are more likely to engage in health activities; passive forms of information seeking, such as television, radio, newspapers, other patients and friends are most commonly used by others,[24] but passive information seeking can prompt the search for further, more focused information.[16,25] While the use of print materials (such as brochures) has a small effect on patients' level of education related to illness,[26] multiple and tailored personalised materials have the greatest effect.[18,23,27,28]

The Cancer Council NSW reported that from October 2005 to June 2006 more than 15,000 calls were logged to the Helpline, with more than 100,000 people visiting the state website per month, and approximately 1000–1500 people per month accessing their 'Cancer Answers' (frequently asked questions) webpage. Additionally, they distributed 10,000 information and support packs and over 216,000 booklets across the state in 2007.[29] The most popular titles were those that addressed psychosocial or practical issues.

3.1 *Using the internet*

One of the most powerful tools to emerge in recent times is the use of the internet to obtain health-related information, as internet usage has grown exponentially in many Western countries. Although available statistics on internet utilisation for the purpose of seeking health information are scant, Eysenbach estimated that on any given day more than 12.5 million health-related computer searches are conducted on the World Wide Web.[30] He estimated that in the developed world 39% of people with cancer use the internet to search for related information (equating to approximately 2.3 million people world wide). A further 15–20% of people with cancer are thought to use the internet 'indirectly' through family and friends.

Bright *et al.* found that in their sample of cancer patients, 48% of those that had searched for information in the past had looked on the internet in the first instance.[31] This is in contrast to only 14% who indicated they would search for books, or access a health care professional (11%). Other research has confirmed this finding: for example, Mayer and colleagues found that over one-third of their sample sought out information from the internet, compared to only 19% who asked health care professionals, or 13% who indicated accessing reference books.[21] Others found that between 36%[32] and 40%[33] of people use internet resources to gather further information.

Cancer patients use the internet for various reasons, including: gathering information, understanding their diagnosis, finding out and making decisions about treatment, making anonymous enquiries, finding information regarding diet and contacting support groups.[34] Other studies have found that up to 65% of people access the internet in search of online support groups,[35] supporting Ziebland and colleagues' conclusion that "the internet may be used not only to gather information and gain support from others, but also to make sense of the experience of cancer (pp. 1792)".[34]

In a longitudinal study (eight weeks) of newly diagnosed cancer patients, Bauerie–Bass *et al.* found an increase in use of the internet to access cancer-related information.[36] Direct users constituted 45% of the sample at baseline, and 57% at follow-up. Indirect users rose from 21% at baseline to 25% at follow-up. They concluded that "being diagnosed with a serious and life-threatening disease such as cancer spurs people to actually go online and seek information (pp. 230)".[36] This is particularly true for women: women have been reported as conducting more focused searches (regarding illness and symptoms), while men tend to search for information relating to prognosis and treatment.[20] As people with chronic conditions and those who face a higher price to obtain information (for example, travel time to doctor) are also more likely to use the internet, Bundorf *et al.* suggest that "for providers, this suggests that internet based resources are likely to become an increasingly important tool in reaching patients; this may include patients with significant health care needs and those in remote areas (pp. 833)".[33]

3.2 The digital divide: Characteristics of offline populations

An underserved population with regards to opportunities to seek health information using the internet has been identified in most countries; it has been termed the 'digital divide'. Generally, people who are younger (under age 65), have higher levels of education (graduates and above), are female, and have higher levels of income are more likely to have access to, and use the internet to retrieve health information.[20,21,31,33,35–38] In Australia, the digital divide disadvantages those with poor English proficiency and lower levels of education or income and those aged over 65 years, Indigenous Australians and people not in the labour force.[39]

3.3 Consequences of accessing online information and support

A number of positive elements regarding information seeking on the internet have been identified: convenience, access to current and up-to-date information, greater access to information and support when required, a greater volume of information available, a variety of perspectives, privacy, independence from constraints of distance and time, offering an intimate form of communication, especially with others who share the same concerns, assisting family and friends to gain knowledge about the illness and greater freedom to access information regarding sensitive matters.[19,21,31,32,40,41] People tend to access a variety of medical sites, cancer-specific organisational sites, patient-run cancer sites, message boards and chat rooms.[32,42,43] Research into the use of message boards indicates that in addition to receiving valuable information, people feel supported. Such interaction facilitates a psychosocial connection with others in a similar situation. Content analysis[3] of message boards has revealed that the main themes involve information regarding treatment, emotional support, and medication/treatment side effects. People who post on message boards "are interested in the experiences of other patients and derive benefit by interacting with them directly (pp. 64)",[43] a finding validated by others.[44,45] Postings in these studies primarily related to cancer types, treatment and procedures, side effects and family and personal issues relating to the illness. They too concluded that message boards were a useful tool for sharing information with others who have similar experiences and were a means by which people could both give and receive emotional support.[44,45]

Seeking information and support from online sources is associated with positive outcomes, including improved communication with health care professionals. Information seekers were more likely to prepare questions for their doctor and to ask more questions per consultation, more likely to share their feelings, had an improved understanding of issues and greater knowledge, improved self-care, enhanced coping strategies and self-efficacy, lower scores on anxiety and depression; furthermore, they tended to actively participate in treatment decisions and felt reassured and more empowered.[19,21,36,37,42,43,46–48]

It can be assumed that increasing access to online health information will serve to educate patients about their illness, motivate them to participate in their care and better evaluate treatment options, and will foster social support and the building of effective coping strategies.[49]

4.   Preferred Sources of Patient Information

Despite newly available communication channels, clinicians remain the most highly trusted information source, and patients express a high level of trust in the information they receive from their treating clinician.[3] In The Health Information National Trends Survey (2005), trust in the internet as a health information source was divided, with about one-fourth expressing a lot of trust and one-fourth expressing no trust in the information that can be gleaned from the internet. Radio was the least trusted health information source.[15]

In the HINTS survey, those in the 18–34 year age range were almost nine times more likely to go to the internet first, before going to their clinician (61.1% vs. 7.1%). An almost equal percentage of persons 65 years and older reported going to the internet first, or consulting their clinician first (21.4% vs. 20.9%).[3] When asked where they preferred going for cancer information, 49.5% reported wanting to go to their clinicians first.

There were strong age-related differences: persons 65 years and older were almost ten times more likely to go to clinicians before going to the internet (75.6% vs. 7.7%), persons aged 35–64 were almost equally split between clinicians and the internet and those aged 18–34 were about nine times more likely to go to the internet first (38.9% vs. 46.6%).[15]

Trust in health information sources was strongly age- and gender-dependent, with persons aged 18 to 64 years and women generally more trusting of most sources. The differences in trust by age are especially pronounced for the internet: adults aged 18 to 34 years were more than ten times as likely, and adults aged 35 to 64 years more than five times as likely as those 65 years or older to report a lot or some trust in the internet.[3]

Information provision by doctors and interactions with health care professionals are highly rated by patients and carers, who greatly value professionals who take time to listen to them, are accessible and willing to provide advice and discuss treatment issues. Although these needs were highly valued, research indicated that they are often not met.[50–53] In a rural sample, 23% of participants indicated a need for more information, with reasons given including the doctor failing to provide sufficient information and insufficient time with the doctor.[54] Those reporting a need tended to be: younger, female, had a previous diagnosis, and were internet users. Others report similar findings, suggesting that other sources of information are important for patients who feel their needs are not met by health care professionals.[42] While most prostate cancer patients were generally satisfied with health professionals' communication, nearly 40% of were less than satisfied with the quality of communication with their medical team.[55] Main sources of dissatisfaction also related to insufficient information or time constraints at the consultation, or feeling that doctors failed to provide information addressing specific questions.[42]

5.   Communication and Patient Satisfaction

A systematic review of 51 studies compared the perceptions of health professionals, patients, and caregivers about the communication of prognostic information.[56] There was a large discrepancy between the amount of information patients/carers and health professionals believed had been provided: health professionals tended to underestimate patients' need for information and overestimate patients' understanding and awareness of their prognosis.[56]

Many people report inadequate information to guide their decision-making. One study reported that while the majority of patients and their clinicians were willing to engage in discussions about psychosocial issues, many patients and clinicians left the initiative of discussing these topics to the other party.[57]

Patients need access to appropriate information in order to participate in clinical decision-making, and geographical and cultural barriers can limit access to information and services. Cultural factors play a role in the major disparities in access to health care and research for minority and underprivileged cancer patients.[58] A heightened awareness about issues of cultural sensitivity and of cultural competence has developed, and is increasingly applied to clinical practice.

Most cancer patients in developed countries want to have as much information as possible about their cancer treatment and prognosis, and many wish to be involved in decision-making, but the attitudes to and use of shared decision-making (SDM) by cancer doctors are not well known. Australian clinicians treating a diverse range of cancers were surveyed, to identify their usual approach to decision-making and their comfort with different decision-making styles, when discussing treatment with patients. Most clinicians (62.4%) reported using SDM and being most comfortable with this approach, with specialisation in breast or urological cancers, a high patient load, and female gender independently associated with an increased likelihood of using SDM.[6]

A recent Australian report sought to measure the patients' experience directly and identify their level of satisfaction with the services provided and areas where more effort is required.[59] Over 4000 cancer outpatients and 600 inpatients completed the survey, which invited patients to reflect on the previous six months of treatment, gathering feedback about the patient journey. Overall the results show a high level of satisfaction by cancer in-patients, with over 90% rating services as excellent, very good or good. Similarly, more than 97% of cancer outpatients also rated services highly. The report identified the level of emotional support they received, and accompanying relevant information as the two main areas of lower consumer satisfaction.[59]

Patients reported the need for staff to do everything to control pain, and wanting more professional help to cope with their anxieties about cancer and its treatment. They wanted more information about their rights and responsibilities, and how their illness and the treatment would affect them once they went home. Receiving more timely information about cancer treatments and their side effects, possible changes in relationships, sexual activity and emotions and a need for counselling or support regarding coping with cancer at home or at work were rated highly. Participants wanted more information from health care providers about complementary, alternative, or non-traditional therapies, and wanted them to take into account family or living situations when planning their treatment.[59]

A survey of patient satisfaction with the National Health Service (NHS) in England noted that while the level of satisfaction with the NHS was high (80% of inpatients surveyed thought that the level of care was good or very good), specific complaints regarding information about their progress were voiced by 25% of inpatients and 31% of out-patients.[60] The authors quoted an earlier study by Abel–Smith, which found that as most users lack the critical ability to appraise the quality of health care they receive, so they defaulted to complaining more about the "hotel" aspect of care, rather than the treatments, the quality of which they were unable to judge.[60]

A recent study commissioned by the Cancer Council NSW surveyed 290 people affected by cancer (patients, carers or family members of people with cancer), to determine their specific information and support needs, and how well they were being met.[61] Regarding information on diagnosis and treatment, respondents ranked highly access to frank and transparent information and being cared for by health professionals with good listening skills, who could provide support and instill confidence and were sensitive to the way they deliver information. Respondents also valued being given opportunities to participate in choices around treatment.[61]

To further identify the specific needs of people with advanced cancer, the Cancer Council NSW sought the views of people affected by pancreatic cancer, using a focus group discussion format. Patients and carers expressed a desire for more comprehensive information on signs and symptoms of disease, treatment options and side effects and more information about complementary and alternative therapies, as well as how to access palliative care in rural areas.[62]

6. Communication About Complementary and Alternative Therapies

Information and communication around the use of complementary and alternative therapies (CAM) is an area where commonly the perceptions of patients and health carers diverge widely.

The increased public access to information, more scientific research in CAM therapies, and increased political activism have changed public and medical perceptions of CAM; Cassileth identifies the acceptance of unconventional therapies by mainstream care in the US as a defining moment for health care in the 1990s.[63]

It is interesting to speculate as to why CAM has been adopted preferentially in developed countries, which are strong promoters of evidence-based practice in health care:

- An aging population and the increased prevalence of chronic diseases (where conventional medicine is perceived as less effective) have led consumers to explore other treatment options.

- CAM has become a social movement, which increased its legitimacy as an alternative health care system.
- The politicisation of health has returned the control of health to the individual and the control of the health care system to the community.
- Traditional medicine has lost some legitimacy in representing the public interest in matters of health care.[64]

CAM use is common among cancer patients, with recent US surveys indicating that from 9–91% of cancer patients used some form of CAM therapy at some point in the disease course (the use of different definitions of what represents CAM in different studies is partly responsible for the wide range of estimates).[65] Australian studies found that from 17–22% of cancer patients used some form of CAM,[66,67] with three-quarters of them using more than one modality.[66]

Although a great deal of information about CAM is readily available to patients, consumers commonly lack the know-how on evaluating the credibility of the information.[63] Patients most commonly receive information on CAM from family and friends,[68,69] from the media,[69] from books and increasingly, from the internet.[70] While consumers can access a large amount of information about CAM (an internet-based search using the keywords "complementary or alternative medicine and cancer" produced 2,680,000 results), the ability to separate reputable sources of information from those selling "bogus cures" is a significant challenge.[63]

A study of websites dedicated to CAM treatments in cancer found that the information presented was often unreliable and at times dangerous,[71] corroborating the findings of the US Federal Trade Commission (FTC), which identified hundreds of websites promoting phoney cures for cancers and other serious conditions.[63]

The extent to which patients disclose CAM use to their physicians remains below 40% in serial US surveys,[72] with slightly higher rates found among breast cancer patients (54%).[73] A survey in New Zealand, found that only 41% of patients had discussed CAM use with their oncologists.[74]

CAM use estimates by doctors are consistently lower than what is found through patient interviews: a US study demonstrated that although 37% of patients treated with radiotherapy also used CAM, their treating doctors estimated the prevalence of CAM to be only 4%.[75] Although in one study approximately half the patients receiving cancer treatment were also using at least one type of CAM, in 75% of cases, their doctors did not know about it.[76] Patients' reasons for non-disclosure included: lack of doctor interest, the expectation of a negative response and the perception that the CAM therapies were not affecting conventional treatments.[72,77]

However, although consumers often equate "natural" with "safe", around 5% of patients experience side effects related to CAM use,[68,78,79] highlighting the need for patients to disclose their use to their practitioners.

Cassileth found that among medical practitioners, CAM was used mostly by family doctors and psychiatrists,[80] a finding confirmed by surveys conducted in the US and Israel.[81] Surveys of primary care providers in the US,[82] Canada[83] and Great Britain[84] found that practitioners viewed some CAM practices as effective and that the majority had referred patients (or influenced referral) for CAM therapies.[85]

Oncologists are generally reluctant to endorse complementary therapies, related to perceptions of their potential to cause harm.[86,87] A cross-sectional survey of Japanese oncologists found that the majority (82%) believed CAM treatments were ineffective, with a lack of reliable information (85%) and concerns about drug interactions (84%) identified as the main reasons they would not endorse their use.[88] A Brazilian survey suggested oncologists were fairly knowledgeable of CAM, but over 80% of them indicated they would not recommend their use, because of a perceived lack of efficacy.[89] Surveys of oncologists' knowledge and utilisation of CAM carried out in Italy, Canada and Australia identified gaps in their knowledge of many non-traditional therapies.[86]

There is a need for medical practitioners to become more familiar with complementary medicines,[90] to support their patients in making informed decisions, advise against dangerous treatments, or identify those with the potential to interact with standard therapies.[91] Some authors suggest that in light of the high prevalence of herbal medicine usage, questions about herbal medicines use should be included in the routine history taking, to adequately identify and advise patients about potential drug-herb interactions.[92] The Australian Expert Committee on Complementary Medicines emphasises the need for all practitioners who use or advise on complementary medicine to acquire and continually update their information through undergraduate, vocational and continuing education,[93] but significant barriers exist in putting this into practice.

In 2004, the Australian Senate commissioned an inquiry into cancer treatment services and complementary therapies, prompted by increasing public demand for a more consumer-focussed approach to cancer care; it identified several key areas in need of improvements/reform, including a need to moving towards integrating mainstream and evidence-based complementary treatments.[94] Progress has been incremental in achieving these outcomes and the recent inception of the National Institute for Complementary Therapies is expected to provide added impetus for strategically directed research into complementary medicine and the translation of evidence into practice.

7.   Summary

Health care and health care decision making have undergone a change in recent decades. Patients are now encouraged to actively participate in their own health care, and to independently seek out knowledge, although the degree to which patients embrace this new ideology is variable. Better targeting health messages to the various groups of information seekers will result in effective communication at both a social and individual level. For a clinician, establishing from the outset how much information their patient would prefer enhances communication for both the clinician the patient.

Although clinicians tend to underestimate the patient's need for information, patients and carers view clinicians as their preferred information source. Also, seeking information and support online is becoming increasingly prevalent. The great public interest in complementary and alternative medicine highlights the importance of enquiring about CAM in all consultations and supporting patients to make informed choices about treatments.

Acknowledgements

The authors wish to thank Angela Pearce, University of Western Sydney, NSW. Australia for assistance with retrieving references and carrying out part of the literature review.

References

1. R. Sanson-Fisher, A. Girgis and A. Boyes, The unmet supportive care needs of patients with cancer, *Cancer* **88**: 226–237 (2000).
2. K. Soothill, S. Morris, C. Thomas *et al.*, The universal, situational, and personal needs of cancer patients and their main carers, *Eur. J. Oncol. Nurs.* **7**: 5–13 (2003).
3. B. Hesse, D. Nelson, G. Kreps, R. Croyle, N. Arora, B. Rimer *et al.*, Trust and Sources of Health Information. The Impact of the internet and its implications for health care providers: Findings from the first health information national trends survey, *Arch. Intern. Med.* **165**: 2618–2624 (2005).
4. R. A. Hiatt and B. K. Rimer, A new strategy for cancer control research, *Cancer Epidemiol. Biomarkers Prev.* **8**: 957–964 (1999).
5. L. F. Rutten, R. P. Moser, E. B. Beckjord, B. W. Hesse and R. T. Croyle, *Cancer Communication: Health Information National Trends Survey* (National Cancer Institute, Washington D.C., 2007).
6. H. Shepherd, M. Tattersall and P. Butow, The context influences doctors' support of shared decision-making in cancer care, *Br. J. Cancer* **97**: 6–13 (2007).
7. D. Spiegel, Health caring. Psychosocial support for patients with cancer, *Cancer* **74**: S1453–S1457 (1994).
8. B. Rehse and R. Pukrop, Effects of psychosocial interventions on quality of life in adult cancer patients: Meta analysis of 37 published controlled outcome studies, *Patient Educ. Couns.* **50**: 179–186 (2003).
9. National Breast Cancer Centre, National Cancer Control Initiative, Clinical practice guidelines for the psychosocial care of adults with cancer. In: *National Breast Cancer Centre*, 1st ed. (Camperdown, NSW, 2003).
10. M. Hagedoorn, R. G. Kuijer, B. P. Buunk, G. M. DeJong, T. Wobbes and R. Sanderman, Marital satisfaction in patients with cancer: Does support from intimate partners benefit those who need it the most? *Health Psychol.* **19**: 274–282 (2000).

11. S. Payne, P. Smith and S. Dean, Identifying the concerns of informal carers in palliative care, *Palliat. Med.* **13**: 37–44 (1999).

12. W. E. Haley, L. A. LaMonde, B. Han, A. M. Burton and R. Schonwetter, Predictors of depression and life satisfaction among spousal caregivers in hospice: Application of a stress process model. *J. Palliat. Med.* **6**: 215–224 (2003).

13. A. B. Matthews, Role and gender differences in cancer-related distress: A comparison of survivor and caregivers' self-reports, *Oncol. Nurs. Forum* **30**(3): 493–499 (2003).

14. J. Bookwala and R. Schulz, A comparison of primary stressors, secondary stressors, and depressive symptoms between elderly caregiving husbands and wives: The Caregiver Health Effects Study, *Psychol. Aging* **15**(4): 607–616 (2000).

15. L. F. Rutten, R. P. Moser, E. B. Beckjord, B. W. Hesse and R. T. Croyle, *Cancer Communication: Health Information National Trends Survey*, ed. Institute NC (National Cancer Institute, Washington D.C., 2007).

16. M. Dutta-Bergman, Acess to the internet in the context of community participation and community satisfaction, *New Media Soc.* **7**(1): 89–109 (2005).

17. R. Czaja, C. Manfredi and J. Price, The determinants and consequences of information seeking among cancer patients, *J. Health Commun.* **8**(6): 529–562 (2003).

18. E. W. Maibach, D. Weber, H. Massett, G. R. Hancock and S. Price, Understanding consumers' health information preferences. Development and validation of a brief screening instrument, *J. Health Commun.* **11**(8): 717–736 (2006).

19. D. J. Bowen, H. Meischke, N. Bush, J. A. Wooldridge, R. Robbins, A. Ludwig *et al.*, Predictors of women's internet access and internet health seeking, *Health Care Women Int.* **24**: 940–951 (2003).

20. S. R. Cotten and S. S. Gupta, Characteristics of online and offline health information seekers and factors that discriminate between them, *Soc. Sci. Med.* **59**: 1795–1806 (2004).

21. D. K. Mayer, N. C. Terrin, G. L. Kreps, U. Menon, K. McCance, S. K. Parsons *et al.*, Cancer survivors information seeking behaviours: A comparison of survivors who do and do not seek information about cancer, *Patient Educ. Couns.* **65**: 342–350 (2007).

22. C. N. Wathen, Health information seeking in context: How women make decisions regarding hormone replacement therapy, *J. Health Commun.* **11**: 477–493 (2006).

23. R. Jones, J. Pearson, S. McGregor, A. J. Cawsey, A. Barrett, N. Craig *et al.*, Randomised trial of personalised computer based information for cancer patients, *Br. Med. J.* **319**: 1241–1247 (1999).

24. M. Carlsson, Cancer patients seeking information from sources outside the health care system, *Support Care Cancer* **8**(6): 453–457 (2000).

25. C. P. Purvis-Cooper, K. P. Mallon and P. C. Leadbetter, Cancer internet search activity on a major search engine, United States 2001–2003, *J. Med. Internet Res.* **7**(3): e36 (2005).

26. T. Milewa, M. Calnan and A. Stephen, Patient education literature and help seeking behaviour: Perspectives from an evaluation in the United Kingdom, *Soc. Sci. Med.* **51**(3): 463–475 (2000).

27. A. C. Marcus, M. Mondi and P. Wolfe, The efficacy of tailored print materials in promoting colorectal cancer screening: Results from a randomized trial involving callers to the national cancer institute's cancer information service, *J. Health Commun.* **10**(Suppl. 1): 83–104 (2005).

28. V. J. Strecher, A. Marcus and K. Bishop, A randomized controlled trial of multiple tailored messages for smoking cessation among callers to the cancer information service, *J. Health Commun.* **10**(Suppl. 1): 105–118 (2005).

29. Cancer Council NSW, *Annual Report* (The Cancer Council NSW, Sydney, 2007).

30. G. Eysenbach, The impact of the internet on cancer outcomes, *CA Cancer J. Clin.* **53**: 356–371 (2003).

31. M. A. Bright, L. Fleischer, C. Thomsen, M. E. Morra, A. Marcus and W. Gehrig, Exploring e-Health usage and interest among cancer information service users: The need for personalized interactions and multiple channels remains, *J. Health Commun.* **10**(35): 35–52 (2005).

32. H. R. Winefield, B. J. Coventry, M. Pradhan,E. Harvey and V. Lambert, A comparison of women with breast cancer who do and do not seek support from the Internet, *Aust. J. Psychol.* **15**(1): 30–34 (2003).

33. M. K. Bundorf, T. H. Wagner, S. J. Singer and L. C. Baker, Who searches the internet for health information? *Health Ser. Res.* **41**(3): 819–836 (2006).

34. S. Ziebland, The importance of being expert: The quest for cancer information on the Internet, *Soc. Sci. Med.* **59**: 1783–1793 (2004).

35. J. Monnier, M. Laken and C. Carter, Patient and caregiver interest in internet-based cancer services. *Cancer Pract.* **10**(6): 305–310 (2002).

36. S. Bauerle-Bass, S. B. Ruzek and T. F. Gordon, Relationship of internet health information use with patient behaviour and self-efficacy: Experiences of newly diagnosed cancer patients who contact the National Cancer Institute's cancer information service, *J. Health Commun.* **11**: 219–236 (2006).

37. S. Fox, *Health Information Online: Technical Report from the Pew Internet and American Life Project* (Pew Research Center, Washington, DC, 2005).

38. R. Hardyman, P. Hardy, J. Brodie and R. Stephens, It's good to talk: Comparison of a telephone helpline and website for cancer information, *Patient Educ. Couns.* **57**: 315–320 (2005).

39. Australian Bureau of Statistics, *National Health Survey 2001*, ed. Commonwealth of Australia (ABS, 2002).

40. G. Eysenbach and G. Kohler, How do consumers search for and appraise health information on the world wide web? Qualitative study using focus groups, usability tests, and in-depth interviews, *Br. Med. J.* **324**(7337): 573–577 (2002).

41. H. Skinner, S. Biscope and B. Poland, Quality of internet access: Barrier behind internet use, *Soc. Sci. Med.* **57**: 875–880 (2003).

42. J. Kivits, Researching the 'informed patient': The case of online health information, *Info. Commun. Soc.* **7**(4): 510–530 (2004).

43. S. P. LaCoursiere, A theory of online social support, *Adv. Nurs. Sci.* **24**(1): 60–77 (2001).

44. W. Marcias, L. S. Lewis and T. Smith, Health-related message boards/chatrooms on the web: Discussion content and implications for — pharmaceutical sponsorships, *J. Health Commun.* **10**: 209–223 (2005).

45. P. N. Schultz, C. Stava, M. L. Beck and R. Vassilopoulou-Sellin, Internet message board use by patients with cancer and their families, *Clin. J. Oncol. Nurs.* **7**(6): 663–667 (2003).

46. S. Andreasen, I. Randers, E. Naslund, D. Stockkeld and A. Mattiasson, Family members' experiences, information needs and information seeking in relation to living with a patient with oesophageal cancer, *Eur. J. Cancer Care* **14**: 426–434 (2005).

47. S. Netttleton, R. Burrows, L. O'Malley and I. Watt, Health e-types? An analysis of the everyday use of the internet for health, *Infor. Commun. Soc.* **7**(4): 531–553 (2004).

48. C. Von Knoop, D. Lovich, M. B. Silverstein and M. Tutty, *Vital Signs: E-Health in the United States* (Boston Consulting Group, Boston, MA, 2003).

49. S. C. Kalichman, E. G. Benotsch, L. Weinhardt, J. Austin, W. Luke and C. Cherry, Health related internet use, coping, social support and health indicators in people living with HIV/AIDS. Preliminary results from a community survey, *Health Psychol.* **22**(1): 111–116 (2003).

50. S. Aranda, P. Schofield, L. Weich, P. Yates, D. Milne, R. Faulkner *et al.*, Mapping the quality of life and unmet needs of urban women with metastatic breast cancer, *Eur. J. Cancer Care* **14**: 211–222 (2005).

51. E. W. Boburg, D. H. Gustafson, R. P. Hawkins, K. P. Offord, C. Koch, K. Y. Wen *et al.*, Assessing the unmet information, support and care delivery needs of men with prostate cancer, *Patient Educ. Couns.* **49**(3): 233–242 (2003).

52. C. F. Grbich, I. Maddocks and D. Parker, Family caregivers, their needs, and home-based palliative cancer services, *J. Fam. Stud.* **7**(2): 171–188 (2001).

53. C. G. Vivar, Informational and emotional needs of long-term survivors of breast cancer, *J. Adv. Nurs.* **51**(5): 520–528 (2005).

54. K. Engleman, D. L. Perpich and D. L. Peterson, Cancer information needs in rural areas, *J. Health Commun.* **10**(3): 199–208 (2005).

55. D. J. Cegala, R. R. Bahnson, S. K. Clinton, P. David, M. C. Gong, J. P. Monk 3rd *et al.*, Information seeking and satisfaction with physician-patient communication among prostate cancer survivors, *Health Commun.* **23**(1): 62–69 (2008).

56. K. Hancock, J. Clayton, S. Parker, S. Walder, P. Butow, S. Carrick *et al.*, Discrepant perceptions about end-of-life communication: A systematic review, *J. Pain Symptom Manag.* **34**(2): 190–200 (2007).

57. S. Detmar, N. Aaronson, L. Wever, M. Muller and J. Schornagel, How are you feeling? Who wants to know? Patients' and oncologists' preferences for discussing health-related quality-of-life issues, *J. Clin. Oncol.* **18**: 3295–3301 (2000).

58. A. Surbone, Cultural aspects of communication in cancer care, *Support. Care Cancer* **16**: 235–240 (2008).

59. G. Heading, N. Mallock, S. Sinclair and J. Bishop, *New South Wales Cancer Patient Satisfaction Survey 2007, Interim Report* (Cancer Institute NSW, Sydney, 2008).

60. J. Allsop, Health policy and the NHS: Towards 2000. Ch 12 The NHS and its users. In: *Longman Social Policy in Britain Series*, 2nd ed. (London, New York, 1995).

61. The Leading Edge, *Segmentation for Opportunity Identification Report* (2008).

62. H. Gooden, C. Saunders, A. Friedsam and M. Robotin, *Recommending Research Priorities in Pancreatic Cancer: Listening to the Consumer Voice* (The Cancer Council NSW, Sydney, 2008).

63. B. Cassileth, G. Deng and A. Vickers, *PDQ Integrative Oncology* (B. C. Decker, Hamilton, Ontario, Canada, 2005).

64. I. D. Coulter and E. M. Willis, The rise and rise of complementary and alternative medicine: A sociological perspective, *Med. J. Aust.* **180**(11): 587–589 (2004).

65. J. D. White, The National Cancer Institute's perspective and agenda for promoting awareness and research on alternative therapies for cancer, *J. Altern. Complement. Med.* **8**(5): 545–550 (2002).

66. S. D. Begbie, Z. L. Kerestes and D. R. Bell, Patterns of alternative medicine use by cancer patients, *Med. J. Aust.* **165**(10): 545–548 (1996).

67. A. Girgis, J. Adams and D. Sibbritt, The use of complementary and alternative therapies by patients with cancer, *Oncol. Res.* **15**(5): 281–289 (2005).

68. I. Hyodo, N. Amano, K. Eguchi, M. Narabayashi, J. Imanishi, M. Hirai *et al.*, Nationwide survey on complementary and alternative medicine in cancer patients in Japan, *J. Clin. Oncol.* **23**(12): 2645–2654 (2005).

69. J. Shen, R. Andersen, P. S. Albert, N. Wenger, J. Glaspy, M. Cole *et al.*, Use of complementary/alternative therapies by women with advanced-stage breast cancer, *BMC Complement. Altern. Med.* **2**: 8 (2002).

70. E. Ernst, The current position of complementary/alternative medicine in cancer, *Eur. J. Cancer* **39**(16): 2273–2277 (2003).

71. E. Ernst and K. Schmidt, 'Alternative' cancer cures via the Internet? *Br. J. Cancer* **87**(5): 479–480 (2002).

72. D. M. Eisenberg, R. B. Davis, S. L. Ettner, S. Appel, S. Wilkey, M. Van Rompay *et al.*, Trends in alternative medicine use in the United States, 1990–1997: Results of a follow-up national survey, *J. Am. Med. Assoc.* **280**(18): 1569–1575 (1998).

73. S. R. Adler and J. R. Fosket, Disclosing complementary and alternative medicine use in the medical encounter: A qualitative study in women with breast cancer, *J. Fam. Pract.* **48**(6): 453–458 (1999).

74. K. Chrystal, S. Allan, G. Forgeson and R. Isaacs, The use of complementary/alternative medicine by cancer patients in a New Zealand regional cancer treatment center, *N. Z. Med. J.* **116**(1168): U296 (2003).

75. G. D. Kao and P. Devine, Use of complementary health practices by prostate carcinoma patients undergoing radiation therapy, *Cancer* **88**(3): 615–619 (2000).

76. C. Laino, *People with Cancer may Hide Supplement Use* (WebMD Medical News, 2005).

77. S. R. Adler, Complementary and alternative medicine use among women with breast cancer, *Med. Anthropol. Q* **13**(2): 214–222 (1999).

78. M. J. Kim, S. D. Lee, D. R. Kim, Y. H. Kong, W. S. Sohn, S. S. Ki *et al.*, Use of complementary and alternative medicine among Korean cancer patients, *Korean J. Intern. Med.* **19**(4): 250–256 (2004).

79. A. Molassiotis, P. Fernadez-Ortega, D. Pud, G. Ozden, J. A. Scott, V. Panteli *et al.*, Use of complementary and alternative medicine in cancer patients: A European survey, *Ann. Oncol.* **16**(4): 655–663 (2005).

80. B. R. Cassileth, E. J. Lusk, T. B. Strouse and B. J. Bodenheimer, Contemporary unorthodox treatments in cancer medicine. A study of patients, treatments, and practitioners, *Ann. Intern. Med.* **101**(1): 105–112 (1984).

81. J. Borkan, J. O. Neher, O. Anson and B. Smoker, Referrals for alternative therapies, *J. Fam. Pract.* **39**(6): 545–550 (1994).

82. B. M. Berman, B. K. Singh, L. Lao, B. B. Singh, K. S. Ferentz and S. M. Hartnoll, Physicians' attitudes toward complementary or alternative medicine: A regional survey, *J. Am. Board Fam. Pract.* **8**(5): 361–366 (1995).

83. M. J. Verhoef and L. R. Sutherland, General practitioners' assessment of and interest in alternative medicine in Canada, *Soc. Sci. Med.* **41**(4): 511–555 (1995).

84. R. A. van Haselen, U. Reiber, I. Nickel, A. Jakob and P. A. Fisher, Providing complementary and alternative medicine in primary care: The primary care workers' perspective, *Complement. Ther. Med.* **12**(1): 6–16 (2004).

85. M. Wetzel, D. M. Eisenberg and T. Kaptchuck, Courses involving complementary and alternative medicine at US medical schools, *J. Am. Med. Assoc.* **280**: 784–787 (1998).

86. I. L. Bourgeault, Physicians' attitudes toward patients' use of alternative cancer therapies, *Can. Med. Assoc. J.* **155**(12): 1679–1685 (1996).

87. S. Newell and R. W. Sanson-Fisher, Australian oncologists' self-reported knowledge and attitudes about non-traditional therapies used by cancer patients, *Med. J. Aust.* **172**(3): 110–113 (2000).

88. I. Hyodo, K. Eguchi, T. Nishina, H. Endo, M. Tanimizu, I. Mikami *et al.*, Perceptions and attitudes of clinical oncologists on complementary and alternative medicine: A nationwide survey in Japan, *Cancer* **97**(11): 2861–2868 (2003).

89. E. S. Samano, L. M. Ribeiro, A. S. Campos, F. Lewin, E. S. Filho, P. T. Goldenstein *et al.*, Use of complementary and alternative medicine by Brazilian oncologists, *Eur. J. Cancer Care* **14**(2): 143–148 (2005).

90. U. Werneke, J. Earl, C. Seydel, O. Horn, P. Crichton and D. Fannon, Potential health risks of complementary alternative medicines in cancer patients, *Br. J. Cancer* **90**(2): 408–413 (2004).

91. B. R. Cassileth and G. Deng, Complementary and alternative therapies for cancer, *Oncologist* **9**(1): 80–89 (2004).

92. A. Sparreboom, M. C. Cox, M. R. Acharya and W. D. Figg, Herbal remedies in the United States: Potential adverse interactions with anticancer agents, *J. Clin. Oncol.* **22**(12): 2489–2503 (2004).

93. Expert Committee on Complementary Medicines in the Health System, Complementary medicines in the Australian health system. In: *Report to the Parliamentary Secretary to the Minister for Health and Ageing* (Commonwalth of Australia, Canberra, 2003).

94. Community Affairs References Committee, The cancer journey: Informing choice. In: *Report into Services and Treatment Options for Persons with Cancer* (The Senate, Commonwealth of Australia, Canberra, 2005).

95. C. L. Bylund, C. M. Sabee, R. S. Imes and A. Aldridge-Sanford, Exploration of the construct of reliance among patients who talk with their providers about Internet information, *J. Health Commun.* **12**: 17–28 (2007).

14

Neurosurgical Involvement with Cancer Patients

Mark A. J. Dexter
and Juyong Cheong

Abstract

A neurosurgeon may be invited into the multidisciplinary team caring for a cancer patient for a variety of reasons — usually when the cancer has spread to the brain or spine. Frequently the involvement occurs at a time of crisis or emergency and is often associated with the development of new or unexpected neurological signs. With advances in imaging and improved screening, neurosurgical involvement is increasingly requested following the diagnosis of asymptomatic metastatic disease.

The neurosurgical team is involved in the management of cancer when the brain, spinal cord or the bony coverings of these structures are invaded. In addition to surgical treatment of metastatic involvement of the central nervous system, neurosurgeons are involved in the assessment and management of associated thromboembolic issues, as well as the longer term consequences of treatment, including the impact on cognition and quality of life.

Keywords: Cerebral metastases, spinal metastases, neurosurgery, deep vein thrombosis, pulmonary embolism, neuro-cognitive outcome.

1.   Introduction

The prospect of neurosurgical intervention in the clinical care of a patient with cancer often "spells the beginning of the end" in the minds of many patients, their families and often other clinicians. The management of central nervous system involvement of systemic cancer should occur in the setting of multidisciplinary teams, as it is one where many clinical boundaries are crossed, occasionally with conflicting treatment objectives. With advances in imaging, surgical techniques, radiotherapy and chemotherapy, effective treatment is often possible.

The neurosurgical involvement may be a simple request to establish a histological diagnosis in a patient presenting with multiple intracranial lesions, without a primary diagnosis of malignancy. Increasingly neurosurgeons are involved in the management of patients presenting with intracranial or spinal mass lesions, where strategies are needed for cytological reduction prior to chemotherapy or radiotherapy, to provide symptomatic improvement or occasionally curative resection.

With improvements in chemotherapy and radiation therapy, the impact and incidence of central nervous system involvement is increasing in patients with disseminated malignancy and it is not uncommon for a neurosurgeon to be involved at multiple points in the therapeutic journey. Patients have increasing expectations regarding their care, both in the pre- and post-operative phases and are now involved in all aspects of the decision making process. Quality of life, cosmesis and reconstruction are important aspects of neurosurgical procedures. Patients are at high risk of thromboembolic complications during the treatment of metastatic disease of the central nervous system. With improved rates of long term survival, late neuropsychological consequences of the treatment of intracranial metastatic disease are of increasing importance to patients and their carers.

2.   Intracranial Metastatic Disease

2.1   Case 1

A 41 year old white male presented to the emergency room with a seven day history of headache, nausea and confusion. His past medical history was benign and non-contributory. Neurological examination demonstrated papilloedema and confusion, but no localising signs. The remainder of the physical examination was normal.

CT imaging of the brain demonstrated multiple contrast enhancing lesions within the cerebrum, cerebellum and brainstem. CT imaging of the chest abdomen and pelvis showed no abnormality outside of the central nervous system.

The patient was commenced on high dose dexamethasone (4mg po qid), with resolution of his headache within 48 hours. A stereotactic "keyhole" right parietal craniotomy was performed and the larger subcortical lesion excised. The patient remained neurologically intact and was discharged home on the second post-operative day. Histological examination demonstrated metastatic small cell lung cancer. The patient went on to have palliative whole brain cranial radiation therapy and systemic chemotherapy. He subsequently developed pulmonary, hepatic and bony lesions. He died of progressive intracranial disease seven months following the original presentation.

2.2   *Epidemiological data*

Intracranial metastases are the most common brain tumours seen clinically by neurosurgeons. Approximately 25% of patients with malignancy will develop metastatic disease; in the United States ten times as many patients will die from metastatic disease than from malignant primary brain tumours.[1,2] There is an apparent increase in the incidence of intracranial metastatic disease, which may be related to the increasing length of survival of cancer patients, an enhanced ability to detect the presence of intracranial metastatic disease due to the widespread availability of MR imaging, and the fact that the blood-brain barrier limits the penetrance of a variety of chemotherapeutic agents into the central nervous system.[3] Cerebral metastases are most commonly due to primary malignancies of lung, breast, gastrointestinal or renal origin, with metastatic melanoma also common in the Australian community. Cerebral metastatic disease may be the presenting symptom in 10–15% of patients with a single intracranial metastasis.[4]

2.3   *Clinical presentation*

Most metastatic spread to the brain is haematogenous and consequently most symptomatic lesions occur in the distribution of the middle cerebral artery, namely the posterior frontal, parietal or temporal lobes. As metastatic cells tend to be trapped at sites of acute arterial narrowing near the brain surface, many metastases are peripherally located at the grey-white junction and are roughly spherical (see Fig. 1). Approximately 50% of symptomatic brain metastases are single and of these, 80% are located in the cerebrum, 16% in the cerebellum and 3% in the brainstem.[5]

Symptoms and signs may be related to increased intracranial pressure and typically include headache, often associated with nausea and vomiting. Headache will be present in 50% of patients at the time of diagnosis. Patients will often describe a headache that progresses over several weeks, is worse in the morning and

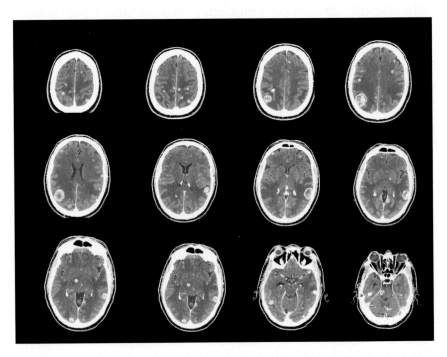

Figure 1.   A 41-year-old Caucasian male is referred with the acute onset confusion. Contrast enhanced CT imaging of the brain demonstrates multiple lesions within the brain, brainstem and cerebellum.

often only partly alleviated with simple analgesia. The elevation of intracranial pressure may be related to the volume of tumour, associated peritumoural white matter oedema, or obstruction of CSF pathways. Obstructive hydrocephalus is most commonly seen with cerebellar metastases, but may occur with any lesion adjacent to the CSF pathway. Cognitive decline, mental status changes and confusion may be manifestations of elevated intracranial pressure, or be due to involvement of the frontal or temporal lobes.

Focal deficits are related to the location of the metastatic deposits within the central nervous system and are site specific. Seizures may be focal or generalised and occur in 15–25% of patients with cerebral metastases.[6] They are more common in patients with multiple brain metastases, patients with haemorrhagic metastases and in secondary melanoma.[7] An abrupt stroke-like presentation may occur in 10% of patients and may result from tumour haemorrhage or occlusion or compromise of local vessels by tumour cells. Haemorrhage into metastatic tumours is particularly common in metastatic melanoma, choriocarcinoma and renal cell carcinoma.[8]

2.4   *Investigation and imaging*

There are no specific clinical features that will distinguish between primary and secondary brain tumours. Often the differential diagnosis may include non-neoplastic processes such as infection, demyelination, trauma, or stroke. When a single supratentorial lesion is identified on CT imaging and the patient has a history of treated cancer, in 93% of instances the lesion will be metastatic. If there is no history of malignancy and the chest X-ray is normal, only 7% will be metastases, 87% will be primary brain tumours and 6% will be non-neoplastic lesions.[4]

In our centre, MRI is the imaging of choice in the evaluation of intracranial metastatic disease, as it is more sensitive in detecting intracranial metastases.[9] MR-spectroscopy can occasionally differentiate between neoplastic and non-neoplastic processes and the MRI data, when acquired in a volumetric sequence, can be loaded into the intra-operative image guidance system to assist minimally invasive surgery. Staging of extracranial disease utilises CT imaging of the chest, abdomen and pelvis, a bone scan and occasionally PET-FDG imaging of the brain and whole body.

2.5 *Medical therapy*

Corticosteroids have an important role in the management of patients with intracranial metastatic disease; not only in palliating the acute presenting symptoms (especially headaches) but also in conjunction with surgery, radiation and chemotherapy. Symptomatic improvement may be seen within hours and maximal benefit is often achieved within the first two days. Neurosurgeons routinely use dexamethasone at a dosage of 4mg qid and adjust the regimen based on the balance between symptomatic improvement and side effects. It can be given orally or intravenously and frequently larger dose are used in the setting of extensive white matter oedema. Their primary role is to reduce peri-tumoural white matter oedema, but occasionally a direct oncolytic action is seen particularly with lymphoma. By reducing the permeability of both normal and oedematous brain, corticosteroids are used to reduce oedema formation in normal and peri-tumoural cortex following surgical trauma, radiation therapy and chemotherapy. Caution is required in patients with diabetes mellitus, as blood sugar levels may rise dramatically following the administration of steroids. Occasionally — particularly in the elderly — high dose steroids may contribute to agitation and the development of an acute organic brain syndrome. H2 antagonists or proton pump inhibitors are used concurrently, to ameliorate gastrointestinal side effects.

The use of anti-convulsants in patients with metastatic disease varies enormously between units and continues to be debated by neurosurgeons and neurologists. While there would be consensus that patients presenting with seizures need anti-convulsants, almost all other issues are open for debate. The majority of neurosurgeons would still commence patients having surgery for supratentorial brain metastases on prophylactic anticonvulsants, although the evidence for this is not compelling.[6,10] Neurosurgeons have traditionally used phenytoin (Dilantin), as it can be administered intravenously or orally at the same dosage, making it convenient to use in patients during the peri-operative period and in patients with altered mental status, who may be at risk of aspiration. However, phenytoin side effects are common and complex drug interactions occur with other medications undergoing hepatic metabolism, particularly chemotherapeutic agents such as temozolamide.[11] There is a trend towards using some of the newer anti-convulsants such as levetiracetam (Keppra), which is now also available intravenously.

2.6   Case 2

A 62-year-old female presents with progressive headache and mild left-sided hemiparesis. Nine years previously she had undergone a left mastectomy, axillary clearance (two positive lymph nodes) and local radiotherapy for a hormone receptor negative breast cancer. CT imaging of the brain demonstrated a right posterior frontal lesion. She was commenced on oral dexamethasone, phenytoin and ranitidine. CT imaging of the chest abdomen and pelvis, as well as a bone scan were normal. MR imaging of the brain confirmed the presence of a right posterior frontal lesion, as well as a second smaller lesion in the left posterior frontal lobe. PET-FDG imaging of the brain demonstrated increased glucose metabolism in the right posterior frontal region. PET-FDG imaging

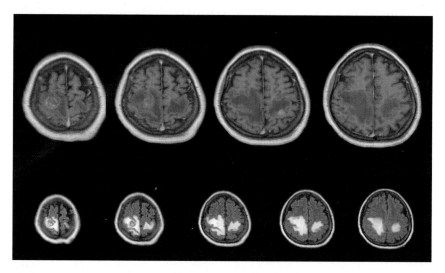

Figure 2.   A 62-year-old female presents with headache and left-sided hemiparesis. MR imaging demonstrates bilateral posterior frontal contrast enhancing lesions (upper row — axial T1 images with Gadolinium) with dramatic associated white matter oedema (lower row — axial FLAIR images).

of the body did not demonstrate metastases outside of the central nervous system.

The patient's headache resolved with dexamethasone and there was a significant improvement in the hemiparesis. She elected to undergo a single neurosurgical procedure, in which both frontal metastases were removed through small bilateral "keyhole" craniotomies. She was discharged home on post-operative day 6 and underwent adjuvant whole brain radiotherapy. She remains well and disease-free three years following the procedure.

2.7   *Neurosurgical procedures*

Neurosurgical procedures for intracranial metastatic disease essentially fall into three categories:

(1) Biopsy which is performed stereotactically to establish a histological diagnosis;
(2) Craniotomy which is used to remove one or more symptomatic lesions; and
(3) Placement of an intraventricular catheter and reservoir (Ommaya or Rickham) for intrathecal chemotherapy, in the setting of disseminated leptomeningeal disease.

The decision making process will depend upon a variety of individual patient and disease related factors and the management plan is individualized in the setting of a multidisciplinary team, taking into account patient preferences. The primary role of neurosurgery is in the treatment of single brain metastases in patients who have controlled or controllable systemic cancer. This group comprises only about 20–25% of patients with systemic cancer. The two major factors that influence survival in patients undergoing surgery and radiation therapy for single metastases are the extent of systemic disease and the patient's condition prior to surgery.[12] In general we recommend surgical excision for single lesions in patients with controlled or controllable systemic disease and minimal or reversible neurological deficits, particularly if the lesion is easily accessible. We feel that a histological diagnosis is important, as 11% of patients with abnormalities on brain CT or MR imaging who have a history of cancer treated in the preceding five years do not have metastases.[13]

The neurosurgical treatment of multiple metastases is more contentious, as generally patients have much worse survival than patients with single lesions.[14] Occasionally a single metastasis is removed to establish a histological diagnosis (as in Case 1). We have also removed a single metastasis in a patient with multiple lesions, where that lesion was clearly symptomatic, or posed a threat to life. This is not an uncommon situation in a patient with a large cerebellar lesion causing hydrocephalus and other small supratentorial lesions. On occasions we have removed more than one metastasis in a single procedure (as in Case 2) as there is some evidence that when a limited number of metastases can be simply and safely excised, survival is comparable to cases where only a single metastasis is present.[15]

Neurosurgical procedures in the modern era are usually performed with the aid of an image guidance system. This has allowed the development of "keyhole" techniques or mini-craniotomies. Patients typically undergo a CT or MRI scan on the day of the procedure. The stereotactic data is loaded into an intra-operative image guidance system, which allows precise positioning of the craniotomy immediately overlying the lesion and intra-operative localisation of the subcortical metastasis. The size of the craniotomy, size of the incision and need for hair shaving are all minimised, improving the safety, efficiency, cosmetic impact and outcomes of the surgery.

On occasion, we are asked to implant a delivery system into the CSF circulation for delivery of intrathecal chemotherapy. Although almost all malignancies have been reported to cause leptomeningeal dissemination of tumour through the CSF pathway, this is more common in patients who have leukaemia, non-Hodgkin lymphoma and breast cancer. These patients often have small ventricular systems due to diffuse cerebral oedema and ventricular catheter placement may be difficult. Essentially a catheter is placed into the ventricular system via a burr hole and a subcutaneous reservoir (Ommaya or Rickham) is attached to lie beneath the skin.

2.8 Adjuvant radiation therapy and chemotherapy in the management of intracranial metastatic disease

While the purpose of this chapter was to focus on specific neuro-surgical issues, the important input from colleagues in radiation therapy and medical oncology needs acknowledgement. The majority of our patients with intracranial metastatic disease have adjuvant radiation therapy and many are continuing with ongoing chemotherapy to control systemic disease.

Stereotactic radiosurgery is an increasingly important tool in the management of patients with central nervous system metastases. It involves delivering a single fraction of radiation therapy to the lesion, with minimal irradiation of adjacent tissues. The treatment is non-invasive, carries minimal morbidity and can be delivered on an out-patient basis. It is being used increasingly in the management of cerebral metastases and has control rates comparable to surgery.[16]

3. Deep Vein Thrombosis and Pulmonary Embolism in Patients with Intracranial Metastatic Disease

Patients with brain tumours have among the highest venous thromboembolism rates of all cancer patients, rivalling the incidence seen in individuals with pancreatic and gynaecologic malignancies.[17] This is another area where neurosurgical management crosses clinical boundaries. Many patients have had or will need intracranial surgery, or may have even presented with intracranial haemorrhage.

The incidence of thromboembolic disease in patients with primary brain tumours ranges from 19 to 29%, and 20% of patients with brain metastases from systemic cancer develop pulmonary emboli.[18] Timely diagnosis and initiation of therapy for thromboembolic disease is essential. Left untreated, nearly 50% of all patients who have symptomatic, proximal deep vein thrombosis will develop pulmonary emboli, with mortality rates ranging from 10 to 34%.[19]

The high incidence of venous thromboembolic disease may be related to the release of circulating brain-derived tissue factors, which activate the systemic coagulation cascade, predisposing to venous thrombosis. Elevated levels of markers of activated coagulation, including D-dimer, thrombin-antithrombin complexes and fibrin monomers are seen in patients with brain tumours, supporting this hypothesis. Abnormalities of the fibrinoloytic system have been also observed amongst brain tumour patients. Moreover, a 'tumour load-incidence of venous thrombo-embolism' relationship has been observed, where larger and more aggressive tumours have been found to release more tissue factors, and also have higher incidence of pulmonary emboli and deep vein thrombosis.[17] There are additional clinical risk factors for thrombo-embolic disease in brain tumour patients, including immobilisation following surgery, neurological deficit, exposure to chemotherapy agents and use of corticosteroids.

Routine lower limb venous duplex ultrasonography in combination with clinical evaluation is used to screen patients for deep vein thrombosis. However, the sensitivity of ultrasound in detecting calf deep vein thrombosis, especially when asymptomatic is low, with one study reporting a sensitivity of only 50%.[20] Standard tests for diagnosis of pulmonary embolism include ventilation-perfusion scans, helical CT and pulmonary angiograms, although these symptoms are used to investigate clinical suspicions, rather than for screening.

Given the high incidence of venous thromboembolism, prophylactic measures including mechanical therapies (early ambulation, compression stockings, and intra-operative calf compressors) and anticoagulation are used in all patients. The greatest concern with the use of anticoagulation is the risk of intracranial hemorrhage. However, a meta-analysis of four clinical trials of thromboprophylaxis in patients with brain tumours found that low molecular weight heparin or unfractionated heparins reduced the risk for VTE from 12.5 to 6.2% and carried a 2% risk of major bleeding.[21] There is still dispute amongst neurosurgeons regarding the use of anticoagulation in patients undergoing intracranial surgery and practice patterns vary. One author has argued that anticoagulation should probably be avoided in patients who have brain metastases from melanoma, choriocarcinoma, or renal or thyroid cancer, as these tumours are associated with an increased rate of haemorrhage.[19] Our practice has been to use prophylactic subcutaneous heparin 5000u subcutaneously bd in patients undergoing treatment for intracranial metastases. The use of unfractionated heparin allows regular monitoring of APTT levels, so as to avoid unanticipated over-anticoagulation.

In established venous thromboembolism, the aim of treatment is to prevent pulmonary embolism, improve lower limb circulation, and reduce oedema and pain. Anticoagulation involving low molecular weight heparin, unfractionated heparin and warfarin are utilised. A number of studies have been performed to compare the efficacies of these treatments.[22–24] Inferior vena caval filters are associated with high rates of complications and are only recommended in cases where anticoagulation is contraindicated. This may include patients who have had recent craniotomy, intracranial haemorrhage, frequent falls, poor compliance, or prolonged thrombocytopenia from chemotherapy.[19] Our preference has been to therapeutically anticoagulate with heparin so that we can monitor the APTT and hopefully avoid over-anticoagulation. It also allows us to rapidly reverse the anticoagulation if intracranial haemorrhage is suspected. We would then systemically anticoagulate with warfarin. Consultation with the vascular surgery service is often helpful in determining the duration of therapy.

4. Neuro-Cognitive Outcomes in Patients with Intracranial Metastatic Disease

Despite many advances in the treatment of cerebral metastases, the prognosis of patients with brain metastasis generally remains poor, with a median survival of one month in untreated patients and four to six months in treated patients.[25–27] Quality of life and the neurocognitive impact of treatment has become an extremely important outcome measure in patients, second only to survival. The recognition and management of neuro-cognitive deficits requires input from neuropsychologists, clinical psychologists, psychiatrists, rehabilitation medicine specialists, neurologists, social workers as well as other health professionals across a spectrum of clinical boundaries.

Neurocognitive function is an important indicator of patient's quality of life. It relates to patient's ability to manage finances, recognise safe and unsafe behaviour, and comply with medication regimes. Hence, any decline in neurocognitive function causes a dramatic decline in functional independence of the patient.[25] In addition, baseline memory, a component of neuropsychological testing, has been found to be an independent predictor of survival in patients with brain metastasis in a multivariate analysis.[28] Patients with brain metastases suffer a certain degree of neurocognitive functional impairment related to multiple factors, including the site and size of the tumour, whole brain radiation therapy, neurosurgical procedures, chemotherapy, and other neurotoxic therapies (including anticonvulsants and steroids) or from paraneoplastic effects induced by the malignancy.[29]

The mechanism by which whole brain radiation therapy causes neurocognitive dysfunction is not clearly understood. The toxicity of cranial irradiation can be divided into three phases: acute, subacute and late.[30] Acute effects occur during the first few weeks of treatment and are due to cerebral oedema. Subacute encephalopathy occurs one to six months after radiotherapy and is secondary to diffuse demyelination. Late (or delayed) effects are due to irreversible white matter damage related to vascular injury, demyelination and necrosis. Of particular interest is the sensitivity of hippocampus to radiation-induced injury.[31]

The treatment for neurocognitive impairment related to radiation therapy is currently limited and remains in the domain of controlled studies. Animal studies have found erythropoietin and non-steroidal anti-inflammatory drug indomethacin to be neuroprotective after radiotherapy.[32,33] A phase II study of donepezil, an acetylcholinesterase inhibitor used to treat Alzheimer's dementia, has shown improved cognitive function and quality of life in irradiated brain tumour patients.[34] Memantine, an NMDA antagonist has also been trialled.[30] Many innovative prophylactic treatments have been suggested and are currently being investigated. With improved rates of survival, mimimisation of late effects of treatment, whether they are related to surgery, radiation therapy or chemotherapy will be of increasing importance.

5. Spinal Metastatic Disease

Malignant spinal cord compression is a devastating complication of metastatic cancer. It occurs in approximately 2.5% of cancer patients, most frequently as metastatic spread from myeloma, prostate, lung, breast, prostate and kidney carcinoma.[35] Occasionally haematological spread to spinal cord occurs, but most intraspinal metastases are located epidurally and derived from vertebral or paravertebral metastases.[36] Untreated they result in progressive pain, paralysis, sensory loss and sphincter dysfunction. Patients with paralysis either at presentation or after treatment have a much shorter life expectancy than ambulatory patients. Spinal cord compression is a neurosurgical emergency that has a dramatic impact upon independence and quality of life,[37] so urgent diagnosis and treatment should transgress all clinical boundaries.

5.1 *Clinical presentation and diagnosis*

Initial symptoms typically include back pain, gait disturbances, leg weakness, and sphincter disturbances. Back pain is the most commonly described symptom, occurring in 50–96% of patients.[36,38–40] It occurs on average three months prior the radiological diagnosis of malignant cord compression, and precedes other symptoms by a median of seven weeks.[38–40] It is usually a severe debilitating pain, frequently present at night and independent of movement, as distinct from degenerative disc disease. It often has a radicular component (79%), most commonly in the thoracic region (hence patients complain of a band-like pain around chest or abdomen), or involves upper lumbar roots (anterior thigh pain). Less commonly, it presents as localised back pain (44%). The pain is most commonly described as sharp, shooting, deep pain, precipitated by coughing, bending and sneezing. The location of pain has no predictive value on the actual location of spinal cord compression, as there is a discordance between the level of pain and the structural level of compression as detected on MR imaging.[38] Hence patients with thoracic compression can complain of lumbar pain. Because of this, regional CT scans and plain films often miss the diagnosis, by imaging the incorrect level. One study found that plain X-rays were able to predict the correct level of compression in only 21% of cases.[38] Other initial symptoms include ataxia (67%), leg weakness (27–40%), sphincter disturbances (5–18%) and sensory changes including sensory levels (25%).[36,40]

There is a significant delay in diagnosis and during this delay period patients frequently develop new symptoms and signs. At the time of diagnosis, 82–90% of patients have moderate to severe motor deficits and gait dysfunction, with 65% being unable to walk. Further, 52–61% of patients have a sensory level and 55% of patients have bladder or bowel dysfunction.[36,38,39]

The mean interval between symptom onset and diagnosis ranged from 40 days to three months.[36,38,40] The delay appears to be multifactorial, including delay in patients reporting their symptoms to health professionals, delay in GP referral to specialists, or delay after referral has been made, mainly due to poor access to MRI outside working hours. As a result, majority of patients are diagnosed far too late and present with moderate-severe motor weakness and gait disturbances. This finding is distressing, as the single most important prognostic factor for ambulation after treatment is ambulatory status at time of diagnosis (other important indicators being the nature of the primary tumour and the speed of onset of motor deficits).[38,41]

A potential solution to this delay problem has been suggested by The Scottish Cord Compression Study Group. They proposed the following protocol:[38]

Emergency Referral (suspected malignant cord compression)

Cancer or suspected cancer + myelopathy (i.e. weakness, sensory loss, urinary retention) → Admit

Urgent Referral (suspected malignant epidural disease)

Cancer + suspicious pain → urgent MRI

Cancers most at risk:

- *Breast, prostate, lung.*
- *Known bone metastases.*

Suspicious pain:

- *Nerve root pain — tingling, burning, shooting, especially anterior thigh, around chest wall and posterior thigh.*
- *Localised back pain — especially thoracic.*

- *Severe, progressive pain, poorly responsive to medicines.*

Talcott *et al.*[42] described a multivariate model, which identified six independent risk factors that predict the possibility of malignant cord compression. The six risk factors are inability to walk, increased deep tendon reflexes, previous compression fracture, previous known bony metastases and age less than 60 years. They have found that patients having none of these risk factors had a 4% chance of malignant cord compression, whilst a patient with five risk factors had an 87% chance of having malignant cord compression.

5.2 Case 3

A 73 year old male presents with neck pain and left brachialgia. He was diagnosed with prostatic adenocarcinoma four years previously, after presenting with urinary frequency and nocturia. He underwent local radiation therapy. His past medical history is significant for previous aortic valve replacement, requiring therapeutic anticoagulation with warfarin and for type 2 diabetes mellitus.

MR imaging demonstrated circumferential epidural metastatic disease at the C3 level. Plain X-rays of the cervical spine performed in flexion and extension did not demonstrate spinal instability. The patient was commenced on dexamethasone 4mg po bd, with resolution of his symptoms. He underwent focused radiation therapy to the cervical spine. He remains well and asymptomatic two years following treatment, with no evidence of disease progression or spinal instability.

5.3 Medical management of spinal metastases

There are currently two systematic reviews related to the use of corticosteroids of malignant spinal compression. The most recent review[37] found two randomised controlled trials, a phase II trial, and one case-control study. The two randomised controlled trials were small. The trial by Sorensen *et al.*[43] involving 57 patients, compared high-dose corticosteroids with no corticosteroids in patients receiving radiotherapy. The rate of ambulation was significantly

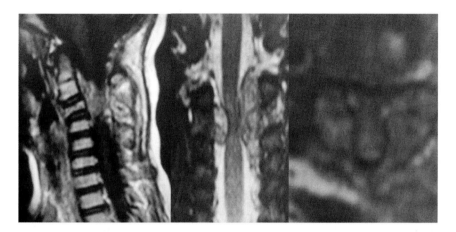

Figure 3. A 73-year-old male with a history of prostate cancer presents with neck pain and left brachialgia. Sagittal, coronal and axial MR imaging confirms the presence of epidural metastatic disease at the C3 level.

higher with corticosteroids (81% vs 63%, p = 0.046), although 11% of patients had significant adverse effects (including psychoses and gastric ulcers requiring surgery). The smaller randomised controlled trial by Vecht *et al.*[44] involving 37 patients, compared high and moderate corticosteroids doses in patients receiving radiation and found no significant difference in neurologic status. The phase 2 trial (in 20 patients) found that corticosteroids may not be necessary for patients with good functional status before radiation therapy.[45] The review concluded that corticosteroids are unnecessary for patients with good motor function. Another systematic review[46] concluded that whilst there is good evidence to support the use of steroids, a potential contraindication to their use in a young patient with an undiagnosed mass is the fact that corticosteroids may cause an oncolytic effect on lymphomas and thymomas, delaying diagnosis and definitive treatment.

5.4 Surgery and radiation therapy in the management of metastatic spine disease

The two modalities of definitive treatment are radiotherapy and surgical decompression. Both treatments are highly effective. In a review of ten uncontrolled observational studies of radiotherapy,

94% (95%CI: 91–96%) of patients who were ambulatory before treatment remained ambulatory after treatment.[37]

A systematic review[37] of two prospective studies, one RCT, and 12 retrospective reviews has recommended surgery should be used when there is spinal instability, bony compression, unknown primary site, single site of cord compression and for radioresistant tumours. Radiotherapy should be used for radiosensitive tumours and in patients with limited survival.[47]

There continues to be debate related to the most appropriate treatment for patients with single area of compression and no spinal instability. Surgery, especially vertebrectomy, is associated with significant morbidity and prolonged hospitalisation. In a review of 17 articles reviewing circumferential spinal cord decompression in patients with metastasis, mortality ranged from 0–31%, and postoperative morbidity ranged from 0–65%.[46] However, a meta-analysis[48] of 24 surgical studies (999 patients) and four radiation studies (543 patients) — mostly uncontrolled cohort studies, often retrospective — found a 1.3 times greater chance of being ambulatory with surgery than with radiation (p < 0.001). The meta-analysis concluded that whilst surgery should be the primary treatment with radiation given as adjuvant therapy, the treatment must take into account patients' neurological status and their overall health, extent of disease (spinal and extraspinal) and primary pathology. Ongoing cooperation between oncologist, radiation oncology and surgeon is an important part of holistic patient care.

6. Conclusion

When cancer involves the neurosurgeon, the prognosis of most patients is poor. However, a small but increasing number of patients can be cured. The disease and its treatment cross many clinical boundaries and mandates input from a variety of clinicians. To minimise the impact of acute disease and treatment related side effects, an understanding of issues such as venous thromboembolism is important. To minimise long term treatment consequences, understanding factors such as potential adverse neuropsychological sequelae are essential. The goal of therapy is always to maintain an acceptable quality of life whilst extending the length of survival. We have found that the collaborative efforts of the multidisciplinary team rarely results in conflict and consensus is invariably achieved.

References

1. C. C. Boring, T. S. Squires and T. Tong, Cancer statistics, *CA: A Cancer J. Clin.* **43**: 7–26 (1993).
2. A. E. Walker, M. Robins and F. D. Weinfeld, Epidemiology of brain tumours: The national survey of intracranial neoplasms, *Neurology* **35**: 219–226 (1985).
3. J. L. Nugent, P. A. Bunn and M. J. Mathews, CNS metastases in small-cell bronchogenic carcinoma: Increasing frequency and changing pattern with lengthening survival, *Cancer* **44**: 1885–1893 (1979).
4. R. M. Voorhies, N. Sundaresan and H. T. Thaler, The single supratentorial lesion. An evaluation of preoperative diagnosis, *J. Neurosurg.* **53**: 364–368 (1980).
5. J. Y. Delattre, G. Krol and H. T. Thaler, Distribution of brain metastases, *Arch. Neurol.* **45**: 741–744 (1988).
6. N. Cohen, G. Strauss and R. Lew, Should prophylactic anticonvulsants be administered to patients with newly diagnosed cerebral metastases? A retrospective study, *J. Clin. Oncol.* **6**: 1621–1624 (1988).
7. I. M. Mendez and R. F. Del Maestro, Cerebral metastases from malignant melanoma, *Can. J. Neurol. Sci.* **15**: 119–123 (1988).
8. D. Kondziolka, M. Bernstein and L. Resch, Significance of haemorrhage into brain tumours: Clinicopathological study, *J. Neurosurg.* **67**: 852–857 (1987).
9. A. P. Mintz, J. G. Cairncross, Treatment of a single brain metastasis. The role of radiation following surgical excision, *J. Am. Med. Assoc.* **280**: 1527–1529 (1998).
10. V. Siomin, L. Angelov, L. Li and M. A. Vogelbaum, Results of a survey of neurosurgical practice patterns regarding the prophylactic use of antiepilepsy drugs in patients with brain tumours. *J. Neurooncol.* **74**(2): 211–215 (2005).
11. K. Y. Yap, W. K. Chui and A. Chan, Drug interactions between chemotherapeutic regimens and antiepileptics, *Clin. Ther.* **30**(8): 1385–1407 (2008).

12. J. H. Galicich, N. Sundaresan and E. Arbit, Surgical treatment of single brain metastasis: Factors associated with survival, *Cancer* **45**: 381–86 (1980).

13. R. A. Patchell, P. A. Tibbs and J. W. Walsh, A randomized trial of surgery in the treatment of single metastasis to the brain, *N. Engl. J. Med.* **322**: 494–500 (1990).

14. L. M. DeAngelis, L. R. Mandell and H. T. Thaler, The role of post-operative radiotherapy after resection of single brain metastasis, *Neurosurgery* **24**: 798–804 (1989).

15. R. K. Bindal, R. Sawaya and M. E. Leavens, Surgical treatment of multiple brain metastasis, *J. Neurosurg.* **79**: 210–216 (1993).

16. A. Mucavic, B. Wowra, A. Siefert, J. C. Tonn, H. J. Steiger and F. W. Kreth, Microsurgery plus whole brain irradiation versus Gamma knife surgery alone for treatment of single metastases to the brain: A randomized controlled multicenter phase III trial, *J. Neurooncol.* **87**: 299–307 (2008).

17. D. E. Gerber, S. A. Grossman and M. B. Streiff, Management of venous thrombo-embolism in patients with primary and metastatic brain tumours, *J. Clin. Oncol.* **24**(8): 1310–1318 (2006).

18. R. Sawaya, M. Zuccarello, M. Elkalliny and H. Nishiyama, Postoperative venous thromboembolism and brain tumours: Part 1. Clinical profile, *J. Neurooncol.* **14**: 119–125 (1992).

19. J. Drappatz, D. Schiff, S. Kesari, A. D. Norden and P. Y. Wen, Medical management of brain tumour patients, *Neurol. Clin.* **25**: 1035–1071 (2007).

20. J. B. Segal, J. Eng, L. J. Tamariz and E. B. Bass, Review of the evidence on diagnosis of deep venous thrombosis and pulmonary embolism, *Ann. Fam. Med.* **5**(1): 63–73 (2007).

21. A. Iorio and G. Agnelli, Low-molecular-weight and unfractionated heparin for prevention of venous thromboembolism in neurosurgery: A meta-analysis, *Arch. Int. Med.* **160**(15): 2327–2332 (2000).

22. P. Mismetti, S. Laporte, J. Y. Darmon, A. Buchmuller and H. Decousus, Meta-analysis of low molecular weight heparin in the prevention of venous thromboembolism in general surgery, *Br. J. Surg.* **88**(7): 913–930 (2001).

23. E. Rocha, M. A. Martinez-Gonzalez, R. Montes and C. Panizo, Do the low molecular weight heparins improve efficacy and safety of the treatment of deep venous thrombosis? A meta-analysis, *Haematologica* **85**(9): 935–942 (2000).

24. A. Y. Lee, M. N. Levine and R. I. Baker, Low-molecular-weight heparin versus a coumarin for the prevention of recurrent venous thromboembolism in patients with cancer, *N. Engl. J. Med.* **349**(2): 146–153 (2003).

25. J. Li, S. M. Bentzen, J. Li, M. Renschler and M. P. Mehta, Relationship between neurocognitive function and quality of life after whole-brain radiotherapy in patients with brain metastasis, *Int. J. Radiat. Oncol. Biol. Phys.* **71**(1): 64–70 (2008).

26. J. T. Sundstrom, H. Minn, K. K. Lertola and E. Nordman, Prognosis of patients treated for intracranial metastases with whole-brain irradiation, *Ann. Med.* **30**(3): 296–299 (1998).

27. S. Zimm, G. L. Wampler, D. Stablein, T. Hazra and H. F. Young, Intracerebral metastases in solid-tumour patients: Natural history and results of treatment, *Cancer* **48**(2): 384–394 (1981).

28. C. A. Meyers, J. A. Smith, A. Bezjak, M. P. Mehta, J. Liebmann, T. Illidge, I. Kunkler, J. M. Caudrelier, P. D. Eisenberg, J. Meerwaldt, R. Siemers, C. Carrie, L. E. Gaspar, W. Curran, S. C. Phan, R. A. Miller and M. F. Renschler, Neurocognitive function and progression in patients with brain metastases treated with whole-brain radiation and motexafin gadolinium: Results of a randomized phase III trial, *J. Clin. Oncol.* **22**(1): 157–165 (2004).

29. C. A. Meyers, Neurocognitive dysfunction in cancer patients, *Oncology* **14**(1): 75–79 (2000).

30. D. Khuntia, P. Brown, J. Li and M. P. Mehta, Whole-brain radiotherapy in the management of brain metastasis. *J. Clin. Oncol.* **24**(8): 1295–1304 (2006).

31. M. L. Monje and T. Palmer, Radiation injury and neurogenesis. *Curr. Opin. Neurol.* **16**(2): 129–134 (2003).

32. B. Adamcio, D. Sargin, A. Stradomska, L. Medrihan, C. Gertler, F. Theis, M. Zhang, M. Muller, I. Hassouna, K. Hannke, S. Sperling, K. Radyushkin, A. El-Kordi, L. Schulze, A. Ronnenberg, F. Wolf, N. Brose, J. S. Rhee, W. Zhang and H. Ehrenreich, Erythropoietin enhances hippocampal long-term potentiation and memory, *BMC Biol.* **6**: 37 (2008).

33. M. L. Monje, H. Toda and T. D. Palmer, Inflammatory blockade restores adult hippocampal neurogenesis, *Science* **302**(5651): 1760–1765 (2003).

34. E. G. Shaw, R. Rosdhal, R. B. D'Agostino Jr., J. Lovato, M. J. Naughton, M. E. Robbins and S. R. Rapp, Phase II study of donepezil in irradiated

brain tumor patients: Effect on cognitive function, mood, and quality of life, *J. Clin. Oncol.* **24**(9): 1415–1420 (2006).

35. D. A. Loblaw, N. J. Laperriere and W. J. Mackillop, A population-based study of malignant spinal cord compression in Ontario, *Clin. Oncol.* **15**: 211–217 (2003).

36. F. Bach, B. H. Larsen, K. Rohde, S. E. Borgesen, F. Gjerris, T. Boge-Rasmussen, N. Agerlin, B. Rasmusson, P. Stjernholm and P. S. Sorensen, Metastatic spinal cord compression, *Acta Neurochir.* **107**: 37–43 (1990).

37. D. A. Loblaw, J. Perry, A. Chambers and N. J. Laperriere, Systematic review of the diagnosis and management of malignant extradural spinal cord compression: The cancer care Ontario practice guidelines initiative's neuro-oncology disease site group, *J. Clin. Oncol.* **23**(9): 2028–2037 (2005).

38. P. Levack, J. Graham, D. Collie *et al.*, Scottish Cord Compression Study Group, Don't wait for a sensory level — Listen to the symptoms: A prospective audit of the delays in diagnosis of malignant cord compression, *Clin. Oncol.* **14**: 472–480 (2002).

39. R. W. Gilbert, J. H. Kim and J. B. Posner, Epidural spinal cord compression from metastatic tumour: Diagnosis and treatment, *Ann. Neurol.* **3**: 40–51 (1978).

40. S. Helweg-Larsen and P. S. Sorensen, Symptoms and signs in metastatic spinal cord compression: A study of progression from first symptom until diagnosis in 153 patients, *Eur. J. Cancer* **30A**(3): 396–398 (1994).

41. D. Rades, F. Heidenreich and J. H. Karstens, Final results of a prospective study of the prognostic value of the time to develop motor deficits before irradiation in metastatic spinal cord compression, *Int. J. Radiat. Oncol. Biol. Phys.* **53**(4): 975–979 (2002).

42. J. A. Talcott, P. C. Stomper, F. W. Drislane, P. Y. Wen, C. C. Block, C. C. Humphrey, C. Lu and F. Jolesz, Assessing suspected spinal cord compression: A multidisciplinary outcomes analysis of 342 episodes, *Suppl. Care Cancer* **7**: 31–38 (1999).

43. S. Sorensen, S. Helweg-Larsen, H. Mouridsen and H. H. Hansen, Effect of high-dose dexamethasone in carcinomatous metastatic spinal cord compression treated with radiotherapy: A randomized trial, *Eur. J. Cancer* **30A**(1): 22–27 (1994).

44. C. J. Vecht, H. Haaxma-Reiche, W. L. van Putten, M. de Visser, E. P. Vries and A. Twijnstra, Initial bolus of conventional versus high-dose

dexamethasone in metastatic spinal cord compression, *Neurology* **39**(9): 1255–1257 (1989).

45. E. Maranzano, P. Latini, S. Beneventi, E. Perruci, B. M. Panizza, C. Aristei, M. Lupattelli and M. Tonato, Radiotherapy without steroids in selected metastatic spinal cord compression patients. A phase II trial, *Am. J. Clin. Oncol.* **19**(2): 179–183 (1996).

46. P. Klimo Jr., J. R. Kestle and M. H. Schmidt, Treatment of metastatic spinal epidural disease: A review of the literature, *Neurosurg. Focus* **15**(5): 1–8 (2003).

47. S. M. Dy, S. M. Asch, A. Naeim, H. Sanati, A. Walling and K. A. Lorenz, Evidence-based standards for cancer pain management, *J. Clin. Oncol.* **26**(23): 3879–3885 (2008).

48. P. Klimo Jr., C. J. Thompson, J. R. Kestle and M. H. Schmidt, A meta-analysis of surgery versus conventional radiotherapy for the treatment of metastatic spinal epidural disease, *Neuro-Oncology* **7**(1): 64–76 (2005).

15

Cancer and the Thoracic Surgeon

Edmund Kassis
and Stephen C. Yang

Abstract

The practice of thoracic surgery is a model of using a multidisciplinary approach to the care of patients, particularly in the area of cancer. These diseases include primary malignancies of the lung, esophagus, pleura, chest wall, airway and mediastinum; less commonly, metastatic deposits to the lung, pleura, chest wall and mediastinum require the thoracic surgeon's attention for diagnosis, for potential curative resection, or for palliative intervention. The optimal and efficient approach to diagnosing, staging, and managing patients with thoracic malignancies is constantly evolving, with the choices available to the patient becoming ever more complex. Yet, the care is moving toward personalization, based on certain factors such as demographics, staging characteristics, and biologic markers. Thus, the traditional roles of the individual disciplines managing these patients are constantly being challenged and are becomes less frequent. As a result of advanced imaging technologies and patient demand for 'minimally invasive' procedures, several disciplines are now providing overlapping services. The input from a wide range of these specialists demonstrates the importance of a multidisciplinary approach to optimize treatments and to streamline care. Weekly conferences are held to discuss these complex patients, and a list of those whose services are often required is listed in Table 1. This chapter will focus on the common diagnostic, staging, and therapeutic modalities that are available to the clinician taking care of the patients with non-small cell lung cancer (NSCLC). In particular the aspects of management that fall 'in-between' disciplines will be the focus of this discussion.

Keywords: Lung cancer, surgery, diagnosis, staging.

1.   Introduction

Evaluation of the solitary pulmonary nodule remains as one of the most common problems presented to the thoracic surgeon. Depending upon the demographics, up to one-third of the U.S. population may have these abnormalities, and obviously only a small fraction represent cancer. The incidence of discovering these nodules is on the rise, due in part to the common availability of

Table 1.   Speciality services involved in the multidisciplinary care of lung cancer.

Service	Role
Thoracic surgery	Surgical evaluation
Pulmonary	Interventional bronchoscopy, preop. evaluation
Gastroenterology	Endoscopic biopsy of mediastinal lymph nodes
Radiology	Diagnostic, nuclear, interventional studies
Radiation therapy	Pre-/postoperative radiation
Medical oncology	Pre-/postoperative chemotherapy
Pathology	Interpretation of histology
Speech pathology	Assessing aspiration risks
Public health	Enrolment into public health trials
Patient advocates	Help patients navigate through medical systems
Cardiologists	Cardiac clearance
Clinical trial coordinators	Enrolment into clinical trials
Anesthesia and critical care	Preoperative clearance
Physical and occupational therapy	Preoperative assessment of exercise tolerance

CT scanning, particularly in this era of CT screening for lung cancer. For the thoracic surgeon, the critical question is to decide if malignancy exists, and thus whether further studies are needed to offer surgery and stage the disease based on patient and nodule characteristics. These occasionally involved the input from the radiologists for study interpretation, and the pulmonologist if interventional diagnostic bronchoscopy is required. Furthermore, if cancer is still suspected or is diagnosed, and at a more advanced stage, then the input of the multiple disciplines is required in order to decide an appropriate treatment strategy for that particular patient.

Lung cancer remains as the leading cause of cancer-related deaths not only in the U.S. adult population, but also in many other parts of the world. It is predicted that the incidence of lung cancer will remain stable or decrease slightly in many developed countries including the United States; but for other countries such as China, the peak incidence has not been seen yet because the delayed effects of smoking are yet to be seen. Unfortunately, only approximately one-quarter of patients present with early stage disease that is amenable to resection. This is due in part to the lack of reliable screening tests, unlike for some other tumors, and the fact that symptoms usually appear late in the disease process. Thus, staging is critical not only to provide prognosis, but mainly to choose the appropriate therapy, which often does not involve surgery. Therefore, given the current available modalities, accurate tumor staging often requires a multidisciplinary approach.

2. Diagnosis

Once clinical or radiographic evaluation raises the suspicion of lung cancer, it is up to the physician to decide if a tissue diagnosis is required, and if so, how to achieve this in the most expeditious, safe, and cost-effective manner. There are several modalities available to aid in the diagnosis of lung cancer, including sputum cytology, flexible bronchoscopy with transbronchial biopsy, image-guided transthoracic biopsy, endobronchial ultrasound (EBUS) with biopsy, video-assisted thoracic surgery (VATS) and thoracotomy. The modality selected to diagnose a suspected lung cancer is based on symptomatology, characteristics of the mass, presence of metastatic disease and the anticipated treatment plan.

2.1 *Sputum cytology*

Numerous studies[1–9] have been performed to assess the sensitivity of sputum cytology in the diagnosis of lung cancer. The sensitivity ranges from 40–90% with specificity ranging from 60–100%. Many — but not all studies — have demonstrated superior sensitivity of sputum cytology for centrally located lesions, compared to peripherally located masses. Patient and lesion characteristics that enhance the sensitivity of sputum cytology for the diagnosis of lung cancer are demonstrated in Table 2.

2.2 *Fiberoptic bronchoscopy*

Fiberoptic bronchoscopy with biopsy, brushing, bronchoalveolar lavage (BAL) and transbronchial needle aspiration (TBNA) is frequently used in the diagnosis and staging of lung cancer. The utility of bronchoscopic procedures has been extensively studied in the literature.[10–27] Fiberoptic bronchoscopy is the diagnostic procedure of choice for central and endobronchial lesions. The diagnostic accuracy of fiberoptic bronchoscopy is highest in conjunction with endobronchial biopsy. The sensitivity of bronchoscopy and biopsy ranges from 50–93%. Bronchial brushings and washings demonstrate a lower sensitivity compared to direct biopsy in nearly all studies looking at this issue. The range in sensitivity for brushings and washings for centrally located lesions is 30–80% and 30–60%, respectively.

In contrast, brushing demonstrated the highest sensitivity for lesions beyond the segmental bronchi, followed by biopsy and BAL. The diagnostic sensitivity and accuracy was significantly higher if the lesion was greater that 2 cm in diameter.

Table 2. Factors that enhance the sensitivity of sputum cytology in diagnosis of lung cancer.

1. Number of sputum specimens collected per patient
2. Bloody sputum
3. Low FEV1
4. Large tumors
5. Centrally located tumors
6. Squamous cell cancer

2.3 Transthoracic Needle Biopsy (TTNB)

The overall sensitivity of TTNB ranges from 60–99%. TTNB is currently the procedure of choice in the diagnosis of peripherally located lesions less than 3cm in size. Several studies have analyzed the impact of lesion size on the diagnostic sensitivity of TTNB.[28–48] These studies have failed to demonstrate a statistically significant improvement in sensitivity of TTNB for larger lesions, compared to smaller nodules. The sensitivity of transthoracic fine needle aspiration (TTFNA) was similar to transthoracic core biopsy (TTCB) for the diagnosis of malignancy. However, TTCB had improved sensitivity for aiding in the specific diagnosis for non-malignant lesions.

2.4 Video-Assisted Thoracic Surgery (VATS)

If sputum cytology and fiberoptic bronchoscopy are non-diagnostic, the physician is left with the decision to proceed with TTNB or surgery to assist in the diagnosis. Swenson and colleagues in 1997[49] described three radiographic and three clinical factors predicting malignancy (Table 3). In patients with these radiographic and/or clinical characteristics, it is reasonable to proceed directly to surgical intervention, since TTNB may only delay definitive therapy. Schmulewitz in 2004[50] described several circumstances where FNA is recommended to avoid surgery: if the patient is a high operative risk, or has low risk of malignancy based on clinical and radiologic characteristics; if a definite benign diagnosis is considered likely; if the patients prefers to have a diagnosis of cancer before proceeding to the operating room; or the patients is not an

Table 3. Clinical and radiographic criteria predicting malignancy in solitary pulmonary nodules.

Radiographic:	Diameter > 2cm
	Spiculation
	Upper lobe lesions
Clinical:	Age > 40 years
	Smoking history
	Cancer history

operative candidate and tissue diagnosis is needed before com-mencing with therapy. However, not every solitary pulmonary nodule is accessible via VATS wedge resection. These lesions optimally should be peripheral, ≤ 3cm in diameter, near the acute angle of the fissure, and not more than 1cm deep to the pleural surface.

3. Staging

After the diagnosis of lung cancer is established, or remains highly suspicious, determining the extent of disease is critical in deter-mining the management strategy and prognosis of the patient. Staging of lung cancer is critical for determining prognosis, selecting appropriate therapy, and comparing the results of clinical trials.

The current staging system is based on data from Mountain and associates.[51] Recently, the International Association for the Study of Lung Cancer (IASLC) has proposed changes[52–56] to the current TNM system. The IASLC proposals were based on data from over 100,000 patients from an international database. Tables 4 and 5 compare the current UICC-6 and the proposed IASLC staging systems.

Probably the most important role of accurate clinical staging of patients with NSCLC is in planning appropriate therapy. The importance of staging is perhaps most evident in distin-guishing patients with clinical stages I and II from stages III and IV. In general patients with clinical stages I and II NSCLC undergo surgical resection followed by systemic chemotherapy, based on final pathologic stage. Several authors have demon-strated a survival advantage in patients with clinical stage IIIA disease undergoing neoadjuvant, rather than postoperative chemotherapy. Additionally, patients clinically staged as IIIB or IV are typically not candidates for surgical intervention and receive definitive chemoradiotherapy. These examples under-score the importance of accurate pre-treatment staging in the management of NSCLC. Staging of lung cancer can be divided into two broad groups: non-invasive and invasive staging.

Table 4. Comparison of T and M stages of UICC-6 (A) and IASLC (B) staging systems.

A. UICC-6 Staging System

Tx: Primary tumor cannot be assessed, *or* tumor proven by the presence of malignant cells in sputum or bronchial washings but not visualized by imaging or bronchoscopy.

T0: No evidence of primary tumor.

Tis: Carcinoma *in situ*.

T1:
Tumor 3 cm or less in greatest dimension, surrounded by lung or visceral pleura, without evidence of invasion more proximal than the lobar bronchus.

T2:
Tumor more than 3 cm in diameter; or tumor with *any* of the following features:
— involves main bronchus, 2 cm or more distal to the carina;
— invades visceral pleura; or
— associated with atelectasis or obstructive pneumonitis that extends to the hilar region but does not involve the entire lung.

T3:
Tumor more than 7 cm or
— direct invasion any of the following: chest wall (including superior sulcus tumours), diaphragm, phrenic nerve, mediastinal pleura, parietal pericardium;
— tumor in the main bronchus less than 2 cm distal to the carina without carinal invasion; or
— associated atelectasis or obstructive pneumonitis of the entire lung.

T4:
Tumor of any size that invades any of the following:
— mediastinum, heart, great vessels, trachea, recurrent laryngeal nerve, esophagus, vertebral body or carina.
Separate tumor nodule(s) in the ipsilateral primary lobe.
Malignant pleural effusion.

M1: Distant metastases.

(Continued)

Table 4.   *(Continued)*

B. IASLC Staging System

Tx: Primary tumor cannot be assessed, *or* tumor proven by the presence of malignant cells in sputum or bronchial washings but not visualized by imaging or bronchoscopy.

T0: No evidence of primary tumor.

Tis: Carcinoma *in situ*.

T1:
Tumor 3 cm or less in greatest dimension, surrounded by lung or visceral pleura, without evidence of invasion more proximal than the lobar bronchus.

T1a: Tumor 2 cm or less in greatest dimension.

T1b: Tumor more than 2 cm but not more than 3 cm in greatest dimension.

T2:
Tumor more than 3 cm but not more than 7 cm;
or tumor with *any* of the following features:
- involves main bronchus, 2 cm or more distal to the carina;
- invades visceral pleura; or
- associated with atelectasis or obstructive pneumonitis that extends to the hilar region but does not involve the entire lung.

T2a: Tumor more than 3 cm but not more than 5 cm in greatest dimension.

T2b: Tumor more than 5 cm but not more than 7 cm in greatest dimension.

T3:
Tumor more than 7 cm or
- direct invasion any of the following: chest wall (including superior sulcus tumours), diaphragm, phrenic nerve, mediastinal pleura, parietal pericardium;
- tumor in the main bronchus less than 2 cm distal to the carina;
- associated atelectasis or obstructive pneumonitis of the entire lung; or
- separate tumor nodule(s) in the same lobe.

(Continued)

Table 4. (*Continued*)

B. IASLC Staging System

T4:

Tumor of any size that invades any of the following: mediastinum, heart, great vessels, trachea, recurrent laryngeal nerve, esophagus, vertebral body or carina. Separate tumor nodule(s) in a different ipsilateral lobe.

M1a: Tumor nodule in contralateral lung, tumor with pleural nodules, malignant effusion.

M1b: Distant metastases.

Table 5. Comparison of TNM stage groupings of IASLC vs UICC-6 staging systems.

	UICC-6	IASLC
Stage IA	T1 N0 M0	T1a N0 M0
		T1b N0 M0
Stage IB	T2 N0 M0	T2a N0 M0
Stage IIA	T1 N1 M0	T1a N1 M0
		T1b N1 M0
		T2a N1 M0
		T2b N0 M0
Stage IIB	T2 N1 M0	T2b N1 M0
	T3 N0 M0	T3 N0 M0
Stage IIIA	T3 N1 M0	T1a N2 M0
	T1-3 N2 M0	T1b N2 M0
		T2a N2 M0
		T2b N2 M0
		T3 N1 M0
		T3 N2 M0
		T4 N0 M0
		T4 N1 M0
Stage IIIB	T4, Any N, M0	T4 N2 M0
	Any T, N3 M0	Any T, N3, M0
Stage IV	Any T, Any N, M1	Any T, Any N, M1 a/b

3.1 Non-invasive staging

3.1.1 Computed Tomography (CT) scanning

Chest CT has become the most widely utilized modality in the non-invasive staging patients with NSCLC. The majority of studies evaluating CT scanning in the staging of mediastinal nodal involvement have used a short axis of $\geq$ 1cm as the threshold for defining abnormal lymph nodes. Toloza et al.[57] have reviewed data from over 20 manuscripts encompassing over 3500 patients. The overall sensitivity and specificity were 60% and 81%, respectively. Although 10% of patients with clinical T1N0 NSCLC will have N2 disease on pathologic stage, conversely 20–40% of patients with malignant appearing nodes on CT (> 1cm) will be negative histologically.[58] However, significant inter observer variation may exist.[59] While the clinician should not rely solely on the CT scan for staging, CT continues to be an important modality in staging patients with NSCLC, as it effectively guides selective biopsy by endobronchial ultrasound (EBUS), mediastinoscopy, VATS, or transthoracic approaches. Any suspicious node identified on CT should be biopsied to prove malignant involvement.

CT scanning has limited sensitivity in distinguishing between T1/T2 tumors and T3/T4 tumors as reported by Webb et al.[60] Additionally, the sensitivity for identification of mediastinal invasion that would preclude surgical resection is 60–80%. In this regard, CT scanning has not demonstrated an ability to avoid futile or non-therapeutic thoracotomies.

3.1.2 Positron Emission Tomography (PET) scanning

PET scanning uses the radiolabeled glucose analog ^{18}F-fluoro-deoxy-D-glucose (FDG) to asses the metabolic activity of tumor cells. In general, cancer cells have increased cellular uptake and metabolic activity compared to normal cells thus cancer cells accumulate the FDG molecule to a greater degree than normal cells.[61] Cellular accumulation is detected on a PET camera, with the intensity of uptake measured and reported as a standard uptake value (SUV). A SUV of greater than 2.5 is considered abnormal.

As previously discussed, the sensitivity and specificity of CT scanning is inadequate in differentiating benign from malignant adenopathy. The addition of PET scanning has increased the overall sensitivity and specificity of non-invasive mediastinal staging. As reported by Toloza,[53] the sensitivity and specificity of PET is 84% and 89%, respectively regarding the involvement of mediastinal lymph nodes. While a negative PET may eliminate the need for invasive mediastinal staging, a positive PET still requires histologic confirmation, as numerous inflammatory and infectious conditions may demonstrate positive PET findings.

3.1.3 Integrated CT-PET

PET demonstrated superior sensitivity and specificity when compared to CT scanning. The recent evaluation of integrated CT-PET has shown that this technology is superior to PET alone in assessing the T or N stage.[63,64] Integrated CT-PET accurately identified the T stage in 88% of patients, compared with 40% of patients with PET alone. For nodal disease, CT-PET correctly identified the nodal stage in 81% of patients, compared to 49% for PET alone.[65]

3.2 Invasive staging

The status of mediastinal lymph nodes is the major factor determining resectability and sequence therapy in patients with NSCLC. Several authors have demonstrated an improvement in survival in patients treated with preoperative chemotherapy in N2/IIIA NSCLC.[66,67] Also, positivity of N3 nodes in NSCLC is a contraindication to surgical resection and definitive chemoradiotherapy is the treatment of choice. Thus, accurate determination of mediastinal nodal involvement is critical to appropriate patient management. There is controversy regarding the need for invasive mediastinal staging on all patients with NSCLC. This argument stems from the fact that approximately 5–15% of patients with stage IA NSCLC will have mediastinal nodal metastases on pathologic staging. The importance of this occult N2 disease however has not been resolved. It is well established however that suspicious mediastinal lymph nodes by CT/PET scanning should be sampled invasively, since up to 40% of these nodes will not harbor malignancy.[64] A variety of invasive tests done almost exclusively by the thoracic surgeon have been utilized to stage the mediastinum in NSCLC and each will be discussed in this section.

3.2.1 *Mediastinoscopy*

Cervical mediastinoscopy allows for the dissection and sampling of bilateral upper and lower paratracheal, pretracheal, and subcarinal lymph nodes (levels 2R, 2L, 4R, 4L, and 7). Ginsberg *et al.*[68] reported data on over 2000 mediastinoscopies and in their analysis the total complication rate was 2%, with no mortality. The sensitivity of mediastinoscopy in detecting metastatic disease in mediastinal lymph nodes is 80–85%, with a false negative rate of 5–12% and a specificity of 100%. The false negative rates are lowest for paratracheal nodes and highest for subcarinal nodes. The false negative rate may reflect the effort of the operator in dissecting and sampling these nodes at mediastinoscopy. Ideally, five nodal stations are sampled at mediastinoscopy (2 R/L, 4 R/L and 7). The high sensitivity and specificity, coupled with a low morbidity, have made mediastinoscopy the gold standard among invasive staging modalities for the mediastinum.[69] These are done routinely now in an outpatient setting.[70,71]

However there are several contraindications to this procedure that may not be apparent to the non-surgeons, especially in this population of patients. A permanent tracheostomy precludes this approach. Other relative contraindications include a prior mediastinoscopy (noting that previous cardiac surgery is not necessarily a contraindication), mediastinal irradiation, high venous pressure or pulmonary hypertension, and aortic or great vessel aneurysms.

3.2.2 *Extended mediastinoscopy and anterior mediastinotomy*

Aortopulmonary window (level 5) and subaortic (level 6) lymph nodes are N2 nodes frequently involved in NSCLC, especially in patients with carcinoma of the left upper lobe. Importantly, these nodal stations are not accessible by standard cervical mediastinoscopy. Two modalities have been developed to access the level 5/6 nodal stations. Classically, access to this region of the mediastinum was performed using the Chamberlain procedure (anterior mediastinotomy).[72] This procedure involves a left parasternal incision, with access to the mediastinum through the second or third intercostal space. Biopsy of the nodes in question is performed through the mediastinoscope. The sensitivity of the Chamberlain procedure is 87%, with a false negative rate of 10%.[73,74] Extended cervical mediastinoscopy is an alternate method used to access the level 5/6 lymph nodes.[75] This procedure is performed in a manner similar to cervical mediastinoscopy. In the extended mediastinoscopy, the mediastinoscope is placed in a plane superolateral to the aorta, between the innominate and carotid arteries. Sensitivity of this procedure ranges from 69 to 83%, with a false negative rate of 9–11% with minimal morbidity and mortality.[76,77]

3.2.3 Transthoracic needle aspiration

Sensitivity of image guided transthoracic biopsies of mediastinal lymph nodes have improved significantly with advances in imaging technology. The sensitivity of this modality has been reported to be as high as 90%; the false negative rate has been reported to range from 20 to 40% and is likely due to sampling error.[78,79] Thus a negative result cannot definitively rule out metastatic involvement. However, this technique this technique is rarely used these days, because of the depth of penetration the needle has to pass through (with associated complications) and the availability of less invasive methods, such as EUS and EBUS (below).

3.2.4 Endoscopic Ultrasound (EUS) and Endobronchial Ultrasound (EBUS)

Several studies have demonstrated that the addition of trans-esophageal endoscopic ultrasound (EUS) to transcervical mediastinoscopy identified a greater proportion of T4 or mediastinal metastases than either modality alone.[80,81] One study[82] reported that the addition of EUS to mediastinoscopy could lead to a 16% reduction in futile thoracotomies. EUS adds the ability to access levels 5, 8 and 9 lymph nodes, which are inaccessible by mediastinoscopy. Eloubeidi et al.[83] performed EUS-FNA on all patients with suspicious nodes at levels 5, 7, 8, and 9 based on PET-CT. A total of

28 patients (14%) had nodal metastases by EUS, unsuspected by imaging. A more recent method to stage the mediastinum is endobronchial ultrasound (EBUS). EBUS provides the ability to sample levels 1–5, 7, 10 and 11. The sensitivity and specificity of EBUS have been reported as 80–95% and 100% respectively.[84–86] A trial is currently underway at MD Anderson Cancer Center to compare transcervical mediastinoscopy to EBUS in patients with clinical N2 disease.

3.2.5 *Video-Assisted Thoracic Surgery (VATS)*

VATS is a minimally invasive alternative that allows access to the entire pleural cavity for both diagnostic and therapeutic purposes. On the left, levels 5, 6, 7, 8 and 9 nodal stations may be easily sampled. VATS mediastinal staging is 100% sensitive and 100% specific, as reported by Landreneau and colleagues.[87] Roviaro and colleagues[88] reported that VATS identified unresectable lesions in 8.3% of cases, thus avoiding unnecessary thoracotomy, due to either invasion into critical non-removable structures (spine, aorta, trachea), pleural involvement, multiple lesions or advanced nodal disease. VATS is limited to assessment of only one side of the mediastinum; unless bilateral exploration is performed.

4.   Preoperative Assessment

In patients offered surgery for either staging purposes or for definitive resection, assessment of their co-morbidities is mandatory to ensure an acceptable surgical outcome. Consultations with the cardiologist and/or pulmonologist may be required to assess cardiopulmonary function and reserve. Up to 25% of lung cancer patients will have some degree of coronary, valvular or myocardial disease. In asymptomatic patients, evaluation of cardiac function is not necessary; however, in patients with symptoms, or who have a history of cardiac disease/surgery, other tests are required, such as echocardiography, exercise/persantin stress tests, nuclear (thallium) scans, and/or right and left heart catheterization are necessary. 'Cardiac clearance' is usually mandated, however, marginal patients are increasingly being offered surgery, due to better peri-operative care and the experience of the surgeon.

Occasionally surgery may be the only option, especially if there are no other alternatives from the pulmonary, radiation, oncology, or radiologic interventional standpoint. Age should not preclude surgical resection: while the mean age of presentation for lung cancer is 72, many older patients remain healthy and can undergo aggressive management.

Several pulmonary function parameters have been implicated in predicting complications after surgery. Classic teaching regarding the use of preoperative pulmonary function tests requires that the predicted postoperative forced-expiratory volume in one second (FEV1) should be greater than 800 cc, or 30% of that predicted, and that preoperative diffusion capacity of carbon monoxide (DLCO) should be greater than 40% of predicted. If these parameters are borderline, then other sophisticated tests, such as arterial blood cases (looking at oxygen and carbon dioxide levels), exercise testing (maximum oxygen consumption, VO2 max, <10–15 mL/min/m^2, predicting complications), evaluation of right and left heart function, and cardiac catheterization should be done. Physical therapy services can be enlisted to determine the six-minute walk tests, assessment of stair climbing abilities, or even to do preoperative pulmonary rehabilitation, to optimize borderline emphysema patients for surgery.

5.   Treatment

Upon completion of a thorough staging evaluation of the patient with NSCLC, attention is turned to management. The appropriate treatment of these patients is ultimately based on the patients' clinical stage. This section will detail the treatments modalities effective for each particular stage of disease. Tables 3 and 4 highlight the TNM classifications and stage groupings for NSCLC.

Patients with stages I and II NSCLC are considered to have early stage disease and demonstrate a 5-year survival as high as 76% and 55%, respectively. Unfortunately, these patients constitute just 20–30% of all patients with NSCLC. Surgery is the mainstay of therapy for these patients with early stage disease. While there are no randomized trials directly comparing surgery alone to either radiation therapy or chemotherapy alone in the treatment of early stage NSCLC, retrospective data indicates that surgery can offer the greatest survival advantage to early stage patients. In a prospective randomized trial, The Lung Cancer Study Group (LCSG) reported significantly increased local and distal recurrence and mortality rates in patients that underwent limited resection, versus those that underwent lobectomy.[90] This trial did demonstrate an increase in pulmonary complications in the lobectomy group. In contrast, Watanabe and colleagues demonstrated no significant difference in 30-day or in-hospital mortality between lobectomy and lesser resections.[91] While lobectomy is the treatment of choice in patients with early stage NSCLC, there remains a role for limited resections. Limited resections (wedge resections and segmentectomies) have been demonstrated to be of benefit in poor pulmonary reserve and N0 disease.[92,93] Currently, the American College of Chest Physicians recommends sublobar resection over non-surgical interventions in patients with co-morbid illness, or compromised pulmonary function that would preclude lobectomy.[94]

Video assisted thoracic surgery (VATS) lobectomy is a valid approach to the management of early stage NSCLC. While randomized trials comparing the VATS to the open approach are lacking, several papers have demonstrated comparable complication rates and 5-year survival for both methods.[95,96]

With respect to multimodality therapy for early stage NSCLC, the use of adjuvant chemotherapy is not recommended for patients with stage IA NSCLC. A significant improvement in survival in patients with stages IB (T > 4 cm) and II NSCLC has been demonstrated treated with adjuvant platinum-based chemotherapy.[97–102]

The role of radiation therapy in the management of stage I and II NSCLC is limited to patients who are not surgical candidates. Local control has been reported with definitive radiotherapy with local recurrence rates of approximately 40%.[103] Radiation therapy in the adjuvant setting for early stage NSCLC is associated with increased mortality and currently has no role in the management of these patients.[104]

Patients that are not surgical candidates secondary to poor cardiopulmonary reserve or extensive unresectable disease are candidates for alternative methods for local control. Stereotactic radiotherapy and radiofrequency ablation (RFA) have been described as alternatives to definitive radiation therapy in these patients. The utility of these modalities has not been established and should only be offered in an investigational setting.

One of the topics of current debate is who should perform these pulmonary resections (general versus thoracic surgeons) and where these should be done (high versus low volume centers, teaching versus non-teaching hospitals). It is generally accepted that thoracic surgeons have improved surgical outcomes, compared to those surgeons who do not specialize in lung cancer resections.[105–107] Though hospital volume has been shown to be a significant factor in better surgical outcomes for certain procedures like esophagectomies and pancreatic resections,[107] the data are mixed regarding pulmonary resections, but somewhat favoring higher volume surgeons.

The peri-operative care of these patients can occasionally be complicated, and this is beyond the scope of this discussion. However, several services are often involved that are critical to the successful outcome of the surgical lung cancer patient. These include: anesthesiologists who are familiar with thoracic surgery; multidisciplinary intensive care teams including board-certified intensivists, nurses, mid-level care providers (nurse practitioners, physician assistants), and pharmacy doctorates; acute pain management teams; specialized nursing care teams and floors dedicate to the care of thoracic surgical patients; and physical and occupational therapists.

6.   Summary

Lung resection remains the best chance of cure for patients with early-stage non-small cell lung cancer. Unfortunately most patients present with advanced stages, but by involving other treatment modalities, patients have improved survival using a multimodality approach. Patients should not be denied surgery based on age, co-morbidities or sub-optimal lung function alone. Critical is the need for assessment of the individual patient by multiple services to accurately diagnose, stage, and assess the patient's candidacy for surgery. Several guidelines exist by the Society of Thoracic Surgeons, the American College of Chest Physicians, and the National Comprehensive Cancer Network in the appropriate treatment of patients with NSCLC. Outside these guidelines, the input of multiple services are required to discuss and offer potentially curative options. The use of these multidisciplinary therapies and teams in lung cancer has served as a model for other thoracic tumors such as esophageal cancer, malignant mesothelioma, and thymic carcinoma.

References

1. J. Benbassat, A. Regev and P. E. Slater, Predictive value of sputum cytology, *Thorax* **42**: 165–172 (1987).
2. A. C. Mehta, J. J. Marty and F. Y. Lee, Sputum cytology, *Clin. Chest Med.* **14**: 69–85 (1993).
3. A. Sing, N. Freudenberg, C. Kortsik *et al.*, Comparison of the sensitivity of sputum and brush cytology in the diagnosis of lung carcinomas, *Acta Cytol.* **41**: 399–408 (1997).
4. W. H. Kern, The diagnostic accuracy of sputum and urine cytology, *Acta Cytol.* **32**: 651–654 (1988).
5. M. Matsuda, T. Horai, O. Doi *et al.*, Diagnosis of squamous-cell carcinoma of the lung by sputum cytology: With special reference to correlation of diagnostic accuracy with size and proximal extent of resected tumor, *Diagn. Cytopathol.* **6**: 248–251 (1990).
6. X. M. Liang, Accuracy of cytologic diagnosis and cytotyping of sputum in primary lung cancer: Analysis of 161 cases, *J. Surg. Oncol.* **40**: 107–111 (1989).
7. H. Kawachi and K. Shimokata, Factors affecting the rate of positivity of sputum cytology in lung cancer, *Jpn. J. Clin. Oncol.* **15**: 451–456 (1985).
8. T. Tanaka, M. Yamamoto, T. Tamura *et al.*, Cytologic and histologic correlation in primary lung cancer: A study of 154 cases with resectable tumors, *Acta Cytol.* **29**: 49–56 (1985).
9. R. S. Fontana, D. R. Sanderson, W. F. Taylor *et al.*, Early lung cancer detection: Results of the initial (prevalence) radiologic and cytologic screening in the Mayo Clinic study, *Am. Rev. Respir. Dis.* **130**: 561–565 (1984).
10. D. A. Schenk, C. L. Bryan, J. H. Bower *et al.*, Transbronchial needle aspiration in the diagnosis of bronchogenic carcinoma, *Chest* **92**: 83–85 (1987).
11. W. A. Baaklini, M. A. Reinoso, A. B. Gorin *et al.*, Diagnostic yield of fiberoptic bronchoscopy in evaluating solitary pulmonary nodules, *Chest* **117**: 1049–1054 (2000).

12. A. Dasgupta, P. Jain, O. A. Minai *et al.*, Utility of transbronchial needle aspiration in the diagnosis of endobronchial lesions, *Chest* **115**: 1237–1241 (1999).

13. J. A. Govert, L. G. Dodd, P. S. Kussin *et al.*, A prospective comparison of fiberoptic transbronchial needle aspiration and bronchial biopsy for bronchoscopically visible lung carcinoma, *Cancer* **87**: 129–134 (1999).

14. S. Bilaceroglu, O. Gunel, U. Cagirici *et al.*, Comparison of endobronchial needle aspiration with forceps and brush biopsies in the diagnosis of endobronchial lung cancer. *Monaldi Arch. Chest Dis.* **52**: 13–17 (1997).

15. J. A. Govert, J. M. Kopita, D. Matchar *et al.*, Cost-effectiveness of collecting routine cytologic specimens during fiberoptic bronchoscopy for endoscopically visible lung tumor, *Chest* **109**: 451–456 (1996).

16. J. Castella, J. Buj, C. Puzo *et al.*, Diagnosis and staging of bronchogenic carcinoma by transtracheal and transbronchial needle aspiration, *Ann. Oncol.* **6**: S21–S24 (1995).

17. J. P. Utz, A. M. Patel and E. S. Edell, The role of transcarinal needle aspiration in the staging of bronchogenic carcinoma, *Chest* **104**: 1012–1016 (1993).

18. G. Buccheri, P. Barberis and M. S. Delfino, Diagnostic, morphologic, and histopathologic correlates in bronchogenic carcinoma: A review of 1,045 bronchoscopic examinations, *Chest* **99**: 809–814 (1991).

19. W. Popp, H. Rauscher, L. Ritschka *et al.*, Diagnostic sensitivity of different techniques in the diagnosis of lung tumors with the flexible fiberoptic bronchoscope: Comparison of brush biopsy, imprint cytology of forceps biopsy, and histology of forceps biopsy, *Cancer* **67**: 72–75 (1991).

20. P. C. Gay and W. M. Brutinel, Transbronchial needle aspiration in the practice of bronchoscopy, *Mayo Clin. Proc.* **64**: 158–162 (1989).

21. S. Saita, A. Tanzillo, C. Riscica *et al.*, Bronchial brushing and biopsy: A comparative evaluation in diagnosing visible bronchial lesions, *Eur. J. Cardiothorac. Surg.* **4**: 270–272 (1990).

22. F. Reichenberger, J. Weber, M. Tamm *et al.*, The value of transbronchial needle aspiration in the diagnosis of peripheral pulmonary lesions, *Chest* **116**: 704–708 (1999).

23. J. F. Aristizabal, K. R. Young and H. Nath, Can chest CT decrease the use of preoperative bronchoscopy in the evaluation of suspected bronchogenic carcinoma? *Chest* **113**: 1244–1249 (1998).

24. J. de Gracia, C. Bravo, M. Miravitlles *et al.*, Diagnostic value of bronchoalveolar lavage in peripheral lung cancer, *Am. Rev. Respir. Dis.* **147**: 649–652 (1993).

25. K. G. Torrington and J. D. Kern, The utility of fiberoptic bronchoscopy in the evaluation of the solitary pulmonary nodule, *Chest* **104**: 1021–1024 (1993).

26. M. Pirozynski, Bronchoalveolar lavage in the diagnosis of peripheral, primary lung cancer, *Chest* **102**: 372–37 (1992).

27. S. I. Rennard, C. Albera, L. Carratu *et al.*, Clinical guidelines and indications for bronchoalveolar lavage (BAL): Pulmonary malignancies, *Eur. Respir. J.* **3**: 956–969 (1990).

28. S. Gasparini, M. Ferretti, E. B. Secchi *et al.*, Integration of transbronchial and percutaneous approach in the diagnosis of peripheral pulmonary nodules or masses: Experience with 1,027 consecutive cases, *Chest* **108**: 131–137 (1995).

29. Y. Lacasse, E. Wong, G. H. Guyatt *et al.*, Transthoracic needle aspiration biopsy for the diagnosis of localised pulmonary lesions: A meta-analysis, *Thorax* **54**: 884–893 (1999).

30. H. Li, P. M. Boiselle, J. O. Shepard *et al.*, Diagnostic accuracy and safety of CT-guided percutaneous needle aspiration biopsy of the lung: Comparison of small and large pulmonary nodules, *Am. J. Roentgenol.* **167**: 105–109 (1996).

31. J. S. Klein, G. Salomon and E. A. Stewart, Transthoracic needle biopsy with a coaxially placed 20-gauge automated cutting needle: Results in 122 patients, *Radiology* **198**: 715–720 (1996).

32. N. Milman, P. Faurschou and G. Grode, Diagnostic yield of transthoracic needle aspiration biopsy following negative fiberoptic bronchoscopy in 103 patients with peripheral circumscribed pulmonary lesions, *Respiration* **62**: 1–3 (1995).

33. M. F. Zakowski, R. M. Gatscha and M. B. Zaman, Negative predictive value of pulmonary fine needle aspiration cytology, *Acta Cytol.* **36**: 283–286 (1992).

34. P. C. Yang, Y. C. Lee, C. J. Yu *et al.*, Ultrasonographically guided biopsy of thoracic tumors: A comparison of large-bore cutting biopsy with fine-needle aspiration, *Cancer* **69**: 2553–2560 (1992).

35. E. G. Cristallini, S. Ascani, R. Farabi *et al.*, Fine needle aspiration biopsy in the diagnosis of intrathoracic masses, *Acta Cytol.* **36**: 416–422 (1992).

36. E. Lopez Hanninen, T. J. Vogl, J. Ricke *et al.*, CT-guided percutaneous core biopsies of pulmonary lesions: Diagnostic accuracy, complications and therapeutic impact, *Acta Radiol.* **42**: 151–155 (2001).

37. F. Laurent, V. Latrabe, B. Vergier *et al.*, CT-guided transthoracic needle biopsy of pulmonary nodules smaller than 20 mm: Results with an automated 20-gauge coaxial cutting needle, *Clin. Radiol.* **55**: 281–287 (2000).

38. M. J. Charig and A. J. Phillips, CT-guided cutting needle biopsy of lung lesions: Safety and efficacy of an out-patient service, *Clin. Radiol.* **55**: 964–969 (2000).

39. J. L. Swischuk, F. Castaneda, J. C. Patel *et al.*, Percutaneous transthoracic needle biopsy of the lung: Review of 612 lesions, *J. Vasc. Interv. Radiol.* **9**: 347–352 (1998).

40. R. C. Larscheid, P. E. Thorpe and W. J. Scott, Percutaneous transthoracic needle aspiration biopsy: A comprehensive review of its current role in the diagnosis and treatment of lung tumors, *Chest* **114**: 704–709 (1998).

41. D. F. Yankelevitz, C. I. Henschke, J. H. Koizumi *et al.*, CT-guided transthoracic needle biopsy of small solitary pulmonary nodules, *Clin. Imag.* **21**: 107–110 (1997).

42. L. Santambrogio, M. Nosotti, N. Bellaviti *et al.*, CT-guided fine needle aspiration cytology of solitary pulmonary nodules: A prospective, randomized study of immediate cytologic evaluation, *Chest* **112**: 423–425 (1997).

43. L. Cattelani, F. Campodonico, M. Rusca *et al.*, CT-guided transthoracic needle biopsy in the diagnosis of chest tumours, *J. Cardiovasc. Surg.* **38**: 539–542 (1997).

44. D. U. Knudsen, S. M. Nielsen, J. Hariri *et al.*, Ultrasonographically guided fine-needle aspiration biopsy of intrathoracic tumors, *Acta Radiol.* **37**: 327–331 (1996).

45. F. Garcia Rio, S. Diaz Lobato, J. M. Pino *et al.*, Value of CT-guided fine needle aspiration in solitary pulmonary nodules with negative fiberoptic bronchoscopy, *Acta Radiol.* **35**: 478–480 (1994).

46. R. Targhetta, J. M. Bourgeois, C. Marty-Double *et al.*, Peripheral pulmonary lesions: Ultrasonic features and ultrasonically guided fine needle aspiration biopsy, *J. Ultrasound Med.* **12**: 369–374 (1993).

47. G. Grode, P. Faurschou and N. Milman, Percutaneous transthoracic fine-needle lung biopsy with 3 different needles: A retrospective

study of results and complications in 224 patients, *Respiration* **60**: 284–288 (1993).

48. C. D. Collins, E. Breatnach and P. H. Nath, Percutaneous needle biopsy of lung nodules following failed bronchoscopic biopsy, *Eur. J. Radiol.* **15**: 49–53 (1992).

49. S. J. Swensen *et al.*, The probability of malignancy in solitary pulmonary nodules. Application to small radiologically indeterminate nodules, *Arch. Intern. Med.* **157**: 849 (1997).

50. N. Schmulewitz, S. Wildi, S. Varadarajulu *et al.*, Accuracy of EUS criteria and primary tumor site for identification of mediastinal lymph node metastasis from non-small-cell lung cancer, *Gastrointest. Endosc.* **59**: 205–212 (2004).

51. C. F. Mountain, Revisions in the international system for staging lung cancer, *Chest* **111**: 1710–1717 (1997).

52. P. A. Groome, V. Bolejack, J. J. Crowley, C. Kennedy, M. Krasnik, L. H. Sobin *et al.*, The IASLC Lung Cancer Staging Project: Validation of the proposals for revision of the T, N, and M descriptors and consequent stage groupings in the forthcoming (seventh) edition of the TNM classification of malignant tumors, *J. Thorac. Oncol.* **2**: 694–705 (2007).

53. R. Rami-Porta, D. Ball, J. Crowley, D. J. Giroux, J. Jett, W. D. Travis *et al.*, The IASLC Lung Cancer Staging Project: Proposals for the revision of the T descriptors in the forthcoming (seventh) edition of the TNM classification of malignant tumors, *J. Thorac. Oncol.* **2**: 593–602 (2007).

54. P. Goldstraw, J. Crowley, K. Chansky, D. Giroux, P. A. Groome, R. Rami-Porta *et al.*, The IASLC Lung Cancer Staging Project: Proposals for the revision of the TNM stage groupings in the forthcoming (seventh) edition of the TNM classification of malignant tumors, *J. Thorac. Oncol.* **2**: 706–714 (2007).

55. V. W. Rusch, J. Crowley, D. J. Giroux, P. Goldstraw, J. G. Im, M. Tsuboi *et al.*, The IASLC Lung Cancer Staging Project: Proposals for the revision of the N descriptors in the forthcoming (seventh) edition of the TNM classification of malignant tumors, *J. Thorac. Oncol.* **2**: 603–612 (2007).

56. P. E. Postmus, E. Brambilla, K. Chansky, J. Crowley, P. Goldstraw, E. F. Patz *et al.*, The IASLC Lung Cancer Staging Project: Proposals for the revision of the M descriptors in the forthcoming (seventh)

edition of the TNM classification of malignant tumors, *J. Thorac. Oncol.* **2**: 686–693 (2007).

57. E. Toloza, L. Harpole and D. C. McCrory, Noninvasive staging of non-small cell lung cancer. A review of the current evidence, *Chest* **123**: 137S (2003).

58. T. C. McLoud, P. M. Bourgouin, R. W. Greenberg *et al.*, Bronchogenic carcinoma: Analysis of staging in the mediastinum with CT by correlative lymph node mapping and sampling, *Radiology* **182**: 319–323 (1992).

59. E. C. M. Bollen, R. Goei, B. E. Hof-Grootenboer *et al.*, Inter-observer variability and accuracy of computed tomographic assessment of nodal status in lung cancer, *Ann. Thorac. Surg.* **58**: 158–162 (1994).

60. W. R. Webb *et al.*, CT and MR imaging in staging non-small cell bronchogenic carcinoma. Report of the Radiologic Diagnostic Oncology Group, *Radiology* **178**: 705 (1991).

61. K. B. Nolop, C. G. Rhodes, L. H. Brudin *et al.*, Glucose utilization *in vivo* by human pulmonary neoplasms, *Cancer* **60**: 2682–2689 (1987).

62. R. I. Wahl, G. D. Hitchins, D. J. Buchsbaum *et al.*, 18F-2 deoxy-2-fluoro-D-glucose uptake into human tumor xenografts: Feasibility studies for cancer imaging with positron-emission tomography, *Cancer* **67**: 1544–1550 (1991).

63. D. Lardinois, W. Weder *et al.*, Staging of non-small cell lung cancer with integrated positron emission tomography and computed tomography, *N. Engl. J. Med.* **348**: 2500 (2003).

64. R. J. Cerfolio, A. S. Bryant *et al.*, Improving the inaccuracies of clinical staging in patients with NSCLC: A prospective trial, *Ann. Thorac. Surg.* **80**: 1207–1214 (2005).

65. R. J. Cerfolio, B. Ojha *et al.*, The accuracy of integrated PET-CT compared with dedicated PET one for the staging of patients with non-small cell lung cancer, *Ann. Thorac. Surg.* **78**: 1017–1023 (2004).

66. J. A. Roth, F. Fossella, R. Komaki *et al.*, A randomized trial comparing perioperative chemotherapy and surgery with surgery alone in resectable stage IIIA non-small-cell lung cancer, *J. Natl. Cancer. Inst.* **86**(9): 673–680 (1994).

67. R. Rosell, J. Maestre, A. Font *et al.*, A randomized trial of mitomycin/ifosfamide/cisplatin preoperative chemotherapy plus surgery versus surgery alone in stage IIIA non-small cell lung cancer, *Semin. Oncol.* **21**(3 Suppl. 4): 28–33 (1994).

68. R. J. Ginsberg, Evaluation of the mediastinum by invasive techniques, *Surg. Clin. North. Am.* **67**: 1025 (1987).
69. Z. T. Hammoud, R. C. Anderson, B. F. Meyers *et al.*, The current role of mediastinoscopy in the evaluation of thoracic disease, *Thorac. Cardiovasc. Surg.* **118**: 894–899 (1999).
70. I. J. Cybulsky and W. F. Bennett, Mediastinoscopy as a routine outpatient procedure, *Ann. Thorac. Surg.* **58**: 176–178 (1994).
71. E. A. Vallières, A. Pagé and A. Verdant, Ambulatory mediastinoscopy and anterior mediastinotomy, *Ann. Thorac. Surg.* **52**: 1122–1126 (1991).
72. T. M. McNeil and J. M. Chamberlain, Diagnostic anterior mediastinotomy, *Ann. Thorac. Surg.* **2**: 532–539 (1966).
73. J. Jiao, P. Magistrelli and P. Goldstraw, The value of cervical mediastinoscopy combined with anterior mediastinotomy in the preoperative evaluation of bronchogenic carcinoma of the left upper lobe, *Eur. J. Cardiothorac. Surg.* **11**: 450–454 (1997).
74. L. A. Best, M. Munichor, M. Ben-Shakhar *et al.*, The contribution of anterior mediastinotomy in the diagnosis and evaluation of diseases of the mediastinum and lung, *Ann. Thorac. Surg.* **43**: 78–81 (1987).
75. R. J. Ginsberg *et al.*, Extended cervical mediastinoscopy. A single staging procedure for bronchogenic carcinoma of the left upper lobe, *J. Thorac. Cardiovasc. Surg.* **94**: 673 (1987).
76. J. Freixinet Gilart, P. G. Garcia, F. R. de Castro *et al.*, Extended cervical mediastinoscopy in the staging of bronchogenic carcinoma, *Ann. Thorac. Surg.* **70**: 1641–1643 (2000).
77. J. Kuzdal, M. Zielinski *et al.*, Transcervical extended mediastinal lymphadenectomy — The new operative technique and early results in lung cancer staging, *Eur. J. Cardiothorac. Surg.* **27**: 384–390 (2005).
78. C. Savage, R. J. Morrison and J. B. Zwischenberger, Bronchoscopic diagnosis and staging of lung cancer, *Chest. Surg. Clin. North Am.* **11**(4): 701–21, vii–viii (2001).
79. H. Kramer and H. J. Groen, Current concepts in the mediastinal lymph node staging of non-small cell lung cancer, *Ann. Surg.* **238**(2): 180–188 (2003).
80. C. G. Micames and D. C. McCrory *et al.*, Endoscopic ultrasound — Guided fine-needle aspiration for non-small cell lung cancer staging: A systematic review and metaanalysis, *Chest* **131**: 539–548 (2007).
81. J. T. Annema, M. I. Versteegh, M. Veselic *et al.*, Endoscopic ultrasound added to mediastinoscopy for preoperative staging of patients with lung cancer, *J. Am. Med. Assoc.* **294**: 931–936 (2005).

82. S. S. Larsen, P. Vilmann, M. Krasnik *et al.*, Endoscopic ultrasound guided biopsy performed routinely in lung cancer staging spares futile thoracotomies: Preliminary results from a randomised clinical trial, *Lung Cancer* **49**: 377–385 (2005).

83. M. A. Eloubeidi, R. J. Cerfolio, V. K. Chen *et al.*, Endoscopic ultrasound-guided fine needle aspiration of mediastinal lymph node in patients with suspected lung cancer after positron emission tomography and computed tomography scans, *Ann. Thorac. Surg.* **79**: 263–268 (2005).

84. K. Yasufuku, M. Chiyo, E. Koh *et al.*, Endobronchial ultrasound guided transbronchial needle aspiration for staging of lung cancer, *Lung Cancer* **50**: 347–354 (2005).

85. F. J. Herth, A. Ernst, R. Eberhardt *et al.*, Endobronchial ultrasound-guided transbronchial needle aspiration of lymph nodes in the radiologically normal mediastinum, *Eur. Respir. J.* **28**: 910–914 (2006).

86. P. Vilmann, M. Krasnik, S. S. Larsen *et al.*, Transesophageal endoscopic ultrasound-guided fine-needle aspiration (EUS-FNA) and endobronchial ultrasound-guided transbronchial needle aspiration (EBUS-TBNA) biopsy: A combined approach in the evaluation of mediastinal lesions, *Endoscopy* **37**: 833–839 (2005).

87. R. J. Landreneau, M. J. Mack, R. D. Dowling *et al.*, The role of thoracoscopy in lung cancer management, *Chest* **113**(1 Suppl.): 6S–12S (1998).

88. G. Roviaro, F. Varoli, C. Rebuffat *et al.*, Videothoracoscopic staging and treatment of lung cancer, *Ann. Thorac. Surg.* **59**(4): 971–974 (1995).

89. H. Poonyagariyagorn and P. J. Mazzone, Lung cancer: Preoperative pulmonary evaluation of the lung resection candidate, *Semin. Respir. Crit. Care Med.* **29**(3): 271–284 (2008).

90. R. J. Ginsberg and L. V. Rubinstein, Randomized trial of lobectomy versus limited resection for T1N0 non-small cell cancer by the Lung Cancer Study Group, *Ann. Thorac. Surg.* **60**: 615–623 (1995).

91. S. Watanabe, H. Asamura, K. Suzuki *et al.*, Recent results of postoperative mortality for surgical resections in lung cancer, *Ann. Thorac. Surg.* **78**: 999–1002 (2004).

92. P. A. Linden, R. Bueno, Y. L. Colson *et al.*, Lung resection in patients with preoperative FEV1 <35% predicted, *Chest* **127**: 1984–1990 (2005).

93. A. E. Martin-Ucar, A. Nakas, J. E. Pilling *et al.*, A case-matched study of anatomical segmentectomy versus lobectomy for stage I lung

cancer in high-risk patients, *Eur. J. Cardiothorac. Surg.* **27**: 675–695 (2005).

94. W. J. Scott, J. Howington, S. Feigenberg *et al.*, Treatment of non-small cell lung cancer stage I and II: ACCP evidence-based clinical practice guidelines (2nd Edition), *Chest* **132**: 234–242 (2007).

95. L. J. Daniels, S. S. Balderson, M. W. Onaitis *et al.*, Thoracoscopic lobectomy: A safe and effective strategy for patients with stage I lung cancer, *Ann. Thorac. Surg.* **74**: 860–864 (2002).

96. R. J. McKenna, W. Houck and C. B. Fuller, Video-assisted thoracic surgery lobectomy: Experience with 1,100 cases, *Ann. Thorac. Surg.* **81**: 421–426 (2006).

97. K. M. W. Pisters and T. Le Chevalier, Adjuvant chemotherapy in completely resected non-small cell lung cancer, *J. Clin. Oncol.* **23**: 3270–3278 (2005).

98. J. P. Pignon, H. Tribodet, G. V. Scagliotti *et al.*, Lung Adjuvant Cisplatin Evaluation (LACE): A pooled analysis of five randomized clinical trials including 4,584 patients, *J. Clin. Oncol.* **26**(21): 3552–3559 (2008).

99. T. L. Winton, R. Livingston, D. Johnson *et al.*, Vinorebline plus cisplatin vs. observation in resected non-small cell lung cancer, *N. Engl. J. Med.* **352**: 2589–2597 (2005).

100. J. Y. Douillard, R. Rosell, M. De Lena *et al.*, Adjuvant vinorelbine plus cisplatin versus observation in patients with completely resected stage IB-IIIA non-small cell lung cancer (Adjuvant Navelbine International Trialist Association [ANITA]): A randomised controlled trial, *Lancet* **7**: 719–727 (2006).

101. G. M. Strauss, J. E. Herndon, M. A. Maddaus *et al.*, Adjuvant chemotherapy in stage IB non-small cell lung cancer: Update of Cancer and Leukemia Group B protocol 9633, *J. Clin. Oncol.* **24**(18S): 7007 (2006).

102. R. Arriagada, B. Bergman, A. Dunant *et al.*, Cisplatin-based adjuvant chemotherapy in patients with completely resected non-small-cell lung cancer, *N. Engl. J. Med.* **350**: 351–360 (2004).

103. X. Qiao, O. Tullgren, I. Lax *et al.*, The role of radiotherapy in treatment of stage I non-small cell lung cancer, *Lung Cancer* **41**: 1–11 (2003).

104. PORT Meta-analysis Trialists Group, *Cochrane Database of Systematic Reviews 2008 Issue 3* (John Wiley & Sons, Ltd., 2008).

105. G. A. Silvestri, J. Handy, D. Lackland *et al.*, Specialists achieve better outcomes than generalists for lung cancer surgery, *Chest* **114**: 675–680 (1998).

106. P. P. Goodney, F. L. Lucas, T. A. Stukel *et al.*, Surgeon speciality and operative mortality with lung resection, *Ann. Surg.* **241**: 179–184 (2005).

107. P. P. Goodney, F. L. Lucas, T. A Stukel and J. D. Birkmeyer, Surgeon speciality and operative mortality with lung resection, *Ann. Surg.* **241**(1): 179–184 (2005).

108. J. D. Birkmeyer, T. A. Stukel, A. E. Siewers *et al.*, Surgeon volume and operative mortality in the United States, *N. Engl. J. Med.* **349**(22): 2117–2127 (2003).

16

Cancer and the Oesophageal Surgeon

Urs Zingg,
Reginald V. Lord and
David I. Watson

Over 95% of all oesophageal cancers are either adeno- or squamous cell carcinomas. With increasing growth they cause dysphagia, weight loss and bleeding. Diagnosis is made with endoscopy and biopsy, and staging is completed by endoscopic ultrasound, abdomino-thoracic CT scan and PET. The UICC TNM classification is used to stage oesophageal tumours, and in gastro-oesophageal junction tumours the anatomical classification described by Siewert is commonly used when planning surgical resection.

Patients with locally resectable tumours and no distant metastases are classified as curative candidates. For these patients the gold standard for treatment is surgery with or without neo-adjuvant radio-chemotherapy. Tumours stage T2 or higher and/or N1 are usually considered for neoadjuvant treatment. Additional to the oncological staging, a risk analysis for each individual patient should be performed as oesophagectomy is associated with significant risks of morbidity and mortality. Co-morbidity, age and the number of surgical procedures performed by the treating institution are important predictors of outcome. Surgery is performed either with open, or minimal invasive techniques. The stomach is most commonly used conduit to replace the oesophagus, with a segment of large bowel an alternative in some individuals. Post-operative morbidity includes anastomotic leak, empyaema, chylothorax, and most importantly respiratory complications. After multimodal treatment, survival is between 20% and 40% at five years.

In patients with locally advanced tumours, metastases, or who are unfit for surgery, definitive radio-chemotherapy is the treatment of choice. Standard treatment regimens include radiotherapy (50 to 60 Gy) and chemotherapy with 5-FU and Cisplatin. If stenosis or obstruction is present, adjuvant interventions such as stent placement, dilatation and argon plasma ablation may be used.

Keywords: Oesophageal cancer, staging, surgery, survival.

1.   Background

1.1   *Epidemiology*

Oesophageal cancer is the seventh most common cause of cancer death in the developed world. Over the last three decades, the incidence of adenocarcinoma has risen by more than 400% in the Western world, whilst the incidence of squamous cell carcinoma (SSC) has remained largely unchanged.[1] The incidence of this tumour is higher in older people, and the mean age at diagnosis is now approximately 65 to 70 years. More than 80% of oesophageal adenocarcinomas now occur in men.

1.2   *Aetiology*

Smoking and alcohol are associated with an increased risk of developing SCC. The combination of these factors has a synergistic effect, with the risk of development of SCC is directly correlated to the number of pack years smoked. Other risk factors are achalasia, oesophageal diverticula, prior radiation, ingestion of caustic fluids and genetic connective tissue diseases such as tylosis (non-epidermolytic palmoplantar keratoderma). Additionally, SCC is clearly associated with low socioeconomic status.[2]

For adenocarcinoma, gastro-oesophageal reflux disease (GORD) is the major risk factor. This is mediated via the development of

Barrett's oesophagus (replacement of normal squamous epithelium with metaplastic columnar epithelium in the distal oesophagus), which develops in up to 10% of patients with GORD. It is associated with a 0.5–2.0% annual risk of neoplastic transformation. Male sex, cigarette smoking, low intake of fruit or vegetables and obesity have been discussed as possible risk factors, whereas *Helicobacter pylori* infection and non-steroidal anti-inflammatory drugs seem to decrease the risk of oesophageal cancer.[3] More recently, evidence has emerged which confirms that obesity, particularly in males, is a major risk factor for the development of this cancer.[4]

1.3   *Pathology*

Over 95% of all oesophageal cancers are either SCC or adenocarcinoma. Leiomyo(sarco)mas, melanomas, lymphomas, gastrointestinal stromal tumours (GIST), neuroendocrine tumours and other carcinomas are rare. In 20% of sufferers, SCC is found in the proximal third of the oesophagus, in 50% it is in the middle third, and in 30% it is in the distal third of the oesophagus. In contrast, most adenocarcinomas arise in the distal third of the oesophagus and the region of the gastro-oesophageal junction. Oesophageal cancers tend to grow circumferentially and longitudinally. Submucosal lymphatic channels allow the spread in the submucosal plane, and this can result in long tumours with the possibility of multiple mucosal lesions. As the lymphatic drainage of the oesophagus is longitudinal as well, draining lymph nodes are widely distributed and skip metastasis is common.[5]

Adenocarcinomas of the gastro-oesophageal junction, defined as being 5 cm either side of the anatomical cardia, can be confusing, with divergent opinions as to whether they arise from the stomach or the esophagus, and whether they are part of the same cancer spectrum, or are different tumours, requiring a different treatment strategy. In reality, the confusion is largely caused by the location of these tumours across the gastro-oesophageal junction. Siewert proposed a classification of tumours of the gastro-oesophageal junction in three types, based on morphologic and anatomical findings as outlined in Table 1.[6] If the tumour is entirely confined to the stomach, the operative strategy usually entails total gastrectomy, whereas any involvement of the lower

Table 1. Classification of tumours of the gastro-oesophageal junction according Siewert *et al.*[6] Tumours of the gastro-oesophageal junction have their centre by definition within 5 cm proximal or distal of the anatomic cardia.

Type I	Adenocarcinoma of the distal oesophagus which usually arises from Barrett's mucosa and which may infiltrate the gastro-oesophageal junction
Type II	True tumour of the gastro-oesophageal junction arising from cardiac epithelium or short segments of intestinal metaplasia
Type III	Sub-cardial gastric carcinoma which infiltrates the gastro-oesophageal junction and distal oesophagus from below

esophagus will usually require esophagectomy if surgical treatment is undertaken. Hence, the surgical strategy is influenced by the anatomical location of the tumour, independent of the tumour biology.

1.4 Clinical appearance

Most patients present late in the course of their disease, due to the insidious nature of this disease, as symptoms are initially non-specific. Dysphagia (>70% of patients), weight loss (>50% of patients) and decreased performance status are the most common clinical findings, but such symptoms develop late in the course of the disease. Dysphagia occurs when over 70% of the oesophageal lumen is occluded. Other symptoms include anaemia, regurgitation, and meat aversion. Invasive growth of the tumour may result in chronic coughing (if involving the trachea or the left bronchus), hoarseness (if involving the recurrent laryngeal nerve) and Horner's syndrome (if involving the sympathetic trunk).

2. Pre-Operative Work-Up

2.1 Diagnosis

Dysphagia and weight loss indicate the need for further investigation. Physical examination normally doesn't reveal any specific signs. Upper gastrointestinal endoscopy with biopsy is the cornerstone of diagnosis. In combination with endoscopic ultrasound

(EUS), it allows accurate locoregional staging, including determination of the length of the tumour and the extent of local invasion. EUS fine needle aspiration of suspicious lymph nodes can be used to more accurately determine lymph node status. The stomach and duodenum can also be inspected for coexisting disease. In the setting of a tumour causing near complete oesophageal obstruction, endoscopic dilatation may be required to enable the passage of the endoscope in order to complete the investigation.

Thoraco-abdominal computed tomography (CT) scan is essential for the assessment of the local extent of tumour and metastatic disease. 2-F-18-fluoro-2-deoxy-D-glucose positron emission tomography (^{18}F-PET), in combination with CT (PET-CT), is increasingly used to rule out distant metastases, and this investigation identifies additional patients with metastatic disease, thereby reducing the proportion of patients who undergo surgical resection. The double contrast barium esophagogram is still sometimes used to determine the exact location of the tumour, as well as its length, although upper GI endoscopy can often provide the same information. Magnetic resonance imaging (MRI) does not provide any advantage over CT in the staging of oesophageal cancer. Bronchoscopy is indicated if there is a suspicion of bronchial or tracheal invasion. Staging laparoscopy, in combination with laparoscopic ultrasound, allows detection of metastatic abdominal lymph nodes and distant metastases, as well as cytologic examination of lavage fluids. This is often used for distal oesophageal adenocarcinoma which extends into the gastric cardia. Its role in the assessment of tumours which are entirely confined to the thoracic oesophagus is more controversial, and there is little consensus between surgeons about whether or not to routinely undertake staging laparoscopy.

2.1.1 *Staging*

Oesophageal cancers are commonly staged using the International Union against Cancer (UICC) TNM Classification of Malignant Tumours, 6th Ed. (Table 2). Both histopathological subtypes are treated as one entity, even though there is evidence that the tumours behave differently in clinical practice. There is some controversy concerning staging of tumours of the gastro-oesophageal junction. These tumours can either be staged according the classification for

Table 2.　UICC TNM stage system.

Tx	Primary tumour cannot be assessed
T0	No evidence of primary tumour
Tis	Carcinoma *in situ*
T1	Tumour invades lamina propria or submucosa
T2	Tumour invades muscularis propria
T3	Tumour invades adventitia
T4	Tumour invades adjacent structures
Nx	Regional lymph nodes cannot be assessed
N0	No regional lymph node metastasis
N1	Regional lymph node metastasis
Mx	Distant metastasis cannot be assessed
M0	No distant metastasis
M1	Distant metastasis

For tumours of the lower thoracic oesophagus

M1a	Metastasis in coelic lymph nodes
M1b	Other distant metastasis

For tumours of the upper thoracic oesophagus

M1a	Metastasis in cervical lymph nodes
M1b	Other distant metastasis

For tumours of the mid-thoracic oesophagus

M1a	Not applicable
M1b	Non-regional lymph node or other distant metastasis

Stage grouping: oesophageal cancer

Stage 0	Tis	N0	M0
Stage I	T1	N0	M0
Stage IIA	T2	N0	M0
	T3	N0	M0
Stage IIB	T1	N1	M0
	T2	N1	M0
Stage III	T3	N1	M0
	T4	Any N	M0
Stage IV	Any T	Any N	M1
Stage IVA	Any T	Any N	M1A
Stage IVB	Any T	Any N	M1B

oesophageal, or that of gastric cancers. However, these staging systems are different, and this can cause confusion. Whereas T1 stage gastric cancer can be subdivided into T1a (limited to the mucosa) and T1b (invasion into the submucosa), the classification of oesophageal cancers does not differentiate this, even though in clinical practice this sub-differentiation is widely used and is clinically useful. Concerning the N-system, the oesophageal TNM system distinguishes only nodal positive and nodal negative disease stage, whereas the gastric system subclassifies according the number of tumour bearing lymph nodes (N1=1–6; N2=7–15; N3≥15). Interestingly, the oesophageal system classifies coeliac lymph nodes as M1a. The pattern of lymphatic spread of tumours of the gastro-oesophageal junction would suggest that Siewert type 1 tumours should be staged according the oesophageal system, and Siewert type 2 & 3 tumours according the TNM system for gastric cancer.[7]

Pre-operative staging of the tumour and the fitness of the actual individual are the most important factors to consider when deciding how to manage each patient. To determine the T stage, EUS is the most accurate method. It has an accuracy of up to 90%, compared to CT's accuracy of 80%. Both methods lack optimal differentiation between T2 and T3 lesions, although EUS is usually able to differentiate T1 from T2 stage. To assess locoregional lymph nodes, EUS again is superior to CT, especially when combined with fine needle aspiration (sensitivity of 85% and 95%, respectively). For locoregional staging, the combination of CT and EUS provides an overall accuracy of over 90%.[8] To assess distant metastatic disease, CT and PET are the primary staging techniques. Metastatic lymph nodes in the abdomen, as well as distant metastases in liver or lungs can be detected with up to 85% accuracy by CT. In case of CT-based suspicion, additional information may be obtained by PET(-CT), with the reported accuracy being up to 90%. PET has the advantage of evaluating the whole body. Furthermore, PET allows restaging after neo-adjuvant treatment, where EUS and CT show less accuracy, due to alteration of the tumour tissue by the radiotherapy.[9] Staging laparoscopy and laparoscopic ultrasound have been used to determine intra-abdominal lymph node metastasis, peritoneal metastatic spread and liver metastases. It is especially useful in tumours of the gastro-oesophageal junction and distal oesophagus. Staging thoracoscopy has been shown to be very accurate, but it has not been widely used so far. In one study, the combination of laparoscopy and thoracoscopy has been shown to change the original CT and EUS assigned stage in up to 30% of individuals.[10]

2.2   Indication for surgery

There is broad consensus that oesophageal resections should only performed with a curative intention. Poor long term survival in patients without complete tumour resection, combined with substantial morbidity and mortality, as well as decreased post-operative quality of life, are the main reasons to avoid palliative resections. The main selection criteria for surgery are locally resectable tumour and absence of distant metastasis. In patients with advanced disease, radio-chemotherapy is often the first-line treatment, followed by restaging. If there has been a significant response, under some circumstances surgery can be reconsidered. In the palliative and obstructive situation, the indication for supportive surgery, such as placement of a feeding jejunostomy should be discussed.

2.3   Neo-adjuvant therapy and restaging

Randomised trials have shown that neo-adjuvant therapy (chemoradiation or chemotherapy alone) moderately increases overall survival, reduces locoregional recurrence and increases the rate of R0 resections.[11,12] The best results have been achieved when chemotherapy and radiotherapy have been administered concurrently, rather than sequentially. Complete pathological response rates of 20% after neo-adjuvant chemoradiation have been described. The main indication for neo-adjuvant therapy is UICC stages IIb, III and possibly IVa. Whether neo-adjuvant therapy is of any benefit in stages I and IIa is unclear, and such patients would not normally be considered by neo-adjuvant therapy outside clinical trials. Most therapy regimes include 5-FU and cisplatin, combined with radiotherapy of 40 to 50 Gy. Restaging with CT and sometimes PET(-CT) determines the clinical response to treatment.

Surgery is performed four to eight weeks after the completion of neo-adjuvant therapy.

2.4　*Risk analysis*

As oesophageal resections remain high risk procedures, with substantial morbidity (up to 60%) and mortality (up to 7%), appropriate selection of patients according their performance status and co-morbidities is necessary.[13] Different risk scores have been developed to predict surgical mortality. Most scores use age, pre-operative therapies, hospital volume and co-morbidities to define post-operative mortality. Age over 80 years increases the risk significantly, with doubled odds ratios (OR) for post-operative mortality, compared to 65 year old patients. Neo-adjuvant pre-treatment has also been associated with increased post-operative mortality following oesophagectomy. Hospital volume is an important factor influencing mortality, with differences of up to 10 % between low (< 0.67 to 1.0 cases/year) and high volume centres (> 2.3 to 2.6 cases/year).[14,15] Co-morbidity is highly predictive, with two-fold increased OR ratios for post-operative mortality. In general, the indication for oesophagectomy in patients over 80 years, or with severely impaired organ function should be evaluated very carefully, as most of these patients will not be selected for oesophagectomy.

2.5　*Preparation for surgery*

Prior to surgery, smoking and alcohol consumption should be ceased. As most patients suffer from considerable malnutrition and weight loss, review by a dietician is advisable to optimise the nutritional status. There is some evidence suggesting that immuno-modulating nutrition enriched with omega-3 fatty acids, arginine and other amino acids decreases the rate of post-operative infections and length of hospital stay.[16] Nutritional support should be initiated well in advance of surgery or neo-adjuvant pre-treatment. Other measures to optimise the performance status of the patient are increasing physical exercise and chest physiotherapy, especially in patients with pulmonary co-morbidity (chronic obstructive pulmonary disease).

As part of the standard work-up, every patient should undergo a formal assessment of pulmonary function (spirometry, chest X-ray), cardiac function (echocardiography, electrocardiography), renal function (creatinine) and hepatic function (alanine amino-transferase, aspartate aminotransferase, INR). Additionally, basic blood tests including type and screen testing should be performed. Significant co-morbidities preclude surgery, and other options should then be considered.

2.6 *Non-surgical treatment options*

If surgery is not an appropriate option for the treatment of oesophageal cancer, definitive radio-chemotherapy (RTC) should be considered. The main reasons for a non-surgical management approach are either metastatic or locally invasive tumours and/or an increased mortality risk for oesophagectomy due to significant co-morbidities. Radiotherapy with up to 60 Gy, and concomitant chemotherapy with 5-FU and cisplatin is currently the standard treatment regimen. Overall, survival rates are between 10 to 20% following this approach.

After completing radio-chemotherapy, patients should be restaged. Depending on the clinical tumour response and whether the primary reason for the non-operative treatment was oncological stage, rather than excessive surgical risk, salvage oesophagectomy can be an option. However, the results of non-randomised studies which have compared definitive RTC with versus without surgery are not consistent, and no survival benefit has been demonstrated for salvage surgery.[17]

3. Surgery

3.1 *Localised disease*

3.1.1 *Open surgery*

The basic principle of surgery is to completely remove the tumour bearing part of the oesophagus including all locally draining lymph nodes. The location of the tumour defines whether a sub-total resection with anastomosis in the chest (for distal tumours and tumours of the gastro-oesophageal junction) is possible, or whether a total oesophagectomy with anastomosis in the neck (for tumours located in the middle third of the oesophagus) is necessary.

For distal tumours, two different techniques, transthoracic or transhiatal, are used, depending on the surgeon's preference. The classic transthoracic procedure is the Ivor Lewis operation, where the stomach and diaphragmatic hiatus are dissected and a gastric tube is formed via a midline or transverse laparotomy, followed by the dissection of the oesophagus through a right-sided thoracotomy. The gastric tube is then used as a substitute for the resected oesophagus and an intra-thoracic anastomosis, either hand sewn or stapled, is performed. The main advantages of this approach are good exposure and access to the locoregional lymph nodes, which can be removed en bloc with the main specimen.

However, it mandates a thoracotomy, which will increase pulmonary morbidity and post-operative pain. Alternatively, a transhiatal approach, where the oesophagus is mobilised through the hiatus and from the cervical wound, can be used. This procedure does not include a thoracotomy and might have a lower morbidity, but a part of the dissection of the thoracic oesophagus is performed bluntly with the fingers, inducing the risk for uncontrollable bleeding or tracheobronchial injury. For this reason, tumours located in the middle third of the oesophagus are usually unsuitable for this approach. Whether the transthoracic or the transhiatal oesophagectomy is associated with a better survival outcome is unclear. A number of studies have addressed this issue, with inconsistent results.[18] Only a handful of randomised trials have been conducted, again with inconsistent results. The largest trial was conducted in the Netherlands. It showed a non-significant 4% 5-year survival advantage following transthoracic oesophagectomy. Other trials, including one with only neo-adjuvant treated patients, have also not demonstrated any significant outcome difference for either technique.[19-22] Pre-treatment has been shown to eliminate lymph node (micro-)metastasis, perhaps rendering radical lymphadenectomy unnecessary. An alternative technique to distal and gastro-oesophageal junction tumours is the left-sided thoraco-abdominal approach, where a continuous incision from the left hemithorax to the upper abdominal midline is used. This technique allows good exposure for distal tumours, whereas the aorta restricts exposure of more proximal tumours.

In patients with middle and upper third tumours, a total oesophagectomy with anastomosis in the neck is usually warranted. This can either be achieved with the three stage technique, where the first step is a right thoracotomy with mobilisation of the oesophagus, followed by a laparotomy with formation of the gastric tube, and finally performing an anastomosis in the neck. Alternatively, a transhiatal approach as described above might be considered for some patients.

Substantial controversy exists about the extent of lymph node dissection required during oesophagectomy. Whereas one group of surgeons is convinced that radical lymph node dissection improves oncological outcome, the other considers lymph node metastasis as a sign of advanced disease, where radical lymph node resection does not offer any survival benefit. The rationale for complete lymph node removal is also more accurate staging, as not only the number of affected lymph nodes, but also the lymph node ratio (number of positive nodes divided by the total number of harvested lymph nodes) is of prognostic importance. Ratios over 10% have been shown to be associated with lower survival, compared to patients with ratios under 10%.[23] At this point in time, however, there are no proven adjuvant therapies for patients who have undergone an oesophagectomy, and hence the prognostic information does not influence therapy in a practical sense.

In patients with high grade dysplasia or early tumours (Tis, T1) where no lymph node dissection is indicated and who are not eligible for endoscopic mucosal resection, vagal sparing oesophagectomy with colonic interposition has been described as an alternative with good functional results.[24] Preservation of the stomach as a reservoir with normal secretory and motor function leads to better alimentation and bowel regulation. The decision whether a transthoracic or transhiatal approach is used will ultimately be dictated by the preference of the operating surgeon. In general, the transhiatal approach is less invasive, as it is not associated with a thoracotomy. However, experienced surgeons can achieve similar morbidity and mortality using a transthoracic approach.

As described above , the stomach is the most commonly used organ for oesophageal replacement. The main advantages of using the stomach are ease of dissection, a good blood supply, and reconstruction requiring only one anastomosis. The disadvantages are the loss of the gastric reservoir, and a substantial risk of post-surgical reflux, which can impact adversely the quality of life. Blood supply for the gastric tube is mainly via through the right gastroepiploic artery, and this must be carefully preserved during dissection. To avoid gastric emptying impairment due to vagal denervation, most surgeons perform a pyloromyotomy or pyloroplasty. As reflux at the location of the anastomosis is a common consequence of oesophagectomy, anti-reflux procedures such as creating a wrap around the anastomosis have been described. This is only feasible when constructing the anastomosis within the thorax.

Alternative organs which can be used are colon or small bowel. The main advantage for these is preservation of the stomach as a reservoir and avoidance of oesophageal reflux. However, the disadvantage is the need for two additional anastomoses and the expansion of what is already a major procedure. In cases of inadequate quality of the stomach (due to previous surgery) or ischaemia or necrosis of a gastric tube, a colonic interposition is the most commonly used replacement. Before using any large bowel, colonoscopy to rule out any intra-luminal pathology and angiography to evaluate the colonic vascular anatomy should be performed. In cases of upper third tumours, where parts of the hypopharynx might have to be included in the resection, free small bowel interpositions are used. Another indication for small bowel interpositions is segmental resections of the distal esophagus (Merendino procedure). A feeding jejunostomy or a nasojejunal tube is commonly placed, as most patients will stay fasting for up to five days, and the time to full oral nutrition will usually take a further 5–7 days.

3.1.2 Minimal invasive surgery

Minimal invasive techniques have been introduced in recent years and gained acceptance in some centres. A number of studies have shown the feasibility and safety of these operations.[25] The main advantage is less post-operative pain, quicker recovery and smaller scars. So far, no study has identified any disadvantage in either morbidity or oncological survival.[26] Basically, two different approaches can be performed, similar to the two above described open techniques. Thoracoscopic mobilisation of the oesophagus with (total minimal invasive) or without (thoracoscopic-assisted) laparoscopic formation of a gastric tube and anastomosis in the neck represents the minimally invasive variant of the transthoracic approach. Alternatively, the laparoscopic dissection of the oesophagus transhiatally similar to the open transhiatal approach can be performed. So far, no significant differences between these techniques have been identified.[27] In both of these techniques, the anastomosis is performed in the neck. Less commonly used is the minimally invasive adaptation of the Ivor Lewis technique with an intra-thoracic anastomosis, where less mobilisation of the gastric tube (shorter distance to bridge as anastomosis is lower) and a lower incidence of recurrent laryngeal nerve injury have been described.[28]

One of the main critical points in minimally invasive oesophagectomy is the fact that the systematic intra-thoracic lymph node dissection is difficult and probably not performed as meticulously as with open transthoracic surgery. However, neo-adjuvant treatment has been shown to have an positive impact on nodal (micro-)metastasis, and this might compensate for any lack of radical lymph node dissection.

3.1.3 *Endoscopic surgery*

Open, as well as minimally invasive oesophagectomy is still associated with a substantial morbidity and mortality. In high grade dysplasia and small superficial lesions not penetrating the muscularis mucosa (intra-mucosal cancer), endoscopic mucosal resection is an alternative treatment.[29] Determination of tumour depth is most important, as lymph node involvement increases with advancing tumour depth, more so in squamous cancer than in adenocarcinoma. In intra-mucosal tumours the prevalence of lymph node metastasis is less than 5% (probably 1 to 2%), whereas in tumours extending into the submucosa the prevalence increases up to 30%.[30] The staging process for patients with early neoplastic lesions is identical to that of more advanced tumours. EUS is the cornerstone in determination of tumour depth.

Photodynamic therapy and ablation with Nd:YAG laser or argon beam are alternative techniques for early neoplastic lesions. However, all these techniques have some important disadvantages. The depth of the therapy is variable and there is no resected specimen and thus no histopathological assessment. Furthermore, fibrotic oesophageal strictures can develop following any of these therapies.

3.2 Metastatic or locally unresectable disease

There is no indication for palliative resection in locally advanced tumours with infiltration in adjoining organs, or in metastatic disease. In these situations, the primary goal of therapy is palliation of dysphagia, weight loss, and pain. Palliation of dysphagia can be achieved by endoscopic dilatation, self-expandable metallic stents, ablation, photodynamic therapy, Argon Plasma Coagulation (APC) and brachytherapy. Dilatation, stents and APC provide fast relief of dysphagia, although dilatation and APC require repeated sessions at 4–6 weeks intervals. Brachytherapy with 6 or 12Gy has been shown to be as effective as stenting in long term outcome.[31] As dysphagia is best treated with endoscopic techniques, the indication for surgery is mainly to ensure adequate nutrition. If the tumour is passable, the least invasive way in a patient not eligible for surgery will be insertion of a PEG tube for enteral feeding. However, some patients with locally advanced tumours might undergo restaging after full dose radio-chemotherapy and, in cases of major response and absence of metastases might become eligible for salvage oesophagectomy. As the stomach is the most commonly used organ for reconstruction, insertion of a feeding jejunostomy might be a better option. This can be either performed with a small laparotomy or laparoscopically.

3.3 Recurrent disease after esophagectomy

Locoregional or distant recurrences generally cannot be treated by surgical approaches, apart from the above mentioned palliative measures. Palliative radiotherapy with or without chemotherapy may be indicated, if no previous radiotherapy has been administered to the site of recurrence.

4.   Post-Operative Management

4.1   General management after oesophagectomy

Generally, all patients after oesophagectomy are admitted to an intensive care unit. Routine ventilation for the first one to two post-operative days is still used in some centres. However, most patients are extubated at the end of surgery. The intra-operatively placed nasogastric tube is left *in situ* for several days. Many surgeons will arrange an X-ray with oral contrast 5–7 days post-operatively, to assess the anastomosis and exclude an anastomotic leak. However, there has been some controversy as to whether routine post-operative contrast studies are necessary, as small leaks might not be detected.[32] Nutrition via the feeding jejunostomy or nasojejunal tube is started on the first post-operative day. Oral nutrition is commenced several days after surgery, when the nasogastric tube is removed. Thoracic and intra-abdominal drains are removed in the first 5–7 days, depending on the amount of fluid produced. Early mobilisation is warranted, as pulmonary morbidity is high in all patients with oesophagectomy. Hospital stay is generally between 10–14 days if no complications occur.

4.2   Surgical complications and management

The most severe complication is anastomotic leakage, which occurs with a frequency of 5–20%. Cervical anastomoses have a higher leak rate compared to intra-thoracic anastomoses. However, most cervical leaks represent a local problem, whereas intra-thoracic leaks can be a life threatening complication, due to the risk of mediastinitis, empyema, and sepsis. The major challenge is to discover the leak early enough to initiate adequate therapy. Slow progression of post-operative recovery, a persistently elevated temperature of 37° to 38°C, and persisting high inflammatory markers should raise the suspicion for an anastomotic leak. An oral contrast swallow, or oral contrast enhanced CT scan are the diagnostic tools of choice. Endoscopy, preferably performed by the surgeon, allows assessment of the anastomotic region.

With cervical leaks, leaving the drain in place or bedside opening of the wound and moist dressing might be a sufficient therapy.

If the gastric conduit is necrotic, takedown of the anastomosis with cervical esophagostomy and delayed reconstruction can occasionally be necessary. With intra-thoracic leaks, the clinical condition of the patient will determine the subsequent management. Contained leaks in non-septic patients with adequate drainage through the chest drains can be managed conservatively. Endoscopic treatment with lavage, debridement, fibrin glue injections and endoclipping in small leaks or stenting in larger ones are possible options.[33] In patients with sepsis, empyema or mediastinitis operative revision is mandatory. The extent of any surgery is dictated by the intra-operative findings and this may include lavage, drainage, closure of a small leak with sutures, patches or muscular flaps. In large leaks, or gastric tube necrosis, formation of a cervical oesophagostomy and blind closure distally might be necessary. In these situations, subsequent reconstruction with colonic or small bowel interposition after recovery is performed. In general, the critical steps in management of an anastomotic leak are ensuring that the leak is well drained, and the provision of ongoing nutrition via a feeding jejunostomy tube (if present), or parental nutrition.

Thoracic duct leaks with chylothorax occur in up to 3% of patients. Untreated, chylothorax has a high mortality (up to 50%), due to severe fat and protein loss and immunodeficiency. If the volume of drainage is low (<500 ml/24 hrs), a conservative approach with a fat-free diet can be undertaken. However, most surgeons opt for early revisional surgery and ligation of the duct, either intra-abdominally or intra-thoracically.[34]

Laryngeal nerve injury occurs predominantly in patients with cervical anastomosis in up to 10%. Hoarseness is transient in approximately 80% of these patients and resolves in two to 12 weeks. Persisting nerve injury requiring additional vocal cord therapy, such as medialisation or Teflon injection occurs in 1–2%.[35] Other complications are post-operative bleeding in 1–2%, wound infection and/or dehiscence in 2–5%.

4.3 Adjuvant therapy

Adjuvant radiotherapy, chemotherapy and combination chemo-radiotherapy have been used for patients after esophagectomy.

The outcome data on these therapies show no definite evidence of any survival benefit. Patients with incomplete resection or high UICC stages (III and above) might benefit from adjuvant radio-therapy. Adjuvant chemotherapy has no definite role in completely resected esophageal cancer. Different randomised studies evaluating cisplatin-based adjuvant chemotherapies in squamous cell cancer have not shown any survival benefit compared to surgery alone.[36] Adjuvant chemotherapy for adenocarcinoma of the gastro-oesophageal junction has been shown to improve survival, but no data on esophageal adenocarcinoma has been reported so far.[37]

5.   Long Term Results

5.1   *Outcome after surgery*

Although the outcome of esophageal cancer treatment has markedly improved with multimodal treatment over the last years, overall survival is still low, with approximately 20 to 40% survival at five years following surgery. Furthermore, over half of all patients have unresectable or metastatic disease at the time of diagnosis. The most important prognostic factors for post-surgical survival are absence of lymph node involvement and complete resection (R0). Survival data varies considerably throughout the literature, as shown in Table 3. Many reasons for these differences in survival should be considered: selection criteria, surgical techniques, multimodal therapy concepts, and the case load of hospitals.

Table 3.   Five-year survival following oesophagectomy versus tumour stage.

			Adenocarcinoma only	Adenocarcinoma and SCC	Adenocarcinoma only
Stage 0	59	100	N/A	N/A	N/A
Stage I	65	100	69	55/66	90
Stage IIa	28	59.1*	17	32/52	60*
Stage IIb	29	N/A	20	17/42	N/A
Stage III	11	36.8	3	10/14	15
Stage IV	10	13.3	0	N/A	0
Reference	35	38	39	40	41

*No distinction between IIa and IIb.

5.2　Long term complications and management

The most common long term complications after oesophagectomy are anastomotic stricture and reflux. Strictures are more common following cervical anastomosis and after anastomotic leaks. Repeated dilatation is the therapy of choice, with good results. Acid (despite vagotomy) and bile reflux is a common problem after oesophagectomy, with a frequency up to 30%. This is seen especially in patients with gastric conduit reconstruction with a pyloric drainage procedure.[42] Conservative management with proton-pump inhibitor and prokinetic medications, and physical measures such as sitting upright after eating are primarily indicated. In the situation of debilitating reflux, biliary diversion with a Roux-en-Y reconstruction has been described. Dumping syndromes after oesophagectomy with pyloroplasty are another problem, best dealt with by dietary modification. In patients without pyloric drainage procedures, delayed gastric emptying may occur. Prokinetic drugs, endoscopic dilatation, botulinum toxin injections and ultimately pyloromyotomy or pyloroplasty are the treatment options, although gastric emptying problems usually resolve spontaneously without intervention by one to two years after surgery.

5.3　Quality of life

Quality of life after oesophagectomy has not been frequently studied in the past. Recent studies show substantial long term impairment, with decreased physical function.[43] The recovery and rehabilitation after esophagectomy takes from several months to one year.[44] No definite differences have been shown between patients undergoing surgery alone or combined treatment with neo-adjuvant therapy. Not only physical factors, such as late complications, fatigue and tension, but also psychological factors determine post-operative quality of life. Social functioning, financial issues, long absence from work and fear of recurrence have a substantial negative effect on quality of life.

5.4　Surveillance

After surgical resection, three monthly to half-yearly clinical reviews are undertaken in most patients. There are no tumour markers presently available to aid follow-up. If a patient develops symptoms of weight loss, reduced performance status, dysphagia, pain, imaging with CT scan and an upper GI endoscopy are indicated. As surgical options for locoregional or metastatic recurrence are limited, a multidisciplinary approach is needed to determine if radiotherapy or chemotherapy are appropriate.

6. Screening for Oesophageal Cancer

There is currently no rationale for offering screening for oesophageal cancer to the general population, except in those parts of the world which have a very high incidence. In most countries, oesophageal cancer is uncommon, and the only adequate screening method is upper gastrointestinal endoscopy, which is not cost-effective. In patients with Barrett's oesophagus, which pre-disposes to esophageal adenocarcinoma, however, regular surveillance endoscopy is the accepted clinical practice. Two yearly interval endoscopies with four quadrant biopsies (at 2 cm intervals) for known Barrett's oesophagus are part of usual clinical practice. If low grade dysplasia is detected in biopsies, the next surveillance endoscopy should be performed after six months and intensive acid suppression should be ensured. If high grade dysplasia is identified, then a further endoscopy with biopsies is required for independent confirmation of the diagnosis. If confirmed, then surgical resection with oesophagectomy is standard treatment in fit patients. Endoscopic ablation or endoscopic mucosal resection can also be considered, according to the individual's fitness for oesophagectomy.[45]

7. The Future in (Surgical) Oesophageal Cancer Treatment

The main goal in oesophageal cancer treatment is to prolong survival. A multimodal approach including medical oncologists, radiooncologists and surgeons is mandatory in every patient. New neo-adjuvant radiochemotherapy protocols might increase the response rates. Reduction of pre-operative risk factors by careful selection of patients and optimal conditioning (quitting smoking and alcohol, immunonutrition, increasing mobility) as well as advances in surgical technique (increased radicality, minimal invasive techniques, robotics) might improve the surgical outcome. However, other approaches than oncological or surgical might be the key to further improvement of outcome. Understanding host immune response and its influence on inhibition of recurrence might be a first step to develop treatment strategies. So far, tumour vaccination has not been evaluated in oesophageal cancer. Chemoprevention and pharmacological intervention to prevent the development of cancer is a new field. Non-steroidal anti-inflammatory drugs have been shown to reduce risk in gastrointestinal cancers. Until today, the cornerstone of curative treatment has been unquestionably surgery, but will this be so in the future?

References

1. J. Falk, H. Carstens, L. Lundell and M. Albertsson, Incidence of carcinoma of the oesophagus and gastric cardia. Changes over time and geographical differences, *Acta Oncol.* **46**: 1070–1074 (2007).
2. P. C. Enzinger and R. J. Mayer, Esophageal cancer, *New Engl. J. Med.* **349**: 2241–2252 (2003).
3. M. Pera, C. Manterola, O. Vidal and L. Grande, Epidemiology of esophageal adenocarcinoma, *J. Surg. Oncol.* **92**: 151–159 (2005).
4. D. C. Whiteman, S. Sadeghi, N. Pandeya, B. M. Smithers, D. C. Gotley, C. J. Bain, P. M. Webb and A. C. Green, Australian Cancer study. Combined effects of obesity, acid reflux and smoking on the risk of adenocarcinomas of the oesophagus, *Gut* **57**(2): 173–180 (2008).
5. S. B. Hosch, N. H. Stoecklein, U. Pichlmeier, A. Rehders, P. Scheunemann, A. Niendorf, W. T. Knoefel and J. R. Izbicki, Esophageal cancer: The mode of lymphatic tumor cell spread and its prognostic significance, *J. Clin. Oncol.* **19**: 1970–1975 (2001).
6. J. R. Siewert and H. J. Stein, Classification of adenocarcinoma of the oesophagogastric junction, *Br. J. Surg.* **85**: 1457–1459 (1998).
7. B. H. Von Rahden, M. Feith and H. J. Stein, Carcinoma of the cardia: Classification as esophageal or gastric cancer? *Int. J. Colorectal Dis.* **20**: 89–93 (2005).
8. W. A. Marsman and P. Fockens, State of the art lecture: EUS for esophageal tumors, *Endoscopy* **38**(S1): S17–S21 (2006).
9. R. Iyer and R. DuBrow, Imaging of esophageal cancer, *Cancer Imag.* **4**: 125–132 (2004).

10. J. D. Luketich, M. Meehan, N. T. Nguyen, N. Christie, T. Weigel, S. Yousem, R. J. Keenan and P. R. Schauer, Minimally invasive surgical staging for esophageal cancer, *Surg. Endosc.* **14**: 700–702 (2000).

11. J. D. Urschel and H. Vasan, A meta-analysis of randomized controlled trials that compared neoadjuvant chemoradiation and surgery to surgery alone for resectable esophageal cancer, *Am. J. Surg.* **185**: 538–543 (2003).

12. I. G. Kaklamanos, G. R. Walker, K. Ferry, D. Franceschi and A. S. Livingstone, Neoadjuvant treatment for resectable cancer of the esophagus and gastroesophageal junction: A meta-analysis of randomized clinical trials, *Ann. Surg. Oncol.* **10**: 754–761 (2003).

13. H. Bartels, H. Stein and J. R. Siewert, Preoperative risk analysis and post-operative mortality of oesophagectomy for resectable oesophageal cancer, *Br. J. Surg.* **85**: 840–844 (1998).

14. E. W. Steyerberg, B. A. Neville, L. B. Koppert, V. E. Lemmens, H. W. Tilanus, J. W. Coeberg, J. C. Weeks and C. C. Earle, Surgical mortality in patients with esophageal cancer: Development and validation of a simple risk score, *J. Clin. Oncol.* **24**: 4277–4284 (2006).

15. J. Ra, E. C. Paulson, J. Kucharczuk, K. Armstrong, C. Wirtalla, R. Rapaport-Kelz, L. R. Kaiser and F. R. Spitz, Postoperative mortality after esophagectomy for cancer: Development of a preoperative risk prediction model, *Ann. Surg. Oncol.* **15**: 1577–1584 (2008).

16. D. N. Moskovitz and Y. I. Kim, Does perioperative immunonutrition reduce postoperative complications in patients with gastrointestinal cancer undergoing operations? *Nutr. Rev.* **62**: 443–447 (2004).

17. Z. Liao, J. D. Cox and R. Komaki, Radiochemotherapy of esophageal cancer, *J. Thorac. Oncol.* **2**: 553–568 (2007).

18. J. B. Hulscher, J. G. Tijssen, H. Obertop, J. J. van Lanschot, Transthoracic versus transhiatal resection for carcinoma of the esophagus: A meta-analysis, *Ann. Thorac. Surg.* **72**: 306–313 (2001).

19. J. B. Hulscher, van J. W. Sandick, A. G. de Boer, B. P. Wijnhoven, J. G. Tijssen, P. Fockens, P. F. Stalmeier, F. J. ten Kate, H. van Dekken H. Obertop, H. W. Tilanus and J. J. van Lanschot, Extended transthoracic resection compared with limited transhiatal resection for adenocarcinoma of the esophagus, *N. Engl. J. Med.* **347**: 1662–1669 (2002).

20. K. M. Chu, S. Y. Law, M. Fok and J. Wong, A prospective randomized comparison of transhiatal and transthoracic resection for lower-third esophageal carcinoma, *Am. J. Surg.* **174**: 320–324 (1997).

21. M. Goldminc, G. Maddern, E. Le Prise, B. Meunier, J. P. Campion and B. Launois, Oesophagectomy by transhiatal approach or thoracotomy: A prospective randomized trial, *Br. J. Surg.* **80**: 367–370 (1993).

22. M. A. Morgan, W. G. Lewis, A. N. Hopper, X. Escofet, T. J. Havard, A. E. Brewster, T. D. Crosby, S. A. Roberts and G. W. Clark, Prospective comparison of transthoracic versus transhiatal esophagectomy following neoadjuvant therapy for cancer, *Dis. Esophagus* **20**: 225–231 (2007).

23. J. A. Hagen, S. R. DeMeester, J. H. Peters, P. Chandrasoma and T. R. DeMeester, Curative resection for esophageal adenocarcinoma: Analysis of 100 *en bloc* esophagectomies, *Ann. Surg.* **234**: 520–530 (2001).

24. F. Banki, R. J. Mason, S. R. DeMeester, J. A. Hagen, N. S. Balaji, P. F. Crookes, C. G. Bremner, J. H. Peters and T. R. DeMeester, Vagal-sparing esophagectomy: A more physiologic alternative, *Ann. Surg.* **236**: 324–336 (2002).

25. B. M. Smithers, D. C. Gotley, I. Martin and J. M. Thomas, Comparison of the outcomes between open and minimally invasive esophagectomy, *Ann. Surg.* **245**: 232–240 (2007).

26. M. S. Kent, M. Schuchert, H. Fernando and J. D. Luketich, Minimally invasive oesophagectomy: State of the art, *Dis. Esophagus* **19**: 137–145 (2006).

27. G. Dapri, J. Himpens and G. B. Cadiere, Minimally invasive esophagectomy for cancer: Laparoscopic transhiatal procedure or thoracoscopy in prone position followed by laparoscopy, *Surg. Endosc.* **22**: 1060–1067 (2008).

28. C. Bizekis, M. S. Kent, J. D. Luketich, P. O. Buenaventura, R. J. Landereau and M. J. Schuchert and M. Alvelo-Rivera, Initial experience with minimally invasive Ivor Lewis esophagectomy, *Ann. Thorac. Surg.* **82**: 402–406 (2006).

29. S. Tanabe, W. Koizumi, K. Higuchi, T. Sasaki, K. Nakatani, N. Hanaoka, T. Ae, K. Ishido, H. Mitomi and K. Saigenji, Clinical outcomes of endoscopic oblique aspiration mucosectomy for superficial esophageal cancer. *Gastrointest. Endosc.* **67**: 814–820 (2008).

30. S. R. DeMeester, Adenocarcinoma of the esophagus and cardia: A review of the disease and its treatment, *Ann. Surg. Oncol.* **13**: 12–30 (2006).

31. M. Y. Homs, E. J. Kuipers and P. D. Siersema, Palliative therapy, *J. Surg. Oncol.* **92**: 246–256 (2005).

32. M. B. Tirnaksiz, C. Deschamps, M. S. Allen, D. C. Johnson and P. C. Pairolero, Effectiveness of screening aqueous contrast swallow in detecting clinically significant anastomotic leaks after esophagectomy, *Eur. Surg. Res.* **37**: 123–128 (2005).

33. D. Schubert, M. Pross, G. Nestler, H. Ptok, H. Scheidbach, J. Fahlke and H. Lippert, Endoscopic treatment of mediastinal leaks, *Zentralbl. Chir.* **131**: 369–375 (2006).

34. S. Merigliano, D. Molena, A. Ruol, G. Zaniotto, M. Cagol, S. Scappin and E. Ancona, Chylothorax complicating esophagectomy for cancer: A plea for early thoracic duct ligation, *J. Thorac. Cardiovasc. Surg.* **119**: 453–457 (2000).

35. M. B. Orringer, B. Marshall, A. C. Chang, J. Lee, A. Pickens and C. L. Lau, Two thousand transhiatal esophagectomies: Changing trends, lessons learned, *Ann. Surg.* **246**: 363–374 (2007).

36. M. M. Mooney, Neoadjuvant and adjuvant chemotherapy for esophageal adenocarcinoma, *J. Surg. Oncol.* **92**: 230–238 (2005).

37. G. Y. Ku and D. H. Ilson, Esophageal cancer: Adjuvant therapy, *Cancer. J* **13**: 162–167 (2007).

38. T. Lerut, P. Nafteux, J. Moons, W. Coosemans, G. Decker, P. De Leyn, D. Van Raemdonck and N. Ectors, Three-field lymphadenectomy for carcinoma of the esophagus and gastroesophageal junction in 174 R0 resections: Impact on staging, disease-free survival and outcome, *Ann. Surg.* **240**: 962–974 (2004).

39. X. Zhang, D. I. Watson, G. G. Jamieson, C. Lally, J. R. Bessell and P. G. Devitt, Outcome of oesophagectomy for adenocarcinoma of the oesophagus and oesophagogastric junction, *ANZ. J. Surg.* **74**: 513–519 (2005).

40. C. Alexiou, O. A. Khan, E. Black, M. L. Field, P. Onyeaka, L. Beggs, J. P. Duffy and D. F. Beggs, Survival after esophageal resection for carcinoma: The importance of the histologic cell type, *Ann. Thorac. Surg.* **82**: 1073–1077 (2006).

41. G. Portale, J. A. Hagen, J. H. Peters, L. S. Chan, S. R. DeMeester, T. A. Gandamihardja and T. R. DeMeester, Modern 5-year survival of resectable esophageal adenocarcinoma: Single institution experience with 263 patients, *J. Am. Coll. Surg.* **202**: 588–596 (2006).

42. D. Palmes, M. Weilinghoff, M. Colombo-Benkmann, N. Senninger and M. Bruewer, Effect of pyloric drainage procedures on gastric passage and bile reflux after esophagectomy with gastric conduit reconstruction, *Langenbecks Arch. Surg.* **392**: 135–141 (2007).

43. P. Lagergren, K. N. Avery, R. Hughes, C. P. Barham, D. Alderson, S. J. Falk and J. M. Blazeby, Health related quality of life among patients cured by surgery for esophageal cancer, *Cancer* **110**: 686–693 (2007).
44. J. V. Reynold, R. McLaughlin, J. Moore, S. Rowley, N. Ravi and P. J. Byrne, Prospective evaluation of quality of life in patients with localized oesophageal cancer treated by multimodality therapy or surgery alone, *Br. J. Surg.* **93**: 1084–1090 (2006).
45. Guidelines for the diagnosis and management of Barrett's columnar lines oesophagus, A report of the working party of the British Society of Gastroenterology, http://www.bsg.org.uk (2005).

17

Abdominal Emergencies in Cancer Patients: Diagnosis and Management

Brian Badgwell
and Barry Feig

Abstract

Surgical oncologists are frequently asked to evaluate cancer patients with symptoms and signs suggestive of acute abdominal pathology. The traditional general surgical differential diagnosis must be considered in addition to conditions specific to the cancer patient. There are many factors unique to the cancer patient that may influence surgical decision making, such as immunosuppression, neutropenia, chemotherapy and radiotherapy, chronic pain and narcotic use, steroid use, and malnutrition. These factors may alter or mask the clinical presentation of these patients, compared to their non-cancer counterparts. As many of these patients and conditions meet the criteria for palliative care, consideration must be given to oncologic prognosis, quality of life, and the potential for symptom improvement; outcomes that are impossible to predict and infrequently reported in studies. This chapter focuses on the more common and unique conditions for which surgical consultations are requested. Bowel perforation may occur more frequently in cancer patients and is a known side effect of some chemotherapeutic agents. Treatment is primarily operative, but comfort care or non-operative treatment may be at times appropriate, as many patients are at extremely high risk for surgical complications and have limited survival. Bowel obstruction in patients with advanced or incurable cancer is another difficult situation which requires a tailored approach and in which controversy remains with regard to contraindications for surgical intervention. Neutropenia and abdominal pain may represent a wide variety of disorders and consideration must be given to neutropenic enterocolitis. This chapter also addresses the diagnosis and management of cholecystitis, biliary obstruction, gastrointestinal bleeding, and appendicitis in the cancer patient.

Keywords: Bowel obstruction, bowel perforation, neutropenic enterocolitis, cholecystitis, biliary obstruction, gastrointestinal bleeding, appendicitis.

1. Bowel Perforation

Bowel perforation may present as pneumoperitoneum (air within the peritoneal cavity), contained leakage of gastrointestinal contents, or a new onset fistula. Cancer patients may be at increased risk for bowel perforation due to chemotherapy, radiotherapy, steroid use, frequent endoscopic procedures, and complications from the primary tumor or metastases. Figure 1 demonstrates pneumoperitoneum in a patient with carcinomatosis and malignant ascites. In addition to these cancer-specific etiologies, cancer patients are prone to the same causes of bowel perforation as their non-cancer counterparts, such as diverticulitis and peptic ulcer disease. In the majority of cases of bowel perforation, the location of the perforation is not at the actual site of the tumor or metastasis. It is therefore often unclear as to how sequelae of the tumor or cancer treatment may have contributed to the perforation. There are many factors unique to the cancer patient that may influence surgical decision making when a patient presents with a perforation, such as neutropenia, side effects of chemotherapy and radiation therapy, chronic pain, and malnutrition. Surgical intervention typically will delay systemic chemotherapy administration for four to six weeks and longer in the event of post-operative complications. In addition, all treatment strategies must take into consideration oncologic prognosis and quality of

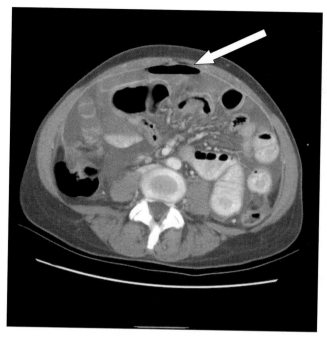

Figure 1. CT scan image demonstrating pneumoperitoneum (marked by arrow) in a patient with carcinomatosis and ascites.

life; outcomes that are impossible to predict and infrequently reported in studies.

There has been a paucity of data on the treatment and outcomes associated with bowel perforation specifically in cancer patients. In a recent study of 124 cases of pneumoperitoneum from M. D. Anderson Cancer Center, the treatment strategy was comfort care (palliative) in 19 patients, non-operative in 33 patients, and operative in 72 patients.[1] Thirty-day mortality rates were 100% in the comfort care group, 12% in the non-operative group, and 15% in the surgical group. Treatment was based on patient, family, and practitioner decisions, in the context of the clinical presentation and with respect to oncologic prognosis. For these reasons, predictors of management strategy were difficult to identify on retrospective analysis; however, factors such as abdominal pain and tenderness were associated with surgical management, as expected.

Surgery is the standard of care for patients with bowel perforation and offers the best chance of survival. However, there is frequently significant morbidity and mortality associated with surgical intervention in high-risk cancer patients. Stage of disease and prognosis are important components of the decision to proceed with non-operative management of bowel perforation. For example, in the 33 patients in the M. D. Anderson study who underwent non-operative management, 70% had stage IV disease and an additional 12% had leukemia refractory to treatment, or glioblastoma multiforme. Future prospective studies should include an evaluation of quality of life, perhaps the most important outcome for patients with advanced or incurable cancer.

Bowel perforation is a rare, but well documented complication of some 'targeted' systemic chemotherapeutic agents. Bevacizumab, for example, is a humanized monoclonal antibody to vascular endothelial growth factor (VEGF) with a reported bowel perforation rate of 1–2%. Another important side effect of bevacizumab to consider prior to proceeding with surgery is delayed wound healing. Scappaticci *et al.* reported a wound complication rate of 13% in patients undergoing surgery while being treated with bevacizumab.[2] We recently reported our management strategy for 24 patients with bevacizumab-associated bowel perforation, utilising a liberal definition for perforation that included enterocutaneous fistula formation and leakage from previous surgical anastomoses.[3] The 60-day mortality rate for this cohort was 25% (6/24). Three patients died within 30 days of presentation and were not surgical candidates, due to advanced carcinomatosis. The three additional deaths occurred between 30 to 60 days of presentation in patients treated non-operatively who recovered from their perforation and were discharged to hospice care without signs of sepsis or active infection. Five patients were treated operatively; one of these patients developed delayed wound healing while another developed anastomotic leakage, requiring further surgery with stoma placement. Other authors have reported significant rates of anastomotic leakage and enterocutaneous fistula formation.[2,4,5] These reports, in addition to ours, support strong consideration for stoma placement in patients requiring a bowel resection in the setting of bevacizumab-associated bowel perforation.

2.   Bowel Obstruction

Bowel obstruction in patients with cancer represents another difficult situation with little prospective data upon which to base decisions. Patients presenting with bowel obstruction and potentially curable cancer represent relatively straightforward management decisions. Treatment is primarily surgical, although patients with rectal obstruction may benefit from expandable rectal stent placement, to allow for bowel preparation and avoidance of a stoma. Patients with advanced or incurable cancer who meet the criteria for palliative care are far more difficult to manage clinically, and there are no clear-cut treatment guidelines or algorithms to follow. The final decision for palliation is ultimately based on multidisciplinary input, typically from medical and surgical oncology, in the context of the family and patients' desires and best attempts at estimating prognosis.

A notable exception to mechanical bowel obstruction, but with a similar clinical presentation is colonic pseudo-obstruction, or 'Ogilvie's syndrome'. Colonic pseudo-obstruction represents a severe form of adynamic ileus typically described in hospitalized, deconditioned patients on bed rest, receiving narcotics and with concomitant electrolyte abnormalities, or in patients recovering from neurosurgical procedures. Initial conservative treatment should consist of nothing by mouth, nasogastric tube decompression, discontinuation of anti-motility agents and limitation of narcotics, electrolyte correction, and rectal tube placement. Patients who fail to respond to conservative treatment, or demonstrate dilatation of the caecum beyond 10–12 cm should be considered for neostigmine administration.[6–8] Patients not responsive to neostigmine may require colonoscopic decompression, or surgery.

The history and physical examination is of critical importance in the evaluation of functional bowel obstruction in the setting of advanced or incurable malignancy, as is the case with bowel obstruction without a history of malignancy. Much of the history is focused on determining whether the obstruction represents a partial versus complete obstruction. Physical exam findings of fever, tachycardia, and significant abdominal tenderness are concerning for ischaemia, as is an elevated white blood cell count on laboratory evaluation. Optimally, surgical intervention should be performed prior to findings suggesting ischemia, but this must be weighed against the approximate 50% chance that the obstruction will resolve without surgery.[9] Radiographic imaging (primarily a CT scan) is more important in patients with a history of cancer than in their counterparts without a malignancy. Additionally, care must be taken to rule out other sites of obstruction distal to the initial obstruction. A barium enema may be helpful in this situation, in order to identify potential areas of distal colonic obstruction. CT imaging may allow the identification of patients at risk for poor outcomes, such as patients with carcinomatosis and small bowel obstruction or ascites.[10,11] The detection of contraindications for surgery in patients with malignant bowel obstruction has been attempted through retrospective reviews which identified factors associated with high morbidity or mortality. Mortality rates of 10–40%, even higher morbidity rates, and the frequency of short-term re-obstruction are reasons to proceed with caution when considering surgical intervention to relieve obstruction in the setting of carcinomatosis.[12–14]

Medical management is critical in patients undergoing surgical intervention, as well as in patients that are not candidates for surgical palliation. Treatment includes analgesics for control of abdominal pain, anti-cholinergics and/or somatostatin analogues to control gastrointestinal secretions, and anti-emetics for nausea/vomiting. Patients with inoperable disease and refractory nausea and vomiting can be considered for percutaneous endoscopic gastrostomy tube placement (PEG tube). PEG tubes are successfully placed in 94–98% of cases and have been described as providing successful control of nausea and vomiting in over 80% of cases.[15–17]

3.   Neutropenia and Abdominal Pain

Neutropenia is a common side effect of systemic chemotherapy. Abdominal pain in the neutropenic cancer patient can represent a wide variety of diagnoses, many with considerable morbidity and even mortality. In an early case series of patients presenting with neutropenia and abdominal pain, the authors assigned 26 different diagnoses to the patient population.[18] Neutropenia can alter the typical presentation of abdominal pain and even mask an intra-abdominal catastrophe. In a study from the Roswell Park Cancer Institute, an attempt was made to correlate clinical diagnoses for patients with neutropenia and abdominal pain with findings at laparotomy or autopsy. Overall, the clinical diagnosis was correct in only 53% of the cases.[19]

Neutropenic enterocolitis is an extremely common clinical finding in patients that are neutropenic from chemotherapy and must be considered in any patient with neutropenia and abdominal pain that does not have another clear cause for their pain. The diagnosis of neutropenic enterocolitis is difficult, as there are no universally accepted criteria for this diagnosis. A recent comprehensive review of the literature proposed the findings of neutropenia (neutrophil count <1000 cells/µl), abdominal pain, fever, and bowel wall thickening on radiographic imaging as clinical criteria for neutropenic enterocolitis.[20] A CT scan image demonstrating evidence of diffuse colonic thickening in a patient diagnosed with neutropenic enterocolitis is shown in Fig. 2. Pathologic diagnostic criteria are also not well established, due to heterogeneity present within the specimens, as well as the lack of specimen availability for pathologic review, as the majority of cases are managed non-operatively. Neutropenic enterocolitis has gone by many terms in the past including agranulocytic/necrotising colitis, typhlitis, and neutropenic enteropathy.

We recently published our experience at the M. D. Anderson Cancer Center with 60 patients requiring evaluation by the surgical

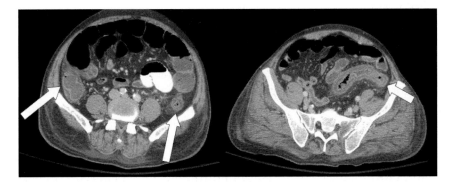

Figure 2. CT scan image demonstrating colonic thickening (marked by arrows) in a patient diagnosed with neutropenic enterocolitis.

Source: With permission from Badgwell *et al.*[21]

Table 1. Study population demographics and diagnoses for patients with neutropenia and abdominal pain ($n = 60$ patients).

Parameter	No. of patients	% of patients
Median age, years (range)	58 (22–84)	
Sex		
Male	31	52
Female	29	48
Malignancy		
Hematologic	43	72
Solid tumor	17	28
Median ANC*, × 1000 cells/µl (range)	0.17 (0–0.99)	
Median duration of neutropenia, days (range)	9 (1–120)	
Cause of abdominal pain		
Neutropenic enterocolitis	17	28
Small-bowel obstruction	7	12
Clostridium difficile colitis	4	7
Diverticulitis	3	5
Appendicitis	3	5
Cholecystitis	2	3
Colonic pseudo-obstruction	2	3
Splenic rupture	1	2
Unclear	21	35

Source: With permission from Badgwell *et al.*[21]
*ANC indicates absolute neutrophil count.

oncology consult service for neutropenia and abdominal pain.[21] Table 1 displays the demographic data for this population and the wide variety of diagnoses found in patients with neutropenia and abdominal pain. Of note is that the most frequent diagnostic category was one in which we were not able to firmly establish a diagnosis. The second most frequent diagnostic category was neutropenic enterocolitis. The diagnostic criteria for neutropenic enterocolitis in this study included neutropenia, abdominal pain and bowel wall thickening on imaging. We did not include fever as part of our inclusion criteria for neutropenic enterocolitis. This was supported by the results of our study, which did not show an association between fever and neutropenic enterocolitis. The 30- and 90-day mortality rates for the entire cohort were high, at 30% and

52%, respectively, which highlights the serious nature of this clinical scenario and the frequent presence of co-morbidities and advanced or incurable malignancy. Surgery was performed in nine patients (15%). Five of these patients underwent deliberate attempts to delay surgery to allow for resolution of neutropenia, reflecting our reluctance to operate in this setting.

The considerable mortality rate associated with surgery in neutropenic patients has been frequently described. An early case series from the National Institutes of Health reported an in-house mortality rate of 57%. Only two patients in our series were neutropenic at the time of surgery and both patients had uncomplicated post-op courses. It is unclear based on the small numbers of this infrequent clinical scenario if the mortality rate with surgery in neutropenic patients has decreased in the current era of colony stimulating factors, white blood cell transfusions, broad spectrum antibiotics, advanced critical care, and improved post-operative care. We continue to recommend delaying surgery, if possible, to allow for the resolution of neutropenia.

Prospective trials of the management of neutropenia and abdominal pain or neutropenic enterocolitis are unlikely to ever be performed. Many clinicians rely on the recommendations for febrile neutropenia proposed by the Infectious Diseases Society of America for management decisions regarding antibiotic and antifungal use and administration of colony stimulating factors. In short, for antibiotic administration, these guidelines recommend monotherapy with either cefepime/ceftazidime/carbapanem/piperacillin-tazobactam, or dual therapy with an antipseudomonal B-lactam and an aminoglycoside. Antifungal administration is recommended for patients who remain febrile, or shows signs of infection concomitantly with neutropenia for over five days. The guidelines for the use of granulocyte colony stimulating factors include patients with high-risk conditions such as pneumonia, profound neutropenia, and sepsis.

4. Cholecystitis and Biliary Obstruction

Cholecystitis in cancer patients may result from cholelithiasis, but may also occur as a complication of local treatments, such as chemoembolization of hepatic neoplasms, radioembolization with microspheres for hepatocellular cancer, or metallic biliary stent placement.[22,23] In addition, cancer patients frequently display immunosuppression, malnutrition, and other factors that may predispose them to acalculous cholecystitis. Cancer patients may also not proceed with elective laparoscopic cholecystectomy for biliary colic in the same manner as their non-cancer counterparts, over concerns related to delaying systemic treatment, or due to the fact that the symptoms of biliary colic may be less significant, compared to prognostic concerns related to their cancer. Abdominal ultrasonography is the most common initial test and has an excellent positive predictive value for non-cancer patients with calculous cholecystitis.[24] However, patients with cancer may have intra-abdominal fluid or ascites that could make identification of peri-cholecystic fluid difficult and often have abdominal pain that could complicate the interpretation of a sonographic Murphy's sign (tenderness when the ultrasound probe is pressed against the abdomen overlying the gallbladder). Hepatobiliary scintigraphy may help confirm the diagnosis of cholecystitis in these situations. Hepatobiliary scintigraphy has demonstrated higher accuracy and specificity for cholecystitis, when compared to abdominal ultrasonography.[25,26]

Treatment for patients without significant comorbidities, or cancer-related risk factors is primarily early laparoscopic cholecystectomy. Percutaneous cholecystostomy tube placement under radiologic guidance is frequently used for patients felt to represent a prohibitive risk for surgical intervention.[27] Interval laparoscopic cholecystectomy remains an option for patients having undergone a cholecystostomy tube, and in a recent series from the Cleveland Clinic, this procedure was performed at a mean of 12 weeks after tube placement, with only one conversion to an open procedure.[28] However, it should be noted that no data exists describing a large series of patients with significant cancer-related issues and cholecystitis upon which to base treatment decisions.

The optimal palliation for patients with biliary obstruction and unresectable pancreatic, gallbladder, or bile duct cancers is a matter of debate. Patients presenting with biliary obstruction as an abdominal emergency are rare, but may present with cholangitis. For patients noted to have unresectable disease prior to surgery, the least invasive option would be endoscopic stent placement.

Metallic expandable wall stents provide a longer duration of biliary drainage than traditional plastic stents. If endoscopic stent placement is unsuccessful, another non-surgical option is a percutaneous biliary drain placed by interventional radiology. Internalising percutaneous drains may be attempted once adequate biliary drainage has been established. After both endoscopic and percutaneous biliary catheter placement, the patients must be followed closely for, and instructed in, the signs and symptoms of cholangitis. Surgical bypass has a higher morbidity, mortality and increased length of hospital stay, when compared to non-surgical approaches.[29,30] However, surgery demonstrates a longer duration of palliation from jaundice and decreased episodes of cholangitis.[31-33] In general, surgical bypass is utilized only in patients found to be unresectable at the time of laparotomy, although further studies are needed to determine the optimal palliative approach. For the purposes of patients presenting with emergent biliary obstruction and cholangitis, the preferred approach would be endoscopic stent placement.

5.   Gastrointestinal Bleeding

Gastrointestinal (GI) bleeding in cancer patients is reported to arise from non-cancer sources in the majority of cases.[34-36] The most common causes are peptic ulcer disease and gastritis, not unlike the non-cancer counterparts of patients presenting with GI bleeding. Patients with gastric lymphoma receiving chemotherapy have traditionally been described as a population at high risk for gastrointestinal bleeding. A recent series of patients receiving chemotherapy for gastric lymphoma found that 11% of patients developed gastric bleeding, although surgery was infrequently required.[37] The workup should proceed according to standard surgical principles and should be based on signs indicating an upper GI versus lower GI source of bleeding. Once stabilized in the intensive care unit, the initial diagnostic and therapeutic procedure for patients with upper GI bleeding is endoscopy. Endoscopic control of malignant upper gastrointestinal bleeding has been found to be efficacious and can provide time for elective surgical intervention.[38] When weighed against the risks of emergent surgery for upper GI bleeding, many clinicians would even consider a second endoscopic procedure prior to proceeding with surgical intervention if the patient is hemodynamically stable. If the source of bleeding is found to be a gastric cancer, the risks of surgical intervention are increased. The postoperative morbidity and mortality rate in patients undergoing emergency surgery for a bleeding gastric cancer are 31% and 8%, respectively.[39]

For patients with signs of lower GI bleeding, the initial procedure after stabilization is again, endoscopy. If the bleeding is found to arise from a colon cancer, endoscopy may allow for control of the hemorrhage, so that bowel preparation may be completed and the patient can undergo a one-stage surgical procedure. Nuclear red blood cell scans and angiography may also assist in the diagnosis of patients without clear findings on endoscopy.

6.   Appendicitis

Delayed appendectomy in adults without cancer is unsafe and has been shown to increase the rate of perforation, abscess, and post-operative complications.[40] However, there are no studies focusing on appendicitis in adult cancer patients upon which to base treatment decisions. There are small case series pertaining to children with chemotherapy-induced neutropenia and attempts at conservative management.[41] The concerns over neutropenia, as previously discussed in this chapter, apply to this clinical scenario as well. Although the indications for laparoscopic appendectomy in the general surgical arena remain controversial,[42,43] it is possible that laparoscopy may help avoid the increased post-operative complications and mortality associated with surgery and neutropenia. There are promising case reports of successful laparoscopic appendectomies in the setting of neutropenia.[44] In our report on patients with neutropenia and abdominal pain, three patients presented with appendicitis; one patient developed post-chemotherapy coagulopathy and appendicitis and expired 24 hours after diagnosis from intra-cerebral hemorrhage, one patient underwent immediate open appendectomy and recovered well, and one patient underwent conservative management with delayed appendectomy at 23 days after diagnosis, once the neutropenia had resolved.[21] In general, as discussed in the section on neutropenia, we have tried to delay surgical intervention in patients with appendicitis and neutropenia until the bone marrow function has adequately recovered, in order to minimize surgical morbidity and mortality. However, patients with signs and symptoms of peritonitis require immediate surgical intervention. The decision-making process for surgical intervention is frequently very complicated in these patients, requiring input from the medical oncologist, surgical oncologist, as well as the patient and family members.

7. Conclusions

The majority of the studies focusing on abdominal emergencies in cancer patients are retrospective chart reviews of relatively small numbers of patients. Given the rarity and heterogeneity of many of these conditions, it is unlikely that many of the questions regarding the treatment of cancer patients with abdominal emergencies can be unequivocally answered in clinical trials. However, future studies might benefit from a prospective analysis and multi-institutional collaboration. As usual in clinical decision making in oncology, multi-disciplinary cooperation is of paramount importance. As many of these patients have symptoms and conditions related to an advanced or incurable cancer, there may also be important quality-of-life and symptom improvement questions that can be addressed, with attention to palliative care. The conditions we have covered help describe many of the abdominal emergencies a surgeon can expect to face as a consultant to an oncologic population. As we move forward into the era of new chemotherapeutic agents, targeted agents, proton beam therapy, and other oncologic advances, attention should be paid to the unique surgical variables in cancer patients; many of which represent complications of cancer treatment.

References

1. B. Badgwell, B. W. Feig, M. I. Ross, P. F. Mansfield, S. Wen and G. J. Chang, Pneumoperitoneum in the cancer patient, *Ann. Surg. Oncol.* **14**: 3141–3147 (2007).
2. F. A. Scappaticci, L. Fehrenbacher, T. Cartwright, J. D. Hainsworth, W. Heim, J. Berlin, F. Kabbinavar, W. Novotny, S. Sarkar and H. Hurwitz, Surgical wound healing complications in metastatic colorectal cancer patients treated with bevacizumab, *J. Surg. Oncol.* **91**: 173–180 (2005).

3. B. D. Badgwell, E. R. Camp, B. Feig, R. A. Wolff, C. Eng, L. M. Ellis and J. N. Cormier, Management of bevacizumab-associated bowel perforation: A case series and review of the literature, *Ann. Oncol.* **19**: 577–582 (2008).

4. J. H. Heinzerling and S. Huerta, Bowel perforation from bevacizumab for the treatment of metastatic colon cancer: Incidence, etiology, and management, *Curr. Surg.* **63**: 334–337 (2006).

5. B. J. Giantonio, D. E. Levy, J. O'Dwyer, P. N. J. Meropol, P. J. Catalano and A. B. Benson, 3rd, A phase II study of high-dose bevacizumab in combination with irinotecan, 5-fluorouracil, leucovorin, as initial therapy for advanced colorectal cancer: Results from the Eastern Cooperative Oncology Group study E2200, *Ann. Oncol.* **17**: 1399–1403 (2006).

6. R. Mehta, A. John, P. Nair, V. V. Raj, C. P. Mustafa, D. Suvarna and V. Balakrishnan, Factors predicting successful outcome following neostigmine therapy in acute colonic pseudo-obstruction: A prospective study, *J. Gastroenterol. Hepatol.* **21**: 459–461 (2006).

7. C. G. Loftus, G. C. Harewood and T. H. Baron, Assessment of predictors of response to neostigmine for acute colonic pseudo-obstruction, *Am. J. Gastroenterol.* **97**: 3118–3122 (2002).

8. R. J. Ponec, M. D. Saunders and M. B. Kimmey, Neostigmine for the treatment of acute colonic pseudo-obstruction, *N. Engl. J. Med.* **341**: 137–141 (1999).

9. J. D. Wayne and R. J. Bold, Oncologic emergencies. In: *The M. D. Anderson Surgical Oncology Handbook*, eds. B. W. Feig, D. H. Berger and G. M. Fuhrman (Lippincott Williams & Wilkins, Philadelphia, 2006), pp. 577.

10. S. L. Blair, D. Z. Chu and R. E. Schwarz, Outcome of palliative operations for malignant bowel obstruction in patients with peritoneal carcinomatosis from nongynecological cancer, *Ann. Surg. Oncol.* **8**: 632–637 (2001).

11. H. Higashi, H. Shida, K. Ban, S. Yamagata, K. Masuda, T. Imanari and T. Yamamoto, Factors affecting successful palliative surgery for malignant bowel obstruction due to peritoneal dissemination from colorectal cancer, *Jpn. J. Clin. Oncol.* **33**: 357–359 (2003).

12. C. Ripamonti, R. Twycross, M. Baines, F. Bozzetti, S. Capri, F. De Conno, B. Gemlo, T. M. Hunt, H. B. Krebs, S. Mercadante, R. Schaerer and P. Wilkinson, Clinical-practice recommendations for the management of bowel obstruction in patients with end-stage cancer, *Support. Care Cancer* **9**: 223–233 (2001).

13. C. I. Ripamonti, A. M. Easson and H. Gerdes, Management of malignant bowel obstruction, *Eur. J. Cancer* **44**: 1105–1115 (2008).
14. S. M. Abbas and A. E. Merrie, Resection of peritoneal metastases causing malignant small bowel obstruction, *World J. Surg. Oncol.* **5**: 122 (2007).
15. E. Campagnutta and R. Cannizzaro, Percutaneous endoscopic gastrostomy (PEG) in palliative treatment of non-operable intestinal obstruction due to gynecologic cancer: A review, *Eur. J. Gynaecol. Oncol.* **21**: 397–402 (2000).
16. E. Campagnutta, R. Cannizzaro, A. Gallo, A. Zarrelli, M. Valentini, M. De Cicco and C. Scarabelli, Palliative treatment of upper intestinal obstruction by gynecological malignancy: The usefulness of percutaneous endoscopic gastrostomy, *Gynecol. Oncol.* **62**: 103–105 (1996).
17. B. Pothuri, M. Montemarano, M. Gerardi, M. Shike, L. Ben-Porat, P. Sabbatini and R. R. Barakat, Percutaneous endoscopic gastrostomy tube placement in patients with malignant bowel obstruction due to ovarian carcinoma, *Gynecol. Oncol.* **96**: 330–334 (2005).
18. H. F. Starnes Jr, F. D. Moore Jr, S. Mentzer, R. T. Osteen, G. D. Steele Jr and R. E. Wilson, Abdominal pain in neutropenic cancer patients, *Cancer* **57**: 616–621 (1986).
19. D. S. Wade, H. Douglass Jr, H. R. Nava and M. Piedmonte, Abdominal pain in neutropenic patients, *Arch. Surg.* **125**: 1119–1127 (1990).
20. M. Gorschluter, U. Mey, J. Strehl, C. Ziske, M. Schepke, I. G. Schmidt-Wolf, T. Sauerbruch and A. Glasmacher, Neutropenic enterocolitis in adults: Systematic analysis of evidence quality, *Eur. J. Haematol.* **75**: 1–13 (2005).
21. B. D. Badgwell, J. N. Cormier, C. J. Wray, G. Borthakur, W. Qiao, K. V. Rolston and R. E. Pollock, Challenges in surgical management of abdominal pain in the neutropenic cancer patient, *Ann. Surg.* **248**: 104–109 (2008).
22. J. Gates, G. G. Hartnell, K. E. Stuart and M. E. Clouse, Chemoembolization of hepatic neoplasms: Safety, complications, and when to worry, *Radiographics* **19**: 399–414 (1999).
23. M. Veerasamy, L. R. Roberts and J. C. Andrews, Clinical challenges and images in GI radiation cholecystitis, *Gastroenterology* **135**: 18, 328 (2008).
24. P. W. Ralls, P. M. Colletti, S. A. Lapin, P. Chandrasoma, W. D. Boswell Jr, C. Ngo, D. R. Radin and J. M. Halls, Real-time sonography in

suspected acute cholecystitis. Prospective evaluation of primary and secondary signs, *Radiology* **155**: 767–771 (1985).

25. S. N. Chatziioannou, W. H. Moore, P. V. Ford and R. D. Dhekne, Hepatobiliary scintigraphy is superior to abdominal ultrasonography in suspected acute cholecystitis, *Surgery* **127**: 609–613 (2000).

26. J. E. Freitas, S. H. Mirkes, D. M. Fink-Bennett and R. L. Bree, Suspected acute cholecystitis. Comparison of hepatobiliary scintigraphy versus ultrasonography, *Clin. Nucl. Med.* **7**: 364–367 (1982).

27. M. F. Byrne, P. Suhocki, R. M. Mitchell, T. N. Pappas, H. L. Stiffler, P. S. Jowell, M. S. Branch and J. Baillie, Percutaneous cholecystostomy in patients with acute cholecystitis: Experience of 45 patients at a US referral center, *J. Am. Coll. Surg.* **197**: 206–211 (2003).

28. E. Berber, K. L. Engle, A. String, A. M. Garland, G. Chang, J. Macho, J. M. Pearl and A. E. Siperstein, Selective use of tube cholecystostomy with interval laparoscopic cholecystectomy in acute cholecystitis, *Arch. Surg.* **135**: 341–346 (2000).

29. A. C. Smith, J. F. Dowsett, R. C. Russell, A. R. Hatfield and P. B. Cotton, Randomised trial of endoscopic stenting versus surgical bypass in malignant low bile duct obstruction, *Lancet* **344**: 1655–1660 (1994).

30. J. R. Andersen, S. M. Sorensen, A. Kruse, M. Rokkjaer and P. Matzen, Randomised trial of endoscopic endoprosthesis versus operative bypass in malignant obstructive jaundice, *Gut* **30**: 1132–1135 (1989).

31. M. C. Taylor, R. S. McLeod and B. Langer, Biliary stenting versus bypass surgery for the palliation of malignant distal bile duct obstruction: A meta-analysis, *Liver Transpl.* **6**: 302–308 (2000).

32. M. K. Hyoty and I. H. Nordback, Biliary stent or surgical bypass in unresectable pancreatic cancer with obstructive jaundice, *Acta Chir. Scand.* **156**: 391–396 (1990).

33. P. C. Bornman, E. P. Harries-Jones, R. Tobias, G. van Stiegmann and J. Terblanche, Prospective controlled trial of transhepatic biliary endoprosthesis versus bypass surgery for incurable carcinoma of head of pancreas, *Lancet* **1**: 69–71 (1986).

34. J. D. Wayne and R. J. Bold, Oncologic emergencies. In: *The M. D. Anderson Surgical Oncology Handbook*, eds. B. W. Feig, D. H. Berger and G. M. Fuhrman (Lippincott Williams & Wilkins, Philadelphia, 2006), pp. 580–581.

35. F. Schnoll-Sussman and R. C. Kurtz, Gastrointestinal emergencies in the critically ill cancer patient, *Semin. Oncol.* **27**: 270–283 (2000).

36. T. A. Stellato and R. R. Shenk, Gastrointestinal emergencies in the oncology patient, *Semin. Oncol.* **16**: 521–531 (1989).
37. G. Spectre, D. Libster, S. Grisariu, N. Da'as, D. B. Yehuda, Z. Gimmon and O. Paltiel, Bleeding, obstruction, and perforation in a series of patients with aggressive gastric lymphoma treated with primary chemotherapy, *Ann. Surg. Oncol.* **13**: 1372–1378 (2006).
38. T. J. Savides, D. M. Jensen, J. Cohen, G. M. Randall, T. O. Kovacs, E. Pelayo, S. Cheng, M. E. Jensen and H. Y. Hsieh, Severe upper gastrointestinal tumor bleeding: Endoscopic findings, treatment, and outcome, *Endoscopy* **28**: 244–248 (1996).
39. H. J. Lee, J. Park do, H. K. Yang, K. U. Lee and K. J. Choe, Outcome after emergency surgery in gastric cancer patients with free perforation or severe bleeding, *Dig. Surg.* **23**: 217–223 (2006).
40. M. F. Ditillo, J. D. Dziura and R. Rabinovici, Is it safe to delay appendectomy in adults with acute appendicitis? *Ann. Surg.* **244**: 656–660 (2006).
41. V. A. Wiegering, C. J. Kellenberger, N. Bodmer, E. Bergstraesser, F. Niggli, M. Grotzer, D. Nadal and J. P. Bourquin, Conservative management of acute appendicitis in children with hematologic malignancies during chemotherapy-induced neutropenia, *J. Pediatr. Hematol. Oncol.* **30**: 464–467 (2008).
42. A. C. Moberg, F. Berndsen, I. Palmquist, U. Petersson, T. Resch and A. Montgomery, Randomized clinical trial of laparoscopic versus open appendicectomy for confirmed appendicitis, *Br. J. Surg.* **92**: 298–304 (2005).
43. S. Olmi, S. Magnone, A. Bertolini and E. Croce, Laparoscopic versus open appendectomy in acute appendicitis: A randomized prospective study, *Surg. Endosc.* **19**: 1193–1195 (2005).
44. C. Ustun, Laparoscopic appendectomy in a patient with acute myelogenous leukemia with neutropenia, *J. Laparoendosc. Adv. Surg. Tech. A* **17**: 213–215 (2007).

18

Peri-operative Management of Patients with GI Malignancy: The Interdisciplinary Approach

Ross C. Smith

Abstract

Improvements in the peri-operative management of gastrointestinal malignancies allows patients to start eating and walking almost immediately after recovery from anaesthesia, and results in earlier discharge in a better state of health. This is termed fast track surgery and results from the judicious use of minimally invasive procedures or better open surgery, and is enhanced by modern anaesthetic protocols, reducing the use of opiate drugs and is predicated by a team effort. When patients present with advanced cancers and a prolonged period of poor food intake, the risk of suffering complications following surgery is increased. Many different nutritional risk assessment tools have been developed and have been shown to be effective in deciding which patients should undergo peri-operative nutritional therapy.

Artificial nutrition reduces the risk of post-operative complications when used selectively on at risk patients. In low risk patients, the complications of enteral nutrition and parenteral nutrition, although uncommon, may be serious and significantly reduce the effectiveness of these therapies. However, in high risk patients significant reductions in mortality and morbidity can be achieved and their benefits can be substantial.

439

Keywords: Enteral nutrition, parenteral nutrition, fast track surgery, gastrointestinal malignancies, perioperative care, malnutrition, nutritional risk assessment, prognostic nutritional index.

1.   Introduction

The trend towards early cancer diagnosis, together with improved diagnostic techniques, modern anaesthetic protocols and more effective antibiotics, are just a few aspects of modern patient care which contributed together to improve outcomes in GI cancer. For smaller sized tumours, specific management protocols, which include laparoscopic techniques, can lead to a quicker return to normality and reduce complication rates. However, some patients still present with advanced symptoms, which compromise their wellbeing and nutritional state. This is particularly the case with gastrointestinal malignancies, where a reduced food intake and an inflammatory response to the tumour can contribute to adverse outcomes. Therefore these patients require special peri-operative care.

2.   Fast-Track Surgery Challenging Traditional Peri-operative Care

"Fast-track surgery" is an evolving concept, whereby a concerted effort is made to help patients recover rapidly with return to good health. This concept has encompassed a number of radically different management protocols and different approaches and involves staff from different disciplines. The key principles of fast track surgery are listed in Table 1 and some of them will be discussed below.

When ill patients are admitted to hospital for diagnostic tests, they frequently have already been through a period of limited nutrition intake. They then have periods of fasting required for X-rays and other tests, may limit their food intake, as hospital food may not be to their liking and this leads to a deterioration of the patient's nutritional status while waiting for surgery.[2]

In the traditional model of surgical care patients are fasted for 12 hours before surgery and after surgery until the wounds are secure and the bowel has started to function. Patients were also kept on bed rest for a week or more.

Table 1. The principles of fast-track surgery.

Allow the patient to take nourishing fluids up to two hours before surgery
No bowel preparation, unless constipated
Use of anaesthetic procedures which allow early recovery
Minimise the use of opiates
Avoiding intravenous fluid overload
Minimal use of naso-gastric tubes
Early return to enteral or oral nutrition
Early mobilisation

Fast tracking patients has challenged traditional management protocols in almost every way. The traditional model of prolonged bed rest has been replaced by early post-operative mobilisation and early introduction of oral nutrition with supplements which usually allows rapid return to normal diet, preventing further weight loss. The principles of fast-tracking have been shown to apply not only to colonic surgery[3] but also to pancreatic surgery[4,5] and prostate surgery.[6] Thus the focus in peri-operative care is to have the patient recovering from surgery as soon as possible, to allow for early discharge and this requires a close collaboration between anaesthetists, surgeons, dietitians, nursing staff and other members of the team.

2.1 *Use of oral pre-operative carbohydrate fluids*

Traditionally patients are fasted before receiving an anaesthetic to prevent vomiting at the time of induction of anaesthesia, which can cause aspiration of acidic gastric fluid and cause severe respiratory distress, but this concept has been challenged by Ljungqvist's group.[7] They have shown that the provision of carbohydrate-rich fluids up to two hours before surgery is safe, as carbohydrates do not stimulate gastric acid production,[8] do not delay gastric emptying[9] and therefore do not put the patient at risk of aspiration. Taking a carbohydrate drink up to two hours before surgery improves sepsis rates after colorectal surgery.[3,10] In a recent randomised trial, whole-body protein balance was better maintained when patients received a carbohydrate-rich beverage before colorectal surgery, due to the suppressive effect of insulin on endogenous glucose release.[11]

2.2　*Bowel preparation prior to surgery*

The practice of bowel preparation prior to surgery has also been challenged. Bowel preparation involves limiting food intake to fluids for a few days before surgery and the taking of aperients. The use of bowel preparation has been shown to increase the risk of infection, rather than to improve the outcome of colorectal surgery,[12] but recent meta-analysis of comparative studies examined 2304 patients who had bowel preparation and 2297 who did not have it and found no difference in infection or anastomotic wound breakdown.[13] As there was no benefit for mechanical bowel preparation before colorectal surgery, it was concluded that this need not be part of routine preparation for surgery, but some surgeons still prefer to operate on an empty colon, which would particularly seem to be important in patients with a tendency to constipation. Therefore the surgeon's preference is important in deciding an individual patient's management.

Constipation is best avoided at the time of surgery. It is certainly more difficult to cope with constipation when a patient has a painful wound. Therefore, although bowel preparation is no longer considered necessary before colonic surgery, it may be wise to consider treating constipation before surgery to avoid this difficulty in the post-operative period.

Other important aspects of fast track management include the use of use of specific anaesthetic agents, early post-operative mobilization, avoidance of naso-gastric tubes and abdominal drains, early post-operative intake of balanced nutritional liquids and solid food, minimising opiates for pain control and the use of bowel stimulating drugs. Using these strategies as a combined pathway leads to earlier discharge at about day four, with a low risk of re-admission within 30 days.[14,15]

2.3　*Early return to normal nutrition*

Under the traditional model of care, patients are maintained on nil by mouth until their wounds are shown to be secure by return to normal bowel function or until X-rays indicate anastomoses to be free of leaks. An important aspect of fast tracking surgical recovery is to commence nutrition more quickly after surgery. This may involve the use of enteral nutrition in the first few hours after surgery, although such a practice would be dangerous in patients with intra-abdominal sepsis, where ileus can result in massive distension and bowel ischaemia. However in the case of elective surgery, there is evidence, from randomised studies, that early return to normal nutrition is of benefit. Han-Geurts *et al.* examined early resumption of oral intake in 128 patients after colorectal and vascular surgery.[16] Although early resumption of oral intake did not diminish the duration of post-operative ileus and it significantly increased the rate of naso-gastric tube reinsertion, the early commencement of an oral diet did not influence gastrointestinal functional recovery. The authors found no reason to withhold oral intake following open colorectal or abdominal vascular surgery, and suggested that post-operative management should include an early resumption of diet.

Furthermore, after upper gastrointestinal surgery, a recent multicentre study compared the strategies of using nil by mouth and enteral tube feeding, or allowing normal oral food intake from the first day after surgery in 453 patients.[17] There was no difference between the groups for the primary outcome variables of mortality (4.4% compared to 5.0%), major complications (33.5% compared with 28.2%) and the frequency of re-operation (15.9% compared with 13.2%). However the post discharge complications were reduced in the "at will" early oral feeding group, mainly due to a reduction in the wound infection rate, which was greater in the enteral tube feeding group (8.1% compared with 2.4%, $p < 0.01$).

3. Management of Patients with More Advanced Symptoms

Patients with cancers of the intestinal tract face special challenges, as tumours of the upper gastrointestinal tract frequently cause anorexia, obstruction, nausea and a feeling of bloatedness, which interfere with nutritional intake, resulting in weight loss and a degree of malnutrition. Anorexia is often severe and disturbs patients and their carers. It can be disease-related, treatment-related, or caused by emotional distress. Patients may have unusual smell or taste sensations, which put them off their food. These tumours also have a propensity to increase metabolic rate and therefore the amount of calories required to maintain health. This situation can be aggravated by poor pancreatic function, leading to reduced absorption of nutrients and associated diarrhoea. Any of these factors working in combination may often be present.

3.1 *Anorexia and metabolic disturbances*

Disease-related anorexia is caused by different metabolic disturbances which vary between patients (see Table 2). An increase in serum lactate or ketosis during fasting have been identified as frequent causes of anorexia.[18] Increased levels of metabolically active peptides including serotonin, parathormone, lipolytic substances, toxohormone-L, bombesin, satietins, glucagon or glucagon-like peptides, Ghrelin, resistin, leptin, adiponectin, IGF-I[19] and certain cytokines are also considered to have a role.[20] An inflammatory bio-moderator, Interleukin-1 (IL-1) is frequently produced during tumour growth and is considered to induce anorexia, by facilitating tryptophan supply to the brain, where it increases serotonin production. Brain levels of serotonin have also been related to anorexia, as are many other substances resulting from the breakdown of large tumour masses. However, some patients feel well despite the presence of large tumours, while others are symptomatic with small tumour masses. The complex causes of anorexia are the reason there is no simple medication which can easily reverse this distressing symptom.

Tumours compete for the body's nutrients and protein stores, and furthermore, they are metabolically inefficient, wasting energy and amino acids, which results in further loss of healthy tissues such as muscle and leads to weakness. In addition, the production of increased levels of cytokines, such as tumor necrosis factor-α (TNF-α) and interleukins (IL-1 and IL-6),[21] increase muscle

Table 2. Reasons for weight loss in patients with GI tract malignancy.

Obstruction of the GI tract
Poor nutritional intake due to nausea and anorexia
Poor food absorption
Tumour competing for energy and protein
Cancer-driven increased metabolic rate

breakdown. Some tumours utilise available fats to make excessive amounts of prostaglandin E2, which also raises the body's metabolic activity, mimicking an inflammatory response to the tumour. Prostaglandin E2 is derived from long chain fatty acids; the amount is modified by the presence of ω-3 fatty acids which are present in fish oil. The increased inflammatory response results in anorexia, reducing nutrition intake, but at the same time increasing the nutrition requirements because of increased protein turnover, which causes a loss of body tissue.

This complex mix of different mediators renders unimodal nutritional interventions unlikely to be very successful. Therefore, clinical trials using combination therapies or immuno-nutrition are required for future success.[22]

Weight loss during the three months leading to the diagnosis is generally graded as moderate (up to 10%), severe (10–20%), and very severe (greater than 20%). When the tumour is advanced, the nutritional deficiency becomes most pronounced and leads to a state of cachexia, where very severe weight loss is associated with a loss of function. Weight loss is not the best measure of the effect of malnutrition (nutritional deficit) on the body, as the illness results in water retention, which conceals the loss of other important nutrients and muscle mass.

3.2   *Malnutrition*

Cancer-associated malnutrition has features indicating a combination of the classical syndromes of Kwashiorkor and Marasmus (see Table 3).[23] The consequence of weight loss is a progressive interference in bodily functions, as reduced serum proteins leads to impaired wound healing, and interferes with the body's immune defences and the gut may lose its resistance to the bacteria which reside in its lumen. Furthermore, weakness causes a reduction in the ability to cough and move and can cause an impairment of renal and hepatic function. This results in loss of body fat and muscle mass, but the plasma proteins are preserved and the immune system remains competent. Such patients have small reserves, which are rapidly depleted by a small insult. When the body protein reserves are exhausted, blood levels of protein are suppressed causing immunological deficiencies.[23]

Table 3. Types of malnutrition and their key features.

Marasmus-like	Proportional loss of fat and muscle
	Normal plasma proteins
	Immune competence maintained
	Poor reserves
	Marked weight loss
Kwashiorkor-like	Loss of body protein
	Loss of muscle mass
	Low plasma proteins
	Immunological failure
	Impaired response to surgery
	Weight may be maintained

Water retention can be a consequence of protein deficiency and this masks the role of weight loss as a guide to malnutrition. This excessive fluid in the tissues is identified by oedema in the legs and ascites in the abdomen. Better measures of malnutrition in this situation include serum albumin, prealbumin, retinol binding protein, lymphocyte count, and measures of immune function. In the nutrition laboratory, we are able to measure body protein and water and fat stores, and a careful study of the influence of illness on these macro components of the body allows the measurement of the influence of malnutrition has in cancer patients.

The micronutrients are also important. Loss of blood from the gastrointestinal tract leads to iron deficiency and therefore anaemia. Anaemia can also result from poor absorption of folic acid and vitamin B12, which may be an important consequence of gastric cancer. Jaundiced patients are frequently deficient in vitamin K, because this substance requires bile salts in the gut for its absorption. However, cancer patients may develop many different trace element and vitamin deficiency states which should be recognised and treated on their merits.

4.   Pre-Operative Assessment of Nutritional Status

It is important to identify patients who have poor nutritional status before surgery, because malnutrition will impair a patient's ability to recover from surgery and because treatments are available to improve the malnourished patient's outcome.

There are many ways of determining the extent of malnutrition and here I will refer to some commonly used tools. Nutritional assessment in cancer patients has recently been undertaken in a multicentre study of 1000 patients with cancer.[24] The authors used the Nutritional Risk Assessment, which relies on different measures of a patient's weight loss, serum protein levels, capacity to function and immune status, and demonstrated that one third of patients had nutritional deficiency. They concluded that weight loss and nutritional risk are frequent in an unselected series of cancer outpatients. The site of primary tumour, its stage and patient performance status appear to be associated, on preliminary analysis, with significant weight loss and nutritional risk. Anorexia and weight loss are closely related, and this supports the concept that nutritional depletion can play a major role in the onset of malnutrition-cachexia.

Many workers have been able to demonstrate the relationship between malnutrition and complications after surgery. Classic studies in the 1940s demonstrated that weight loss was related to the death rate after gastrectomy. In the 1970s, Mullen described a complex method of measuring malnutrition (the Prognostic Nutritional Index)[25] and subsequently many workers have described simplified methods of assessing the relationship between malnutrition and the complication rate after surgery. These have been compared by Kylie et al.[26] and Kuzu et al.[27]

Notably, all methods demonstrate an association between nutritional status and complications, but it has been difficult to demonstrate an advantage of one assessment method over the other. Although many methods have enabled improved outcomes after surgery since that decade, malnutrition continues to be prevalent in hospitalised patients and its relationship with poor post-operative outcomes continues to be demonstrable.[28]

4.1 *Subjective global assessment (SGA)*

SGA is widely used because it can be assessed by the bedside, using history and physical examination and because it has been frequently shown to be predictive of post-operative complications.

SGA has been demonstrated to be as effective as the more sophisticated measures in predicting outcomes. It subjectively classifies patients as SGA A, B or C, by considering the amount and duration of weight loss, dietary intake, gastrointestinal symptoms of greater than two weeks' duration, functional effects of the illness, nutritional demands of the stress and the physical effects of the illness (loss of fat, muscle wasting, ankle oedema, sacral oedema and ascites). Although the SGA is simple in principle, it requires a specific commitment by the admitting physician to document these factors in the patient's record. In a recent study which used a nutritional risk score similar to the SGA, 40% of patients presenting with malignancy were found to have increased risk of malnutrition, compared to 8% of patients presenting with benign disorders. Furthermore, the risk of complications following surgery was 54% in patients shown to have high risk, compared to 15% for those with low risk of post-operative complications.[28]

4.2   Malnutrition related complication score (MRCS)

Because the task of nutritional assessment on all patients admitted to hospital can be very time-consuming and labour-intensive, it is infrequently undertaken. A new method of screening patients for the risk of malnutrition-related complications is available, which requires the entry of six values which have categorical cut off values and can be obtained from the hospital's pathology reporting system. If the first three clinical questions were written on the patient's first blood request form, the score could be available for every patient being admitted to hospital. The method can also be used at the bedside.[28,29]

The three bedside questions are:

- Does, or will, the patient have a wound?
- Has the patient had a poor oral intake?
- Does the patient have a malnutrition-related admission diagnosis?

The cut-off value for three blood measures are:

- Serum albumin <31.5 g/L
- Lymphocyte count <1202 × 10^9/L
- Haemoglobin <99.5 g/L.

If one or none of these factors is abnormal, the risk of complications is very low and the proposed surgical procedure can be undertaken safely. If two blood tests are abnormal, the risk of complication is increased in up to 37% of patients, and special nutritional care should be offered. The MRCS uses a sophisticated program to rank the order of combinations of these factors to give a more precise assessment of risk of complications and can be calculated by writing a program in the hospital's pathology software system.

4.3 *Prevention of malnutrition-related complications*

Prevention is always better than cure. The most effective means of preventing malnutrition in cancer patients is to recognise the tumour early, before malnutrition sets in. One of the most pleasing changes over the last 30 years in my experience is that there are significantly fewer patients presenting with severe malnutrition. It is now relatively rare for patients to present with the most severe form, where operative surgery would carry prohibitive risk and yet the cancer is still at a sufficiently early stage, such that resection could provide a significant chance of cure. This improvement is the result of earlier diagnosis through the wider use of endoscopy and CT scanning. Nonetheless, many patients still present with advanced cancer, when curative surgery is not possible, but when palliative surgery to overcome obstructions can provide improved quality of life.

4.4 *Fasting for tests*

When ill patients are admitted to hospital for tests there are several reasons for poor nutrition input. They are frequently fasted prior to having X-rays and other investigations, hospital food may not be to their liking or they may already be suffering anorexia as a result of their disease. A famous study by Muller, published in the *Lancet* in 1982,[2] examined the influence of ten days of pre-operative parenteral nutrition (PPN) on the post-operative complication rate for gastrointestinal carcinoma. Fifty-nine patients (controls) received the regular hospital diet and 66 received PPN. The rates of post-operative wound infection, pneumonia, major complications, and mortality were generally lower in the PPN group. The results can be explained by the improvement in various indices of humoral and cellular immuno-competence and protein status in the PPN group and their deterioration in the control group during the pre-operative course.[2] In follow-up reviews of this paper the deterioration of nutritional status in the control group was considered to be the predominant effect in the results of the study. These papers emphasise the importance of nutrition in cancer patients requiring surgery. In a subsequent study by the same group, the complication rate had become so low that a very large study would be required to prove the benefit for giving pre-operative parenteral nutrition, because of the reduced incidence of complications in the modern clinical setting.

5.   The Concept of Peri-Operative Nutritional Support

A patient's nutritional status is an important factor influencing the complications associated with surgery and it is therefore logical that nutritional therapy will improve the outcome of the malnourished patient. Nutritional therapy is considered to be an important concept, which enhances recovery and quality of life.[30] Peri-operative nutritional therapy can be given in three ways: supplemental nutritional drinks, enteral nutrition or parenteral nutrition. Nutritional therapy should start before surgery and continue throughout the post-operative period, until the patient has fully recovered.

The European Society of Parenteral and Enteral Nutriton (ESPEN) developed guidelines using evidence-based recommendations for the treatment of surgical patients.[31] They were developed by an interdisciplinary expert group and discussed and accepted in a consensus conference. The group considered that enteral nutrition was indicated even in patients without obvious under-nutrition, if it is anticipated that the patient will be unable to eat for a period exceeding seven days post-operatively. Clearly if the patient is unable to tolerate enteral nutrition, parenteral nutrition is required. Supplementary nutritional support is indicated if a patient cannot maintain oral intake above 60% of recommended intake for more than ten days. In these situations nutritional support should be initiated without delay. Delay of surgery for pre-operative nutritional therapy should be considered if the patient has severe nutritional risk, defined by the presence of at least one of the following criteria: weight loss > 10–15% over six months, BMI < 18.5 kg/m^2,[32] Subjective Global Assessment Grade C, or serum albumin < 30 g/L (with no evidence of hepatic or renal dysfunction). The surgical team should develop a focus on prevention of severe undernutrition by the use of nutritional support.[33]

5.1 Nutritional supplements

Pre-operative immunotherapy is an enteral nutrition formula containing added amounts of nutrients considered to have the effect of enhancing the immune system. One of these formulae, Impact® (Novartis), contains added amounts of glutamine, arginine, ω-3 fatty acids and nucleotides. This has been studied in a meta-analysis which examined 17 randomised studies combining the results of 2304 patients. A dosage of 0.5–1 L/day for five to seven days before elective gastrointestinal surgery improved post-operative morbidity. This was considered to be a cost effective way of improving surgical outcomes. No study compared the role of Impact® (Novartis) with a standard protein-rich formula, so it is difficult to be sure that the immune enhancing formula is important for this finding, or whether nutrition in general is important. Good nutrition should be balanced, whereas large amounts of a nutrient in an unbalanced formulation will frequently aggravate deficiencies in other nutrients. It will be important to study the question of whether the benefits are due to nutritional supplements in general, or to the specific effect of the immune enhancing agents.

6. Enteral Nutrition

Enteral nutrition relates to the method of providing nutrition into the gut via a fine-bore tube, which may be placed through the nose into the stomach. Because these tubes are soft and of a fine caliber, they are easily tolerated and do not interfere with swallowing or breathing. However, over the longer term they become uncomfortable and in some groups of patients with motility disorders or head and neck tumours, a percutaneous endoscopic gastrostomy (PEG) is placed whereby a tube is guided through the abdominal wall into the stomach and held by a balloon or flange. A similar technique can be used to guide a tube directly into the jejunum.[34] These tubes can also be placed at surgery. When there is a partial blockage of the outlet of the stomach, the fine-bore tube can be placed beyond the stomach directly into the small bowel, as enteral nutrition is easily absorbed through the small intestine. A recent study[35] examining enteral feeding after oesophageal surgery, compared the use of naso-jejunal tubes with surgical jejunostomy as a means of access. They concluded that naso-jejunal tubes were safe and efficient and although there were complications with the tubes in both groups, one patient developed a life-threatening leak, in the jejunostomy group required a re-operation. Others have emphasized the importance of complications from the feeding jejunostomy procedure and indicated the importance of using this selectively.[36] Although these complications are rare, they are serious and can be life-threatening when they occur.

However, feeding jejunostomies are very valuable for patients when it is evident that long term nutritional support will be required, as in this situation the benefits are greater than the risks. Patients can receive their nutritional requirements for full recovery from surgery and for repletion of their depleted nutritional status.[37] When the jejunostomy is established, the feeding should be gradually increased towards goal rates over about three days to ensure there is no abdominal distension, pain or severe diarrhoea. The procedure is successful in about 80% of patients and 60–80% of the goal rate can generally be achieved.

Enteral nutrition may be given in boluses, but this may be associated with a feeling of fullness, nausea and sometimes diarrhoea and bolus nutrition tends to suppress appetite. These adverse symptoms are minimised by feeding slowly over 24 hours, which has the added advantage of not suppressing the appetite.

If patients are mobile, the feeding can be stopped intermittently and the tube capped. In some patients who can cope with some other nutritional fluids and food, supplemental nocturnal feeding is all that is required to maintain weight.

A recent meta-analysis examined the literature for studies comparing enteral nutrition (EN) with parenteral nutrition (PN). 29 suitable trials published from 1979 to 2001, examined outcomes of 2552 patients who had been randomised to have EN or PN. They found that EN was superior to PN in terms of reducing complications, although the mortality rate (3% compared to 4%) was not significantly different. The year of publication and type of PN were also factors affecting outcome.[37]

7.   Parenteral Nutrition

7.1   *Pre-operative parenteral nutrition*

When the gastrointestinal tract is not functioning and a patient is severely malnourished, a period of PN can reverse the immune deficiency,[38] improve protein levels and have a good influence on the outcome of surgery, but this has been a hotly debated topic for many years. A meta-analysis of many of these studies has demonstrated little improvement in mortality but improvement in complications.[39]

PN poses several difficult questions. How much nutrition should be administered? How long does it take to reverse the nutritional deficit? Is it enough to see improvement in muscle function with the patient being able to walk and cough vigorously? There are no good randomised studies specifically addressing these questions, however, a number of studies has demonstrated improvement in some of these measures after seven to 14 days of nutritional therapy. Although these questions remain unanswered, what is important is that there should be a greater emphasis on providing nutritional support for patients who are malnourished at the time of presentation for surgery. Because the half-life of albumin is about 21 days, the level of serum albumin is not a satisfactory marker of recovery. Therefore, the operation should be undertaken as soon as the patient has recovered physiological function.

7.2   *Post-operative parenteral nutrition*

PN may become an important therapy when patients are not tolerating sufficient EN to provide nutritional needs. Patients undergoing major surgery frequently have a central line in place from the time of the anaesthetic. If this is not in place, it may be possible to use a peripherally placed midline or a peripherally inserted central venous catheter (PICC) for this treatment.[40] The PN provided currently is a compound containing glucose, lipid and amino acids in a number of standard formulations. To enhance the tolerance of peripheral veins, the lipid to glucose ratio may be 66%:33%, although many prefer the lipid component to be less than 50% of the non-protein calories.[41] The amount of PN required to prevent catabolism after surgery is about 35 kcal/kg/day and about 0.3 gN/kg/day.[42] Good pain control with epidural analgesia improves the efficacy of the PN.[41] Vigilant prevention of sepsis is important for the treatment to be successful and TPN teams are a valuable resource in maintaining good practice to achieve this in the complex hospital environment.

It frequently takes more than two weeks for a patient to recover from a major surgical procedure, to the point where normal nutritional intake can recommence. In this case, there is further deterioration of the patient's protein stores. We have demonstrated that fasting after a Whipple's procedure results in a loss of 1.5 kg protein, which is equivalent to a loss of 4.5 kg of muscle (see Fig. 1).[41] This is a large proportion of a patient's muscle mass and adds to the patient's weakness resulting from surgery. There is a concurrent loss of fat tissue, but because of excess water retention, the loss of weight does not reflect the extent of loss of functioning tissue. Therefore if a patient is unable to be nourished by the gastrointestinal tract, it is important to provide nutrition by the intravenous route. Body composition studies are the best way of determining how much nutrition is required to prevent the loss of body tissue, demonstrating the

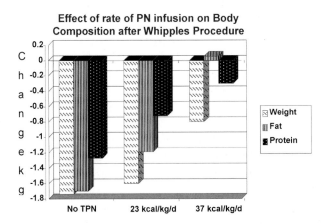

Figure 1. Losses of body tissues in the first two weeks after a Whipple's procedure when given different amounts of parenteral nutrition. The 1.3 kg protein loss in patients without nutrition is equivalent to a loss of 4 kg muscle is prevented when a full nutrition protocol is used providing 37 kcal/kg/d.[1]

importance of providing about 0.3 gN/kg/day and 35 kcal/kg/day to prevent this loss. It is more common to provide less than this in standard formulations of PN, which may provide 0.15–0.23 gN/kg/day and 23 kcal/kg/day.[42] Patients who are unlikely to return to oral intake in the first week after surgery should be given parenteral nutrition to provide full nutritional requirements.

7.3 Nutritional therapy reduces the risk of complications after surgery

A large and important study undertaken by the Veterans Hospitals in America[43] was undertaken to establish the role of pre-operative parenteral nutrition, but their results were interpreted as indicating a negative finding. The complexity of the patients studied confused the surgical community for some time. Their study included patients with normal nutritional status, mild malnutrition and severe malnutrition. Patients with normal nutritional status were disadvantaged by the pre-operative intravenous nutrition, because there were septic complications of the nutritional therapy. In patients with severe malnutrition, complications were reduced by the provision of parenteral nutrition. Careful consideration of their data clarified the place of nutritional care in the peri-operative period. Patients with normal nutritional status should not have their surgery delayed, but should be scheduled for surgery as soon as practical. However, patients with severe malnutrition would benefit significantly by a period of preoperative nutritional support. This demonstrates the importance of determining the nutritional status of patients before surgery to determine which protocol should be used.

In a randomised controlled study, Wu et al.[44] entered 468 patients who were malnourished as SGA B (300 patients) or C (168 patients) to receive peri-operative nutrition. The treatment protocol delivered nutrition to provide 24.6 kcal/kg/d and 1.5 g protein/kg/d for seven days before and seven days after surgery. The nutrition was given enterally in 32% of patients and parenterally in 68% of patients. The control group received isotonic intravenous dextrose solution and some amino acid infusion after surgery. About half of the patients had gastric cancer and half had colorectal cancer. The results demonstrate the importance of balanced nutritional therapy with significant differences in the post-operative complication rate

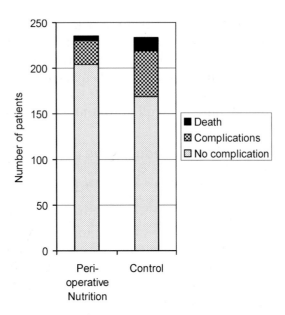

Figure 2. Results from Wu *et al.*[43] indicating reduced morbidity and mortality with peri-operative nutrition.

($P < 0.003$) and mortality rate ($P < 0.012$) (Fig. 2). Median hospital stay was 29 days in the control group and 22 days in the peri-operative nutrition group, indicating a significant economic advantage for the role of peri-operative nutrition. It is important to consider how this study of patients from Shanghai relates to the treatment of patients in Australia. In 1986, Katelaris *et al.*[45] demonstrated that 32% of patients presenting for major cancer surgery had three or more abnormal measures related to nutritional stress, and a recent study demonstrated 32 of 143 patients presenting to a general surgical ward were SGA B or C and had significantly increased odds of having complications of 2.4.[28] Therefore, 30% of patients are likely to be undernourished and should be considered for treatment.

7.4 Choosing the mode of post-operative nutritional support

There is a general rule that nutrition should be given through the gastrointestinal tract in preference to the intravenous route whenever possible. For this reason, fine bore tubes are very useful and can be placed at the time of surgery either through the nose or the abdominal wall to lie in the stomach or small bowel. A feeding jejunostomy can also be positioned into the jejunum at the end of an operation, providing a route for enteral nutrition directly into the small bowel. Because this is beyond the stomach it is unusual, although not impossible, to have vomiting when the jejunostomy is used to provide enteral nutrition. Many recommend the placement of jejunostomy tubes at the end of major operations, while the bowel is exposed, for convenience. Although feeding jejunostomies are preferred by many surgeons, they have been associated with specific complications and so their benefits are diminished for patients having straightforward surgical procedures. However, if a patient is expected to have a complicated course, a feeding jejunostomy may be very valuable and a problem-free means of providing nutrition. A recent randomised controlled study has demonstrated similar benefits for naso-jejunal tubes compared to surgically introduced fine bore jejunostomies after an oesophagectomy for carcinoma of the oesophagus.[35]

Peripheral parenteral nutrition has many benefits in the post-operative period. It has been shown to have a reduced incidence of sepsis compared with central parenteral nutrition.[46] It is simple to administer and does not require placement of risky central lines or uncomfortable nasal tubes or jejunostomies, which also carry risk. Furthermore, peripherally administered parenteral nutrition can provide sufficient nutrition to prevent the loss of muscle mass, which would otherwise occur with major surgery.[41,42] This work has been recently confirmed in patients undergoing oesophageal surgery, where there was evidence of reduced mortality in a small randomised trial.[47]

The surgeon has to make a judgement on which is the best method to provide nutrition for the individual case — see Table 4.

7.5   *Long term outcome in malnourished patients*

In an interesting study undertaken by Aslani *et al.*, the patient's nutritional status was measured before surgery and compared with the patient's survival. Nitrogen index (NI) was used to determine if a patient had a normal body protein store. Of 27 patients

Table 4. A comparison between jejunostomy feeding and parenteral intuition.

	Jejunostomy feeding	Parenteral nutrition
Requires functioning gut	Yes	No
Requires a separate procedure	Yes	No
Abdominal complications	5%	No
Peripheral sepsis	No	Yes
Complications treated by simple cessation of treatment	No	Yes

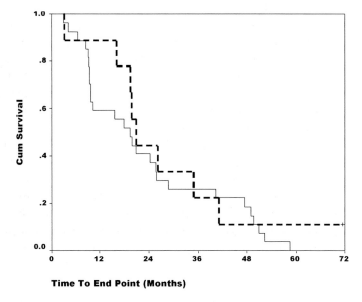

Figure 3. Kaplan-Meier survival curves for patients undergoing a Whipple's procedure with protein deficient patients with a low nitrogen index of <0.95 represented by dotted line and those with normal body protein represented by solid line.

undergoing a Whipple's procedure for pancreatic malignancy, 6 had low NI (<85% of expected value for height and weight). Some of these patients had values as low as 70% of the expected value, which is in the extreme level of protein deficiency. These six patients were able to undergo resection with nutritional support during the peri-operative period and had similar survival expectation to those with a normal NI at the time of surgery. Therefore it is important to first determine the resectability of the tumour, and if a patient has malnutrition, this can be treated to allow the surgery that is necessary to achieve the best patient outcomes. In other words, a poor nutritional state should not deny a patient the necessary surgery that may produce a good long term outcome (Aslani PhD thesis, University of Sydney).

8. Conclusion

Improvements in outcome following surgery for gastrointestinal neoplasms have been observed and are due to many factors. Traditional management has been challenged and now patients can expect to take nourishment up to a few hours before surgery, and to start drinking shortly after surgery when the operation has been uncomplicated. Early mobilisation, better pain management and home support systems use the skills of a number of different paramedical professionals but result in an earlier discharge and a more rapid return to independence. Treatment needs to be individualised in the more major surgical cases. We have learnt much about the nutritional management of these patients and it is important to identify the at risk patient and to utilise enteral nutrition or parenteral nutrition when indicated. Nutritional support will improve the morbidity and mortality arising from surgery in patients selected because they are in the high risk group. Long term outcome can be successful in malnourished patients if their neoplasm remains localised and surgically resectable.

References

1. A. Aslani and R. C. Smith, *In vivo* body composition in cancer and surgery, *Int. J. Body Compos. Res.* **2**(2): 83–90 (2004).
2. J. M. Muller, U. Brenner, C. Dienst and H. Pichlmaier, Preoperative parenteral feeding in patients with gastrointestinal carcinoma, *Lancet* **1**: 68–71 (1982).
3. S. E. Noblett, D. S. Watson, H. Huong, B. Davison, P. J. Hainsworth and A. F. Horgan, Pre-operative oral carbohydrate loading in colorectal surgery: A randomized controlled trial, *Colorectal Dis.* **8**: 563–569 (2006).
4. M. W. Wichmann, M. Roth, K. W. Jauch and C. J. Bruns, A prospective clinical feasibility study for multimodal "fast track" rehabilitation in elective pancreatic cancer surgery, *Rozhl. Chir.* **85**: 169–175 (2006).

5. P. O. Berberat, H. Ingold, A. Gulbinas, J. Kleeff, M. W. Muller, C. Gutt, M. Weigand, H. Friess and M. W. Buchler, Fast track — Different implications in pancreatic surgery, *J. Gastrointest. Surg.* **11**: 880–887 (2007).

6. O. Gralla, F. Haas, N. Knoll, D. Hadzidiakos, M. Tullmann, A. Romer, S. Deger, V. Ebeling, M. Lein, A. Wille, B. Rehberg, S. A. Loening and J. Roigas, Fast-track surgery in laparoscopic radical prostatectomy: Basic principles, *World J. Urol.* **25**: 185–191 (2007).

7. J. Hausel, J. Nygren, A. Thorell, M. Lagerkranser and O. Ljungqvist, Randomized clinical trial of the effects of oral preoperative carbohydrates on postoperative nausea and vomiting after laparoscopic cholecystectomy, *Br. J. Surg.* **92**: 415–421 (2005).

8. J. Nygren, A. Thorell, H. Jacobsson, S. Larsson, P. O. Schnell, L. Hylen and O. Ljungqvist, Preoperative gastric emptying. Effects of anxiety and oral carbohydrate administration, *Ann. Surg.* **222**: 728–734 (1995).

9. J. Hausel, J. Nygren, M. Lagerkranser, P. M. Hellstrom, F. Hammarqvist, C. Almstrom, A. Lindh, A. Thorell and O. Ljungqvist, A carbohydrate-rich drink reduces preoperative discomfort in elective surgery patients, *Anesth. Analg.* **93**: 1344–1350 (2001).

10. S. Fasting, E. Soreide and J. C. Raeder, Changing preoperative fasting policies. Impact of a national consensus, *Acta Anaesthesiol. Scand.* **42**: 1188–1191 (1998).

11. M. Svanfeldt, A. Thorell, J. Hausel, M. Soop, O. Rooyackers, J. Nygren and O. Ljungqvist, Randomized clinical trial of the effect of preoperative oral carbohydrate treatment on postoperative whole-body protein and glucose kinetics, *Br. J. Surg.* **94**: 1342–1350 (2007).

12. J. C. Santos Jr., J. Batista, M. T. Sirimarco, A. S. Guimaraes and C. E. Levy, Prospective randomized trial of mechanical bowel preparation in patients undergoing elective colorectal surgery, *Br. J. Surg.* **81**: 1673–1676 (1994).

13. C. E. Pineda, A. A. Shelton, T. Hernandez-Boussard, J. M. Morton and M. L. Welton, Mechanical bowel preparation in intestinal surgery: A meta-analysis and review of the literature, *J. Gastrointest. Surg.* **12**: 2037–2044 (2008).

14. Y. Kariv, W. Wang, A. J. Senagore, J. P. Hammel, V. W. Fazio and C. P. Delaney, Multivariable analysis of factors associated with hospital readmission after intestinal surgery, *Am. J. Surg.* **191**: 364–371 (2006).

15. L. Basse, J. D. Hjort, P. Billesbolle, M. Werner and H. Kehlet, A clinical pathway to accelerate recovery after colonic resection, *Ann. Surg.* **232**: 51–57 (2000).

16. I. J. Han-Geurts, W. C. Hop, N. F. Kok, A. Lim, K. J. Brouwer and J. Jeekel, Randomized clinical trial of the impact of early enteral feeding on postoperative ileus and recovery, *Br. J. Surg.* **94**: 555–561 (2007).

17. K. Lassen, J. Kjaeve, T. Fetveit, G. Trano, H. K. Sigurdsson, A. Horn and A. Revhaug, Allowing normal food at will after major upper gastrointestinal surgery does not increase morbidity: A randomized multicenter trial, *Ann. Surg.* **247**: 721–729 (2008).

18. W. L. Dills Jr., Nutritional and physiological consequences of tumour glycolysis, *Parasitology* **107**(Suppl.): S177–S186 (1993).

19. M. Kerem, Z. Ferahkose, U. T. Yilmaz, H. Pasaoglu, E. Ofluoglu, A. Bedirli, B. Salman, T. T. Sahin and M. Akin, Adipokines and ghrelin in gastric cancer cachexia, *World J. Gastroenterol.* **14**: 3633–3641 (2008).

20. S. S. Yeh, K. Blackwood and M. W. Schuster, The cytokine basis of cachexia and its treatment: Are they ready for prime time? *J. Am. Med. Dir. Assoc.* **9**: 219–236 (2008).

21. D. Zhang, Y. Zhou, L. Wu, S. Wang, H. Zheng, B. Yu and J. Li, Association of IL-6 gene polymorphisms with cachexia susceptibility and survival time of patients with pancreatic cancer, *Ann. Clin. Lab. Sci.* **38**: 113–119 (2008).

22. R. J. Skipworth and K. C. Fearon, The scientific rationale for optimizing nutritional support in cancer, *Eur. J. Gastroenterol. Hepatol.* **19**: 371–377 (2007).

23. G. Bovio, R. Bettaglio, G. Bonetti, D. Miotti and P. Verni, Evaluation of nutritional status and dietary intake in patients with advanced cancer on palliative care, *Minerva Gastroenterol. Dietol.* **54**: 243–250 (2008).

24. F. Bozzetti and on behalf of the SCRINIO Working Group, Screening the nutritional status in oncology: A preliminary report on 1,000 outpatients, *Support. Care Cancer* **17**: 279–284 (2009).

25. J. L. Mullen, G. P. Buzby, D. C. Matthews, B. F. Smale and E. F. Rosato, Reduction of operative morbidity and mortality by combined preoperative and postoperative nutritional support, *Ann. Surg.* **192**: 604–613 (1980).

26. U. G. Kyle, M. P. Kossovsky, V. L. Karsegard and C. Pichard, Comparison of tools for nutritional assessment and screening at hospital admission: A population study., *Clin. Nutr.* **25**: 409–417 (2006).

27. M. A. Kuzu, H. Terzioglu, V. Genc, A. B. Erkek, M. Ozban, P. Sonyurek, A. H. Elhan and N. Torun, Preoperative nutritional risk assessment in predicting postoperative outcome in patients undergoing major surgery, *World J. Surg.* **30**: 378–390 (2006).

28. R. C. Smith, J. P. Ledgard, G. Doig and D. Cheshire, An effective automated nutrition screen for hospitalised patients, *Nutrition* **25**: 309–315 (2009).
29. L. Brugler, A. K. Stankovic, M. Schlefer and L. Bernstein, A simplified nutrition screen for hospitalized patients using readily available laboratory and patient information, *Nutrition* **21**: 650–658 (2005).
30. M. Marin, M. Caro, A. Laviano and C. Pichard, Nutritional intervention and quality of life in adult oncology patients, *Clin. Nutr.* **26**: 289–301 (2007).
31. A. Weimann, M. Braga, L. Harsanyi, A. Laviano, O. Ljungqvist, P. Soeters, K. W. Jauch, M. Kemen, J. M. Hiesmayr, T. Horbach, E. R. Kuse and K. H. Vestweber, ESPEN guidelines on enteral nutrition: Surgery including organ transplantation, *Clin. Nutr.* **25**: 224–244 (2006).
32. Y. Kariv, C. P. Delaney, A. J. Senagore, E. A. Manilich, J. P. Hammel, J. M. Church, J. Ravas and V. W. Fazio, Clinical outcomes and cost analysis of a "fast track" postoperative care pathway for ileal pouch-anal anastomosis: A case control study, *Dis. Colon Rectum* **50**: 137–146 (2007).
33. A. Weimann, M. Braga, L. Harsanyi, A. Laviano, O. Ljungqvist, P. Soeters, K. W. Jauch, M. Kemen, J. M. Hiesmayr, T. Horbach, E. R. Kuse and K. H. Vestweber, ESPEN Guidelines on Enteral Nutrition: Surgery including organ transplantation, *Clin. Nutr.* **25**: 224–244 (2006).
34. K. F. Chin, S. Townsend, W. Wong and G. V. Miller, A prospective cohort study of feeding needle catheter jejunostomy in an upper gastrointestinal surgical unit, *Clin. Nutr.* **23**: 691–696 (2004).
35. I. J. Han-Geurts, W. C. Hop, C. Verhoef, K. T. Tran and H. W. Tilanus, Randomized clinical trial comparing feeding jejunostomy with naso-duodenal tube placement in patients undergoing oesophagectomy, *Br. J. Surg.* **94**: 31–35 (2007).
36. R. S. Date, W. D. Clements and R. Gilliland, Feeding jejunostomy: Is there enough evidence to justify its routine use?, *Dig. Surg.* **21**: 142–145 (2004).
37. T. Mazaki and K. Ebisawa, Enteral versus parenteral nutrition after gastrointestinal surgery: A systematic review and meta-analysis of randomized controlled trials in the English literature, *J. Gastrointest. Surg.* **12**: 739–755 (2008).

38. R. C. Smith and R. Hartemink, Improvement of nutritional measures during preoperative parenteral nutrition in patients selected by the prognostic nutritional index: A randomized controlled trial, *J. Parenter. Enteral. Nutr.* **12**: 587–591 (1988).

39. D. K. Heyland, M. Montalvo, S. MacDonald, L. Keefe, X. Y. Su and J. W. Drover, Total parenteral nutrition in the surgical patient: A meta-analysis, *Can. J. Surg.* **44**: 102–111 (2001).

40. S. R. Kohlhardt, R. C. Smith, C. R. Wright and K. A. Sucic, Fine-bore peripheral catheters versus central venous catheters for delivery of intravenous nutrition, *Nutrition* **8**: 412–417 (1992).

41. S. M. Barratt, R. C. Smith, A. J. Kee, L. E. Mather and M. J. Cousins, Multimodal analgesia and intravenous nutrition preserves total body protein following major upper gastrointestinal surgery, *Reg. Anesth. Pain Med.* **27**: 15–22 (2002).

42. A. Sevette, R. C. Smith, A. Aslani, A. J. Kee, R. Hansen, S. M. Barratt and R. C. Baxter, Does growth hormone allow more efficient nitrogen sparing in postoperative patients requiring parenteral nutrition? A double-blind, placebo-controlled randomised trial, *Clin. Nutr.* **24**: 943–955 (2005).

43. The Veterans Affairs Total Parenteral Nutrition Cooperative Study Group, Perioperative total parenteral nutrition in surgical patients, *N. Engl. J. Med.* **325**: 525–532 (1991).

44. G. H. Wu, Z. H. Liu, Z. H. Wu and Z. G. Wu, Perioperative artificial nutrition in malnourished gastrointestinal cancer patients, *World J. Gastroenterol.* **12**: 2441–2444 (2006).

45. P. H. Katelaris, G. B. Bennett and R. C. Smith, Prediction of post-operative complications by clinical and nutritional assessment, *Aust. NZ. J. Surg.* **56**: 743–747 (1986).

46. S. R. Kohlhardt, R. C. Smith and C. R. Wright, Peripheral versus central intravenous nutrition: Comparison of two delivery systems, *Br. J. Surg.* **81**: 66–70 (1994).

47. S. C. Cooper, C. M. Hulley, C. E. Grimley, J. Howden, K. McCluskey, R. N. Norton and C. U. Nwokolo, Perioperative peripheral parenteral nutrition for patients undergoing esophagectomy for cancer: A pilot study of safety, surgical, and nutritional outcomes, *Int. Surg.* **91**: 358–364 (2006).

19

Management Challenges Following Rectal Cancer Treatment

Margaret Schnitzler

Abstract

The treatment of rectal carcinoma is usually multidisciplinary, involving surgery, radiation therapy and chemotherapy. Appropriate surgical technique to ensure adequate mesorectal excision and clear margins provides the best prospect for cure and prevention of local recurrence. Adjuvant chemoradiotherapy is effective in reducing local recurrence, and where indicated by accurate staging, is usually given pre-operatively.

There may be significant physical and psychological consequences after treatment of rectal carcinoma. Bowel function is altered in the majority of patients after rectal resection, with increased stool frequency, urgency and incontinence commonly experienced. These symptoms are more likely in patients who are treated with radiotherapy, either pre or post-operatively. Many patients also experience impairment of urinary function and sexual dysfunction. Some patients will require a stoma, which may be temporary or permanent. This can be associated with complications and may have effects on body image and sexual function.

Local recurrence occurs in a proportion of patients despite optimal surgery and adjuvant therapy, and is a cause of considerable morbidity. In selected patients, aggressive surgical treatment of local recurrence can achieve cure.

Keywords: Rectal cancer, psychological consequences, bowel function, sexual dysfunction, stoma.

1.   Background

The current management of rectal carcinoma usually involves multiple treatment modalities, namely surgery, radiotherapy and chemotherapy. Patients often experience significant alterations in bowel function after treatment, and many will require a temporary or permanent stoma. Following treatment there may also be effects on sexual function, body image and quality of life. Even though the patient is be cured of the carcinoma, the effects of treatment may be life-long, and require input from clinicians in various disciplines.

2.   Treatment of Rectal Carcinoma

2.1   *Pre-operative radiation and chemotherapy*

Improvements in pre-operative staging have made it possible to select patients who are most likely to benefit from pre-operative radiation and chemotherapy. Endorectal ultrasound and magnetic resonance imaging allow for accurate determination of the local extent of the tumour, and can also identify node positive disease in many patients.[1] While acknowledging that there are false positives and negatives with all staging modalities, it is desirable to stage the tumour as accurately as possible in order to select patients who are likely to benefit from pre-operative therapy. There are advantages in providing pre-operative rather than post-operative adjuvant therapy in terms of improved local control and reduced toxicity.[2–4] Both long course (usually 50G in 25 fractions) and short course (25G in 5 fractions) radiotherapy have been evaluated in the treatment of rectal carcinoma.[5] The addition of chemotherapy has also been shown to have benefits in terms of reducing the rate of local recurrence in patients with stage T3 or T4 rectal cancer, whether given pre-operatively or post-operatively.[6]

It has been demonstrated that pre-operative radiotherapy significantly reduces the rate of local recurrence after surgical treatment with total mesorectal excision (TME), even though recurrence rates with TME are substantially lower than those achieved with non-TME surgery.[7] The benefit of such therapy is greatest in those with more advanced disease, while in patients with early stage rectal carcinoma, surgical treatment alone can provide high rates of local control and cure.[8] However even in more advanced or node-positive disease, high-quality standardised surgery can provide acceptably low rates of local recurrence.[9] In view of this, the benefits of chemoradiotherapy must be balanced with its side-effects and morbidity, so that patients can make informed decisions about their treatment.

2.2 *Surgery*

Surgery remains the mainstay of rectal cancer treatment and the quality of the surgery has a larger effect on local recurrence rates than any other factor. Pathological studies of the pattern of nodal spread have highlighted the importance of achieving clear circumferential margins.[10] This knowledge, combined with improved understanding of the fascial planes around the rectum led to the development of total mesorectal excision.[11] Although the nuances of surgical technique are still debated in the literature, it is clear that surgery that removes the rectum with an adequate amount of attached mesorectum and clear circumferential resection margins will result in lower rates of local recurrence than surgery that does not achieve these outcomes.[8,12] The consequence of this more complex surgery is that the level of anastomosis is often low, with a resultant increase in post-operative complications in some studies.[8,13] A majority of patients will have a defunctioning temporary loop ileostomy after a low rectal anastomosis, and this is also associated with specific complications, particularly after stoma closure.[14,15]

The rate of permanent colostomy formation associated with abdominoperineal resection (APR) of the rectum has declined as advances in surgical technique have facilitated lower rectal anastomoses and rates of permanent colostomy formation of 12 to 15% are achievable.[16,17] In most experienced surgical units, APR is necessary only if the tumour involves or abuts the anal sphincter. It is usually possible to perform a low or ultra-low anastomosis and achieve a restorative resection. Such low resections are achieved at the cost of an increased rate of anastomotic leakage, and more significant alterations in bowel function.[8,18] Various surgical techniques have been developed in an attempt to reduce these adverse consequences, including the formation of a colonic pouch or coloplasty procedure.[19,20]

Local excision of rectal carcinoma has a small role in curative treatment of this disease. In early stage tumours with no adverse histological features, acceptable rates of local control and cure have been reported, although in some series high rates of local recurrence and reduced overall survival have been described.[21,22] Local excision may be combined with radiotherapy in certain patients.[22]

2.3 Post-operative radiotherapy

There has been a trend towards pre-operative radiotherapy as discussed in Sec. 2.1 because it is associated with a reduced incidence of functional consequences, and because patients are more likely to complete the course of treatment if this is given pre-operatively.[4] Studies of post-operative radiotherapy have confirmed that it is effective in reducing local recurrence rates.[23,24] Even with the best pre-operative staging there will be patients in whom advanced local disease or involved lymph nodes may not be accurately identified, and they are treated with surgery alone. In these groups there is still a role for post-operative radiation therapy.

2.4 Post-operative chemotherapy

Patients with node-positive colonic carcinoma have improved survival with adjuvant chemotherapy, but the evidence for a similar benefit in patients with rectal carcinoma is less clear. Adjuvant chemotherapy is associated with improved local control after rectal cancer surgery, but improved disease-free survival has not been convincingly established.[6,25] In patients with stage II disease, it has been shown that adjuvant fluorouracil-based therapy improves local control and survival after rectal cancer surgery, although the absolute benefits of this treatment are small.[26]

3. Effects of Treatment

3.1 *Bowel function*

Rectal cancer treatment has the potential to significantly alter bowel function. The functional consequences are thought to be due to a combination of factors including loss of the rectal reservoir, shortened colonic transit time, reduction in the anorectal pressure gradient and sensory changes. The effects are more pronounced with low or ultra-low resections, especially if the anastomosis is in the anal canal or handsewn rather than stapled.[18,27]

The term 'anterior resection syndrome' has been used to describe the constellation of symptoms that may be experienced by patients who have had rectal resection.[28] These include increased stool frequency, urgency, stool clustering and faecal incontinence.

Particularly in the early weeks and months after surgery, these symptoms may be distressing and result in impaired quality of life.[29,30] Symptoms are often particularly troublesome in patients undergoing post-operative chemotherapy, when loose stools exacerbate the problems of frequency, urgency and incontinence.

Temple and colleagues have developed a validated instrument to evaluate bowel function after sphincter-preserving surgery for rectal cancer.[18] They analysed data from 127 patients and found that only 50% were satisfied with their bowel function. The majority of patients reported incomplete evacuation, stool clustering, loose stool and flatus incontinence at a mean time of 28 months post-operatively. The median number of bowel movements was 3.5 per day. Symptoms were more pronounced in those who were irradiated and those who had a coloanal anastomosis, particularly if this was handsewn.

Improvements in bowel function can be expected for up to two years after completion of therapy, but many patients continue to experience problems throughout their lives.[31] In an attempt to reduce the functional effects of rectal surgery, surgical techniques such as the colonic pouch and coloplasty have been developed. Formation of a colonic J-pouch has been shown to significantly reduce stool frequency, nocturnal defaecation and the need for anti-diarrhoeal medications.[20,32] However, it may be technically difficult to create a satisfactory pouch, particularly in patients with a thick short mesocolon or a narrow pelvis. The technique of coloplasty was developed in attempt to overcome these problems.[19] This involves a linear colotomy which is closed transversely, allowing an increase in capacity of the neo-rectum, without the need for pouch formation. Both pouch creation and coloplasty techniques appear to result in a similar improvement in bowel function when compared with straight anastomosis after low anterior resection.[32,33]

3.1.1 Management of bowel dysfunction

Early post-operative bowel dysfunction can be improved by measures which improve stool consistency, delay transit time and reduce urgency. Diet plays a role, but there is considerable individual variability in this regard. Many patients are able to identify particular foods which worsen their bowel function and to avoid them. The use of a fibre supplement such as psyllium is sometimes helpful by improving stool bulk and reducing the tendency for stools to be loose.[34] Loperamide is very effective in many patients, as it significantly reduces transit time and decreases the urgency which is often a major concern.[35,36]

In some cases, particularly when a colonic pouch has been created, patients may experience difficultly in emptying the rectum. The use of a glycerol suppository or self-administered enema is often beneficial in this situation.

3.1.2 Management of incontinence

As outlined above, it is important to ensure that the stool consistency is not too loose as this will exacerbate incontinence. Loperamide helps to improve continence, both by its effects on colonic transit and also because of a small direct effect on the anal sphincter.[35] Formal assessment of continence with anorectal physiology studies can identify patients who might benefit from biofeedback therapy, although this has not been formally evaluated in patients who have had rectal cancer therapy. There are reports of improvement in continence with the use of sacral nerve stimulation in a small number of patients with faecal incontinence after anterior resection.[37,38]

3.2 Stomas

Formation of a stoma, either temporary or permanent, is frequently required in the management of rectal carcinoma. This is often a source of anxiety and distress for the patient, and the involvement of a stomal therapist is an essential component of education, management and support.

3.2.1 Defunctioning loop ileostomy

A loop ileostomy is often formed at the time of anterior resection. Performance of a defunctioning stoma significantly reduces the rate of symptomatic or clinically relevant anastomotic leakage after low anterior resection.[39,40] Despite this benefit, the closure itself is associated with a significant incidence of complications, in particular small bowel obstruction, anastomotic leak and wound infection.[14,15,41] It is usual for closure to be carried out several weeks or months after rectal surgery, although it has been shown that closure can be performed in the early post-operative period with acceptable morbidity.[42,43] The risk of complications such as small bowel obstruction is increased if ileostomy closure is performed less than two months post-operatively.[14] However it is known that the presence of a temporary loop ileostomy has a detrimental effect on quality of life, particularly in regard to physical and role function, so patients are often keen to have the stoma closed as early as possible.[44,45] The timing of stoma closure may be affected in patients who are receiving chemotherapy, and overall is delayed as compared with patients who do not have post-operative therapy.[41] In some patients closure is deferred until after chemotherapy is completed (i.e. more than six months after surgery), or alternatively a break in treatment is scheduled to allow for the procedure to be performed. This can be a difficult period for the patient who must adjust to the likely alteration in bowel function exacerbated by loose stools and other possible side effects of chemotherapy.

Incontinence can be a particularly distressing symptom, having a significant adverse effect on overall quality of life, as well as social and sexual function. It is important to determine the pre-operative continence of the patient, as those who already have some impairment are likely to experience worsening of their symptoms after rectal cancer treatment. The pre-treatment continence of the patient can be a factor which influences the choice of therapy, particularly with regards to the performance of a low anastomosis, which may be associated with poor post-operative function. Consideration should be given to the performance of an abdominoperineal resection in these patients, as quality of life is adversely affected by faecal incontinence after rectal cancer treatment.[30]

3.2.2   Permanent colostomy

For many patients diagnosed with carcinoma of the rectum, the possible need for a permanent colostomy is a major concern. Several studies have demonstrated that patients treated with APR experience negative effects on body image and sexual function.[46–48] Guren and colleagues compared 90 patients who had undergone APR with 229 who had a low rectal resection and found that quality of life was better preserved in patients who had undergone anterior resection, despite the fact that bowel function was worse in this group.[48]

Other studies have found no difference in quality of life between patients treated with APR or anterior resection,[46] and some have concluded that there is worse quality of life after anterior resection because of disordered bowel function and impaired social functioning.[49] A recent meta-analysis of outcomes for 1443 patients found no significant differences in the general quality of life or global health scores between those treated with APR and those who had a restorative resection.[50] While the choice of surgical procedure will depend on many elements, including tumour location, technical factors and patient preference, it seems likely that overall quality of life is good regardless of whether a permanent stoma is performed and patients can be reassured by this information.

3.3   Radiotherapy effects

The benefit of a reduction in local control comes at the cost of substantial functional consequences after radiotherapy for rectal cancer. These effects are more pronounced in patients treated with post-operative radiotherapy, presumably due at least in part to the fact that irradiated colon is used to create the neorectum.[51] Radiation therapy is associated with significant long term impairment of function, as well as manometric and ultrasound evidence of sphincter dysfunction.[52,53] Prolonged pudendal nerve terminal motor latency has been demonstrated in patients treated with pre-operative radiotherapy in a dose of 45G, and this may also contribute to disturbances in bowel function and continence.[54] In a follow-up to the Dutch rectal cancer study of pre-operative short course radiotherapy and TME, 597 patients completed a questionnaire about their bowel function. There was a significantly greater incidence of faecal incontinence (62% vs. 38%) in the irradiated group, and these patients reported reduced satisfaction with their bowel function.[55]

Similar findings were obtained from a detailed long term study of sixty-four patients randomised to either low anterior resection only or in combination with short course pre-operative radiotherapy in the Stockholm trial. There was a significant increase in the incidence of faecal incontinence (57 vs. 26%), flatus incontinence (71 vs. 46%) and stool frequency (20 vs. 10%) in the irradiated group. In addition these patients had significantly lower resting and squeeze anal pressure manometrically, and more scarring of the anal sphincters. The patients were studied at a mean time of 14 years after treatment, indicating that these effects on the anal sphincter are likely to be permanent.[53]

An increased incidence of small bowel obstruction has been identified in patients treated with post-operative radiotherapy, when compared with those who had pre-operative treatment.[56] In a long term follow-up of patients treated in the Stockholm rectal cancer trials, there was an increased incidence of cardiovascular disease in the patients who were irradiated pre-operatively, although the number of patients with vascular complications within the pelvis or lower limbs was too small for meaningful analysis.[57]

3.4   *Sexual function*

It is important to assess the patient's sexual function prior to therapy for rectal cancer, so that they can be counseled appropriately about the possible consequences of treatment, and also because the patient's feelings about this issue may influence their choice of treatment.

Rectal cancer treatment can affect sexual function adversely in many ways, due to a combination of physical and psychological factors. Surgery and radiotherapy can result in impotence or retrograde ejaculation in men, although it is important to note that these problems may exist prior to treatment. In a detailed questionnaire survey of 99 men, Hendren *et al.* found that 19% of men had some degree of erectile dysfunction pre-operatively, compared with 54% after treatment. Ejaculatory disorders were reported by 10% pre-operatively and 43% post-operatively.[58] Breukink and colleagues objectively assessed male sexual function before and after laparoscopic total mesorectal excision and short course radiotherapy, and found that there was a significant deterioration in erectile function and intercourse satisfaction after treatment.[59] When compared with surgery alone, the addition of short-course pre-operative radiotherapy significantly worsens sexual function in both men and women.[60] Unfortunately, problems with sexual function do not improve and may actually deteriorate over time.[60,61]

Referral to a urologist with expertise in the management of sexual dysfunction is appropriate, so that the patient receives thorough evaluation and advice. There are numerous treatment options available for the management of impotence, but few have been specifically evaluated in patients who have had rectal cancer. One randomised controlled trial examined the use of sildenafil (Viagra) in patients who had undergone rectal resection and found that it improved erectile dysfunction in 79% of men.[62]

While female sexual dysfunction after rectal surgery has been less well-studied, almost one third of a group of 81 women surveyed at a median of 52 months post-operatively said that surgery made their sexual lives worse.[58] These investigators found evidence of reduced arousal, decreased orgasms and dyspareunia in a substantial proportion of women after rectal cancer surgery.

As discussed above, the presence of a stoma, whether temporary or permanent, is known to impair sexual function in both males and females.[47]

3.5   *Fertility*

In view of the age distribution of rectal carcinoma, the effect of treatment on fertility is not a major concern for most patients. For younger women and some men of any age, however, the effects of surgery, chemotherapy and radiotherapy on fertility are important considerations. It seems likely that issues of fertility are not adequately discussed with patients prior to treatment, suggesting that clinicians lack awareness of the importance of this matter.[62] Involvement of obstetricians and gynaecologists with expertise in the field should be considered prior to treatment so that patients receive advice about options for preserving fertility. Pelvic radiotherapy is likely to result in ovarian failure and premature menopause in women, and there is also evidence that rectal surgery for benign disease adversely affects fertility.[64,65] Options such as ovarian transposition, embryo cryop-reservation and ovarian cryopreservation may be used to provide the option of future fertility after treatment.[66,67]

There is also evidence that irradiation for rectal carcinoma can result in permanent testicular dysfunction, as indicated by reduced levels of testosterone and increased gonadotropins compared to men who were treated with surgery alone.[68]

3.6   *Urinary function*

Alterations in urinary function are common after rectal cancer treatment. Symptoms such as poor flow, urinary frequency, emptying difficulty and incontinence are reported and are associated with impaired social functioning.[29] In a large study of 785 patients surveyed after treatment for rectal cancer with TME with or without pre-operative short-course radiotherapy, there was a significant rate of post-treatment urinary dysfunction.[68] Nearly 40% of patients reported urinary incontinence and 30% had difficulty with bladder emptying after surgery, although some patients had these symptoms pre-operatively. Women were more likely to develop incontinence, while difficulty emptying was more likely to occur in patients who had peri-operative blood loss, or recognised autonomic nerve injury. In this study, radiotherapy was not associated with an increased risk of urinary dysfunction, but others have found a significantly higher rate of urinary incontinence in those who had pre-operative short course radiotherapy (45% vs. 27% in those who had surgery alone).[57] It has been consistently found that urinary dysfunction persists over time, and in fact is likely to worsen, particularly in women, presumably due to age-related factors.

3.7 Quality of life

It is apparent from the above that treatment for rectal carcinoma can have major effects on various aspects of physical functioning. Many of these factors have been examined in isolation, but it is perhaps more important to assess the effect of treatment on overall quality of life. In the early post-operative period of up to three months, most measurements of quality of life show a drop below baseline levels.[61,70] Over time, however, quality of life improves and in many domains returns to pre-treatment levels, comparable to that of the general population.[29,60] Social functioning is impaired in patients with bowel or urinary dysfunction.[29] There is also some evidence to suggest that women are more likely than men to experience impaired physical functioning and reduced global health.[70,71] Global quality of life and physical functioning are also worse in those over the age of 70 than in younger patients.[71,72]

4. Local Recurrence

A major aim of neoadjuvant therapy and surgery for rectal carcinoma is the prevention of local recurrence. Even in some recently published series, local recurrence rates in the order of 40% have been reported,[73] and in a review of more than 10,000 patients treated with surgery alone, the median local recurrence rate was 18.5%.[74] In some of the early multi-centre trials of adjuvant radiotherapy, local recurrence rates of more than 20% were reported in the surgery alone groups.[3] These studies have been criticised because optimal treatment, particularly in relation to surgical technique, can result in local recurrence rates of less than 5%.[8,12] A number of factors are known to be associated with an increased risk of local recurrence. These include anastomotic leakage, abdominoperineal, rather than anterior resection, low level of the tumour or anastomosis and involved resection margins.[10,75–78]

4.1 Diagnosis

Approximately 50% of patients who present with locally recurrent disease do so within two years of their original surgery, but recurrences may present up to many years later.[79] The majority of patients have pain at the time of diagnosis, and this is a poor prognostic factor.[79,80] In those who have had anterior resection, other symptoms include alteration in bowel habit and rectal bleeding, while patients who have had abdominoperineal resection are more likely to present with pain or an elevated carcino-embryonic antigen.[81] Rarely the tumour fungates through the anus, or involves the perianal skin. Anastomotic recurrence may be detected at the pre-symptomatic stage by routine clinical examination, while extra-luminal recurrence is detected on imaging studies. The outcome of resectional surgery is better in those patients whose recurrence is detected at the pre-symptomatic stage.[79,80] In approximately 50% of cases, the recurrence is localised, while in the remainder it is associated with distant metastatic disease.[74] Positron emission tomography (PET) has a useful role in detecting distant or unresectable disease and thus in preventing inappropriate surgery.[82]

4.2   Treatment

The development of local recurrence is a poor prognostic feature, but in selected patients further treatment can result in excellent palliation or cure. Pre-operative radiotherapy may improve survival but may not be feasible, depending on previous radiation treatment.[80] Intra-operative radiotherapy has been used to overcome the dose-limitation problems of external beam therapy in some patients.[79] The addition of chemotherapy to pre-operative radiotherapy improves local control and survival in this group of patients.[83] In well-selected groups of patients, more than 75% of those undergoing operation are able to have the recurrence resected.[79,81,84] The achievement of microscopically clear margins of resection is a significant prognostic factor, and is possible in 45–82% of patients.[79,84,85] Surgical treatment usually involves abdomino-perineal resection and, depending on the nature and extent of the recurrence, *en bloc* resection of other structures including bladder, prostate, vagina and sacrum. The morbidity of this major surgery is considerable but if microscopically clear margins are achieved, long term disease-free survival rates of 20–35% can be expected.[79,81,84–86]

5. Conclusion

Significant physical and psychological consequences can occur after treatment of rectal carcinoma. Alterations in bowel function, impairment of urinary function and sexual dysfunction can occur, and the need for a stoma in some patients can be associated with complications and may have effects on body image and sexual function.

Local recurrence occurs in a proportion of patients with rectal cancer, despite optimal surgery and adjuvant therapy, and is a cause of considerable morbidity. With multidisciplinary collaboration between surgeons, radiation oncologists and medical oncologists cure can be achieved in selected patients with local recurrences.

References

1. N. K. Kim, M. J. Kim, J. K. Park, S. I. Park and J. S. Min, Preoperative staging of rectal cancer with MRI: Accuracy and clinical usefulness, *Ann. Surg. Oncol.* **7**(10): 732–737 (2000).
2. L. Påhlman and B. Glimelius, Pre- or postoperative radiotherapy in rectal and rectosigmoid carcinoma. Report from a randomized multi-center trial, *Ann. Surg.* **211**(2): 187–195 (1990).
3. G. J. Frykholm, B. Glimelius and L. Påhlman, Preoperative or postoperative irradiation in adenocarcinoma of the rectum: Final treatment results of a randomized trial and an evaluation of late secondary effects, *Dis. Colon Rectum* **36**(6): 564–572 (1993).
4. R. Sauer, H. Becker, W. Hohenberger, C. Rödel, C. Wittekind, R. Fietkau, P. Martus, J. Tschmelitsch, E. Hager, G. F. Hess, J. H. Karstens, T. Liersch, H. Schmidberger and R. Raab, German Rectal Cancer Study Group. Preoperative versus postoperative chemoradiotherapy for rectal cancer, *N. Engl. J. Med.* **351**(17): 1731–1740 (2004).
5. C. Ortholan, E. Francois, O. Thomas, D. Benchimol, J. Baulieux, J. F. Bosset and J. P. Gerard, Role of radiotherapy with surgery for T3 and resectable T4 rectal cancer: Evidence from randomized trials, *Dis. Colon Rectum* **49**(3): 302–310 (2006).
6. J. F. Bosset, L. Collette, G. Calais, L. Mineur, P. Maingon, L. Radosevic-Jelic, A. Daban, E. Bardet, A. Beny and J. C. Ollier, EORTC Radiotherapy Group Trial 22921. Chemotherapy with preoperative radiotherapy in rectal cancer, *N. Engl. J. Med.* **355**(11): 1114–1123 (2006).

7. E. Kapiteijn, C. A. Marijnen, I. D. Nagtegaal, H. Putter, W. H. Steup, T. Wiggers, H. J. Rutten, L. Pahlman, B. Glimelius, J. H. van Krieken, J. W. Leer and C. J. van de Velde, Dutch Colorectal Cancer Group. Preoperative radiotherapy combined with total mesorectal excision for resectable rectal cancer, *N. Engl. J. Med.* **345**(9): 638–646 (2001).

8. W. L. Law and K. W. Chu, Anterior resection for rectal cancer with mesorectal excision: A prospective evaluation of 622 patients, *Ann. Surg.* **240**(2): 260–268 (2004).

9. T. D. Cecil, R. Sexton, B. J. Moran and R. J. Heald, Total mesorectal excision results in low local recurrence rates in lymph node-positive rectal cancer, *Dis. Colon Rectum* **47**(7): 1145–1149 (2004).

10. K. F. Birbeck, C. P. Macklin, N. J. Tiffin, W. Parsons, M. F. Dixon, N. P. Mapstone, C. R. Abbott, N. Scott, P. J. Finan, D. Johnston and P. Quirke, Rates of circumferential resection margin involvement vary between surgeons and predict outcomes in rectal cancer surgery, *Ann. Surg.* **235**(4): 449–457 (2002).

11. J. K. MacFarlane, R. D. Ryall and R. J. Heald, Mesorectal excision for rectal cancer, *Lancet* **341**(8843): 457–460 (1993).

12. R. J. Heald, B. J. Moran, R. D. Ryall, R. Sexton and J. K. MacFarlane, Rectal cancer: The Basingstoke experience of total mesorectal excision, 1978–1997, *Arch. Surg.* **133**(8): 894–899 (1998).

13. C. Laurent, S. Nobili, A. Rullier, V. Vendrely, J. Saric and E. Rullier, Efforts to improve local control in rectal cancer compromise survival by the potential morbidity of optimal mesorectal excision, *J. Am. Coll. Surg.* **203**(5): 684–691 (2006).

14. R. O. Perez, A. Habr-Gama, V. E. Seid, I. Proscurshim, A. H. Sousa Jr., D. R. Kiss, M. Linhares, M. Sapucahy and J. Gama-Rodrigues, Loop ileostomy morbidity: Timing of closure matters, *Dis. Colon Rectum* **49**(10): 1539–1545 (2006).

15. A. Thalheimer, M. Bueter, M. Kortuem, A. Thiede and D. Meyer, Morbidity of temporary loop ileostomy in patients with colorectal cancer, *Dis. Colon Rectum* **49**(7): 1011–1017 (2006).

16. E. W. Chuwa and F. Seow-Choen, Outcomes for abdominoperineal resections are not worse than those of anterior resections, *Dis. Colon Rectum* **49**(1): 41–49 (2006).

17. S. B. Lim, S. C. Heo, M. R. Lee, S. B. Kang, Y. J. Park, K. J. Park, H. S. Choi, S. Y. Jeong and J. G. Park, Changes in outcome with sphincter preserving surgery for rectal cancer in Korea, 1991–2000, *Eur. J. Surg. Oncol.* **31**(3): 242–249 (2005).

18. L. K. Temple, J. Bacik, S. G. Savatta, L. Gottesman, P. B. Paty, M. R. Weiser, J. G. Guillem, B. D. Minsky, M. Kalman, H. T. Thaler, D. Schrag and W. D. Wong, The development of a validated instrument to evaluate bowel function after sphincter-preserving surgery for rectal cancer, *Dis. Colon Rectum* **48**: 1353–1365 (2005).

19. C. R. Mantyh, T. L. Hull and V. W. Fazio, Coloplasty in low colorectal anastomosis: Manometric and functional comparison with straight and colonic J-pouch anastomosis. *Dis. Colon Rectum* **44**(1): 37–42 (2001).

20. N. Dehni, E. Tiret, J. D. Singland, C. Cunningham, R. D. Schlegel, M. Guiguet and R. Parc, Long-term functional outcome after low anterior resection: Comparison of low colorectal anastomosis and colonic J-pouch-anal anastomosis, *Dis. Colon Rectum* **41**(7): 817–822 (1998).

21. A. Mellgren, J. Goldberg and D. A. Rothenberger, Local excision: Some reality testing, *Surg. Oncol. Clin. N. Am.* **14**(2): 183–196 (2005).

22. J. A. Greenberg, D. Shibata, J. E. Herndon 2nd, G. D. Steele Jr., R. Mayer and R. Bleday, Local excision of distal rectal cancer: An update of cancer and leukemia group B 8984, *Dis. Colon Rectum* **51**(8): 1185–1191 (2008).

23. N. Wolmark, H. S. Wieand, D. M. Hyams, L. Colangelo, N. V. Dimitrov, E. H. Romond, M. Wexler, D. Prager, A. B. Cruz Jr., P. H. Gordon, N. J. Petrelli, M. Deutsch, E. Mamounas, D. L. Wickerham, E. R. Fisher, H. Rockette and B. Fisher, Randomized trial of postoperative adjuvant chemotherapy with or without radiotherapy for carcinoma of the rectum: National Surgical Adjuvant Breast and Bowel Project Protocol R-02, *J. Natl. Cancer Inst.* **92**(5): 388–396 (2000).

24. Colorectal Cancer Collaborative Group, Adjuvant radiotherapy for rectal cancer: A systematic overview of 8,507 patients from 22 randomised trials, *Lancet* **358**(9290): 1291–1304 (2001).

25. M. Braendengen, K. M. Tveit, A. Berglund, E. Birkemeyer, G. Frykholm, L. Påhlman, J. N. Wiig, P. Byström, K. Bujko and B. Glimelius, Randomized phase III study comparing preoperative radiotherapy with chemoradiotherapy in nonresectable rectal cancer, *J. Clin. Oncol.* **26**(22): 3687–3694 (2008).

26. Quasar Collaborative Group, R. Gray, J. Barnwell, C. McConkey, R. K. Hills, N. S. Williams and D. J. Kerr, Adjuvant chemotherapy versus observation in patients with colorectal cancer: A randomised study, *Lancet* **370**(9604): 2020–2029 (2007).

27. N. D. Karanjia, D. J. Schache and R. J. Heald, Function of the distal rectum after low anterior resection for carcinoma, *Br. J. Surg.* **79**(2): 114–116 (1992).
28. M. E. Williamson, W. G. Lewis, P. J. Holdsworth, P. J. Finan and D. Johnston, Decrease in the anorectal pressure gradient after low anterior resection of the rectum. A study using continuous ambulatory manometry, *Dis. Colon Rectum* **37**(12): 1228–1231 (1994).
29. J. H. Vironen, M. Karialuoma, A.-M. Aalto and I. H. Kellokumpu, Impact of functional resuls on quality of life after rectal cancer surgery, *Dis. Colon Rectum* **49**: 568–578 (2006).
30. A. Murata, C. J. Brown, M. Raval and P. T. Phang, Impact of short-course radiotherapy and low anterior resection on quality of life and bowel function in primary rectal cancer, *Am. J. Surg.* **195**(5): 611–615 (2008).
31. M. E. Williamson, W. G. Lewis, P. J. Finan, A. S. Miller, P. J. Holdsworth and D. Johnston, Recovery of physiologic and clinical function after low anterior resection of the rectum for carcinoma: Myth or reality? *Dis. Colon Rectum* **38**(4): 411–418 (1995).
32. F. H. Remzi, V. W. Fazio, E. Gorgun, M. Zutshi, J. M. Church, I. C. Lavery and T. L. Hull, Quality of life, functional outcome, and complications of coloplasty pouch after low anterior resection, *Dis. Colon Rectum* **48**(4): 735–743 (2005).
33. C. J. Brown, D. S. Fenech and R. S. McLeod, Reconstructive techniques after rectal resection for rectal cancer, *Cochrane Database Syst. Rev.* **16**(2): CD006040 (2008).
34. D. Z. Bliss, H. J. Jung, K. Savik, A. Lowry, M. LeMoine, L. Jensen, C. Werner and K. Schaffer, Supplementation with dietary fiber improves fecal incontinence. *Nurs. Res.* **50**(4): 203–213 (2001).
35. M. Read, N. W. Read, D. C. Barber and H. L. Duthie, Effects of loperamide on anal sphincter function in patients complaining of chronic diarrhea with fecal incontinence and urgency, *Dig. Dis. Sci.* **27**(9): 807–814 (1982).
36. K. R. Palmer, C. L. Corbett and C. D. Holdsworth, Double-blind cross-over study comparing loperamide, codeine and diphenoxylate in the treatment of chronic diarrhea, *Gastroenterology* **79**(6): 1272–1275 (1980).
37. B. Holzer, H. R. Rosen, W. Zaglmaier, R. Klug, B. Beer, G. Novi and R. Schiessel, Sacral nerve stimulation in patients after rectal resection — Preliminary report, *J. Gastrointest. Surg.* **12**(5): 921–925 (2008).

38. C. Ratto, E. Grillo, A. Parello, M. Petrolino, G. Costamagna and G. B. Doglietto, Sacral neuromodulation in treatment of fecal incontinence following anterior resection and chemoradiation for rectal cancer, *Dis. Colon Rectum* **48**(5): 1027–1036 (2005).

39. P. Matthiessen, O. Hallböök, J. Rutegård, G. Simert and R. Sjödahl, Defunctioning stoma reduces symptomatic anastomotic leakage after low anterior resection of the rectum for cancer: A randomized multicenter trial, *Ann. Surg.* **246**(2): 207–214 (2007).

40. N. Hüser, C. W. Michalski, M. Erkan, T. Schuster, R. Rosenberg, J. Kleeff and H. Friess, Systematic review and meta-analysis of the role of defunctioning stoma in low rectal cancer surgery, *Ann. Surg.* **248**(1): 52–60 (2008).

41. J. T. Lordan, R. Heywood, S. Shirol and D. P. Edwards, Following anterior resection for rectal cancer, defunctioning ileostomy closure may be significantly delayed by adjuvant chemotherapy: A retrospective study, *Colorectal Dis.* **9**(5): 420–422 (2007).

42. O. Krand, T. Yalti, I. Berber and G. Tellioglu, Early vs. delayed closure of temporary covering ileostomy: A prospective study, *Hepatogastroenterology* **55**(81): 142–145 (2008).

43. R. Bakx, O. R. Busch, D. van Geldere, W. A. Bemelman, J. F. Slors and J. J. van Lanschot, Feasibility of early closure of loop ileostomies: A pilot study, *Dis. Colon Rectum* **46**(12): 1680–1684 (2003).

44. A. Tsunoda, Y. Tsunoda, K. Narita, M. Watanabe, K. Nakao and M. Kusano, Quality of life after low anterior resection and temporary loop ileostomy, *Dis. Colon Rectum* **51**(2): 218–222 (2008).

45. J. Engel, J. Kerr, A. Schlesinger-Raab, R. Eckel, H. Sauer and D. Hölzel, Quality of life in rectal cancer patients: A four-year prospective study, *Ann. Surg.* **238**(2): 203–213 (2003).

46. C. E. Schmidt, B. Bestmann, T. Küchler, W. E. Longo and B. Kremer, Prospective evaluation of quality of life of patients receiving either abdominoperineal resection or sphincter-preserving procedure for rectal cancer, *Ann. Surg. Oncol.* **12**(2): 117–123 (2005).

47. C. E. Schmidt, B. Bestmann, T. Küchler, W. E. Longo and B. Kremer, Ten-year historic cohort of quality of life and sexuality in patients with rectal cancer, *Dis. Colon Rectum* **48**(3): 483–492 (2005).

48. M. G. Guren, M. T. Eriksen, J. N. Wiig, E. Carlsen, A. Nesbakken, H. K. Sigurdsson, A. Wibe and K. M. Tveit, Norwegian Rectal Cancer Group, Quality of life and functional outcome following anterior or

abdominoperineal resection for rectal cancer, *Eur. J. Surg. Oncol.* **31**(7): 735–742 (2005).

49. M. M. Grumann, E. M. Noack, I. A. Hoffmann and P. M. Schlag, Comparison of quality of life in patients undergoing abdominoperineal extirpation or anterior resection for rectal cancer, *Ann. Surg.* **233**(2): 149–156 (2001).

50. J. A. Cornish, H. S. Tilney, A. G. Heriot, I. C. Lavery, V. W. Fazio and P. P. Tekkis, A meta-analysis of quality of life for abdominoperineal excision of rectum versus anterior resection for rectal cancer, *Ann. Surg. Oncol.* **14**(7): 2056–2068 (2007).

51. P. Gervaz, N. Rotholtz, S. D. Wexner, S. Y. You, N. Saigusa, E. Kaplan, M. Secic, E. G. Weiss, J. J. Nogueras and B. Belin, Colonic J-pouch function in rectal cancer patients: Impact of adjuvant chemoradiotherapy, *Dis. Colon Rectum* **44**(11): 1667–1675 (2001).

52. K. Ammann, W. Kirchmayr, A. Klaus, G. Mühlmann, R. Kafka, M. Oberwalder, A. De Vries, D. Ofner and H. Weiss, Impact of neoadjuvant chemoradiation on anal sphincter function in patients with carcinoma of the midrectum and low rectum, *Arch. Surg.* **138**(3): 257–261 (2003).

53. J. Pollack, T. Holm, B. Cedermark, B. Holmström and A. Mellgren, Long-term effect of preoperative radiation therapy on anorectal function, *Dis. Colon Rectum* **49**(3): 345–352 (2006).

54. J. F. Lim, J. J. Tjandra, R. Hiscock, M. W. Chao and P. Gibbs, Preoperative chemoradiation for rectal cancer causes prolonged pudendal nerve terminal motor latency, *Dis. Colon Rectum* **49**(1): 12–19 (2006).

55. K. C. Peeters, C. J. van de Velde, J. W. Leer, H. Martijn, J. M. Junggeburt, E. K. Kranenbarg, W. H. Steup, T. Wiggers, H. J. Rutten and C. A. Marijnen, Late side effects of short-course preoperative radiotherapy combined with total mesorectal excision for rectal cancer: Increased bowel dysfunction in irradiated patients — A Dutch colorectal cancer group study, *J. Clin. Oncol.* **23**(25): 6199–6206 (2005).

56. N. N. Baxter, L. K. Hartman, J. E. Tepper, R. Ricciardi, S. B. Durham and B. A. Virnig, Postoperative irradiation for rectal cancer increases the risk of small bowel obstruction after surgery, *Ann. Surg.* **245**(4): 553–559 (2007).

57. J. Pollack, T. Holm, B. Cedermark, D. Altman, B. Holmström, B. Glimelius and A. Mellgren, Late adverse effects of short-course

preoperative radiotherapy in rectal cancer, *Br. J. Surg.* **93**(12): 1519–1525 (2006).

58. S. K. Hendren, B. I. O'Connor, M. Liu, T. Asano, Z. Cohen, C. J. Swallow, H. M. Macrae, R. Gryfe and R. S. McLeod, Prevalence of male and female sexual dysfunction is high following surgery for rectal cancer, *Ann. Surg.* **242**(2): 212–223 (2005).

59. S. O. Breukink, M. F. van Driel, J. P. Pierie, C. Dobbins, T. Wiggers and W. J. Meijerink, Male sexual function and lower urinary tract symptoms after laparoscopic total mesorectal excision, *Int. J. Colorectal Dis.* **23**(12): 1199–1205 (2008).

60. C. A. Marijnen, C. J. van de Velde, H. Putter, M. van den Brink, C. P. Maas, H. Martijn, H. J. Rutten, T. Wiggers, E. K. Kranenbarg, J. W. Leer and A. M. Stiggelbout, Impact of short-term preoperative radiotherapy on health-related quality of life and sexual functioning in primary rectal cancer: Report of a multicenter randomized trial, *J. Clin. Oncol.* **23**(9): 1847–1858 (2005).

61. J. Camilleri-Brennan and R. J. Steele, Prospective analysis of quality of life and survival following mesorectal excision for rectal cancer, *Br. J. Surg.* **88**(12): 1617–1622 (2001).

62. I. Lindsey, B. George, M. Kettlewell and N. Mortensen, Randomized, double-blind, placebo-controlled trial of sildenafil (Viagra) for erectile dysfunction after rectal excision for cancer and inflammatory bowel disease, *Dis. Colon Rectum* **45**(6): 727–732 (2002).

63. M. Strong, W. Peche and C. Scaife, Incidence of fertility counseling of women of child-bearing age before treatment for colorectal cancer, *Am. J. Surg.* **194**(6): 765–767 (2007).

64. K. Ø. Olsen, S. Juul, S. Bülow, H. J. Järvinen, A. Bakka, J. Björk, T. Oresland and S. Laurberg, Female fecundity before and after operation for familial adenomatous polyposis, *Br. J. Surg.* **90**(2): 227–231 (2003).

65. A. Waljee, J. Waljee, A. M. Morris and P. D. Higgins, Threefold increased risk of infertility: A meta-analysis of infertility after ileal pouch anal anastomosis in ulcerative colitis, *Gut* **11**: 1575–1580 (2006).

66. C. P. Spanos, A. Mamopoulos, A. Tsapas, T. Syrakos and D. Kiskinis, Female fertility and colorectal cancer, *Int. J. Colorectal Dis.* **8**: 735–743 (2008).

67. K. B. Clough, F. Goffinet, A. Labib, C. Renolleau, F. Campana, A. de la Rochefordiere and J. C. Durand, Laparoscopic unilateral ovarian

transposition prior to irradiation: Prospective study of 20 cases, *Cancer* **77**(12): 2638–2645 (1996).

68. K. Bruheim, J. Svartberg, E. Carlsen, S. Dueland, E. Haug, E. Skovlund, K. M. Tveit and M. G. Guren, Radiotherapy for rectal cancer is associated with reduced serum testosterone and increased FSH and LH, *Int. J. Radiat. Oncol. Biol. Phys.* **70**(3): 722–727 (2008).

69. M. M. Lange, C. P. Maas, C. A. Marijnen, T. Wiggers, H. J. Rutten, E. K. Kranenbarg and C. J. van de Velde, Cooperative Clinical Investigators of the Dutch Total Mesorectal Excision Trial. Urinary dysfunction after rectal cancer treatment is mainly caused by surgery, *Br. J. Surg.* **95**(8): 1020–1028 (2008).

70. C. E. Schmidt, B. Bestmann, T. Küchler, W. E. Longo, V. Rohde and B. Kremer, Gender differences in quality of life of patients with rectal cancer. A five-year prospective study, *World J. Surg.* **29**(12): 1630–1641.

71. S. Pucciarelli, P. Del Bianco, P. Toppan, S. Serpentini, F. Efficace, L. M. Pasetto, M. L. Friso, G. L. De Salvo and D. Nitti, Health-related quality of life outcomes in disease-free survivors of mid-low rectal cancer after curative surgery, *Ann. Surg. Oncol.* **15**(7): 1846–1854 (2008).

72. C. E. Schmidt, B. Bestmann, T. Kuchler, W. E. Longo and B. Kremer, Impact of age on quality of life in patients with rectal cancer, *World J. Surg.* **29**(2): 190–197 (2005).

73. A. Chiappa, R. Biffi, A. P. Zbar, F. Luca, C. Crotti, E. Bertani, F. Biella, G. Zampino, R. Orecchia, N. Fazio, M. Venturino, C. Crosta, G. C. Pruneri, C. Grassi and B. Andreoni, Results of treatment of distal rectal carcinoma since the introduction of total mesorectal excision: A single unit experience, 1994–2003, *Int. J. Colorectal Dis.* **20**(3): 221–230 (2005).

74. J. L. McCall, M. R. Cox and D. A. Wattchow, Analysis of local recurrence rates after surgery alone for rectal cancer, *Int. J. Colorectal Dis.* **10**(3): 126–132 (1995).

75. S. H. Jung, C. S. Yu, P. W. Choi, D. D. Kim, I. J. Park, H. C. Kim and J. C. Kim, Risk factors and oncologic impact of anastomotic leakage after rectal cancer surgery, *Dis. Colon Rectum* **51**(6): 902–908 (2008).

76. R. Marr, K. Birbeck, J. Garvican, C. P. Macklin, N. J. Tiffin, W. J. Parsons, M. F. Dixon, N. P. Mapstone, D. Sebag-Montefiore, N. Scott, D. Johnston, P. Sagar, P. Finan and P. Quirke, The modern abdominoperineal excision: The next challenge after total mesorectal excision, *Ann. Surg.* **242**(1): 74–82 (2005).

77. F. A. Bonadeo, C. A. Vaccaro, M. L. Benati, G. M. Quintana, X. E. Garione and M. T. Telenta, Rectal cancer: Local recurrence after surgery without radiotherapy, *Dis. Colon Rectum* **44**(3): 374–379 (2001).

78. A. Wibe, A. Syse, E. Andersen, S. Tretli, H. E. Myrvold and O. Søreide, Norwegian Rectal Cancer Group. Oncological outcomes after total mesorectal excision for cure for cancer of the lower rectum: Anterior vs. abdominoperineal resection, *Dis. Colon Rectum* **47**(1): 48–58 (2004).

79. D. Hahnloser, H. Nelson, L. L. Gunderson, I. Hassan, M. G. Haddock, M. J. O'Connell, S. Cha, D. J. Sargent and A. Horgan, Curative potential of multimodality therapy for locally recurrent rectal cancer, *Ann. Surg.* **237**(4): 502–528 (2003).

80. N. Saito, K. Koda, N. Takiguchi, K. Oda, M. Ono, M. Sugito, K. Kawashima and M. Ito, Curative surgery for local pelvic recurrence of rectal cancer, *Dig. Surg.* **20**(3): 192–199 (2003).

81. J. C. Salo, P. B. Paty, J. Guillem, B. D. Minsky, L. B. Harrison and A. M. Cohen, Surgical salvage of recurrent rectal carcinoma after curative resection: A 10-year experience, *Ann. Surg. Oncol.* **6**(2): 171–177 (1999).

82. A. J. Watson, S. Lolohea, G. M. Robertson and F. A. Frizelle, The role of positron emission tomography in the management of recurrent colorectal cancer: A review, *Dis. Colon Rectum* **50**(1): 102–114 (2007).

83. M. Braendengen, K. M. Tveit, A. Berglund, E. Birkemeyer, G. Frykholm, L. Påhlman, J. N. Wiig, P. Byström, K. Bujko and B. Glimelius, Randomized phase III study comparing preoperative radiotherapy with chemoradiotherapy in nonresectable rectal cancer, *J. Clin. Oncol.* **26**(22): 3687–3694 (2008).

84. A. G. Heriot, C. M. Byrne, P. Lee, B. Dobbs, H. Tilney, M. J. Solomon, J. Mackay and F. Frizelle, Extended radical resection: The choice for locally recurrent rectal cancer, *Dis. Colon Rectum* **51**(3): 284–291 (2008).

85. P. Schurr, E. Lentz, S. Block, J. Kaifi, H. Kleinhans, G. Cataldegirmen, A. Kutup, C. Schneider, T. Strate, E. Yekebas and J. Izbicki, Radical redo surgery for local rectal cancer recurrence improves overall survival: A single center experience, *J. Gastrointest. Surg.* **12**(7): 1232–1238 (2008).

86. F. Lopez-Kostner, V. W. Fazio, A. Vignali, L. A. Rybicki and I. C. Lavery, Locally recurrent rectal cancer: Predictors and success of salvage surgery, *Dis. Colon Rectum* **44**(2): 173–178 (2001).

20

Management of Nutritional Issues After Major Pancreatic Resections

Nam Q. Nguyen,
Neil D. Merrett and
Andrew V. Biankin

Pancreatic resection is associated with a number of long term gastrointestinal complications that can lead to malnutrition and a consequent reduction in the quality of life. These are predominantly the manifestation of exocrine and endocrine insufficiency, gastrointestinal dysmotility, biliary dysfunction and bacterial overgrowth. Such sequelae can lead to reduced oral intake, macro- and micronutrient malabsorption, and impaired glucose homeostasis, which adversely impact on the patient's well-being. In order to minimise these complications after major pancreatic resection, it is imperative to identify these deficiencies and closely monitor the patient's energy consumption, symptoms and nutritional status. The management needs to be coordinated using a multi-disciplinary approach and in each case treatment individualised and based on an understanding of the anatomical, physiological and nutritional sequelae caused by the loss of pancreatic parenchyma through surgical resection.

Keywords: Pancreatic cancer, pancreatectomy, pancreatic insufficiency, gastrointestinal dysmotility, malabsorption, nutritional management, quality of life.

1. Introduction

Surgical resection offers the only possibility of cure for patients with peri-ampullary and pancreatic cancer.[1-3] The classic Whipple's procedure[2] and the pylorus-preserving pancreatico-duodenectomy (PPPD)[4,5] are the two most common operative techniques used for carcinoma in the pancreatic head. For tumours located toward the body/tail of the pancreas, left-sided pancrea-tectomy is preferable. Although the operative mortality rate of these procedures is below 5% in high-volume surgical centres,[1,6,7] the operative morbidity related to pancreatic fistulae, sepsis, and delayed gastric emptying (DGE) remains high at 30 to 40%.[8-10] Furthermore, as the pancreas plays a vital role in food digestion and glucose homeostasis, long-term survivors after pancreatoduo-denectomy are at risk of pancreatic exocrine insufficiency and malabsorption.[11] The presence of symptoms such as diarrhoea, flatulence, tenesmus, and steatorrhoea may substantially affect the quality of life of these individuals, and can lead to progressive weight loss and malnutrition.[12,13] Gastrointestinal dysmotility can also be a significant clinical problem in a small proportion of patients and may lead to symptoms such as DGE, early satiety and entero-gastric reflux.[14,15] Together, these long-term complications of exocrine insufficiency and GI dysmotility after major pancreatic resection can adversely affect the oral intake and GI absorptive function of these patients and predispose them to significant malnutrition.

Although the morbidity and mortality benefits of pre-operative nutritional support have been well demonstrated,[16,17] especially in malnourished patients, the impact of nutrition on long term out-comes of patients who have had a pancreatic resection are yet to be defined. Overall, current data suggest that pancreatic resection causes a notable reduction in global quality of life.[18,19] The current chapter reviews the anatomical and physiological impact of major pancreatic resection on gastrointestinal (GI) function, subsequent nutrition and discussed relevant issues in the management of these patients.

2. Management of Pancreatic Insufficiency After Pancreatectomy

2.1 *Exocrine insufficiency*

The degree of alteration in the digestive function of the pancreas after resection depends on the amount of pancreatic parenchyma resected and the functional capacity of the residual pancreas (Table 1). Clinically, this relates to the type of surgical procedure carried out and the presence of underlying pancreatic atrophy or pancreatitis. In a cohort of approximately 700 patients, pancreatic parenchymal volume was strongly correlated with body weight, exocrine and endocrine function.[20] The presence of partial gastrectomy or antrectomy further disrupts post-prandial synchrony of digestion, by impairing the release of gastrin, pancreatic polypeptide and cholecystokinin.[21,22] The type of pancreatico-enterostomy is also important and can influence post-operative exocrine function.

Due to the early deactivation of pancreatic enzymes by gastric acid, deterioration in pancreatic exocrine function in patients who

Table 1. Impact of major pancreatic resection on upper gastrointestinal tract function.

Pancreatic function
- Pancreatic exocrine insufficiency from reduced function.
  - Degree of insufficiency correlates with extent of parenchymal resection and functional state of the residual pancreas.
- Diabetes mellitus from reduced endocrine function.

Gastric function
- Delayed gastric emptying; most improve within six months.
- Inadequate acid buffering leading to peptic ulceration.

Biliary function
- Recurrent cholangitis from either strictures or bacterial overgrowth.

Small intestinal function
- Disturbed jejunal migrating motor complex (MMC) phase III and reduced feed pattern.
- Entero-gastric reflux.
- Diarrhoea and malabsorption from bacterial overgrowth (blind loop syndrome).

have undergone PPPD with pancreatico-gastrostomy is greater,[11,23] and can be overcome with the administration of acid suppressive therapy.[24] Compared to patients with a normal residual pancreas, pancreatic function of those with chronic pancreatic disease such as chronic pancreatitis or atrophy is often impaired, even before any type of resection is carried out. In these patients, exocrine and endocrine pancreatic function deteriorates progressively after a major resection and aggressive replacement is required.[11]

Management

As pancreatic enzymes play a major role in food digestion and absorption, appropriate replacement to correct exocrine insufficiency is essential and reduces malnutrition, normalises biochemical indices of malnutrition, assists patients in recovering much of the original body weight and improves quality of life.[25,26] Because patients have different degrees of exocrine insufficiency, the dosage of pancreatic enzymes has to be adjusted to the individual.[25,27,28] All patients should be monitored and screened for symptoms and signs of inadequate replacement, which includes loss of body weight, diarrhoea or steatorrhoea, dyspeptic symptoms with gaseous distension and a stool fat excretion greater than 15 g/day.[25]

Amongst the pancreatic enzymes, lipases have significantly shorter intra-luminal survival time because they are most susceptible to acidic and proteolytic denaturation[25,29] and the aim of successful pancreatic enzyme replacement is to achieve sufficient lipase activity in the intestine.[29] Contrary to general belief, there is not a linear relationship between the dose of pancreatic enzymes and the symptoms of mal-digestion. In general, the required amount of lipase to be delivered to the duodenum with each meal is of the order of 25,000 to 40,000 units to achieve lipase activity of 40–60 units/ml of chyme.[25,29] As the unprotected enzyme is rapidly destroyed by gastric acid, co-administration of acid suppression therapy is a useful adjunct therapy and is recommended especially if severe steatorrhoea continues with adequate dosing with pancreatic enzymes.[25,29,30]

More recently, pH-sensitive pancreatic lipase microsphere preparations have become increasingly popular and have been recommended by some authors as the treatment of choice.[27–29,31] This preparation however may be ineffective in patients who underwent PPPD because the microspheres are retained in the stomach.[32] In these patients, conventional powdered pancreatic enzyme preparations may improve the efficacy of treatment.[32] If symptoms and signs of mal-digestion persist despite the above therapeutic measures, trials of pH-sensitive enteric-coated microspheres, restricting the amount of dietary fat and/or replacing fat with medium chain triglycerides should be considered.[22,25,33,34]

2.2   *Endocrine insufficiency*

Approximately 20 to 50% of patients who have major pancreatic resection for malignancy develop diabetes mellitus,[11,35] and the incidence is significantly higher in patients who have a left-sided pancreatectomy than after a Whipple's procedure (57% versus 36%, respectively).[36] Similar to exocrine insufficiency, a greater degree of endocrine insufficiency is seen in patients with a compromised residual pancreas from pre-existing chronic pancreatitis or atrophy.[36–38]

Management

It is important to note that the glucose homeostasis and response to insulin treatment in these patients with secondary diabetes mellitus is different to those with idiopathic diabetes mellitus. As glucagon secretion is simultaneously reduced in these patients, they are 'hyper-sensitive' to the effects of insulin, exposing the patients to higher risk of recurrent attacks of hypoglycaemia and a substantial number of deaths and brain-injury.[11,39] Previously, this complication was considered to be a major issue for these patients, having been reported, especially in those who with alcoholic chronic pancreatitis.[40] Until recently, short-acting insulin preparations given repeatedly before meals and according to pre-prandial glucose levels have been the mainstay of therapy. This required intensive monitoring with slow dosage titration, to avoid hypoglycaemic complications. The recent advances in long-acting formulations of insulin have substantially reduced this problem, improving overall glycaemic control.

3. Management of Upper Gastrointestinal Dysfunction After Pancreatectomy

3.1 *Upper gastrointestinal dysfunction*

Although delayed gastric emptying (DGE) occurs in up to 50% of patients during the early post-operative period, only a small proportion of patients have persistent symptoms beyond six months post-operatively.[41–43] In more recent studies, the incidence of DGE fell to less than 10% and this improvement is most likely related to the advances in surgical technique, increased surgical experience, and improvements in post-operative intensive care management.[44–52] Currently, known risk factors for delayed gastric emptying after pancreatic resection include: pre-operative cholangitis, post-operative leakage and sepsis, pancreatico- and biliary-enteric anastomosis via the retro-mesenteric route and radical pancreatico-duodenectomy.[44–52] Whilst there has been much debate surrounding the higher incidence of DGE after PPPD compared to the classical Whipple's procedure, the most recent meta-analysis failed to demonstrate a difference in the rate of DGE between the two procedures[2] and the current rates of DGE following pancreatic resection are significantly lower (3–7%) than historically reported.[44–52] The reasons that underlie the controversy are multi-factorial and are most likely related to the variation in the definition of DGE between trials,[53] increased surgical experience and advances in post-operative intensive care management.[44–52]

Dysmotility of the upper jejunum with slower phase III of the migrating motor complex (MMC) and a reduced feed pattern are also frequently observed, leading to problems with entero-gastric reflux and bacterial growth in a small proportion of patients.[15,54,55] Entero-gastric reflux is more frequently observed in patients after Whipple's resection compared to those with PPPD, as the retained pylorus is competent to prevent entero-gastric reflux.[15] Recent data, however, suggest the use of undivided Roux-en-Y reconstruction following Whipple's procedures may decrease the incidence of entero-gastric reflux and thus, eliminating problems due to bile reflux gastritis and ulceration.[56]

Division of the vagus nerve and removal of the duodenal pacemaker by duodenectomy have been proposed as neuro-hormonal mechanisms involved in the pathogenesis of upper gastrointestinal dysfunction after major pancreatic resection, leading to a loss of coordination of gastrointestinal motility and an alteration in plasma concentrations of gastrointestinal peptides and hormones important for regulation of normal gastric motility such as motilin, pancreatic polypeptide, glucagon-like peptide-1, and peptide YY.[54,57–60]

Peptic ulceration occurs infrequently after pancreatic surgery (5%), particularly with Whipple's resection,[43] and is related to inadequate acid buffering from the fall in pancreatic bicarbonate secretion and the impaired mixing of bicarbonate secreted into the ascending loop with the 'acidic' chyme.[11,43]

Management

It is important to treat delayed gastric emptying promptly and effectively as this post-operative complication significantly increases the length of hospital stay, the number of days with a naso-gastric tube, and the number of days until solid food is tolerated.[52] More importantly, measures such as meticulous care during the operation to prevent post-operative leakage and sepsis, as well as avoiding the retro-mesenteric route for pancreato- or biliary-enteric anastomosis should be taken to reduce the risk of DGE.[61–63] Centralisation of pancreatic resections in high-volume centres with recent advances in operative techniques and post-operative care have not only reduced the need for re-operation but also lowered the incidence of DGE to an extremely low level.[1,15,64]

Prokinetic therapy should be the initial treatment for upper gastrointestinal tract dysmotility. The currently used prokinetic agents to improve upper gastrointestinal dysmotility in clinical practice are erythromycin, metoclopramide and domperidone. Low doses of erythromycin (a motilin agonist, 1 mg/kg/d) induce antral contraction and initiate premature gastric phase 3 activity of the MMC that migrates through the small intestine,[65–67] and has been shown to reduce the incidence of DGE by 50–75% with a shorter duration of naso-gastric drainage, and earlier resumption of eating.[68,69] Although no major adverse effects of erythromycin were observed in these trials,[68,69] care must be taken to avoid drugs that can interact and cause a prolonged QT interval and related cardiac arrhythmias. Despite their frequent uses in clinical practice, efficacy data of dopamine antagonists such as metoclopramide and domperidone for improving delayed gastric emptying in patients with pancreato-duodenectomy are lacking. Although cisapride (a 5-HT4 receptor antagonist) has been shown to accelerate gastric emptying in patients with DGE after PPPD with a Billroth I type duodeno-jejunostomy,[70,71] its clinical use has been restricted to highly specialised centres for refractory cases, because of the risk of cardiac arrhythmia when used in combination with other prokinetic agents such as erythromycin.[72,73]

Approximately 2–6% of patients experience prolonged upper gastrointestinal dysmotility despite prokinetic therapy,[71,74-78] and treatment of these persistent cases proves challenging, with the role of prokinetic agents being controversial. Although switching to another prokinetic agent or adding a second agent with a different mechanism of action is frequently adopted in clinical practice, the efficacy data for these approaches in these persistent cases are lacking. Furthermore, the major concern of prolonged uses of these prokinetic agents is associated tachyphylaxis. Recently, the role of electrical stimulation or pacing was investigated and preliminary data in patients with gastroparesis from Roux-en-Y gastric bypass suggested that electric gastric pacing improved both gastric emptying as well as nausea and vomiting in the majority of patients.[79]

3.2   Biliary dysfunction

Motility changes in the small bowel loop used for the entero-biliary anastomosis may result in bacterial overgrowth and hence recurrent bouts of cholangitis without any evidence of anastomostic stricture. Recurrent attacks of cholangitis may also occur in the small subset of patients who develop entero-biliary anastomostic strictures.

Management

Entero-biliary anastomostic strictures need to be excluded in all patients, as these strictures can be promptly treated with the combination of antibiotic therapy and endoscopic intervention. Occasionally, radiological and/or surgical interventions are required when endoscopic intervention has failed due to alteration in the upper gastrointestinal anatomy.[80] If recurrent cholangitis occurs in the absence of anastomotic stricture, combinations of prokinetic and long term, low dose antibiotic prophylaxis may prevent recurrence.[11]

3.3 Bacterial overgrowth

Bacterial overgrowth is common after both types of pancreatic resection, especially in the entero-pancreatico-biliary loop. The presence of excessive bacteria results in de-conjugation of bile acids with consequent failure of micelle formation and decreases lipid uptake further impairing fat absorption and causing more steatorrhoea,[15,54,55] leading to malabsorption of both macro- and micro-nutrients.[11] The syndrome should be considered if steatorrhoea persists despite adequate pancreatic enzyme replacement with appropriate acid suppressive therapy.

Management

The diagnosis should be confirmed by hydrogen breath tests prior to treatment with a combination of intermittent antibiotic therapy such as ciprofloxacin or metronidazole and prokinetic agents.[11]

4. Management of Other Nutritional-Related Issues After Pancreatectomy

Loss of muscle mass, impairment of voluntary muscle function and respiratory function can be seen as early as the third post-operative day.[81] Dual energy X-ray absorptiometry (DEXA) detects a small, but significant reduction in mid-arm circumference and total body fat during the first post-operative week.[82] Patients who have undergone a Whipple's resection are more likely to restrict their intake of fat, and to a lesser extent, carbohydrate due to heartburn, dyspepsia and steatorrhoea.[13] Consequently, up to one-third of these patients were found to have deficiencies in the intake of micronutrients and minerals such as iron, zinc, calcium, vitamin D and selenium.[11,13,82] Although the body mass index (BMI) of most patients is often well below their pre-illness level,[64] the overall body weight remains stable and ongoing weight loss is more often a sign of recurrent disease.[11]

Management

In addition to pancreatic enzyme replacement and treatment of upper gastrointestinal dysfunction,[83,84] specific dietary modification

Table 2. Key issues in the management of patients after major pancreatic resection.

- Understanding the nature of the surgical resection.
- Individualising the dosage of pancreatic enzymes, as patients have different degree of exocrine pancreatic insufficiency.
- The presence of weight loss, diarrhoea or steatorrhoea, dyspeptic symptoms with strong meteorism and a stool fat excretion greater than 15 g/day indicates inadequate replacement.
- Co-administration of acid suppression therapy is recommended, especially if severe steatorrhoea continues with adequate dosing of pancreatic enzyme.
- In patients with endocrine insufficiency, glucagon secretion is simultaneously reduced and the dosage of insulin needs to be titrated slowly to avoid hypoglycaemic complications.
- Specific dietary modification to a high carbohydrate, protein and fat moieties meals is recommended.
- Temporary enteral nutritional support is recommended for patients with debilitating gastric stasis, significant abdominal pain or ongoing weight loss despite apparently adequate dietary intake.
- Neither short or long term parenteral nutritional support are recommended.
- Correct the associated upper GI dysmotilities with prokinetic therapy to improve oral intake.
- If steatorrhoea persists despite adequate pancreatic enzyme replacement with appropriate acid suppressive therapy, intestinal bacterial overgrowth should be considered and treated if present.

is essential to ensure that the intake of both macronutrients and micronutrients is adequate (Table 2). Frequent small meals with high carbohydrate and protein (1.0–1.5 g/kg) content are recommended, and up to 30% of calories of the meal can be given as fat in these patients. Aggressive post-operative nutritional support reduces loss of muscle mass, enhances voluntary muscle and respiratory function during the first few weeks after the surgery,[85] and facilitates normalisation of these parameters at six months following surgery.[12,13]

In patients who fail to gain or maintain adequate body weight, and/or experience persistent steatorrhoea, the amount of dietary fat should be minimized. Medium chain triglycerides (MCT) can be trialed because of the lipase independent absorption property of MCT.[83,86] However, MCTs are poorly tolerated by most patients and may induce side effects such as abdominal pain, nausea and diarrhoea.[86] In addition, the amount of fibre in the diet should be low, as fibres absorb enzymes and this may lead to reduce intake of nutrients. In view of recent data on micronutrients and mineral deficiencies,[87,88] it is important to replace these essential vitamins and micronutrients adequately in this group of patients.

In patients who have debilitating gastric stasis, significant abdominal pain or ongoing weight loss despite apparently adequate dietary intake, enteral nutrition is indicated and is best delivered temporarily via a jejunal feeding tube to correct the malnourishment prior to definitive treatment of any underlying cause.[16,84,89] Enteral formulae that are peptide or amino acid based are recommended and may be given overnight. However, enteral infusion of fat and protein activates neurohumoral feedback mechanisms that can potentially impair gastric emptying and prolong post-operative gastroparesis. Cyclic enteral feeding is preferable and is associated with a shorter period of enteral nutrition, a faster return to a normal diet and a shorter hospital stay than those fed continuously.[90] Currently, the role of immuno-nutrition in these patients remains controversial. Whilst earlier studies suggested that immune-enhanced enteral nutrition decreases infectious complications by 13%,[91,92] this has not been reproduced.[93] Data on long-term enteral nutritional therapy is not available.

Routine use of parenteral nutrition is not recommended post-operatively, either short term or long term usage, due to the concerns of septic complications.[16] Overall, administration of post-operative parenteral nutrition in these patients is associated with a greater intestinal permeability, an increased infective complication rate, with no improvement in mortality and higher health care costs.[94–99] Recent studies failed to show any differences in the rate of diarrhoea, abdominal distension or vomiting, whether post-operative parenteral or enteral nutrition was used.[95,96,98]

5.   Summary and Conclusions

In summary, major pancreatic resection impairs not only the pancreatic exocrine and endocrine function, but also the function of the gastrointestinal tract. A better understanding of the anatomical and physiological sequelae after pancreatectomy is imperative to ensure optimal nutritional support in these patients. Given the adverse impact of malnutrition on well-being and health related quality of life, nutritional status should be closely monitored and treated appropriately.

References

1. M. W. Buchler, M. Wagner, B. M. Schmied *et al.*, Changes in morbidity after pancreatic resection: Toward the end of completion pancreatectomy, *Arch. Surg.* **138**(12): 1310–1314; discussion 1315 (2003).
2. M. K. Diener, H. P. Knaebel, C. Heukaufer *et al.*, A systematic review and meta-analysis of pylorus-preserving versus classical pancreaticoduodenectomy for surgical treatment of periampullary and pancreatic carcinoma, *Ann. Surg.* **245**(2): 187–200 (2007).
3. C. J. Yeo, J. L. Cameron, K. D. Lillemoe *et al.*, Pancreaticoduodenectomy for cancer of the head of the pancreas. 201 patients, *Ann. Surg.* **221**(6): 721–731; discussion 731–733 (1995).
4. L. W. Traverso, The surgical management of chronic pancreatitis: The Whipple procedure, *Adv. Surg.* **32**: 23–39 (1999).
5. L. W. Traverso, The pylorus preserving Whipple procedure for the treatment of chronic pancreatitis, *Swiss Surg.* **6**(5): 259–263 (2000).
6. M. Trede, G. Schwall and H. D. Saeger, Survival after pancreatoduodenectomy. 118 consecutive resections without an operative mortality, *Ann. Surg.* **211**(4): 447–458 (1990).
7. C. J. Yeo, J. L. Cameron, T. A. Sohn *et al.*, Six hundred fifty consecutive pancreaticoduodenectomies in the 1990s: Pathology, complications, and outcomes, *Ann. Surg.* **226**(3): 248–257; discussion 257–260 (1997).
8. C. Bassi, M. Falconi, R. Salvia *et al.*, Management of complications after pancreaticoduodenectomy in a high volume centre: Results on 150 consecutive patients, *Dig. Surg.* **18**(6): 453–457; discussion 458 (2001).
9. D. J. Gouma, R. C. van Geenen, T. M. van Gulik *et al.*, Rates of complications and death after pancreaticoduodenectomy: Risk factors and the impact of hospital volume, *Ann. Surg.* **232**(6): 786–795 (2000).
10. A. Richter, M. Niedergethmann, J. W. Sturm *et al.*, Long-term results of partial pancreaticoduodenectomy for ductal adenocarcinoma of the pancreatic head: 25-year experience, *World J. Surg.* **27**(3): 324–329 (2003).
11. S. Kahl and P. Malfertheiner, Exocrine and endocrine pancreatic insufficiency after pancreatic surgery, *Best Pract. Res. Clin. Gastroenterol.* **18**(5): 947–955 (2004).

12. R. S. McLeod, Quality of life, nutritional status and gastrointestinal hormone profile following the Whipple procedure, *Ann. Oncol.* **10**(Suppl. 4): 281–284 (1999).

13. R. S. McLeod, B. R. Taylor, B. I. O'Connor *et al.*, Quality of life, nutritional status, and gastrointestinal hormone profile following the Whipple procedure, *Am. J. Surg.* **169**(1): 179–185 (1995).

14. J. Closset and M. Gelin, Delayed gastric emptying after pancreatoduodenectomy, *Acta Chir. Belg.* **103**(3): 338–339 (2003).

15. R. C. Williamson, N. Bliouras, M. J. Cooper and E. R. Davies, Gastric emptying and enterogastric reflux after conservative and conventional pancreatoduodenectomy, *Surgery* **114**(1): 82–86 (1993).

16. K. S. Goonetilleke and A. K. Siriwardena, Systematic review of perioperative nutritional supplementation in patients undergoing pancreaticoduodenectomy, *J. Pancreas* **7**(1): 5–13 (2006).

17. C. H. Su, Y. M. Shyr, W. Y. Lui and F. K. P'Eng, Factors affecting morbidity, mortality and survival after pancreaticoduodenectomy for carcinoma of the ampulla of Vater, *Hepatogastroenterology* **46**(27): 1973–1979 (1999).

18. C. Bloechle, J. R. Izbicki, W. T. Knoefel *et al.*, Quality of life in chronic pancreatitis — Results after duodenum-preserving resection of the head of the pancreas, *Pancreas* **11**(1): 77–85 (1995).

19. J. R. Izbicki, B. DC, C. F. Eisenberger *et al.*, Pancreatic and small bowel surgery — Effects of postoperative quality of life, *Pancreatology* **1**(S1): 62–70 (2001).

20. Y. Nakamura, S. Higuchi and K. Maruyama, Pancreatic volume associated with endocrine and exocrine function of the pancreas among Japanese alcoholics, *Pancreatology* **5**(4–5): 422–431 (2005).

21. P. Malfertheiner, M. Buchler, B. Glasbrenner *et al.*, Adaptive changes of the exocrine pancreas and plasma cholecystokinin release following subtotal gastric resection in rats, *Digestion* **38**(3): 142–151 (1987).

22. H. Friess, J. Bohm, M. W. Muller *et al.*, Maldigestion after total gastrectomy is associated with pancreatic insufficiency, *Am. J. Gastroenterol.* **91**(2): 341–347 (1996).

23. J. Y. Jang, S. W. Kim, S. J. Park and Y. H. Park, Comparison of the functional outcome after pylorus-preserving pancreatoduodenectomy: Pancreatogastrostomy and pancreatojejunostomy, *World J. Surg.* **26**(3): 366–371 (2002).

24. N. Toyota, T. Takada, H. Yasuda *et al.*, The effects of omeprazole, a proton pump inhibitor, on early gastric stagnation after a

pylorus-preserving pancreaticoduodenectomy: Results of a randomized study, *Hepatogastroenterology* **45**(22): 1005–1010 (1998).

25. M. Braga, M. Cristallo, R. De Franchis *et al.*, Pancreatic enzyme replacement therapy in post-pancreatectomy patients, *Int. J. Pancreatol.* **5**(Suppl.): 37–44 (1989).

26. L. Czako, T. Takacs, P. Hegyi *et al.*, Quality of life assessment after pancreatic enzyme replacement therapy in chronic pancreatitis, *Can. J. Gastroenterol.* **17**(10): 597–603 (2003).

27. P. Layer, J. Keller and P. G. Lankisch, Pancreatic enzyme replacement therapy, *Curr. Gastroenterol. Rep.* **3**(2): 101–108 (2001).

28. J. D. Morrow, Pancreatic enzyme replacement therapy, *Am. J. Med. Sci.* **298**(5): 357–359 (1989).

29. M. Ferrone, M. Raimondo and J. S. Scolapio, Pancreatic enzyme pharmacotherapy, *Pharmacotherapy* **27**(6): 910–920 (2007).

30. F. Marotta, S. J. O'Keefe, I. N. Marks *et al.*, Pancreatic enzyme replacement therapy. Importance of gastric acid secretion, H2-antagonists, and enteric coating, *Dig. Dis. Sci.* **34**(3): 456–461 (1989).

31. H. Anthony, C. E. Collins, G. Davidson *et al.*, Pancreatic enzyme replacement therapy in cystic fibrosis: Australian guidelines. Pediatric Gastroenterological Society and the Dietitians Association of Australia, *J. Paediatr. Child Health* **35**(2): 125–129 (1999).

32. M. J. Bruno, J. J. Borm, F. J. Hoek *et al.*, Comparative effects of enteric-coated pancreatin microsphere therapy after conventional and pylorus-preserving pancreatoduodenectomy, *Br. J. Surg.* **84**(7): 952–956 (1997).

33. G. Dobrilla, Management of chronic pancreatitis. Focus on enzyme replacement therapy, *Int. J. Pancreatol.* **5**(Suppl.): 17–29 (1989).

34. H. Friess, J. Bohm, M. Ebert and M. Buchler, Enzyme treatment after gastrointestinal surgery, *Digestion* **54**(Suppl. 2): 48–53 (1993).

35. W. M. Stone, M. G. Sarr, D. M. Nagorney and D. C. McIlrath. Chronic pancreatitis. Results of Whipple's resection and total pancreatectomy, *Arch. Surg.* **123**(7): 815–819 (1988).

36. Y. S. Shan, M. L. Tsai, N. T. Chiu and P. W. Lin, Reconsideration of delayed gastric emptying in pancreaticoduodenectomy, *World J. Surg.* **29**(7): 873–879; discussion 880 (2005).

37. C. F. Frey and K. L. Mayer. Comparison of local resection of the head of the pancreas combined with longitudinal pancreaticojejunostomy (frey procedure) and duodenum-preserving resection of

the pancreatic head (beger procedure), *World J. Surg.* **27**(11): 1217–1230 (2003).

38. S. Maartense, M. Ledeboer, W. A. Bemelman *et al.*, Effect of surgery for chronic pancreatitis on pancreatic function: Pancreatico-jejunostomy and duodenum-preserving resection of the head of the pancreas, *Surgery* **135**(2): 125–130 (2004).

39. R. F. Martin, R. L. Rossi and K. A. Leslie, Long-term results of pylorus-preserving pancreatoduodenectomy for chronic pancreatitis, *Arch. Surg.* **131**(3): 247–252 (1996).

40. A. G. Patel, M. T. Toyama, A. M. Kusske *et al.*, Pylorus-preserving Whipple resection for pancreatic cancer. Is it any better? *Arch. Surg.* **130**(8): 838–842; discussion 842–843 (1995).

41. J. G. Hunter and T. W. White, Gastrostomy and jejunostomy using a transgastric tube for early enteral nutrition after pylorus-preserving pancreaticoduodenectomy, *Surg. Gynecol. Obstet.* **173**(4): 316–318 (1991).

42. A. L. Warshaw and D. L. Torchiana, Delayed gastric emptying after pylorus-preserving pancreaticoduodenectomy, *Surg. Gynecol. Obstet.* **160**(1): 1–4 (1985).

43. P. A. Grace, H. A. Pitt and W. P. Longmire, Pylorus preserving pancreatoduodenectomy: An overview, *Br. J. Surg.* **77**(9): 968–974 (1990).

44. C. M. Schmidt, E. S. Powell, C. T. Yiannoutsos *et al.*, Pancreaticoduodenectomy: A 20-year experience in 516 patients, *Arch. Surg.* **139**(7): 718–725; discussion 725–727 (2004).

45. S. Sriussadaporn, S. Prichayudh, K. Kritayakirana and R. Pak-art, Pylorus preserving pancreaticoduodenectomy with low incidence of early delayed gastric emptying, *J. Med. Assoc. Thai.* **90**(1): 82–88 (2007).

46. E. Lermite, P. Pessaux, O. Brehant *et al.*, Risk factors of pancreatic fistula and delayed gastric emptying after pancreaticoduodenectomy with pancreaticogastrostomy, *J. Am. Coll. Surg.* **204**(4): 588–596 (2007).

47. C. M. Kang, J. Y. Kim, G. H. Choi *et al.*, Pancreaticoduodenectomy of pancreatic ductal adenocarcinoma in the elderly, *Yonsei Med. J.* **48**(3): 488–494 (2007).

48. M. Tani, H. Terasawa, M. Kawai *et al.*, Improvement of delayed gastric emptying in pylorus-preserving pancreaticoduodenectomy: Results of a prospective, randomized, controlled trial, *Ann. Surg.* **243**(3): 316–320 (2006).

49. K. I. Paraskevas, C. Avgerinos, C. Manes *et al.*, Delayed gastric emptying is associated with pylorus-preserving but not classical Whipple pancreaticoduodenectomy: A review of the literature and critical reappraisal of the implicated pathomechanism, *World J. Gastroenterol.* **12**(37): 5951–5958 (2006).

50. X. M. Bu, J. Xu, X. W. Dai *et al.*, Is delayed gastric emptying so terrible after pylorus-preserving pancreaticoduodenectomy? Prevention and management, *World J. Gastroenterol.* **12**(39): 6382–6385 (2006).

51. M. Tanaka, Gastroparesis after a pylorus-preserving pancreatoduodenectomy, *Surg. Today* **35**(5): 345–350 (2005).

52. L. Strommer, S. Raty, R. Hennig *et al.*, Delayed gastric emptying and intestinal hormones following pancreatoduodenectomy, *Pancreatology* **5**(6): 537–544 (2005).

53. M. N. Wente, C. Bassi, C. Dervenis *et al.*, Delayed gastric emptying (DGE) after pancreatic surgery: A suggested definition by the International Study Group of Pancreatic Surgery (ISGPS), *Surgery* **142**(5): 761–768 (2007).

54. E. Naslund, P. Gryback, L. Backman *et al.*, Distal small bowel hormones: Correlation with fasting antroduodenal motility and gastric emptying, *Dig. Dis. Sci.* **43**(5): 945–952 (1998).

55. H. T. Debas and T. Yamagishi, Evidence for pyloropancreatic reflux for pancreatic exocrine secretion, *Am. J. Physiol.* **234**(5): E468–E471 (1978).

56. M. Wayne, I. Jorge and A. M. Cooperman, Alternative reconstruction after pancreaticoduodenectomy, *World J. Surg. Oncol.* **6**(1): 9 (2008).

57. T. Ueno, A. Tanaka, Y. Hamanaka *et al.*, A proposal mechanism of early delayed gastric emptying after pylorus preserving pancreatoduodenectomy, *Hepatogastroenterology* **42**(3): 269–274 (1995).

58. M. Tanaka and M. G. Sarr, Total duodenectomy: Effect on canine gastrointestinal motility, *J. Surg. Res.* **42**(5): 483–493 (1987).

59. M. Tanaka and M. G. Sarr, Role of the duodenum in the control of canine gastrointestinal motility, *Gastroenterology* **94**(3): 622–629 (1988).

60. P. Malfertheiner, M. G. Sarr, M. P. Spencer and E. P. DiMagno, Effect of duodenectomy on interdigestive pancreatic secretion, gastrointestinal motility, and hormones in dogs, *Am. J. Physiol.* **257**(3 Pt. 1): G415–G422 (1989).

61. C. J. Yeo, Management of complications following pancreaticoduodenectomy, *Surg. Clin. North Am.* **75**(5): 913–924 (1995).

62. C. J. Yeo, The Johns Hopkins experience with pancreaticoduodenectomy with or without extended retroperitoneal lymphadenectomy for

periampullary adenocarcinoma, *J. Gastrointest. Surg.* **4**(3): 231–232 (2000).

63. C. J. Yeo and J. L. Cameron, Improving results of pancreaticoduo-denectomy for pancreatic cancer, *World J. Surg.* **23**(9): 907–912 (1999).

64. R. E. Jimenez, C. Fernandez-del Castillo, D. W. Rattner *et al.*, Outcome of pancreaticoduodenectomy with pylorus preservation or with antrectomy in the treatment of chronic pancreatitis, *Ann. Surg.* **231**(3): 293–300 (2000).

65. V. Annese, J. Janssens, G. Vantrappen *et al.*, Erythromycin accelerates gastric emptying by inducing antral contractions and improved gastroduodenal coordination, *Gastroenterology* **102**(3): 823–828 (1992).

66. B. Coulie, J. Tack, T. Peeters and J. Janssens, Involvement of two different pathways in the motor effects of erythromycin on the gastric antrum in humans, *Gut* **43**(3): 395–400 (1998).

67. J. Tack, J. Janssens, G. Vantrappen *et al.*, Effect of erythromycin on gastric motility in controls and in diabetic gastroparesis, *Gastroenterology* **103**(1): 72–79 (1992).

68. S. Ohwada, Y. Satoh, S. Kawate *et al.*, Low-dose erythromycin reduces delayed gastric emptying and improves gastric motility after Billroth I pylorus-preserving pancreaticoduodenectomy, *Ann. Surg.* **234**(5): 668–674 (2001).

69. C. J. Yeo, M. K. Barry, P. K. Sauter *et al.*, Erythromycin accelerates gastric emptying after pancreaticoduodenectomy. A prospective, randomized, placebo-controlled trial, *Ann. Surg.* **218**(3): 229–237; discussion 237–238 (1993).

70. M. Feldman and H. J. Smith, Effect of cisapride on gastric emptying of indigestible solids in patients with gastroparesis diabeticorum. A comparison with metoclopramide and placebo, *Gastroenterology* **92**: 171–174 (1987).

71. T. Takeda, J. Yoshida, M. Tanaka *et al.*, Delayed gastric emptying after Billroth I pylorus-preserving pancreatoduodenectomy: Effect of postoperative time and cisapride, *Ann. Surg.* **229**(2): 223–229 (1999).

72. M. R. Glessner and D. A. Heller, Changes in related drug class utilization after market withdrawal of cisapride, *Am. J. Manag. Care* **8**(3): 243–250 (2002).

73. A. Walker, P. Szneke and L. Weatherby, The risk of serious cardiac arrhythmias among cisapride users in the United Kingdom and Canada, *Am. J. Med.* **107**: 356–362 (1999).

74. B. W. Miedema, M. G. Sarr, J. A. van Heerden *et al.*, Complications following pancreaticoduodenectomy. Current management, *Arch. Surg.* **127**(8): 945–949; discussion 949–950 (1992).

75. H. Riediger, F. Makowiec, W. D. Schareck *et al.*, Delayed gastric emptying after pylorus-preserving pancreatoduodenectomy is strongly related to other postoperative complications, *J. Gastrointest. Surg.* **7**(6): 758–765 (2003).

76. I. Kobayashi, M. Miyachi, M. Kanai *et al.*, Different gastric emptying of solid and liquid meals after pylorus-preserving pancreatoduodenectomy, *Br. J. Surg.* **85**(7): 927–930 (1998).

77. W. Kozuschek, H. B. Reith, H. Waleczek *et al.*, A comparison of long term results of the standard Whipple procedure and the pylorus preserving pancreatoduodenectomy, *J. Am. Coll. Surg.* **178**(5): 443–453 (1994).

78. L. G. Lupo, O. C. Pannarale, D. F. Altomare *et al.*, Is pyloric function preserved in pylorus-preserving pancreaticoduodenectomy? *Eur. J. Surg.* **164**(2): 127–132 (1998).

79. J. R. Salameh, R. E. Schmieg, J. M. Runnels Jr and T. L. Abell, Refractory gastroparesis after Roux-en-Y gastric bypass: Surgical treatment with implantable pacemaker, *J. Gastrointest. Surg.* **11**(12): 1669–1672 (2007).

80. B. J. Ammori, S. Joseph, M. Attia and J. P. Lodge, Biliary strictures complicating pancreaticoduodenectomy, *Int. J. Pancreatol.* **28**(1): 15–21; discussion 21–22 (2000).

81. R. Gupta, R. Thurairaja, C. D. Johnson and J. N. Primrose, Body composition, muscle function and psychological changes in patients undergoing operation for hepatic or pancreatic disease, *Pancreatology* **1**(2): 90–95 (2001).

82. R. Gupta and H. Ihmaidat, Nutritional effects of oesophageal, gastric and pancreatic carcinoma, *Eur. J. Surg. Oncol.* **29**(8): 634–643 (2003).

83. D. Silk, Diet following resections of the small intestine and the pancreas, *Pancreatology* **1**(S1): 27–34 (2001).

84. R. F. Meier and C. Beglinger, Nutrition in pancreatic diseases, *Best Pract. Res. Clin. Gastroenterol.* **20**(3): 507–529 (2006).

85. M. I. van Berge Henegouwen, T. M. Moojen, T. M. van Gulik *et al.*, Postoperative weight gain after standard Whipple's procedure versus pylorus-preserving pancreatoduodenectomy: The influence of tumour status, *Br. J. Surg.* **85**(7): 922–926 (1998).

86. S. Caliari, L. Benini, C. Sembenini *et al.*, Medium-chain triglyceride absorption in patients with pancreatic insufficiency., *Scand. J. Gastroenterol.* **31**(1): 90–94 (1996).

87. T. Armstrong, L. Strommer, F. Ruiz-Jasbon *et al.*, Pancreaticoduodenectomy for peri-ampullary neoplasia leads to specific micronutrient deficiencies, *Pancreatology* **7**(1): 37–44 (2007).

88. T. Armstrong, E. Walters, S. Varshney and C. D. Johnson, Deficiencies of micronutrients, altered bowel function, and quality of life during late follow-up after pancreaticoduodenectomy for malignancy, *Pancreatology* **2**(6): 528–534 (2002).

89. R. Meier, J. Ockenga, M. Pertkiewicz *et al.*, ESPEN guidelines on enteral nutrition: Pancreas, *Clin. Nutr.* **25**(2): 275–284 (2006).

90. M. I. van Berge Henegouwen, L. M. Akkermans, T. M. van Gulik *et al.*, Prospective, randomized trial on the effect of cyclic versus continuous enteral nutrition on postoperative gastric function after pylorus-preserving pancreatoduodenectomy, *Ann. Surg.* **226**(6): 677–685; discussion 685–687 (1997).

91. F. Bozzetti and V. Bozzetti, Efficacy of enteral and parenteral nutrition in cancer patients, *Nestle Nutr. Workshop Ser. Clin. Perform. Programme,* **10**: 127–139; discussion 139–142 (2005).

92. L. Gianotti, M. Braga, O. Gentilini *et al.*, Artificial nutrition after pancreaticoduodenectomy, *Pancreas* **21**(4): 344–351 (2000).

93. S. Jo, S. H. Choi, J. S. Heo *et al.*, Missing effect of glutamine supplementation on the surgical outcome after pancreaticoduodenectomy for periampullary tumors: A prospective, randomized, double-blind, controlled clinical trial, *World J. Surg.* **30**(11): 1974–1982; discussion 1983–1984 (2006).

94. M. Braga, L. Gianotti, O. Gentilini *et al.*, Feeding the gut early after digestive surgery: Results of a nine-year experience, *Clin. Nutr.* **21**(1): 59–65 (2002).

95. M. Braga, L. Gianotti, O. Gentilini *et al.*, Early postoperative enteral nutrition improves gut oxygenation and reduces costs compared with total parenteral nutrition, *Crit. Care Med.* **29**(2): 242–248 (2001).

96. F. Bozzetti, M. Braga, L. Gianotti *et al.*, Postoperative enteral versus parenteral nutrition in malnourished patients with gastrointestinal cancer: A randomised multicentre trial, *Lancet* **358**(9292): 1487–1492 (2001).

97. S. Aiko, Y. Yoshizumi, Y. Sugiura *et al.*, Beneficial effects of immediate enteral nutrition after esophageal cancer surgery, *Surg. Today* **31**(11): 971–978 (2001).

98. R. L. Koretz, Enteral nutrition led to fewer postoperative complications than did parenteral feeding in gastrointestinal cancer, *ACP J. Club* **136**(3): 93 (2002).

99. R. L. Koretz, T. O. Lipman and S. Klein, AGA technical review on parenteral nutrition, *Gastroenterology* **121**(4): 970–1001 (2001).

Management Decisions in Primary and Secondary Liver Cancer

Mark E. Brooke-Smith and
Robert T. A. Padbury

Abstract

Management of liver neoplasia is a multidisciplinary endeavour. In the non-cirrhotic liver resectional surgery has a well-defined place in the management of primary liver tumours. In the cirrhotic liver, the approach to treatment of hepatocellular carcinoma depends on the severity of underlying liver disease and the size of the tumour. The best long term results are achieved with transplantation regardless of severity of liver failure, but the number and size of lesions is important. Liver resection can be used in any size lesion, but the extent of resection possible is dependent on the severity of liver disease. As with ablative methods, the tumour volume is an important prognostic factor. Colorectal cancer is the most common secondary liver cancer with a chance of cure following surgical resection. Surgical resection is becoming more aggressive, as more sophisticated techniques and increasing chemotherapeutic options allow removal of more advanced tumours. The role and timing of surgery, local ablation, chemotherapy and adjuvant chemotherapy are explored in the setting of both synchronous and metachronous disease. Surgical resection and the chance of cure is possible in a subset of patients with neuroendocrine liver metastases, but pharmacological and chemotherapeutic therapies are available if resection is not possible. Surgery is less applicable in non-colorectal, non-neuroendocrine tumours, but in some circumstances, it may be of benefit.

Keywords: Hepatocellular carcinoma, ablation, surgery, chemotherapy, colorectal liver metastases, cholangiocarcinoma, sarcoma, neuroendocrine liver metastases.

1.   Introduction

Multidisciplinary teams are particularly important in managing liver neoplasia. The surgeon, oncologist, radiation oncologist, radiologist, hepatologist, pathologist, palliative care physician and general practitioner are among the clinicians routinely involved in managing patients with liver lesions. In addition, oncology and surgical nurses, transplant coordinators, pharmacists, dieticians, social workers, and allied health professionals are required to address many organisational, psychosocial and paraclinical issues. The following chapter seeks to underline the importance of involving a number of disciplines to provide the best patient outcomes, focussing on areas where new evidence or controversy exists.

2.   Primary Liver Cancer in the Cirrhotic Patient

2.1   *Hepatocellular carcinoma*

2.1.1   *Epidemiology*

Hepatocellular carcinoma (HCC) is the most common primary cancer of the liver, and most commonly occurs in the cirrhotic patient. HCC is implicated in approximately 500,000 deaths per year and internationally is the 5th most common solid organ malignancy.[1-3] HCC is associated with chronic liver disease and the disease is much more common in geographic areas where hepatitis B or C is endemic.[4] In many countries, including Australia, where the incidence has been relatively low, HCC incidence is increasing, and this has been attributed to a rise in the prevalence of chronic hepatitis B and C infections.[5,6] HCC is also more commonly associated with alcohol-related cirrhosis,[7] non-alcoholic fatty liver disease (NAFLD)[8,9] and other genetic conditions affecting the liver, such as haemochromatosis.[10]

2.1.2   Diagnosis of hepatocellular carcinoma

The investigation and diagnosis of liver lesions has been haphazard, potentially compromising the many treatment strategies that have become available. In response to this, the European Association for the Study of the Liver (EASL) produced a consensus statement to set criteria for the diagnosis of HCC in cirrhotics to prevent inappropriate treatment or prevent unnecessary biopsy, compromising potential curative treatments like surgical resection.[11] For lesions greater than 2 cm, the criteria in Table 1 have become widely accepted as sufficient for the diagnosis of HCC, and non-invasive assessment alone has an accuracy of 99.6%.[12,13] Typical distinguishing radiological features on ultrasonography, computer tomography and magnetic resonance imaging of common liver lesions are summarised in Table 2. It should be noted that HCC often has a variable appearance, and does not always show vascular contrast enhancement.[14] If a lesion is smaller than 1 cm, the risk of malignancy is less than 50%.[3] For lesions between 1 and 2 cm the diagnosis of HCC is more difficult and cytopathological confirmation has been recommended.[11] Unfortunately there is a false negative rate of between 30 and 40% and a risk of needle tract seeding of 2%, with ultrasound guided needle aspiration biopsy.[15]

Alphafeto protein (AFP) levels of greater than 400 ng/ml are considered diagnostic for HCC.[3,11,17] The specificity for this level of AFP is 99%, but the sensitivity is only 15%.[18] In patients undergoing liver transplantation for HCC, or found to have HCC, only 15% had an AFP of greater than 400 ng/ml.[18] AFP can also be raised in conditions such as chronic active hepatitis, and so mildly elevated levels do not necessarily confirm an underlying HCC, but suspicion is increased. Ultrasonography is associated with a sensitivity of between 35–84%.[19] In a recent randomised controlled trial, AFP and ultrasound were combined and performed at six-monthly intervals, to demonstrate improved detection of HCC and improved survival.[16]

Table 1. Non-invasive diagnostic criteria for hepatocellular carcinoma.

- Mass >2 cm in a cirrhotic liver
- Identified by means of 2 coincident imaging techniques ultrasonography, spiral computed tomography, magnetic resonance imaging, angiography
- One imaging study must have contrast enhancement

2.1.3 Staging and management

The severity of the underlying liver dysfunction in cirrhotics with HCC is critical in the management of these patients. Patients with greater hepatic reserve can better tolerate therapies where a larger amount of liver is compromised. Similarly the size, location, and biology of the tumour are determinants of the type of therapies that can be offered. Several prognostic systems have been proposed, suggesting that there is not yet a perfect staging system. These systems use tumour factors (size, vascular invasion, extrahepatic spread and AFP) and liver factors (performance status, Child-Pugh Score, bilirubin and albumin levels, portal hypertension, ascites) to aid in clinical decision making and prognostication.[20–23]

2.1.4 Ablative and 'non-invasive' therapies

A number of ablative therapies have been used to treat liver lesions, with ethanol injection and radiofrequency ablation (RFA) as the most widely used. Other 'non-invasive' therapies have been described, including systemic chemotherapy, targeted chemo- or radiotherapy, for example transarterial chemo-embolisation (TACE), and external beam radiotherapy. The applicability of the latter technique has been limited by the relative sensitivity of the liver to radiation damage.

The limitation of ablative techniques is largely due to the tumour size and location. Percutaneous ethanol injection (PEI) is performed under ultrasound guidance and absolute alcohol is injected until the lesion becomes hyperechoic on ultrasound. The rate of tumour necrosis varies according to the size of the lesion, with 90% complete necrosis in lesions <2 cm, 70% in 3 cm tumours

Table 2. Radiological differentiation of liver tumours.

	Morphology	Ultrasound	CT	MRI	Contrast enhancement
Cysts	Well-defined Smooth	An-echoic	Hypodense	T1: Hypointense T2: Bright	Nil
Haemangioma	Well-defined Smooth No cirrhosis	Echogenic (70%)	Hypodense	T1: Hypointense T2: Bright	Early: Peripheral Nodular Late: Complete fill-in
Focal fatty infiltration	Adjacent to porta hepatis, falciform or gallbladder fossa	Echogenic	Hypodense	T1 & T2: Iso-intense	Nil
Focal nodular hyperplasia	Most <5 cm Central scar Homogeneous No capsule	Iso-echoic	Iso-intense	T1 & T2: Iso-intense with vascular central scar	Early: Intense homogeneous Delayed: Rapid washout, scar enhancing late
Hepatic adenoma	Most >5 cm Capsule associated haemorrhage No scar	Iso-echoic	Iso-intense	T1 & T2: Iso-intense	Early: Intense homogeneous Delayed: Rapid washout

(Continued)

Table 2. *(Continued)*

	Morphology	Ultrasound	CT	MRI	Contrast enhancement
Fibrolamellar HCC	Most >10 cm Heterogenous Central scar Calcium and nodes in 2/3 No cirrhosis	Heterogenous	Heterogenous	T1: Hypo-intense T2: Hyperintense	Early: Hypervascular, but heterogenous
HCC	Cirrhosis Vascular invasion	Variable	Variable	Variable	Hypervascular
Metastases	Poorly defined margins Heterogenous No scar No capsule No cirrhosis	Hypo-echoic	Hypodense	T1: Hypo-intense T2: Mildly hyperintense	Early: Enhances more than normal liver Peripheral ring common

and 50% in 5 cm tumours.[24,25] PEI has the advantage of being relatively cheap. In contrast RFA requires more expensive equipment, but has the advantage of ablating a margin of liver around the tissue. Slightly larger lesions can be managed with RFA, but in common with PEI, complete necrosis rates fall as tumours exceed 4 cm. RFA does result in an increase in local tumour control when compared with PEI.[26] The only evidence of improved overall survival comes from case-control series where 4-year survival was improved from 61% to 68% in Child's A and B patients.[27] These excellent survival data were achieved because most tumours were less than 3 cm in size. Tumour size is an important determinant of overall survival, with tumours larger than 4–5 cm having less than 30% 5-year survival rate, compared with 50% in 3–4 cm tumours and 70% in tumours less than 2 cm in size for Child's A and B cirrhotics.[27] RFA is less effective if tumours are adjacent to larger blood vessels, as a heat-sink effect occurs and tissue heating, on which RFA relies, is significantly reduced.

Both PEI and RFA are associated with potential complications. Pain and fever occur with both methods. PEI is rarely associated with ethanol injection into portal triad structures, resulting in cholangitis or thrombosis. Mortality from both PEI and RFA is low. A review of complications of RFA found a mortality rate of 0.5% and significant complication rate of 9%, from abscess formation, intraperitoneal bleeding, hepatic decompensation and perforation of adjacent organs. In addition there is the risk of needle tract seeding, perhaps slightly higher with RFA, due to the larger probe size, but coagulation of the needle tract on removal may decrease this.

TACE can be applied to larger tumours than is possible with other ablative techniques. A meta-analysis of randomised controlled trials has shown that TACE improves survival in unresectable HCC.[28] TACE involves direct intra-arterial injection of a chemotherapeutic agent (for example, doxorubicin) combined with lipiodol, which is retained in HCC, and allows an increased dose of chemotherapeutic agents to be delivered. This is usually combined with embolisation of the tumour, as HCC are generally supplied almost exclusively by the hepatic artery. As part of the blood supply to the liver is compromised, the technique is less applicable in patients with decompensated liver disease. In Child's A cirrhosis the mortality is less than 2%, but rises to 37% in Child's C patients.[29] HCC has a propensity to invade the portal vein as it enlarges, and clearly if both the portal vein and hepatic artery are occluded, these patients will decompensate, so TACE cannot be used. Other side effects include fever, abdominal pain and a rise in serum transaminases. Other less common and more severe complications can include liver decompensation, cholecystitis, and duodenal or gastric wall necrosis, due to inadvertent embolisation of other arterial branches. Patients are usually prescribed proton-pump inhibitors to address the latter complication. Hypervascular tumours at baseline, tumour uptake of lipiodol and repeated administration of TACE are variables associated with improved survival.[30,31]

All local ablative techniques are best suited to lesions less than 3 cm in size. More recently, a randomised controlled trial of 291 patients has demonstrated that combining modalities such as RFA and TACE can result in improved survival.[32] This paper has subsequently been retracted due to fraudulent reporting, though the institution of origin does perform TACE plus RFA. Surgical resection can result in 5-year survivals of up to 55%, though it is difficult to compare directly, as TACE and RFA are usually reserved for patients with larger tumours and poorer liver function.[33]

2.1.5 Surgical resection

In many centres, surgical resection of HCC is the mainstay of treatment, as resection is associated with the highest long term survival figures of all treatment modalities except transplantation. However the best surgical candidates are also the best candidates for loco-regional therapies. Surgical resection can be offered for larger lesions, but the ability of the liver to cope with liver volume loss and regenerate becomes a limiting factor as the severity of liver failure increases. Many HCC are associated with multi-focal disease, which can limit the feasibility of liver resection. Also, as with other less invasive therapies, recurrence can occur in up to 80% of patients at five years.[34]

With improved patient selection and better peri-operative management, in-hospital mortality for surgical resection in cirrhotics has fallen to between 0 and 5%.[35] Conventional wisdom is that major resection in cirrhotic liver should only be undertaken with Child's A disease, and generally in patients without portal hypertension.[36-38] However, some Child-Pugh A patients may undergo major liver resection (of three or more segments) in the presence of portal hypertension with acceptable mortality. In a recent series, mortality was not statistically increased in Child-Pugh A patients with portal hypertension, compared to those without (11% versus 5%).[39] Lesser liver resection may be carried out in Child-Pugh B patients, however Child-Pugh C patients are at significant risk of decompensation with any liver resection. Dynamic tests of liver function, such as clearance of intravenously injected indocyanine green can be used to aid the assessment of hepatic reserve.[35,38] The volume of liver remnant remaining should also be assessed. In non-cirrhotics, up to 75% of the liver can be removed safely, however in cirrhotics, even with good hepatic reserve, resection of 50–60% of liver volume can precipitate liver decompensation.[36,40]

2.1.6 *Portal vein embolisation*

Portal vein embolisation (PVE) has been used in an attempt to increase the volume of the remnant liver and therefore decrease the risk of post-operative liver failure. PVE can be achieved radiologically via a percutaneous transhepatic approach. Regeneration of the liver remnant is usually achieved in two to four weeks. Prospective studies have shown that PVE results in an increased resectability rate, decreased post-operative complications and decreased length of hospital and intensive care stay, provided that hypertrophy of the liver remnant is achieved.[40,41] Therefore in the two to six weeks following PVE, further imaging should be done to re-assess liver volume. If no increase in residual liver volume is achieved, this reflects an inability of the liver to regenerate and resection should not be performed.

2.1.7 *Adjuvant therapy*

The high rate of HCC recurrence has led to the investigation of adjuvant therapies. A number of randomised controlled trials have failed to show a survival benefit, or decreased recurrence for systemic chemotherapy, hepatic arterial chemotherapy, or hepatic arterial chemo-embolisation.[42] However there is emerging data from a small randomised controlled trial and case-controlled studies with five to ten year follow-up, suggesting that ^{131}I-labelled lipiodol is likely to improve recurrence rates and disease-free survival post-resection and should be considered.[43,44] Despite these promising results, monitoring resected patients is important, as many may benefit from re-resection, other loco-regional therapies or transplantation.[45]

2.1.8 *Liver transplantation*

The advantage of liver transplantation in the treatment of HCC is that it is the only modality that addresses both the underlying liver disease and the tumour, and is the only potentially curative therapy that can be delivered in patients with advanced liver disease. However, initial results for liver transplantation in HCC were poor, with five-year survival ranging between 18 and 40%.[46] Mazzaferro *et al.* found that a subgroup of patients with HCC (less than three tumours less than 3 cm in size, or a single tumour less than 5 cm) had long term survival figures similar to non-tumour patients.[47] Given the shortage of organ donors and to maximise organ utility, these (Milan) criteria have been widely applied and have resulted in five-year survivals over 70%, which is no different from patients transplanted without HCC.[48–50] When compared to resection of HCC, transplantation gives an additional five-year survival in 20–30% of patients.[51–54]

Encouraged by the excellent results from the implementation of the Mazzaferro (or Milan) criteria, expanded (UCSF) criteria for liver transplantation have been proposed. With a single tumour less than 6.5 cm, or with two to three tumours, all <4.5 cm and a total diameter of all tumours <8 cm, five-year survivals of 75% can be expected.[49,55] Adopting these criteria results in approximately

10% more patients being offered transplantation, but long term survival in the group is unchanged.[55,56]

The supply of donor organs falls short of demand; therefore, in many centres, Child's A patients are offered resection before transplantation, which does not appear to hamper the long term survival in patients who meet the Milan criteria.[57] Disease progression and dropout from the waiting list occurs in 9%, 19% and 32% of patients at 90, 180 and 365 days after listing (United Network for Organ Sharing- UNOS- database figures).[58] Many studies comparing primary resection to transplantation have failed to take this into account, but when results of liver resection are examined using an intention to treat analysis, results are more favourable because of the shortage of organ donors and increasing waiting times.

There is however a regional difference in the result of liver resection and salvage transplantation. In Asia, where Hepatitis B is the most common aetiology, resection with a view to salvage transplantation for recurrence, up to 80% are transplantable if disease recurs.[56,59] However in Europe, where HCV replaces HBV as the most common viral aetiology, less than 40% are eligible for salvage transplantation if HCC recurs.[60] Many patients who are resected have a sufficient long term survival to fall outside age guidelines for transplantation when disease recurs.[61] Furthermore, liver transplantation is also more difficult following liver resection.[62] Due to the complex nature of decision making in this area, those with transplantable HCC should be managed by a transplant team.

To reduce disease progression on the transplant waiting list, bridging therapies have been employed; most commonly these are RFA and TACE. A recent meta-analysis on TACE as a bridging therapy did not find any convincing evidence that it prevented dropout from the waiting list, but it was safe and randomised controlled trials are needed.[63] There are also no randomised controlled trials of RFA, but compared to historical controls, dropout rates range from 0–6%, compared to 32%, with complication rates of 5–8%.[64–66] These bridging treatments should be used in patients in danger of progressing beyond transplant criteria, or who are likely to have a prolonged wait.

2.1.9 Chemotherapy

There is a limited role for systemic chemotherapy in the treatment of HCC. The exception to this is sorafenib, which inhibits tumour cell proliferation, tumour angiogenesis and increases the rate of tumour cell apoptosis.[67] A phase 3 randomised controlled trial has shown a modest increased median survival in patients with advanced HCC and Child-Pugh A cirrhosis treated with sorafenib, when compared to a placebo.[68] It remains to be seen whether this translates into a benefit in patients with more advanced liver disease, or when used as adjuvant therapy to surgery or ablative therapies.

3. Primary Liver Cancer in the Non-Cirrhotic Patient

The main difficulty in the non-cirrhotic liver is the diagnosis of liver lesions. The disease may be incidental, which presents a diagnostic conundrum, or it presents late, decreasing the possibility of curative resection. Common radiological findings are summarised in Table 2, however the availability of a multidisciplinary team meeting of radiologists, surgeons and oncologists allows difficult cases to be discussed and junior members to be educated.

3.1 Hepatocellular carcinoma

HCC is uncommon in the normal liver and the main differential diagnoses include benign lesions, such as focal nodular hyperplasia, which can be treated expectantly, and adenoma, which often requires resection. HCC in normal livers is often associated with underlying liver diseases, such as hepatitis B, haemachromatosis and NAFLD. Ultrasound, triple phase contrast enhanced computed tomography (CT) and contrast enhanced MRI are complementary modalities. In contrast to HCC in cirrhotic livers, the serum AFP is often normal in the non-cirrhotic liver with HCC.

Unlike the cirrhotic liver, treatment of HCC in the normal liver is more straightforward. Resection is associated with low morbidity (15%) and mortality (1%) and a five-year survival of more than 50%.[69-71] Liver transplantation with cadaveric donors is generally not indicated for this group, but in unresectable cases, living related liver transplantation is being explored.[72]

Fibrolamellar carcinoma is a rare variant of HCC which occurs in the normal liver and 85% have a normal AFP. The tumours are usually large and solitary; five-year survival following resection may exceed 65% and the results are comparable to liver transplantation.[73]

3.2 Cholangiocarcinoma

Cholangiocarcinoma may be divided into central (infiltrating), gallbladder and peripheral (intrahepatic, mass-forming) subtypes. In all subtypes surgical resection offers the only hope of cure, although new chemotherapeutic agents such as gemcitabine are offering some response in those patients without resectable disease. Peripheral cholangiocarcinomas are often diagnosed fortuitously, or are very large at the time of diagnosis. They may be associated with a raised serum CA 19.9 or CA 125. The radiological findings on CT usually demonstrate a lesion with late contrast enhancement and associated with capsular retraction. Many central cholangiocarcinomas are associated with atrophy of liver segments, due to the involvement of vascular and biliary pedicles, but rarely invade the portal vein. The long term (five-year) survival following resection of intra-hepatic mass-forming cholangiocarcinoma may be as high as 50%, but many Western series including patients with central cholangiocarcinomas have five-year survival rates of 20% with resection.[74] Patients with hilar/central infiltrating cholangiocarcinoma should have a right or left hepatectomy or trisectionectomy with resection of the caudate lobe. Once there is separation of the second order bile ducts on imaging, the likelihood of curative resection is low and this is generally regarded as a contraindication to surgery. Involvement of the portal vein does not necessarily preclude resection, but if reconstruction of the hepatic artery is involved, operative mortality is significantly increased, and long term survival lessened.[75,76] Central resection is employed in higher risk patients, but is associated with a higher incidence of positive margins.[77–79]

Gallbladder cancer may be suspected preoperatively or found incidentally following 1% of cholecystectomies.[80] Patients with T1 disease (confined to the muscular layer) discovered at cholecystectomy have a 90–100% five-year survival and do not require further surgery.[81] In patients who have T2 disease (not breaching serosa) on the post-cholecystectomy specimen, overall survival is improved from at least 20 to 60% with extended resection.[81,82] For those with T3 or T4 disease, where the tumour invades into the liver and/or other adjacent organs or vascular structures, the decision for extended resection is more controversial, although five-year survival of approximately 28–45% is possible, provided there are no distant metastases and the N2 (peripancreatic and celiac) nodes are clear of tumour.[82,83] Patients with suspected resectable gallbladder cancer pre-operatively should undergo cholecystectomy by a surgeon expecting to perform an extended resection, including partial segmentectomy of segments 4 and 5 and nodal clearance.

3.3   *Other primary liver tumours*

Sarcomas of the liver, though rare, are generally associated with a poor prognosis. Angiosarcomas are rapidly growing and associated with median survivals of six months, but long term survival is possible with resection.[84,85] Other sarcomas, in particular leiomyosarcoma, are associated with a better prognosis and resection should be attempted if possible.[86]

Epithelioid hemangioendothelioma is a rare tumour arising from the sinusoidal endothelial cells, occurring in young adults. It usually has a multifocal distribution and MRI and biopsy are often required to make the diagnosis.[87] Resection is often not possible, due to its multi-focal nature and therefore liver transplantation offers the only hope of disease control with five-year survival of 50–70% even in patients with limited extra-hepatic disease.[88–91]

Chemotherapy, with agents such as thalidomide, 5-fluorouracil, doxorubicin, vincristine and TACE, and radiotherapy have also been used to treat these patients.[89]

4.   Secondary Liver Cancer

4.1   *Colorectal liver metastases*

4.1.1   *Epidemiology*

Colorectal liver metastases may be present in 25% of patients at the time of diagnosis or resection of the primary tumour (synchronous disease) and 25% of patients may develop liver metastases (metachronous disease) at a median time of one and half years after resection of the primary tumour.[92,93] The natural history of colorectal liver metastases is variable, with a five-year survival of almost 0% without treatment.[94–97] Availability of more recent chemotherapy regimens, combined with surgical resection in selected patients has improved survival to 30% or more at five years.[98]

4.1.2 Presentation

Liver metastases may be discovered on pre-operative staging investigations, such as CT, and on inspection and palpation of the liver at the time of laparotomy. During the follow-up period, colorectal metastases can be discovered following the detection of a rising serum carcino-embryonic antigen (CEA) concentration, or planned CT surveillance. A meta-analysis and Cochrane review have demonstrated a survival benefit with intensive follow-up regimes that include CEA and CT surveillance, with a median eight month earlier detection of recurrence and a higher likelihood of curative surgery being performed.[99,100] No conclusions about the timing of follow-up investigations could be drawn, but given that the median time to recurrence is one and a half years, CT scanning at one to two years, with CEA monitoring, would seem a minimum, but is the subject of ongoing trials.

4.1.3 Imaging

Triple phase contrast enhanced CT and ultrasonography are the most common imaging modalities to detect metastatic colonic cancer. The typical findings can be found in Table 2. In addition to these modalities, magnetic resonance imaging (MRI), positron emission tomography (PET), intra-operative ultrasound (IOUS) and CT arterial portography (CTAP) are used to further characterise and evaluate intra- and extra-hepatic disease.

CTAP has been used for characterisation of lesions less than 1 cm in size on CT, as it has a sensitivity of 80–90%.[101,102] There is a false positive rate of 15–35%, which limits its usefulness for planning surgery, so this modality has been superseded by multislice triple phase CT scanning.[102,103] New liver-specific contrast agents have been used with MRI and these increase sensitivity and specificity, compared to conventional MRI, including lesions less than 1 cm in size.[102,104,105] These agents increase the contrast between normal liver and non-liver tissue and include superparamagnetic iron oxide particles (for example, resovist), which is taken up by the reticuloendothelial system of normal liver and dampens the signal intensity, and gadoxetic acid (primovist), which is taken up by hepatocytes and increases their signal intensity. Liver-specific contrast enhanced MRI has been shown to alter surgical management in 17% of patients.[102] PET and PET/CT are useful for the detection of extra-hepatic disease, but are less sensitive and specific compared to liver-specific contrast enhanced MRI for the hepatic staging of colorectal metastases.[106]

Ideally, patients presenting with colorectal liver metastases and being considered for surgery should have both PET/CT and liver-specific contrast enhanced MRI or multislice CT. Intra-operative ultrasound should be performed at the time of liver surgery, as this modality provides additional information in one in five patients and changes the surgical strategy in 17%.[107]

4.1.4 Chemotherapy

Chemotherapy alone is not yet a curative strategy, but with newer agents improved survival is being achieved. The antimetabolite, 5-fluorouracil (5-FU) has been the most widely used agent in the adjuvant and palliative setting for colorectal cancer. Capecitabine is an oral analogue of 5-FU and has the same toxicity profile. When capecitabine is compared to bolus infusion of 5-FU, there is a better response rate, but no overall improvement in survival.[108] Continuous infusion of 5-FU appears to be superior to bolus 5-FU with regard to a slight improvement in survival and a reduced side effect profile.[109] Folinic acid (leucovorin) has been combined with 5-FU to double response rates and improve overall survival.[110]

More recently agents such as irinotecan (a topoisomerase I inhibitor) and oxaliplatin (a platinum analogue) have become available and show a survival benefit in treatment of colorectal cancer metastases. A number of studies have looked at these agents in combination with 5-FU (Irinotecan — FOLFIRI; oxaliplatin — FOLFOX), and demonstrated an improved response rate compared to 5-FU alone.[111-114] FOLFOX regimes may be better tolerated,[115] and Irinotecan requires dose adjustment in patients with impaired liver function.[116]

Two mono-clonal antibodies have been evaluated in the treatment of advanced colorectal cancer. Cetuximab targets an endothelial growth factor receptor, and while it has been associated with improved response following irinotecan, a randomised controlled trial failed to show any improvement in survival in this setting.[117] Cetuximab has been shown to improve overall survival when other treatments have failed.[118] Bevacizumab targets vascular endothelial growth factor, and when added to 5-FU and leucovorin, demonstrated an improvement in median survival from 15 to 20 months.[119] Bevacizumab has also shown improved response when combined with FOLFIRI and FOLFOX regimes.[120,121]

4.1.5   *Patient selection for surgery*

Liver resection offers the only chance of cure and prolonged survival advantage. The boundaries for resection have increased in recent years, limited mainly by the need to preserve arterial and portal venous inflow and hepatic venous outflow to 30% of functioning parenchyma.

A few series have examined the additive effect of potential adverse pre-operative factors, perhaps the best known reported by the Memorial Sloan-Kettering group.[122,123] A scoring system has been developed, which demonstrates the impact of these factors on longevity and can be useful when discussing the role of surgery with individual patients.[122] The negative prognostic factors are node positive disease, a disease-free interval of less than 12 months, more than one tumour, a tumour greater than 5 cm or a CEA greater than 200 ng/ml.[122,123] If none of these are present, median survivals of 74 months can be achieved, whereas if all five are present the median survival is 22 months with resection.[122] Additional factors have been added and have led to the development of a nomogram for prognostic information following resection.[123] Recently Rees *et al.* confirmed the findings of the Memorial Sloan-Kettering group in a large series of patients.[124]

The single most important prognostic factor is the ability to achieve clear margins at resection. Traditionally a margin of more than one centimetre has been sought, but it is now evident that a margin of 1–2 mm is adequate if a larger margin cannot be obtained.[125,126]

Apart from patient fitness for surgery, other factors are important in determining whether a patient should undergo surgery. These include the volume and health of the liver remnant, as discussed above for HCC. Patients who have received oxaliplatin-based chemotherapy can develop a sinusoidal injury and those that receive irinotecan can develop steatosis, which decreases the volume of liver that can be safely resected and significantly increases the morbidity from surgery.[127,128] FOLFOX does not appear to significantly impact on the mortality, though, if six cycles or less are given (over three months).[127,128]

Generally if the metastatic disease is resectable, liver surgeons would prefer to operate prior to chemotherapy. The sinusoidal injury following oxaliplatin can lead to increased blood loss and if there are a number of small metastases, and these radiologically disappear after chemotherapy, identifying them at the time of surgery can be problematic.

4.1.6 *Adjuvant chemotherapy*

Adjuvant treatment with 5-FU and leucovorin has been shown to improve five-year disease free survival and a trend towards overall survival.[129] Trials of adjuvant FOLFOX compared with 5FU have demonstrated the superiority of FOLFOX for adjuvant chemotherapy in primary colorectal cancer.[130,131] Therefore it was surprising to find that neo-adjuvant chemotherapy with three cycles of FOLFOX prior to surgical resection, followed by three cycles after resection, did not show any statistically significant benefit in three-year progression free survival over surgery alone in the intention to treat analysis of a multicentre randomised controlled trial.[128] There was a statistically significant benefit in the progression-free survival when only the eligible and resected patients were analysed, but this came at the cost of increased complications following surgery after chemotherapy, though there was no increase in mortality.[128] In the neoadjuvant setting, bevacizumab has been combined with capecitabine and oxaliplatin, but was ceased five weeks pre-operatively, and it did not demonstrate a significant adverse effect on mortality, bleeding, wound healing or liver regeneration.[132]

4.1.7 Downstaging chemotherapy to increase resectability

As surgery offers the best chance of cure and long term survival, modalities that safely increase the resectability of colorectal metastases should also be explored. Pre-operative chemotherapy may downsize tumours so as to make initially non-resectable disease resectable.[133] Treatment with FOLFOX regimes downstages disease, to allow resection in an additional 20–50% of patients who were initially not resectable.[134-136] More recently FOLFOX has been combined with irinotecan (FOLFOXIRI) in unresectable liver metastatic disease and has shown a significant increase in R0 resection rates from 6 to 15% and an improvement in overall survival, compared to FOLFIRI in a phase III trial.[137]

4.1.8 Portal vein embolisation to increase resectability

If the remnant liver volume is less than 25% in a healthy liver, consideration should be given to portal vein embolisation (PVE) of the liver to be resected. When PVE is employed, and initially non-resectable disease is resected, similar operative mortality and five-year survival rates can be achieved.[40,138] Some authors have found that PVE may lead to increased growth of tumours in the non-embolised liver, and in one series there was no difference in overall survival in the embolised group.[139,140] It is difficult to compare groups in these non-randomised series, as for example in one of the studies, 50% fewer patients in the PVE group received post-operative chemotherapy.[139,140]

4.1.9 Other strategies to increase resectability

The location, number and size of liver lesions determine resectability, although strategies such as staged resections combined with chemotherapy in initially non-resectable disease, can lead to meaningful survival benefits.[127,141,142] Oxaliplatin-based chemotherapy can be given between resections to increase the resectability and control the non-resected disease, whilst post-operative recovery and liver regeneration occurs. Resection can be combined with RFA to improve the resectability of colorectal liver metastases with successful outcomes.[143–146] The presence of extra-hepatic disease is also important in determining resectability, yet if the extrahepatic deposits are localised and can be resected, this does not preclude the resection of liver lesions.[147] Re-resection also plays a role if disease recurs in the liver, with equivalent five-year survival figures possible in patients requiring a second or third resection.[147]

4.1.10 *Local ablation*

Radiofrequency ablation is an attractive technique for the management of colorectal liver metastases as it preserves normal liver parenchyma and is potentially less invasive, though the best results have been achieved at open operation.[146,148] A percutaneous approach appears to be inferior to the laparoscopic approach, which in turn is less successful at tumour control than the open approach (Table 3).[146,148–154] Complete tumour ablation can be achieved in two-thirds of cases, however as with other liver lesions, the best responses are in smaller tumours that are not adjacent to vascular or biliary structures.[148,155,156] It is difficult to offer this modality to patients with resectable disease and so there are no randomised controlled trials comparing RFA to surgery. Treatment site recurrence rates following RFA range from 5–39%.[157–159] Apart from local recurrence, studies have also examined liver recurrence and found

Table 3. Colorectal metastases treatment site recurrence after RFA via open, laparoscopic and percutaneous approaches.

Series	Access	Recurrence (%)	Length of follow-up
Elias *et al.* (2004)[148]	Open	6	28 months
Abdalla *et al.* (2004)[146]	Open	9	21 months
Siperstein *et al.* (2000)[151]	Laparoscopic	39	?
Berber *et al.* (2005)[149]	Laparoscopic	46	?
Solbiati *et al.* (2001)[153]	Percutaneous	55	? (2–3 years)
Livraghi *et al.* (2003)[150]	Percutaneous	40+	33 months
White *et al.* (2004)[154]	Percutaneous	39+	17 months

that compared to surgery, RFA is associated with higher local recurrence and a much greater development of new liver lesions.[146] The increase in new liver lesions after RFA alone compared to surgery has been postulated to be responsible for the poorer long term survival.[160] However in the era of more effective chemotherapy agents, when surgical resection is not possible, five-year survivals in the order of 18% can be achieved with RFA alone and can be combined with surgery in otherwise non-resectable disease.[143,144] RFA also plays a role in the treatment of recurrence following surgery.

4.1.11 *Approach to synchronous liver metastases*

With so many options for treatment available, it is difficult to know what the best approach is for a patient with a primary colorectal tumour and synchronous liver-only resectable metastases. These metastases may be discovered at the time of primary resection, or may have been detected pre-operatively.

For patients with known resectable liver metastases prior to colorectal surgery, the option of synchronous resection of the primary and liver secondaries exists. Initial poor results dampened the enthusiasm for this approach, however, more recent data suggests no adverse effect on survival, along with a reduction in total hospitalisation with a synchronous resection of the primary and liver secondaries.[161–165] Some of these studies found that identifying more than six positive lymph nodes was an adverse prognostic marker, but this is difficult to apply pre-operatively.[162,166] More recently, patients undergoing synchronous liver resection with a T4 primary tumour and 4 or more liver metastases appear to have poorer overall survival, compared to those undergoing delayed resection and therefore should be considered for neo-adjuvant chemotherapy and delayed resection.[161] A case can be made for resection of the liver secondary first if there is a risk of the liver metastasis becoming non-resectable, for example in patients requiring pelvic radiotherapy prior to the resection of their primary. A recent series found improved survival in patients treated with chemotherapy, liver resection and then removal of the colorectal primary in non-obstructing colorectal cancers.[167–169]

For those with liver metastases discovered at the time of resection for the primary tumour, the choice is between neo-adjuvant chemotherapy and resection or immediate resection followed by adjuvant chemotherapy. It was believed that response to chemotherapy was a prognostic indicator,[170] but a number of studies have demonstrated similar overall survival between synchronous and delayed resection of liver metastases, regardless of response to chemotherapy.[162–166] With little data to guide decision making, a sensible approach would be to offer immediate resection to patients who are fit, consented, have easily resectable disease and access to a liver surgeon, as their disease may be more difficult to resect after chemotherapy. For those patients who are not able to undergo immediate major surgery, reassessment following the colorectal resection should occur. In light of the histopathology of the primary tumour, a more meaningful discussion can occur about resection followed by adjuvant chemotherapy, or three months/ six cycles of neo-adjuvant chemotherapy, restaging and resection.

4.2. Other liver metastases

4.2.1 Neuroendocrine liver metastases

Neuroendocrine metastases to the liver are associated with a 30% five-year survival without treatment.[171,172] Surgery in resectable lesions with curative intent offers five-year survivals of 50–79%,[173–177] although 85–90% are multifocal and bilobar.[177,178] Carcinoid tumours appear to have a better prognosis compared with other neuroendocrine tumours.[179] Prior to surgery imaging to look for extrahepatic disease should be carried out. Somatostatin scintigraphy is best for the detection of bone and lung metastases, and somatostatin scintigraphy combined with CT or MRI detects 96% of liver metastases.[179,180] In preparation for surgery, pharmacological therapy is instituted one month pre-operatively.[179] Patients who have more than 50–75% of liver involvement rarely have a curative resection and the indications for surgery are rare.[177,181] There is emerging evidence that long acting octreotide can improve survival and debulking surgery may have a therapeutic role in neuroendocrine tumours of gastric, pancreatic, small intestinal or colonic origin.

For neuroendocrine tumours that are not resectable, a number of different treatment strategies exist. The aims of treatment are to control symptoms and extend survival. Pharmacological therapy is usually employed as first-line therapy, for example with proton pump inhibitors for gastrinomas, or somatostatin analogues for gastrinomas. Systemic chemotherapy with agents such as streptozocin combined with other agents has been used, but is associated with variable and short-lived responses and significant side-effects.[179,182] I[131]-metaiodobenzylguanidine (MIBG) has been shown to improve five-year survival in 42–85% of patients, but only 50% have receptors and a complete response is rare and relapse inevitable.[183–186] Hepatic artery chemoembolisation is associated with relief of symptoms in 64–90%,[187–189] and up to 79% have a tumour response, but there is no evidence of improved overall survival.[190–193] Liver transplantation has been used in highly selected cases, where the liver disease is not resectable, a six-month disease-stable period following resection of the primary has occurred, the histologically proven carcinoid or well-differentiated neuroendocrine tumour has arisen from an area drained by the portal system and liver involvement is less than 50% and age less than 55 years.[194,195]

4.2.2 *Non-colorectal, non-neuroendocrine liver metastases*

The role for surgery in non-colorectal, non-neuroendocrine liver metastases is less well-defined. Generally these tumours have less favourable tumour biology if they have arisen from the gastrointestinal tract or are the result of systemic arterial spread, rather than portal haematogenous spread, and so the chance of cure is much lower. There are some exceptions where five-year survivals approach those achievable with resection of colorectal secondaries. These include tumours where there is a long disease-free interval, for example two years, and a negative margin can be achieved.[173,196,197] Margin-free resection of reproductive tract tumour liver metastases (for testicular, ovarian, endometrial, cervical, fallopian tube cancer) and sarcoma metastases are also associated with five-year survival of up to 30%, independent of the disease-free interval.[173,198]

References

1. H. B. El Serag and A. C. Mason, Rising incidence of hepatocellular carcinoma in the United States, *N. Engl. J. Med.* **340**: 745–750 (1999).

2. D. M. Parkin, F. Bray, J. Ferlay and P. Pisani, Estimating the world cancer burden: Globocan 2000, *Int. J. Cancer* **94**: 153–156 (2001).

3. J. M. Llovet, A. Burroughs and J. Bruix, Hepatocellular carcinoma, *Lancet* **362**: 1907–1917 (2003).

4. W. H. Caselmann and M. Alt, Hepatitis C virus infection as a major risk factor for hepatocellular carcinoma, *J. Hepatol.* **24**: 61–66 (1996).

5. M. G. Law *et al.*, Primary hepatocellular carcinoma in Australia, 1978–1997: Increasing incidence and mortality, *Med. J. Aust.* **173**: 403–405 (2000).

6. S. K. Roberts, W. Kemp, S. K. Roberts and W. Kemp, Hepatocellular carcinoma in an Australian tertiary referral hospital 1975–2002: Change in epidemiology and clinical presentation, *J. Gastroenterol. Hepatol.* **22**: 191–196 (2007).

7. T. R. Morgan, S. Mandayam and M. M. Jamal, Alcohol and hepatocellular carcinoma, *Gastroenterology* **127**: S87–S96 (2004).

8. J. A. Marrero *et al.*, NAFLD may be a common underlying liver disease in patients with hepatocellular carcinoma in the United States, *Hepatology* **36**: 1349–1354 (2002).

9. S. H. Caldwell *et al.*, Obesity and hepatocellular carcinoma, *Gastroenterology* **127**: S97–S103 (2004).

10. K. V. Kowdley and K. V. Kowdley, Iron, hemochromatosis, and hepatocellular carcinoma, *Gastroenterology* **127**: S79–S86 (2004).

11. J. Bruix *et al.*, Clinical management of hepatocellular carcinoma. Conclusions of the Barcelona-2000 EASL conference. European association for the study of the liver, *J. Hepatol.* **35**: 421–430 (2001).

12. J. H. Lim *et al.*, Detection of hepatocellular carcinomas and dysplastic nodules in cirrhotic livers: Accuracy of helical CT in transplant patients, *Am. J. Roentgenol.* **175**: 693–698 (2000).

13. G. Torzilli *et al.*, Accurate preoperative evaluation of liver mass lesions without fine-needle biopsy, *Hepatology* **30**: 889–893 (1999).

14. A. M. Lutz, J. K. Willmann, K. Goepfert, B. Marincek and D. Weishaupt, Hepatocellular carcinoma in cirrhosis: Enhancement patterns at dynamic gadolinium- and superparamagnetic iron oxide-enhanced T1-weighted MR imaging, *Radiology* **237**: 520–528 (2005).

15. F. Durand *et al.*, Assessment of the benefits and risks of percutaneous biopsy before surgical resection of hepatocellular carcinoma, *J. Hepatol.* **35**: 254–258 (2001).

16. B. H. Zhang, B. H. Yang and Z. Y. Tang, Randomized controlled trial of screening for hepatocellular carcinoma, *J. Cancer Res. Clin. Oncol.* **130**: 417–422 (2004).

17. F. Trevisani *et al.*, Serum alpha-fetoprotein for diagnosis of hepatocellular carcinoma in patients with chronic liver disease: Influence of HBsAg and anti-HCV status, *J. Hepatol.* **34**: 570–575 (2001).

18. N. Snowberger *et al.*, Alpha fetoprotein, ultrasound, computerized tomography and magnetic resonance imaging for detection of hepatocellular carcinoma in patients with advanced cirrhosis, *Aliment. Pharmacol. Ther.* **26**: 1187–1194 (2007).

19. M. S. Peterson and R. L. Baron, Radiologic diagnosis of hepatocellular carcinoma, *Clin. Liver Dis.* **5**: 123–144 (2001).

20. S. Chevret *et al.*, A new prognostic classification for predicting survival in patients with hepatocellular carcinoma. Groupe d'Etude et de Traitement du Carcinome Hepatocellulaire, *J. Hepatol.* **31**: 133–141 (1999).

21. A new prognostic system for hepatocellular carcinoma: A retrospective study of 435 patients: The Cancer of the Liver Italian Program (CLIP) investigators, *Hepatology* **28**: 751–755 (1998).

22. I. Levy and M. Sherman, Staging of hepatocellular carcinoma: Assessment of the CLIP, Okuda, and Child-Pugh staging systems in a cohort of 257 patients in Toronto, *Gut* **50**: 881–885 (2002).

23. J. M. Llovet *et al.*, Natural history of untreated nonsurgical hepatocellular carcinoma: Rationale for the design and evaluation of therapeutic trials, *Hepatology* **29**: 62–67 (1999).

24. R. Lencioni *et al.*, Long-term results of percutaneous ethanol injection therapy for hepatocellular carcinoma in cirrhosis: A European experience, *Eur. Radiol.* **7**: 514–519 (1997).

25. T. Livraghi *et al.*, Hepatocellular carcinoma and cirrhosis in 746 patients: Long-term results of percutaneous ethanol injection, *Radiology* **197**: 101–108 (1995).

26. R. A. Lencioni *et al.*, Small hepatocellular carcinoma in cirrhosis: Randomized comparison of radio-frequency thermal ablation versus percutaneous ethanol injection, *Radiology* **228**: 235–240 (2003).

27. M. Omata, R. Tateishi, H. Yoshida and S. Shiina, Treatment of hepatocellular carcinoma by percutaneous tumor ablation methods: Ethanol injection therapy and radiofrequency ablation, *Gastroenterology* **127**: S159–S166 (2004).

28. J. M. Llovet and J. Bruix, Systematic review of randomized trials for unresectable hepatocellular carcinoma: Chemoembolization improves survival, *Hepatology* **37**: 429–442 (2003).

29. H. Bismuth *et al.*, Primary treatment of hepatocellular carcinoma by arterial chemoembolization, *Am. J. Surg.* **163**: 387–394 (1992).

30. H. S. Lee *et al.*, Therapeutic efficacy of transcatheter arterial chemoembolization as compared with hepatic resection in hepatocellular carcinoma patients with compensated liver function in a hepatitis B virus-endemic area: A prospective cohort study, *J. Clin. Oncol.* **20**: 4459–4465 (2002).

31. S. Katyal *et al.*, Prognostic significance of arterial phase CT for prediction of response to transcatheter arterial chemoembolization in unresectable hepatocellular carcinoma: A retrospective analysis, *Am. J. Roentgenol.* **175**: 1665–1672 (2000).

32. B. Q. Cheng *et al.*, Chemoembolization combined with radiofrequency ablation for patients with hepatocellular carcinoma larger than 3 cm: A randomized controlled trial, *J. Am. Med. Assoc.* **299**: 1669–1677 (2008).

33. N. Shimozawa and K. Hanazaki, Longterm prognosis after hepatic resection for small hepatocellular carcinoma, *J. Am. Coll. Surg.* **198**: 356–365 (2004).

34. J. Belghiti, Y. Panis, O. Farges, J. P. Benhamou and F. Fekete, Intrahepatic recurrence after resection of hepatocellular carcinoma complicating cirrhosis, *Ann. Surg.* **214**: 114–117 (1991).

35. S. T. Fan *et al.*, Hepatectomy for hepatocellular carcinoma: Toward zero hospital deaths, *Ann. Surg.* **229**: 322–330 (1999).

36. P. A. Clavien, H. Petrowsky, M. L. DeOliveira and R. Graf, Strategies for safer liver surgery and partial liver transplantation, *N. Engl. J. Med.* **356**: 1545–1559 (2007).

37. J. C. Emond, B. Samstein and J. F. Renz, A critical evaluation of hepatic resection in cirrhosis: Optimizing patient selection and outcomes, *World J. Surg.* **29**: 124–130 (2005).

38. R. T. Poon and S. T. Fan, Assessment of hepatic reserve for indication of hepatic resection: How I do it, *J. Hepatobiliary Pancreat. Surg.* **12**: 31–37 (2005).

39. L. Capussotti *et al.*, Portal hypertension: Contraindication to liver surgery? *World J. Surg.* **30**: 992–999 (2006).

40. D. Azoulay *et al.*, Percutaneous portal vein embolization increases the feasibility and safety of major liver resection for hepatocellular carcinoma in injured liver, *Ann. Surg.* **232**: 665–672 (2000).

41. O. Farges *et al.*, Portal vein embolization before right hepatectomy: Prospective clinical trial, *Ann. Surg.* **237**: 208–217 (2003).

42. J. D. Schwartz, M. Schwartz, J. Mandeli and M. Sung, Neoadjuvant and adjuvant therapy for resectable hepatocellular carcinoma: Review of the randomised clinical trials, *Lancet Oncol.* **3**: 593–603 (2002).

43. W. Y. Lau *et al.*, Adjuvant intra-arterial iodine-131-labeled lipiodol for resectable hepatocellular carcinoma: A prospective randomized trial-update on 5-year and 10-year survival, *Ann. Surg.* **247**: 43–48 (2008).

44. E. Boucher *et al.*, Adjuvant intraarterial injection of 131I-labeled lipiodol after resection of hepatocellular carcinoma: Progress report of a case-control study with a 5-year minimal follow-up, *J. Nucl. Med.* **49**: 362–366 (2008).

45. R. T. Poon, S. T. Fan, C. M. Lo, C. L. Liu and J. Wong, Intrahepatic recurrence after curative resection of hepatocellular carcinoma: Long-term results of treatment and prognostic factors, *Ann. Surg.* **229**: 216–222 (1999).

46. B. Ringe, R. Pichlmayr, C. Wittekind and G. Tusch, Surgical treatment of hepatocellular carcinoma: Experience with liver resection and transplantation in 198 patients, *World J. Surg.* **15**: 270–285 (1991).

47. V. Mazzaferro *et al.*, Liver transplantation for the treatment of small hepatocellular carcinomas in patients with cirrhosis, *N. Engl. J. Med.* **334**: 693–699 (1996).

48. S. Jonas *et al.*, Vascular invasion and histopathologic grading determine outcome after liver transplantation for hepatocellular carcinoma in cirrhosis, *Hepatology* **33**: 1080–1086 (2001).

49. F. Y. Yao *et al.*, Liver transplantation for hepatocellular carcinoma: Expansion of the tumor size limits does not adversely impact survival, *Hepatology* **33**: 1394–1403 (2001).

50. J. Figueras *et al.*, Survival after liver transplantation in cirrhotic patients with and without hepatocellular carcinoma: A comparative study, *Hepatology* **25**: 1485–1489 (1997).

51. U. Cillo *et al.*, Partial hepatectomy as first-line treatment for patients with hepatocellular carcinoma, *J. Surg. Oncol.* **95**: 213–220 (2007).

52. J. M. Bigourdan *et al.*, Small hepatocellular carcinoma in Child A cirrhotic patients: Hepatic resection versus transplantation, *Liver Transpl.* **9**: 513–520 (2003).

53. M. Shabahang *et al.*, Comparison of hepatic resection and hepatic transplantation in the treatment of hepatocellular carcinoma among cirrhotic patients, *Ann. Surg. Oncol.* **9**: 881–886 (2002).

54. J. Figueras *et al.*, Resection or transplantation for hepatocellular carcinoma in cirrhotic patients: Outcomes based on indicated treatment strategy, *J. Am. Coll. Surg.* **190**: 580–587 (2000).

55. J. Y. Leung *et al.*, Liver transplantation outcomes for early-stage hepatocellular carcinoma: Results of a multicenter study, *Liver Transpl.* **10**: 1343–1354 (2004).

56. S. Hwang, S. G. Lee, J. W. Joh, K. S. Suh and D. G. Kim, Liver transplantation for adult patients with hepatocellular carcinoma in Korea: Comparison between cadaveric donor and living donor liver transplantations, *Liver Transpl.* **11**: 1265–1272 (2005).

57. J. Belghiti *et al.*, Resection prior to liver transplantation for hepatocellular carcinoma, *Ann. Surg.* **238**: 885–892 (2003).

58. R. B. Freeman, E. B. Edwards and A. M. Harper, Waiting list removal rates among patients with chronic and malignant liver diseases, *Am. J. Transpl.* **6**: 1416–1421 (2006).

59. R. T. Poon, S. T. Fan, C. M. Lo, C. L. Liu and J. Wong, Long-term survival and pattern of recurrence after resection of small hepatocellular carcinoma in patients with preserved liver function: Implications for a strategy of salvage transplantation, *Ann. Surg.* **235**: 373–382 (2002).

60. J. Belghiti and F. Durand, Hepatectomy vs. liver transplantation: A combination rather than an opposition, *Liver Transpl.* **13**: 636–638 (2007).

61. C. Margarit *et al.*, Resection for hepatocellular carcinoma is a good option in Child-Turcotte-Pugh class A patients with cirrhosis who are eligible for liver transplantation, *Liver Transpl.* **11**: 1242–1251 (2005).

62. R. Adam *et al.*, Liver resection as a bridge to transplantation for hepatocellular carcinoma on cirrhosis: A reasonable strategy? *Ann. Surg.* **238**: 508–518 (2003).

63. M. Lesurtel, B. Mullhaupt, B. C. Pestalozzi, T. Pfammatter and P. A. Clavien, Transarterial chemoembolization as a bridge to liver transplantation for hepatocellular carcinoma: An evidence-based analysis, *Am. J. Transpl.* **6**: 2644–2650 (2006).

64. D. S. Lu *et al.*, Percutaneous radiofrequency ablation of hepatocellular carcinoma as a bridge to liver transplantation, *Hepatology* **41**: 1130–1137 (2005).

65. R. J. Fontana *et al.*, Percutaneous radiofrequency thermal ablation of hepatocellular carcinoma: A safe and effective bridge to liver transplantation, *Liver Transpl.* **8**: 1165–1174 (2002).

66. V. Mazzaferro *et al.*, Radiofrequency ablation of small hepatocellular carcinoma in cirrhotic patients awaiting liver transplantation: A prospective study, *Ann. Surg.* **240**: 900–999 (2004).

67. Y. S. Chang *et al.*, Sorafenib (BAY 43-9006) inhibits tumor growth and vascularization and induces tumor apoptosis and hypoxia in RCC xenograft models, *Cancer Chemother. Pharmacol.* **59**: 561–574 (2007).

68. J. M. Llovet *et al.*, Sorafenib in advanced hepatocellular carcinoma, *N. Engl. J. Med.* **359**: 378–390 (2008).

69. C. H. Chang *et al.*, Long-term results of hepatic resection for hepatocellular carcinoma originating from the noncirrhotic liver, *Arch. Surg.* **139**: 320–325 (2004).

70. S. Iwatsuki *et al.*, Hepatic resection versus transplantation for hepatocellular carcinoma, *Ann. Surg.* **214**: 221–228 (1991).

71. J. Belghiti *et al.*, Seven hundred forty-seven hepatectomies in the 1990s: An update to evaluate the actual risk of liver resection, *J. Am. Coll. Surg.* **191**: 38–46 (2000).

72. K. Slater, T. E. Bak, I. Kam and M. E. Wachs, Living donor liver transplant for fibrolamellar hepatocellular carcinoma using a deceased donor graft to reconstruct inferior vena cava, *Liver Transpl.* **10**: 555–556 (2004).

73. B. Ringe, C. Wittekind, A. Weimann, G. Tusch and R. Pichlmayr, Results of hepatic resection and transplantation for fibrolamellar carcinoma, *Surg. Gynecol. Obstet.* **175**: 299–305 (1992).

74. Y. Tajima *et al.*, An intraductal papillary component is associated with prolonged survival after hepatic resection for intrahepatic cholangiocarcinoma, *Br. J. Surg.* **91**: 99–104 (2004).

75. J. K. Sicklick, M. A. Choti, J. K. Sicklick and M. A. Choti, Controversies in the surgical management of cholangiocarcinoma and gallbladder cancer, *Sem. Oncol.* **32**: S112–S117 (2005).

76. M. Miyazaki *et al.*, Recent advance in the treatment of hilar cholangiocarcinoma: Hepatectomy with vascular resection, *J. Hepatobiliary Pancreat. Surg.* **14**: 463–468 (2007).

77. M. Nagino *et al.*, Segmental liver resections for hilar cholangiocarcinoma, *Hepatogastroenterology* **45**: 7–13 (1998).

78. M. Miyazaki *et al.*, Segments I and IV resection as a new approach for hepatic hilar cholangiocarcinoma, *Am. J. Surg.* **175**: 229–231 (1998).

79. Y. Kawarada *et al.*, S4a + S5 with caudate lobe (S1) resection using the Taj Mahal liver parenchymal resection for carcinoma of the biliary tract, *J. Gastrointest. Surg.* **3**: 369–373 (1999).

80. Y. Fong, N. Heffernan and L. H. Blumgart, Gallbladder carcinoma discovered during laparoscopic cholecystectomy: Aggressive reresection is beneficial, *Cancer* **83**: 423–427 (1998).

81. M. Shoup and Y. Fong, Surgical indications and extent of resection in gallbladder cancer, *Surg. Oncol. Clin. N. Am.* **11**: 985–994 (2002).

82. Y. Fong, W. Jarnagin and L. H. Blumgart, Gallbladder cancer: Comparison of patients presenting initially for definitive operation with those presenting after prior noncurative intervention, *Ann. Surg.* **232**: 557–569 (2000).

83. H. Onoyama, M. Yamamoto, A. Tseng, T. Ajiki and Y. Saitoh, Extended cholecystectomy for carcinoma of the gallbladder, *World J. Surg.* **19**: 758–763 (1995).

84. O. Farges and J. Belghiti, Primary malignant tumours of the liver. In: *A Companion to Specialist Surgical Practice: Hepatobiliary and Pancreatic Surgery*, ed. O. J. Garden (Elsevier Sanders, The Netherlands, 2005), pp. 67–96.

85. G. Y. Locker, J. H. Doroshow, L. A. Zwelling and B. A. Chabner, The clinical features of hepatic angiosarcoma: A report of four cases and a review of the English literature, *Medicine (Baltimore)* **58**: 48–64 (1979).

86. J. L. Poggio *et al.*, Surgical treatment of adult primary hepatic sarcoma, *Br. J. Surg.* **87**: 1500–1505 (2000).

87. I. D. Lyburn *et al.*, Hepatic epithelioid hemangioendothelioma: Sonographic, CT, and MR imaging appearances, *Am. J. Roentgenol.* **180**: 1359–1364 (2003).

88. A. Garcia-Botella *et al.*, Epithelioid hemangioendothelioma of the liver, *J. Hepatobiliary Pancreat. Surg.* **13**: 167–171 (2006).

89. A. Mehrabi *et al.*, Primary malignant hepatic epithelioid hemangioendothelioma: A comprehensive review of the literature with emphasis on the surgical therapy, *Cancer* **107**: 2108–2121 (2006).

90. W. Zhang *et al.*, Orthotopic liver transplantation for epithelioid haemangioendothelioma, *Eur. J. Surg. Oncol.* **33**: 898–901 (2007).

91. J. P. Lerut *et al.*, The place of liver transplantation in the treatment of hepatic epitheloid hemangioendothelioma: Report of the European liver transplant registry, *Ann. Surg.* **246**: 949–957 (2007).

92. T. Sato *et al.*, The time interval between primary colorectal carcinoma resection to occurrence of liver metastases is the most important factor for hepatic resection. Analysis of total course following primary resection of colorectal cancer, *Int. Surg.* **83**: 340–342 (1998).

93. V. P. Khatri, N. J. Petrelli and J. Belghiti, Extending the frontiers of surgical therapy for hepatic colorectal metastases: Is there a limit? *J. Clin. Oncol.* **23**: 8490–8499 (2005).

94. P. C. Simmonds, Palliative chemotherapy for advanced colorectal cancer: Systematic review and meta-analysis. Colorectal cancer collaborative group, *Br. Med. J.* **321**: 531–535 (2000).

95. R. Stangl, A. Altendorf-Hofmann, R. M. Charnley and J. Scheele, Factors influencing the natural history of colorectal liver metastases, *Lancet* **343**: 1405–1410 (1994).

96. R. Goslin, G. Steele Jr, N. Zamcheck, R. Mayer and J. MacIntyre, Factors influencing survival in patients with hepatic metastases from adenocarcinoma of the colon or rectum, *Dis. Colon Rectum* **25**: 749–754 (1982).

97. E. A. Bakalakos, J. A. Kim, D. C. Young and E. W. Martin Jr, Determinants of survival following hepatic resection for metastatic colorectal cancer, *World J. Surg.* **22**: 399–404 (1998).

98. P. C. Simmonds *et al.*, Surgical resection of hepatic metastases from colorectal cancer: A systematic review of published studies, *Br. J. Cancer* **94**: 982–999 (2006).

99. M. Jeffery, B. E. Hickey and P. N. Hider, Follow-up strategies for patients treated for non-metastatic colorectal cancer, *Cochrane Database Syst. Rev.* CD002200 (2007).

100. A. G. Renehan, M. Egger, M. P. Saunders and S. T. O'Dwyer, Impact on survival of intensive follow up after curative resection for colorectal cancer: Systematic review and meta-analysis of randomised trials, *Br. Med. J.* **324**: 813 (2002).

101. R. C. Karl, S. S. Morse, R. D. Halpert and R. A. Clark, Preoperative evaluation of patients for liver resection. Appropriate CT imaging, *Ann. Surg.* **217**: 226–232 (1993).

102. R. Hammerstingl *et al.*, Diagnostic efficacy of gadoxetic acid (Primovist)-enhanced MRI and spiral CT for a therapeutic strategy: Comparison with intraoperative and histopathologic findings in focal liver lesions, *Eur. Radiol.* **18**: 457–467 (2008).

103. P. Soyer, D. Lacheheb and M. Levesque, False-positive CT portography: Correlation with pathologic findings, *Am. J. Roentgenol.* **160**: 285–289 (1993).

104. T. J. Vogl *et al.*, Magnetic resonance imaging of focal liver lesions. Comparison of the superparamagnetic iron oxide resovist versus gadolinium-DTPA in the same patient, *Invest. Radiol.* **31**: 696–708 (1996).

105. T. J. Vogl *et al.*, Preoperative evaluation of malignant liver tumors: Comparison of unenhanced and SPIO (Resovist)-enhanced MR imaging with biphasic CTAP and intraoperative US, *Eur. Radiol.* **13**: 262–272 (2003).

106. E. D. Rappeport and A. Loft, Liver metastases from colorectal cancer: Imaging with superparamagnetic iron oxide (SPIO)-enhanced MR imaging, computed tomography and positron emission tomography, *Abdom. Imaging* **32**: 624–634 (2007).

107. G. Mazzoni *et al.*, Intra-operative ultrasound for detection of liver metastases from colorectal cancer, *Liver Int.* **28**: 88–94 (2008).

108. J. K. McGavin and K. L. Goa, Capecitabine: A review of its use in the treatment of advanced or metastatic colorectal cancer, *Drugs* **61**: 2309–2326 (2001).

109. Meta-analysis Group in Cancer, Efficacy of intravenous continuous infusion of fluorouracil compared with bolus administration in advanced colorectal cancer, *J. Clin. Oncol.* **16**: 301–308 (1998).

110. P. Thirion *et al.*, Modulation of fluorouracil by leucovorin in patients with advanced colorectal cancer: An updated meta-analysis, *J. Clin. Oncol.* **22**: 3766–3775 (2004).

111. J. Y. Douillard *et al.*, Irinotecan combined with fluorouracil compared with fluorouracil alone as first-line treatment for metastatic colorectal cancer: A multicentre randomised trial, *Lancet* **355**: 1041–1047 (2000).

112. S. Giacchetti *et al.*, Phase III multicenter randomized trial of oxaliplatin added to chronomodulated fluorouracil-leucovorin as first-line treatment of metastatic colorectal cancer, *J. Clin. Oncol.* **18**: 136–147 (2000).

113. L. B. Saltz *et al.*, Irinotecan plus fluorouracil and leucovorin for metastatic colorectal cancer. Irinotecan Study Group, *N. Engl. J. Med.* **343**: 905–914 (2000).

114. A. de Gramont *et al.*, Leucovorin and fluorouracil with or without oxaliplatin as first-line treatment in advanced colorectal cancer, *J. Clin. Oncol.* **18**: 2938–2947 (2000).

115. R. M. Goldberg *et al.*, A randomized controlled trial of fluorouracil plus leucovorin, irinotecan, and oxaliplatin combinations in patients with previously untreated metastatic colorectal cancer, *J. Clin. Oncol.* **22**: 23–30 (2004).

116. E. Raymond *et al.*, Dosage adjustment and pharmacokinetic profile of irinotecan in cancer patients with hepatic dysfunction, *J. Clin. Oncol.* **20**: 4303–4312 (2002).

117. D. Cunningham *et al.*, Cetuximab monotherapy and cetuximab plus irinotecan in irinotecan-refractory metastatic colorectal cancer, *N. Engl. J. Med.* **351**: 337–345 (2004).

118. D. J. Jonker *et al.*, Cetuximab for the treatment of colorectal cancer, *N. Engl. J. Med.* **357**: 2040–2048 (2007).

119. H. Hurwitz *et al.*, Bevacizumab plus irinotecan, fluorouracil, and leucovorin for metastatic colorectal cancer, *N. Engl. J. Med.* **350**: 2335–2342 (2004).

120. H. S. Hochster, A. Grothey and B. H. Childs, Use of calcium and magnesium salts to reduce oxaliplatin-related neurotoxicity, *J. Clin. Oncol.* **25**: 4028–4029 (2007).

121. C. S. Fuchs *et al.*, Randomized, controlled trial of irinotecan plus infusional, bolus, or oral fluoropyrimidines in first-line treatment of metastatic colorectal cancer: Results from the BICC-C study, *J. Clin. Oncol.* **25**: 4779–4786 (2007).

122. Y. Fong, J. Fortner, R. L. Sun, M. F. Brennan and L. H. Blumgart, Clinical score for predicting recurrence after hepatic resection for metastatic colorectal cancer: Analysis of 1001 consecutive cases, *Ann. Surg.* **230**: 309–318 (1999).

123. M. W. Kattan *et al.*, A nomogram for predicting disease-specific survival after hepatic resection for metastatic colorectal cancer, *Ann. Surg.* **247**: 282–287 (2008).

124. M. Rees *et al.*, Evaluation of long-term survival after hepatic resection for metastatic colorectal cancer: A multifactorial model of 929 patients, *Ann. Surg.* **247**: 125–135 (2008).

125. Z. Z. Hamady *et al.*, Resection margin in patients undergoing hepatectomy for colorectal liver metastasis: A critical appraisal of the 1 cm rule, *Eur. J. Surg. Oncol.* **32**: 557–563 (2006).

126. T, M. Pawlik, J. N. Vauthey, T. M. Pawlik and J. N. Vauthey, Surgical margins during hepatic surgery for colorectal liver metastases: Complete resection not millimeters defines outcome, *Ann. Surg. Oncol.* **15**: 677–679 (2008).

127. H. Nakano *et al.*, Sinusoidal injury increases morbidity after major hepatectomy in patients with colorectal liver metastases receiving preoperative chemotherapy, *Ann. Surg.* **247**: 118–124 (2008).

128. B. Nordlinger *et al.*, Does chemotherapy prior to liver resection increase the potential for cure in patients with metastatic colorectal cancer? A report from the European Colorectal Metastases Treatment Group, *Eur. J. Cancer* **43**: 2037–2045 (2007).

129. G. Portier *et al.*, Multicenter randomized trial of adjuvant fluorouracil and folinic acid compared with surgery alone after resection of colorectal liver metastases: FFCD ACHBTH AURC 9002 trial, *J. Clin. Oncol.* **24**: 4976–4982 (2006).

130. J. P. Kuebler *et al.*, Oxaliplatin combined with weekly bolus fluorouracil and leucovorin as surgical adjuvant chemotherapy for stage II and III colon cancer: Results from NSABP C-07, *J. Clin. Oncol.* **25**: 2198–2204 (2007).

131. T. Andre *et al.*, Oxaliplatin, fluorouracil, and leucovorin as adjuvant treatment for colon cancer, *New. Engl. J. Med.* **350**: 2343–2451 (2004).

132. B. Gruenberger *et al.*, Bevacizumab, capecitabine, and oxaliplatin as neoadjuvant therapy for patients with potentially curable metastatic colorectal cancer, *J. Clin. Oncol.* **26**: 1830–1835 (2008).

133. G. Mentha *et al.*, Neoadjuvant chemotherapy and resection of advanced synchronous liver metastases before treatment of the colorectal primary, *Br. J. Surg.* **93**: 872–878 (2006).

134. S. R. Alberts *et al.*, Oxaliplatin, fluorouracil, and leucovorin for patients with unresectable liver-only metastases from colorectal cancer: A North Central Cancer Treatment Group phase II study, *J. Clin. Oncol.* **23**: 9243–9249 (2005).

135. R. Adam *et al.*, Five-year survival following hepatic resection after neoadjuvant therapy for nonresectable colorectal, *Ann. Surg. Oncol.* **8**: 347–353 (2001).

136. S. Giacchetti *et al.*, Long-term survival of patients with unresectable colorectal cancer liver metastases following infusional chemotherapy with 5-fluorouracil, leucovorin, oxaliplatin and surgery, *Ann. Oncol.* **10**: 663–669 (1999).

137. A. Falcone *et al.*, Phase III trial of infusional fluorouracil, leucovorin, oxaliplatin, and irinotecan (FOLFOXIRI) compared with infusional fluorouracil, leucovorin, and irinotecan (FOLFIRI) as first-line treatment for metastatic colorectal cancer: The Gruppo Oncologico Nord Ovest, *J. Clin. Oncol.* **25**: 1670–1676 (2007).

138. D. Elias, A. Cavalcanti, T. De Baere, A. Roche and P. Lasser, Long-term oncological results of hepatectomy performed after selective portal embolization, *Ann. Chir.* **53**: 559–564 (1999).

139. D. Elias *et al.*, During liver regeneration following right portal embolization the growth rate of liver metastases is more rapid than that of the liver parenchyma, *Br. J. Surg.* **86**: 784–788 (1999).

140. N. Kokudo *et al.*, Proliferative activity of intrahepatic colorectal metastases after preoperative hemihepatic portal vein embolization, *Hepatology* **34**: 267–272 (2001).

141. H. Bismuth *et al.*, Resection of nonresectable liver metastases from colorectal cancer after neoadjuvant chemotherapy, *Ann. Surg.* **224**: 509–520 (1996).

142. R. B. Adams *et al.*, Improving resectability of hepatic colorectal metastases: Expert consensus statement by Abdalla *et al.*, *Ann. Surg. Oncol.* **13**: 1281–1283 (2006).

143. A. E. Siperstein, E. Berber, N. Ballem and R. T. Parikh, Survival after radiofrequency ablation of colorectal liver metastases: 10-year experience, *Ann. Surg.* **246**: 559–565 (2007).

144. T. M. Pawlik, F. Izzo, D. S. Cohen, J. S. Morris and S. A. Curley, Combined resection and radiofrequency ablation for advanced hepatic malignancies: Results in 172 patients, *Ann. Surg. Oncol.* **10**: 1059–1069 (2003).

145. D. Elias *et al.*, Hepatectomy plus intraoperative radiofrequency ablation and chemotherapy to treat technically unresectable multiple colorectal liver metastases, *J. Surg. Oncol.* **90**: 36–42 (2005).

146. E. K. Abdalla *et al.*, Recurrence and outcomes following hepatic resection, radiofrequency ablation, and combined resection/ablation for colorectal liver metastases, *Ann. Surg.* **239**: 818–825 (2004).

147. R. Adam *et al.*, Repeat hepatectomy for colorectal liver metastases, *Ann. Surg.* **225**: 51–60 (1997).

148. D. Elias *et al.*, Local recurrences after intraoperative radiofrequency ablation of liver metastases: A comparative study with anatomic and wedge resections, *Ann. Surg. Oncol.* **11**: 500–505 (2004).

149. E. Berber *et al.*, Predictors of survival after radiofrequency thermal ablation of colorectal cancer metastases to the liver: A prospective study, *J. Clin. Oncol.* **23**: 1358–1364 (2005).

150. T. Livraghi *et al.*, Percutaneous radiofrequency ablation of liver metastases in potential candidates for resection: The "test-of-time approach", *Cancer* **97**: 3027–3035 (2003).

151. A. Siperstein *et al.*, Local recurrence after laparoscopic radio-frequency thermal ablation of hepatic tumors, *Ann. Surg. Oncol.* **7**: 106–113 (2000).

152. L. Solbiati *et al.*, Radiofrequency thermal ablation of hepatic metastases, *Eur. J. Ultras.* **13**: 149–158 (2001).

153. L. Solbiati *et al.*, Percutaneous radio-frequency ablation of hepatic metastases from colorectal cancer: Long-term results in 117 patients, *Radiology* **221**: 159–166 (2001).

154. T. J. White *et al.*, Percutaneous radiofrequency ablation of colorectal hepatic metastases — Initial experience. An adjunct technique to systemic chemotherapy for those with inoperable colorectal hepatic metastases, *Dig. Surg.* **21**: 314–320 (2004).

155. T. F. Wood *et al.*, Radiofrequency ablation of 231 unresectable hepatic tumors: Indications, limitations, and complications, *Ann. Surg. Oncol.* **7**: 593–600 (2000).

156. S. A. Curley *et al.*, Radiofrequency ablation of unresectable primary and metastatic hepatic malignancies: Results in 123 patients, *Ann. Surg.* **230**: 1–8 (1999).

157. L. Solbiati *et al.*, Percutaneous radio-frequency ablation of hepatic metastases from colorectal cancer: Long-term results in 117 patients, *Radiology* **221**: 159–166 (2001).

158. D. A. Iannitti, D. E. Dupuy, W. W. Mayo-Smith and B. Murphy, Hepatic radiofrequency ablation, *Arch. Surg.* **137**: 422–426 (2002).

159. T. J. White *et al.*, Percutaneous radiofrequency ablation of colorectal hepatic metastases — Initial experience. An adjunct technique to systemic chemotherapy for those with inoperable colorectal hepatic metastases, *Dig. Surg.* **21**: 314–320 (2004).

160. A. McKay, E. Dixon and M. Taylor, Current role of radiofrequency ablation for the treatment of colorectal liver metastases, *Br. J. Surg.* **93**: 1192–1201 (2006).

161. L. Capussotti *et al.*, Timing of resection of liver metastases synchronous to colorectal tumor: Proposal of prognosis-based decisional model, *Ann. Surg. Oncol.* **14**: 1143–1150 (2007).

162. S. Fujita, T. Akasu and Y. Moriya, Resection of synchronous liver metastases from colorectal cancer, *Jpn. J. Clin. Oncol.* **30**: 7–11 (2000).

163. J. C. Weber, P. Bachellier, E. Oussoultzoglou and D. Jaeck, Simultaneous resection of colorectal primary tumour and synchronous liver metastases, *Br. J. Surg.* **90**: 956–962 (2003).

164. H. K. Chua *et al.*, Concurrent vs. staged colectomy and hepatectomy for primary colorectal cancer with synchronous hepatic metastases, *Dis. Colon Rectum* **47**: 1310–1316 (2004).

165. S. Lyass *et al.*, Combined colon and hepatic resection for synchronous colorectal liver metastases, *J. Surg. Oncol.* **78**: 17–21 (2001).

166. E. de Santibanes *et al.*, Simultaneous colorectal and hepatic resections for colorectal cancer: Postoperative and longterm outcomes, *J. Am. Coll. Surg.* **195**: 196–202 (2002).

167. C. Verhoef, J. J. Nuytens, A. S. Planting and J. H. de Wilt, Neoadjuvant chemotherapy and resection of advanced synchronous liver metastases before treatment of the colorectal primary, *Br. J. Surg.* **94**: 250 (2007) (Comment in *Br. J. Surg.* **93**: 872–878 (2006)).

168. T. R. O'Rourke, F. K. Welsh, T. John and M. Rees, Neoadjuvant chemotherapy and resection of advanced synchronous liver metastases before treatment of the colorectal primary (*Br. J. Surg.* **93**: 872–878 (2006)) *Br. J. Surg.* **93**: 1434 (2006).

169. G. Mentha *et al.*, Neoadjuvant chemotherapy and resection of advanced synchronous liver metastases before treatment of the colorectal primary, *Br. J. Surg.* **93**: 872–878 (2006).

170. R. Adam *et al.*, Tumor progression while on chemotherapy: A contraindication to liver resection for multiple colorectal metastases? *Ann. Surg.* **240**: 1052–1061 (2004).

171. O. Soreide *et al.*, Surgical treatment as a principle in patients with advanced abdominal carcinoid tumors, *Surgery* **111**: 48–54 (1992).

172. C. G. Moertel, Karnofsky memorial lecture. An odyssey in the land of small tumors, *J. Clin. Oncol.* **5**: 1502–1522 (1987).

173. A. W. Hemming *et al.*, Hepatic resection of noncolorectal nonneuroendocrine metastases, *Liver Transpl.* **6**: 97–101 (2000).

174. F. G. Que, D. M. Nagorney, K. P. Batts, L. J. Linz and L. K. Kvols, Hepatic resection for metastatic neuroendocrine carcinomas, *Am. J. Surg.* **169**: 36–42 (1995).

175. H. Chen, J. M. Hardacre, A. Uzar, J. L. Cameron and M. A. Choti, Isolated liver metastases from neuroendocrine tumors: Does resection prolong survival? *J. Am. Coll. Surg.* **187**: 88–92 (1998).

176. A. Benevento, L. Boni, L. Frediani, A. Ferrari and R. Dionigi, Result of liver resection as treatment for metastases from noncolorectal cancer, *J. Surg. Oncol.* **74**: 24–29 (2000).

177. R. S. Chamberlain *et al.*, Hepatic neuroendocrine metastases: Does intervention alter outcomes? *J. Am. Coll. Surg.* **190**: 432–445 (2000).

178. I. Ihse *et al.*, Neuroendocrine metastases of the liver, *World J. Surg.* **19**: 76–82 (1995).

179. R. Sutcliffe *et al.*, Management of neuroendocrine liver metastases, *Am. J. Surg.* **187**: 39–46 (2004).

180. F. Gibril *et al.*, Somatostatin receptor scintigraphy: Its sensitivity compared with that of other imaging methods in detecting primary and metastatic gastrinomas. A prospective study, *Ann. Intern. Med.* **125**: 26–34 (1996).

181. J. G. Touzios *et al.*, Neuroendocrine hepatic metastases: Does aggressive management improve survival? *Ann. Surg.* **241**: 776–783 (2005).

182. L. M. Veenendaal, R. I. Borel, C. J. Lips and R. van Hillegersberg, Liver metastases of neuroendocrine tumours; early reduction of tumour load to improve life expectancy, *World J. Surg. Oncol.* **4**: 35 (2006).

183. S. D. Safford *et al.*, Iodine-131 metaiodobenzylguanidine treatment for metastatic carcinoid. Results in 98 patients, *Cancer* **101**: 1987–1993 (2004).

184. M. S. Sywak *et al.*, 131I-meta-iodobenzylguanidine in the management of metastatic midgut carcinoid tumors, *World J. Surg.* **28**: 1157–1162 (2004).

185. M. R. Castellani, A. Chiti, E. Seregni and E. Bombardieri, Role of 131I-metaiodobenzylguanidine (MIBG) in the treatment of neuroendocrine tumours. Experience of the National Cancer Institute of Milan, *Q. J. Nucl. Med.* **44**: 77–87 (2000).

186. J. J. Mukherjee *et al.*, Treatment of metastatic carcinoid tumours, phaeochromocytoma, paraganglioma and medullary carcinoma of the thyroid with (131)I-meta-iodobenzylguanidine [(131)I-mIBG], *Clin. Endocrinol.* **55**: 47–60 (2001).

187. A. S. Ho *et al.*, Long-term outcome after chemoembolization and embolization of hepatic metastatic lesions from neuroendocrine tumors, *Am. J. Roentgenol.* **188**: 1201–1207 (2007).

188. C. H. Carrasco *et al.*, The carcinoid syndrome: Palliation by hepatic artery embolization, *Am. J. Roentgenol.* **147**: 149–154 (1986).

189. S. R. Schell, E. R. Camp, J. G. Caridi and I. F. Hawkins Jr, Hepatic artery embolization for control of symptoms, octreotide requirements, and tumor progression in metastatic carcinoid tumors, *J. Gastrointest. Surg.* **6**: 664–670 (2002).

190. S. Dominguez *et al.*, Hepatic arterial chemoembolization with streptozotocin in patients with metastatic digestive endocrine tumours, *Eur. J. Gastroenterol. Hepatol.* **12**: 151–157 (2000).

191. L. J. Perry, K. Stuart, K. R. Stokes and M. E. Clouse, Hepatic arterial chemoembolization for metastatic neuroendocrine tumors, *Surgery* **116**: 1111–1116 (1994).

192. P. Ruszniewski and D. Malka, Hepatic arterial chemoembolization in the management of advanced digestive endocrine tumors, *Digestion* **62** (Suppl. 1): 79–83 (2000).

193. E. Rivera and J. A. Ajani, Doxorubicin, streptozocin, and 5-fluorouracil chemotherapy for patients with metastatic islet-cell carcinoma, *Am. J. Clin. Oncol.* **21**: 36–38 (1998).

194. Y. P. Le Treut *et al.*, Predictors of long-term survival after liver transplantation for metastatic endocrine tumors: An 85-case French multicentric report, *Am. J. Transpl.* **8**: 1205–1213 (2008).

195. V. Mazzaferro *et al.*, Neuroendocrine tumors metastatic to the liver: How to select patients for liver transplantation? *J. Hepatol.* **47**: 460–466 (2007).

196. L. E. Harrison *et al.*, Hepatic resection for noncolorectal, nonneuroendocrine metastases: A fifteen-year experience with ninety-six patients, *Surgery* **121**: 625–632 (1997).

197. C. Laurent, E. Rullier, A. Feyler, B. Masson and J. Saric, Resection of noncolorectal and nonneuroendocrine liver metastases: Late metastases are the only chance of cure, *World J. Surg.* **25**: 1532–1536 (2001).

198. R. P. DeMatteo *et al.*, Results of hepatic resection for sarcoma metastatic to liver, *Ann. Surg.* **234**: 540–547 (2001).

22

Cancer and the Gynaecological Oncologist

D. E. Marsden

Abstract

Gynaecological oncology is now a generally accepted subspecialty of obstetrics and gynaecology, dealing with pre-alignant and malignant diseases of the female reproductive system. A number of medical disciplines have always been involved in treating such conditions, but coordination and cooperation were not always optimal. This paper will present a broad historical perspective on the development of the subspecialty and the evolution of modern approaches to managing three of the diseases and the problems of the women who suffer from them. From this it is hoped that the reader will gain an understanding of some of the cross-disciplinary issues in the area of gynaecological oncology and the ways modern units are dealing with them.

Keywords: Oophorectomy, hysterectomy, cervical cancer, radical hysterectomy, debulking surgery, vulvar cancer, vulvectomy, ovarian cancer.

1.   The Origins of Gynaecological Oncology

Surgery for gynaecological tumours, both benign and malignant, has a long history. Ephraim McDowell of Kentucky is generally credited as the pioneer of oophorectomy, performing his first operation in 1809. Oophorectomy subsequently became a widely practiced procedure with the Atlee brothers in the United States reporting 219 cases in 1852, Spencer Wells in Britain 500 cases in 1872 and Emmett in the United States over 100 cases in 1880.[1] It is of interest that although cancer was a well recognised entity by the time these series were reported, only seven cases of ovarian cancer were included in over 800 cases in these series, an extremely low figure by modern standards. Oophorectomy was among the earliest safe abdominal surgical procedures, and helped the development of abdominal surgery in general. Radical hysterectomy and lymphadenectomy was one of the first abdominal operations to offer the chance of cure for malignant disease, with the first such procedure being reported by Clark in the United States in 1895,[2] although the commonest eponym for the operation is that of Wertheim who performed his first radical hysterectomy in 1898, but was able to report 270 cases by 1905.[3] A French surgeon, Basset, outlined the principles of radical surgery for vulvar cancer in 1912,[4] although the procedure was not widely practised for some years. Such were the origins of gynaecological oncology, although, as will be detailed later, the treatment of gynaecological malignancies was not the sole domain of surgeons, even at its beginnings.

The specialty of gynaecology itself was a disputed area, with one of its earliest practitioners, Howard Kelly of Johns Hopkins, in 1922, questioning whether gynaecology would remain "a spinster all her days" and going on to envisage the specialty "on one hand courted by her obstetrical ancestor, who seeks to draw her once more into an unholy, unfruitful alliance" or on the other hand "wooed by a vigorous manly suitor, General Surgery, seeking to allure her from her autonomy into his own house, under his own name, obliterating her identity."[5] It is interesting that the issue of linking gynaecological surgery with obstetrics rather than keeping it linked with the Royal College of Surgeons, caused one of the greatest British gynaecological surgeons in both benign and malignant disease, Victor Bonney, to refused to join the College of Obstetricians and Gynaecologists when it was formed in 1929, although he later accepted an Honorary Fellowship.[6]

The management of gynaecological cancer had always involved either cooperation or sometimes competition between practitioners of different disciplines. A number of excellent training programs had long existed to prepare doctors to practice in this field, but the training and certification of gynaecological oncologists was first addressed in a formalised way in the USA, with the recognition of gynaecological oncology as a subspecialty of obsterics and gynaecology, and in 1972 the first subspecialists were recognised by the American Board of Obstetrics and Gynecology.[7]

Lewis summarises the concept behind the subspecialty as follows: "The decision was made that, ideally, a gynecologic oncologist should be a clinician who has acquired knowledge and skills sufficient to utilise all of the effective forms of therapy of gynecologic malignancies. The specialist should have training, skills and knowledge not only in radical pelvic surgery but also in radiation therapy, chemotherapy and pathology. He should also possess the general medical knowledge required to care for the multiple problems of patients with gynecologic malignancies. This individual's activities should be organised in a clinical service which utilises all of the effective forms of therapy of gynecologic malignancies."[8] It should be added that quality research, both in the laboratory and clinical settings, was seen to be an essential role of the gynaecological oncologist.

After a rather long, and sometimes bitter, debate the then Royal Australian College of Obstetrics and Gynaecology recognised the subspecialty, developed a curriculum for training, and after 'grandfathering' a number of existing gynaecological oncologists, recognised training centres and set up an examination process for subsequent subspecialists. Currently there are about 40 certified gynaecological oncologists in Australia and New Zealand and ten recognised training centres in Australia and one in New Zealand. Recognised gynaecological oncology units must be able to demonstrate the presence not only of certified gynaecological oncologists, but medical and radiation oncologists with special expertise in gynaecological malignancy, pathologists specialising in gynaecological pathology, nurses with special training in gynaecological oncology and other specialised staff. Multidisciplinary Tumour Boards are mandatory.

Commenting on surgery in the early 20th century, Porter makes the following, somewhat cynical but nonetheless perceptive comment:

> "... the ambitious surgeon was beguiled into believing that all manner of diseases could be cured or checked by chloroforming the patient and plying the knife and needle. The potential of surgery became almost a matter of faith: if patients failed to improve after an operation, didn't this show that further lesions remained to be excised, yet more fixing up to be done?"[9]

Gynaecological surgeons, the predecessors of today's gynaecological oncologists, may have included a number who fitted Porter's description, but it would be fair to say from the very beginnings of the treatment of gynaecological malignancies, there was a recognition of the role of disciplines other than surgery in their management.

This Chapter will address the treatment of gynaecological cancers over the past century and highlight the multidisciplinary approach that has developed to a large extent by evolution over this period of time. It will be readily apparent that gynaecological cancer almost always crosses disciplinary borders and can only be optimally treated in a dedicated centre by a multidisciplinary team. The development of treatment for three of the gynaecological cancers will be used to illustrate this point.

2.   Cervical Cancer

In 1883, the American gynaecologist Jackson described the available surgical approaches to cervical cancer as "little more than antemortem examinations."[10] The operative mortality was of the order of 70% and virtually all the women who survived surgery died of the disease "as if no operation had been performed." There were several reasons for this dismal situation, relating to both surgical issues and to the late detection of the disease. Munde, in 1884, addressed the latter issue, hoping that "the inculcation of a wholesome fear" of cervical cancer might lead women to seek attention for symptoms such as inter-menstrual, post-coital or post-menopausal bleeding allowing earlier, more effective treatment. His modest hope that this might allow "one quarter of the cases … to be healthy after two years" indicates how dismal were the survival statistics of the time.[11]

As already mentioned, the modern approach to the surgery of cervical cancer began with the radical hysterectomy and lymph node dissection developed in the 1890s. This operation had a significant mortality rate and even though the indications were considerably more liberal than they are now the more advanced cases were not generally amenable to surgery. But the 1890s also saw the development of radiotherapy, following the discovery of radium by the Curies and X-rays by Roentgen. The tumoricidal capacity of both these modes of radiation were rapidly recognised and both were soon being used in the treatment of cervical cancer. The first use of radium to treat cervical cancer was reported by Cleaves of New York in 1903.[12] In 1919 the Institute of Radium of Paris set up a multidisciplinary unit for the treatment of cancer with surgeons, urologists, and radiotherapists seeing cancer patients in consultation.[13] There were numerous developments in techniques for the primary treatment of cervical cancer with radiotherapy leading to the current approach which involves use of external beam radiation and brachytherapy. In 1927, Heyman from the Radiumhemmet in Sweden, claimed that using this combined approach the "absolute results obtained in respect to the treatment of cancer of the uterine cervix is superior to operative treatment."[14]

Radiation became the main modality for treating cervical cancer in most centres around the world. Not only did it avoid the need for highly skilled surgeons and the mortality associated with radical surgery, but it was applicable to all stages of the disease. In the days before antibiotics and blood transfusion, radical surgery was a serious undertaking. Nevertheless, there were a number of surgeons who continued to perform radical surgery. One of these was Bonney from England who, in a paper published in 1941, enumerated what he saw to be the relative advantages of radiotherapy and of surgery.[15] He saw as the three main advantages of radiotherapy a low immediate mortality, a shorter recovery period than that of surgery, and a lesser effect on sexual functionality. He also recognised that there were advanced cases where radiation could offer a cure, but surgery could not. On the other hand, he gave three reasons for preferring surgery, the first of which was the ease of concealing from the patient the nature of her disease! The second was that having conducted the surgery the surgeon has "shot all his bolts" and recurrence in such cases is incurable, so no follow-up, which could make the patient suspicious of her diagnosis, was needed! The final advantage was that surgery could cure a proportion of cases with positive lymph nodes whereas radiation, in his opinion, could not. Bonney believed that the only reliable way to determine operability was to open the abdomen and assess the ability to get clear surgical margins. He therefore had to abandon the proposed surgery in a proportion of cases. He estimated that he operated on over 60% of patients referred to him overall, and around 80% of those first seen in his private rooms. Of the 500 patients operated on from 1907, the overall five-year recurrence free survival rate was 40%. When the lymph nodes were negative (as they were in 60% of cases), the five-year recurrence free survival rate was 58%, while for those with involved nodes it was 23%. The operative mortality rate was 10% in the node negative group and 20% where the nodes were positive.

Taussig in the United States looked at ways of combining radiation with surgery for advanced stage cervical cancer. In 1934 he published a paper describing the surgical removal of the pelvic lymph nodes, but with radiotherapy rather than surgery for the primary tumour.[16] His series was small, but it was to greatly influence later surgeons.

It is Meigs, of the USA, who is often credited with the recognition of the appropriate role of radical surgery in the treatment of cervical cancer. In a paper published in 1945 he reported on the use of the operation in 65 patients with no operative deaths.[17] Of the 65 patients, 53 had negative nodes and these women had a survival rate of 96% — a remarkable figure. He advised that patients should be preferably less than 50 years of age, thin and in good physical condition. Involvement of the upper vagina did not preclude surgery, but fixation of the cervix by infiltration into the lateral parametrium did. He believed that clinically apparent lymph node metastases did not preclude surgery if other factors were favourable, citing his own experience and that of Bonney and Taussig in support of the view that disease with nodal involvement could not be cured by radiation.

Surgeons often tend to forget the major advances made in radiotherapy, both in terms of equipment and technique over the years, which have led to higher success rates with treatment and markedly less morbidity. These advances include better techniques for delivering brachytherapy and the development of high energy linear accelerators, which can deliver higher doses of radiation to the target tissues with less damage to normal tissues. More recently techniques of conformal and intensity modulated radiotherapy for cervical cancer have been developed to allow even more precise targeting of therapy.[18]

The modern treatment of cervical cancer generally involves the use of radical hysterectomy and pelvic lymphadenectomy as the primary treatment for frankly invasive cancer clinically confined to the cervix, and radical radiotherapy for more advanced disease. There are, however, many areas of controversy. Where the primary tumour is clinically confined to the cervix, but is 4cm or greater in diameter (Stage IB2), there is vigourous debate as to whether radiation or surgery is the appropriate primary therapy. One of the approaches is to perform a radical hysterectomy and lymph node dissection as the initial therapy and then tailor radiotherapy on the basis of the lymph node status. There has only been one randomised controlled trial comparing radical surgery with primary radiotherapy for Stage I B and II A cervical cancer; it showed that for tumours greater than 4 cm in diameter pelvic relapse occurred in 30% of those treated with primary radiation, compared to 20% of those treated with primary surgery followed by radiation. The distant relapse rate was 13%.[19] Where there is no lymph node involvement, the concern is of central recurrence and so some units recommend the use of 'small field' pelvic radiation using a linear accellerator.[20] The small field reduces the amount of bowel exposed to radiation, thus reducing side effects. This approach is not accepted by a large number of units who believe that primary radiation offers better results. The controversy is likely to continue for some time. On the other hand a recent study suggests that the primary surgical approach followed by tailored radiotherapy is an effective choice.[21]

Another area of controversy is the management of grossly enlarged positive nodes discovered at the time of surgery, or on pre-treatment imaging. Some would suggest that if such nodes are detected at the time of radical hysterectomy the enlarged nodes should be removed, but the radical hysterectomy abandoned, and radiotherapy used as the primary treatment. Others would remove the macroscopically enlarged nodes (often taking 2 cm as the minimum size for removal, on the assumption that nodes larger than this are difficult to sterilise with radiation) but complete the radical hysterectomy and treat the patient with post-operative external beam radiotherapy. Resection of bulky positive nodes followed by radiation has been shown to allow survival rates comparable to those achieved in patients with only micrometastases.[22] Most authors would avoid complete lymphadenectomies where post-operative external beam radiation is to be used to reduce the risk of potentially debilitating lymphoedema.

In the past it was felt that where extrapelvic nodal spread of cervical cancer had occurred, the chance of cure was very low. However, where bulky positive nodes have been surgically debulked and post-operative radiation used, including extended field radiation to cover the pelvis and para-aortic regions, extremely good survival rates can be achieved.[23]

For some years there has been interest in concomitant chemo-radiation as both a primary treatment of advanced stage cervical cancer and as adjuvant therapy for patients considered at high risk for recurrence after primary surgery, most commonly due to node positivity. One such regime involves the use of standard radiation doses with weekly cisplatin chemotherapy at relatively low doses. There appears to be little increase in morbidity but significantly improved recurrence free intervals compared to standard radiation alone.[24]

3.   Vulvar Cancer

Morgagni in 1769 was the first to publish a description of vulvar cancer,[25] but there was virtually no discussion of it in the medical literature until Rothschild of Freiburg presented a dissertation in 1912 describing over 300 cases.[26] The French surgeon, Basset, laid the foundation for the modern approach to the condition.[27] On the basis of anatomical studies of cadavers he postulated that early, bilateral, nodal involvement occurred through two lymphatic pathways, one following the round ligaments to the external iliac nodes, and the other directly to the inguino-femoral nodes. The surgical technique he proposed emphasised the importance of removing the inguinal, femoral and distal iliac nodes en bloc bilaterally, together with a radical excision of the entire vulva:

> "One should in every case strive to remove in a single mass all the tissues to be extirpated. It will always be preferable to start with the nodes and lymphatic pedicles on each side carrying out removal of the tumour only as the last step."[27]

Of the 176 cases of vulvar cancer reviewed by Basset, 27% survived for a year or more, with most of those who died suffering from nodal recurrences. Although Basset did not personally perform his proposed operation, he believed that with earlier diagnosis and the use of his approach, far better outcomes could be achieved.

One of the most important figures in the development of surgical treatment for vulvar cancer was Taussig from the USA, who published his first paper in 1917, describing the treatment of 15 cases of vulvar cancer and who, in 1940, published his results in 155 cases treated with between 1911 and 1940.[28] In his series, vulvectomy alone gave a five-year survival of 8%, vulvectomy combined with superficial or incomplete nodal dissection resulted in a five-year survival of 29%, but where the complete Basset type approach was used it was 59%, even though 41% of these patients had positive lymph nodes. The operative mortality was 7%. Taussig described a modification of the Basset procedure to improve wound healing by using separate incisions in some cases for the vulvectomy and each of the groin dissections and did not record any recurrences in the skin bridges. It was many years before such an approach was generally accepted.

Another important figure in the development of surgical treatments for vulvar cancer was Stanley Way from Britain. In his Hunterian Lecture in 1948 he outlined the principles underlying his radical approach to surgery for vulvar cancer.[29] After discussing the lymphatic drainage of the vulva, he reviewed the results of a range of treatments applied in Newcastle up to 1940. Simple vulvectomy with local excision of tumour gave a 24% five-year survival, diathermy coagulation 10%, excision of the vulva or hemivulvectomy with unilateral groin dissection 23%, and vulvectomy with bilateral superficial groin dissection 21%. Radiotherapy alone gave a 13% five-year survival. Way read of Taussig's results at what he described as "a time of despondency concerning the treatment of carcinoma of the vulva." He concluded that:

> "... we require an operation which will remove the vulva very widely and include a removal of all the pre-malignant lesion; which will remove the nodes up to and including the external iliacs on both sides and which will take away the lymphatic anastomosis situated in the mons veneris."

His lymph node dissection aimed to remove all the affected groups of nodes and the group of nodes beyond them. Initially Way believed that closure of the vulvar wound was impossible and that even if it could be achieved, local recurrence was certain to occur. Later he described how, by binding the patient's legs together at the knees and holding the knees in a flexed position post-operatively, primary closure of the vulva could be achieved in most cases and the post-operative stay reduced from around 90 days to 23 days.[30] In the early years the operative mortality was of the order of 12%, but by 1971 it had fallen to 3%. The application of this surgical approach in 367 cases between 1938 and 1975 led to an overall corrected five-year survival rate of 58%, and when the nodes were negative it was 91%.

The widespread adoption of radical vulvectomy with groin and pelvic lymph node dissection resulted in a dramatic improvement in overall survival of women, but the radicality of the procedure, and the physical and psychological morbidity, were causes for great concern, and in recent years there has been considerable research which has led to major advances in the treatment of the disease.

The modern treatment of vulvar cancer lays greater emphasis on more conservative surgery and the use of multimodality treatment. It is important that the newer approaches to treatment are delivered in the setting of a tertiary referral centre. A British study reviewed the records of 411 patients treated at 35 different hospitals, half of which treated on average one case or less per year.[31] Fifteen different operations were used, most commonly simple vulvectomy, in 35% of cases, followed by radical vulvectomy with bilateral groin node dissection in 34%. Only 1% of patients had a hemivulvectomy. Less than half the patients had lymphadenectomy performed and unilateral node dissection was used in only 2% of patients. When the results were compared with those reported by the Gynecologic Oncology Group for tertiary referral centres in the United States,[32] the survival was dramatically poorer for all stages: 78% compared to 98% for stage I, 53% versus 85% for stage II, 27% versus 74% for stage III and 13% versus 31% for stage IV. Failure to perform a lymph node dissection was the single most important poor prognostic factor, but surgery in a centre treating less than 20 cases in total was also significant. A study from the Netherlands reported similar results, with older patients rarely being referred to gynaecologic oncology units and only 20% of women treated in community hospitals undergoing groin node dissection.[33]

Surgery is still the main modality of treatment for vulvar cancer, but it is in general more conservative, and more frequently used in association with radiation and sometimes chemotherapy to allow less radicality.

The use of the en bloc radical vulvectomy is no longer advocated. For smaller lateralised lesions, radical local excision of the lesion, with a surgical margin of at least 1 cm but with vulvar conservation, and ipsilateral groin node dissection through a separate groin incision, is the commonly accepted treatment.

The single most important prognostic factor for women with vulvar cancer is the status of the groin nodes. It is now recognised that with tumours of less than 2 cm in diameter and invading less than 1mm, nodal involvement is extremely rare and groin dissection can be omitted.[34] For larger or more deeply invasive lesions, inguinofemoral node dissection is recommended on the ipsilateral side in lateralised lesions, and bilaterally for lesions close to the midline. Groin node dissection is associated with a risk of lymphoedema of the order of 60%.[35] Lymphoedema can be a debilitating condition affecting the function and mobility of the limb and often being associated with significant lymphangitis. One strategy to reduce the incidence and severity of this problem is the use of sentinel node biopsy, and this strategy is being investigated in a number of centres. As recurrences in undissected groins are almost always lethal,[36] the key issue with sentinel node biopsy is its false negative rate in various circumstances. At present there is insufficient evidence to support its routine use for vulvar cancer.

A study by the Gynecologic Oncology Group looked at the management of women with positive groin nodes.[37] Patients with positive groin nodes were randomised to have either an ipsilateral pelvic node dissection or bilateral groin and pelvic radiation. The important findings were that the radiated group had a significantly higher two-year survival rate, compared to the group undergoing pelvic node dissection (68% vs. 54%), but that the benefit was limited to those with clinically evident nodes or more than two positive nodes. The incidence and severity of lymphoedema was reduced in the radiated group.

In view of the above findings, many units would now utilise frozen sections of any macroscopically involved groin nodes, and if the nodes prove positive, remove only the grossly enlarged nodes, but not perform a full groin dissection, and rely on radiation to deal with micrometastases, to reduce the combined morbidity of extensive surgery and radiotherapy.

For locally advanced vulvar cancers involving the vagina, rectum or other midline structures vulvectomy, groin node dissection and some form of exenterative procedure provided survival rates of approximately 50%,[38] but the cost in terms of physical and psychosexual morbidity was extremely high. As early as 1973, Boronow had advocated the use of radiotherapy to reduce tumour size and allow more conservative surgery for such patients, but the approach was slow to gain acceptance. In 1987 Boronow reported on the effectiveness of preoperative radiotherapy in 37 cases of locally advanced vulvar cancers and 11 cases of recurrent disease with five-year survival rates of 76% for primary disease and 63% for recurrent disease.[39] The Gynecologic Oncology Group undertook a study of chemoradiation in 73 women with vulvar cancer considered to require exenterative surgery to remove their tumours. Of these patients, 69 achieved sufficient tumour response for more conservative surgery, and all but three of them maintained urinary and faecal continence.[40] Numerous subsequent studies have confirmed the utility of pre-operative radiotherapy followed by more conservative surgery in patients with locally advanced vulvar cancer to avoid exenterative surgery. The addition of concurrent chemotherapy adds to the morbidity of the treatment and it is not clear whether it improves the control rates and survival.

4.   Ovarian Cancer

Epithelial ovarian cancer is the most lethal of the common gynaecological malignancies. The lifetime risk of a woman in a developing country is of the order of 1:70.[41] One of the most problematic aspects of the disease is that in at least two-thirds of patients there is spread of the disease outside the pelvic cavity at the time of diagnosis. To further compound the problem, even when the disease is confined to the ovaries, there is a significant group of patients whose cancer will recur after the surgical removal of their disease.

The development of our current approach to the treatment of ovarian cancer is detailed in a series of papers of which Munnel was the senior author.[42–44] In this series of papers he reports the results of patients treated between 1922 and 1961. There was no improvement in survival between 1922 and 1951, but in the period from 1951 to 1961 there was a marked improvement which was credited to the use of more aggressive surgery together with adjuvant radiotherapy. He advocated total hysterectomy, bilateral salpingoophorectomy, omentectomy and resection of as much tumour as possible, even if that required bowel resections. He also advocated the routine use of post-operative radiotherapy whenever the disease had spread beyond the ovaries.

The problem with radiotherapy as adjuvant therapy for ovarian cancer is that patterns of spread and recurrence of ovarian cancer demand the treatment of the entire peritoneal cavity and the ability to deliver cytotoxic doses is limited by the relative intolerance of the liver and kidneys.

Modern chemotherapy had its beginnings in the 1940s when the Department of Defense in the United States commissioned the pharmacologists, Goodman and Gilman, to look into possible therapeutic uses of agents used in chemical warfare. It had been long known that soldiers exposed to mustard gas had severe bone marrow suppression. After demonstrating that lymphomas in a mouse model responded to mustard agents, in 1946 Goodman used that the newly developed drug mustine in a patient with non Hodgkin's lymphoma, producing a dramatic, albeit short term reduction in the patient's tumour masses, and subsequently used variations of the drug in other malignancies.[45] A range of other chemotherapeutic agents were developed in subsequent years.

The earliest report of the use of chemotherapy in the treatment of ovarian cancer was published in 1952.[46] In 1985 a review article on the treatment of epithelial ovarian cancer concluded that advanced ovarian cancer responded, in varying degrees, to single agent alkylating agents in up to 65% of cases, with no obvious advantage to any particular drug. The responses were said to translate to improved survival.[47] Because the malignancy frequently relapsed if chemotherapy was ceased, the alkylating agents were used continuously until it was recognised, in 1977, that they could cause non-lymphocytic leukaemia. A number of other chemotherapeutic agents had been developed that were also active, as single agents, against ovarian cancer, including fluorouracil, methotrexate, doxorubicin and hexamethylmelamine. In 1965 the concept of combination chemotherapy for various malignancies using several drugs with different modes of action was proposed. The first combination regimen shown in a randomised controlled trial to be superior to single agent alkylating agents in advanced ovarian cancer was hexamethylmelamine, cyclophosphamide, methotrexate and 5 Fluorouracil (HexaCAF).[48] A number of other trials of combination chemotherapy produced conflicting results, possibly due to heterogeneity within the study population and differences in the aggressiveness of the surgical approach. The next major breakthrough in chemotherapy for ovarian cancer was the serendipitous discovery of the platinum-based cytotoxics by Rosenberg in the United States. In 1976, Wiltshaw and Kronor from Great Britain, published a report of the effectiveness of the first platinum drug, cisplatin, in refractory ovarian cancer.[49] Given that the new drug could produce responses in refractory disease it was soon trialled in combination with alkylating agents and demonstrated improved progression-free survival than with alkylating agents alone.[50]

For some time the treatment of choice for advanced ovarian cancer was radical 'debulking' surgery followed by the three-drug combination of cisplatin, cyclophosphamide and adriamycin, although the cardiotoxicity of the adriamycin later led to it being dropped from the regimen in most centres. The next major development in chemotherapy was the use of the taxane drugs, the commonest being paclitaxel. Initial randomised trials comparing the combinations of cisplatin and cyclophosphamide with cisplatin and paclitaxel suggested that the latter combination produced significant increases in progression free survival (18 months vs. 13 months) and overall survival (37 months vs. 24 months).[51,52] The major problem with this regimen was that both cisplatin and paclitaxel are neurotoxic, but it was soon found that the cisplatin analogue, carboplatin, was equally effective as the original drug, and the combination of carboplatin and paclitaxel or one of the other taxanes is the standard of care in most units.

The standard treatment of epithelial ovarian cancer is normally initial surgery to confirm the diagnosis, determine the extent of the disease and to resect as much of the disease as is technically feasible. This process is best carried out by trained gynaecological oncologists in specialised units. The surgery may be quite complex, but the extent of residual disease is an important determinant of outcome for patients with ovarian cancer. Pathological examination of the resulting specimens by a specialised gynaecological pathologist is essential. Only in selected cases of early disease is chemotherapy omitted. Chemotherapy needs to be administered by experienced medical oncologists in units with trained nursing staff.

Not all patients are fit for initial surgery due to age, extent of disease or other co-morbidities. The fitness of a patient for surgery needs to be assessed by a physicians and anaesthetists familiar with the nature of the disease and the effects of the surgery if optimal results are to be achieved. Where patients have massive ascites, large pleural effusions, or are for other reasons considered unsuitable for primary surgery, the use of neoadjuvant chemotherapy is considered. As already implied, the decision to use neoadjuvant chemotherapy must be based on appropriate multidisciplinary consultations, with all participants being aware of the risks and benefits of surgery. Schwartz *et al.* reported that patients treated with neoadjuvant chemotherapy followed by interval debulking did as well as an historical group treated by primary surgery followed by chemotherapy.[53] Others have advocated neoadjuvant chemotherapy both to 'chemically debulk' large tumours and claim equivalent survival to those obtained by primary surgical debulking, but at a lower cost. Overall however, the consensus is that best results are obtained by primary debulking followed by chemotherapy in a multidisciplinary unit.

While the advent of effective chemotherapy dramatically reduced the role of radiotherapy in ovarian cancer, it still has a role in the management of carefully selected patients. In some patients with advanced, unresectable and chemoresistant tumours, radiation may effectively palliate symptoms such as vaginal or rectal bleeding, pain and other symptoms.[54,55]

For the majority of patients, their ovarian cancer will recur at some stage. The management of such recurrences depends on many factors and requires close consultation in a multidisciplinary team setting. Since the advent of the tumour marker Ca125, recurrence is detected in many asymptomatic women. When Ca125 levels rise significantly and there is no clinical evidence of disease, it is the practice in our unit to perform a CT of the abdomen and pelvis together with a chest X-ray to look for radiological evidence of disease. If none is found we choose the well tolerated drug tamoxifen and monitor the Ca 125 levels. About 20% of patients respond to this treatment for a variable period of time.[56–58]

Where scans show potentially resectable disease after a treatment-free interval of 12 months or more, there may be a role for secondary cytoreduction in carefully selected patients.[59,60] Once again, multidisciplinary discussion is critical in selecting patients for this approach.

Where surgery is not considered appropriate, numerous second-line drugs are now available for chemotherapy, the choice depending more on the preference of the oncologist than any other factor. Side effect profiles need to be taken into consideration in this situation.

Surgery in end stage ovarian cancer is a consideration that requires good clinical judgement and very careful consideration. An exhaustive review of the literature concludes that it is not possible to provide clear answers to the questions of who will benefit from surgery, by how much and for how long.[61] This is an area where the true skill of the surgeon is not in the performance of a procedure but in a holistic assessment of the situation in the light of all available information.

Given the very high mortality rate for epithelial ovarian cancer and the importance of symptomatic care both during active treatment and during the terminal phase of the disease, it is wise to involve palliative medical specialists from early in the disease to ensure adequate community linkages and avoid last minute, desperate referrals in a time of crisis.[62] Ideally palliative medicine physicians will participate in all multidisciplinary meetings.

5. Conclusions

While this paper has dealt primarily with three modalities of treatment, namely surgery, radiation and chemotherapy, it should be readily apparent that numerous other disciplines, including other medical disciplines, skilled nurses, psychologists and social workers are essential parts of the team, though space precludes a more detailed discussion of their roles.

The optimal outcome for all women with gynaecological cancer can only be achieved in specialised centres with a full team of health professionals working in concert for the good of the woman.

References

1. J. D. Woodruff, The pathogenesis of ovarian neoplasia, *Johns Hopkins Med. J.* **144**: 117–120 (1979).
2. J. G. Clark, More radical method of performing hysterectomy for cancer of the uterus, *Johns Hopkins Hosp. Bull.* **6**: 120–127 (1895).
3. E. Wertheim, Discussion on the diagnosis and treatment of cancer of the uterus, *Br. Med. J.* **2**: 689–695 (1905).
4. A. Basset, [*L'epitheliome Primitive du Clitoris: Son Reteissment Ganglionaire et son Traitement Operatoire*], No. 180 (G. Steinheil, Paris, 1912).
5. F. H. Garrison, *Introduction to the History of Medicine*, 3rd ed. (W. B. Saunders, Philadelphia, 1922), p. 652.
6. E. E. Philipp, Victor Bonney: The gynaecological surgeon of the twentieth century, *J. R. Soc. Med.* **94**: 311–312 (2001).

7. H. E. Averette, A. Wrennick and R. Angioli, History of gynecologic oncology subspecialty, *Surg. Clin. N. Am.* **81**: 747–751 (2001).

8. J. L. Lewis Jr., Training of the gynecologic oncologist. In: *Gynecologic Oncology. Fundamental Principles and Clinical Practice*, 2nd ed., ed. M. Coppleson (Churchill Livingstone, Edinburgh, 1992), p. 3.

9. R. Porter, *The Greatest Benefit to Mankind: A Medical History of Humanity from Antiquity to the Present* (London, Fontana Press, 1999), p. 599.

10. A. R. Jackson, quoted in H. Speert, *Obstetrics and Gynecology in America. A History* (American College of Obsterics and Gynecology, Chicago, 1980), p. 57.

11. P. Munde, quoted in H. Speert, *Obstetrics and Gynecology in America. A History* (American College of Obsterics and Gynecology, Chicago, 1980), p. 58.

12. M. A. Cleaves, Radium therapy, *Med. Record* **64**: 602–612 (1903).

13. A. Lacassagne, [Evolution et orientation des techniques en radiotherapie des epitheliomas cervico-uterins], *IV Internationaler Radiologenkongress, Zurich* **2**: 44–61 (1934).

14. J. Heyman, Radiological or operative treatment of cancer of the uterus, *Acta Radiol.* **8**: 363–409 (1927).

15. V. Bonney, The results of 500 cases of Wertheim's operation for carcinoma of the cervix, *J. Obstet. Gynaecol. Br. Empire.* **48**: 421–435 (1941).

16. F. J. Taussig, Iliac lymphadenectomy with irradiation in the treatment of cancer of the cervix, *Am. J. Obstet. Gynecol.* **28**: 650–667 (1934).

17. J. V. Meigs, The Wertheim operation for carcinoma of the cervix, *Am. J. Obstet. Gynecol.* **49**: 542–549 (1945).

18. A. Taylor and M. Powell, Conformal and intensity modulated radiotherapy for cervical cancer, *Clin. Oncol.* **20**: 417–425 (2008).

19. F. Landoni, A. Maneo, A. Colombo *et al.*, Randomised study of radical surgery versus radiotherapy for stage IB — IIA cervical cancer, *Lancet* **350**: 535–540 (1997).

20. F. J. Kridelka, D. O. Berg, M. Neuman *et al.*, Adjuvant small field radiation for patients with high risk stage IB node negative cervical cancer after radical hysterectomy and pelvic lymph node dissection: A pilot study, *Cancer* **86**: 2059–2065 (1999).

21. K. Ohara, H. Tsunoda, M. Nishida *et al.*, Use of small pelvic field instead of whole pelvic field in postoperative radiotherapy for node negative, high risk stage I and II cervical squamous carcinoma, *Int. J. Gynecol. Cancer* **13**: 170–176 (2003).

22. J. A. Cosin, J. M. Fowler, M. D. Chen *et al.*, Pretreatment staging of patients with cervical carcinoma: The case for lymph node debulking, *Cancer* **82**: 2241–2248 (1998).

23. N. F. Hacker, G. V. Wain and J. L. Nicklin, Resection of bulky positive lymph nodes in patients with cervical cancer, *Int. J. Gynecol. Cancer* **5**: 250–256 (1995).

24. P. G. Rose, B. Bundy, E. B. Watkins *et al.*, Concurrent cisplatin based radiotherapy and chemotherapy for locally advanced cervical cancer, *N. Engl. J. Med.* **340**: 1144–1153 (1999).

25. J. B. Morgagni, *The Seats and Causes of Diseases Investigated by Anatomy*, Vol. 3 (Millar Cadell Johnson and Payne, London, 1769), p. 70.

26. F. J. Taussig, *Diseases of the Vulva* (Appleton & Co, New York, 1912), p. 142.

27. A. Basset, [Traitment chirurgical operatoire de l'epitheliomaq primitive du clitoris]. *Rev. Chir.* **32**: 546–570 (1912).

28. F. J. Taussig, Cancer of the vulva: An analysis of 155 cases (1911–1940). *Am. J. Obstet. Gynecol.* **40**: 764–779 (1940).

29. S. Way, The anatomy of the lymphatic drainage of the vulva and its influence on the radical operation for carcinoma, *Ann. R. Coll. Surg. Engl.* **3**: 187–209 (1948).

30. S. Way, The surgery of vulval carcinoma: An appraisal, *Clin. Obstet. Gynecol.* **5**: 623–628 (1978).

31. C. A. Rhodes, C. Cummings and M. I. Schafi, The management of squamous cell vulval cancer: A population based retrospective study of 411 cases, *Br. J. Obstet. Gynaecol.* **105**: 200–205 (1998).

32. H. D. Homesley, B. N. Bundy, A. Sedlis *et al.*, Assessment of current International Federation of Gynecology and Obstetrics staging of vulvar cancer relative to prognostic factors for survival: A Gynecologic Oncology Group study, *Am. J. Obstet. Gynecol.* **164**: 997–1004 (1991).

33. J. van der Velden, A. C. van Lindert, C. H. Gimbere *et al.*, Epidemiological data on vulvar cancer: Comparison of hospital and community based data, *Gynecol. Oncol.* **62**: 373–383 (1996).

34. N. F. Hacker, Radical resection of vulvar malignancies: A paradigm shift in surgical approaches, *Curr. Opin. Obstet. Gynecol.* **11**: 61–64 (1999).

35. M. Ryan, M. C. Stainton, E. K. Slaytor, C. Jaconelli, S. Watts and P. Mackenzie, Aetiology and prevalence of lower limb lymphoedema following treatment for gynaecological cancer, *Aust. N. Z. J. Obstet. Gynaecol.* **43**: 148–151 (2003).

36. D. E. Marsden and N. F. Hacker, Contemporary management of primary carcinoma of the vulva, *Surg. Clin. N. Am.* **81**: 799–811 (2001).

37. H. D. Homesley, B. N. Bundy, A. Sedlis *et al.*, Radiation therapy versus pelvic node resection for carcinoma of the vulva with positive groin nodes, *Am. J. Obstet. Gynecol.* **68**: 733–740 (1986).

38. D. Cavanagh and J. Shepherd, The place of pelvic exenteration in the primary management of advanced carcinoma of the vulva, *Gynecol. Oncol.* **13**: 318–324 (1982).

39. R. C. Boronow, B. T. Hickman, M. T. Reagan *et al.*, Combined therapy as an alternative to exenteration for locally advanced vulvovaginal cancer: II. Results, complications and dosimetric and surgical considerations, *Am. J. Clin. Oncol.* **10**: 171–181 (1987).

40. D. H. Moore, G. M. Thomas, G. S. Montana *et al.*, Preoperative chemoradiation for advanced vulvar cancer: A phase II study of the Gynecologic Oncology Group, *Int. J. Radiat. Oncol. Biol. Phys.* **42**: 79–85 (1998).

41. D. Marsden, M. Friedlander and N. Hacker, Current management of epithelial ovarian carcinoma: A review, *Semin. Surg. Oncol.* **19**: 11–19 (2000).

42. E. W. Munnell and H. C. Taylor Jr., Ovarian carcinoma. A review of 200 primary and 51 secondary cases, *Am. J. Obstet. Gynecol.* **58**: 943–952 (1949).

43. E. W. Munnell, H. W. Jacox and H. C. Taylor Jr., Treatment and prognosis in cancer of the ovary. With a review of a new series of 143 cases treated in the years 1944–1951, *Am. J. Obstet. Gynecol.* **74**: 1187–1191 (1957).

44. E. W. Munnell, The changing prognosis and treatment in cancer of the ovary. A report of 235 patients with primary ovarian carcinoma 1952–1961, *Am. J. Obstet. Gynecol.* **100**: 790–805 (1968).

45. L. S. Goodman, M. M. Wintrobe, W. Dameshek *et al.*, Nitrogen mustard therapy. Use of methyl-bis(betachloroethyl)amine hydrochloride and tris(beta chloroethyl)amine hydrochloride for Hodgkin's disease, lymphosarcoma, leukaemia and certain allied and miscellaneous disorders, *J. Am. Med. Assoc.* **105**: 475–476 (1946).

46. R. W. Rundles and W. B. Burton, Triethylene melamine in the treatment of malignant diseases, *Blood* **7**: 483–489 (1952).

47. G. S. Richardson, R. E. Scully, N. Nikrui and J. H. Nelson Jr., Common epithelial cancer of the ovary, *N. Engl. J. Med.* **312**: 474–483 (1985).

48. R. C. Young, B. A. Chabner, S. P. Hubbard *et al.*, Advanced ovarian adenocarcinoma. A prospective clinical trial of melphalan (L-PAM) versus combination chemotherapy, *N. Engl. J. Med.* **299**: 1261–1266 (1978).

49. E. Wiltshaw and T. Kronor, Phase II study of cis-dichlorodiamine platinum (II) (NSC-119875) in advanced adenocarcinoma of the ovary, *Cancer Treast. Rep.* **60**: 55–60 (1976).

50. D. G. Decker, T. R. Fleming, G. D. Malkasian Jr. *et al.*, Cyclophosphamide plus cis-platinum in combination: Treatment program for stage III or IV ovarian carcinoma, *Obstet. Gynecol.* **60**: 481–487 (1982).

51. W. P. McGuire, W. J. Hoskins, M. F. Brady *et al.*, Cyclophosphamide and cisplatin compared with pacltaxel and cisplatin in patients with stage III or IV ovarian cancer, *N. Engl. J. Med.* **334**: 1–6 (1996).

52. C. Trope, M. J. Piccart, G. Stuart *et al.*, Improved survival with paclitaxel-cisplatin compared to cyclophosphamide-cisplatin in advanced ovarian cancer after a median follow up of 39 months: Update of the EORTC, NOCOVA, NCIC, Scottish intergroup study, *Int. J. Gynecol. Cancer.* **9**(Suppl. 1): 57 (1999).

53. P. E. Schwarz, T. J. Rutherford, J. T. Chambers, E. I. Kohorn and R. P. Thiel, Neoaduvant chemotherapy for advanced ovarian cancer: Long term survival, *Gynecol. Oncol.* **72**: 93–99 (1999).

54. B. W. Corn, R. M. Lanciano, M. Boente *et al.*, Recurrent ovarian cancer. Effective radiotherapeutic palliation after chemotherapy failure, *Cancer* **74**: 2979–2983 (1994).

55. D. Gelblum, B. Mychalczak, L. Almadrones *et al.*, Palliative benefit of external beam radiation in the management of platinum refractory epithelial ovarian carcinoma, *Gynecol. Oncol.* **69**: 36–41 (1998).

56. A. M. Myers, G. E. Moore and F. J. Major, Advanced ovarian cancer response to antiestrogen therapy, *Cancer* **48**: 2368–2370 (1981).

57. P. E. Schwarz, G. Keating, N. MacLuskey *et al.*, Tamoxifen therapy for advanced ovarian cancer, *Obstet. Gynecol.* **59**: 583–588 (1982).

58. J. van der Velden, G. Gitsch, G. V. Wain *et al.*, Tamoxifen in patients with advanced epithelial ovarian cancer, *Int. J. Gynecol. Cancer* **5**: 301–305 (1995).

59. S. M. Eisenkop, R. L. Friedman and N. M. Spirtos, The role of secondary cytoreductive surgery in the treatment of patients with recurrent epithelial ovarian carcinoma, *Cancer* **88**: 144–153 (2000).

60. E. H. Tay, P. T. Grant, V. Gebski and N. F. Hacker, Secondary cytoreductive surgery for recurrent epithelial ovarian cancer, *Obstet. Gynecol.* **100**: 1359–1360 (2002).
61. D. J. Feuer, E. K. Broadley, J. H. Shepherd and D. P. Barton, Systematic review of surgery in malignant bowel obstruction in advanced gynaecological and gastrointestinal cancer, *Gynecol. Oncol.* **75**: 313–322 (1999).
62. The Committee on Care at the End of Life, *Approaching Death: Improving Care at the End of Life* (Institute of Medicine, National Academy Press, Washington, DC, 2000).

23

Orthopedic Emergencies in Oncology

Valerae O. Lewis and
Jeffrey T. Luna

Abstract

The management and treatment of orthopedic emergencies that develop in patients with cancer is diverse and often complex. Although treatment algorithms exist, treatment must be tailored to each patient. For the two most common orthopedic emergencies encountered, namely pathologic fracture and spinal cord compression, the primary goals of treatment in both cases are pain relief and early restoration of function. Surgical stabilization of a pathologic fracture and surgical fixation with decompression of a spinal cord compression is often performed to improve the patient's quality of life. In less commonly seen orthopedic emergencies, such as abscesses, necrotizing fasciitis, and acute compartment syndrome, aggressive surgical intervention is warranted, to prevent the compounding complications that may arise if inadequately treated. However, the patient's life expectancy must be considered when planning any type of treatment, since the disease stage may be advanced at the time the patient presents with an orthopedic oncologic emergency. In terminally ill patients, orthopedic surgical treatment should only be considered if there is reasonable evidence that an intervention will improve the patient's quality of life.

Keywords: Pathologic fracture, impending fracture, infection in cancer patients, orthopedic oncologic emergency, spinal cord compression, acute compartment syndrome, amputation.

Background

Managing orthopedic oncologic emergencies is complex, and treatment decisions are often difficult. In treating the diverse orthopedic oncologic emergencies that may arise, the orthopedic surgeon must consider the histology and natural history of the underlying cancer, the acuity of the patient's symptoms, the disease stage, and overall prognosis. In terminally ill patients, treatment should be administered only when there is reasonable evidence that an intervention will improve the patient's quality of life.[1]

This chapter reviews approaches for treating both common and uncommon orthopedic oncologic emergencies, specifically impending and pathologic fractures, spinal cord compression (SCC), infections, and acute compartment syndrome (ACS). The role of amputation in the surgical management of cancer patients with orthopedic emergencies is also reviewed.

1. Fractures

Cancer metastasizes to bone in 50% of patients[2] and the most frequent orthopedic oncologic emergency seen in cancer patients is a pathologic fracture. Pathologic fractures can represent the first sign of metastasis from a known cancer, and in some instances, a pathologic fracture is the first evidence of an unknown/silent cancer. In the cases where a lytic lesion is the first sign of cancer, the management should be directed towards identifying the primary cancer.[1]

Rougraff *et al.*[3] developed a cost-effective and efficient evaluation strategy for the management of the patient who presents with an impending or pathologic fracture due to a metastasis from an unknown primary cancer. This strategy starts with a thorough medical history and physical examination. As breast, lung, prostate, kidney and thyroid cancers are the most common cancers that metastasize to bone, both the history and physical examination should include these areas. The work up should includes routine laboratory analysis, to include: complete blood count, erythrocyte sedimentation rate, C-reactive protein, electrolyte panel, urinalysis, free thyroxine (T4), thyroid stimulating hormone, alkaline phosphatase, prostate specific antigen (PSA) (for males), blood urea nitrogen, creatinine and urine and serum protein electrophoresis. Plain radiographs of the involved extremity and the lungs, as well as computed tomography (CT) scans of the chest, abdomen, and pelvis should be obtained. Once the work-up is completed and reviewed, a biopsy of the most accessible lesion can be performed to confirm the diagnosis. A complete work-up may not only reveal a more accessible lesion to biopsy, but may also (as can be in the case of multiple myeloma) obviate the need for biopsy. For 85% of patients presenting with metastases from an unknown primary tumor, this diagnostic approach will identify the primary tumor site.[3]

To specifically evaluate the osseous involvement, full-length radiographs in two orthogonal planes of the involved bone should first be obtained. These radiographs are necessary to not only identify local boney architecture, but also to identify synchronous lesions within the bone (Fig. 1). A bone scan will identify additional sites of osseous involvement, and multifocal radionuclide uptake is suggestive of metastatic disease. Other imaging studies, such as CT scans, magnetic resonance imaging (MRI) and angiography, can be performed to further evaluate the extent of bone involvement. Computed tomography is useful in evaluating the integrity of bone, while MRI is useful in delineating both the intraosseous extent of the disease and the soft tissue involvement. MRI is particularly useful in evaluating back pain and is the most sensitive investigation for evaluating epidural extension of disease and spinal cord compression.[4] With the advances in CT and MRI, angiography is rarely used as a diagnostic tool. However, its use is vital as a therapeutic adjuvant for highly vascular tumors, such as multiple myeloma, thyroid and renal cell carcinoma, in order to reduce intra-operative blood loss (Fig. 2).[5–7]

Pain from an impending or pathologic fracture is the most common reason why cancer patients with bone metastases present to the emergency room. If the radiographs reveal that the presenting pain is related to a pathologic fracture, the first step initiated in the emergency room should be immobilization of the fractured extremity (Fig. 3). Immobilizing the fractured extremity and

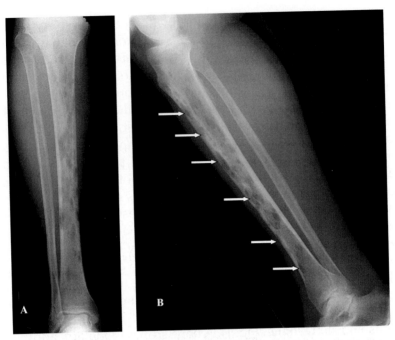

Figure 1. (A) Anteroposterior view of the tibia with metastatic non-small-cell lung carcinoma. (B) Lateral view showing multiple synchronous lytic lesions (arrows) along the tibial shaft.

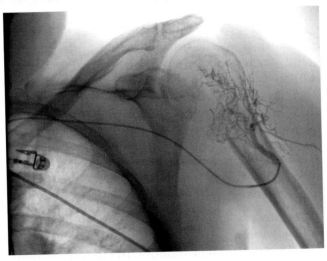

Figure 2. Pre-operative angiography and embolization of a metastatic thyroid carcinoma in the left proximal humerus.

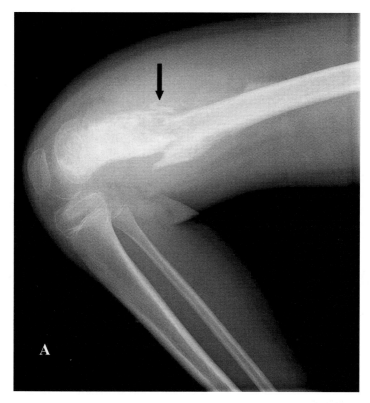

Figure 3. (A) Lateral radiograph of a femur with a pathologic fracture (arrow) secondary to an osteosarcoma. (B) Immobilization of the extremity with a long leg cast.

administering intravenous narcotics will provide the patient with pain relief.[8,9] Furthermore, immobilization not only relieves pain, but also controls the bleeding by reducing the motion of the fractured bone ends. In the case of impending pathological fractures, immobilization not only provides pain relief, but may prevent progression to fracture. This is particularly important for those patients who may have a primary sarcoma of bone. Bramer *et al.*[10] found that overall survival was worse in patients with a fracture resulting from osteosarcoma, or chondrosarcoma.

Immobilization of fractures around the shoulder area, including the proximal humerus, may initially be done with the use of a sling. Middle and distal arm, forearm and hand fractures are best immobilized with splints. If a cast is applied, swelling must be monitored

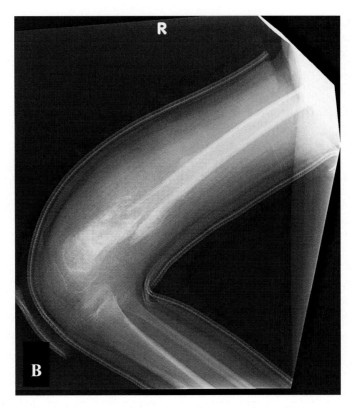

Figure 3. (*Continued*)

closely and the arm should be elevated above the heart. Hip and femur fractures can be immobilized with Buck's traction; however, if there is a contraindication to traction, the extremity can be placed in a comfortable position supported by pillows. More distal fractures of the lower extremities (i.e. tibia and fibula) are best immobilized with splints. Hospitalization is indicated in patients presenting with fractures associated with hemodynamic compromise, neurologic deficits, irreducible fractures, fractures of the hip or femur, or in those patients in whom pain control is not achieved.[1]

1.1 *Impending fractures*

The primary concern regarding bone metastases is the progression of the lesions to a pathologic fracture, i.e. a fracture that results from normal physiologic loading. Pain generally is the first sign of a metastatic bone lesion. Furthermore, pain with weight bearing is the most significant indicator of an impending fracture, since it reflects weakened structural integrity of the bone.[1,11,12] There are several potential benefits to prophylactic stabilization of impending pathologic fractures. These benefits include pain control, maintenance of quality of life, simplicity of the procedure (compared to the fractured state), decrease in operative time, decrease in blood loss, decrease in narcotic use and decrease in hospitalization.[13]

There are several scoring systems that have been developed to assess the risk of developing a pathological fracture. Although new systems utilizing advanced imaging techniques (i.e. CT) are being developed, the Mirels scoring system[11,12,14] and Harrington's[15] classic definition of impending fractures with bone metastases are most commonly used. Both scoring systems are based on the use of radiographs. The Mirels 12-point scoring system for evaluating the risk of pathologic fractures takes into account the site of the bone lesion (upper or lower extremity or peritrochanteric region), associated pain (mild, moderate, or severe), tumor type (blastic, mixed, or lytic), and lesion size (involvement of < 1/3, 1/3–2/3, or > 2/3 of the diameter of the bone). The system then allots 1, 2, or 3 points to each risk factor according to the degree of risk, and provides a maximum score of 12. Patients with a score of 9 or greater are at high risk of developing a pathologic fracture and thus would benefit from prophylactic stabilization. Patients with a score of 7 or less are at a low risk for fracture and can be treated non-operatively, with protected weight bearing and radiation therapy. Harrington's definition of an impending pathologic fracture specifically takes into account the size and location of the lesion, and the lesion's response to radiation treatment. According to Harrington, osseous lesions involving 50% or more of the bone diameter, lesions involving the proximal femur, or that coexist with fractures of the lesser trochanter, and lesions that have failed to respond to radiotherapy are all at high risk for pathologic fracture. Although both of these scoring systems can be helpful, treatment should be individualized and the surgeon must weigh the benefits of prophylactic fixation with the probability of fracture and patient status.

For osseous lesions considered to be at low risk for progressing to a pathologic fracture, non-surgical management can be employed. Management is directed towards pain relief and fracture prevention. Activity modifications, radiotherapy, hormonal and bisphosphonate therapy are excellent options.[2] For the upper extremity, adequate immobilization (functional bracing) and in the lower extremity, protected weight-bearing with the use of crutches, a walker or a wheelchair should be initiated. By administering the appropriate nonsurgical management to patients at low risk of pathologic fracture, pain relief is achieved and the likelihood of progression to a pathologic fracture is minimized.

Early identification of patients with osseous lesions at risk for a pathologic fracture (impending pathologic fracture) is important. Progression of an impending fracture to an actual fracture can be devastating. Prophylactic surgical stabilization is advised to avoid the trauma and disability that may arise from a completed fracture. However, in the treatment of any patient with a bone lesion at risk of pathologic fracture, several considerations must be taken into account.

The patient's diagnosis must be definitively established before treatment can be undertaken.[16] Unless histologic confirmation of metastatic disease or myeloma has been established, a biopsy of a solitary lesion of bone is necessary. This is true even in the setting of an impending fracture, or with a known history of cancer. As previously stated, a biopsy should only be performed after a thorough work-up has been completed. The work-up may not only reveal other lesions requiring surgical attention, but it may reveal the need for neo-adjuvant therapies as well. It has been shown that optimal results are obtained when a surgeon who is experienced with managing both primary and metastatic bone tumors performs the biopsy.[17]

Once the diagnosis is established, operative planning can commence. There are several tumors that are highly vascular. Pre-operative embolization is an important surgical adjuvant. Embolization is advisable before open biopsy and prophylactic stabilization for patients with myeloma, renal thyroid carcinomas, and other highly vascular tumors.[5-7,16] Excessive bleeding may result during stabilization, and uncontrollable hemorrhage may even result in death. Pre-operative embolization has been shown to be a safe and reliable method of reducing intra-operative blood loss at the time of surgical stabilization.

The expected length of survival of the patient should be considered. A patient with metastatic disease should have an expected length of survival that is longer than the expected period of recovery from the surgical procedure. In general, surgical stabilization should be considered in patients with fractures through weight-bearing bones (lower extremity) who have more than four weeks to live, while for patients who have fractures through non-weight bearing bones (upper extremity), surgical stabilization should be considered when they have more than 12 weeks to live.[1,2,16]

Lastly, the role of resection of an isolated metastasis, particularly from a renal cell carcinoma, should be considered. Resection of the isolated metastasis may be advisable to control local disease that is relatively resistant to radiotherapy and it has been shown in select histologies (renal cell carcinoma) to possibly improve overall length of survival.[2,16]

Once the clinical situation has been fully assessed, several prophylactic stabilization techniques are available for impending fractures. The preferred prophylactic stabilization method for diaphyseal lesions at risk for pathologic fracture is locked intramedullary nail fixation (Fig. 4). For the femur, the preferred method of fixation is a reconstruction nail which provides protection of the femoral neck as well.[16] For larger lesions involving significant bone loss, curettage and cementation of the lesion, in addition to intramedullary fixation of the bone should be considered. When the epiphyseal and metaphyseal areas are involved, standard intramedullary prophylactic fixation devices will not provide adequate stabilization. In these cases, resection of the diseased and compromised bone, followed by immediate endoprosthetic reconstruction is the better treatment option.[2,16,18,19] In the proximal humerus and distal femur, alternative treatments such as curettage and cementation may be appropriate for small, well-contained lesions.

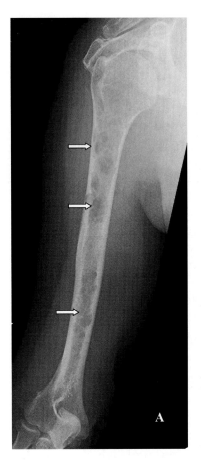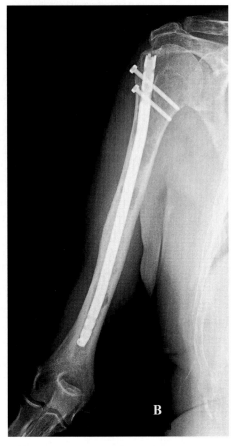

Figure 4. (A) Anteroposterior radiographic view of a humerus with multiple myelomatous lytic lesions along the diaphysis (arrows) at risk for pathologic fracture. (B) Prophylactic fixation with a statically locked intramedullary nail.

When choosing the type of surgical stabilization for impending fractures, the status of the involved bone, the presence of single or multiple metastases, the site of the bone lesion, and the general condition of the patient, should all be considered.[20] The overall goal of prophylactic surgical treatment is to improve the stability of the bone, preventing the actual occurrence of a pathologic fracture, allowing patients to regain early mobilization and restoring their quality of life as early as possible.[18,21]

1.2 *Pathologic fractures*

Pathologic fractures can develop in any patient when there is a change in the bony architecture and hence a change in the strength of the bone, due to a benign or malignant process.[22–24] Pathologic fractures have been noted to occur in 9–29% of patients with bone metastases.[25] They are most frequently seen in the long bones, with the femur being the most common site involved.[26–28] The signs and symptoms of pathologic fractures include pain at the fracture site, decreased range of motion, deformity and inability to bear weight or ambulate. Patients may also present with point tenderness over the involved site, ecchymosis, extremity shortening, edema, and joint effusion.[26]

The decision on whether to treat pathologic fractures surgically or non-surgically is multifactorial and depends on the type and location of the fracture, the tissue diagnosis and the overall condition of the patient. As previously stated, surgical stabilization should be considered in patients who have fractures through weight-bearing bones and have more than one month to live, and in patients who have upper extremity fractures (non-weight-bearing bones) and have more than three months to live. In some cases, immobilization and radiotherapy can be used as definitive treatment. For example, in patients with myeloma or lymphoma, a non-displaced pathologic fracture on a non-weight-bearing bone may respond well to immobilization and radiotherapy.

Approximately 20% of bone metastases occur in the upper extremity.[2] The primary goal of surgical fixation of pathologic fractures in the upper extremity is to provide pain relief and improve the functional status of the patient. Pathologic fractures involving the scapula and glenoid are generally treated non-surgically, since there are few reconstructive options for lesions in these areas.[2,16] Immobilization of the shoulder area and, depending on the tumor type, radiotherapy, radiofrequency ablation, hormonal therapy and bisphosphonates may provide pain relief, without compromising function.[2,9,13]

Pathologic fractures of the proximal humerus (epiphyseal and/or metaphyseal) are amenable to resection and reconstruction with a proximal humeral prosthesis (Fig. 5). Resection and reconstruction of the proximal humerus can provide local oncologic

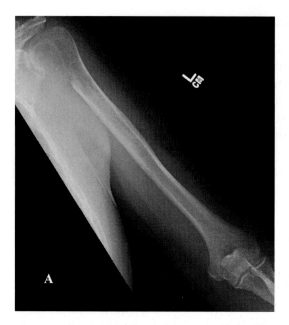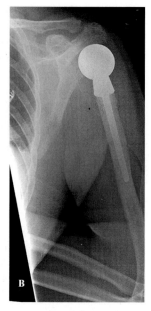

Figure 5. (A) Anteroposterior radiograph of a humerus with a metastatic lytic thyroid cancer lesion (arrow) in the proximal humerus. (B) The proximal humerus was resected and reconstructed with an endoprosthesis.

control and pain relief. However, a full range of motion at the shoulder can be difficult to achieve after such a procedure. On the other hand, the use of a modular prosthesis is particularly beneficial, since it can be converted to a total humeral prosthesis if there is distal progression of the disease.

Humeral shaft pathologic fractures may be treated with plate or intramedullary nail fixation, with or without cementation. Intramedullary nailing, however, is the preferred form of fixation for pathologic fractures involving the humeral diaphysis, since the intramedullary rod spans the entire shaft of the humerus and thus provides excellent stabilization of the entire diaphyseal portion. Curettage and cementation using polymethylmethacrylate (PMMA) of the diaphyseal lesion may provide additional stability and local tumor control. For large, lytic and segmental defects that are amenable to resection, reconstruction with an intercalary metal spacer can be considered. The intercalary spacer not only provides the benefit of spanning the defect but also allows for early return to function.[2,29]

Pathologic fractures involving the distal humeral diaphysis or metadiaphysis are amenable to plating with PMMA augmentation, flexible retrograde nailing with or without cementation, or resection with endoprosthetic reconstruction. Although the use of two perpendicular plates, one placed laterally and the other posteromedially, augmented with PMMA has been shown to result in stronger reconstruction when compared to single plating or flexible nailing,[2] the use of flexible intramedullary nails, with or without PMMA augmentation has several advantages. First, flexible retrograde nails are placed percutaneously under fluoroscopy, thus the surgical exposure is limited small, with little or no manipulation of the radial nerve. Second, flexible retrograde intramedullary nailing stabilizes the entire bone. Third, flexible retrograde nailing maintains the native joint above and below the lesion, which allows for excellent functional recovery. The addition of open curettage and cementation of distal humeral lesions provide stability and local tumor control. Resection and endoprosthetic reconstruction should be reserved for those lesions with large cortical defects affecting the distal humerus not amenable to standard fixation devices.

Metastatic disease below the elbow is rare. If a pathologic fracture occurs in the radius or ulna, the location of the fracture usually dictates what type of fixation is to be used and whether fixation is possible. Treatment options include flexible nailing, plates and screws with PMMA augmentation, resection, and functional bracing.

Although flexible nailing requires limited surgical exposure and provides stabilization of the entire bone, it does not provide rotational control. The addition of curettage and cementations in the surgical treatment not only reconstitutes the bony defect, but also affords rotational control and internal fixation. In contrast to flexible nailing, open reduction with plate and screw fixation can restore the length of the bone and provide adequate rotational control. However, this procedure requires a more extensile approach. If the location precludes stable fixation with the use of standard fixation devices, then functional bracing with adjuvant therapy, such as radiation or radiofrequency ablation, are excellent options for treating forearm fractures. Resection of the bone or creation of a one-bone forearm can be considered if functional reconstruction is not possible.

Metastatic disease in the hand is rare. Resection and functional reconstruction of a pathologic fracture in the hand is often not possible. Therefore, the mainstay of treatment for lesions involving the metacarpal bones and phalanges is intralesional curettage and cementation if there is viable bone stock, versus amputation.[2]

In the lower extremity, a pathologic fracture involving the pelvis and lower extremity has a significant effect on the patient's quality of life. The high physiologic stresses placed on the lower extremity, especially on the hip and proximal femur during activities of daily living, make pain and pathologic fracture more common and non-surgical treatment of impending or completed pathologic fractures more difficult. The goals of palliative treatment (to minimize pain, maintain function and increase mobility) are difficult to achieve in these patients. An untreated lower extremity pathologic fracture in patients will increase morbidity and hasten death, by increasing the need for narcotic medication and requiring bed confinement, thereby increasing the risk for bed sores, pneumonia, urinary tract infection and deep venous thrombosis. Surgery and contemporary reconstructive techniques can result in a high rate of pain control and allow for early mobilization.[19]

Acetabular and proximal femur pathologic fractures can be best treated with surgery, with carefully planned reconstructive procedures. As previously stated, it is important to take into account the patient's overall prognosis and disease status when planning an operative or reconstructive procedure.[19,25] Operative management of periacetabular and proximal femur fractures should provide immediate stabilization, and thus allow early return to weight bearing and independence. Fortunately, improved surgical techniques, advancement in fixation devices, and the supplemental use of polymethyl methacrylate (PMMA), have enabled immediate post-operative weight-bearing and early restoration of function.[18,19,30]

Reconstructive options for the hip area depend on the degree of acetabular dome and medial wall insufficiency. The Harrington classification system[31] and its contemporary adaptation[19] describe specific acetabular anatomic defects and possible reconstruction techniques for each type of defect. Wunder et al.[32] reviewed the results of several published series of reconstruction for acetabular bone metastases. The operative morbidity rate was acceptable, and pain relief with improvement of ambulation was achieved with extensive reconstruction in selected patients.

Femoral head and neck pathologic fractures are best treated with arthroplasty.[19,21,30] Any synchronous metastatic lesions along the femur should be bypassed using a long-stem femoral component. The treatment of pathologic fractures involving the intertrochanteric area depends on the extent of the disease. These fractures can be treated with PMMA to reconstruct the area of bone loss and with internal fixation using a reconstruction-type intramedullary device. However, if bone loss is significant, then resection and reconstruction with a proximal femoral prosthesis may be necessary.

Fixation of subtrochanteric pathologic fracture is often amenable to fixation with an intramedullary nail. Plate fixation in this area has been associated with high failure rates, due to the higher stresses placed on these constructs. PMMA can help re-establish cortical integrity and thus, for cases with substantial bone involvement, its use has been advocated. However, in cases where substantial bone loss precludes the use of a nail fixation device, a long-stem buttressed hemiarthroplasty with PMMA reconstruction of the defective cortex is often necessary. Alternatively, proximal femur replacement may be performed on patients with extensive bone loss. Because of the higher rate of complications associated with the procedure, proximal femoral replacement is reserved for those patients with such extensive bone loss that a long stem traditional or calcar replacement component combined with PMMA reconstruction would likely fail to allow satisfactory pain relief, immediate weight bearing, and early return to function.[19]

Pathologic fractures involving the femoral diaphysis are generally treated with statically locked, large-diameter, intramedullary reconstruction nails. The choice of an open or closed technique depends on the size of the lesion. Closed intramedullary nailing may be performed with small lesions, particularly with radiosensitive tumors. Larger defects may require open curettage with PMMA augmentation. Reconstruction-type intramedullary nails should be used to protect the femoral neck and intertrochanteric area.

Pathologic fractures of the distal femoral metaphysis are often treated with curettage and PMMA reconstruction, followed by a screw-plate fixation device. This form of reconstruction is particularly useful in situations where the fracture is too distal to be fixed by an intramedullary nail. Condylar plates with multiple screw fixations, blade plates and dynamic condylar screws are all viable options in stabilizing pathologic fractures of the distal femur. However, in cases with extensive cortical destruction or epiphyseal and joint involvement, screw and plate fixation is often inadequate. For this reason, extensive involvement of the distal femur and knee joint are best managed with resection and reconstruction.

The surgical approach to pathologic fractures of the tibial diaphysis is similar to that of the femoval diaphysis. As in the femur, a large diameter intramedullary nail is used to treat tibial diaphyseal pathologic fractures. The intramedullary nail should be statically locked to provide a stable fixation around the pathologic fracture site. Again, open or closed nailing depends on the degree of cortical involvement. Significant cortical defects may require curetting and PMMA reinforcement. For smaller lesions involving the tibial diaphysis, closed intramedullary nailing can provide adequate treatment.

Pathologic fractures involving the proximal and distal tibial metaphysis are best treated with plate and screw fixation, with PMMA reinforcement. This form of reconstruction provides adequate bone stability allowing for early mobilization and weight bearing. On the other hand, extensive involvement of the proximal tibia that prevents the use of standard fixation is best treated with resection and reconstruction with endoprosthesis.

Surgical reconstruction of pathologic fractures in the foot can be very difficult. Pathologic fractures in the foot secondary to a metastatic lesion, commonly from a lung or genitourinary carcinoma, usually present in the advanced stage of the disease. Furthermore, surgical reconstruction of the foot rarely allows for immediate weight bearing. These fractures may be best managed non-operatively, with immobilization and radiation therapy; however, if surgery is required, digit or ray amputation may be the best option.

Post-operative treatment of pathologic fractures usually involves aggressive rehabilitation and radiotherapy. Post-operative radiation should include the entire surgical field. For cases of intramedullary nailing, intramedullary reaming and manipulation with implant placement can spread microscopic tumor deposits throughout the canal; therefore, the entire length of the internal fixation and surgical field should be irradiated.

2.   Spinal Cord Compression

Spinal cord compression (SCC) is a well-known oncologic emergency in cancer patients. It is estimated that up to 30% of cancer patients develop spinal metastases, and 10–20% of these patients develop SCC.[33] The incidence of spinal metastasis varies depending on the cancer type: 90% percent of patients with prostate cancer, 75% with breast cancer, 55% with melanoma, 45% with lung cancer, and 30% with renal cell carcinoma develop spinal metastases.[34] Spinal metastases from multiple myeloma and non-Hodgkin lymphoma are also relatively frequent, occurring in 5–10% of cases.[33] The sites of metastases along the spine have also been correlated with tumor histology. Patients with lung or breast cancer often develop thoracic lesions, whereas patients with prostate cancer are more likely to develop lumbar metastatic lesions.[34] The likelihood of symptomatic dural compression from spinal metastases is also related to tumor histology. Symptomatic dural compression from a spinal metastatic lesion occurs in 22% of patients with breast cancer, 20% with kidney cancer, 15% with lung cancer, and 10% with prostate cancer.[34]

Diagnosing SCC resulting from spinal metastases requires a high index of suspicion. Patients with spinal metastases usually present with gradual and progressive onset of back pain. A common error in the evaluation of patients with cancer is to assume that the onset of back pain is related to a degenerative disease, or osteoporosis. Irrespective of the time interval since the diagnosis of the primary cancer, the possibility of a spinal metastasis must be ruled out before attributing the back pain to a degenerative process or osteoporosis.

The type of pain experienced by the patient with metastatic disease is dependent on the tumor mechanism of pain production. The main tumor mechanisms that cause pain are bone infiltration, neural compression, and pathologic fracture. When the tumor infiltrates a vertebra without obvious pathologic fracture or neural impingement, the pain develops gradually and is commonly located in the central spine area. The pain progresses with time and may be aggravated by coughing, bending or sneezing. In addition, pain from bone infiltration is generally non-mechanical (i.e. not related to position), and is usually worse at night.[33,34]

Neural compression may either be central, or peripheral. Pain resulting from a central neural compression in the absence of a myelopathy, usually presents with non-radicular central pain. It may be difficult to differentiate this type of pain from pain symptoms produced by a tumor infiltrating the vertebral body. On the other hand, peripheral neural compression produces radicular symptoms often in a dermatomal distribution. Cervical radiculopathy is easily recognizable because of its distinct dermatomal distribution to the shoulder and upper extremity. Pain in the thoracic area is often described as chest tightness or pain along the ribs. Patients with lumbar involvement usually experience low back pain that radiates down the thigh and leg.[34] Aside from pain, patients may also complain of autonomic dysfunction, such as urinary retention, constipation, or sexual difficulties. Weakness and/or sensory deficits of the extremities may also be apparent upon clinical examination.[33,35]

A pathologic vertebral fracture due to metastatic spinal disease can also produce a significant amount of back pain. Pain from pathologic fractures of the spine usually manifests as sudden onset of centralized pain with or without radiculopathy. Symptoms may be positional, with the patient more comfortable when lying down and a change in position can produce severe pain. Most vertebral pathologic fractures are not associated with any specific incident of trauma. When the tumor affects both the anterior and posterior aspect of the spine, fracture-dislocations and translational or angular displacement can occur. This can produce acute onset of motor and sensory deficits.

New onset back or neck pain in a patient with cancer should alert a physician of the need for prompt evaluation for SCC, even if there are no other signs or symptoms, in order to assess the reason for the pain and to choose the most effective treatment modality. A careful evaluation of the involved vertebral segments is necessary. Diagnostic imaging studies, including plain radiography, MRI, and CT scan should be performed to confirm the diagnosis, evaluate the extent of the disease, and formulate a treatment plan. If the clinical situation permits, standing flexion/extension plain radiographs are obtained, to assess any instability or fracture, as well as the structural integrity of the spine. In cases where little structural involvement is evident, an MRI is used. MRI is the preferred imaging technique as it can assess the presence of vertebral involvement, differentiate tumor form fracture epidural compression, and elements of tumor invasion. On the other hand, CT of the spine may occasionally be necessary, to evaluate the extent of bone destruction.[34] Ideally, the diagnosis of SCC should be established before neurological deficits develop, or when these are still mild and are not causing functional limitation.[33,36]

Early identification of SCC and prompt treatment result in better outcomes.[36-38] As in the treatment of pathological fractures elsewhere in the body, the main objectives of treatment are to relieve pain, preserve or improve neurologic function, and preserve or improve quality of life. Temporary pain relief can be achieved in the emergency room with the use of narcotic or non-narcotic analgesics and corticosteroids. However, care in administering narcotic medications is necessary because these drugs may mask the progression of neurologic deficits.[1,4,35]

Corticosteroids have been noted to improve both the pain and the clinical outcomes of cancer patients with SCC, by decreasing peritumoral edema. Although positive results have been documented, the exact mechanism of action still remains unclear.[33] Dexamethasone is the most commonly used steroid for SCC.[33] Loblaw and Laperriere[39] recommended all patients should receive dexamethasone 10 mg IV X 1 dose, then 4 mg IV every six hours on diagnosis of SCC. Patients should be switched to oral dose when stable and then tapered as tolerated. Earlier studies comparing high-dose steroids with low-dose steroids for SCC showed no significant difference, so lower doses of dexamethasone (10 mg bolus, followed by 4 mg every six hours) are generally used and provide good outcomes and symptom control.[33,34] On the other hand, steroid treatment should be avoided in patients without a histologically established cancer diagnosis. It has been noted that steroids may have a potent oncolytic effect in certain malignancies, such as lymphoma and thymoma.[38]

For years, external-beam radiotherapy has been considered the mainstay in treating spinal metastases. Radiotherapy is generally used as a form of primary treatment for spinal metastases in patients with radiosensitive tumors (e.g. patients with lymphoma, small-cell lung cancer, breast cancer, prostate cancer, multiple myeloma, seminoma, neuroblastoma, or Ewing's sarcoma) who have a contraindication to surgery, short life expectancies, high surgical risk, multilevel or diffuse spinal involvement, subclinical SCC, or total neurologic deficits below the level of compression lasting more than 24–48 hours.[40] Patients who present with SCC without severe myelopathy or radiculopathy may benefit from external-beam radiotherapy for pain control, using fractionation schemes varying from one 800cGy dose to ten 300cGy doses, with similar response rates recorded for the different fractionation schemes.[34] Alternative techniques of delivering radiation, such as intra-operative radiation, three-dimensional conformal radiotherapy, intensity-modulated radiotherapy and stereotactic radiosurgery, are still under investigation. The rationale for these new modalities is to provide higher doses of radiation to the tumor site while minimizing the effects on the surrounding normal tissue.[33]

Although radiotherapy has been the primary therapy for managing spinal metastases, surgery that decompresses the spinal cord followed by reconstruction and immediate stabilization has also been proven effective.[33,34,36,38] Surgery is generally indicated for patients with SCC who present with spinal instability, retropulsed bones or spinal deformities causing spinal compression, radiation-resistant tumors (e.g. sarcoma, non-small-cell lung cancer, colon cancer, renal cell carcinoma, or melanoma), intractable pain non-responsive to medical treatment, an unknown primary tumor (preventing histologic diagnosis), or rapid progression of neurologic deficits. In a meta-analysis performed by Klimo et al.,[40] they found better outcomes in patients who underwent surgery followed by radiotherapy than patients who underwent radiation alone. In that study, patients who underwent surgery plus radiotherapy were two times more likely to regain ambulatory function than patients treated with radiation alone. The overall ambulatory success rates for surgery plus radiation versus radiation alone were 85% and 64%, respectively.

The timing of surgery has a vital role in the neurological outcome of patients presenting with SCC, as a shorter duration of symptoms is associated with a better chance of regaining function or ambulatory ability.[41] Furstenberg *et al.*[42] analyzed the influence of the timing of surgery on the neurological outcome and restoration of mobility in incomplete tetrapelgic and paraplegic SCC patients with metastatic disease. They reported that surgical treatment performed within 48 hours from the onset of neurologic symptoms resulted in better neurological outcomes, when compared to surgery done after 48 hours.

Appropriate patient selection for each treatment modality is important to optimize outcome and avoid unnecessary morbidity. In patients who are good surgical candidates and meet the criteria for surgery, the role of radiation is relegated to an adjuvant to surgical therapy. On the other hand, in patients who are poor surgical candidates or otherwise do not meet the criteria for surgery, radiation should be the primary treatment.[38,40]

3.   Orthopedic Infections

Infections are not uncommon in immunocompromised cancer patients, and a thorough search for a potential source of infection should be performed in febrile neutropenic patients. If the source of infection is identified in the extremity, it should be treated aggressively with local antibiotics, irrigation and debridement, or a combination of these treatment modalities, under adequate anesthesia. In patients suspected of having a joint or extremity infection, it is important to obtain adequate specimens for microbiological studies prior to initiation of empiric antibiotics.

3.1   *Septic arthritis*

Acute septic arthritis is considered to be a medical and surgical emergency.[43] Prompt diagnosis and early treatment are mandatory to prevent debilitating consequences. In cancer patients, immuno-suppression, especially after chemotherapy and organ transplanta-tion, is an important risk factor for the development of septic arthritis. Other common risk factors include history of intravenous drug abuse, hemoglobinopathy, and rheumatoid arthritis.

Septic arthritis may occur through hematogenous spread or direct inoculation by contiguous spread from an infected wound.[44] The pathogenesis of septic arthritis involves bacterial joint inocula-tion followed by infiltration of polymorphonuclear leukocytes (PMNLs). The low oxygen tension of this environment impedes the bactericidal activity of the PMNLs. The bacterial toxins produced result in cell death, and the eventual release of proteolytic enzymes leads to the degradation of the articular cartilage.

Patients with septic arthritis present with pain, swelling, and a decreased range of motion (active and passive) in the affected joint. On physical examination, patients with septic arthritis typically have fever, joint effusion with erythema and increased warmth, and joint guarding (including an antalgic gait when lower extremity joints are involved). The involved joint is often held in slight flexion to decrease intra-articular pressure and minimize pain. However, in the immunocompromised patient population some signs and symptoms such as fever and marked joint guarding may be absent.[1] For this reason, radiographs and blood laboratories must always be performed in all patients suspected to have septic arthritis. Radiography can show joint effusion in the early stages of septic arthritis and joint destruction in the later stages. Laboratory studies often show an elevated white blood cell count, erythrocyte sedimentation rate, and C-reactive protein level.

All suspected septic joints should be aspirated.[45] The synovial fluid specimens should be examined microscopically for the presence of crystals and microorganisms. A synovial fluid analysis demonstrating a white blood cell count greater than 50,000 cells/ml with predominance of PMNs, low glucose levels, and high protein content is indicative of joint sepsis. After adequate synovial fluid and blood culture specimens are obtained, empiric antibiotics can be started.

Empiric antibiotics should be directed towards the most common pathogens encountered in septic arthritis. The most common organisms isolated from a septic joint are *Staphylococcus aureus* and *Streptococcus*.[43–45] However, unusual causes of septic arthritis, such as gram-negative organisms, *Mycobacterium*, and fungi, may also be seen in immunocompromised patients.[1] A change to another antibiotic may be indicated once cultures and sensitivity assays are known.

A trial of needle aspiration using a large-bore needle and saline irrigation may be warranted in some patients with joint sepsis, especially in those patients who are severely immunocompromised, or medically unstable, and are therefore poor surgical candidates.[1] This is especially helpful in smaller joints. The maximum amount of fluid is removed, thereby decompressing the joint and reducing the bacterial load. If the joint is technically difficult to aspirate and in adequately decompressed, or if the patient does not have clinical signs of improvement within 24–48 hours after initial joint decompression, surgical drainage done arthroscopically or through an open technique is indicated.[46–48]

The larger joints, such as the knees, hips and shoulders, often cannot adequately be treated with aspiration. Generally, these joints should be surgically drained. Surgical treatment requires a formal arthrotomy of the involved joint. The capsule should be opened and additional specimens should be collected for microbiological studies. Once adequate specimens are collected, the joint can be thoroughly irrigated.

Once the acute symptoms of septic arthritis have improved, range-of-motion exercises for the involved joint should be initiated. Antibiotics should be continued for four to six weeks. Van der Heijen *et al.*[49] demonstrated the persistence of bacterial DNA three weeks after initiation of antibiotic treatment for septic arthritis, despite sterile cultures being obtained after three days of treatment. After an initial two to four weeks of intravenous antibiotics and once the clinical signs of septic arthritis have resolved, oral antibiotic administration may be appropriate.

3.2   *Necrotizing fasciitis*

Necrotizing fasciitis is an invasive infection characterized by progressive destruction of the skin, subcutaneous fat and fascia. Because fasciitis and cellulitis have similar presenting features, distinguishing between cellulitis and fasciitis is critical, for the treatment and prognosis of these two conditions are dramatically different. Patients with necrotizing fasciitis usually present with fever and tachycardia. As the disease progresses, tachypnea and hypotension may occur. In addition, marked induration, intense pain, excessive tenderness, and crepitus upon palpation of the site are often present. Imaging studies may facilitate diagnosis. Radiography or CT reveals air in the soft tissues, and free air in the subcutaneous tissue and fascial planes is in fact pathognomonic for polymicrobial infection.[1,50]

Most patients with necrotizing fasciitis have polymicrobial infections caused by anaerobic, aerobic, gram-positive, and/or gram-negative organisms. The most common causative organisms, however, are group A streptococci, which have surface receptors and exotoxins that contribute to their virulence.

Necrotizing fasciitis rapidly progresses, often within hours. As the infection spreads along the fascial layers, devascularization of the skin ensues once penetrating vessels thrombose. The skin eventually necroses, forming bullae, and becomes anesthetic in the later stages of the infection. Leukocytosis is apparent in most patients with necrotizing fasciitis, but can be absent in immunocompromised patients.[51,52]

Prompt initiation of treatment is essential. The mortality rate of patients with necrotizing fasciitis has been reported to be between 9% and 26%. Management includes treatment of systemic symptoms, prompt surgical debridement, and broad-spectrum antibiotic coverage, consisting of penicillin, an aminoglycoside, or a third-generation cephalosporin and either clindamycin or metronidazole. Multiple debridements are usually necessary. Serial wound exploration every 12–24 hours ensures the adequacy of debridement, and this aggressive surgical intervention often allows for limb preservation. Amputation, on the other hand, may be necessary in extreme cases to prevent the spread of infection.[50]

3.3. Extremity abscesses

Staphylococci and *streptococci* are the most common causes of extremity abscesses, but gram-negative bacteria and anaerobes can also cause abscesses in immunocompromised patients.[1] In febrile cancer patients, a thorough search for an infection in the extremities should be performed. Peripheral and central venous access sites in the extremities are commonly involved areas, and recrudescence of a partially treated cellulitis or osteomyelitis should also be considered.

Patients with extremity abscesses usually present with fever and pain associated with erythema, fluctuence, and tenderness over the involved site. Needle aspiration can confirm the abscess diagnosis, decompress the abscess, relieve pain and reduce the bacterial load. In a medically stable patient, prompt drainage under aseptic precautions and suitable anesthesia should be performed. Once specimens are collected and submitted for culture and sensitivity assays, antibiotics should be empirically initiated the antibiotic spectrum can be changed once the results of the cultures and sensitivity assays are final. Antibiotics should be continued until all signs and symptoms of infection have subsided.

4.   Acute Compartment Syndrome (ACS)

ACS is a limb-threatening condition considered to be a surgical emergency. ACS is caused by an increase in pressure within a closed fascial plane, thereby compromising the circulation and function of the tissues within that space.[53,54] Because of the unyielding nature of the fascial envelope, an increase in the intra-compartmental pressure (ICP) within the limb reduces the capillary blood inflow, eventually leading to arteriolar compression and muscle and nerve ischemia, progressing to muscle infarction and nerve damage if prompt decompression of the limb compartment is not performed.

Any form trauma to the extremity such as fractures, soft tissue crush injuries, vascular injuries, ischemic reperfusion injuries, prolonged limb compression after tourniquet application, or from malpositioning the patient on a bed or operating table, can cause ACS. A high index of clinical suspicion is required to diagnose this pathologic process, especially in the non-traumatic setting. Clinical suspicion should be high if a patient presents with a swollen and tense limb, and is associated with the 5 P's: pain, paresthesia, paralysis, pallor, and pulselessness.[54–56]

In a conscious and aware patient, a hallmark in the clinical presentation of ACS is pain disproportionate to the size of the injury. This pain, which is usually a result of nerve ischemia, is only partially relieved by the usual analgesics and is different from the acute pain experienced by the patient after the precipitating traumatic injury. An important early clinical finding is pain on passive stretching or compression of the ischemic muscles in the involved limb.[54,56] Another early clinical sign of nerve ischemia is paresthesia, which results from a disordered cell membrane function in the nerves running through the affected compartment.[54] When left untreated, the paresthesia can progress to anesthesia which may eventually lead to paralysis.

Pallor can confirm whether there is a compromised blood supply to the limb, but this can be an unreliable sign. Another clinical sign of compromised circulation is the absence of a pulse resulting from direct arterial injury. When there is a delay in the diagnosis of ACS, the rising ICP reaches approximately the mean arterial pressure level; the main axial arteries are then occluded further compromising the blood supply to the limb.

Laboratory parameters, such as creatinine phosphokinase (CPK) levels, may have a role in identifying ACS in the absence of clinical signs. Seriously elevated CPK levels may indicate severe muscle damage or ischemia. However, CPK levels are not helpful for the early detection of ACS since in the early stages of ACS, muscle damage may not be apparent.

Aside from the clinical observation and the laboratory parameters, it is important to objectively measure the ICP. This is especially true if the clinical signs are unclear, or if the patient's level of consciousness is impaired. It is also important to measure the ICP in all compartments in a limb with suspected ACS. Several techniques for measuring ICP are available and include the simple needle and central venous pressure manometry techniques, wick and slit catheter techniques, side-ported needle technique, fiber-optic transducer technique, near-infrared spectroscopy, and laser Doppler flowmetry.[54,56]

ICP levels ranging from 30 mmHg to 50 mmHg have been proposed as critical levels of pressure, above which the viability of a compartment is compromised. More reliable than the absolute compartment pressures, a delta pressure, (which is a difference between the diastolic pressure and the ICP) of 30 mmHg or less is currently used to diagnose ACS. It has been demonstrated that at a delta pressure cutoff of 30 mmHg, many unnecessary fasciotomies were avoided. Furthermore, patients who had an increased ICP sufficient to cause obvious tissue compromise, as observed at the time of fasciotomy, were correctly identified.[54,56,57]

The goals of treating patients with ACS are to decrease tissue pressure and restore blood flow, thereby minimizing tissue damage and related functional loss. Therefore, once ACS is suspected, all circumferential dressings should be removed, the blood pressure should be normalized, and supplemental oxygen should be given to improve tissue oxygenation. The affected extremity should not be elevated but instead kept at heart level to maintain perfusion in the compartment.

If the clinical signs of ACS are present and/or the delta pressure is below 30 mmHg, an expedient fasciotomy of all relevant compartments should be performed. It is also important to remember that there is a dynamic relationship between the ICP level and the duration of the elevated pressure. The longer the treatment and fasciotomy are delayed, the worse the outcome, with poor results inevitable if treatment is delayed more than 12 hours. Thus, it is necessary to educate caregivers of patients at risk for ACS about early detection of the clinical signs and symptoms. Although fasciotomies may have significantly associated morbidities, a fasciotomy is still preferable to the outcome of a missed ACS.

5. Role of Amputation

An emergency amputation may be indicated in certain oncologic situations, and when indicated, amputation may improve the patient's quality of life and may be curative in some cases.[58] Complications related to tumor fungation, or a pathologic fracture through a bone sarcoma are the most common indications for an emergency amputation in patients with cancer. Tumor fungation in an extremity is unsightly and painful and often renders the extremity useless. An emergency amputation is performed when a secondary bacterial infection leads to sepsis, or when the fungating tumor causes uncontrollable hemorrhaging. The amputation treats the infection or bleeding, provides pain relief, and restores early function.[59]

Amputation is the most common surgery performed for pathologic fractures secondary to a sarcoma. However, recent advances in medical treatment and effective healing responses of pathologic fractures during chemotherapy have encouraged some practitioners to attempt limb-sparing surgery for highly selected patients.[23,24] In some of these patients, a wide excision, combined with chemotherapy, can be curative. However, if limb salvage is not possible, an amputation can improve quality of life by providing pain relief and by promoting early restoration of function.[58,59]

In conclusion, patients with orthopedic oncologic emergencies must be treated individually. The patient's diagnosis and life expectancy, as well as their desires, should be considered before initiating treatment. The goal of palliative treatment is to minimize pain, restore function, and prevent the complications associated with prolonged immobilization. Patients with end stage disease should be treated only when there is reasonable evidence that the treatment will provide palliation of symptoms. Needless suffering can be avoided through judiciously planned, prompt intervention.

References

1. H. H. Manglani, R. A. W. Marco, A. Picciolo and J. H. Healy, Orthopedic emergencies in cancer patients, *Semin. Oncol.* **27**: 299–310 (2000).

2. V. O. Lewis, Surgical management of upper extremity metastatic disease. In: *Orthopaedic Knowledge Updates Musculoskeletal Tumors 2*, ed. H. E. Schwartz (American Academy of Orthopaedic Surgeons, Rosemont IL, 2007), pp. 375–381.

3. B. T. Rougraff, J. S. Kneisl and M. A. Simon, Skeletal metastasis of unknown origin. A prospective study of a diagnostic strategy, *J. Bone Joint Surg. Am.* **75**: 1276–1281 (1993).

4. D. Vanel, J. Bittoun and A. Tardivon, MRI of bone metastases, *Eur. Radiol.* **8**: 1345–1351 (1993).

5. S. Boruban, T. Sancak, Y. Yildiz, and Y. Saglik, Embolization of benign and malignant bone and soft tissue tumors of the extremities, *Diagn. Interv. Radiol.* **13**(3): 164–167 (2007).

6. C. Rossi, S. Ricci, S. Boriani, R. Biagini *et al.*, Percutaneous transcatheter arterial embolization of bone and soft tissue tumors, *Skeletal Radiol.* **19**: 555–560 (1990).

7. M. W. Roscoe, R. J. McBroom, E. St. Louis *et al.*, Preoperative embolization in the treatment of osseous metastases from renal cell carcinoma, *Clin. Orthop. Relat. Res.* **238**: 302–307 (1989).

8. S. Mercadante, Malignant bone pain: Pathophysiology and treatment, *Pain* **69**: 1–18 (1997).

9. F. J. Frassica, D. A. Frassica and F. H. Sim, Management of severe cancer pain: Supportive measures for patients. In: *Surgery for Bone and Soft-Tissue Tumors*, eds. M. L. Simon and D. Springfield (Lippincott-Raven, Philadelphia PA, 1998), p. 628.

10. J. A. M. Bramer, A. A. Abudu, R. J. Grimer, S. R. Carter and R. M. Tillman, Do pathological fractures influence survival and local recurrence rate in bony sarcomas?, *Eur. J. Cancer* **43**: 1941–1955 (2007).

11. H. Mirels, The classic. Metastatic disease in long bones. A proposed scoring system for diagnosing impending pathologic fractures, *Clin. Orthop. Relat. Res.* **415S**: S4–13 (2003).

12. H. Mirels, Metastatic disease in long bones. A proposed scoring system for diagnosing impending pathologic fractures, *Clin. Orthop. Relat. Res.* **249**: 256–264 (1989).

13. C. D. Reich, Advances in the treatment of bone metastases, *Clin. J. Oncol. Nurs.* **7**(6): 641–646 (2003).

14. A. R. Evans, J. Bottros, W. Grant, B. Y. Chen and T. A. Damron, Mirels' rating for humerus lesions is both reproducible and valid, *Clin. Orthop. Relat. Res.* **466**(6): 1279–1284 (2008).

15. K. D. Harrington, Impending pathologic fractures from metastatic malignancy: Evaluation and management, *Instr. Course Lect.* **35**: 357–381 (1986).

16. T. A. Damron, Treatment principles and prediction of impending pathologic fracture. In: *Orthopaedic Knowledge Updates Musculoskeletal Tumors 2*, ed. H.E. Schwartz (American Academy of Orthopaedic Surgeons, Rosemont IL, 2007), pp. 369–374.

17. H. J. Mankin, T. A. Lange and S. S. Spanier, The hazards of biopsy in patients with malignant primary bone and soft tissue tumors, *J. Bone Joint Surg. Am.* **64**: 1121–1127 (1982).

18. F. J. Hornicek, The role of resection and amputation in metastatic disease. In: *Orthopaedic Knowledge Updates Musculoskeletal Tumors 2*,

ed. H. E. Schwartz (American Academy of Orthopaedic Surgeons, Rosemont IL, 2007), pp. 407–416.

19. R. H. Quinn, Surgical management of lower extremity metastatic disease. In: *Orthopaedic Knowledge Updates Musculoskeletal Tumors 2*, H. E. Schwartz (American Academy of Orthopaedic Surgeons, Rosemont IL, 2007), pp. 383–391.

20. J. Manabe, N. Kawaguchi, S. Matsumoto and T. Tanizawa, Surgical treatment of bone metastasis: Indications and outcomes, *Int. J. Clin. Oncol.* **10**: 103–111 (2005).

21. K. L. Weber, R. L. Randall, S. Grossman, and J. Parvizi, Management of lower extremity bone metastasis, *J. Bone Joint Surg. Am.* **88**(4): 11–19 (2006).

22. W. F. Jackson, T. N. Theologis, C. L. Gibbons, S. Mathews and G. Kambouroglou, Early management of pathological fractures in children, *Injury* **38**: 194–200 (2007).

23. S. P. Scully, H. T. Temple, R. J. O'Keefe *et al.*, The surgical treatment of patients with osteosarcoma who sustain a pathologic fracture, *Clin. Orthop. Relat. Res.* **324**: 227–232 (1996).

24. S. P. Scully, M. A. Ghert, D. Zurakowski, R. C. Thompson and M. C. Gebhardt, Pathologic fracture in osteosarcoma: Prognostic importance and treatment implications, *J. Bone Joint Surg. Am.* **84**(4): 49–57 (2002).

25. D. Buggay and K. Jaffe, Metastatic bone tumors of the pelvis and lower extremity, *J. Surg. Orthop. Adv.* **12**(4): 192–199 (2003).

26. W. G. Ward, S. Holsenbeck, F. Dorey, J. Spang and D. Howe, Metastatic disease of the femur: Surgical treatment, *Clin. Orthop. Relat. Res.* **415**: S230–S244 (2003).

27. D. K. Narazaki, C. C. De Neto Alverga, A. M. Baptista, M. T. Caiero and O. P. De Camargo, Prognostic factors in pathologic fractures secondary to metastatic tumors, *Clinics* **612**(4): 313–320 (2006).

28. A. Lipton, Management of bone metastases in breast cancer, *Curr. Treat. Options Oncol.* **6**(2): 161–171 (2005).

29. D. M. Thai, Y. Kitagawa and P. F. Choong, Outcome of surgical management of bony metastases to the humerus and shoulder girdle: A retrospective analysis of 93 patients, *Int. Semin. Surg. Oncol.* **3**: 5 (2006).

30. S. K. Johnson and M. T. Knobf, Surgical interventions for cancer patients with impending or actual acute pathologic fractures, *Orthop. Nurs.* **27**(3): 160–171 (2008).

31. K. D. Harrington, The management of acetabular insufficiency secondary to metastatic malignant disease, *J. Bone Joint Surg. Am.* **63**: 653–664 (1981).

32. J. S. Wunder, P. C. Fergusson, A. M. Griffin, A. Pressman and R. S. Bell, Acetabular metastases: Planning for reconstruction and review of results, *Clin. Orthop. Relat. Res.* **415S**: S187–S197 (2003).

33. M. Penas-Prado and M. E. Loghin, Spinal cord compression in cancer patients: Review of diagnosis and treatment, *Curr. Oncol. Rep.* **10**: 78–85 (2008).

34. A. M. Levine and D. R Desser, Evaluation and treatment of metastasis to the spine. In: *Orthopaedic Knowledge Updates Musculoskeletal Tumors 2*, ed. H. E. Schwartz (American Academy of Orthopaedic Surgeons, Rosemont IL, 2007), pp. 393–406.

35. J. D. Avery and J. A. Avery, Malignant spinal cord compression: A hospice emergency, *Home Healthc. Nurs.* **26**(8): 457–461 (2008).

36. D. Schiff, Spinal cord compression, *Neurol. Clin.* **21**: 67–86 (2003).

37. S. Helweg-Larsen, P. S. Sorensen and S. Kreiner, Prognostic factors in metastatic spinal cord compression: A prospective study using multivariate analysis of variables influencing survival and gait function in 153 patients, *Int. J. Radiat. Oncol. Biol. Phys.* **46**: 1163–1169 (2000).

38. M. H. Bilsky, E. Lis, J. Raizer *et al.*, The diagnosis and treatment of metastatic spinal tumor, *Oncologist* **4**: 459–469 (1999).

39. D. A. Loblaw and N. J. Laperriere, Emergency treatment of malignant extradural spinal cord compression: An evidenced-based guideline, *J. Clin. Oncol.* **16**: 1613–1624 (1998).

40. P. Klimo Jr., C. J. Thompson, J. R. Kestle and M. H. Schmidt, A meta-analysis of surgery versus conventional radiotherapy for the treatment of metastatic spinal epidural disease, *Neuro-oncol.* **7**: 64–76 (2005).

41. K. L. Chaichana, G. F. Woodworth, D. M. Sciubba, M. J. McGirt *et al.*, Predictors of ambulatory function after decompressive surgery for metastatic epidural spinal cord compression, *Neurosurgery* **62**: 683–692 (2008).

42. C. H. Fürstenberg, B. Wiedenhöfer, H. J. Gerner and C. Putz, The effect of early surgical treatment on recovery in patients with metastatic compression of the spinal cord, *J. Bone Joint Surg. Br.* **91**(2): 240–244 (2009).

43. H. K. Kim, B. Alman and N. G. Cole, A shortened course of parenteral antibiotic therapy in the management of acute septic arthritis of the hip, *J. Pediatr. Orthop.* **20**: 44–47 (2000).

44. W. Petty and M. C. Fajgenbaum, Infection of synovial joints. In: *Surgery of the Musculoskeletal System,* ed. E. C. McCollister (Churchill Livingston, New York, 1990), pp. 4399–4427.

45. C. J. Matthews and G. Coakley, Septic arthritis: Current diagnostic and therapeutic algorithm, *Curr. Opin. Rheumatol.* **20**(4): 457–462 (2008).

46. H. Yuan, K. Gong, C. Chen, R. Tang and B. Hwang, Characteristics and outcome of septic arthritis in children, *J. Microbiol. Immunol. Infect.* **39**: 342–347 (2006).

47. I. Jeon, C. Choi and J. Seo, Arthroscopic management of septic arthritis of the shoulder joint, *J. Bone Joint Surg.* **88-A**(8): 1802–1806 (2006).

48. C. Kirchhoff, V. Braunstein, S. Buhmann, T. Oedokoven, W. Mutschler and P. Biberthaler, Stage-dependant management of septic arthritis of the shoulder, *Int. Orthop.,* July 4 [Epub ahead of print] (2008).

49. I. M van der Heijden, B. Wilbrink, A. E. Vije, L. M. Schouls, F. C. Breedveld and P. P. Tak, Detection of bacterial DNA in serial synovial samples obtained during antibiotic treatment from patients with septic arthritis, *Arthritis Rheum.* **42**: 2198–2203 (1999).

50. R. A. Fontes, C. M Oglivie and T. Miclau, Necrotizing soft tissue infections, *J. Am. Acad. Orthop. Surg.* **8**: 151–158 (2000).

51. D. L. Stevens, M. H. Tanner, J. Winship *et al.,* Severe group A streptococcal infections associated with a toxic-like syndrome and scarlet fever toxin A, *N. Engl. J. Med.* **321**: 1–7 (1989).

52. R. G. Ward and M. S. Walsh, Necrotizing fasciitis: 10 Years' Experience in a district general hospital, *Br. J. Surg.* **78**: 488–489 (1991).

53. F. Matsen, R. Winquist and R. Krugmire, Diagnosis and management of compartmental syndromes, *J. Bone Joint Surg. Am.* **62**: 286 (1980).

54. S. Gourgiotis, C. Villias, S. Germanos, A. Foukas and M. P. Ridolfini, Acute limb compartment syndrome: A review, *J. Surg. Educ.* **64**(3): 178–186 (2007).

55. S. Mubarak and A. Hargens, Acute compartment syndromes, *Surg. Clin. North Am.* **63**: 539–565 (1983).

56. W. K. Kostler, P. C. Strohm and N. P. Sudkamp, Acute compartment syndrome of the limb, *Injury* **35**: 1221–1227 (2004).

57. M. M. McQueen and C. M. Court-Brown, Compartment monitoring in tibial fractures. The pressure threshold for decompression, *J. Bone Joint Surg. Br.* **78**: 99–104 (1996).

58. O. Merminsky, Y. Kollender, M. Inbar *et al.*, Palliative major amputation and quality of life in cancer patients, *Acta Oncol.* **36**: 151–157 (1997).
59. J. C. Wittig, J. Bickels, Y. Kollender, K. L. Kellar-Graney, I. Meller and M. M. Malawer, Palliative forequarter amputation for metastatic carcinoma to the shoulder girdle region: Indications, preoperative evaluation, surgical technique, and results, *J. Surg. Oncol.* **77**(2): 105–113 (2001).

24

Recognition, Treatment and Management of Post-cancer Treatment Lymphoedema

Neil Piller

Abstract

About 30% of patients treated for their cancer will develop lymphoedema, most within the first two years of their treatment. Early attention to tissue and limb changes and acknowledging patients' comments about how the limb feels are crucial to control the onset of lymphoedema and/or reduce its severity. Both treatment-related (extent of surgery, radiotherapy and wound management) and patient-related (arm dominance, age, skin condition weight) risk factors need attention. The management of issues such as CCF, and hypertension may help reduce lymph loads, while improving skin care and undertaking physical activity can help improve lymph flow. In order to halt or reverse lymphoedema progression, it is critical to reduce the lymphatic load to below the lymphatic transport capacity. Involvement of a lymphoedema therapist at this stage may help with risk management and be able to provide enhanced lymph flow as part of their treatment.

For patients with lymphoedema, treatment should be targeted and sequenced, beginning with an intensive phase, followed by a maintenance phase. Compression garments and bandaging are still the mainstay of treatment, but compliance issues arise in hot climates. For some patients the main problem is not the size of the affected limb, but how the limb feels, so dealing with subjective issues is equally important. There are many new treatment options available for its treatment and lymphoedema therapists will be aware of those suitable for your patient.

Keywords: Lymphoedema, early and differential diagnosis, treatment options, outcome expectations.

1.   Introduction

In dealing with the lymphatic system, clinicians need to be aware that lymphoedema risk and its outcomes are influenced both by current and past events along the lymphatic drainage pathway. Lymph from the legs, groins, abdominal and thoracic areas, the left arm and the left side of the head normally drain into the left subclavian vein, while that from the right thoracic area, right arm and right side of the head normally drain into the right subclavian vein.

The distant drainage points of the lymphatics into the vascular system suggest that a whole-body assessment approach can often provide answers to difficult questions about sites of potential disruption to lymph flow, and direct and determine treatment options.

While there are many differing opinions and guidelines regarding the definition of lymphoedema and on how to assess its presence and determine treatment, there are some sound international consensus management guidelines with a reasonably strong evidence base. The guidelines include those of the Lymphoedema Framework "Best practice for the management of Lymphoedema"[1] and the International Society for Lymphology consensus for "The diagnosis and treatment of Peripheral Lymphoedema".[2] There are also regional consensus documents, for example from Holland[3] and Italy.[a]

---

[a] Boccado, personal communication (2008).

2.   Lymphoedema

Lymphoedema occurs when the transport capacity of the lymphatic system is reduced (through its malformation (dysplasia), or a surgical/radiotherapeutical intervention), in the presence of a normal lymph load (determined by the amount of fluids and their contents which leave or are removed by the vascular system). A high lymph load, in the presence of a normally functioning lymphatic system leads to the development of oedema, which may suggest problems within the vascular system (hypertension, high CVP, CCF etc), infection or inflammation. If the lymphatic system's transport capacity has been reduced at the same time as there is an increased lymph load, this is has been termed "Safety Valve Failure"[4] which, if detected, needs aggressive management to reduce lymph load to within normal range.

2.1   *Failure of the lymphatic system*

Lymphatic system failure can result in:

- progressive accumulation of extracellular fluids, together with an increasing concentration of cytokines and inflammatory mediators and other components educed tissue oxygenation levels;
- increased distances between the vascular and lymphatic capillaries;
- altered functionality of cells, such as adipocites, macrophages and fibroblasts, leading to changes in cell types, their ratios and products; and/or
- excessive deposition of adipose tissue in the area of slow or poor lymph flow.

While the development of lymphoedema is a continuum, with the rate of progress varying between individuals, it can be divided into two distinct phases. In the first latent, or hidden phase, the subtle changes that may have occurred are noted by patients (but are often missed in a clinical assessment), while in the clinically manifest phase, a distinct circumference and volume difference can be noted. The term 'lymphoedema' is applied to the latter, although there are still significant debates about the criteria used for its diagnosis. Lymphoedema of the extremities is signalled by a swelling of the tissues above the deep fascia, with few if any sub-fascial changes; the presentation is different when lymphoedema involves the groin, abdominal or thoracic areas, where the process affects the deep lymphatic system.

2.2   Development of clinically manifest lymphoedema

While the figures are variable, the literature suggests that on average, most leg and arm lymphoedemas become clinically apparent within the first two years after the triggering intervention. Review of risk factors and reaction to them in this period is crucial if the development of lymphoedema is to be prevented or its severity minimised.

If patients present with no clinically discernible limb swelling (measured by limb circumference differences), but complain that the limb feels different (described as heaviness, tension, or bursting pains), they may be experiencing the latent phase of lymphoedema. Detecting subtle changes, using tools such a Bio-impedance Spectroscopy and initiating an appropriate form of management (Manual Lymphatic Drainage, exercise or activity program) at this stage may save them from developing clinically manifest lymphoedema.

2.3   Types of lymphoedemas

While some causes of lymphoedema are infrequently encountered, awareness of the diversity of aetiological factors is important, as an apparently simple secondary lymphoedema may have several underlying aetiologies, both lymphatic and cardiovascular. While characteristics and appearance may be similar, the rate of progression however depends on the functional status of the lymphatic system.

2.4   Secondary lymphoedema

Secondary lymphoedema appears when the lymphatic transport capacity from a given area is reduced by the surgical and/or radiotherapeutic treatment of cancers. The number of lymph collectors damaged depends on the original number and location of these vessels and on the extent of the surgery.

The ability of the remaining system to handle any fluid load is influenced by post-operative events such as the healing process, the location and direction of the scar, and whether post-operative complications such as seroma or wound infection developed.

Locoregional radiotherapy is likely to damage remaining deep and superficial lymph collectors and the dense network of superficial lymph capillaries. The subsequent fibrosis will also strongly inhibit any regrowth of new lymph capillaries. There is however some evidence that a window of opportunity exists 10–14 days post radiotherapy and surgery, when some interventions may reduce scarring and may assist the regrowth of lymph capillaries in these areas.[4,5] Generally the end point is both a local concentrated build-up of fibre at the surgical site and a more diffuse build-up of fibre in the irradiated area, which can significantly compromise lymphatic transport.

Some research has indicated that at rest and under a normal lymph load, the lymphatic system is working only at about 5–10% of its maximal capacity, which would suggests that a potential 90% destruction or reduction in the lymphatic transport capacity would be needed for even subtle tissue changes to occur; but as lymph loads are rarely normal, this research has yet to be substantiated by good quality scientific investigation.[6]

3.   Other Reasons for a Swollen Limb

Not every swollen arm or leg or part is due to a lymphatic issue, so it is important that the non-lymphatic system issues are dealt with by other experts, as they may increase the risk of developing lymphoedema at a later stage, or worsening its outcome if already present. It is beyond the scope of this chapter to deal in details with other reasons for a swollen limb, which may be due to:

• an increased leakage (from) or poor absorption (into) the vascular system;

- hyper or hypo active thyroid; or
- lipoedema (in the lower limbs).

4.   Incidence and Prevalence of Lymphoedema

Lymphoedema rates are very difficult to determine in the absence of an agreed definition of this condition, and depend on a range of variable measurement strategies to determine its presence. Best estimates sourced from a 2008 review of evidence on secondary lymphoedema indicate that about one in five patients treated for breast cancer will develop lymphoedema. This rate increases with the duration of follow-up, with some studies indicating that some 40–60% will present with the condition six months post-surgery and up to 70–80% at 12 months. However when all rates from all grades of cancer are considered, the incidence figures are estimated at 20%.[7]

Lymphoedema following treatment for gynaecological malignancies in retrospective studies, averaged 18%, ranging from 7% for ovarian cancer to almost 40% for cancer of the vulva.[7] Leg lymphoedema is significantly influenced by other issues, such as lipodystrophy, papillomatous lesions, poor wound healing, ulcers, fistulas and vascular insufficiency, all of which are significant risk factors, irrespective of the nature of the surgical/ radiotherapeutical intervention.

A large-scale study in 1997 indicated an overall lymphoedema incidence of 24% following treatment of breast cancer.[5] In the group receiving modified radical mastectomy without radiation, the incidence was about 19%, while the addition of radiation increased this to almost 29%.[5] An overall incidence rate of about 30% has been quoted by others.[8]

In addition to limb swelling, at least another 30% of patients suffer from problems of heaviness, tension bursting pains, range of movement problems, which impact on patients' daily living activities and on their quality of life.

Lymphoedemas are generally slow to progress (unless an infection is involved) and first develop in the distal ends of the extremity or in the medial upper thigh or upper arm territories, thus making these sites a worthwhile first point of examination, along with the fingers/toes.

5.   Risk Factors for Lymphoedema

These have not all been well established by epidemiological studies and there are yet still many difficulties linking a patient's pre-disposition to actual risk; furthermore, some factors are just difficult to identify. Categorising risk factors into major groups has been suggested and these relate to: 1) cancer treatment, 2) disease status, 3) patient characteristics, and 4) to post-treatment events. The most established risk factors are the extent (level) of nodal clearance in the axilla or groin, with more nodes removed representing a greater risk, and radiotherapy to the root of an extremity.

Known factors that reduce lymphatic transport capacity are:

- surgery and radiotherapy;
- fibrous tissues build-up, as a consequence of the progression of lymphoedema;
- excessive body mass, in the form of excessive amounts of fatty subcutaneous tissues;
- lack of variation in tissue pressures, due to immobility or lack of activity; and
- too much superficial pressure on a small area, especially at the root of an extremity, as might occur with the use of tight underwear or clothes.

Known factors that place an increased load on the lymphatic system include:

- high capillary blood pressures;
- low blood colloidal osmotic pressure;
- injured blood vessels;
- structurally weak capillaries and blood vessels;
- raised central venous pressure;
- increased numbers of active blood capillaries;
- infection;
- sunburn;
- superficial heating of the skin;
- superficial blood capillary dilatation;
- poor quality skin care; and
- not warming down after strenuous exercise.

5.1 Links between lymphatic system function and obesity

Many countries are currently faced with an obesity epidemic and the question often arises as to the relevance of increasing weight gains and the associated epifascial adiposity and its impact not only on the lymphatic load, but also on the ability of the superfical lymphatic collectors to pulsate and carry the load optimally. In 2005 Harvey *et al.* indicated a strong link existed between defects in the lymphatic system and adult onset obesity (albeit in mice).[9] Schneider *et al.* suggested slower lymph flow was also a possible contributing factor.[10]

Keypoint: Reversible risk factors must be identified, eliminated or reduced in order to impact on the risk of developing or progression of lymphoedemas.

---

6. Signs of Impending Lymphoedema and Recognising the Group at Risk

While a patient may complain of feelings of heaviness, tension, bursting etc. in the limb at risk, one of the first signs of a failing lymphatic system is the accumulation of extracellular fluids in the tissues. This may initially be isolated to a single lymphatic territory, but may later involve a whole limb or organ.

When an axillary or groin clearance is undertaken, it is generally the medial territories of the roots of the limbs that show the first changes, although in the case of a groin clearance, the calf territory (which drains into the deeper system via the popliteal nodes) may also be involved.

While most studies indicate that cases of clinically manifest lymphoedema appear within the first two years after treatment,[7] this may occur as far as 20 years later, when the patient may no longer be followed up by their surgeon or radiation oncologist, so unfortunately it is thus often left up to the patient to detect and recognise these early and subtle signs of impending lymphoedema. While patients may know how their limb feels, often due to a lack of information, the condition is diagnosed when the limb becomes swollen, which can often be too late for a favourable outcome.

A specialist and the GP can play an important role in its early recognition and in directing the patient towards the right management or treatment program, as they are most likely to be frequently seeing the patient.

6.1   *Early detection*

For patients at risk of lymphoedema, it is crucial to be able to recognise risk factors (and know how to remove or reduce them), and to detect and respond to the subtle tissue changes detected. Ideally some form of simple measurement of the condition would be beneficial, but due to different forms of measurement, slightly different figures of incidence may be observed.[11,12] Perhaps one of the best means of the early detection of sub-clinical lymphoedema (as well as for the impact of treatment on clinically manifest lymphoedema) is Bio-impedance Spectroscopy (BIS), which has been shown to detect subtle changes in tissue fluids up to ten months earlier than by other means.[13,14]

6.2   *A holistic picture*

For those who have had treatment for lower body cancer, a history of prior abdominal or thoracic trauma, or surgery (especially on the left side), radiotherapy or post-operative wound infections or seroma should be elicited, as they may impact on lymphatic transport capacity. Events such as peritonitis and hernias may also influence lymphatic transport through the abdominal area, as may seemingly less significant events, such as abdominal adiposity, bloating, or chronic constipation. These all can exert external pressure on the lymphatic collectors, slowing lymph flow from the legs and pelvic area. A question about any recurrent infections and an exploration of their possible sources (such as gum disease, other abscesses or skin conditions such as psoriasis, eczema) is also useful.

> **Keypoint:** The swelling may not always be a consequence of a damaged lymphatic system. All aspects of a patient's life-time medical, surgical and familial history should be reviewed.

7.　Measuring and Monitoring Lymphoedema or Its Risk

There are a range of tools and strategies relevant to the early detection of lymphoedema; they are also very useful for monitoring the progress of treatment in the clinically manifest phase of the condition.[15,16] All of the measurements/tests are a reflection of changes to the functional status of the lymphatic system, with the exception of lymphoscintigraphy, which can measure functional changes in the lymphatic system and can often provide a clear indication of future risk of lymphoedema development and of dysfunctional (and functional) lymphatic collector pathways.[17]

7.1　Lymphoscintigraphy

This can detect a reduced lymphatic transport capacity. After the radio-opaque tracer has been administered, the patient should be encouraged to undertake mild exercise to help stimulate uptake and passage of the tracer along the lymph collectors. Rapidity of the tracer's arrival at the axilla or groin and the counts in the region of interest are the best indicators of functional status. Both the quantitative and qualitative aspects of lymphoscintigraphy can provide useful information — especially with respect to targeting and directing treatment in cases which have not responded well to prior treatment. While there are no specific standards for this, there are a range of protocols to ensure good diagnostic outcomes from its use.[17]

Lymphoscintigraphy is also useful in determining lymph transport before surgery in high-risk cases and may be able to indicate areas that need to be protected during the treatment of the patient's cancer.

7.2　Bio-impedance spectroscopy (BIS)

This tool is emerging as a simple and easy strategy for the early detection of subtle changes in extracellular fluids that indicate a failing lymphatic system and some reports have indicated that it can detect subtle changes in the fluids of the epifascial tissues up to ten months prior to other techniques.[13] BIS involves the passing of a very slight electrical current through the tissues and recording the tissues' resistance to its passage.

The technique has been validated as an early detection tool for post-mastectomy lymphoedemas and is able to accurately indicate changes in the extra-cellular/intra cellular fluid ratios in affected areas as small as a forearm or a breast.[18] Bio-impedance instruments range in size from the small hand-held units (Impedimed, Queensland, Australia) suitable for small clinics and individual patients, to the larger stand-on whole-body units (Bio-Space, Seoul, Korea). Absolute and relative changes in extracellular fluids can be detected, but the most salient measurements are the differences between pre- and post-treatment fluid ratios, and those between the affected (or at risk limb) and the contralateral normal one.

7.3   Tonometry

The fibres that form in the superficial tissues can be detected by a technique called tonometry as well as by MRI and ultrasound (as described above).

With tonometry, a weighted plunger is placed on the midpoints (most often) of the lymphatic territories and the resistance to compression is measured, with a higher resistance indicating an increased fibrotic induration of the tissues.

It is only possible to compare indicated resistances to compression with contralateral limb territories, or to measure and record changes over time. Tonometry is useful to detect the build-up of fibrous tissue, not only as a consequence of the progression of the lymphoedema, but also from the surgical and radiotherapeutical scarring.[15,18]

If a tonometer is unavailable, an indication of the extent of fibrotic induration can be gained by a gentle pinch and roll test. The skin is held and rolled between the thumb and forefinger and the rolling resistance is felt and the separation measured. Again, comparison with the contralateral limb territory is essential to detect differences. At the base of the toes/fingers, the inability to pick up a fold of skin is used at a means of detecting superficial lymphatic system changes and is reflective of stage 2 or worse lymphoedema. This sign, called a 'Stemmer sign', is a very simple and widely used indicator of lymphoedema.

8.   Treatment and Management Options

Generally with lymphoedema, treatment is what the health professional or lymphoedema therapist will undertake, while management is what the patient, or their partner or carer will be able to do. In broad terms, treatment will be directed at improving lymph transport/flow, while management will be directed at reducing lymph load. Recent systematic reviews of the range of common conservative therapies for lymphoedema are also a very useful tool to help in the determination of treatments and their options.[7,19]

8.1   *Major aims of treatment*

8.1.1   *Reducing lymph load*

The major strategies here revolve around improving the structural integrity of the vascular system, reducing hypertension, reducing elevated venous pressures, improving the skin as a barrier, encouraging better wound care and rapidly responding to infection, reducing body mass and the use of support garments.

8.1.2   *Increasing lymph transport*

These strategies can be divided into lymphostimulatory (aimed at increasing lymph flow) and lymphogenic (aimed at encouraging the formation and development of new lymph vessels).

Strategies that increase lymph flow are aimed at increasing the entry of extracellular fluids and their contents (inflammatory mediators, cytokines etc) into the lymph capillaries and improving the flow of lymph along the larger lymph collectors.

The very simple way to improve lymph flow is to ensure that there are optimal pressure variations within the superficial (epifascial) tissues, the site of the lymphoedema. There are many ways of facilitating this, ranging from simple movement, to exercise programs through massage, vibratory treatments and electrical stimulation of the musculature of the body and lymphatics.[16,18] Generally, treatments will involve one of more of the following modalities.

8.2 Types of treatment for lymphoedema

8.2.1 Antibiotic therapy

In view of compromised specific and non-specific defence systems in patients whose nodes have been removed and who have lymphoedema and the rather high frequency of occurrence of cellulitis in lymphoedema patients,[20,21] either prophylactic antibiotics, or at very least a rapid response to a suspected infection, is essential.

8.2.2 Exercise machines

It is reasonably clear that any variation in tissue pressures, particularly in the epifascial compartment will help in the loading of the lymphatic system as well as in lymph transport. There are a range of exercise/activity promoting machines/aids which may help facilitate these actions and this help reduce a lymphoedematous limb, some of which have been evaluated more rigorously than others.[22]

8.2.3 Aromatherapy

Lymphatic drainage massage combined with aromatherapy may have a benefit. Essential oils, such as lavender have been shown to have antibacterial properties, as has tea-tree oil. A range of small trials are in progress in this area, but additional research needs to be undertaken.

8.2.4 Benzopyrones

Experimental studies have shown that the use of benzopyrones (such as Paroven and Lymphodran) is associated with the stimulation of macrophages and the destruction of bacteria, as well as improvement in lymphatic system function. Paroven seems to be particularly useful when there are symptoms of pain, heaviness, aches, etc, associated with underlying vascular factors. However, poor or adverse outcomes from some benzopyrone (Loedema) treatment have also been documented and thought to be related to poor CYP2A enzymatic activity,[23] and the current evidence suggests that the effectiveness of these and related groups in lymphoedema treatment is limited and needs further high quality scientific investigation.[23,24]

8.2.5 Compression bandaging

Compression using low-stretch/inelastic bandages slows fluid entering the tissues and can maintain any previous reduction in swelling.[25] Bandages are applied after lymphatic drainage massage and worn overnight for five to ten days. The use of the correct pressure and pressure gradients are essential, so bandaging must be done by a trained professional, although partners of patients can be taught the technique. The greatest danger is too much pressure or a tourniquet effect on an area of the limb. Some work indicates that it is compression which achieves the best outcomes for lymphoedema patients.[4]

8.2.6 Compression garments

Reduced swelling can be maintained by using a compression garment and repeat sessions may be necessary at six to 12-month intervals if the limb cannot be well controlled by other techniques. Selecting the correct compression is crucial for good control and care must be taken to avoid a tourniquet effect on the limb. Standards[26] and templates for best practice exist[27] and can help decide the best strategy.

Garments come in made-to-measure and off-the-shelf forms and it is deemed wise to have a spare garment. They may last from three to six months depending on use, the patient's skin and use of creams. Garments seem to work better with a mild exercise regimen, and a good compression garment can be beneficial if worn on a long air flight, but individual circumstances can greatly determine outcomes. A qualified lymphoedema therapist can be very effective in providing advice and treatment, so referrals and follow-ups can significantly improve results.

8.2.7　Compression pumps

A large range of devices that supply a sequential external compression force or wave, with between one and 12 or more chambers are available. Their aim is to vary the external pressure, helping fluids move into and along the lymph collectors. Forcing fluids into the area of the groin if lymphatics are incompetent and if the fluids are not first cleared by lymphatic massage may be a problem, but views regarding compression pumps, their roles and their effectiveness are very polarised.[4,5,28]

8.2.8　Diet

Diets rich in long-chain fatty acids or triglycerides impose a higher load on the lymph vessels in the abdominal area, which may slow lymph flow from the lower limbs and, in cases of a compromised lymphatic system, may exacerbate lymph clearance. Retrograde flow of this lymph into the vessels draining the reproductive organs (the lymphatic territory of the medial thighs) is possible, sometimes culminating in chyle-filled papillomatous lesions or tags, which leak the fatty lymph. Additional subcutaneous fatty tissues place a greater load on the lymphatic system, and the pressure of these tissues on the lymph collectors may reduce their transport ability.

8.2.9　Diuretics

Most of the lymphology literature indicates that diuretics are not beneficial in the treatment of lymphoedema per se, but they have acknowledged benefit if there is an associated oedema or in the case of rapid-onset malignant lymphoedema.[4] Rapid withdrawal of diuretics in lymphoedema patients who have been wrongly prescribed them is not recommended.

8.2.10　Elevation

For early stage (pitting) lymphoedemas, the value and simplicity of elevation should not be underestimated. Elevation can facilitate movement of fluid from a limb along the functioning lymph vessels and it works best when combined with deeper inspirations and gentle contraction of the muscles.[29] This variation will help the additional extracellular fluids move into the lymphatics and along them and it is estimated that an early stage lymphoedema may improve by 5–8% with elevation.

8.2.11 *Exercise*

In their review of the literature, Moseley and Piller[18] highlighted the importance of different forms of exercise for patient at risk of or with lymphoedema. While the lymphatics pulsate normally about six to ten times per minute, lymph flow is enhanced if the skeletal muscles are contracted and relaxed intermittently. This moves the fluid from the interstitium into the initial lymphatics and then to the collecting ones, where the inherent pulsing carries the lymph towards the nodes. Recent reviews have shown significant benefits of exercise not for cancer survival and management of its sequelae,[30] but also for managing lymphoedemas.[19]

8.2.12 *Hydrotherapy*

The external water pressure in hydrotherapy supports the limb and has a squeezing effect, which supplements the muscle action. There are many programs across the world, with some such as the Encore program widely run through the YWCA targeting women with breast cancer who have arm problems. Many public pools and gyms have mild exercise and limb mobility programs and any water-based exercise seems to have benefits, as long as there are warm up and warm down procedures and if the water temperature is not too high.[18]

8.2.13 *Laser treatments*

There is an increasing recognition of the potential role of laser therapy, but only a good few clinical trials of low-level laser therapy for the management of lymphoedema have been reported[31] and to date only one double blinded crossover trial of low level laser reported.[32,33] Experimental evidence is widespread and generally indicates a systemic photo stimulatory effect, as well as specific local effect on cells such as macrophages and fibroblasts. The wavelength, duration and timing of treatment seem to be important for best outcomes. Laser may also help lymph vessels grow and it has been shown to make them pump faster or more effectively when their function has been compromised. Clinical evidence shows removal of fluid and a softening of the tissues.[31,33] To date, no adverse effects of laser have been reported in the scientific literature.

8.2.14 *Lymphatic massage*

There are many forms of massage and many different schools of thought on what works best for lymphoedema patients. For many of these forms the evidence is anecdotal, although or recent some high quality clinical trials have been conducted,[34] as well as quantitative evaluations of the impact of treatments on individuals.[35] A recent review of the range of physical therapies and of their effectiveness is useful to determine which might be most appropriate,[36] although the availability of a trained therapist is crucial. Irrespective of the technique used, the principles of lymphatic drainage are based around four main areas: improve the uptake of excessive extracellular fluids and its contents into the lymphatic capillaries, facilitate flow of this fluid along lymph collectors, help vary tissue pressures so these event outcomes are optimised, and to open anastomoses and bypass blocked areas of the lymphatic system.[6,28] Lymphatic drainage massage is gentle and always involves the movement of fluid from the more distal sites to previously emptied proximal sites and is usually combined with inelastic bandaging[37] and fitted support garments.

8.2.15 *Massage pads and massage devices*

A range of massage devices are available for home use, but only a few have been clinically trialled, so its often a difficult decision to advise patients with lymphoedema or at risk of it about which or what might be best for them. Generally speaking, any form of vibration (as long as not of a high frequency) can be beneficial for lymphatic drainage. As with massage (a slow form of vibration), massage pads or units change the tissue pressures, helping to load excessive fluids and their contents into the lymphatics and then move along them, to be cleared hopefully into the exit points of the lymphatic system into the blood vascular system. The selection and recommendations for use of the above aids is best managed by a qualified lymphoedema therapist.

8.2.16 *Skin care*

Generally, patients with a compromised lymphatic function have dry, scaly skin; this seems to be related to poor lymphatic and perhaps altered subcutaneous vascular inflow and outflow. Due to a slowed lymphatic function and due to the removal of lymph-nodes at the root of extremities, those limbs are at higher risk of infection should the superficial barrier of the skin be breached.[38] The major reasons for this higher risk are reduced activity and responsiveness of the mononuclear phagocytic system, and slower responses to the mounting of a specific response to the invading bacteria or its products. Protecting the integrity of the skin as a superficial barrier is thus paramount, since its breaching by bacteria will mean a higher risk of cellulitis, which once present can be hard to control, even with intravenous antibiotic administration.

8.2.17 *T'ai Chi and Qi Gong*

These mild forms of exercise are ideally suited to older people. They are particularly beneficial for those with upper limb problems, for which there is some reasonable evidence of effectiveness.[19,29] The exercises facilitate a change in muscle pressure, believed to help the extracellular fluids enter the initial lymphatics and help the lymph move along the collectors.

The link with respiration is important, because the negative intra-thoracic pressure helps establish a pressure gradient between the extremities and the larger thoracic vessels; one clinical trial has shown this to be effective in patients with post-mastectomy lymphoedemas.

8.2.18 *Other treatments*

There are many other conservative treatments (such as magnetic therapies, ultrasound, microwaves, vibration, autologous lymphocyte injection, electrical stimulation of lymphatics[39] and therapist controlled tissue massage units,[40] associated with a range of levels of evidence for their efficacy. There is also a range of surgical techniques, including microsurgical correction, the removal of lymphoedematous tissues by excisional operations, and liposuction (the latter is gaining strong acceptance when conservative therapies fail).[41]

9. Where to Refer Patients who have or are at Risk of Lymphoedema

This varies from area to area, but most capitals and larger cities have a lymphoedema clinic or centre associated with the major teaching hospitals or private health care systems. There are also many physiotherapists, nurses, occupational and massage therapists, as well as other health professionals who are trained in manual lymphatic drainage, complex physical therapy or other courses. Breast care nurses are becoming more informed about lymphoedemas — particularly the hitherto underestimated breast lymphoedema — and are a good resource. The various lymphatic drainage massage schools, such as Dr Vodder, Foeldi, Norton, Close, Casley-Smith, Leduc and other groups, have web sites from which trained professionals can be selected.

10. Summary

Irrespective of whether the patient is at risk of lymphoedema or has already developed it:

- acknowledge factors such as hypertension, vascular fragility, infection, body mass that may put an unnecessary load on the lymphatic system;
- deal with factors that may reduce lymph outflow, but are not immediately associated with the lymphatic dysfunction, i.e. constrictive clothes, underwear, immobility, high body mass;

- respond to the detection of any fibrotic tissues associated with the surgical wound, the area of radiotherapy or the general induration of the lymphatic system, and consider recommending low-level laser or frictional massage or even surgical excision;
- suggest strategies to improve lymphatic transport, e.g. lymphatic massage, mild exercise, respiratory movements;
- encourage patient and partner (or carer) involvement in the maintenance program, i.e. self-massage, skin care, wound management, exercise and mobility programs, fitting a sleeve, and using home-based aids;
- involve the patient and their partner (or carer) in limb monitoring;
- review as necessary, usually at about six to 12-monthly intervals; and
- find a qualified lymphoedema therapist to achieve a good outcome for you're your patient.

References

1. Lymphoedema Framework, *Best Practice for the Management of Lymphoedema*, International Consensus, London MEP Ltd. (2006).
2. M. Bernas *et al.*, The diagnosis and treatment of peripheral lymphoedema, *Lymphology* **41**: 1–5 (2008).
3. R. Damstra and C. Kaandorp, Multi-disciplinary guidelines for early diagnosis and management: Lymphoedema, *J. Lymphoedema* **2**(1): 57–65 (2007).
4. M. Foeldi, E. Foeldi and S. Kubik, eds., *Textbook of Lymphology for Physicians and Lymphoedema Therapists* (Urban and Fisher Munich, 2003).
5. H. Schunemann and N. Willich, Lymphoedema nach Mammakarzinom, Eine Studie uber 5868 falle Dtsche med Wschr **122**, 536–541 (1997), referred to in H. Weissleder and C. Schuchardt, eds., *Lymphoedema, Diagnosis and Therapy*, 4th ed. (Viavital Verlag GmbH Essen, Germany, 2008).
6. S. Modi, A. W. Stanton, W. E. Svenson, A. M. Peters, P. Mortimer and J. R. Levick, Human lymphatic pumping measured in healthy and lymphoedematous arms by lymphatic congestion lymphoscintigraphy, *J. Physiol.* **583**(1): 271–285 (2007).
7. S. Hayes, Review of research evidence on secondary lymphoedema: Incidence, prevention, risk factors and treatment, NBOCC, Surry Hills NSW, Australia, March 2008 Centre report.

8. P. Franks, C. J. Moffatt, D. Doherty, A. Williams, E. Jeffs and P. Mortimer, Assessment of health related quality of life in patients with lymphoedema of the lower limb, *Wound Repair Regen.* **14**: 110–118 (2005).

9. N. L. Harvey, S. Srinivasan, M. E. Dillard *et al.,* Lymphatic vascular defects promoted by Prox1 haploinsufficieiency cause adult onset obesity, *Nature Genet.* **37**(10): 1072–1081 (2005).

10. M. Schneider, E. Conway and P. Carmeliet, Lymph makes you fat, *Nature Genet.* **37**(10): 1023–1024 (2005).

11. J. M. Armer, M. E. Radina, D. Prock and S. D. Culbertson, Predicting breast cancer-related lymphoedema using self report symptoms, *Nurs. Res.* **52**: 370–379 (2003).

12. S. Hayes, M. Janda, B. Cornish, D. Battistutta and B. Newman, Lymphoedema secondary to breast cancer: How choice of measure influences diagnosis, prevalence and identifiable risk factors, *Lymphology* **41**(1): 18–28 (2008).

13. S. Rockson, Bio-impedance analysis in lymphoedema diagnosis and management, *J. Lymphoedema* **2**(1): 44–49 (2007).

14. L. Ward, Bio-electrical impedance analysis: Proven utility in lymphoedema risk assessment and therapeutic monitoring lymphatic, *Res. Boil.* **4**(1): 51–56 (2006).

15. N. B. Piller, To measure or not to measure? What and when is the question, *J. Lymphoedema* **2**(2): 39–47 (2007).

16. N. B. Piller, Lymphoedema in the new millennium, *J. Lymphoedema* **1**(1): 60–65 (2006).

17. V. Keeley, The use of lymphoscintigraphy in the management of chronic oedema, *J. Lymphoedema* **1**(1): 42–57 (2006).

18. A. L. Moseley and N. B. Piller, Reliability of bio-impedance spectroscopy and tonometry after breast conserving cancer treatment, *Lymphatic Res. Biol.* **6**(2): 85–87 (2008).

19. A. L. Moseley and N. B. Piller, Exercise for limb lymphoedema: Evidence that it is beneficial, *J. Lymphoedema* **3**(1): 51–56 (2008).

20. P. Mortimer, Lymphoedema. In: *Oxford Textbook of Medicine*, eds. D. A. Warrell, T. M. Cox and J. D. Firth (Open University, Oxford, 2003), pp. 1202–1208.

21. C. Badger, K. Seers, N. Preston and P. Mortimer, Anti-biotics/anti-inflammatories for reducing acute inflammatory episodes in lymphoedema of the limbs, *Cochrane Database Syst. Rev.* (**2**): CD003143 (2004).

22. N. B. Piller and A. L. Mosley, A new patient focused home based therapy for people with chronic secondary leg lymphoedema, *Lymphology* **37**(2): 53–61 (2004).

23. N. Farinola and N. B. Piller, CYP2A6 polymorphism: Is there a role for pharmacodynamics in preventing coumarin induced hepatotoxicity? *Pharmacogenomics* **8**(2): 151–158 (2007).

24. C. Badger, N. Preston, K. Seers and P. Mortimer, Benzopyrones for reducing and controlling lymphoedema of the limbs, *Cochrane Database Syst. Rev.* (**2**): CD003140 (2004).

25. H. Partsch, Assessing the effectiveness of multilayer inelastic bandaging, *J. Lymphoedema* **2**(2): 55–61 (2007).

26. H. Partsche, M. Clark, Bassez *et al.*, Measurement of lower leg compression *in vivo*. Recommendations for the performance of measurements of interface pressure and stiffness. A consensus statement, *Dermatol. Surg.* **32**: 229–238 (2006).

27. The Lymphoedema Framework, *Template for Practice: Compression Hosiery in Lymphoedema* (London, MEP, 2006).

28. J. R. Casley-Smith and J. R. Casley-Smith, *Modern Treatment of Lymphoedema*, 5th ed. (Lymphoedema Association of Australia, Adelaide, 1997).

29. A. L. Moseley, N. B. Piller and C. Carati, The effect of gentle arm exercise and deep breathing on secondary arm lymphoedema, *Lymphology* **38**(3): 136–146 (2005).

30. S. Hayes and B. Newman, Exercise in cancer recovery. An overview of the evidence, *Cancer Forum* **31**: 13–17 (2006).

31. N. B. Piller and A. Thelander, Treatment of chronic post mastectomy lymphoedema with low level laser. A 2.5 year follow-up, *Lymphology* **31**(2): 74–86 (1998).

32. C. Carati, B. Gannon and N. B. Piller, Low level laser as a treatment option for post mastectomy lymphoedema, *Am. J. Oncol. Rev.* **3**(5): 255–260 (2004).

33. C. Carati, S. Anderson, B. Gannon *et al.*, Treatment of post mastectomy lymphoedema with low level laser. A double blind placebo controlled trial, *Cancer* **98**: 1114–1122 (2003).

34. K. Johansson and N. B. Piller, Weight bearing exercise and its impact on arm lymphoedema, *J. Lymphoedema* **2**(1): 15–22 (2007).

35. R. Harris and N. B. Piller, The effectiveness of manual lymphatic drainage on patients with primary and secondary lymphoedema

using objective measurement tools, *J. Bodyw. Mov. Ther.* **7**(4): 213–221 (2003).

36. C. Badger, N. Preston, K. Seers and P. Mortimer, Physical therapies for reducing and controlling lymphoedema of the limbs, *Cochrane Database Syst. Rev.* (**4**): CD003141 (2004).

37. H. Partsch and M. Junger, Evidence for the use of compression hosiery in lymphoedema. In: *The Lymphoedema Framework: Template for Practice: Compression Hosiery for Lymphoedema* (London MEP, 2006), pp. 5–9.

38. UK Dermatology Clinical Trials PATCH study group, Prophylactic antibiotics for the prevention of cellulitis, *J. Lymphoedema* **2**(1): 34–37 (2007).

39. N. B. Piller J. Douglass, B. Heidenreich, C. Mundy and A. Moseley, Placebo controlled trial of mild electrical lymphatic stimulation supplemented with compression garments for chronic secondary leg lymphoedema, *J. Lymphoedema* **4**(2), in press (2009).

40. A. L. Moseley and N. B. Piller, A comparison of the effectiveness of MLD and LPG techniques, *J. Lymphoedema* **2**(2): 30–38 (2007).

41. H. Brorson, K. Ohlin and B. Svensson, The facts about liposuction as a treatment for lymphoedema, *J. Lymphoedema* **3**(1): 38–47 (2008).

25

Diagnostic and Management Challenges Following Radical Prostatectomy

Manish I. Patel

Abstract

Diagnostic and management challenges after radical prostatectomy pertain to both cancer recurrence and management of complications. The risk of cancer recurrence after radical prostatectomy can be estimated using nomograms based on validated prognostic factors. Follow-up can then be tailored to a patient's risk. The diagnosis of recurrence after radical prostatectomy is made when the PSA is greater than 0.2ng/ml. After recurrence, the great dilemma is to determine whether the recurrence is localised or systemic. This can be determined by a variety of imaging modalities and examination of prostatectomy pathologic characteristics and PSA kinetics. Management of a recurrence can be expectant, or using salvage radiotherapy, or androgen ablation therapy, depending on the likelihood of localised disease, patient health and expectations.

Management of complications of radical prostatectomy can be difficult. The risk of incontinence is determined by patient age, ability to perform a nerve-sparing operation, likelihood of developing anastomotic contracture and surgical experience. Management of post-operative incontinence focuses primarily on pelvic floor exercises. Surgical avenues include injection with periurethral bulking agents, slings and artificial sphincter placement. Erectile dysfunction after radical prostatectomy is also common and depends on pre-surgery erectile function, degree of nerve sparing and surgeon's experience. Following surgery, early penile rehabilitation with intra-cavernosal injections and PDE5 inhibitors have been shown to improve the return of erectile function.

Keywords: Prostate cancer, radical prostatectomy, recurrence, diagnosis, complications, erectile dysfunction, incontinence.

1. Diagnosis and Management of Cancer Recurrence After Radical Prostatectomy

Approximately 40% of men diagnosed with prostate cancer in the United States will undergo radical prostatectomy.[1] Of these, 15% to 46% will manifest an asymptomatic PSA rise post-operatively, suggesting recurrence of the cancer (biochemical recurrence).[2] This chapter reviews the prognostication, definition, investigation and management of a recurrence of prostate cancer. The second part of this chapter reviews common complications occurring during or after radical prostatectomy, their risks and management.

Radical prostatectomy can be performed using an open retropubic approach, a perineal approach, a laparoscopic or a robot assisted laparoscopic approach. Interestingly, the management of recurrence and management of complications is the same irrespective of the type of radical prostatectomy performed.

1.1 *Prognostication and estimation of the risk of recurrence following radical prostatectomy*

Following radical prostatectomy, the ability to predict a risk of recurrence for a particular patient is of vital importance as this will serve to counsel the patient, determine follow-up regimens, and inform the decisions to offer adjuvant therapy or enrolment into a clinical trial. The most common methods for predicting risk of recurrence is by placing the patient into a risk category based on a number of variables known to increase recurrence risk. An alternative method is using a nomogram with algorithms incorporating

Table 1. Prognostic variables associated with recurrence after radical prostatectomy.

Factor
Gleason score in pathological specimen
Pathologic stage
Pre-surgery PSA
Seminal vesical invasion
Lymph node invasion

Table 2. Models for the prediction of biochemical recurrence after radical prostatectomy.

Reference	Year	Prediction instrument	Prediction variables
Kattan et al.[3]	1999	Nomogram	PSA, Gleason score, ECE, SM, SVI, LNI
Partin et al.[46]	1995	Risk catagorisation	PSA, Gleason score, ECE
D'Amico et al.[47]	1998	Probability graph	PSA, Stage, Gleason score, SM
Blute et al.[48]	2001	Risk catagorisation	Adjuvant therapy, Gleason score, PSA, SVI, SM
Moul et al.[49]	2001	Risk catagorisation	PSA, race, stage, Gleason score
Freedland et al.[50]	2004	Risk catagorisation	Gleason score, % positive cores, PSA

ECE: Extra capsular extension, SM: surgical margin, SVI: seminal vesical involvement, LNI: lymph node invasion.

multiple variables to calculate a probability of achieving a particular end point such as biochemical recurrence. Both methods however use similar prognostic variables which increase risk of recurrence. These are outlined in Table 1.

There are at least 16 models for predicting the likelihood of biochemical recurrence after radical prostatectomy. Some of the commonly used prediction tools are given in Table 2. The most widely used is the Kattan nomogram,[3] which is available online (http://www.mskcc.org/mskcc/html/10088.cfm) or on PDA.

This useful application will give a patient the likelihood of freedom from progression for two, five, seven and ten years.

1.2   Follow-up strategies following radical prostatectomy

The percentage of men with biochemical recurrence after radical prostatectomy varies with different series but overall is approximately 30–40% at five years.[4,5] The risk of relapse after five years is greatly reduced, but not insignificant,[6] suggesting follow-up should be continued for a longer time. Follow-up is important after radical prostatectomy as salvage therapies are available and because of a number of non-cancer related complications, which will be discussed later in this chapter.

Follow-up entails regular visits, where a thorough history related to cancer recurrence and complications of radical prostatectomy should be taken. Physical examination also includes a rectal exam, as rarely a palpable tumour may be the first sign of recurrence. The follow-up should also include a PSA test. The measurement of PSA is the cornerstone of follow-up after radical prostatectomy. PSA recurrence almost always precedes clinical recurrence, in many cases by many years; it is however still possible to get a recurrence without a PSA rise.[7,8]

The schedule of post-prostatectomy follow-up has not been well studied and there is no consensus on the correct timings. A common schedule used by many urologists is three-monthly visits for the first year, six-monthly for the next four years and then yearly after that. Men at low risk for recurrence could have six-monthly visits for the first year as well.

1.3   Making the diagnosis of cancer recurrence after radical prostatectomy

1.3.1   Definition of biochemical recurrence

There has been considerable debate as to what level of PSA constitutes a true biochemical failure. Most urologists will use a cut-off value ranging from 0.2 to 0.5ng/ml.[9,10] At values below these cut-offs, detectable PSA has a reduced likelihood of continuing to rise (consistent with disease progression). For example, a post-operative PSA between 0.11 to 0.2ng/ml has only a 64% likelihood of rising further within a year.[10] The half-life of PSA in the serum is 3.15 days,[11] so serum PSA should fall to undetectable levels by 30 days post-surgery. The first PSA level should not be taken prior to this. If the first PSA determination post-operatively is greater than 0.4ng/ml, the presence of systemic disease is quite possible. In rare cases, the PSA after prostatectomy will fail to reach undetectable levels, but remains *stable* at a level below 0.4ng/ml. It is quite possible that this PSA is not due to cancer recurrence, but from retained benign prostate tissue.[12]

Ultrasensitive PSA assays are capable of detection thresholds of 0.001 to 0.01ng/ml. They are not recommended for routine post-operative surveillance as they are yet of unproven value.[9] These assays may detect minute amounts of PSA originating from non-malignant prostatic sources[13] and generate problems with false positive results.

1.3.2 *Local versus systemic disease*

Once a PSA recurrence has been established, one of the most problematic aspects of evaluating patients is to determine whether the source of PSA is from localised or metastatic disease. The distinction is important because the presence of localised disease only, allows for salvage therapy directed at the prostatic fossa with an intent to cure. In contrast, metastatic disease is treated palliatively with androgen ablation therapy initially. The incidence of isolated localised disease in men presenting with PSA recurrence after prostatectomy ranges from 4 to 53%.[14–16]

Table 3 outlines various diagnostic modalities and their usefulness in distinguishing between local and systemic cancer recurrence.

Digital rectal exam is very limited in its diagnostic utility. The prostatic fossa palpation is highly variable after radical prostatectomy and there is often post-operative scarring, making the diagnosis of local recurrence difficult. It should not be used alone to determine a management decision.

Ultrasound guided biopsy of the prostatic fossa is not recommended routinely as there are substantial problems associated

Table 3. Diagnostic modalities for distinguishing between local and systemic spread in patients with biochemical recurrence after radical prostatectomy.

Diagnostic modality	Clinical usefulness
Digital rectal exam	None
Ultrasound-guided biopsy	None
Computed tomography	Marginal, consider if PSA > 10ng/ml or PSADT < 6 months
MRI	Under investigation
Bone scan	Marginal, consider if PSA > 10ng/ml or PSADT < six months
Radio-labelled PSMA antibody	Potentially useful. Further trials required.
Positron emission tomography	Under investigation.

with it. Firstly, with the prostate absent, the exact site to biopsy is not known. The true sensitivity and the true false negative rate is also not known.[9] Additionally, if a local recurrence of prostate cancer is identified, it does not exclude the presence of concomitant systemic disease as well. Finally, results of salvage radiation therapy to the prostatic fossa are equivalent whether the biopsies are positive or negative.[17]

In asymptomatic men, the utility of computed tomography and bone scans has been poor for men with PSA recurrence after radical prostatectomy.[18] Its use has been recommended by some when the PSA is greater than 10ng/ml or when the PSA doubling time (PSADT) is less than six months.

ProstaScint, is a radio-labelled monoclonal antibody to prostate specific membrane antigen (PSMA). PSMA is increased in poorly differentiated and metastatic prostate cancer. Detection of metastatic disease using this imaging method has a sensitivity of approximately 62%.[19] Further larger studies are needed, however, to establish its true sensitivity and specificity.

Currently, the most common method of distinguishing local from systemic prostate cancer recurrence following radical prostatectomy, when PSA levels are still low, is to use a combination of various pathological and PSA variables. Table 4 outlines the variables associated with local and systemic recurrence.

Table 4. Pathological and PSA variables for distinguishing between local and systemic spread in patients with biochemical recurrence after radical prostatectomy.

Variable	Local recurrence	Systemic recurrence
Gleason score	≤ 7	> 7
Lymph node invasion	No	Yes
PSA doubling time	≥ 3–12 months	< 3–12 months
PSA velocity at 1 year	< 0.75 ng/ml/yr	≥ 0.75 ng/ml/yr
Seminal vesical invasion	No	Yes
Time to PSA recurrence	> 1–2 years	≤ 1–2 years

1.3.3 *Natural history of biochemical recurrence*

The natural history of progression to bony metastasis and then to death after biochemical recurrence is highly variable, but generally prolonged. In a study where 304 men with biochemical recurrence after radical prostatectomy were followed for up to 15 years, only 34% developed bone metastases at a median of eight years. These men with bone metastases were treated with androgen deprivation therapy and median time to death from prostate cancer was 5 years later.[20]

The real challenge is to identify the men with biochemical recurrence who will progress rapidly and die early, so early treatment can be instituted. The Gleason score in the prostatectomy specimen and PSA kinetics have been useful for estimating time to developing metastases in men with biochemical recurrence. Table 5 shows the effect of Gleason score, time to PSA recurrence and PSADT on metastasis free survival at three and five years. Clearly a Gleason grade > 7, PSA recurrence earlier than two years and a PSADT of < ten months portrays a poor prognosis.

Once men have developed bone metastases, a large proportion will die of prostate cancer. Freedland *et al.* have demonstrated that the PSADT is strongly predictive of death from prostate cancer (Fig. 1).[21] This data shows that if the PSADT is > 15 months, no patients over a 15-year period died from prostate cancer.

Table 5. Estimation of metastasis-free survival following biochemical recurrence after radical prostatectomy.

	% Metastasis-free	
	Three years	Five years
All patients	78	63
Gleason score 5–7		
Recurrence > two years		
PSADT > 10 m	95	86
PSADT ≤ 10 m	82	69
Recurrence ≤ two years		
PSADT > 10 m	79	76
PSADT < 10 m	81	35
Gleason score 8–10		
Recurrence > two years		
PSADT > 10 m	77	60
Recurrence ≤ two years		
PSADT ≤ 10 m	53	31

Adapted from Pound *et al.*[20] and Laufer *et al.*[14]

1.4 Treatment options for cancer recurrence following radical prostatectomy

Unfortunately, to date there has been no prospective randomised control trial data showing that treatment of PSA recurrence, at any level or by any modality, improves survival. Common treatments undertaken after a PSA recurrence include expectant management, salvage radiotherapy and androgen deprivation therapy. The treatment option chosen depends on the patient's likelihood of:

(1) local versus systemic disease;
(2) cancer characteristics and rate of growth (PSA);
(3) patient's co-morbidities and life expectancy;
(4) side effects of treatment; and
(5) patient's wishes.

1.4.1 Expectant management

As there is no definitive evidence that treatment of a PSA recurrence alone improves survival, and as only half the men will develop

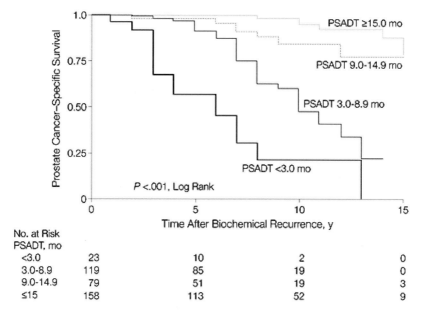

Figure 1. Fifteen-year actuarial Kaplan-Meier prostate cancer–specific survival curves by PSADT. Biochemical recurrence segregated by prostate-specific antigen doubling time among patients who experienced a biochemical recurrence. PSADT indicates prostate-specific antigen doubling time.[21]

a bone metastasis at eight years or later,[20] close monitoring is a very reasonable option for elderly men or those with multiple co-morbidities. If during this time men develop metastases, they can start androgen deprivation therapy.

1.4.2 *Salvage radiotherapy*

Salvage radiotherapy is treatment of the prostatic bed with the aim of curing a man who has a PSA recurrence. It should only be given to men who have a reasonable chance of having only localised disease based on tumour characteristics, PSA kinetics and imaging.

While there are no studies that show that salvage radiotherapy will improve survival, PSA response to salvage radiotherapy is generally about 50%.[22] There is however a large range of responses, (12–77%) depending on the post-prostatectomy pathology and PSA kinetics.[22] PSA responses are better if the Gleason score is less than 8 (less likihood of systemic disease), the surgical margin status is positive (higher likelihood of a local source of PSA), the PSADT is long (less chance of metastatic disease) and the salvage radiotherapy is given at a low PSA, preferable < 1.0ng/ml (low tumour burden).[22] A man with a Gleason 6 prostate cancer with positive surgical margins, PSADT > ten months and starting salvage radiotherapy with a PSA < 2.0ng/ml has a 77% chance of PSA response. A man with a Gleason score of 8, starting salvage therapy with a PSA > 2.0ng/ml has a 12% chance of PSA response. In summary, salvage radiotherapy is effective if given early to someone who has a high likelihood of localized recurrence.[22]

Side effects of salvage radiotherapy are generally well tolerated. Approximately 20% of men previously continent will become mildly incontinent.[23] Approximately 50% of potent men will suffer declines in erectile function and a number of men may also develop urethral strictures or bladder neck contractures.

1.4.3 *Androgen deprivation therapy*

Androgen deprivation therapy (ADT) or 'hormonal therapy' is often used to treat men with PSA recurrence, or men who have established metastases from prostate cancer. Treatment by this method can either be by bilateral orchidectomy, LHRH agonists or anti-androgens such as cyproterone acetate or high dose biclutamide. The treatments all have the final effect of reducing prostate cancer growth and inducing apoptosis by stopping testosterone induced prostate cancer growth. While this therapy is palliative only, as the PSA and cancer will eventually begin to grow, many men can experience prolonged survival following institution of ADT. Once men have developed bone metastases and then start ADT, they will live on average five years.[20] Men with PSA recurrence only will live much longer than this on average.

The timing of commencement of ADT in men that have PSA recurrence is the subject of a number of on-going clinical trials. Retrospective data does suggest that select men with aggressive disease who receive early androgen deprivation therapy for PSA recurrence do experience a delay in developing bone metastases.[24] There is no data however to show this improves survival.[24]

1.5   Summary

PSA is a highly sensitive marker for the detection of recurrence after radical prostatectomy. When the PSA reaches between 0.2 to 0.5ng/ml, a patient is considered to have a recurrence.

The patient's prognosis and likelihood of localised verses systemic disease is highly dependent on the prostatectomy pathology as well as the time to PSA recurrence after prostatectomy and PSADT.

If a patient is likely to have localised recurrence, he is eligible for salvage radiotherapy. If the patients have a high likelihood of systemic disease, androgen deprivation therapy or expectant management may be a more reasonable approach to treatment.

2.   Diagnosis and Management of Complications of Radical Prostatectomy

An anatomic approach to radical perineal prostatectomy was described in 1905,[25] followed by the retropubic approach 40 years later.[26] Historically both approaches were associated with significant morbidity and mortality. In the modern era, with an anatomic approach to sparing the cavernous nerves, greater surgical experience and training, younger patients with fewer co-morbidites and better anaesthetic techniques, significantly less morbidity and mortality has been experienced. This section focuses on the prevention and management of complications following radical prostatectomy.

2.1   General complications

Cardiovascular complications associated with radical prostatectomy include myocardial infarction, cerebrovascular accidents, cardiac arrhythmias, pulmonary embolus and DVT. These complications may occur intraoperatively or post-operatively, but are rarely experienced, for example in a large series the rate of myocardial infarction was observed to be 0.1–0.4% and pulmonary embolus 0–2%.[27,28]

A detailed preoperative review of systems, social, family history as well as cardiovascular risk factors should be performed.

The presence of erectile dysfunction may be an indicator of occult cardiovascular disease. Men with known cardiovascular disease or high risk factors should undergo evaluation. These men often have a reduced life expectancy as well as increased surgical risks and should not be offered a surgical cure for their cancer.

Pulmonary embolus represents the most common life-threatening thromboembolic event associated with radical prostatectomy. The role of prophylaxis has been controversial; however, most centers will use various combinations of graduated compression stockings, mechanical compression boots and pharmacological prophylaxis with heparin or low molecular weight heparin. Minimisation of pelvic vein manipulation, quick surgical procedures, early ambulation and short hospital stays are important factors that minimise the occurrence.[27]

2.2 Intraoperative complications that may impact of long-term functioning

2.2.1 Rectal injury

The rate of rectal injury during surgery is approximately 0.5%.[29] The injury usually occurs when dissecting the apex of the prostate, particularly with small prostate glands. The risk increases in men who have had prior radiotherapy, inflammatory bowel disease or a large number of needle biopsies.

When the injury is identified intra-operatively, it can be repaired by a two layer closure with omental interposition and copious irrigation, provided the rectum had been prepared pre-operatively.[30] If it is not recognised intra-operatively, it will present post-operatively as an abscess or recto-urethral fistula. A temporary colostomy will be required until the injury heals in these situations.

2.2.2 Obturator nerve injury

Obturator injury can occur during lymphadenectomy. It can be avoided by always identifying the nerve prior to ligating the lymph node packet. If injury does occur, it results in a loss of sensation over the medial aspect of the thigh and in ability to adduct the leg. The injury spontaneously resolves over time. Physiotherapy often helps with the muscular weakness.

2.2.3 *Ureteral injury*

This is a rare injury and occurs between 0.05 to 0.2% of cases.[27,28] Injury can occur at many points during the operation, but usually when dissecting the seminal vesicles, dividing the prostate-vesical junction or reconstructing the bladder neck. The injury may be identified intra-operatively or post-operatively with flank pain, a rise in the serum creatinine or urine in the drain fluid. It may also be remain asymptomatic and present years later as an incidental finding of hydronephrosis. Depending on the site and degree of injury, treatment is usually surgical and entails reimplantation into the bladder.

2.3 *Long term complications*

2.3.1 *Bladder neck contracture*

Bladder neck contracture is the narrowing of the bladder neck by scar tissue, at the site of the urethro-vesical anastamosis and occurs in approximately 8% of radical prostatectomy cases.[31] It usually occurs in the first six months after surgery and presents as a gradual slowing of the urinary flow, worsening incontinence or dysuria.

The vast majority of bladder neck contractures will resolve with simple dilatation. Occasionally the contracture will need to be incised to open it sufficiently. Contractures can be kept open by regular intermittent self-dilatation for a few months after cystoscopic dilatation.

2.3.2 *Incontinence*

Between 2.5% and 87% (depending on definition of continence, timing of reporting and surgeon's expertise) will fail to regain continence after radical prostatectomy.[32] Centers of expertise however will report that approximately 96% of men will be continent using validated questionnaires.[33]

Incontinence following radical prostatectomy is almost always caused by damage to the striated (rhabdo) sphincter. In addition to intra-operative sphincter damage, incontinence is related to a number of factors. These are: patient age, degree of neurovascular bundle sparing performed during surgery and the presence of anastomotic contracture.[34] Pre-operative strengthening of the pelvic floor with specific exercises have also been shown to improve continence after surgery.[35]

After surgery, all men should be on a program of pelvic floor exercises.

Approximately 80% of men should be continent at three months.[33] If they are not, then urine infection and bladder neck contracture need to be excluded. They should then be started on a biofeedback program. Continence can continue to improve over one year. If incontinence persists after a year, men should undergo urodynamic studies to quantitate the degree of sphincteric weakness and identify and other contributing factors, such as co-existent bladder instability, which can be treated with anti-cholinergic medication. If a man has mild incontinence, he can undergo a procedure aimed at bulking the urinary sphincter with bulking agents, such as contigen or macroplastique. If a man has moderate incontinence, then a male sling is the most common recommendation. If however the incontinence is severe, an artificial urinary sphincter is usually the best option.

2.3.3 Erectile dysfunction

Erectile dysfunction (ED) is the most common complication following radical prostatectomy and has a profound effect on the quality of life after radical prostatectomy.[36] The likelihood of preserving sexual function depends on patient's age, pre-operative sexual function and degree of neurovascular bundle preservation.[37] The quality of the neurovascular bundle preservation is also highly dependent on surgeon expertise and surgical technique. Potency results following nerve sparing prostatectomy range from 9% to 86% in the literature.[38] Such differing reported results are due to a number of factors, including the type of questionnaire used, definition of potency, surgeon expertise and time of measurement.

Patients often experience ED following a nerve sparing prosta-tectomy. This is usually related to neurapraxia and occurs even with the most skilled of surgeons. The lack of early post-prostatectomy erections results in poor corporeal oxygenation and can lead to cor-poral fibrosis, which ultimately leads to veno-occusive dysfunction[39] and permanent ED.

To avoid poor corporeal oxygenation, it is important to gain erections as early as possible after surgery. Early (four weeks) use of intracavernosal injections of alprostadil has been shown to greatly improve the recovery of erections, compared to observation alone.[40] This should ideally be started as soon as possible after the procedure at an initial dose of 5 µg approximately 2–3 times per week. This early use of Alprostadil also avoids the dysfunctional sexual dynamic that occurs as men lose confidence and withdraw sexually.[41] The intracavernosal injection of a combination of phen-tolamine and papaverine has equal efficacy[42] and causes less pain upon injection, but requires a compounding chemist to make the solution.[43]

Phosphodiesterase inhibitors (PDE5I) have also been shown to increase the quality of erections following radical prostatectomy. Vardenafil (Levitra) and tadalafil (Cialis) have both been shown to improve the quality of erections following radical prostatectomy, when randomised to drug verses placebo. Men who had a bilat-eral nerve sparing operation had a 52% vaginal penetration rate when treated with 20mg tadalafil daily, compared to 26% for the placebo group ($p < 0.05$).[44] Following bilateral nerve sparing radi-cal prostatectomy, men randomised to daily vardenafil 20mg experienced a 74% successful intercourse rate, compared to 49% in the placebo group.[45]

A common practical approach to penile rehabilitation follow-ing radical prostatectomy is to start men on medication within the first month post-operatively. If men are experiencing partial erec-tions, they may start with PDE5Is. If however they are not experiencing any erections, response to PDE5I therapy will be poor and these men are started on intracavernosal injections until they develop partial erections, at which time they can be changed to PDE5I therapy. The dose of PDE5I can be gradually weaned as spontaneous erections improve with time. Research has shown that men experience gradual improvements in erectile function for up to three years following surgery.

3. Summary

Complications following radical prostatectomy can range from general medical problems to intra-operative technical difficulties to long term function problems that can significantly deteriorate quality of life. The key is to fully evaluate and counsel pre-operatively to reduce the likelihood of unforeseen problems. Urinary incontinence is the most disabling long term complication. Pelvic floor exercises pre-operatively and post-operatively are the mainstay of treatment. Surgical treatments with periurethral bulking agents, urethral slings and artificial sphincters, have a high likelihood of salvaging any remaining degree of incontinence. ED after surgery is also disabling, but meticulous surgery and early post-operative aggressive penile rehabilitation will improve ED in most men following nerve sparing surgery.

References

1. T. L. Krupski *et al.*, Geographic and socioeconomic variation in the treatment of prostate cancer, *J. Clin. Oncol.* **23**(31): 7881–7888 (2005).
2. M. N. Simmons, A. J. Stephenson and E. A. Klein, Natural history of biochemical recurrence after radical prostatectomy: Risk assessment for secondary therapy, *Eur. Urol.* **51**(5): 1175–1184 (2007).
3. M. W. Kattan, T. M. Wheeler and P. T. Scardino, Postoperative nomogram for disease recurrence after radical prostatectomy for prostate cancer, *J. Clin. Oncol.* **17**(5): 1499–1507 (1999).
4. P. C. Walsh, A. W. Partin and J. I. Epstein, Cancer control and quality of life following anatomical radical retropubic prostatectomy: Results at 10 years, *J. Urol.* **152**(5 pt. 2): 1831–1836 (1994).
5. P. Kupelian *et al.*, Correlation of clinical and pathologic factors with rising prostate-specific antigen profiles after radical prostatectomy alone for clinically localized prostate cancer, *Urology* **48**(2): 249–260 (1996).
6. F. J. Bianco, P. T. Scardino and J. A. Eastham, Jr., Radical prostatectomy: Long-term cancer control and recovery of sexual and urinary function ("trifecta"), *Urology* **66**(5 Suppl.): 83–94 (2005).

7. W. R. Morgan *et al.*, Prostate specific antigen values after radical retropubic prostatectomy for adenocarcinoma of the prostate: Impact of adjuvant treatment (hormonal and radiation), *J. Urol.* **145**(2): 319–323 (1991).

8. M. G. Oefelein *et al.*, The incidence of prostate cancer progression with undetectable serum prostate specific antigen in a series of 394 radical prostatectomies, *J. Urol.* **154**(6): 2128–2131 (1995).

9. P. W. Swindle, M. W. Kattan and P. T. Scardino, Markers and meaning of primary treatment failure, *Urol. Clin. N. Am.* **30**(2): 377–401 (2003).

10. S. J. Freedland *et al.*, Defining the ideal cutpoint for determining PSA recurrence after radical prostatectomy. Prostate-specific antigen, *Urology* **61**(2): 365–369 (2003).

11. A. W. Partin and J. E. Oesterling, The clinical usefulness of prostate specific antigen: Update 1994, *J. Urol.* **152**(5 pt. 1): 1358–1368 (1994).

12. J. W. Moul, Variables in predicting survival based on treating "PSA-only" relapse, *Urol. Oncol.* **21**(4): 292–304 (2003).

13. E. P. Diamandis and H. Yu, Nonprostatic sources of prostate-specific antigen, *Urol. Clin. N. Am.* **24**(2): 275–282 (1997).

14. M. Laufer *et al.*, Management of patients with rising prostate-specific antigen after radical prostatectomy, *Urology* **55**(3): 309–315 (2000).

15. M. Han *et al.*, Long-term biochemical disease-free and cancer-specific survival following anatomic radical retropubic prostatectomy. The 15-year Johns Hopkins experience, *Urol. Clin. N. Am.* **28**(3): 555–565 (2001).

16. J. A. Connolly *et al.*, Local recurrence after radical prostatectomy: Characteristics in size, location, and relationship to prostate-specific antigen and surgical margins, *Urology* **47**(2): 225–231 (1996).

17. T. M. Koppie *et al.*, Is anastomotic biopsy necessary before radiotherapy after radical prostatectomy? *J. Urol.* **166**(1): 111–115 (2001).

18. O. T. Okotie *et al.*, Predictors of metastatic disease in men with biochemical failure following radical prostatectomy, *J. Urol.* **171**(6 pt. 1): 2260–2264 (2004).

19. J. C. Quintana and M. J. Blend, The dual-isotope ProstaScint imaging procedure: Clinical experience and staging results in 145 patients, *Clin. Nucl. Med.* **25**(1): 33–40 (2000).

20. C. R. Pound *et al.*, Natural history of progression after PSA elevation following radical prostatectomy, *J. Am. Med. Assoc.* **281**(17): 1591–1597 (1999).

21. S. J. Freedland *et al.*, Risk of prostate cancer-specific mortality following biochemical recurrence after radical prostatectomy, *J. Am. Med. Assoc.* **294**(4): 433–439 (2005).

22. A. J. Stephenson *et al.*, Salvage radiotherapy for recurrent prostate cancer after radical prostatectomy, *J. Am. Med. Assoc.* **291**(11): 1325–1332 (2004).

23. M. S. Katz *et al.*, Predictors of biochemical outcome with salvage conformal radiotherapy after radical prostatectomy for prostate cancer, *J. Clin. Oncol.* **21**(3): 483–489 (2003).

24. J. W. Moul *et al.*, Early versus delayed hormonal therapy for prostate specific antigen only recurrence of prostate cancer after radical prostatectomy, *J. Urol.* **171**(3): 1141–1147 (2004).

25. H. H. Young, VIII. Conservative perineal prostatectomy: The results of two years' experience and report of seventy-five cases, *Ann. Surg.* **41**(4): 549–557 (1905).

26. T. Millin, The surgery of the malignant prostate, *Br. J. Urol.* **30**(4): 407–410; discussion 411–414 (1958).

27. H. Lepor and L. Kaci, Contemporary evaluation of operative parameters and complications related to open radical retropubic prostatectomy, *Urology* **62**(4): 702–706 (2003).

28. W. J. Catalona *et al.*, Potency, continence and complication rates in 1,870 consecutive radical retropubic prostatectomies, *J. Urol.* **162**(2): 433–438 (1999).

29. H. Lepor, A. M. Nieder and M. N. Ferrandino, Intraoperative and postoperative complications of radical retropubic prostatectomy in a consecutive series of 1,000 cases, *J. Urol.* **166**(5): 1729–1733 (2001).

30. R. N. Borland and P. C. Walsh, The management of rectal injury during radical retropubic prostatectomy, *J. Urol.* **147**(3 pt. 2): 905–907 (1992).

31. S. P. Elliott *et al.*, Incidence of urethral stricture after primary treatment for prostate cancer: Data from CaPSURE, *J. Urol.* **178**(2): 529–534; discussion 534 (2007).

32. J. Foote, S. Yun and G. E. Leach, Postprostatectomy incontinence. Pathophysiology, evaluation, and management, *Urol. Clin. N. Am.* **18**(2): 229–241 (1991).

33. H. Lepor and L. Kaci, The impact of open radical retropubic prostatectomy on continence and lower urinary tract symptoms: A prospective assessment using validated self-administered outcome instruments, *J. Urol.* **171**(3): 1216–1219 (2004).

34. J. A. Eastham *et al.*, Risk factors for urinary incontinence after radical prostatectomy, *J. Urol.* **156**(5): 1707–1713 (1996).

35. C. Sueppel, K. Kreder and W. See, Improved continence outcomes with preoperative pelvic floor muscle strengthening exercises, *Urol. Nurs.* **21**(3): 201–210 (2001).

36. J. P. Meyer *et al.*, The effect of erectile dysfunction on the quality of life of men after radical prostatectomy, *Br. J. Urol. Int.* **92**(9): 929–931 (2003).

37. F. Rabbani *et al.*, Factors predicting recovery of erections after radical prostatectomy. *J. Urol.* **164**(6): 1929–1934 (2000).

38. A. L. Burnett *et al.*, Erectile function outcome reporting after clinically localized prostate cancer treatment, *J. Urol.* **178**(2): 597–601 (2007).

39. R. B. Moreland, Is there a role of hypoxemia in penile fibrosis: A viewpoint presented to the Society for the Study of Impotence, *Int. J. Impot. Res.* **10**(2): 113–120 (1998).

40. F. Montorsi *et al.*, Recovery of spontaneous erectile function after nerve-sparing radical retropubic prostatectomy with and without early intracavernous injections of alprostadil: Results of a prospective, randomized trial, *J. Urol.* **158**(4): 1408–1410 (1997).

41. A. R. McCullough, Prevention and management of erectile dysfunction following radical prostatectomy, *Urol. Clin. N. Am.* **28**(3): 613–627 (2001).

42. F. Montorsi *et al.*, Effectiveness and safety of multidrug intracavernous therapy for vasculogenic impotence, *Urology* **42**(5): 554–558 (1993).

43. P. Gontero *et al.*, Is there an optimal time for intracavernous prostaglandin E1 rehabilitation following nonnerve sparing radical prostatectomy? Results from a hemodynamic prospective study, *J. Urol.* **169**(6): 2166–2169 (2003).

44. F. Montorsi *et al.*, Tadalafil in the treatment of erectile dysfunction following bilateral nerve sparing radical retropubic prostatectomy: A randomized, double-blind, placebo controlled trial, *J. Urol.* **172**(3): 1036–1041 (2004).

45. G. Brock *et al.*, Safety and efficacy of vardenafil for the treatment of men with erectile dysfunction after radical retropubic prostatectomy, *J. Urol.* **170**(4 pt. 1): 1278–1283 (2003).

46. A. W. Partin *et al.*, Selection of men at high risk for disease recurrence for experimental adjuvant therapy following radical prostatectomy, *Urology* **45**(5): 831–838 (1995).

47. A. V. D'Amico *et al.*, The combination of preoperative prostate specific antigen and postoperative pathological findings to predict prostate

specific antigen outcome in clinically localized prostate cancer, *J. Urol.* **160**(6 pt. 1): 2096–2101 (1998).

48. M. L. Blute *et al.*, Use of Gleason score, prostate specific antigen, seminal vesicle and margin status to predict biochemical failure after radical prostatectomy, *J. Urol.* **165**(1): 119–125 (2001).

49. J. W. Moul *et al.*, Predicting risk of prostate specific antigen recurrence after radical prostatectomy with the Center for Prostate Disease Research and Cancer of the Prostate Strategic Urologic Research Endeavor databases, *J. Urol.* **166**(4): 1322–1327 (2001).

50. S. J. Freedland *et al.*, Preoperative model for predicting prostate specific antigen recurrence after radical prostatectomy using percent of biopsy tissue with cancer, biopsy Gleason grade and serum prostate specific antigen, *J. Urol.* **171**(6 pt. 1): 2215–2220 (2004).

26

Plastic and Reconstructive Surgery in Oncological Surgery

Sean Nicklin
and Mohammad Rahnavardi

Abstract

This chapter attempts to give a brief overview of the breadth of plastic and reconstructive surgery as it applies to oncological surgery. A broad description of the principles on which reconstructive decision making is based is presented and some details on specific techniques are provided. As the head and neck region and the breast are common sites that are presented to plastic surgeons for reconstruction after cancer resection, a more detailed account of reconstructive options and approach at these sites is presented.

Keywords: Plastic surgery, reconstruction, graft, flap, microsurgery, cancer/oncology.

1. Principles of Reconstructive Surgery

Reconstructive surgery for defects created by oncological resection aims to provide a functional construct that is stable and strong enough to allow primary wound healing. The reconstructed tissues should ideally be functionally competent and aesthetically acceptable. Any decision about management should be holistic and take into account other factors like general health and occupation of the patient, any co-morbidity (especially those that compromise wound healing), the likelihood of success, and the risks of surgery and anaesthesia.

Traditionally most reconstructive surgeons have adopted a step-wise approach in planning the management of surgical wounds and reconstructing tissue defects. This is based on the use of the simplest means possible to achieve wound closure. This is described as a "reconstructive ladder" progressing from the simplest (primary closure) to the more complex (free tissue transfer). In recent years, however, the frequency and decreased morbidity associated with more complex reconstructive options has led to a different approach. Mathes and Nahai[1] coined the term "reconstructive triangle" which suggested flaps, microsurgery and tissue expansion as the three points in the reconstructive triangle. Similar to Gottlieb and Krieger's "reconstructive elevator",[2] the reconstructive triangle champions the use of the best means available to achieve the optimal functional and aesthetic result.

1.1   *Primary closure*

Primary closure is the simplest option for reconstruction of the soft tissue and is used when the size of the defect created by resection is small enough to close the wound without tension. If precise approximation of the wound edges cannot be done without tension, a more complex reconstructive method should be the choice. Although sutures are the most common material used for primary closure, they are not always the best option and other materials such as staples, skin tapes, or wound adhesives are also useful in certain situations.

1.2   *Healing by secondary intention*

Occasionally, it is appropriate to allow a wound to heal by secondary intention using extended dressings. Advancement in technology of dressings has allowed for safe management of wounds over an extended period of time with minimal morbidity. The introduction of the vacuum-assisted wound closure therapy over recent years has helped significantly in management of complex wounds.[3] This is a foam dressing with a suction pump attached to it that helps maintain a moist wound environment and encourages granulation tissue. This dressing can be used as definitive management, as a prelude to skin grafting, or to stabilise a wound prior to a more complex reconstruction. However, the wound acts as an ongoing source of potential infection. Furthermore, extracellular fluid and proteins may be lost from the wound in significant quantity to affect the patient systemically and the wound dressings may be uncomfortable for the patient. All of these factors result in the very limited use of dressings as definitive management of complex wounds.

1.3   *Skin grafting*

Skin grafting is a relatively simple option for closing defects that are too large for a tensionless skin apposition. A graft is a tissue that is removed from one part of the body, is completely devascularised, and is replaced in another location to acquire its blood supply from the underlying wound bed. A skin graft consists of epidermis and some (split-thickness) or all (full-thickness) of the dermis. Whereas hair follicles are transferred with a full-thickness skin graft, split-thickness skin grafts, especially thin split-thickness skin grafts, are usually hairless. Skin grafts are innervated by ingrowth of nerve fibres from the recipient bed. A healthy, uninfected, vascularised bed is essential for revascularisation of the graft. The graft should receive nutrients and subsequently revascularises from the recipient bed. Skin grafting will seldom be successful in exposed bone, cartilage, or tendon devoid of their periosteum, perichondrium, or paratenon. Immobilisation of the graft is essential and survival of the graft will be compromised if hematomas or seromas develop under the graft. Multiple mechanical incisions on the graft result in a meshed skin graft allowing drainage through the numerous holes, as well as immediate expansion of the graft. However, meshed skin grafts may be aesthetically unacceptable. An appropriate tie-over or vacuum dressing can reduce dead space and splinting the site helps the graft to remain in place.

The donor site for a skin graft can be anywhere on the body. Nevertheless, the colour, contour, thickness of the dermis, vascularity, and donor site morbidity are important factors to consider before selecting the appropriate donor site. The donor site of a split-thickness skin graft heals by re-epithelialisation in seven to 14 days from remaining dermal adnexal structures. In contrast, the dermis never regenerates and full-thickness skin graft donor sites must be closed primarily. Full-thickness skin grafts are generally harvested from sites that are easily concealed like groin or posterior auricular region. On occasion, specific sites may be used for a particular skin quality, for example, nasolabial fold to replace nasal skin, or upper eyelid to replace lower eyelid skin.

Skin grafts should not be used for reconstruction of defects where adjuvant radiation treatment will be used. They should also be avoided in areas of high friction or over joints. Skin grafts may be used to obtain rapid wound healing with a plan for revision of the skin grafted site with a flap as a delayed procedure. Generally, flap reconstruction will give a better aesthetic and more durable long term result.

1.4   *Tissue expansion*

Tissue expansion is a method of increasing the amount of locally available skin. This creates more tissue which has similar characteristics to the defect in skin colour texture and hair bearing quality. It also allows for easy closure of the donor site.

The first use in the modern era was by Neumann.[4] A rubber balloon was placed beneath the temporal scalp and behind the auricular skin, to create skin for ear reconstruction post-trauma. The technique was used minimally until Radovan presented its use for breast reconstruction in the 1970s. Since that time the use of tissue expansion has become more widespread.

Tissue expansion requires placement of a tissue expander beneath the skin adjacent to the defect. Modern expanders are made of silicone elastomers and come in multiple shapes and sizes. They all have ports for injection of saline to expand the implant and expand the overlying soft tissues, and over a period of time, significant gain in soft tissue can be achieved. The expanded soft tissue can then be moved into the defect as a flap and the donor site closed primarily. Meticulous planning is required and multiple expanders may be used to achieve an optimal result. The need for multi-stage surgery is a significant drawback.

1.5   *Flaps*

A flap, unlike a graft, has its own vascular supply while transferred from a donor to a recipient site, and it may include muscle, skin, fascia, fat, nerve and bone. Flaps are usually the choice for covering poorly vascularised recipient defects, vital structures and body prominences, as well as reconstructing the full thickness of the eyelids, lips, ears, nose and cheeks. Muscle flaps may also act as a functional motor unit, or as a means of infection control in the recipient site. Flaps can be categorised according to their special relationship to the defect (local, regional, or distant), their component parts (e.g. cutaneous, musculocutaneous, osseocutaneous), the nature of their blood supply (random versus axial), or by the movement placed on the flap to fill an associated defect (e.g. advancement, pivot, transposition).

1.5.1   *Local flaps*

Local flaps generally describe the use of tissue adjacent to the defect to be reconstructed. These flaps can be transposition, rotation or advancement flaps. A transposition flap is a rectangle or square flap that is rotated about a pivot point into an immediately adjacent defect. A rotation flap is rotation of a semicircular flap into a triangular defect and thus spreads the tension of closure over a larger area by differential suturing. Advancement flaps are moved directly forward into a defect without any rotation or lateral movement. The choice of flap is dictated by a number of factors; generally, the donor site is selected in such a fashion to position scar within the natural crease lines of the skin (Langer's lines). A significant advantage of local flaps is that they use surrounding skin which has the same characteristics of the area for reconstruction. This is particularly useful on the face, where anatomically distinct areas have skin of a specific colour and texture. The nasal area is a site where local flaps can give an excellent reconstruction. Another area of the face where local flaps are particularly useful is hair bearing areas such as eyebrows, hairlines or the beard. Local flaps can transport in hair that is an excellent match for the defect, whereas hair bearing flaps or grafts from other sites give an inferior result.

Local flaps are generally dependent on a random pattern of blood supply, so are limited in their dimension and also in the ease with which they can be mobilised. However, some local flaps can be raised on an axial blood supply and thus all skin attachments can be divided, allowing a greater degree of mobility. These flaps are sometimes described as loco-regional flaps. It is sometimes necessary to undertake the procedure in two stages, leaving the flap attached by its pedicle and inserting it into the defect. After two to three weeks there would have been enough vessel in growth from the tissues surrounding the original defect and the pedicle can be divided. This type of procedure is commonly used for nasal reconstruction and lip reconstruction. For defects that are too large or do not have adequate surrounding skin two or more flaps may be used. This may also be the case for composite defects requiring a multilayered reconstruction or for flaps crossing anatomical boundaries of the face (Figs. 1a and 1b).

Whenever a flap is mobilised, there is a donor site or a secondary defect. Often the flap is designed in such a way to allow primary closure of this defect, e.g. V-Y advancement flaps. In other situations, a skin graft may be used, usually positioning the skin graft in a less anatomically or aesthetically sensitive site, e.g. forehead flap for nasal reconstruction (Figs. 1a and 1b). Another technique is the use of another flap to distribute tension more widely, e.g. bilobed flap or a transposition flap from an area of laxity (Figs. 2a and 2b).

Larger defects, still, may require the introduction of tissue from a more distant site either regionally or distant.

1.5.2 *Regional flaps*

These are flaps that are harvested from the same anatomical region as the defect to be reconstructed. They are generally axial pattern flaps that are often isolated on their feeding vessels, with complete

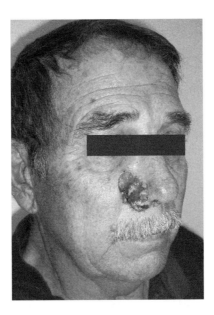

(a)

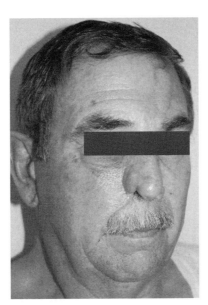

(b)

Figure 1. **(a)** A large BCC involving the cheek and nose. **(b)** Result at two weeks after cheek flap and two-stage forehead flap reconstruction.

(a)

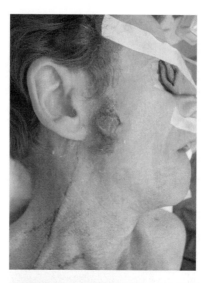

(b)

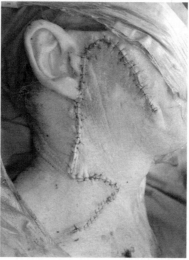

Figure 2. **(a)** A large SCC of the right pre-auricular area. **(b)** Reconstruction with a cervico-facial flap and a z-plasty in the neck for closure of the secondary defect.

division of any skin attachment. This makes them much more versatile for reconstruction than local flaps may be. A greater volume and length of flap can be raised by including the underlying fascia, with or without muscle, and a perforating blood vessel. Isolating the flap on this vascular pedicle allows even greater mobility and versatility of insertion into the tissue defect. This is a so-called pedicled flap. There is a bewildering array of flaps described that can be raised as pedicled flaps and used for regional reconstruction. Most reconstructions rely on a handful of reliable flaps, but it is beyond the scope of this text to describe individual flaps.

Pedicled flaps can be raised from areas quite distant from the defect, being limited only by the pedicle length. A good example is the use of the *latissimus dorsi* muscle flap from the back to reconstruct a breast after mastectomy. The flap pedicle arises in the axilla, thus facilitating the repositioning on the anterior chest wall from the posterior chest wall without division of the flap pedicle. The *latissimus dorsi* flap is a very versatile flap, which can be used as a pedicled flap over most of the upper torso, both anteriorly and posteriorly.

Almost any tissue that can be raised reliably as a pedicled flap can also be raised as a free flap for more distant transfer.

1.5.3 *Free flaps*

A free flap is an autogenous tissue transfer to a distant recipient bed and is of growing importance in oncoplastic surgery. The flap is detached from the vessels at the donor site and re-attached to vessels at the recipient site by microsurgical anastomosis. Free tissue transfer is a demanding technique that requires special microsurgical skills. Free flaps facilitate one-stage transfer of required tissue flaps from a distant site, give better choice of donor site, and allow specialised structures to be transferred, such as sensory or glabrous skin. However, the operation can be time-consuming and there is the possibility of flap failure. The experience of the surgeon, the general condition of the patient, an appropriate choice of a flap, with largest possible diameter and longest possible length of pedicle vessels, appropriate thrombosis prevention, careful flap elevation with early identification of the pedicle and avoiding compression of the pedicle and tight skin closure, are important factors in the success of free flap operations.

Since the first free tissue transfers were performed in the early 1970s, free flaps have become increasingly popular and commonly used in reconstructive surgery. Although an initially very demanding surgery and limited in its application, free tissue transfer is now utilised by an expanding number of surgical disciplines. For many years now the free flap has not been the sole domain of the plastic and reconstructive surgeon.

In recent years, there has been a refinement in techniques of free tissue transfer, which has allowed for improvements in outcomes. Advances have been made, which allow tailoring of tissue to the requirements of the defect and also limiting donor site morbidity. The more recent development of "super microsurgery" (vessels of 1 mm or less diameter) has made tissue from almost anywhere in the body available for transfer as a free flap.

There have also been developments in the understanding of vascular anatomy. This has paved the way for the so-called "perforator" flap. These are flaps which include the necessary vasculature and tissue required without any tissue which may contribute to donor site morbidity. This has given significant improvements in donor site morbidity. The standardisation of techniques and the almost routine nature of microvascular surgery have led to an improved array of free flaps that can significantly improve donor site morbidity and also improve reconstructive outcomes.

It is beyond the scope of this text to discuss the multitude of oncological defects and the reconstructive options. Below is a review of reconstructive approaches to more common sites that the reconstructive plastic surgeon is called upon to reconstruct after ablative surgery, the head and neck region and breast reconstruction.

2.   Head and Neck Reconstructive Surgery

2.1   Introduction

The goals of head and neck reconstruction are to restore the patient functionally and aesthetically in an expeditious manner and with minimal surgical morbidity.[5] Reliable primary wound healing is the key to successful head and neck reconstruction in these patients, who are often debilitated by their disease. Even in situations where long term survival is unrealistic, it is still a worthwhile goal to aim to optimise the quality of life. Specific functions for consideration in the head and neck region include speech, mastication, deglutition and the sensations of taste, touch and smell. All of these functions play a crucial role in communication and social interaction. Historically, little regard was given to the finer detail of these functions, with reconstruction focussed on primary wound healing. Improvement in reconstructive options has led to an increased awareness of these functions and modification of reconstructive techniques to attempt to restore such complex functions partially or completely.

In recent times, priorities in head and neck cancer surgery have changed. The survival rates for most head and neck cancers have changed little in the last 30 years. Local control of head and neck cancer can be compromised, as standard wide excision with 1 cm to 3 cm margins are either impossible, or can significantly affect or expose neighbouring vital structures in the head and neck, resulting in local recurrence and metastasis with relatively poor survival rates.[6] The focus has now shifted, with an expectation of poor survival in many of these cases, and more emphasis is now placed on quality of life following surgery.

The head and neck region presents a significant challenge for the reconstructive plastic surgeon. The intricate anatomy, aesthetic importance, and crucial role of head and neck in human's speech, respiration, and alimentation, make reconstruction of this anatomical region highly demanding. Often malignancies presenting in the head and neck region, particularly, squamous cell carcinoma of the upper aerodigestive tract, are aggressive in nature. This necessitates radical ablative surgery, which will usually result in exposure of critical anatomical structures, and can further compound the difficulty of reconstruction at this site. This also means that many reconstructive options low on the reconstructive ladder (skin graft or local flap) are not appropriate. In many circumstances, free tissue transfer is the reconstruction of first choice.[7–10]

Traditional approaches with the use of regional or pedicled flaps often produces significant donor site morbidity and also increased rates of delayed wound healing (Figs. 3 and 4). These flaps are often bulky, presenting difficulties in inset into the head and neck region. The pedicle for the flap can produce an aesthetically unacceptable result and often impaired functional outcome (Figs. 3 and 4).[11] Aforementioned factors have led to an increased

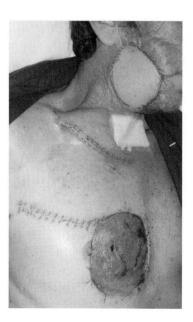

Figure 3. A pectoralis major flap reconstruction for an upper neck to cheek defect. The donor site has been skin grafted.

utilisation of free tissue transfer as a first option in head and neck reconstruction.

Although there are a multitude of flaps available for free tissue transfer, only a small subset of them are most frequently used for head and neck reconstruction. There is some variation between institutions, but the most common flaps are radial forearm and *rectus abdominis* flaps for soft tissue reconstruction, and radial forearm and fibula flaps for bony reconstruction.[7–10,12,13] The lateral arm is often used for soft tissue reconstruction in the author's institution. In recent years, the anterolateral thigh flap has become more popular and is increasingly used in the author's institution. Raising of a large skin island (up to 9 cm diameter) with or without fascia is possible with direct closure of the donor site. This greatly limits donor site morbidity. Unfortunately, the anterolateral thigh region may frequently be too fat in a western population for this flap to be used. The lateral arm flap serves as a reasonable alternative for bony reconstruction; once again primary closure of the donor site is possible with flaps up to 6 cm in diameter.

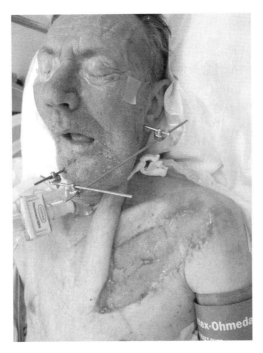

Figure 4. A deltopectoral flap for reconstruction of a composite intra-oral mandibular defect. The external frame stabilises the jaw

2.2 Specific anatomic sites

2.2.1 Intraoral

Intraoral defects can involve oral cavity, tongue, floor of mouth, buccal mucosa, oropharynx, hypopharynx, larynx and cervical oesophagus. Speech and swallowing may be severely affected by surgery at these sites. Swallowing is most severely affected by tongue and pharyngeal resections; however, speech is also profoundly affected by such surgery.[14] When possible, the intraoral defect should be closed primarily as this produces the best possible outcome. This is, however, usually not possible except on the tongue and buccal mucosa. Tissue must be introduced from elsewhere, with qualities that allow freedom of movement of the tongue (i.e. being pliable and non-tethering). The *pectoralis major* flap was the flap of choice for many years, but its pedicled blood supply and bulk limit its usefulness (Fig. 3). Thus, a free tissue transfer is indicated. The free tissue transfer gives great flexibility of insertion, allowing more accurate three-dimensional reconstructions. The radial forearm flap is ideally suited to this as it is soft and pliable. Unfortunately, there are some issues with the donor site morbidity associated with the radial forearm free flap. This has led to the increasing use of the lateral arm flap in our institution.

Defects of the tongue up to 50% in volume can be closed primarily, but larger defects need tissue bulk for best functional outcome.[15] Maintaining the mobility of the remaining tongue is of greatest importance. Even larger defects that leave little functional tongue elements require a flap that can largely fill the oral cavity and give some contact with the roof of the mouth for speech and deglutition. There have been some attempts to create a functional replacement for a tongue in total glossectomy,[16-18] but there is little evidence of the efficacy of these techniques.

Circumferential defects of the oropharynx, hypopharynx and cervical oesophagus require tissue shaped as a tube for reconstruction. Once again free tissue transfer is the first choice for these defects. Free jejunal transfer is most frequently used as the free flap of choice, as it provides a ready-made tube with peristaltic function and mucosal lining for rapid healing, it has a relatively low rate of complications and provides good swallowing function. The main downfall of this flap is the poor quality of alaryngeal speech that is attainable.[19,20] Reconstruction with a tubed fasciocutaneous flap provides a more rigid tube that allows good swallowing function and also more satisfactory speech. The anterolateral thigh flap lends itself perfectly to this reconstruction, with a 9.5 cm wide flap (with primary closure of donor site) being turned on itself into a tube of 3 cm in diameter. This is the choice of flap for these defects in the author's institution.

2.2.2 Mandible

Defects in the mandible may arise from invasion from soft tissue tumours, or from primary tumours of the mandible. Small defects of the mandible without soft tissue loss may be reconstructed with metal plates, with or without non-vascularised bone graft. Composite defects, irradiated fields, defects in the central mandible and any impairment of well vascularised soft tissue envelope require the use of a vascularised bone containing flap. Vascularised flaps can be successfully used for both large and small bony defects in both irradiated and non-irradiated fields. Use of non-vascularised bone grafts, should be limited to small non-irradiated structural defects with normal perfusion.[21] Particularly for lateral defects, it may be possible to reconstruct the mandible with a reconstruction plate only and no bone implantation. Such recon-structions are contraindicated in the central portion of the mandible which is subject to much greater forces.[22]

The fibula free-flap is widely accepted as the gold standard for reconstruction of the mandible. It is possible to harvest a great length of bone that can be used to reconstruct defects in any region of the mandible and for subtotal mandibular reconstruction. Soft tissue can also be included to increase the versatility of this flap. The bone quality of fibula free-flap is excellent, can be safely osteotomised and the pedicle vessels are large. The skin paddle has been reported as unreliable, but initial concerns are largely unfounded, as clinical experience has shown the skin paddle to be quite satisfactory.[23] Other options for bony reconstruction include the lateral arm flap, radial forearm flap, deep circumflex iliac artery flap and scapular flap.

2.2.3 *Midface*

The midface forms the centre point of the aesthetic face, but also contains the confluence of many of the supporting buttresses of the facial skeleton and important structures, such as the nose, orbits, maxilla, sinuses and palatal structures. Thus, defects in this area are often composite and present a significant three-dimensional reconstructive challenge. Tumours that present in this area often require adjuvant radiotherapy to maximise local control; therefore, well vascularised stable soft tissue cover is essential. There are very limited locoregional or pedicled flap options and free tissue trans-fer is the choice in the vast majority of defects. To achieve primary wound healing, close dead space and prevent central nervous system contamination or infection, a muscle containing flap is often used for defects involving the maxilla. The *rectus abdominis* free flap is the most frequently used free flap. Similar principles apply to bony reconstruction as delineated for mandibular reconstruction. However, many areas of the midfacial skeleton may not require formal bony reconstruction.

2.2.4 *Skull base*

The priority in skull base reconstruction is to achieve a stable barrier between the central nervous system and the external environment. Well vascularised tissue between these two environments helps prevent acute and chronic cross-contamination. Local flaps, such as temporoparietal fascia or pericranial flaps, have been used extensively in this area. The utilisation of free tissue transfer has allowed more aggressive ablative surgery and more reliable soft tissue cover and thus decreased infection rates.[24-26] The *rectus abdominis* free flap is the flap used in the vast majority of cases for similar reasons as for midfacial reconstruction. The muscle fills the dead space and seals the defect to the central nervous system and the pedicle is long and of good calibre. It may be necessary to use free fascial grafts (*fascia lata*) for dural reconstruction.

2.2.5 *Cutaneous and soft tissue*

Simple cutaneous defects can be managed with local flaps, or locoregional options as described previously. Local flaps provide the best skin colour and texture match. Larger composite defects may still require free flap reconstruction. This tends to give an inferior result in terms of matching to facial skin colour and texture. Free tissue transfer can provide necessary bulk where the fat pads of the face have been ablated.

2.3 *Summary*

Head and neck reconstruction in the modern era has become largely dependent on the utilisation of microvascular free tissue transfers. Surgery is complicated and prolonged, and pre-operative planning in a multidisciplinary environment is crucial to a satisfactory outcome.

3. Breast Reconstructive Surgery

3.1 *Introduction*

Modern day breast reconstruction is ideally coordinated and administered within a multidisciplinary environment. Plastic and reconstructive surgeons work within this team and need an understanding of the basic principles governing overall care of the patient with breast cancer. Changes in the management of breast cancer in recent years have impacted on the reconstructive options that can be used. The increased diagnosis of high risk patients has also led to an increased number of women having prophylactic mastectomy. There is a constantly evolving understanding and acceptance of breast reconstruction, which has a significant impact on the number of women considering reconstruction. An increasing quality of life and expectation has led to an increase in breast reconstruction in older age patients. All of these factors suggest that breast reconstruction will be increasingly sought after and will become a more integral part of breast cancer management in coming years.

Breast reconstruction involves the use of implants alone, autologous tissue alone or a combination of both. However, the options for breast reconstruction are usually complex, involving multistage surgery and consideration of surgery for the contralateral breast. A brief overview of some of the options available and an approach to decision making is outlined below.

3.2 *Pre-operative assessment*

Ideally women considering breast reconstruction would consult a reconstructive surgeon prior to their ablative procedure. This allows for a discussion of immediate or delayed breast reconstruction. In any discussion, prior to breast reconstruction surgery it is important to gain an in-depth understanding of patients' desires and expectations. Appropriate delineation of expected outcomes and possible complications is essential. Often, women will have negative perceptions regarding implant reconstructions, due to media reports of adverse outcomes from such materials.[27] This can be addressed with the provision of strong medical evidence to show this is not the case.[28]

At the initial assessment, an understanding of the planned or completed breast cancer treatment is important. The plan for adjuvant therapies may impact significantly on decision making in breast reconstruction. If there is a high likelihood of radiation therapy post-mastectomy, it is often better to delay reconstruction. It has been demonstrated about 28% of patients having immediate flap reconstructions will require secondary reconstruction due to radiation effects.[29] Attitudes to surgery for the contralateral breast need to be explored. Often, women will choose to have prophylactic mastectomies if risk factors are felt to be significant enough.

An overall assessment for potentially prolonged surgery and evidence of any peripheral vascular disease may make some patients less suitable for free flap breast reconstruction. Otherwise, general pre-operative work up is appropriate.

3.3 *Immediate versus delayed reconstruction*

Immediate reconstructions permit skin-sparing mastectomies and reduce the total number of procedures and associated costs needed for the final outcome.[30,31] There is some evidence that avoidance of time spent with a mastectomy deformity, by using immediate breast reconstruction can have psychological benefits.[32] However, immediate reconstructions are associated with a two-fold risk of having at least one peri-operative complication.[33] Furthermore, women having delayed reconstructions have a greater improvement in quality of life measures and satisfaction rates than women having immediate reconstruction.[34] Immediate reconstruction may not be a viable option for some women, dependent on the availability of surgeons and facilities, time for recovery, time for decision making and potential planned radiation therapy. Immediate reconstruction is considered by many to be contraindicated if post-mastectomy radiotherapy is planned.[35]

3.4 *Options for breast reconstruction*

3.4.1 *Implant*

Generally implant reconstructions are performed in two stages, with the use of a tissue expander as the first stage. The tissue expander is placed underneath the *pectoralis* muscle at the time of mastectomy (immediate) or at a later date (delayed). This is then expanded with saline through a special port over a period of weeks to months, with weekly or bi-weekly injections. Once the expander is at the correct size (approximately 30% greater than the planned implant volume) inflation is ceased and the tissues allowed to consolidate before the second stage, three months or more later. At the second stage, the expander is removed and replaced with a permanent implant, usually silicone cohesive gel.

Implant reconstruction is associated with shortened operating times and reduced surgical morbidity. There is also no donor site morbidity to consider. However, implants can migrate, leak or ripple. They also form a capsule which can contract and require secondary surgery. Generally, implant reconstructions are less natural to look and feel than autologous reconstructions.

3.4.2   *Autologous tissue and implant*

In an attempt to overcome some of the limitations of "implant alone" breast reconstruction, autologous tissue as an adjunct has been utilised. The reconstruction can then be performed in one stage. The implant is given more soft tissue cover and therefore may have a more natural feel and less obvious implant edges or ripples. At the same time the transferred tissue does not need to supply all of the volume for the breast and is therefore associated with less complex surgery. This may contribute to decreased surgical morbidity. A combination of implant and *latissimus dorsi* muscle transfer can give excellent breast reconstructive results (Fig. 5), while limiting the shortcomings of "implant only" or "autologous only" reconstructions.

3.4.3   *Autologous*

Autologous reconstructions involve the transfer of tissue from other parts of the body as either pedicled flaps (which remain attached) or free flaps (detached and re-attached by microvascular surgery). The most commonly used flaps use the abdominal skin and fat and are based on the deep superior or inferior epigastric vessels. This flap is termed the Transverse Rectus Abdominis

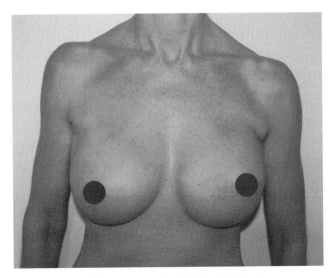

Figure 5. Result 3 months after bilateral breast reconstruction with *latissimus dorsi* flaps and implants undertaken immediately after mastectomy.

Myocutaneous (TRAM) flap. It can be transferred without inclusion of the *rectus abdominis* muscle, when it is termed the Deep Inferior Epigastric Perforator (DIEP) flap after the blood vessel on which it is based. There are a number of other donor sites described, but these are infrequently used.

Pedicled TRAM (Fig. 6)

Blood vessels from the deep superior and inferior epigastric blood vessels pass through the *rectus abdominis* muscle to supply the skin and fat of the abdominal apron. Scheflan *et al.*[36] described a transversly oriented skin ellipse based on these vessels to increase the volume of tissue available and to improve cosmesis of the donor site. A large volume of infraumbilical skin and subcutaneous tissue can be transferred, allowing the reconstruction of a good volume breast in most women. The pedicled TRAM flap relies on preservation of the deep superior epigastric blood vessel. The flap is raised and tunnelled subcutaneously to be positioned on the chest wall at the site of the new breast. The flap is dependent on the non-dominant vascular system and thus lesser volumes of tissue can be

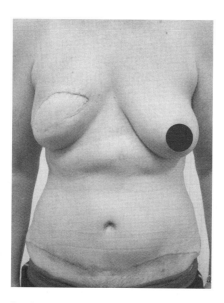

Figure 6. Result 6 weeks after unilateral immediate breast reconstruction with a pedicled TRAM flap.

transferred and there is a higher chance of partial flap loss, compared to free TRAM flap transfer. The pedicled TRAM flap requires complete sacrifice of all of the *rectus abdominis* muscle on that side, which increases the chances of abdominal wall complications.

Free TRAM

The free TRAM flap uses the same skin and subcutaneous tissue as the pedicled TRAM flap, but based on the deep inferior epigastric blood vessels. This is the dominant blood supply for this area and thus greater volumes of tissue can be transferred more reliably. The flap was first described by Holmstrom and requires complete detachment of the flap and then microvascular anastomosis of the vessels to the thoracodorsal vessels in the axilla, or the internal mammary vessels retrosternally. This increases the complexity of the procedure and operating time compared to pedicled TRAM. There is also the possibility of complete flap failure, in up to 1% of cases.[37] The free TRAM flap offers the ability to preserve some or all of the *rectus abdominis* muscle. In the so-called DIEP flap, the small perforators are dissected from the muscle and all the muscle is preserved. This can help decrease morbidity at the level of the abdominal wall. The complete separation of the flap also allows more flexibility for flap shaping and positioning, which is proposed as an advantage over pedicled TRAM flap reconstruction. Although the free TRAM flap is a more complex and demanding technique, requiring microvascular skills that may not be available, it is considered to be the technique that gives the most consistently high quality reconstructive outcomes.

3.5 *Nipple reconstruction*

Many women will wish to have a nipple reconstructed at the appropriate site on the reconstructed breast. This is usually the final stage of breast reconstruction and may be combined with other procedures. There is a bewildering array of techniques described, but the most common ones rely on manipulation of local skin as flaps to create and project an island of skin as a nipple. Many women then choose to have tattooing to create the areolar colouring.

3.6 *Summary*

Breast reconstruction is a field of plastic surgery that is both technically and intellectually demanding. Patients require lengthy detailed consultations to come to a decision and often need a lot of support to cope with the multi-stage surgery that may be required. The results that can be achieved and the satisfaction that patients can get make this surgery a greatly rewarding experience for the patient and the reconstructive surgeon.

References

1. S. J. Mathes and F. Nahai, *Reconstructive Surgery: Principles, Anatomy and Technique* (Churchill Livingstone, London, 1997), pp. 11–12.
2. L. J. Gottlieb and L. M. Krieger, From the reconstructive ladder to the reconstructive elevator, *Plast. Reconstr. Surg.* **93**: 1503–1504 (1994).

3. A. K. Deva, G. H. Buckland, E. Fisher, S. C. Liew, S. Merten, M. McGlynn, M. P. Gianoutsos, M. A. Baldwin and P. G. Lendvay, Topical negative pressure in wound management, *Med. J. Aust.* **7**(173): 128–131 (2000).

4. C. G. Neumann, The expansion of an area of skin by progressive distension of a subcutaneous balloon, *Plast. Reconstr. Surg.* **19**: 124 (1957).

5. S. S. Kroll, An overview of head and neck reconstruction. In: *Reconstructive Plastic Surgery for Cancer,* 1st ed., ed. S. S. Kroll (Mosby, St. Louis, 1996).

6. E. A. Blair and D. L. Callender. Head and neck cancer. The problem, *Clin. Plast. Surg.* **21**: 1–7 (1994).

7. T. Nakatsuka, K. Harii, H. Asato, A. Takushima, S. Ebihara, Y. Kimata, A. Yamada, K. Ueda and S. Ichioka, Analytic review of 2372 free flap transfers for head and neck reconstruction following cancer resection, *J. Reconstr. Microsurg.* **19**: 363–368 (2003).

8. J. D. Suh, J. A. Sercarz, E. Abemayor, T. C. Calcaterra, J. D. Rawnsley, D. Alam and K. E. Blackwell, Analysis of outcome and complications in 400 cases of microvascular head and neck reconstruction, *Arch. Otolaryngol. Head Neck Surg.* **130**: 962–966 (2004).

9. B. H. Haughey, E. Wilson, L. Kluwe, J. Piccirillo, J. Fredrickson, D. Sessions and G. Spector, Free flap reconstruction of the head and neck: Analysis of 241 cases, *Otolaryngol. Head Neck Surg.* **125**: 10–17 (2001).

10. J. J. Disa, A. L. Pusic, D. H. Hidalgo and P. G. Cordeiro, Simplifying microvascular head and neck reconstruction: A rational approach to donor site selection, *Ann. Plast. Surg.* **47**: 385–389 (2001).

11. K. A. Hurvitz, M. Kobayashi and G. R. Evans, Current options in head and neck reconstruction, *Plast. Reconstr. Surg.* **118**: 122e–133e (2006).

12. E. Rosenthal, W. Carroll, M. Dobbs, J. Scott Magnuson, M. Wax and G. Peters, Simplifying head and neck microvascular reconstruction, *Head Neck* **26**: 930–936 (2004).

13. R. B. Smith, J. C. Sniezek, D. T. Weed and M. K. Wax, Microvascular Surgery Subcommittee of American Academy of Otolaryngology — Head and Neck Surgery. Utilization of free tissue transfer in head and neck surgery, *Otolaryngol. Head Neck Surg.* **137**: 182–191 (2007).

14. G. C. Gurtner and G. R. Evans, Advances in head and neck reconstruction, *Plast. Reconstr. Surg.* **106**: 672–682 (2000).

15. J. Teichgraeber, J. Bowman and H. Goepfert, Functional analysis of treatment of oral cavity cancer, *Arch. Otolaryngol. Head Neck Surg.* **112**: 959–965 (1986).

16. N. J. Yousif, W. W. Dzwierzynski, J. R. Sanger, H. S. Matloub and B. H. Campbell, The innervated gracilis musculocutaneous flap for total tongue reconstruction, *Plast. Reconstr. Surg.* **104**: 916–921 (1999).

17. A. H. Salibian, G. R. Allison, W. B. Armstrong, M. E. Krugman, V. V. Strelzow, T. Kelly, J. J. Brugman, P. Hoerauf and B. L. McMicken, Functional hemitongue reconstruction with the microvascular ulnar forearm flap, *Plast. Reconstr. Surg.* **104**: 654–660 (1999).

18. B. H. Haughey, J. C. Beggs, J. Bong, E. M. Genden and A. Buckner, Microneurovascular allotransplantation of the canine tongue, *Laryngoscope* **109**: 1461–1470 (1999).

19. P. Gullane, T. Havas, A. Patterson, T. Todd and B. Boyd, Pharyngeal reconstruction: Current controversies, *J. Otolaryngol.* **16**: 169–173 (1987).

20. C. R. Bradford, R. M. Esclamado and W. R. Carroll, Monitoring of revascularized jejunal autografts, *Arch. Otolaryngol. Head Neck Surg.* **118**: 1042–1044 (1992).

21. R. D. Foster, J. P. Anthony, A. Sharma and M. A. Pogrel, Vascularized bone flaps versus nonvascularized bone grafts for mandibular reconstruction: An outcome analysis of primary bony union and endosseous implant success, *Head Neck* **21**: 66–71 (1999).

22. J. B. Boyd, R. S. Mulholland, J. Davidson, P. J. Gullane, L. E. Rotstein, D. H. Brown, J. E. Freeman and J. C. Irish, The free flap and plate in oromandibular reconstruction: Long-term review and indications, *Plast. Reconstr. Surg.* **95**: 1018–1028 (1995).

23. M.A. Schusterman, G. P. Reece, M. J. Miller and S. Harris, The osteocutaneous free fibula flap: Is the skin paddle reliable? *Plast. Reconstr. Surg.* **90**: 787–793 (1992).

24. G. L. Clayman, F. DeMonte, D. M. Jaffe, M. A. Schusterman, R. S. Weber, M. J. Miller and H. Goepfert, Outcome and complications of extended cranial-base resection requiring microvascular free-tissue transfer, *Arch. Otolaryngol. Head Neck Surg.* **121**: 1253–1257 (1995).

25. P. C. Neligan, S. Mulholland, J. Irish, P. J. Gullane, J. B. Boyd, F. Gentili, D. Brown and J. Freeman, Flap selection in cranial base reconstruction, *Plast. Reconstr. Surg.* **98**: 1159–1166 (1996).

26. J. J. Disa, V. M. Rodriguez and P. G. Cordeiro, Reconstruction of lateral skull base oncological defects: The role of free tissue transfer, *Ann. Plast. Surg.* **41**: 633–639 (1998).

27. M. Palcheff-Wiemer, M. J. Concannon, V. S. Conn and C. L. Puckett, The impact of the media on women with breast implants, *Plast. Reconstr. Surg.* **92**: 779–785 (1993).

28. P. Tugwell, G. Wells, J. Peterson, V. Welch, J. Page, C. Davison, J. McGowan, D. Ramroth and B. Shea, Do silicone breast implants cause rheumatologic disorders? A systematic review for a court-appointed national science panel, *Arthritis Rheum.* **44**: 2477–2484 (2001).

29. N. V. Tran, D. W. Chang, A. Gupta, S. S. Kroll and G. L. Robb, Comparison of immediate and delayed free TRAM flap breast reconstruction in patients receiving postmastectomy radiation therapy, *Plast. Reconstr. Surg.* **108**: 78–82 (2001).

30. C. E. Desch, L. T. Penberthy, B. E. Hillner, M. K. McDonald, T. J. Smith, A. L. Pozez and S. M. Retchin, A sociodemographic and economic comparison of breast reconstruction, mastectomy, and conservative surgery, *Surgery* **125**: 441–447 (1999).

31. A. Khoo, S. S. Kroll, G. P. Reece, M. J. Miller, G. R. Evans, G. L. Robb, B. J. Baldwin, B. G. Wang and M. A. Schusterman, A comparison of resource costs of immediate and delayed breast reconstruction, *Plast. Reconstr. Surg.* **101**: 964–968 (1998).

32. E. E. Elder, Y. Brandberg, T. Björklund, R. Rylander, J. Lagergren, G. Jurell, M. Wickman and K. Sandelin, Quality of life and patient satisfaction in breast cancer patients after immediate breast reconstruction: A prospective study, *Breast* **14**: 201–208 (2005).

33. A. K. Alderman, E. G. Wilkins, H. M. Kim and J. C. Lowery, Complications in postmastectomy breast reconstruction: Two-year results of the Michigan breast reconstruction outcome study, *Plast. Reconstr. Surg.* **109**: 2265–2274 (2002).

34. D. M. Harcourt, N. J. Rumsey, N. R. Ambler, S. J. Cawthorn, C. D. Reid, P. R. Maddox, J. M. Kenealy, R. M. Rainsbury and H. C. Umpleby, The psychological effect of mastectomy with or without breast reconstruction: A prospective, multicenter study, *Plast. Reconstr. Surg.* **111**: 1060–1068 (2003).

35. S. J. Kronowitz, Immediate versus delayed reconstruction, *Clin. Plast. Surg.* **34**: 39–50 (2007).

36. M. Scheflan, C. R. Hartrampf and P. W. Black, Breast reconstruction with a transverse abdominal island flap, *Plast. Reconstr. Surg.* **69**: 908–909 (1982).
37. J. C. Selber, J. E. Kurichi, S. J. Vega, S. S. Sonnad and J. M. Serletti, Risk factors and complications in free TRAM flap breast reconstruction, *Ann. Plast. Surg.* **56**: 492–497 (2006).

27

Cancer and the ENT Surgeon

Timothy P. Makeham,
Julia Crawford,
Mark Smith,
Meville Da Cruz
and Carsten E. Palme

Abstract

Tumours in the head and neck region are diverse in nature and arise within cutaneous, mucosal, glandular, and mesenchymal tissues. They may cause either specific or systemic symptoms directly due to disturbance of upper aerodigestive tract function, indirectly via invasion of local structures, or due to distant metastases. Tumours in this region can be difficult to manage, because they are often advanced at the time of presentation and treatment must strike a balance between limiting morbidity and achieving cure. The challenge for the treating physician is to find the optimal balance between disease specific and overall survival, quality of life, and morbidity for each individual patient. Treatment administration and planning therefore should take place within the setting of a multidisciplinary team, where the appropriate combination of surgery, external beam radiotherapy, and/or chemotherapy for each individual patient can be achieved. Ear, nose and throat surgeons play a central and pivotal role in this setting, as they are uniquely trained in the anatomy, physiology, histopathology, clinical assessment, and surgical management of neoplasms arising within the head and neck region.

Keywords: Head neck cancer, ENT surgeon, multidisciplinary team.

1. Epidemiology

The worldwide incidence of head and neck cancer is thought to be increasing, with an estimated 644,000 new cases of head and neck cancers diagnosed each year.[1] There is a discrepancy between the rate of head and neck cancer in Western countries and developing nations. Head and neck cancer is the fifth most common tumour in the West, while it is the most common tumour in Central Asia.[2,3] The majority of head and neck squamous cell carcinomas (HNSCC) occur in the sixth to seventh decade of life, with men affected more frequently than women.[4] The incidence of HNSCC among women, particularly in the larynx and oropharynx, is thought to be increasing, as more women smoke.[5]

2. Aetiology

The aetiology of tumours within the head and neck vary with the site and tissue of origin. HNSCC is the most common malignant neoplasm in this region and there are several well established risk factors. Cancers of the skin, thyroid, and salivary glands have there own specific risk factors.[6,7]

Development of HNSCC is thought to be the result of a series of genetic events that are influenced by chemical exposure, dietary factors, viral infection, radiation exposure, occupational exposure, and mechanical factors. The concept of field cancerisation, which stipulates that cancers arise from a broadly dysplastic epithelium, is important when considering HNSCC.[7] The appearance of dysplastic epithelium may vary, and it can take the form of leuko-plakia which is a descriptive term meaning white lesion, or erythroplakia meaning red lesion. The concept of multifocal field carcinogenesis partly explains why second or multiple primaries develop in 15% to 25% of patients.[8]

The majority of head and neck cancers are associated with the use of tobacco and alcohol.[9,10] The effect of tobacco and alcohol in HNSCC is multiplicative: HNSCC is six times greater in smokers and as much as 200 times greater in heavy drinkers and smokers. Alcohol in any form increases the risk of HNSCC and a recent study has shown alcohol-containing mouth wash preparations potentially increasing the risk of oral cavity SCC.[11]

Betel nut chewing, which is common in many parts of Asia is associated with HNSCC and is synergistic with tobacco and alcohol use.[12]

Viral infections including Epstein-Barr virus (EBV) and human papilloma virus (HPV) have been linked with certain types of head and neck malignancies. Nasopharyngeal carcinoma (NPC), which is prevalent in northern Africa and Asia is associated with EBV infection. HPV is implicated in up to 35% of all HNSCC and in the subsites of the oral cavity, oropharynx and tonsil are implicated in 50% to 72% of tumours.[13] In one study of oropharyngeal malignancy DNA from HPV subtypes 16, 33, and 35 were found in 40% of tumours. The presence of HPV DNA appears to correlate with tumour sensitivity to chemotherapy and radiotherapy and is a favourable predictor of survival.[14]

There are a number of associations between occupation and head and neck malignancy. The strongest association is that of sinonasal adenocarcinoma in hard wood workers, while exposure to formaldehyde is associated with NPC. Exposure to ionizing radiation is a well established risk factor for developing mesenchymal tumors such as sarcoma and thyroid carcinoma. Gastroesophageal reflux disease is now thought to be a significant risk factor for cancer of the larynx, predominantly that of the anterior two-thirds of the vocal cords.

3. Pathology

Head and neck cancers present a complex heterogenous group of malignancies. There are ten anatomic sites: oral cavity, oropharynx, larynx, hypopharynx, trachea, nasopharynx, nasal cavity and paranasal sinuses, skin and lymphatics, salivary glands, and thyroid glands. Most of these sites have several subsites. Squamous cell carcinoma is the most frequent histological subtype; other tumours are classified as carcinomas (undifferentiated, anaplastic epithelial), adenocarcinoma (adenoid cystic, mucoepidermoid, salivary duct), esthesioneuroblastoma, sarcoma or lymphoma.[15] Table 1 shows a differential diagnosis for an isolated neck lump, which is a common presentation of head and neck malignancies.[16]

Table 1.   Differential diagnosis of the solitary neck mass.

Congenital		Vascular malformation Branchial apparatus abnomality Thyroglossal duct cyst Epidermoid cyst, dermoid, teratoma
Acquired	Inflammatory	Viral, bacterial, fungal Granulomatous: Mycobacterial/ sarcoidosis

	Benign	Salivary gland
		   Pleomorphic adenoma
		   Warthin's tumour
		Thyroid
		Schwannoma
		Fibroma
		Lipoma
		Glomus tumour

	Malignant	Salivary gland
		   Mucoepidermoid, adenoid cystic
		   carcinoma
		Thyroid
		   Papillary, follicular, medullary,
		   Hurthle cell, anaplastic
		   carcinoma
		Sarcoma, lymphoma

	Secondary	SCC (upper aerodigestive
		   tract, skin, unknown primary)
		Adenocarcinoma (GIT, urogenital,
		   lung, breast)
		Salivary gland
		Thyroid

	Traumatic	Haematoma Pseudoaneurysm Neuroma

Modified from Palme *et al.* (2004).[16]

4. Clinical

4.1 *Presentation*

With few exceptions, head and neck malignancies present late, because the early symptoms, if present are indistinguishable from common benign illnesses. Upper aerodigestive tract symptoms such as: epistaxis, nasal obstruction, sore throat, and or globus pharyngeus (foreign body sensation in throat) are common in general practice and are usually due to benign, self-limiting conditions and only occasionally are they due to malignancy.[17]

Tumours of the glottis, oral cavity, lip, and skin are more likely to present at an early stage, as they either symptoms early. Malignancies at other subsites such as the base of tongue, supraglottis, hypopharynx, sinonasal cavity, temporal bone and nasopharynx however can remain notoriously clinically silent for a long time, until they have become significantly advanced. These tumors may then cause symptoms by mass effect on surrounding structures leading to upper aerodigestive tract function impairment, invasion of nearby nerves or bone, lymph node spread, or distant metastases.

Different subsites have particular patterns of presentation, as shown in Table 2.[16] Nasopharyngeal carcinoma presents as a neck mass in up to 90% of cases and/or with a unilateral middle ear effusion when the Eustachian tube is obstructed. Cancers of the oropharynx and hypopharynx produce relatively few symptoms and are not apparent until they cause airway obstruction, odynophagia, dysphagia, trismus, limitations of tongue movement and palpable cervical lymphadenopathy. Sinonasal and anterior skull base tumours may present with symptoms similar to rhinosinusitis and include nasal blockage, discharge and pain. Similarly patients who suffer from temporal bone malignancies may experience hearing loss, pain and discharge which are symptoms commonly seen by the local practitioner.

4.2 *Physical examination*

The purpose of physical examination is to define the diagnosis, stage the tumour if one is clinically present, and provide the grounds for planning further investigations and treatment. With

Table 2. Symptoms and signs according to side of origin in head and neck region.

Site of origin	Symptoms	
Nasopharynx	Early	Hearing loss, tinnitus, epistaxis, nasal obstruction, neck mass
	Late	Headache, cranial nerve abnormalities, trismus, weight loss
Oral cavity	Early	Dysphagia, odynophagia, denture malposition, mouth bleeding
	Late	Pain from bone invasion, cranial nerve abnormalities, tongue tethering, trismus, palpable lymph nodes, weight loss, skin infiltration
Glottic larynx	Early	Dysphonia (hoarseness)
	Late	Dyspnoea (airway obstruction), neck mass
Supraglottis/ orophaynx/ hypopharynx	Early	Dysphagia, unilateral otalgia (earache), neck mass
	Late	Dyspnoea (airway obstruction), odynophagia, palpable lymph nodes, weight loss
Paranasal sinus	Early	Non-healing ulcer, epistaxis, facial dysaesthesia, poor fitting denture
	Late	Unilateral nasal obstruction, headache, diplopia, proptosis, unilateral vision loss

Modified from Kalish and Palme (2008).[17]

the aid of good lighting, basic tongue depressors, otoscope, gloves and a cooperative patient, it should be within the capacity of all physicians to perform a basic head and neck examination which includes careful evaluation of the oral cavity, oropharynx (Tonsil region and soft palate), performing otoscopy and anterior rhinoscopy, through examination of the neck and cranial nerve assessment. The specific skills of the ENT surgeon are required in the assessment of the less accessible subsites, such as the ear, sinonasal cavity, the nasopharynx, larynx and oropharynx. Thorough examination requires the use of a laryngeal mirror, a fibreoptic nasal endoscope or an operating microscope.

Head and neck carcinomas not infrequently present as a solitary neck mass and all who present in this manner should be reviewed by an ENT surgeon. All neck lumps should be assessed in terms of their site, size, shape, colour, contour, consistency, skin attachment and pulsation. Valuable information can be gained, which in the majority of cases will lead to the correct diagnosis. In metastatic disease, the location of the node (as defined in Table 3) can be a clue to the location of the primary tumour. For example, oral cavity tumours spread to level I lymph nodes, tumours of the nasopharynx classically present as level V or posterior triangle lymph node (the jugulodigastric node is the most frequently involved lymph node in NPC), and laryngeal cancers spread most commonly to levels II and III. Supraclavicular lymphadenopathy may suggest a primary arising below the clavicle which includes malignancies such as breast, renal cell, pancreas or bowel.[16]

5.   Management

The aim of investigation of a patient with a suspected malignancy includes confirming the diagnosis, staging, and obtaining all information required to plan appropriate treatment.[18] The decision making process is illustrated in Fig. 1. Confirmation of the diagnosis by histological means is imperative in the management of all suspected tumours. Investigation with plain X-ray, ultrasound, computed tomography, magnetic resonance imaging, and PET scanning are used to stage a tumour and define its extent and respectability. The management of patients with head and neck cancer requires thorough assessment by other medical specialists, including the anaesthetist. This is due to both specific and systemic problems that are unique to this patient population. Head and neck cancer may significantly interfere with normal upper aerodigestive tract function (including the airway) and therefore provide a major challenge when considering general anaesthesia, complex surgery (including ablation and reconstruction), rehabilitation and prolonged recovery. In addition these patients are often elderly and life long smokers, which are associated with significant comorbidities including heart and pulmonary disease.

Table 3. Definition of cervical lymph node levels.

Level I	Submental and submandibular nodes.
Level I A	Submental nodes, between the medial margins of the anterior bellies of the digastric muscles.
Level I B	Submandibular nodes, lateral to level I A nodes and anterior to the back of the submandibular salivary gland.
Level II	Upper internal jugular nodes, posterior to the back of the submandibular salivary gland, anterior to the back of the sternocleidomastoid muscle and above the level of the bottom of the body of the hyoid bone.
Level III	Middle jugular nodes, between the level of the bottom of the body of the hyoid bone and the level of the bottom of the cricoid arch, anterior to the back of the sternocleidomastoid muscle.
Level IV	Low jugular nodes, between the level of the bottom of the cricoid arch and the level of the clavicle, anterior to a line connecting the back of the sternocleidomastoid muscle and the posterolateral margin of the anterior scalene muscles; they are lateral to the carotid arteries.
Level V	Posterior triangle nodes, posterior to the back of the sternocleidomastoid muscle, and posterior to the line described in level IV.
Level V A	Above the level of the bottom of the cricoid arch.
Level V B	Between the level of the bottom of the cricoid atch and the level of the clavicle.
Level VI	Upper visceral nodes, between the carotid arteries from the level of the bottom of the body of the hyoid bone to the level of the top of the manubrium.
Level VII	Superior mediastinal nodes, between the carotid arteries below the level of the top of the manubrium and above the innominate vein.
Supraclavicular nodes	Nodes at, or caudal to, the level of the clavicle and lateral to the carotid artery.
Retropharyngeal nodes	Nodes behind the pharynx, medial to the internal carotid artery, from the skull base down to the level of the hyoid bone.

From Som *et al.* (1999).[43]

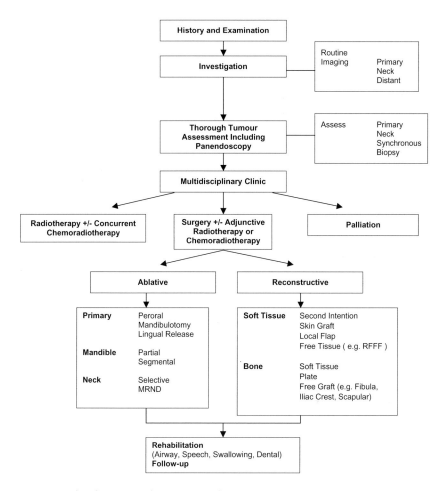

Figure 1. The decision making process for patients with head and neck carcinoma. The overall approach is the same for all patients but with the modality of treatment varying with the type of carcinoma and patient comorbidities. (Modified from Palme *et al.*[18]).

5.1 *Histological diagnosis*

A histological diagnosis can be obtained by a fine needle aspiration (FNA) biopsy, incisional biopsy, or an excisional biopsy. The role of FNA is greatest in the assessment of neck lumps including cervical lymph nodes, salivary gland tumours, and thyroid nodules.[19] FNA is easy to obtain and can be performed under ultrasound or CT guidance, where a lesion is close to vital structures. A non-diagnostic FNA should be repeated and if the subsequent FNA is non-diagnostic an incisional or excisional biopsy should be performed.

Incisional biopsies of the oral cavity and skin can generally be safely performed under a local anaesthetic. Biopsies of all other sites should be performed in an operating theatre, with the surgeon and theatre team prepared to manage all possible airway and haemorrhagic complications. This includes being prepared to perform a surgical tracheostomy under local anaesthetic prior to the biopsy if the patient has an advanced upper aerodigestive tract tumour.

Excisional biopsy can be performed on lymph nodes, skin lesions, and small oral cavity lesions. Excised lymph nodes should be sent to the pathology laboratory fresh and evaluated for amongst other things, lymphoma, tuberculosis, and metastatic carcinoma. Excisional biopsy is a useful strategy in skin lesions, such as melanoma, where a more complex wide local excision may need to be planned.

5.2   Imaging

The use of the various imaging modalities is directed by the location of the tumour and the medical status of the patient. The most common imaging modalities used include chest X-ray, ultrasound, CT, MRI and an orthopantomograph (OPG). A chest X-ray should be performed on all patients with HNSCC, to screen for pulmonary metastases, evidence of aspiration, and chronic lung disease. An OPG is routinely used for assessing mandibular/maxillary involvement and the state of the dentition. Ultrasound is used to characterise neck masses, lesions of the major salivary glands, and thyroid nodules. It also helps facilitate FNA biopsies in a way which is quick, safe, cheap, and radiation free.

Computed tomography scanning provides high resolution three-dimensional assessment of the structures of the head and neck. CT scanning has greater sensitivity and specificity for the detection of cervical lymphadenopathy over physical examination.[20] CT is useful for assessing bone structures, such as the skull base, while MRI provides invaluable information on the soft tissue host tumor interface, neurovascular structures, and fascial planes. This greatly enhances the pre-operative assessment of the surgical resectability of a given tumour.

Positron emission tomography CT (PET CT) is increasingly used in the staging of head and neck cancer, screening for tumour recurrence, evaluation of metastatic carcinoma of unknown primary site, and evaluating tumour response to treatment.

5.3   *Examination under anaesthesia (EUA)*

The mucosa of the upper aerodigestive tract should be thoroughly evaluated at the time the patient is having a biopsy, to obtain a histological diagnosis. The reasons for performing an EUA is to perform a biopsy, to accurately assess the tumour with regard to stage and resectability, and to exlude the presence of a second primary tumour. An EUA involves microlaryngsocopy, oesophagoscopy and bronchoscopy.

5.4   *Staging*

Tumours of the head and neck are staged using the American Joint Commission on Cancer (AJCC) TMN staging system.* The tumour stage is used in the allocation of treatment, measurement of outcomes, determining prognosis, and in research.[21] However, the current staging system is limited, in that it does not account for several important factors, including tumour histopathology and heterogeneity, or patient factors such as age. For example HPV positive oropharyngeal tumours have a better prognosis and response to treatment than HPV negative tumours, suggesting that a less morbid treatment strategy can be utilised. Further the true extent of disease may only become apparent after the surgical resection and the exact histopathological characteristics are known.

---

* T refers to the tumour size and extent at the primary site. The T stage is specific to each individual subsite. N refers to the size and extent of cervical lymph node metastases and is common to all sites except the nasopharynx and cutaneous cancer. M refers to the presence or absence distant metastatic disease.

5.5 *Treatment*

The aims in head and neck cancer treatment are to achieve locoregional control (eradication of the tumour from the site of origin and from the draining lymph nodes), and survival, while maintaining the patients' quality of life. Ideally the treatment is with a single modality (surgical resection or external beam radiotherapy), however, this may not be possible for advanced stage head and neck carcinomas. The treatment for an individual depends on tumour factors, patient factors, institutional/surgeon experience and philosophy, and the availability of health care (health economics). The poor overall prognosis of many advanced stage head and neck cancers, the quality of patient life, and the significant distress and suffering that comes with uncontrolled locoregional disease must all be considered in arriving at an appropriate treatment strategy.

The concept of a multidisciplinary treatment team (MDT) is import in the field of head and neck cancer, as it is best placed to strike a balance between the treatment goals of disease eradication and the patient's quality of life. Further this ensures the patient has access to the appropriate rehabilitation, psychological support, and medical staff to help manage the treatment and treatment related morbidity. Treatments can be painful and deforming and the related morbidity affects many of the basic activities of daily living, such as verbal and non-verbal communication and eating. As such, an MDT involves a wide variety of specialists including the ENT surgeon, reconstructive surgeon, medical oncologist, radiation oncologist, specialist nurse, speech therapist, dietician, occupational therapist, and social worker.

Depending on the overall picture of the patient, the aim of treatment may be curative or palliative. Even in palliative treatment of head and neck cancers, management of the local tumour can be of paramount importance, as uncontrolled disease can lead to significant upper aerodigestive tract dysfunction, in terms of the airway, swallowing, speech, smell, sight, and taste.

The choice of curative treatment depends on many factors, but importantly the stage of the malignancy. Early disease will typically involve one treatment modality, either surgery or radiotherapy.

Late disease usually requires a combined therapy approach, including primary surgery with adjuvant radiotherapy or neoadjuvant/concurrent chemoradiotherapy.

6. Subsites of Head and Neck Pathology

6.1 *Malignant lesions of the temporal bone*

Tumours involving the temporal bone are rare, and present with symptoms similar to inflammatory ear disease, often mistaken for chronic otitis externa. Temporal bone cancer tends to affect the 50- to 60-year-old age group predominantly and gender proportion is near equal. Exposure to ultraviolet light is the most common aetiological factor in laterally arising lesions. Chronic inflammation is thought to cause those that arise more medially.

Squamous cell carcinoma is the most frequent type of malignancy arising in the temporal bone. Adenocarcinoma, melanoma, and mesenchymal tumours are rarer causes of temporal bone malignancy. The symptoms of pain, discharge and hearing loss are commonly associated with benign, as well as malignant disease. Severe pain, bleeding and facial palsy are relatively uncommon in chronic inflammatory disease and point to a more sinister cause.

Treatment of temporal bone malignancy is a major undertaking and necessitates specialist resources for surgical resection and reconstruction, as well as post-operative radiotherapy and rehabilitation. There is currently no role for external beam radiotherapy as a single modality treatment, or for chemotherapy in treatment of temporal bone malignancy except in a palliative setting.[22]

6.2 *Mucosal squamous cell carcinoma*

The topic of head and neck cancer is dominated by the heterogeneous group of mucosal squamous cell carcinomas, which can arise from any portion of the upper aerodigestive tract. Treatment of this condition must take into consideration the following factors:

- tumour site,
- tumour stage,

- function of the site in which the tumour arises, and
- histopathological tumour factors — margin status, depth of tumour invasion, tumour grade, perineural and perivascular spread of the tumour.

Tumour site is defined by the anatomical units of the upper aerodigestive tract and includes the oral cavity, oropharynx, larynx, hypopharynx, nasopharynx and sinonasal cavity. The tumours within each of these regions are further considered in terms of separate subsites. These regions are considered separately, on the grounds that tumour presentation, incidence, aetiology, behaviour, and treatment are significantly influenced by the individual anatomic and physiologic characteristics of each region.

6.2.1 *Oral cavity carcinoma*

Oral cavity cancers are primarily managed with surgical resection and/or adjuvant external beam radiotherapy. Consideration for adding chemotherapy is given in those cases that are deemed high risk however no prospective data exists currently as to its benefit. In general early stage disease (Stage I/II) is managed with surgical resection only, while those with advanced disease require a multimodality approach.[18]

The most important prognostic factor in the management of oral cavity cancer is the status of the lymph nodes. While later stage (T3/T4) disease will require treatment of the cervical lymph nodes, the detection and management of occult lymph node metastases in early stage (T1/T2) tumours provide a significant management dilemma. It is generally accepted that the neck nodes should be treated where the risk of occult nodal metastases is greater than 20%. The subsite involved, the size of the primary, and high risk features such as perineural spread, perivascular spread, or tumour thickness greater than 5 mm predict the presence of occult lymph node metastases. Tumours of the hard palate, upper gum, and lip have low rates of metastatic disease, while buccal mucosal, floor of mouth, and oral tongue cancers have higher rates of nodal metastases and a poorer prognosis.

The decision to manage the neck with surgery, radiotherapy, or combined modality depends on the treatment of the primary, need for reconstruction, and the histopathological characteristics of both the tumour and neck lymphatics.

6.2.2 *Oropharyngeal carcinoma*

The oropharynx consists of the soft palate, tonsil, and tongue base, with the prognosis and treatment being site dependent. The stage related prognosis for each subsite is shown in Table 4. Soft palate carcinoma tends to behave in a relatively indolent manner and presents generally at an early stage. The risk of occult nodal metastases is high and may be predicted by the thickness of the primary tumour, with low rates seen where the thickness is less than 3 mm.[23] Treatment of early stage disease can be either surgical, or with radiotherapy (either external beam, or brachytherapy).

Tonsillar carcinoma has an association with previous HPV infection (particularly subtype 16). Survival and locoregional control rates are comparable between surgery and radiotherapy for Stages I and II disease. Simple transoral surgical excision may be adequate for Stage I disease, however, later stage disease requires more radical surgery and free flap reconstruction. The treatment decision in late stage oropharyngeal tumours depends on many factors but most significantly on morbidity of treatment and the quality of life of the patient. For this reason most tumours are primarily managed with concurrent chemoradiotherapy.

Tumours of the tongue base tend to be advanced at the time of presentation, due to its silent location and the propensity for early nodal spread (70% of T1 tongue base tumours have nodal

Table 4. Five-year survival statistics for oropharyngeal carcinoma.

Stage	Soft palate[40] (%)	Tonsil[41] (%)	Tongue base[42] (%)
I	83	100	65
II	78	86	54
III	38	82	44
IV	26	IVa 63	30
		IVb 22	

metastases). The functional status is superior for early tumours treated with radiotherapy, rather than surgery. For advanced stage disease surgery is unacceptably morbid, often requiring total glossectomy, including total laryngectomy. Concurrent chemoradiotherapy has become treatment of choice for these complex tumours, with comparable outcomes to radical surgery.

6.2.3 Laryngeal carcinoma

The larynx is subdivided into the glottis, supraglottis, and subglottis, each of which have different lymphatic drainage characteristics, metastatic potential, and management strategies.

More than 90% of laryngeal carcinomas are of squamous cell type, for which the risks factors include smoking, alcohol, HPV infection, gastroesophageal reflux, and exposure to inhaled toxins. The remaining tumours arise in the minor salivary glands (adenoid cystic and mucoepidermoid carcinoma) or mesenchymal tissues (such as chondrosarcoma).

Symptoms will vary depending of the location of the tumour. Glottic tumours are more likey to present at an early stage with a hoarse voice, as even small changes in the contour, thickness or vibratory characteristics of the vocal cord produce a perceived change in phonation. Tumours of the subglottis and supraglottis do not produce functional impairment until they are larger, so they present in a more advanced stage. Late symptoms include airway obstruction, unilateral otalgia, odynophagia and or dysphagia.

Careful clinical assessment of the tumour by direct visualisation using a flexible nasendoscope, or in the operating theatre is required to determine which treatment approach is best suited to the patient. The management of the neck nodes in early larynx carcinoma is subsite dependent. With the exception of locally recurrent T1 or T2 glottic carcinomas, or those involving the anterior commissure, the risk of nodal metastases is low and approximately 0%–7%. For all other laryngeal subsites the risk is higher and treatment of the neck with surgery or radiotherapy is generally required.

The treatment goals of early stage laryngeal carcinoma are to cure the primary tumour while preserving upper aerodigestive tract function (airway, protection, phonation, deglutition) and quality of life. The strategies available include transoral laser resection, primary external beam radiotherapy, and partial laryngeal surgery. The expectation should be local control rates in excess of 90% (better for T1N0 carcinomas), preservation of upper aerodigestive tract function and acceptable quality of life.[24]

Locally advanced laryngeal tumours have a much poorer prognosis than early stage disease and voice preservation is a secondary treatment goal to curative intent. Organ preserving concurrent chemoradiotherapy protocols may be recommended in patients with T3 tumours (fixed vocal cord). Where the primary tumour is more advanced, with cartilage invasion or extralaryngeal spread, total laryngectomy and adjunctive external beam radiotherapy is the best treatment. Overall survival does not appear to differ significantly between either an organ preserving, or the more traditional approach of radical surgery followed by external beam radiotherapy. Regardless of the treatment strategy employed, speech therapy and rehabilitation is critical to achieving good outcomes.

6.2.4 Hypopharyngeal carcinoma

The hypopharynx is a rare site for tumours and occurs predominantly in males. Tumours of this region present in advanced stages and have poor survival rates with any treatment modality. Primary treatment options include external beam radiotherapy, surgery, chemotherapy or combination. Early stage tumours are most commonly managed using single modality, whereas advanced tumours require a more radical approach. This includes total laryngopharyngectomy, adjuvant external beam radiotherapy or concurrent chemoradiotherapy as an attempt at organ preservation. Despite these measures, disease specific and overall survival at five years, are well less then 50%.

6.2.5 Nasopharyngeal carcinoma

Nasopharyngeal carcinoma (NPC) arise within the nasopharynx, which is located in the upper part of the pharynx behind the nose. NPC has a regional preponderance and is endemic in south east China, some regions in the Middle East, Mediterranean and North Africa. This condition has other genetic associations, which include HLA types A2, B14, B46, B Sin2, or haplotypes Aw19, Bw46.[25] The condition is strongly associated with the Epstein-Barr virus, and to a lesser extend to smoking and possibly to the consumption of salt cured fish which contain carcinogenic nitrosamines.[25]

Surgery has a limited role in the primary treatment of this condition and may be reserved for salvage of the neck and rarely to the primary site. The mainstay of management includes external beam radiotherapy for early stage disease and concurrent chemoradiotherapy for later stage disease. Long term follow-up with direct visualisation of the nasopharynx is important and has been greatly facilitated by modern endoscopes.

6.2.6 Squamous cell carcinoma of unknown primary site

Carcinoma presenting as metastatic nodal neck disease in the absence of a symptomatic primary tumour is an infrequent but not uncommon presentation. The cervical lymph nodes are the most common site for metastatic squamous cell carcinoma of unknown primary site. Evaluation of these patients includes histological evaluation of the metastatic node via an FNA, and a thorough evaluation of the potential primary sites (most commonly the oropharynx or nasopharynx). A thorough evaluation includes endoscopic evaluation of the nasopharynx, larynx, bronchii, and oesophagus. Tonsillectomy with blind biopsies of the nasopharynx and tongue base should also be performed if there is no obvious primary on panendoscopy. A tonsil primary is detected in up to 25% of patients with cervical nodal disease and in approximately 5% the primary is in the tonsil contralateral to the nodal metastases. CT-PET scanning can localise the primary in a quarter of patients and can detect previously unrecognised distant metastatic disease. The FNA specimen can be analysed for EBV and HPV DNA to help localise the primary site and direct treatment. Detection of EBV DNA implies a nasopharyngeal primary and which should be included in the radiotherapy treatment field. Management of the neck nodal disease can be with surgery (neck dissection), radiotherapy, or concurrent chemoradiotherapy. Neck dissection offers the same overall survival as radiotherapy. Adjunctive radiotherapy following neck dissection should be strongly considered where the neck disease demonstrates high risk features such as extracapsular extension, multiple positive nodes, or poorly differentiated tumour histology. The radiotherapy field should involve the contralateral neck as there is a lower risk of recurrent disease. Survival does not appear to be improved by irradiation of potential primary sites. Concurrent chemoradiotherapy may offer a survival benefit over single modality treatment, though this is yet to be conclusively demonstrated. About 50% of patients who undergo single modality treatment are alive and free of disease at 5 years, while this rate is as high as 70% in preliminary studies of concurrent chemoradiotherapy protocols. Approximately 10% of patients will develop a head and neck primary following treatment, while a further 10% will develop distant metastatic disease.

6.3   *Sinonasal carcinoma*

Diagnosis, treatment and monitoring of sinonasal carcinoma has evolved and changed greatly with the improvement of endoscopic equipment, imaging technology and surgical techniques. Tumours in this region are uncommon and the histological subtypes include squamous cell carcinoma, adenocarcinoma (particuarly in patients exposed to hardwood dust), olfactory neuroblastoma, adenoid cystic carcinoma, sarcoma and mucosal melanoma. Patients with these conditions have a broad number of presentations that coincide with more benign and common pathologies.

The modalities utilised include surgery, radiotherapy, and concurrent chemoradiotherapy. The selection of an appropriate treatment strategy is influenced by tumour, patient and institutional treatment factors.[26] Surgery can be used as a primary treatment modality, or as a salvage option after radiotherapy/concurrent chemoradiotherapy; there are a broad number of surgical procedures and strategies possible, including craniofacial resection. These procedures, which benefit greatly from advances in real time three-dimensional imaging technologies, require an experienced team comprising an ENT surgeon, neurosurgeon, and reconstructive surgeon.

6.4   *Thyroid carcinoma*

Cancer of the thyroid is rare, representing only 1% of all cancers, but includes several distinct tumour types which are each associated with their own distinct epidemiological, clinical and prognostic features. There are four main pathologies encountered in thyroid cancer: papillary, follicular, medullary and anaplastic.

Unlike most head and neck tumours, thyroid cancer is more common in women. For differentiated and anaplastic thyroid carcinomas, the female to male ratio is 3:1 and for medullary carcinoma the ratio is 4:3. The most important risk factor in differentiated thyroid carcinoma is previous irradiation. Other factors include genetic predisposition, geographical distribution, Hashimoto's disease and iodine content of the diet.[27]

Presentation of thyroid neoplasms is similar to benign lesions; any solitary thyroid lump needs to be treated with suspicion. Recent growth, or evidence of hoarseness, dysphagia or obstruction should raise the possibility of a neoplastic growth.[28] All thyroid nodules need to be investigated with routine thyroid function tests, ultrasound and a fine needle aspiration biopsy.

The treatment of papillary and follicular carcinoma involves either hemi or total thyroidectomy. After undergoing a total thyroidectomy, a significant number of patients receive radioiodine (I^{131}) to ablate the remnant thyroid bed and decrease the likelihood of recurrent disease.[29] Patients with medullary thyroid carcinoma should undergo total thyroidectomy with regional lymph node dissection. Patients with anaplastic carcinoma have a grave prognosis and treatment is supportive — focusing on maximising the quality of the remaining life.

6.5   *Carcinoma of the salivary glands*

The major and minor salivary glands of the head and neck are the site of a diverse group of benign and malignant neoplasms. Malignant salivary neoplasms account for 7% of head and neck cancers. Tumours most commonly occur in the parotid gland. The risk of a tumour being malignant is inversely proportional to the size of the gland in which it arises. Forty per cent of submandibular gland tumours are malignant and the majority of minor salivary gland tumours are malignant, however, the parotid gland is the most common site for malignant neoplasms. Malignant tumours of the parotid gland in Australia are most commonly metastatic cutaneous SCC.[30] The most common primary malignancy is mucoepidemoid carcinoma, except in the location of the lingual gland, where 40% to 60% of tumours are adenoid cystic.

Salivary gland tumours may present as a mass in the upper aerodigestive tract (hard palate), or more commonly as a mass within one of the major salivary glands. Features that suggest a malignant pathology include nerve palsy, pain, tethering to nearby structures, and rapid growth. The presence of a facial nerve palsy in association with a parotid tumour is strongly suggestive of a malignant tumour and carries a poor overall prognosis.[31]

Treatment of salivary gland tumours is with primary surgery and adjunctive radiotherapy. Primary treatment with radiotherapy or chemoradiotherapy occurs where the tumour is unresectable, or the patient is not suitable for a general anaesthetic.

7.   Role of ENT Surgery in Head and Neck Cancer

Otolaryngology head and neck surgeons (otherwise known as ENT surgeons) are the natural custodians of the field of head and neck cancer management and the evolution of the specialty is closely linked with the treatment of head and neck cancer. The role of the ENT surgeon incorporates the accurate diagnosis and assessment of a patient's cancer, co-ordination of the patient's treatment within the setting of a multidisciplinary treatment team, surgical treatment, research and evaluation of treatment strategies, and advocacy of needs of patients afflicted by head and neck cancer to health authorities and the broader community. Thus, the role of the ENT surgeon extends from primary care giver and primary prevention to the tertiary treatment of head and neck cancer.

7.1   *History of head and neck surgery*

State-of-the-art contemporary management of head and neck cancer has become possible given the significant advances and evolution of diagnostic techniques, anaesthetic techniques, surgical instruments, surgical techniques, reconstructive techniques, and radiotherapy techniques. In considering this history it is also important to recognise the importance of the expanding knowledge base of the conditions we treat. The recognition of important aetiological factors and education of the broader community with regard to such things as the risk posed by smoking has changed significantly over the last 150 years.

Surgical excision and reconstruction using pedicled flaps for cutaneous malignancies have been utilised for a long time. Shushrata described a forehead flap for nasal carcinomas 2000 years ago and Tagliacozzi used pedicled flaps from the upper arm for facial defects in the 16th century.[32] Due to the inaccessibility of the laryngeal and pharyngeal pathology, diagnosis and management of these pathologies stalled until the development of modern endoscopic techniques. The larynx was initially visualised by Manuel Patricio Rodriquez Garcia of the Paris conservatory using a dental mirror, but it was the development of direct endoscopy by Dr. Chevalier Jackson that permitted accurate assessment of the upper aerodigestive tract.[33] Detailed assessment of tumours allowed the planning of therapeutic interventions and the first partial laryngectomy in 1867 by Dr. Solis-Cohen, followed by the first total laryngectomy performed by Billroth in 1874.[34] These procedures remain in the armamentarium of modern head and neck surgeons and have been greatly improved by advances in technology, anaesthesia, post-operative care, radiotherapy, and voice rehabilitation.

Recognition of the pathways of cancer spread from its primary site to the cervical lymph nodes and treatment of these metastatic deposits with surgical dissection has improved locoregional control of head and neck cancers. Crile described radical neck dissection in 1906 and modified radical neck dissection was described by Bocca in 1967. Treatment of the cervical nodes is an important focus for the treatment of many head and neck cancers and the surgical approaches include selective dissection of the cervical nodes, comprehensive dissection of all the cervical nodes, and modified radical neck dissection (which includes the sacrifice of the internal jugular vein, sternocleidomastoid muscle, and accessory nerve).

Organ preserving surgery and treatment has become the focus in the current management of head and neck cancer. The operating microscope in combination with the development of microsurgical instruments allowed the microsurgical treatment of selected laryngeal tumours — which was first reported in the 1960s by Kleinsaser.[35] Strong and Jako reported the treatment of early laryngeal tumours with carbon dioxide laser in 1972. Advances in these techniques have provided an important alternative to primary radiotherapy in the treatment of early stage laryngeal tumours. Surgical treatment outcomes have also benefited from the development of microvascular surgical techniques, which have allowed free tissue grafting to better reconstruct the defects of surgical resections with lower rates of complications and morbidity.[36]

Paralleling the development of surgical instruments and techniques there have been major advances the development of anaesthetic agents, monitoring, and techniques allowing longer, more complex operations. Additionally, the advent of CT scanning, MRI, and CT PET scanning have allowed improved patient selection for treatment. Skull base surgery has greatly benefitted from the improved diagnostic capacity, as well as the development of image guidance systems that greatly enhance the accuracy and safety of surgery in this anatomically complex area.

7.2   *ENT surgeon as the primary care physician*

Ear nose and throat (ENT) surgery is a broad surgical specialty that has at its core a general ENT training programme from which surgeons sub-specialise. The sub-specialty divisions include head and neck surgery, neurotology and skull base surgery, rhinology and anterior skull base surgery, reconstructive surgery, and facial plastic surgery. The presentation of malignant diseases of the head and neck can mimic many benign diseases and it is the role of all ENT surgeons to accurately differentiate between diagnoses and thoroughly examine the upper aerodigestive tract.

Common presenting symptoms of cancers in this region are the cause of many referrals to ENT surgeons and include hoarseness, oral ulceration, sore throat, otalgia, bleeding, nasal obstruction, dysphagia or globus sensation and or cervical lymphadenopathy.[17] Secondary symptoms include deafness (due to intracranial skull base tumours or Eustachian tube obstruction from nasopharyngeal tumours), aspiration pneumonia, facial nerve palsy, or sinusitis. Where the ENT surgeon is the primary point of contact, the role of the surgeon is to diagnose the condition, provide counseling and support for the patient, act as a contact point for the patient's general practitioner, and ensure appropriate and prompt referral to an appropriate treatment centre.

7.3 ENT surgeon as the tertiary care physician

Head and neck oncological treatment occurs within a tertiary setting, owing to the complexity of the conditions being treated, the intensity of the hospital resource requirements, and the requisite coordination of large number of specialists and therapies involved in treatment and rehabilitation of patients. The collaboration of medical specialists and allied health professionals is broadly termed the multidisciplinary team (MDT). Within this context the ENT surgeon plays a central role and the role in treatment depends on the sub-specialty interest of the ENT surgeon.

Head and neck services have, prior to the advent of MDT's, evolved in a fragmented manner, alongside the surgical sub-specialties of otolaryngology, maxillofacial surgery, plastic surgery, and general surgery. The single specialty units or single clinician-based practises, therefore, delivered a heterogeneous collective of treatments with wide variations in standards and workload.[37] MDT's allow the patient to a broad range of treatment options in a coordinated and timely fashion, tailoring treatment to the patient and disease specific factors. MDT's are now the standard of care across the world in the treatment of head and neck cancer and this approach has been shown to correlate with improved patient outcomes and survival.[38] Further, the MDT approach has been shown to increase patient satisfaction with the treatment experience and fosters a collegiality among the staff of the team.

7.3.1 The role of the ENT surgeons in MDT

Arising from the Calman-Heine report, it was proposed that all patients with cancer should be seen by surgeons who specialised in their type of cancer and worked with colleagues in multidisciplinary teams that included diagnostic specialist and nurses.[39]

7.3.2 *The purpose and benefits of MDT*

The difficulty in treating head and neck malignancy effectively is that the disease is relatively uncommon, involves multiple organ sites, pathological subtypes, and specialised resources are required. A multidisciplinary team is a group composed of members with varied but complementary experience, qualifications and skills that contribute to the achievement of specific objectives. For the treatment of head and neck pathology the team will include an ENT surgeon, radiation oncologist, medical oncologist, MDT co-ordinator and allied health staff including a speech pathologist, dietitian, psychologist, dentist and dedicated MDT nursing staff. The purpose of the MDT is to establish a diagnosis for patients, classify the disease according to a recognised system and plan appropriate treatment based on best available evidence base and institutional factors.[39]

There are many benefits to an MDT in the management of patients with head and neck carcinoma. Not only does it allow the synergistic involvement of a diverse range of medical professionals, but it also aides in focusing a broad range of treatments on the specific needs of an individual patient. It also facilitates medical research, auditing of outcomes, and more cost effective treatment.[39]

7.4 *ENT surgeon as innovator, educator and researcher*

The progression, evolution, and maintenance of treatment standards of the specialty of ENT in the treatment of head and neck cancer has occurred from the process of recursively evaluating treatment outcomes and incorporating new technologies and scientific discoveries into treatment. Technological advances in medical imaging, histopathological assessment and the delivery of radiotherapy have continued to mould treatments and outcomes, as have advances in the understanding of the molecular mechanism of cancer and tumour targeted therapies, such as protein kinase receptor antibodies and human papilloma virus vaccines becoming available. Research allows rigorous evaluation of these new stategies and helps define their role in the overall treatment paradigm. Research can also be focused on a spectrum of end points including novel imaging techniques for staging and treatment evaluation, therapeutic approaches including organ preservation strategies, rehabilitation, quality of life and prognostic factors.[39]

MDT's with centralised treatment allows an increased recruitment into clinical trials investigating new techniques and innovations in treatment. Larger treatment bases increase the opportunity for audit of current treatment outcomes. The publishing of research arising from each unit, combined with the presentation of the results at national and international meetings ensures that there is worldwide collaboration and advances in treatment are widespread.

The ENT surgeon must be an educator of peers, trainees, other medical and allied health specialties, and of the broader community. In the community, much of the pathology that the ENT surgeon deals with has a basis in common behaviours like smoking and alcohol consumption, which are preventable causes of disease. Primary prevention and early recognition are critical in many fields of cancer management in terms of reducing the community wide disease burden. Head and neck cancer is no different and early appropriate referral by general practitioners, dentists, and community health workers can lead to better outcomes through treatment of early stage disease, as no effective screening programmes for head and neck cancer are currently avalible.

8.   Conclusion

The ENT surgeon with an intimate knowledge of the head and neck region plays an important and integral role in head and neck malignancy from the point of diagnosing the condition, through examination to planning and executing treatment, followed by surveillance after treatment, which is usually life-long. In addition ENT surgeons, working within a multidisciplinary team can contribute to a number of adjunctive roles including ongoing research and education.

References

1. S. Marur and A. A. Forastiere, Head and neck cancer: Changing edidemiology, diagnosis, and treatment, *Mayo Clin. Proc.* **83**(4): 489–501 (2008).

2. P. H. Rhys Evans, P. Q. Montgomery and P. J. Guillane, *Principles and Practice of Head and Neck Oncology* (Martin Dunitz, United Kingdom, 2003).

3. D. M. Parkin, P. Pisani and J. Ferlay, Global cancer statistics, *CA Cancer J. Clin.* **49**: 33–64 (1999).

4. A. G. Sikora, P. Toniolo and M. D. Delacure, The changing demographics of head and neck squamous cell carcinoma in the United States, *Laryngoscope* **114**: 1915–1923 (2004).

5. C. H. Shiboski, B. L. Schmidt and R. C. Jordan, Tongue and tonsil carcinoma: Increasing trends in the U.S. population ages 20–44 years, *Cancer* **103**(9): 1843–1849 (2005).

6. M. J. Veness, S. Porceddu, C. E. Palme and G. J. Morgan, Cutaneous head and neck squamous cell carcinoma metastatic to parotid and cervical lymph nodes, *Head Neck* **29**(7): 621–631 (2007).

7. D. P. Slaughter, H. W. Southwick and W. Smejkal, Field cancerization in oral stratified squamous epithelium: Clinical implications of multicentric origin, *Cancer* **6**: 963–968 (1953).

8. B. H. Haughey, G. A. Gates, C. L. Arfken *et al.*, Meta-analysis of second malignant tumors in head and neck cancer: The case for an endoscopic screening protocol, *Ann. Otol. Rhinol. Laryngol.* **101**: 105–112 (1992).

9. M. R. Spitz, Epidemiology and risk factors for head and neck cancer, *Semin. Oncol.* **21**: 281–288 (1994).

10. R. Wight, V. Paleri and P. Arullendran, Current theories for the development of nonsmoking and nondrinking laryngeal carcinoma, *Curr. Opin. Otolaryngol. Head Neck Surg.* **11**: 73–77 (2003).

11. M. McCullough and C. S. Farah, The role of alcohol in oral carcinogenesis with particular reference to alcohol-containing mouthwashes, *Aust. Dent. J.* **53**(4): 302–305 (2008).

12. D. Goldenberg, J. Lee, W. M. Koch *et al.*, Habitual risk factors for head and neck cancer, *Otolaryngol. Head Neck Surg.* **131**: 986–993 (2004).

13. J. Mork, K. Lie, E. Glatte *et al.*, Human papilloma virus infection as a risk for squamous cell carcinomas of the head and neck, *N. Engl. J. Med.* **344**: 1125–1131 (2001).

14. C. Fakhry, W. Westra, S. Li *et al.*, Prognostic significance of Human Papilloma Virus (HPV) tumor status for patients with head and neck squamous cell carcinoma (HNSCC) in a prospective multicenter clinical trial, *J. Clin. Oncol.* **25**: 299s (2007).

15. J. Giralt, S. Benavente and M. Arguis, Optimizing approaches to head and neck cancer: Strengths and weaknesses in multidisciplinary treatments of locally advanced disease, *Ann. Oncol.* **19**(7): 195–199 (2008).

16. C. E. Palme, P. J. Gullane and J. Irish, Solitary neck mass. In: *Current Surgical Therapy*, 8th edn., ed. J. L. Cameron (Elsevier, Mosby, Philadelphia, 2004), pp. 1061–1066.

17. L. Kalish and C. E. Palme, Globus pharyngeus and an approach to dysphagia, *Mod. Med.* **9**(5): 28–38 (2008).

18. C. E. Palme, P. J. Gullane and R. W. Gilbert, Current treatment options in squamous cell carcinoma of the oral cavity, *Surg. Oncol. Clin. N. Am.* **13**(1): 47–70 (2004).

19. X. Punthakee, C. E. Palme, J. H. Franklin, I. Zhang, J. L. Freeman and Y. C. Bedard, Fine-needle aspiration biopsy findings suspicious for papillary thyroid carcinoma: A review of cytopathological criteria, *Laryngoscope* **115**(3): 433–436 (2005).

20. R. M. Merritt, M. F. Williams, T. H. James *et al.*, Detection of cervical metastasis, *Arch. Otolaryngol. Head Neck Surg.* **123**: 149–152 (1997).

21. C. E. Palme, S. G. MacKay, I. Kalnins, G. J. Morgan and M. J. Veness, The need for a better prognostic staging system in patients with metastatic cutaneous squamous cell carcinoma of the head and neck, *Curr. Opin. Otolaryngol. Head Neck Surg.* **15**(2): 103–106 (2007).

22. D. A. Moffat, J. A. Chiossone-Kendel and M. Da Cruz, Squamous cell carcionoma. In: *Principles and Practice of Head and Neck Oncology*, eds. P. H. Rhys-Evans, P. Q. Montgomeny and P. J. Gullane (Martin Dunitz — an imprint of the Taylor and Francis Group, London, 2003), pp. 355–375.

23. S. Baredes, D. J. Leeman, T. S. Chen and M. A. Mohit-Tabatabai, Significance of tumour thickness in soft palate carcinoma, *Laryngoscope* **103**: 389–393 (1993).

24. W. Steiner, P. Ambrosch, C. E. Palme *et al.*, Laser microsurgical resection of T1a glottic carcinoma: Results of 333 cases, presented at the *126th Annual Meeting of the American Laryngological Association, Boca Raton, FL, May 13–14, 2005* [abstract].

25. E. T. Chang and H. O. Adami, The enigmatic epidemiology of nasopharyngeal carcinoma, *Cancer Epidemiol. Biomarkers Prev.* **15**(10): 1765–1777 (2006).

26. N. Oddone, G. J. Morgan, C. E. Palme, L. Perera, J. Shannon, E. Wong, V. Gebski and M. J. Veness, Metastatic cutaneous squamous cell

carcinoma of the head and neck: The immunosuppression, treatment, extranodal spread, and margin status (ITEM) prognostic score to predict outcome and the need to improve survival, *Cancer* **115**: 1883–1891 (2009).

27. S. N. Raza, M. D. Shah, C. E. Palme, F. T. Hall, S. Eski and J. L. Freeman, Risk factors for well-differentiated thyroid carcinoma in patients with thyroid nodular disease, *Otolaryngol. Head Neck Surg.* **139**(1): 21–26 (2008).

28. J. L. Freeman and C. E. Palme, Thyroid nodular evaluation and treatment in elderly patients, *Geriatr. Ageing* **6**(1): 18–22 (2003).

29. S. L. Cushing, C. E. Palme, N. Audet, S. Eski, P. G. Walfish and J. L. Freeman, Prognostic factors in well-differentiated thyroid carcinoma, *Laryngoscope* **114**(12): 2110–2115 (2004).

30. C. E. Palme, C. J. O'Brien, M. J. Veness, E. B. McNeil, L. P. Bron and G. J. Morgan, Extent of parotid disease influences outcome in patients with metastatic cutaneous squamous cell carcinoma, *Arch. Otolaryngol. Head Neck Surg.* **129**(7): 750–753 (2003).

31. N. Audet, C. E. Palme, P. J. Gullane, R. W. Gilbert, D. H. Brown, J. Irish and P. Neligan, Cutaneous metastatic squamous cell carcinoma to the parotid gland: Analysis and outcome, *Head Neck* **26**(8): 727–732 (2004).

32. J. P. Shah, The making of a specialty, *Am. J. Surg.* **176**: 398–403 (1998).

33. K. Fung, The role of ENT surgeons in head and neck surgery, *Hong Kong Med. Diary* **12**(7): 9–10 (2007).

34. S. Zeitels and J. da Silva Solis-Cohen, America's first head and neck surgeon, *Head Neck* **19**(4): 342–346 (1997).

35. E. Helidonis, The history of otolaryngology from ancient to modern times, *Am. J. Otolaryngol.* **14**(6): 382–393 (1993).

36. C. E. Palme and P. J. Gullane, Principles of oral cavity reconstruction. In: *Oral Cavity Reconstruction*, eds. T. Day and D. A. Girod (Taylor and Francis Pty Ltd., New York, 2006), pp. 1–9.

37. J. Jeannon *et al.*, Implementing the national institute of clinical excellence improving outcome guidelines for head and neck cancer: Developing a business plan with reorganization of head and neck cancer services, *Clin. Otolaryngol.* **33**: 116–151 (2008).

38. P. J. Bradley, B. Zutshi and C. M. Nutting, An audit of clinical resources available for the care of head and neck cancer patients in England, *Clin. Oncol.* **17**: 604–609 (2005).

39. T. Westin and J. Stalfors, Tumour boards/multidiscinplinary head and neck cancer meetings: Are they of value to patients, treating staff or a political additional drain on healthcare resources? *Curr. Opin. Otolaryngol. Head Neck Surg.* **16**: 103–107 (2008).

40. R. J. Amdur, W. M. Medenhall, T. T. Parsons *et al.*, Carcinoma of the soft palate treated with irradiation: Analysis of results and complications, *Radiother Oncol.* **9**: 185–194 (1987).

41. W. M. Mendenhall, R. J. Amdur, S. P. Stringer *et al.*, Radiation therapy for squamous cell carcinoma of the tonsillar region: A preferred alternative to surgery? *J. Clin. Oncol.* **18**: 2219–2225 (2000).

42. W. Zhen, L. H. Karnell, H. T. Hoffman *et al.*, The National Cancer Data Base report on squamous cell carcinoma of the base of tongue, *Head Neck* **26**: 660–674 (2004).

43. P. M. Som, H. D. Curtin and A. A. Mancuso, An imaging-based classification for the cervical nodes designed as an adjunct to recent clinically based nodal classifications, *Arch. Otolaryngol. Head Neck Surg.* **125**: 388–396 (1999).

28

Thyroid Cancer and the Endocrinologist

Nirusha Arnold
and Howard C. Smith

Abstract

Differentiated thyroid carcinoma (DTC) is the most common endocrine malignancy and its incidence is increasing worldwide. It is an indolent disease with a good prognosis. The individual patient's risk of mortality and morbidity, as determined by clinicopathological characteristics at presentation and response to therapy guides the intensity of treatment and surveillance. The endocrinologist uses various aspects of normal thyroid physiology in the management of DTC. Standard therapeutic options include surgery, radioactive iodine and thyroid hormone suppressive therapy. External beam radiation therapy may be useful in high risk patients or for palliation. Chemotherapy has doubtful benefits and is therefore rarely employed. The most sensitive tool for surveillance is thyroglobulin (a tumour marker found in blood) with neck ultrasound, radioactive iodine whole body scans and sometimes PET scanning used as adjunctive investigations. There remain a number of unresolved issues in regards to management of DTC due to the lack of evidence from prospective randomised controlled trials.

Keywords: Thyroid neoplasm, radioactive iodine, thyroglobulin, thyroid hormone.

Patients with differentiated thyroid carcinoma (DTC), from diagnosis to treatment and subsequent surveillance, are managed primarily by endocrinologists, nuclear medicine physicians and surgeons. Due to marked similarities between neoplastic and normal thyroid tissue, the clinician can manipulate thyroid hormone physiology to treat and follow up DTC. The goal of treatment is to remove or ablate all disease, thereby reducing mortality and recurrence. Thereafter surveillance has to balance the identification of ongoing disease at the earliest stage, without imposing a disease burden on patients who are mostly at low risk of recurrent or persistent cancer.

Thyroid carcinoma is the most common endocrine malignancy. Although it is characterised by an indolent course, low morbidity and low mortality, it still remains the most common cause of death from endocrine cancers. The incidence of DTC is steadily rising, with the largest increases in women with papillary carcinomas smaller than one centimetre in diameter.[1-3] The average annual adjusted incidence in the US has increased from 5/100,000 population in the period from 1974–1978 to 8.3/ 100,000 population in the period 1999–2003. As to whether this increase is due to more widespread use of neck ultrasonography, more extensive histological examination of surgical specimens or other factors is yet to be determined.

Differentiated thyroid carcinoma is a term encompassing papillary, follicular and hurthle cell carcinomas. These histological subtypes have similar clinical characteristics and prognosis (see Table 1). Their cells retain properties unique to thyroid epithelium, which are utilised in the management of DTC. Iodine is taken up almost exclusively by DTC cells and the residual thyroid via a sodium iodide symporter. Radioactive iodine (RAI) therefore selectively destroys these cells and localises disease (on post-dose whole body scans). Thyroglobulin (Tg) is another protein produced specifically by thyroid-derived cells and used as a tumour marker following initial therapy. Manipulation of TSH levels enables the endocrinologist to alter the expression of these proteins and the growth of DTC. Of note, DTC does not include anaplastic and medullary cell carcinomas.

Table 1. Histological subtypes of thyroid carcinoma derived from thyroid epithelial cells.

	Papillary	Follicular	Hurthle cell	Anaplastic
Median age at diagnosis	30–40 years	40–50 years	40–50 years, 60–70 years	> 50 years
% of DTC population	60–70%	10–20%	3–5%	< 2%
Ten-year survival rates	92–95%	80–85%	76%	13%
Histological characteristics	• Tumour cells arranged around a fibovascular core • Nuclei have ground glass appearance • Intracellular inclusions • Psammoma bodies • Can have areas of follicular differentiation • 20% multicentric	• Cells arranged in follicles • Can be very similar to normal thyroid tissue except with vascular or capsular invasion or metastatic spread • Solid sheets of cells • Nuclear atypia, vesicular nuclei	• Large eosinophillic granular cells • Abundant cytoplasm	• Small cells or large cells or carcinosarcomas • Little resemblance to normal thyroid cells or architecture
Spread	Cervical and upper mediastinal lymph nodes	Local invasion or distally to lung or bone	Locally invasive or to cervical lymph nodes, pulmonary metastases	Local invasion and distant metastases

1.   Prognosis of Differentiated Thyroid Cancer

Differentiated Thyroid Carcinoma usually presents at an early stage, with 75–85% of patients classified as low risk (MCAIS < 6, AMES Criteria).[4] Disease is confined to the thyroid at initial presentation in approximately 60% of cases, with cervical lymph nodes involved in 20–90% (depending on the extent of surgical dissection and microscopic examination). Distant metastases have been reported in 2–5% of patients at presentation.[5,6]

Despite increases in incidence, mortality rates have been stable in patients with DTC, indicating improved survival.[5] Studies have reported ten-year mortality rates as low as 1.7%.[7] The major causes of death in DTC are respiratory insufficiency due to pulmonary metastases, haemorrhage and airway obstruction from local tumour extension and circulatory failure from inferior vena caval compression.[8]

Clinically evident recurrence is found in 15–30% of patients with DTC, sometimes 30–40 years after they were considered disease-free. Over two-thirds of recurrences in case series are local (in either cervical lymph nodes or the thyroid bed), with an associated mortality of 8%. Distant recurrences occur in less than 8% of patients, with an associated mortality of 50%.[9–13] In the Mayo clinic series, patients treated from 1940 to 1990 had adjusted survival rates at 20 years of 96% in low risk patients and 50% in high risk patients ($p = 0.001$). In low risk patients, the risk of recurrence was 5%, with 27% of these patients dying from their disease (mostly with pulmonary metastases). In the high risk population, 31% of patients experienced recurrent disease and 75% of these patients died of thyroid carcinoma.[4] The current tools for surveillance, such as thyroglobulin and ultrasound, have vastly improved in accuracy and reproducibility. It is therefore possible that many of these recurrences may now be detected earlier (or more accurately be reclassified as persistent disease), resulting in improved survival.

Adverse prognostic features at presentation include male gender, advanced age,[9] locally advanced disease,[10] the presence of distant metastases, large primary lesions above 2 to 4 cm, poorly differentiated tumours and incomplete surgical resection.[9] The presence of lymph node metastases correlates with recurrent or persistent disease but not uniformly with mortality.[5] Younger children can have recurrence rates as high as 40%, but still maintain low mortality rates (1–2% at 30 years). Elderly male patients with large lesions represent a particularly worrisome group, with aggressive tumours that are unresponsive to radioactive iodine (RAI). In the Mayo Clinic cohort, elderly patients with distant metastases had five-year survival rates of only 56%.[13] In addition, certain subtypes of papillary carcinoma such as the tall cell and columnar cell variant confer a worse prognosis. Minimally invasive follicular carcinoma and sclerosing variant of papillary carcinoma, on the contrary, are associated with better outcomes. The above mentioned properties are used to predict the risk of death and recurrence, and therefore, guide treatment and follow-up.

2.   Initial Treatment

The most rational approach to management is a matter of debate. It is not feasible to conduct a prospective randomised controlled trial adequately powered to show significant differences in mortality.[14] Management is therefore based on multivariate analyses of uncontrolled retrospective studies.[14] In addition, numerous and changing approaches to therapy, various definitions of recurrence and dissimilar patient populations have led to non-uniform results from clinical trials. Initial treatment can incorporate surgery, thyroid remnant ablation (TRA) with radioactive iodine and thyroid hormone suppression therapy (THST). Radiotherapy may be useful for undifferentiated tumours or locally invasive disease that is not amenable to RAI.

2.1 *Surgery*

Total or near total thyroidectomy aimed at removing all macroscopic disease and thyroid tissue has been shown to reduce cancer specific mortality and recurrence rates, compared to more limited surgery.[9,11,15–17] Unilateral thyroidectomy may be considered for small unifocal papillary carcinomas without unfavourable histology, or minimally invasive follicular carcinomas in patients under 45 years of age.[3,5,6] Even in the setting of metastatic disease, excision of the thyroid and locoregional disease has been shown to improve outcomes.[18] Emerging evidence suggests that prophylactic central lymph node dissection may result in a survival benefit and lead to lower or undetectable thyroglobulin (Tg) levels. This approach however can lead to increased surgical complications.[5,6]

Complications unique to thyroid surgery are recurrent laryngeal nerve palsy and hypoparathyroidism. Recurrent laryngeal nerve palsy is often temporary and resolves in one to six months. Permanent damage, and rarely, aspiration pneumonia occur in less than 2% of patients in the hands of experienced thyroid surgeons.[3] Transient hypoparathyroidism may occur in one-third of patients, but persists for more than 3 months in less than 2%.[3] Supplementation with calcium and 1,25 hydroxy vitamin D derivatives therefore may be required within a few days of surgery.[3]

2.2 Radioactive iodine therapy

Following surgery, the endocrinologist needs to decide on the value of thyroid remnant ablation (TRA) with RAI. Radioactive Iodine is taken in the form of an oral capsule. When a dose of more than 1000 MBq (37 megabecquerels is equivalent to 1 millicurie unit) is administered, the patient needs to be isolated in a lead-lined room with closed circuit ventilation for approximately four to seven days, until radiation has fallen to safe levels.

The optimal dose of RAI for TRA has been challenged, with some studies suggesting 1100 MBq to have similar efficacy to the traditionally used 3700 MBq.[6] A recent systematic review, however, concluded that the success of ablation was probably greater with higher doses.[6,19] More studies are needed to trial smaller doses of RAI in remnant ablation. In the setting of a large thyroid remnant or metastatic disease, higher doses of 4000–6000 Mbq are necessary.[20]

2.2.1 Preparation for RAI

Prior to RAI, a low iodine diet (< 50 µg/day) for three weeks has been shown to increase iodine uptake and therefore the radiation dose delivered.[5] Thyrotropin (TSH) also stimulates the uptake of iodine through increased expression of the sodium-iodide symporter on the surface of thyroid cells. The patient is rendered hypothyroid by withholding thyroid hormone (LT4) replacement for a minimum of three weeks. This permits the TSH to rise above the required 30 mIU/L in 90% of cases.[3,6] Triiodothyronine (LT3) may be used in the interim to reduce the period of symptomatic hypothyroidism. This, however, also needs to be withdrawn two weeks before treatment in order to increase TSH adequately.[3,6] Most patients will experience symptoms of hypothyroidism during this time, with unpublished studies documenting days of missed work.[21]

Recombinant thyrotropin (rhTSH), alternatively, can be used to increase TSH without hypothyroidism. It is particularly useful when hypothyroidism may be contraindicated (as in psychiatric disturbances or congestive cardiac failure), or in pituitary disease where there is impairment of endogenous TSH secretion. Recombinant TSH is administered in two injections (0.9 mg) on two consecutive days followed by administration of RAI on the third day and measurement of Tg and WBS on the fifth day. It has been shown to have similar efficacy to thyroid hormone withdrawal (THW) in TRA in regards to reducing the occurrence of recurrent or persistent disease in the future.[6,22]

The practice of performing diagnostic RAI whole body scans (WBSs) looking for absence of uptake in the neck to avoid unnecessary TRA is not done routinely, as fewer than 1% of patients have negative WBSs.[5] In addition, this may lead to stunning (the therapeutic dose is not taken up after a diagnostic dose) if TRA is subsequently required. Stunning is reduced when I-123 (as opposed to I-131) is used, however this isotope is more expensive and unstable.[6]

2.2.2 Side effects of radioactive iodine

Side effects are generally dose related.[6] Radiation thyroiditis, especially with large thyroid remnants, causes neck pain and swelling and may require corticosteroid therapy. Nausea and vomiting within one to two days of the dose is effectively treated with antiemetic drugs. Nasolacrimal gland obstruction[6] and salivary gland swelling and pain may develop immediately or some months later. In addition consequent sialoadinitis, xerostomia, taste alterations, infection, dental caries, facial nerve involvement, stomatitis, candidiasis, and neoplasia in the salivary glands do occur. Hydration, lollies, amifostine, and cholinergic agents can hasten transit time through the salivary glands, however, studies have not demonstrated a clinical benefit. Treatment may include gland massage, antibiotics, botulinum toxin injections and surgery.[6]

Second primary malignancies such as breast, bone and soft tissue, colorectal, melanoma, salivary gland cancers and leukaemia[23-25] have been associated with RAI and DTC. A recent multicentre study showed a 30% increase in the risk of second primary malignancies in DTC patients[26] and a linear relationship between the risk of these cancers with the cumulative dose of RAI. Authors suggested (by extrapolation) that cumulative doses as little as 3.7 GBq (as used in TRA) could lead to increased risks of second malignancies; however clinical evidence suggests an increased risk only when the cumulative dose of RAI exceeds 22 GBq.[3]

Gonadal exposure is reduced with good hydration, frequent micturition, and avoidance of constipation. Radioactive iodine does not affect future fertility, offspring birthweight, the incidence of congenital malformations or prematurity in either men or women.[6] Amenorrhoea and increased risk of miscarriage are reported in the first year after RAI. Therefore, RAI should not be administered to pregnant or breastfeeding women.[3] Menopause may also occur at an earlier age.[6] In men, increases in FSH reflecting impaired spermatogenesis and decreases in testosterone have been observed for six to 12 months after RAI. Testicular atrophy and azoospermia have been observed with higher cumulative doses of RAI and therefore when more than 15 Gbq is administered to a patient, it is recommended that sperm cryostorage be considered.[6]

Rare side effects of RAI such as pulmonary fibrosis occurs especially in the presence of pulmonary metastases. Transient changes are observed in white blood cells and platelet counts after a treatment dose, however, permanent effects are seen if the dose to the bone marrow exceeds 200 cGy.[6]

2.2.3 Thyroid remnant ablation

Thyroid remnant ablation aims to reduce local disease recurrence and cancer-related mortality by ablating all residual thyroid tissue and DTC after surgery.[3,5] Studies examining the value of TRA have yielded differing results. In Sawka's recent meta-analysis, TRA showed a benefit in one of seven studies on mortality, three of six studies on overall recurrence, three of three studies looking at locoregional recurrence and two of three studies with data on distant metastases.[7] The pooled analysis showed a 69% reduction in locoregional recurrence (4% absolute risk reduction) and 50% reduction in metastatic disease (2% absolute risk reduction). The studies that showed benefit had the biggest patient populations and most prolonged follow-up, therefore supporting TRA.

Patients with more advanced disease have a clearer treatment benefit. The evidence supporting the use of TRA in patients less than 45 years of age, with small primary tumours under 1.5 cm and no local invasion or lymph node involvement is less definitive. American and European Guidelines therefore have recommended its use in patients with primary tumours over 1–2 cm, especially if older than 45 years, and selected patients that may have other poor prognostic factors, such as local invasion, metastases and aggressive histology.[3,6]

Thyroid remnant ablation has the added benefit of assisting clinicians in follow-up. Post-therapeutic WBSs are more sensitive than diagnostic WBSs in detecting disease and total ablation improves the specificity of Tg.[3,5]

2.3 Thyroid hormone suppressive therapy (THST)

Thyrotropin is a known growth factor for normal and neoplastic thyroid cells. Therefore TSH is suppressed (through negative feedback) by treating patients with supraphysiological doses of LT4. Most studies agree that TSH suppression below 0.1 mIU/L may benefit patients with high risk or persistent disease.[5,6,27] Indeterminate results pertain mostly to low risk tumours and patients who have been disease-free for a number of years. A recent meta-analysis concluded that TSH suppression is likely to reduce the overall number of major adverse clinical events (RR 0.73, $p < 0.05$).[28] The degree and duration of TSH suppression is also debated. The increased risks of atrial fibrillation, osteoporosis in post-menopausal women, exacerbation of angina in patients with ischaemic heart disease and symptoms of thyroid hormone excess have to be weighed up against the potential benefits of THST.[29]

Recent American guidelines suggest that patients with persistent or high risk disease should have their TSH suppressed to < 0.1 mIU/L. Patients who had high risk disease initially, but are currently clinically-free from disease and low risk patients should maintain their TSH between 0.1–0.5 mIU/L. Low risk patients that are free of disease can have TSH levels in the low normal range (0.3–2 mIU/L).[6] The British and European guidelines recommend that all patients should have their TSH suppressed to < 0.1 mIU/L, however, higher levels may be acceptable once the patient has been disease-free for several years.[3]

3. Follow-Up

An understanding of the accuracy and pitfalls of follow-up tests allows clinicians to appropriately interpret these investigations and treat patients. As mentioned, there continues to be a minority of low risk patients who unpredictably die from disease, necessitating long term, diligent follow-up for all patients.

3.1 *Tools for disease surveillance*

3.1.1 *Thyroglobulin (Tg)*

Thyroglobulin measurements have become the cornerstone of DTC surveillance. Its levels are determined by the volume of thyroid-derived tissue, their degree of differentiation and TSH values. Unfortunately false negative and false positive results impair its accuracy.

Thyrotropin increases Tg production from DTC or the thyroid. Increasing TSH at the time of measurement (by rendering the patient hypothyroid or administering rhTSH) will increase the sensitivity of Tg for detecting disease. In eight studies comprising 1028 low risk patients, 76% had a Tg of less than 1 mcg/L on THST.

In this patient group, 21% had significant increases in Tg after TSH stimulation with 36% found to have metastatic disease. Of those found to have metastatic disease, one-third had distant metastases.[3] Therefore many authors caution against relying solely on Tg measurements on THST.[30]

Thyroglobulin is measured by radioimmunometric assay, where lower limits of detection should be at least 1 mcg/L.[3] Different laboratories and assays have different cut-off values and therefore serial Tg measurements should be made in the same laboratory.[5] It is generally agreed that Tg levels after surgical and RAI ablation should be undetectable on THST, < 10 mcg/L after THW and < 2 mcg/L after rhTSH to consider the patient free of disease.[31,32] Thyroid hormone withdrawal produces higher Tg levels than rhTSH, due to more prolonged hypothyroidism.[33] Recombinant TSH is as effective as THW in detecting metastatic disease (when Tg is > 2 mcg/L) and ruling out residual cancer (when Tg is < 1 mcg/L).[31] After partial thyroidectomy or in the absence of TRA, these cut-off levels cannot be used with certainty,[34] therefore trends in Tg measurements should guide treatment.

Thyroglobulin antibodies are present in about 20–25% of patients with thyroid carcinoma and 10% of the general population.[6] They decrease dramatically after total thyroidectomy.[35] Thyroglobulin antibodies (even in low titres) may lead to false negative Tg results.[31] Thyroglobulin antibodies should therefore be measured with each Tg measurement and results should be considered invalid if they are present. Interestingly Tg antibodies can be a surrogate tumour marker of DTC, as concentrations reflect circulating Tg antigen.[3,31] A study of 228 patients found recurrence rates amongst patients with persistent Tg antibodies to be 49% (vs. 3.4% in Tg antibody negative patients $p < 0.0001$) and levels decreased after successful treatment.[36]

False negative Tg results occur with poorly differentiated tumours (that lose the capacity to produce Tg) and those with metastatic cervical lymph nodes or low volume disease.[3,5,6]

3.1.2 *Neck ultrasonography*

Cervical lymph nodes are the most common site of recurrence, where disease can exist without elevation or indeterminate levels of Tg.[37,38] Schlumberger found false negative Tg levels in 20% of patients with cervical lymph node metastases.[39] Neck ultrasound is therefore complementary, even when Tg is negative, and facilitates the localisation of disease for fine needle aspiration. Lymph nodes as small as 2–3 mm in diameter can be detected.[3] Ultrasound features suspicious of malignancy include hypoechogenicity, lack of an echogenic central line, a round shape, microcalcifications, a cystic component and hypervascularisation on colour Doppler.[21] Unlike the other investigations it can be performed without TSH stimulation.

Neck ultrasound has gained popularity in America and Europe, where centres have reported a sensitivity and specificity of more than 96% and 99% respectively for detecting persistent or recurrent disease when combined with Tg.[38,40] Unfortunately these results may not be replicated in other centres, due to the lack of dedicated and experienced personnel with inadequate time and resources available to examine multiple lymph node groups and biopsy suspicious lesions. A clinician may therefore receive more indeterminate or even erroneous results. Specificity may be improved when used to investigate a patient with detectable Tgs, or when serial examinations reveal progressive lesions.

3.1.3 *Radioactive iodine whole body scans*

Whole body scans (WBS) identifying and localising disease can be performed after therapeutic (3700–6000 Mbq) or diagnostic doses (approximately 200 MBq) of RAI. Recombinant TSH and THW are equivalent in preparing patients for these WBSs,[41,42] with the exception of sporadic cases of metastatic DTC leading to the recommendation for its use in patients who otherwise do not have evidence of persistent disease.[3]

Previously diagnostic WBSs were performed as part of the standard follow-up of DTC. Due to their relative insensitivity when compared to Tg and the possibility of stunning they have recently lost favour. In six studies looking at TSH stimulated Tg as levels and diagnostic WBSs in over 780 patients, 91% with unsuspected metastases were identified by an elevated Tg as compared to only 19% identified by a positive WBS.[31] Six other studies looking at

750 cases found no patient with an undetectable Tg had a positive diagnostic WBS.[43] In Pacini's study of 340 consecutive patients with DTC, TSH-stimulated diagnostic WBSs had a sensitivity of only 21% and a NPV of 89%.[38] The combination of TSH-stimulated Tg levels and WBS had a sensitivity of 92.7% and a NPV of 99%. Diagnostic scans may be of more value in patients with Tg antibodies where Tg levels are unreliable.

3.1.4   [18F]-2-fluoro-2-deoxy-d-glucose positron emission tomography (FDG-PET)

Positron Emission Tomography (PET) identifies disease that is metabolically active, but not RAI avid. Where patients have a negative post-therapeutic WBS and positive Tgs, FDG-PET scanning can localise disease requiring resection, EBRT or close observation, therefore changing clinical management and outcome.[44–46] Even in the setting of other positive imaging it can detect additional sites of metastases.[45] The sensitivity of PET scanning is improved with TSH stimulation and CT fusion.[6] It is more likely to be positive with higher thyrolgobulin levels.[47,48] In the setting of minimal residual disease in cervical nodes, however, FDG-PET does not differentiate small inflammatory cervical nodes from cancerous nodes.[32,44,49]

FDG-PET positivity identifies a group of patients that are less likely to respond to RAI.[50] Disease-free survival in these patients is less than two to three years.[51] Survival correlates with the number of FDG avid lesions, the glycolytic rate of the bigger lesions and Tg levels.[5]

3.2   Protocols for follow-up

Guidelines for the follow-up of DTC have recently been published in Europe and America.[3,6,32] In addition to the prognostic variables described above, response to initial treatment and results of follow-up investigations are also incorporated into these protocols to predict the risk of recurrence and thereby guide the intensity of follow-up.[32]

At TRA an undetectable Tg and uptake in the neck only on the WBS confers a good prognosis.[52] An elevated Tg at this time is of indeterminate significance,[21,53,54] and uptake outside the neck signifies metastatic disease and a need for close follow-up and further treatment. Thyrotropin takes at least three months to reach a steady state, and therefore TSH and thyroglobulin are measured at that time.[3] Thyroid function tests (to assess adequacy of TSH suppression) and clinical examination need to be repeated at three- to four-monthly intervals in the first year. Thyroglobulin should also be measured on at least one occasion on THST in the first year.[3] An undetectable Tg at this time is a good prognostic indicator.[55] The American and European guidelines also recommend neck ultrasounds twice in the first year. In the presence of a suspicious neck examination or an elevated Tg, neck ultrasounds and other imaging should be performed and further treatment considered.

A TSH stimulated Tg should then be measured, ideally six to 12 months after initial treatment. This Tg level has a sensitivity up to 100% and specificity of 90–95% for identifying tumour presence.[54] In addition, imaging studies are recommended. The European and American guidelines once again recommend neck ultrasounds. For intermediate to high risk patients, however, a diagnostic WBS should also be considered. When rhTSH is not available, diagnostic WBSs are still performed in patients taking advantage of the elevated TSH required for Tg measurements.

When a patient has an undetectable Tg, and imaging and clinical examination are negative in the first year, they can be classified as low risk, or disease-free. Clinicians can then take a minimalistic approach to disease surveillance and follow a patient with clinical examination, annual Tg levels on THST and neck ultrasounds every three to five years. The value of ongoing TSH stimulated Tg levels and WBSs in this situation is controversial. It is thought that clinically significant disease will become apparent by rising Tg levels even on THST.[3] Patients who do not have total thyroidectomy or radioablation are by nature low risk patients and therefore follow-up can be similar to low risk patients.

If disease is persistent or high risk, further TSH stimulated Tg levels, imaging, RAI therapy and other appropriate treatment may be necessary and follow-up should be intensified.[38,56] If a high risk patient then becomes disease-free, the clinician will have to decide when they can be downgraded to low risk.

4.   Treatment of Recurrent or Persistent Disease

Surgery and/or RAI are the first line treatments for recurrent or persistent disease followed by EBRT. In general EBRT is reserved for local control of unresectable lesions or non-iodine avid disease. Some studies have shown benefits of EBRT in patients at high risk of local recurrence (i.e. over 45 years old, microscopic residual disease, extrathyroidal extension or poorly differentiated disease).[6] It also has a role in palliation or symptom control of bone, CNS, pelvic and mediastinal metastases.[57,58] Disease may partially respond to chemotherapy but remission is rare. Chemotherapy may be used as a last resort, to which disease at best may partially respond. Imaging to identify the source of ongoing disease consists of WBS, neck ultrasounds, Computer Tomography (especially for pulmonary, abdominal and CNS disease) MRI scans, FDG PET scans, Bone scans (bone metastases) and Sestamibi scans. When undifferentiated disease is found or suspected (as in older patients with extensive local invasion or disseminated disease on presentation), FDG-PET is particularly helpful.

Local disease especially when bulky is best treated with surgery.[50] This includes lymph nodes larger than 1 cm, enlarging lymph nodes six months after RAI, and invasion of the aerodigestive tract.[6] Radioactive Iodine, by itself, is unlikely to fully ameliorate this disease. It is often used as an adjunct following surgery. External beam radiotherapy is another therapeutic option, especially with macroscopic residual disease following surgery and poorly differentiated disease that does not take up RAI.[5] In patients who have recently had RAI the decision to treat may be deferred for six months till the full therapeutic effect can be assessed.

Distant metastases occur most commonly in the lung, followed by bone.[59] Disease-specific survival rates are estimated to be 30–60% at ten to 20 years. Survival is related to age, RAI uptake, degree of differentiation and extent of disease. Complete response to RAI is associated with a good outcome with 15-year survival rates reported to be 89% (compared with 8%) in a study of 2200 patients with metastatic disease.[60]

Pulmonary disease is found in 4–6% of patients with DTC with survival rates of around 50% at 20 years.[59,61,62] These patients are more likely to be male, older, have higher post-operative Tgs and larger thyroid remnants. Survival in one study was 91% for patients with a normal X-ray and positive diagnostic WBSs, compared with 63% for those with a positive chest X-ray and micronodules, and 11% in those with macronodules.[31] Schlumberger reported a 100% ten-year survival in patients with an elevated Tg, negative diagnostic WBS and positive post-therapeutic WBSs.[31] He recommended administration of RAI every six to 12 months till resolution for responsive patients. Pineda found that Tg decreased in 81% after the first dose, in 90% after the second dose and in 100% after the third treatment.[63] Radioactive iodine is less effective in macronodular disease and non-iodine avid disease.[64] Other therapeutic options may include metastectomy, EBRT (especially in mediastinal disease for symptom control) and endobronchial laser ablation. Bone metastases can be treated with surgery, RAI, EBRT (for pain management and patients at risk of a pathological fracture), bone seeking radioisotopes or bisphosphonates.[3,6] Cerebral metastases should firstly be considered for surgical removal, with EBRT and RAI also having beneficial effects especially where neurological deficits are likely.[6]

5. Therapeutic Dilemmas

5.1 *Low detectable thyroglobulin*

A low detectable Tg is < 1–2 mcg/L on THST, < 10 mcg/L after THW, or < 2 mcg/L after rhTSH. Thyroglobulin levels may take several years after RAI therapy to decline, requiring the clinician to cautiously observe and reassess six to 12 months later.[32,65] The positive predictive value of a TSH stimulated Tg, six to 12 months after surgery, of above 10 mcg/L is 53% (thought to be low because of low recurrence rates). The positive predictive value, however, of increasing TSH stimulated Tg values is 83%.[66] Treatment should therefore be reserved for those with evidence of progressive disease. Neck ultrasounds may be useful to identify diseased cervical lymph nodes which commonly present in this manner.[38,67]

5.2 Thyroglobulin positive, whole body scan negative patients

A patient with a positive Tg and negative diagnostic WBS should be assessed with clinical examination and neck ultrasounds. A chest X-ray and CT scan should also be performed, as lung metastases have been reported in 5–55% of these patients.[61,68,69] The CT scan should be done without iodinated contrast (although this may help identify mediastinal disease), as I-131 therapy may be necessary.[6] Further to these investigations FDG-PET scans can also be useful.

If imaging is negative, it is arguable that patients should be treated empirically with RAI. Post-therapeutic scans have been found to show additional foci of disease in 10–26% of patients, and[70] changed disease stage and management in 10–15% of patients.[6,71] Studies have also demonstrated higher rates of conversion to undetectable or decreased Tgs and negative post-therapeutic WBS after a therapeutic dose of RAI.[61,72,73] There is no evidence, however, that this approach improves survival and opposing studies reveal that Tg may become undetectable without treatment, especially when other imaging studies are negative.[62]

De-differentiation therapy is also useful in this setting. Tumours (either initially or during progression of disease) can become less differentiated, thereby losing their capacity to take up iodine. Retinoic acids are active metabolites of Vitamin A that interact with nuclear receptors to regulate growth and differentiation. *In vitro* retinoic acid (RA) increases the expression of thyroid specific proteins and their ability to take up RAI. There is also good evidence for its anti-proliferative effects. *In vivo*, RA has been shown to increase RAI uptake, and induce tumour stabilisation or regression.[74] Studies have shown response rates of 20 to 50% for RA.[74] Side effects are common and include dry skin, nausea, epistaxis, changes in blood count, cough and liver function test abnormalities. Other chemotherapeutic agents, such as histone deactylase inhibitors and methyltransferase inhibitors, have shown favourable effects on DTC cell lines but are yet to be tested in clinical trials.

6. Concluding Remarks

Differentiated thyroid carcinoma has a good prognosis and effective treatments. Despite this a significant minority of patients can develop recurrent and/or fatal disease, sometimes after many years of being disease-free, necessitating life-long surveillance. Patients at high risk of recurrence, benefit most from receiving a combination of surgery, RAI treatment, THST and close follow-up. The advantages of such an intensive regimen for low risk patients is uncertain. The endocrinologist has to therefore employ a risk stratified approach to management, balancing the side-effects and benefits of treatment and surveillance. In the future, further case series may assist us in deciding on more appropriate management strategies for the growing population of low risk patients who are long term survivors of DTC, as well as on novel therapies for patients unresponsive to the standard therapeutic options.

References

1. M. J. Hayat, N. Howlader, M. E. Reichman and B. K. Edwards, Cancer statistics, trends, and multiple primary cancer analyses from the Surveillance, Epidemiology, and End Results (SEER) Program, *Oncologist* **12**(1): 20–37 (2007).
2. L. Davies and H. G. Welch, Increasing incidence of thyroid cancer in the United States, 1973–2002, *J. Am. Med. Assoc.* **295**(18): 2164–2167 (2006).
3. F. Pacini, M. Schlumberger, H. Dralle, R. Elisei, J. W. Smit and W. Wiersinga, European consensus for the management of patients with differentiated thyroid carcinoma of the follicular epithelium, *Eur. J. Endocrinol.* **154**(6): 787–803 (2006).
4. L. E. Sanders and B. Cady, Differentiated thyroid cancer: Re-examination of risk groups and outcome of treatment, *Arch. Surg.* **133**(4): 419–425 (1998).
5. R. M. Tuttle, R. Leboeuf and A. J. Martorella, Papillary thyroid cancer: Monitoring and therapy, *Endocrinol. Metab. Clin. North Am.* **36**(3): 753–778, vii (2007).
6. D. S. Cooper, G. M. Doherty, B. R. Haugen, R. T. Kloos, S. L. Lee, S. J. Mandel *et al.*, Management guidelines for patients with thyroid nodules and differentiated thyroid cancer, *Thyroid* **16**(2): 109–142 (2006).

7. A. M. Sawka, K. Thephamongkhol, M. Brouwers, L. Thabane, G. Browman and H. C. Gerstein, Clinical review 170: A systematic review and metaanalysis of the effectiveness of radioactive iodine remnant ablation for well-differentiated thyroid cancer, *J. Clin. Endocrinol. Metab.* **89**(8): 3668–3676 (2004).

8. Y. Kitamura, K. Shimizu, M. Nagahama, K. Sugino, O. Ozaki, T. Mimura *et al.*, Immediate causes of death in thyroid carcinoma: Clinicopathological analysis of 161 fatal cases, *J. Clin. Endocrinol. Metab.* **84**(11): 4043–4049 (1999).

9. N. A. Samaan, P. N. Schultz, R. C. Hickey, H. Goepfert, T. P. Haynie, D. A. Johnston *et al.*, The results of various modalities of treatment of well differentiated thyroid carcinomas: A retrospective review of 1599 patients, *J. Clin. Endocrinol. Metab.* **75**(3): 714–720 (1992).

10. L. J. DeGroot, E. L. Kaplan, M. McCormick and F. H. Straus, Natural history, treatment, and course of papillary thyroid carcinoma, *J. Clin. Endocrinol. Metab.* **71**(2): 414–424 (1990).

11. E. L. Mazzaferri and S. M. Jhiang, Long-term impact of initial surgical and medical therapy on papillary and follicular thyroid cancer, *Am. J. Med.* **97**(5): 418–428 (1994).

12. E. L. Mazzaferri, An overview of the management of papillary and follicular thyroid carcinoma, *Thyroid* **9**(5): 421–427 (1999).

13. I. D. Hay, G. B. Thompson, C. S. Grant, E. J. Bergstralh, C. E. Dvorak, C. A. Gorman *et al.*, Papillary thyroid carcinoma managed at the Mayo Clinic during six decades (1940–1999): Temporal trends in initial therapy and long-term outcome in 2444 consecutively treated patients, *World J. Surg.* **26**(8): 879–885 (2002).

14. J. B. Wong, M. M. Kaplan, K. B. Meyer and S. G. Pauker, Ablative radioactive iodine therapy for apparently localized thyroid carcinoma. A decision analytic perspective, *Endocrinol. Metab. Clin. North Am.* **19**(3): 741–760 (1990).

15. N. F. Esnaola, S. B. Cantor, S. I. Sherman, J. E. Lee and D. B. Evans, Optimal treatment strategy in patients with papillary thyroid cancer: A decision analysis, *Surgery* **130**(6): 921–930 (2001).

16. I. D. Hay, E. J. Bergstralh, C. S. Grant, B. McIver, G. B. Thompson, J. A. van Heerden *et al.*, Impact of primary surgery on outcome in 300 patients with pathologic tumor-node-metastasis stage III papillary thyroid carcinoma treated at one institution from 1940 through 1989, *Surgery* **126**(6): 1173–1181; discussion 1181–1182 (1999).

17. Y. Ito and A. Miyauchi, Lateral and mediastinal lymph node dissection in differentiated thyroid carcinoma: Indications, benefits, and risks, *World J. Surg.* **31**(5): 905–915 (2007).

18. B. M. Stephenson, M. H. Wheeler and O. H. Clark, The role of total thyroidectomy in the management of differentiated thyroid cancer, *Curr. Opin. Gen. Surg.* **12**: 53–59 (1994).

19. A. Hackshaw, C. Harmer, U. Mallick, M. Haq and F. A. Franklyn, 131I activity for remnant ablation in patients with differentiated thyroid cancer: A systematic review, *J. Clin. Endocrinol. Metab.* **92**(1): 28–38 (2007).

20. P. W. Rosario, A. L. Barroso, L. L. Rezende, E. L. Padrao, M. A. Borges, T. A. Fagundes *et al.*, Ablative treatment of thyroid cancer with high doses of 131I without pre-therapy scanning, *Nucl. Med. Commun.* **26**(2): 129–132 (2005).

21. M. Schlumberger, F. Pacini, W. M. Wiersinga, A. Toft, J. W. Smit, F. Sanchez Franco *et al.*, Follow-up and management of differentiated thyroid carcinoma: A European perspective in clinical practice, *Eur. J. Endocrinol.* **151**(5): 539–548 (2004).

22. R. M. Tuttle, M. Brokhin, G. Omry, A. J. Martorella, S. M. Larson, R. K. Grewal *et al.*, Recombinant human TSH-assisted radioactive iodine remnant ablation achieves short-term clinical recurrence rates similar to those of traditional thyroid hormone withdrawal, *J. Nucl. Med.* **49**(5): 764–770 (2008).

23. A. Y. Chen, L. Levy, H. Goepfert, B. W. Brown, M. R. Spitz and R. Vassilopoulou-Sellin, The development of breast carcinoma in women with thyroid carcinoma, *Cancer* **92**(2): 225–231 (2001).

24. C. Rubino, F. de Vathaire, M. E. Dottorini, P. Hall, C. Schvartz, J. E. Couette *et al.*, Second primary malignancies in thyroid cancer patients, *Br. J. Cancer* **89**(9): 1638–1644 (2003).

25. M. E. Dottorini, G. Lomuscio, L. Mazzucchelli, A. Vignati and L. Colombo, Assessment of female fertility and carcinogenesis after iodine-131 therapy for differentiated thyroid carcinoma, *J. Nucl. Med.* **36**(1): 21–27 (1995).

26. T. C. Sandeep, M. W. Strachan, R. M. Reynolds, D. H. Brewster, G. Scelo, E. Pukkala *et al.*, Second primary cancers in thyroid cancer patients: A multinational record linkage study, *J. Clin. Endocrinol. Metab.* **91**(5): 1819–1825 (2006).

27. P. W. Wang, S. T. Wang, R. T. Liu, W. Y. Chien, S. C. Tung, Y. C. Lu *et al.*, Levothyroxine suppression of thyroglobulin in patients with differentiated thyroid carcinoma, *J. Clin. Endocrinol. Metab.* **84**(12): 4549–4553 (1999).

28. N. J. McGriff, G. Csako, L. Gourgiotis, C. G. Lori, F. Pucino and N. J. Sarlis, Effects of thyroid hormone suppression therapy on adverse clinical outcomes in thyroid cancer, *Ann. Med.* **34**(7–8): 554–564 (2002).

29. A. D. Toft, Clinical practice. Subclinical hyperthyroidism, *N. Engl. J. Med.* **345**(7): 512–516 (2001).

30. M. Schlumberger, Is stimulation of thyroglobulin (Tg) useful in low-risk patients with thyroid carcinoma and undetectable Tg on thyroxin and negative neck ultrasound?, *Clin. Endocrinol. (Oxf.)* **62**(2): 119–120 (2005).

31. E. L. Mazzaferri, R. J. Robbins, C. A. Spencer, L. E. Braverman, F. Pacini, L. Wartofsky *et al.*, A consensus report of the role of serum thyroglobulin as a monitoring method for low-risk patients with papillary thyroid carcinoma, *J. Clin. Endocrinol. Metab.* **88**(4): 1433–1441 (2003).

32. R. M. Tuttle and R. Leboeuf, Follow up approaches in thyroid cancer: A risk adapted paradigm, *Endocrinol. Metab. Clin. North Am.* **37**(2): 419–435 (2008).

33. F. Pacini, E. Molinaro, F. Lippi, M. G. Castagna, L. Agate, C. Ceccarelli *et al.*, Prediction of disease status by recombinant human TSH-stimulated serum Tg in the postsurgical follow-up of differentiated thyroid carcinoma, *J. Clin. Endocrinol. Metab.* **86**(12): 5686–5690 (2001).

34. M. Ozata, S. Suzuki, T. Miyamoto, R. T. Liu, F. Fierro-Renoy and L. J. DeGroot, Serum thyroglobulin in the follow-up of patients with treated differentiated thyroid cancer, *J. Clin. Endocrinol. Metab.* **79**(1): 98–105 (1994).

35. L. Chiovato, F. Latrofa, L. E. Braverman, F. Pacini, M. Capezzone, L. Masserini *et al.*, Disappearance of humoral thyroid autoimmunity after complete removal of thyroid antigens, *Ann. Intern. Med.* **139**(5 pt. 1): 346–351 (2003).

36. J. K. Chung, Y. J. Park, T. Y. Kim, Y. So, S. K. Kim, D. J. Park *et al.*, Clinical significance of elevated level of serum antithyroglobulin antibody in patients with differentiated thyroid cancer after thyroid ablation, *Clin. Endocrinol. (Oxf.)* **57**(2): 215–221 (2002).

37. M. Torlontano, U. Crocetti, L. D'Aloiso, N. Bonfitto, A. Di Giorgio, S. Modoni *et al.*, Serum thyroglobulin and 131I whole body scan after recombinant human TSH stimulation in the follow-up of low-risk patients with differentiated thyroid cancer, *Eur. J. Endocrinol.* **148**(1): 19–24 (2003).

38. F. Pacini, E. Molinaro, M. G. Castagna, L. Agate, R. Elisei, C. Ceccarelli *et al.*, Recombinant human thyrotropin-stimulated serum thyroglobulin

combined with neck ultrasonography has the highest sensitivity in monitoring differentiated thyroid carcinoma, *J. Clin. Endocrinol. Metab.* **88**(8): 3668–3673 (2003).

39. M. J. Schlumberger, Papillary and follicular thyroid carcinoma, *N. Engl. J. Med.* **338**(5): 297–306 (1998).

40. A. Frasoldati, M. Pesenti, M. Gallo, A. Caroggio, D. Salvo and R. Valcavi, Diagnosis of neck recurrences in patients with differentiated thyroid carcinoma, *Cancer* **97**(1): 90–96 (2003).

41. B. R. Haugen, F. Pacini, C. Reiners, M. Schlumberger, P. W. Ladenson, S. I. Sherman *et al.*, A comparison of recombinant human thyrotropin and thyroid hormone withdrawal for the detection of thyroid remnant or cancer, *J. Clin. Endocrinol. Metab.* **84**(11): 3877–3885 (1999).

42. R. J. Robbins, R. M. Tuttle, R. N. Sharaf, S. M. Larson, H. K. Robbins, R. A. Ghossein *et al.*, Preparation by recombinant human thyrotropin or thyroid hormone withdrawal are comparable for the detection of residual differentiated thyroid carcinoma, *J. Clin. Endocrinol. Metab.* **86**(2): 619–625 (2001).

43. M. Schlumberger, G. Berg, O. Cohen, L. Duntas, F. Jamar, B. Jarzab *et al.*, Follow-up of low-risk patients with differentiated thyroid carcinoma: A European perspective, *Eur. J. Endocrinol.* **150**(2): 105–112 (2004).

44. W. Wang, H. Macapinlac, S. M. Larson, S. D. Yeh, T. Akhurst, R. D. Finn *et al.*, [18F]-2-fluoro-2-deoxy-D-glucose positron emission tomography localizes residual thyroid cancer in patients with negative diagnostic (131)I whole body scans and elevated serum thyroglobulin levels, *J. Clin. Endocrinol. Metab.* **84**(7): 2291–2302 (1999).

45. B. O. Helal, P. Merlet, M. E. Toubert, B. Franc, C. Schvartz, H. Gauthier-Koelesnikov *et al.*, Clinical impact of (18)F-FDG PET in thyroid carcinoma patients with elevated thyroglobulin levels and negative (131)I scanning results after therapy, *J. Nucl. Med.* **42**(10): 1464–1469 (2001).

46. N. Lee and M. Tuttle, The role of external beam radiotherapy in the treatment of papillary thyroid cancer, *Endocr. Relat. Cancer* **13**(4): 971–977 (2006).

47. M. Zoller, S. Kohlfuerst, I. Igerc, E. Kresnik, H. J. Gallowitsch, I. Gomez *et al.*, Combined PET/CT in the follow-up of differentiated thyroid carcinoma: What is the impact of each modality? *Eur. J. Nucl. Med. Mol. I.* **34**(4): 487–495 (2007).

48. L. A. Zimmer, B. McCook, C. Meltzer, M. Fukui, D. Bascom, C. Snyderman *et al.*, Combined positron emission tomography/

computed tomography imaging of recurrent thyroid cancer, *Otolaryngol. Head Neck Surg.* **128**(2): 178–184 (2003).

49. W. Wang, S. M. Larson, R. M. Tuttle, H. Kalaigian, K. Kolbert, M. Sonenberg *et al.*, Resistance of [18f]-fluorodeoxyglucose-avid metastatic thyroid cancer lesions to treatment with high-dose radioactive iodine, *Thyroid* **11**(12): 1169–1175 (2001).

50. R. T. Kloos, Approach to the patient with a positive serum thyroglobulin and a negative radioiodine scan after initial therapy for differentiated thyroid cancer, *J. Clin. Endocrinol. Metab.* **93**(5): 1519–1525 (2008).

51. R. J. Robbins, A. Driedger and J. Magner, Recombinant human thyrotropin-assisted radioiodine therapy for patients with metastatic thyroid cancer who could not elevate endogenous thyrotropin or be withdrawn from thyroxine, *Thyroid* **16**(11): 1121–1130 (2006).

52. F. Pacini, M. Capezzone, R. Elisei, C. Ceccarelli, D. Taddei and A. Pinchera, Diagnostic 131-iodine whole-body scan may be avoided in thyroid cancer patients who have undetectable stimulated serum Tg levels after initial treatment, *J. Clin. Endocrinol. Metab.* **87**(4): 1499–1501 (2002).

53. T. Y. Kim, W. B. Kim, E. S. Kim, J. S. Ryu, J. S. Yeo, S. C. Kim *et al.*, Serum thyroglobulin levels at the time of 131I remnant ablation just after thyroidectomy are useful for early prediction of clinical recurrence in low-risk patients with differentiated thyroid carcinoma, *J. Clin. Endocrinol. Metab.* **90**(3): 1440–1445 (2005).

54. K. A. Heemstra, Y. Y. Liu, M. Stokkel, J. Kievit, E. Corssmit, A. M. Pereira *et al.*, Serum thyroglobulin concentrations predict disease-free remission and death in differentiated thyroid carcinoma, *Clin. Endocrinol. (Oxf.)* **66**(1): 58–64 (2007).

55. L. Giovanella, L. Ceriani, S. Suriano, A. Ghelfo and M. Maffioli, Thyroglobulin measurement before rhTSH-aided (131)I ablation in detecting metastases from differentiated thyroid carcinoma, *Clin. Endocrinol. (Oxf.)* **69**(4): 659–663 (2008).

56. A. F. Cailleux, E. Baudin, J. P. Travagli, M. Ricard and M. Schlumberger, Is diagnostic iodine-131 scanning useful after total thyroid ablation for differentiated thyroid cancer?, *J. Clin. Endocrinol. Metab.* **85**(1): 175–178 (2000).

57. P. C. Wilson, B. M. Millar and J. D. Brierley, The management of advanced thyroid cancer, *Clin. Oncol. (R. Coll. Radiol.)* **16**(8): 561–568 (2004).

58. R. W. Tsang, J. D. Brierley, W. J. Simpson, T. Panzarella, M. K. Gospodarowicz and S. B. Sutcliffe, The effects of surgery, radioiodine, and external radiation therapy on the clinical outcome of patients with differentiated thyroid carcinoma, *Cancer* **82**(2): 375–388 (1998).

59. M. Shoup, A. Stojadinovic, A. Nissan, R. A. Ghossein, S. Freedman, M. F. Brennan *et al.*, Prognostic indicators of outcomes in patients with distant metastases from differentiated thyroid carcinoma, *J. Am. Coll. Surg.* **197**(2): 191–197 (2003).

60. M. Schlumberger, C. Challeton, F. De Vathaire, J. P. Travagli, P. Gardet, J. D. Lumbroso *et al.*, Radioactive iodine treatment and external radiotherapy for lung and bone metastases from thyroid carcinoma, *J. Nucl. Med.* **37**(4): 598–605 (1996).

61. J. D. Lin, T. C. Chao, S. C. Chou and C. Hsueh, Papillary thyroid carcinomas with lung metastases, *Thyroid* **14**(12): 1091–1096 (2004).

62. S. Ilgan, A. O. Karacalioglu, Y. Pabuscu, G. K. Atac, N. Arslan, E. Ozturk *et al.*, Iodine-131 treatment and high-resolution CT: Results in patients with lung metastases from differentiated thyroid carcinoma, *Eur. J. Nucl. Med. Mol. I.* **31**(6): 825–830 (2004).

63. J. D. Pineda, T. Lee, K. Ain, J. C. Reynolds and J. Robbins, Iodine-131 therapy for thyroid cancer patients with elevated thyroglobulin and negative diagnostic scan, *J. Clin. Endocrinol. Metab.* **80**(5): 1488–1492 (1995).

64. F. Pacini, L. Agate, R. Elisei, M. Capezzone, C. Ceccarelli, F. Lippi *et al.*, Outcome of differentiated thyroid cancer with detectable serum Tg and negative diagnostic (131)I whole body scan: Comparison of patients treated with high (131)I activities versus untreated patients, *J. Clin. Endocrinol. Metab.* **86**(9): 4092–4097 (2001).

65. E. L. Mazzaferri and R. T. Kloos, Clinical review 128: Current approaches to primary therapy for papillary and follicular thyroid cancer, *J. Clin. Endocrinol. Metab.* **86**(4): 1447–1463 (2001).

66. E. Baudin, C. Do Cao, A. F. Cailleux, S. Leboulleux, J. P. Travagli and M. Schlumberger, Positive predictive value of serum thyroglobulin levels, measured during the first year of follow-up after thyroid hormone withdrawal, in thyroid cancer patients, *J. Clin. Endocrinol. Metab.* **88**(3): 1107–1111 (2003).

67. A. Bachelot, S. Leboulleux, E. Baudin, D. M. Hartl, B. Caillou, J. P. Travagli *et al.*, Neck recurrence from thyroid carcinoma: Serum thyroglobulin and high-dose total body scan are not reliable criteria

for cure after radioiodine treatment, *Clin. Endocrinol. (Oxf.)* **62**(3): 376–379 (2005).

68. M. Schlumberger, M. Tubiana, F. De Vathaire, C. Hill, P. Gardet, J. P. Travagli *et al.*, Long-term results of treatment of 283 patients with lung and bone metastases from differentiated thyroid carcinoma, *J. Clin. Endocrinol. Metab.* **63**(4): 960–967 (1986).

69. F. Pacini, F. Lippi, N. Formica, R. Elisei, S. Anelli, C. Ceccarelli *et al.*, Therapeutic doses of iodine-131 reveal undiagnosed metastases in thyroid cancer patients with detectable serum thyroglobulin levels, *J. Nucl. Med.* **28**(12): 1888–1891 (1987).

70. V. Fatourechi, I. D. Hay, H. Javedan, G. A. Wiseman, B. P. Mullan and C. A. Gorman, Lack of impact of radioiodine therapy in Tg-positive, diagnostic whole-body scan-negative patients with follicular cell-derived thyroid cancer, *J. Clin. Endocrinol. Metab.* **87**(4): 1521–1526 (2002).

71. M. Schlumberger, F. Mancusi, E. Baudin and F. Pacini, 131I therapy for elevated thyroglobulin levels, *Thyroid* **7**(2): 273–276 (1997).

72. J. M. Koh, E. S. Kim, J. S. Ryu, S. J. Hong, W. B. Kim and Y. K. Shong, Effects of therapeutic doses of 131I in thyroid papillary carcinoma patients with elevated thyroglobulin level and negative 131I whole-body scan: Comparative study, *Clin. Endocrinol. (Oxf.)* **58**(4): 421–427 (2003).

73. K. M. van Tol, P. L. Jager, E. G. de Vries, D. A. Piers, H. M. Boezen, W. J. Sluiter *et al.*, Outcome in patients with differentiated thyroid cancer with negative diagnostic whole-body scanning and detectable stimulated thyroglobulin, *Eur. J. Endocrinol.* **148**(6): 589–596 (2003).

74. S. M. Coelho, M. Vaisman and D. P. Carvalho, Tumour re-differentiation effect of retinoic acid: A novel therapeutic approach for advanced thyroid cancer, *Curr. Pharm. Des.* **11**(19): 2525–2531 (2005).

29

The Effects of Cancer Therapy on Gonadal Function and Fertility

Howard C. Smith

Abstract

Effective treatment and survival are the prime focus of oncologists and patients with cancer. With longer survival for many patients, the preservation or restoration of the opportunity to have biological children is an important aspect of their management. Impaired fertility can be the result of the cancer or its treatment. In women delay in the opportunity to conceive caused by cancer or treatment may be a significant contribution to their distress. Adult males have the option of sperm cryopreservation, but this may not be possible for adolescent boys and is not available for pre-pubertal boys. Embryo cryopreservation is the most successful option for women with a male partner. Mature oocyte or ovarian tissue cryopreservation currently provides only a slim opportunity of a later pregnancy for single women and prepubertal girls.

Keywords: Fertility preservation or restoration, cryopreservation, spermatogenesis, premature ovarian failure, embryo, oocyte, sex hormones.

1. Background — Significance and Recognition of Infertility after Cancer

For patients of reproductive age, the loss of reproductive function from cancer treatment is easily underestimated, as potential infertility is a significant issue among cancer patients. The diagnosis of a cancer did not influence the desire for pregnancy in 71% of women and 68% of men.[1–3] The concerns about loss of fertility are more pronounced in patients who do not have children prior to cancer diagnosis: three quarters (76%) of cancer survivors (women and men) without children voiced fertility concerns, compared to just over a quarter (31% of women and 26% of men) of cancer survivors who already had children.[1,4] The stress associated with infertility alone, as assessed by standardised methods, is equivalent to that experienced by patients with heart disease or cancer.[5] In a web-based survey of potentially fertile women with breast cancer (mean age 32.9 years), 57% recalled substantial concern at the time of diagnosis about becoming infertile with treatment and 29% reported that infertility concerns influenced treatment decisions.[6]

Surveys of oncologists completed several years ago showed that while most agreed that sperm banking should be offered to all men at risk of testicular damage from cancer treatment, 48% usually did not bring up the topic with their patients.[4] This may have partially reflected the knowledge of some oncologists at that time, as a study completed in 1999 found that only 26% of oncologists were aware that the application of intra-cytoplasmic sperm injection, in which sperm obtained by testicular aspiration, if necessary, could allow men previously considered infertile to become biologic fathers. In women a similar situation existed, as outlined in a study of breast cancer patients.[6] In this study, 72% of women discussed fertility concerns with their doctor, but only 51% felt their concerns were addressed adequately. This situation has now changed, as reflected by the position statement of the American Society of Clinical Oncology which now recommends that: "oncologists should discuss with patients the possibility of infertility when treated during their reproductive years" and "oncologists should be prepared to discuss possible fertility preservation options or to refer appropriately".[7] Guidelines on fertility preservation developed by both American and British Colleges underline the importance of informing patients affected by cancer prior to or during their reproductive lifespan about the possibility of fertility impairment due to cancer treatment and the available options to preserve fertility.[8,9]

Physicians managing patients with recently diagnosed cancer face several challenges and conflicts in dealing with cancer and fertility at the same time. Counselling has to be offered within the small timeframe between diagnosis and the start of treatment. In addition to decisions concerning treatment strategies, patients have to make an additional decision with regard to fertility preservation at a time of life crisis.[8] They must aim for the treatment with the highest therapeutic efficiency and at the same time the lowest negative impact on testicular or ovarian function. They may need to decide between treatment commencing as soon as possible — perhaps associated with hormone suppressive agents (to somewhat reduce the impact on the gonad) — and a treatment delay, to allow multiple semen collections or ovarian stimulation for egg harvesting and fertilisation. An additional conflict occurs in the management of children with cancer, when parents may wish preservation of germ cells and there is lack of informed consent from the child or adolescent. Oncologists and fertility specialists must inform and educate patients about treatment options and at the same time assess the emotional, cognitive and physical state of the patient. Their decisions will also take into account an assessment of the probable chance for cure or the impact on disease-free survival in individual patients.

Gonadal function is decreased or permanently impaired by the direct effects of many chemotherapeutic drugs and endocrine altering agents, by radiotherapy involving the testes, ovaries, uterus and other parts of the reproductive tract and pituitary gland and, particularly in women, by treatment which delays the opportunity to conceive, so that advancing female age significantly reduces the chances of pregnancy.

2. Direct Effects of Cancer Therapy

2.1 *Effect of cytotoxic therapies on the ovary*

Female reproductive lifespan is established during foetal life, when the foetal ovary becomes populated by more than one million primordial follicles. Post-natally these are progressively depleted until the age of the menopause. The best markers of ovarian age include the early follicular phase serum FSH, the ovarian follicle count assessed by pelvic ultrasound and the serum AMH (Anti-Mullerian Hormone) concentration.[9] AMH is produced by pre-antral and small antral follicles, which also contain the majority of oocytes within the ovary. AMH is perhaps the most sensitive indicator of ovarian age, as AMH concentrations in the circulation normally decline with age[10] and become undetectable several years prior to the menopause. AMH reasonably predicts the ovarian response to controlled ovarian stimulation with exogenous FSH.[11,12]

It has been recognised for many years that chemotherapy depletes the ovary of growing follicles. This was well documented in a morphological study of the ovaries of girls with leukaemia.[13] Chemotherapy causes depletion of the primordial follicle pool in a drug and dose-dependent manner.[14–16] Ovarian failure following chemotherapy is also dependent on the age of the woman, as well as the chemotherapeutic regimen used.[17,18] Changes in ovarian function following ovarian cancer therapy are most easily observed when acute ovarian failure occurs during or soon after cancer treatment, however, significant follicle depletion may occur despite maintenance of regular menstrual cycles.[19,20] Hence chemotherapy may either cause rapid onset of secondary amenorrhoea, or shorten the duration of subsequent ovarian function and a premature menopause. A recent study of ovarian biopsy samples from young women before and after chemotherapy showed a deterioration in ovarian follicle quality after chemotherapy, with an increased number of abnormal granulosa cell nuclei and oocyte nuclear vacuolisation.[21] Chemotherapy therefore can be considered to cause a form of accelerated ovarian ageing. Reduced serum AMH concentrations have been found in young women treated for cancer during childhood, in whom menstrual cycles are maintained and other markers of ovarian function, e.g. FSH and Inhibin B, are not altered.[19]

The risk of chemotherapy induced ovarian failure varies with specific drug regimens, with alkylating and platinum-based agents having the greatest potential to damage the ovary.[22,23] Several studies have attempted to categorise chemotherapy drugs

Table 1. Gonadotoxic potential of chemotherapeutic agents.[15,30,70]

Cytotoxic substances with a high risk of premature ovarian failure (POF)
- Cyclophosphamide
- Chlorambucil
- Melphalan
- Busulfan
- Procarbazine
- Nitrosourea
- Mechlorethamine (nitrogen mustard)
- Cytarabine (cytosine arabinoside)
- Ifosfamide
- Thiotepa

Cytotoxic substances with an intermediate risk of POF
- Cisplatin
- Doxorubicin
- Epirubicin

Cytotoxic substances with a low or no risk of POF
- Methotrexate
- 5-Fluorouracil
- Vincristine
- Vinblastine
- Bleomycin
- Actinomycin D
- Mitomycin C

Substances with an as yet unknown risk of POF
- Taxanes
- Oxaliplatin
- Irinotecan
- Monoclonal antibodies (e.g. Trastuzumap)
- Tyrosine kinase (EGFR) inhibitor (e.g. Erlotinib)

according to their potential to cause premature ovarian failure (see Table 1).

2.2   *Radiotherapy and the ovary*

Radiotherapy to the ovaries is also a significant risk factor for acute ovarian failure,[24] with more than 70% of young women exposed to

2000cGy during treatment of leukaemia or lymphoma becoming amenorrhoeic. From observations of children and adolescents who received total body irradiation, Wallace *et al.* have calculated the LD$_{50}$ of the human oocyte to be < 2 Gy.[25] Smaller doses of irradiation were also capable of causing ovarian failure, if associated with other factors, such as concomitant exposure to an alkylating agent, or an older age at diagnosis.[26]

Subtle disorders of ovarian function are also seen in survivors of childhood cranial irradiation for acute lymphoblastic leukaemia.[27] Luteal phase length was shorter and ovarian production of both oestrogen and progesterone less than in a control group. The abnormalities were attributed to alterations in hypothalamic-pituitary secretion of gonadotrophins, particularly LH.

Uterine development and function may also be a casualty of cancer treatment. After total body irradiation, reduced uterine volume, undetectable uterine blood supply and absent endometrium were seen.[28] After three months of physiological sex steroid replacement treatment, uterine blood supply and endometrial responses were not significantly different from controls, and uterine volume improved, but remained significantly smaller than controls and correlated with age at total body irradiation.

2.3   *Effect of cytotoxic therapies on the testis*

In males direct testicular irradiation as well as many chemotherapeutic agents are gonadotoxic, causing azoospermia, or reduced sperm counts. The effects on the testis depend on the underlying disease, the patient's age, the type and dose of drug used, and the duration of treatment (see Tables 2 and 3).[29–31] Some drugs are well recognised to cause infertility; for example, a total cumulative dose of cyclophosphamide of > 300 mg/kg, or cisplatin > 400 mg/m^2 causes irreversible impairment of spermatogenesis in > 80% of men.[32,33] Although available data is limited, it is estimated that about half of the males treated with a combination of chemotherapeutic drugs remain permanently oligoazoospermic.

Chemotherapy which does not result in complete loss of spermatogenesis may cause mutagenic changes in the sperm, such as a transient increase in sperm aneuploidy,[34] or loss of sperm DNA

Table 2. Fertility in men following different chemotherapy treatment regimes.[29]

Diagnosis	Treatment	Post-treatment fertility
Hodgkin lymphoma	Mustine Vincristine Procarbazine Prednisolone	Azoospermia in > 90%
Hodgkin's lymphoma	Other regimes	Temporary azoospermia Normal sperm concentration after 18 months
Non-Hodgkin lymphoma	Cyclophosphamide Doxorubin Vincristine Prednisolone	Permanent azoospermia in about 30%
Testicular cancer	Cisplatin/ carboplatin-based chemotherapy	Normospermia • 50% at two years • 80% in five years

Table 3. Testicular damage with cancer treatment.[31]

	Regiments	Azoospermia (%)
Hodgkin disease	MOPP, MVPP, COPP, CVPP ABVD/MOPP	85–100 0–50
Non-Hodgkin lymphoma	With cyclophosphamide	50–100
Sarcoma	Depends on cyclophosphamide dose	30–90
Testicular cancer	Depends on cisplatinum dose	0–55
Sarcoma	Depends on cisplatinum dose	5–55

integrity. DNA fragmentation in sperm can now be measured in several laboratory tests.[35–37] These changes in sperm DNA reduce the probability of pregnancy without medical assistance. Use of sperm previously exposed to chemotherapy in an assisted reproduction treatment programme is associated with a lower *in vitro* fertilisation rate, poorer embryo development and quality and lower pregnancy rates.

Questions arise about the safety of a spontaneous pregnancy after cancer treatment in men. These include whether there is an increased risk of genetic abnormalities in offspring and if the risk is indefinite, or whether there a washout period. Many oncologists advise couples to use birth control measures for 18 months after chemotherapy. When assisted reproduction treatment is needed, some have advocated that pre-implantation genetic screening (PGS) of embryos be used to help exclude genetic abnormalities which may arise because of the poor sperm quality. To date a follow-up of offspring of post cancer treated men has shown no increase in the risk of gross chromosomal abnormalities.[38]

2.4 *Radiotherapy and the testis*

Direct irradiation of the prostate or testes may also impair testicular function. A dose of 100–300cGy directed to the testis can reduce spermatogenesis, however, full recovery from the effects of this dose is possible. Following radiotherapy spermatogenesis may gradually improve over a period of up to five years, even if the man remains azoospermic after one year.[39] A dose of more than 400cGy may cause permanent azoospermia.[34]

Within the testis, the germinal epithelium is more sensitive than the interstitial cells to chemotherapy. Therefore adult men with cancer may retain normal serum testosterone concentrations, while becoming azoospermic after chemotherapy or radiotherapy. Loss of gonadal function in pre-pubertal cancer survivors requires that these patients be given hormone replacement, to achieve development milestones and adult bone strength.

3. Sex Hormone Production, Cancer and Gonadotoxic Therapy

Oestrogen production in women is directly linked to cyclical oocyte maturation. Loss of oocytes therefore means a loss of the ability of the ovary to produce the usual premenopausal concentrations of oestradiol. In men testosterone production may occur in the absence of spermatogenesis. However in both sexes, cancer and its treatment may cause loss of sex steroid production by the gonad. As well as acute symptoms such as vasomotor instability and emotional changes, loss of these hormones impairs sexual function, long term quality of life, and increases the risk of premature degenerative disease such as osteoporosis and cardiovascular disease.

4. Fertility Preservation Options for Patients with Cancer

The prime focus of physicians and patients is effective treatment and survival from cancer. Many patients now have a longer life expectancy after cancer treatment, therefore it is becoming more important to consider their quality of life. This includes the possibility of a successful pregnancy. Providing options for preserving fertility in men, women and children is a quality of life issue, as well as a future reproductive issue.

The options for retaining the possibility of becoming a parent are limited. Initial consideration should be given to any measures which may protect the reproductive organs while cancer treatment is being administered. Because these have limited effectiveness, collection and cryostorage of sperm and oocytes should also be considered. Adult men usually have the option of cryopreservation of sperm for later use. This is not an option for pre-pubertal boys, or even for many post-pubertal adolescents. Cryopreservation of oocytes for a female of any age is not a proven option, although significant progress has been made in the successful freeze-thawing of mature oocytes from postpubertal females. The only reliable option for women is collection of mature oocytes for creation of embryos *in vitro* which may be cryopreserved. This is not an option for single women and pre-pubertal girls.

4.1 *Protection of the gonads during cancer treatment*

4.1.1 *Ovarian transposition before radiation*

Radiation treatment of leukaemia or lymphoma located in the lower abdomen or inguinal region may expose the ovary to megavoltage radiotherapy. As already described, this may cause acute and permanent ovarian failure, depending on the total dose of radiotherapy. Ovarian function following pelvic radiation is further impaired if the patient has also received chemotherapy.[40]

During radiotherapy the gonads should be shielded whenever possible, or removed from the field of therapy. The whole ovary may be relocated prior to radiation therapy during a laparoscopic procedure. Several techniques have been described, including relocation behind the uterus,[41] to the lateral wall of the pelvis,[42] or under the right lobe of the liver.[43] To maintain ovarian blood supply, the fimbrial end of the Fallopian tube is relocated together with the ovary. When fertility is desired at a later date in this situation, the ovaries need to be relocated in the pelvis, to allow for easy oocyte collection for an IVF procedure.

4.1.2 Use of gonadotrophin releasing hormone (GnRH) analogues and oral contraceptives to protect the ovary during chemotherapy

Ovarian function is preserved in most long-term survivors of lymphoma treated pre-pubertally. Only a minority of those treated post-pubertally with a similar treatment protocol retain ovarian function.[44] This observation creates the rationale for the use of GnRH analogues, or oral contraceptives, to create a temporary pre-pubertal state in women of reproductive age during chemotherapy. Both of these agents suppress FSH, which is responsible for stimulating the recruitment of small ovarian follicles, making them more susceptible to chemotherapy. A recent meta-analysis of nine retrospective studies using either or both GnRH analogues and oral contraceptives found a partially protective effect of these agents, when used prior to and during chemotherapy. Use of a GnRH analogue reduced the risk of premature ovarian failure (POF) from 55.5% to 11.1%, while oral contraceptive use was associated with a 13.2% rate of POF, compared with 29.8% in the control group.[45] Two of the studies found no benefit from the use of an oral contraceptive alone. The value of GnRH analogue treatment appears chemotherapy-drug dose dependent and is of no significant benefit in association with high dose chemotherapy used prior to bone marrow transplantation.

A protective benefit of GnRH analogues has not been reported for men, or for gonadal damage induced by irradiation of the gonads.[46]

4.2 Cryopreservation to maintain the possibility of a pregnancy

4.2.1 Collection and cryopreservation of fertilised oocytes or embryos

Oocyte collection, *in vitro* fertilisation, and cryostorage of fertilised oocytes are widely available and relatively successful components of all Assisted Reproduction Treatment (ART) programmes. Since 1978 more than three million babies have been born worldwide following this treatment. It involves simultaneous stimulation of multiple ovarian follicles with a daily subcutaneous injection for approximately twelve days of FSH (follicle stimulating hormone), while using a GnRH analogue to prevent a premature LH (luteinizing hormone) surge. During this time, the ovarian response is monitored by serum measurement of oestradiol and pelvic ultrasound scanning. Follicle maturation leading to ovulation is triggered by a single injection of either LH or hCG (human chorionic gonadotrophin). Oocytes are collected by transvaginal ultrasound guided needle aspiration, just prior to the expected time of ovulation. (Fig. 1) The oocytes are fertilised *in vitro* with the partner's sperm and this may involve direct sperm injection into oocytes if semen quality is poor. A fertilised oocyte or embryo is placed into the uterus between two and five days later and the remaining embryos which continue to grow *in vitro* may be preserved by freezing for later use by the couple.

This process is now regarded as a proven treatment option for sub-fertile couples throughout the world. Completion of an ART treatment cycle with cryopreservation of all fertilized oocytes is therefore an option prior to chemo or radiotherapy for cancer patients who have a long-term partner. Freeze-thaw survival rates are approximately 75% and clinical pregnancy rates per embryo are approximately 30% for women less than age 38 years, with lower success rates for older women. This process may not be relevant to single women, those patients who need urgent chemotherapy, or whose disease process may be aggravated by increased concentrations of oestrogen. ART treatment cycles are commenced in accordance with the woman's menstrual cycle. For women with cancer this may mean an extra delay in commencing cancer treatment. A recent study however demonstrated that ovarian follicle

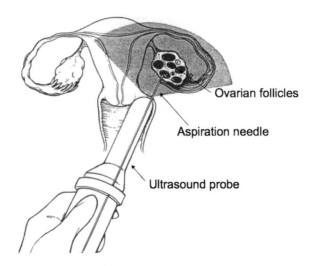

Figure 1.   Ultrasound-guided needle aspiration of ovarian follicles.

stimulation could be commenced at short notice at any time in the woman's menstrual cycle, without decreasing the expectation of obtaining fertilising oocytes for cryopreservation.[47]

During ART the woman's serum concentration of oestradiol increases rapidly, in accordance with the number of growing follicles. This may mean she experiences more than a ten-fold increase in oestradiol. Because of the concern this may promote the growth of oestrogen sensitive cancer cells, Oktay *et al.*[48] investigated the use of ART, which included the use of an aromatase inhibitor, during the phase of follicle stimulation. This agent effectively blocks the production of oestrogens from androgens within the granulosa cells of the ovarian follicle and prevents the major increase in the serum concentration of oestrogen. Oocyte quality as judged by the fertilisation rate and embryo cleavage rate is not influenced by blocking oestrogen production.

There have been very few published reports of the long term health of women who completed an ovarian stimulation cycle prior to chemotherapy. In 2008, Azim *et al.* published the outcome of a study of 79 women who received ovarian stimulation combined with an aromatase inhibitor, compared with 136 women who received no ovarian stimulation treatment prior to chemotherapy.

This group found no adverse effect of the stimulation treatment after more than two years of follow up.[49]

4.2.2 Mature oocyte and ovarian cortical tissue cryopreservation

Other means of attempting to preserve fertility options include cryopreservation of mature metaphase II oocytes or ovarian cortical tissue biopsy samples. As both of these have so far been associated with very little success in eventually achieving a pregnancy, they must still be regarded as very uncertain options.

Mature human oocytes are particularly susceptible to cryoinjury causing disruption of the meiotic cell spindle. The process of oocyte cryopreservation has improved recently by both the conventional slow programmed cryopreservation process and the use of vitrification technology. With these improvements to date, approximately 600 babies have been born worldwide from the use of frozen-thawed oocytes.[50,51] Collection of mature oocytes requires the same ovarian stimulation treatment used in an ART cycle and therefore causes the same risks and inconveniences as the process leading to embryo cryopreservation.

Ovarian cortical tissue transplantation was first reported to result in a live birth by Donnez *et al.* in 2004.[52] Since then however only six live births, two biochemical pregnancies and two clinical miscarriages have been reported worldwide.[53–55] The probability of a successful outcome with this approach is not known, as there is no accurate data on the number of transplantation attempts that have been made. Collection of the ovarian tissue sample requires an operative procedure under general anaesthetic. Because the density of primordial and small growing follicles remaining in the ovary declines with female age and because the freeze thawing process may further deplete the sample of viable follicles, this option is probably of little value for women over the age of 30 years.[56]

UK Criteria for Selection of Women for Ovarian Cryopreservation[56]

- Age < 30 yrs

- No previous chemotherapy or radiotherapy (patients < 15 yrs considered if previous chemotherapy was low risk)
- Realistic chance of long term survival
- High risk of treatment-induced immediate ovarian failure (estimate at > 50%)
- Informed consent from patient
- Negative HIV and hepatitis serology
- No existing children

It is important to consider that ovarian tissue sample transplantation carries the theoretical risk of re-implanting tumour cells contained in the biopsy sample. Current research is focussed on identifying tumour cell markers in the tissue samples before transplantation.[57]

4.2.3 Cryopreservation options for men

The most widely available standard procedure for post-pubertal males able to ejaculate is cryopreservation of ejaculated sperm. The opportunity for a future pregnancy may be increased if more than one sample is stored. Freeze-thawing of semen results in a decrease in the number of motile sperm recovered from the sample, which means that most cryostored samples are not suitable for simple insemination and may only be used to achieve a pregnancy in conjunction with IVF.

Current assisted reproduction techniques include the *in vitro* use of ICSI (Intra-Cytoplasmic Sperm Injection). Using this procedure, a single sperm may be injected into the cytoplasm of a mature oocyte, to create an embryo for cryopreservation and replacement into the uterus at a future date. Therefore any semen sample which contains sperm, even if extremely few in number, should be cryopreserved.

Semen should be cryopreserved before cancer treatment begins, or shortly after starting treatment.[58] It is well recognised that acute and chronic illness including cancer may increase DNA damage to sperm,[59] and that both chemotherapy and radiotherapy may further increase sperm aneuploidy rate[60] and sperm DNA fragmentation.[61] Despite this, to date there have been no reports of increased chromosomal congenital abnormalities in children born with sperm from men undergoing, or having had chemotherapy.

When it is not possible to obtain an ejaculate, or when the semen contains no sperm because of previous damage to spermatogenesis or obstruction of the vas deferens, it may be possible to obtain sperm by direct testicular or epididymal aspiration or biopsy (Fig. 2). Sperm suitable for use in ICSI may also be extracted from orchidectomy specimens from men with testicular cancer. This may also be possible for peri-pubertal boys.[62] Testicular tissue biopsy samples from pre-pubertal boys have been cryopreserved in the expectation of successful future transplantation.

5. Stem Cell Therapy for Germ Line Replacement

The existence of spermatogonial stem cells in the testis offers the possibility of cryopreservation and subsequent restoration of fertility in a man rendered infertile by cancer therapy. Infusion of these stem cells into rodent and primate testes has been shown to restore spermatogenesis;[63] however, to date this has not been reported in humans. Efforts are concentrated on methods to deplete testicular tissue samples of tumour cells, while increasing the concentration of stem cell spermatogonia. Germ cell transplantation, germ cell maturation *in vitro* and stem-cell to germ-cell maturation have been successful in some animal studies.[62]

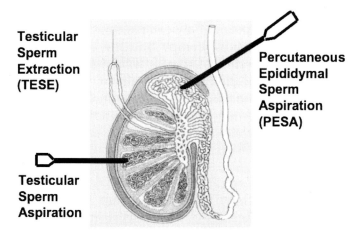

Figure 2. Surgical sperm recovery.

6. Treatment of Cancer of the Cervix, Endometrium, Ovaries and Subsequent Fertility

6.1 *Cervical cancer*

The standard treatment for invasive cervical cancer is hysterectomy. A recent literature review estimated that 43% of women with cervical cancer are aged less than 45 years,[64] so fertility-sparing surgery may be an option for women with stage 1 cervical cancer.[65] Pregnancies after such surgery are associated with an increased risk of premature birth.[66]

6.2 *Endometrial cancer*

Approximately 5% of women with endometrial cancer are less than age 40 years at the time of diagnosis and successful pregnancies have been recorded in a selected number of these women after hormonal treatment of their cancer.[67] The treatment options include high dose megestrol acetate, or medroxyprogesterone acetate, MIRENA, GnRH analogues, or aromatase inhibitors combined with hysteroscopic resection of the endometrial cancer. Concomitant ovarian tumour or myometrial invasion demonstrated by MRI and sonography excludes the possibility of fertility conserving treatment in more than 50% of these women. Hormonal treatment for endometrial cancer, which allows conservation of the uterus, may be allowed in these women, when there is a well differentiated carcinoma, absence of suspicious pelvic or para-aortic lymph nodes, no contraindication to medical therapy, and the patient understands and accepts that as hormonal therapy is not standard treatment, close follow-up is essential.[68] This usually means repeat uterine curettage every three months, unless pregnant. Chiva *et al.* reported that only 51% of women selected by these criteria had a lasting and complete response to hormonal treatment.[68]

6.3 *Ovarian cancer*

Borderline ovarian tumours account for up to 20% of ovarian tumours and the average age of diagnosis is ten years earlier than for ovarian epithelial tumours. When diagnosed in a potentially fertile woman, conservative surgery which respects one ovary and the uterus may allow the woman the opportunity of pregnancy. The risk of recurrent cancer after this fertility-sparing surgery is increased, but survival rates are not altered.[69]

7. Sex Hormone Replacement Therapy

Sex hormone therapy should be given to post-pubertal patients who do not have a sex hormone sensitive cancer, to alleviate symptoms of deficiency and to prevent long term health problems. These include osteoporosis and vascular disease. The aim of this therapy is hormonal replacement to restore normal physiology. In discussion with patients this should be clearly distinguished from pharmacological doses of testosterone in men or post-menopausal therapy in women.

Pre-pubertal boys and girls who lose gonadal or pituitary gland function because of cancer or cancer treatment require sex hormone treatment to complete pubertal development, as well as for long term health.

8. Summary

Fertility may be a casualty of cancer or its treatment. Population studies suggest that the ability to have their own children is of great importance to many people. Therefore any physician managing patients of reproductive age or younger with cancer should address the potential for treatment-related infertility with them or their parents.

The probability of permanent infertility or compromised fertility after cancer treatment varies and depends on many factors related to the individual patient, the cancer itself, as well as the type dose duration and method of administration of treatments. In both sexes fertility may be transiently or permanently affected by cancer treatments. In women the effects may only become manifest some time later, by the occurrence of premature menopause; the resumption of regular menses does not guarantee normal fertility.

The American Society of Clinical Oncology practice guidelines recommends that:

"As part of education and informed consent before cancer therapy, oncologists should address the possibility of infertility with

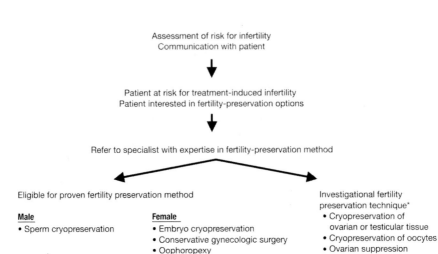

Figure 3. American Society of Clinical Oncologists — recommendations 2005.[7]

patients treated during their reproductive years and be prepared to discuss possible fertility preservation options or refer appropriate and interested patients reproductive specialists. Clinical judgement should be employed in the timing of raising this issue, but discussion at the earliest possible opportunity is encouraged. Sperm and embryo cryopreservation are considered standard practice and are widely available; other available fertility preservation methods should be considered investigational and be performed in centers with the necessary expertise."[7]

A management plan recommended by the American Society of Clinical Oncologists for patients whose fertility is threatened by cancer or its treatment is described in Fig. 3.

References

1. L. R. Schover, Psychosocial aspects of infertility and decisions about reproduction in young cancer survivors: A review, *Med. Pediatr. Oncol.* **33**(1): 53–59 (1999).
2. L R. Schover, K. Brey, A. Lichtin, L. I. Lipshultz and S. Jeha, Knowledge and experience regarding cancer, infertility, and sperm banking in younger male survivors, *J. Clin. Oncol.* **20**(7): 1880–1889 (2002).

3. V. Zanagnolo, E. Sartori, E. Trussardi, B. Pasinetti and T. Maggino, Preservation of ovarian function, reproductive ability and emotional attitudes in patients with malignant ovarian tumors, *Eur. J. Obstet. Gynecol. Reprod. Biol.* **123**(2): 235–243 (2005).

4. L. R. Schover, K. Brey, A. Lichtin, L. I. Lipshultz and S. Jeha, Oncologists' attitudes and practices regarding banking sperm before cancer treatment, *J. Clin. Oncol.* **20**(7): 1890–1897 (2002).

5. T. M. Cousineau and A. D. Domar, Psychological impact of infertility, *Best. Pract. Res. Clin. Obstet. Gynaecol.* **21**(2): 293–308 (2007).

6. A. H. Partridge, S. Gelber, J. Peppercorn, E. Sampson, K. Knudsen, M. Laufer *et al.*, Web-based survey of fertility issues in young women with breast cancer, *J. Clin. Oncol.* **22**(20): 4174–4183 (2004).

7. S. J. Lee, L. R. Schover, A. H. Partridge, P. Patrizio, W. H. Wallace, K. Hagerty *et al.*, American Society of Clinical Oncology recommendations on fertility preservation in cancer patients, *J. Clin. Oncol.* **24**(18): 2917–2931 (2006).

8. K. W. Brown, A. R. Levy, Z. Rosberger and L. Edgar, Psychological distress and cancer survival: a follow-up 10 years after diagnosis, *Psychosom. Med.* **65**(4): 636–643 (2003).

9. A. de Vet, J. S. Laven, F. H. de Jong, A. P. Themmen and B. C. Fauser Antimullerian hormone serum levels: A putative marker for ovarian aging, *Fertil. Steril.* **77**(2): 357–362 (2002).

10. I. A. van Rooij, F. J. Broekmans, G. J. Scheffer, C. W. Looman, J. D. Habbema, F. H. de Jong *et al.*, Serum antimullerian hormone levels best reflect the reproductive decline with age in normal women with proven fertility: A longitudinal study, *Fertil. Steril.* **83**(4): 979–987 (2005).

11. R. Fanchin, L. M. Schonauer, C. Righini, N. Frydman, R. Frydman and J. Taieb, Serum anti-Mullerian hormone dynamics during controlled ovarian hyperstimulation, *Hum. Reprod.* **18**(2): 328–332 (2003).

12. R. Fanchin, L. M. Schonauer, C. Righini, J. Guibourdenche, R. Frydman and J. Taieb, Serum anti-Mullerian hormone is more strongly related to ovarian follicular status than serum inhibin B, estradiol, FSH and LH on day 3, *Hum. Reprod.* **18**(2): 323–327 (2003).

13. R. Himelstein-Braw, H. Peters and M. Faber, Morphological study of the ovaries of leukaemic children, *Br. J. Cancer* **38**(1): 82–87 (1978).

14. R. M. Chapman, S. B. Sutcliffe, L. H. Rees, C. R. Edwards and J. S. Malpas, Cyclical combination chemotherapy and gonadal function. Retrospective study in males, *Lancet* **1**(8111): 285–289 (1979).

15. M. Sonmezer and K. Oktay, Fertility preservation in female patients, *Hum. Reprod. Update* **10**(3): 251–266 (2004).
16. G. L. Warne, K. F. Fairley, J. B. Hobbs and F. I. Martin, Cyclophosphamide-induced ovarian failure, *N. Engl. J. Med.* **289**(22): 1159–1162 (1973).
17. J. Bines, D. M. Oleske and M. A. Cobleigh, Ovarian function in premenopausal women treated with adjuvant chemotherapy for breast cancer, *J. Clin. Oncol.* **14**(5): 1718–1729 (1996).
18. D. Meirow and J. G. Schenker, The current status of sperm donation in assisted reproduction technology: Ethical and legal considerations, *J. Assist. Reprod. Genet.* **14**(3): 133–138 (1997).
19. L. E. Bath, W. H. Wallace, M. P. Shaw, C. Fitzpatrick and R. A. Anderson, Depletion of ovarian reserve in young women after treatment for cancer in childhood: Detection by anti-Mullerian hormone, inhibin B and ovarian ultrasound, *Hum. Reprod.* **18**(11): 2368–2374 (2003).
20. E. C. Larsen, J. Muller, C. Rechnitzer, K. Schmiegelow and A. N. Andersen, Diminished ovarian reserve in female childhood cancer survivors with regular menstrual cycles and basal FSH <10 IU/l, *Hum. Reprod.* **18**(2): 417–422 (2003).
21. R. Abir, A. Ben-Haroush, C. Felz, E. Okon, H. Raanani, R. Orvieto *et al.*, Selection of patients before and after anticancer treatment for ovarian cryopreservation, *Hum. Reprod.* **23**(4): 869–877 (2008).
22. T. Maltaris, H. Koelbl, R. Seufert, F. Kiesewetter, M. W. Beckmann, A. Mueller *et al.*, Gonadal damage and options for fertility preservation in female and male cancer survivors, *Asian J. Androl.* **8**(5): 515–533 (2006).
23. Y. X. Su, J. W. Zheng, G. S. Zheng, G. Q. Liao and Z. Y. Zhang, Neoadjuvant chemotherapy of cisplatin and fluorouracil regimen in head and neck squamous cell carcinoma: A meta-analysis, *Chin. Med. J. (Engl.)* **121**(19): 1939–1944 (2008).
24. W. Chemaitilly, A. C. Mertens, P. Mitby, J. Whitton, M. Stovall, Y. Yasui *et al.*, Acute ovarian failure in the childhood cancer survivor study, *J. Clin. Endocrinol. Metab.* **91**(5): 1723–1728 (2006).
25. W. H. Wallace, A. B. Thomson and T. W. Kelsey, The radiosensitivity of the human oocyte, *Hum. Reprod.* **18**(1): 117–121 (2003).
26. C. C. Lushbaugh and G. W. Casarett, The effects of gonadal irradiation in clinical radiation therapy: A review, *Cancer* **37**(2 Suppl.): 1111–1125 (1976).
27. L. E. Bath, R. A. Anderson, H. O. Critchley, C. J. Kelnar and W. H. Wallace, Hypothalamic-pituitary-ovarian dysfunction after

prepubertal chemotherapy and cranial irradiation for acute leukaemia, *Hum. Reprod.* **16**(9): 1838–1844 (2001).

28. H. O. Critchley and W. H. Wallace, Impact of cancer treatment on uterine function, *J. Natl. Cancer Inst. Monogr.* **2005**(34): 64–68 (2005).

29. S. J. Howell and S. M. Shalet, Testicular function following chemotherapy, *Hum. Reprod. Update* **7**(4): 363–369 (2001).

30. W. H. Wallace, R. A. Anderson and D. S. Irvine, Fertility preservation for young patients with cancer: Who is at risk and what can be offered? *Lancet Oncol.* **6**(4): 209–218 (2005).

31. D. J. Handelsman and J. D. Zajac, Androgen deficiency and replacement therapy in men, *Med. J. Aust.* **180**(10): 529–535 (2004).

32. S. A. Rivkees and J. D. Crawford, The relationship of gonadal activity and chemotherapy-induced gonadal damage, *J. Am. Med. Assoc.* **259**(14): 2123–2125 (1988).

33. M. Brydoy, S. D. Fossa, O. Klepp, R. M. Bremnes, E. A. Wist, T. Wentzel-Larsen *et al.*, Paternity following treatment for testicular cancer, *J. Natl. Cancer Inst.* **97**(21): 1580–1588 (2005).

34. K. L. Schmidt, E. Carlsen and A. N. Andersen, Fertility treatment in male cancer survivors, *Int. J. Androl.* **30**(4): 413–418; discussion 418–419 (2007).

35. A. Edelstein, H. Yavetz, S. E. Kleiman, R. Hauser, A. Botchan, G. Paz *et al.*, Effect of long-term storage on deoxyribonucleic acid damage and motility of sperm bank donor specimens, *Fertil. Steril.* **90**(4): 1327–1330 (2008).

36. M. Meseguer, R. Santiso, N. Garrido and J. L. Fernandez, The effect of cancer on sperm DNA fragmentation as measured by the sperm chromatin dispersion test, *Fertil. Steril.* **90**(1): 225–227.

37. J. R. Spermon, L. Ramos, A. M. Wetzels, C. G. Sweep, D. D. Braat, L. A. Kiemeney *et al.*, Sperm integrity pre- and post-chemotherapy in men with testicular germ cell cancer, *Hum. Reprod.* **21**(7): 1781–1786 (2006).

38. F. Belva, S. Henriet, E. Van den Abbeel, M. Camus, P. Devroey, J. Van der Elst *et al.*, Neonatal outcome of 937 children born after transfer of cryopreserved embryos obtained by ICSI and IVF and comparison with outcome data of fresh ICSI and IVF cycles, *Hum. Reprod.* **23**(10): 2227–2238 (2008).

39. S. J. Howell and S. M. Shalet, Spermatogenesis after cancer treatment: Damage and recovery, *J. Natl. Cancer Inst. Monogr.* **2005**(34): 12–17 (2005).

40. R. S. Williams, R. D. Littell and N. P. Mendenhall, Laparoscopic oophoropexy and ovarian function in the treatment of Hodgkin disease, *Cancer* **86**(10): 2138–2142 (1999).

41. S. M. Scott and W. Schlaff, Laparoscopic medial oophoropexy prior to radiation therapy in an adolescent with Hodgkin's disease, *J. Pediatr. Adolesc. Gynecol.* **18**(5): 355–357 (2005).

42. M. Bisharah and T. Tulandi, Laparoscopic preservation of ovarian function: An underused procedure, *Am. J. Obstet. Gynecol.* **188**(2): 367–370 (2003).

43. L. A. Farber, J. W. Ames, S. Rush and D. Gal, Laparoscopic ovarian transposition to preserve ovarian function before pelvic radiation and chemotherapy in a young patient with rectal cancer, *Med. Gen. Med.* **7**(1): 66 (2005).

44. T. T. Ortin, C. A. Shostak and S. S. Donaldson, Gonadal status and reproductive function following treatment for Hodgkin's disease in childhood: The Stanford experience, *Int. J. Radiat. Oncol. Biol. Phys.* **19**(4): 873–880 (1990).

45. Z. Blumenfeld and M. von Wolff, GnRH-analogues and oral contraceptives for fertility preservation in women during chemotherapy, *Hum. Reprod. Update* **14**(6): 543–552 (2008).

46. Z. Blumenfeld, Gender difference: Fertility preservation in young women but not in men exposed to gonadotoxic chemotherapy, *Minerva Endocrinol.* **32**(1): 23–34 (2007).

47. M. von Wolff, C. J. Thaler, T. Frambach, C. Zeeb, B. Lawrenz, R. M. Popovici *et al.*, Ovarian stimulation to cryopreserve fertilized oocytes in cancer patients can be started in the luteal phase, to appear in *Fertil. Steril.* (16 October 2008) [Epub ahead of print].

48. K. Oktay, A. Hourvitz, G. Sahin, O. Oktem, B. Safro, A. Cil *et al.*, Letrozole reduces estrogen and gonadotropin exposure in women with breast cancer undergoing ovarian stimulation before chemotherapy, *J. Clin. Endocrinol. Metab.* **91**(10): 3885–3890 (2006).

49. A. A. Azim, M. Costantini-Ferrando and K. Oktay, Safety of fertility preservation by ovarian stimulation with letrozole and gonadotropins in patients with breast cancer: A prospective controlled study, *J. Clin. Oncol.* **26**(16): 2630–265 (2008).

50. M. Antinori, E. Licata, G. Dani, F. Cerusico, C. Versaci and S. Antinori, Cryotop vitrification of human oocytes results in high survival rate and healthy deliveries, *Reprod. Biomed. Online* **14**(1): 72–79 (2007).

51. E. Porcu, R. Fabbri, G. Damiano, S. Giunchi, R. Fratto, P. M. Ciotti *et al.*, Clinical experience and applications of oocyte cryopreservation, *Mol. Cell Endocrinol.* **169**(1–2): 33–37 (2000).

52. J. Donnez, M. M. Dolmans, D. Demylle, P. Jadoul, C. Pirard, J. Squifflet *et al.*, Livebirth after orthotopic transplantation of cryopreserved ovarian tissue, *Lancet* **364**(9443): 1405–1410 (2004).

53. R. A. Anderson, Fertility preservation techniques: Laboratory and clinical progress and current issues, *Reproduction* **136**(6): 667–669 (2008).

54. R. A. Anderson, W. H. Wallace and D. T. Baird, Ovarian cryopreservation for fertility preservation: Indications and outcomes, *Reproduction* **136**(6): 681–689 (2008).

55. C. Y. Andersen, M. Rosendahl, A. G. Byskov, A. Loft, C. Ottosen, M. Dueholm *et al.*, Two successful pregnancies following autotransplantation of frozen/thawed ovarian tissue, *Hum. Reprod.* **23**(10): 2266–2272 (2008).

56. Report of a Working Party of the Royal College of Physicians, Royal College of Radiologists and Royal College of Obstetricians and Gynaecologists. In: *The Effects of Cancer Treatment on Reproductive Functions: Guidance on Management* (Royal College of Physicians, London, 2007).

57. D. Meirow, I. Hardan, J. Dor, E. Fridman, S. Elizur, H. Ra'anani *et al.*, Searching for evidence of disease and malignant cell contamination in ovarian tissue stored from hematologic cancer patients, *Hum. Reprod.* **23**(5): 1007–1013 (2008).

58. K. Chung, J. Irani, G. Knee, B. Efymow, L. Blasco and P. Patrizio, Sperm cryopreservation for male patients with cancer: An epidemiological analysis at the University of Pennsylvania, *Eur. J. Obstet. Gynecol. Reprod. Biol.* **113**(Suppl. 1): S7–11 (2004).

59. C. O'Flaherty, F. Vaisheva, B. F. Hales, P. Chan and B. Robaire, Characterization of sperm chromatin quality in testicular cancer and Hodgkin's lymphoma patients prior to chemotherapy, *Hum. Reprod.* **23**(5): 1044–1052 (2008).

60. G. Fait, L. Yogev, A. Botchan, G. Paz, J. B. Lessing and H. Yavetz, Sex chromosome aneuploidy in sperm cells obtained from Hodgkin's lymphoma patients before therapy, *Fertil. Steril.* **75**(4): 828–829 (2001).

61. H. Kobayashi, K. Larson, R. K. Sharma, D. R. Nelson, D. P. Evenson, H. Toma *et al.*, DNA damage in patients with untreated cancer as measured by the sperm chromatin structure assay, *Fertil. Steril.* **75**(3): 469–475 (2001).

62. A. Revel and S. Revel-Vilk, Pediatric fertility preservation: Is it time to offer testicular tissue cryopreservation? *Mol. Cell Endocrinol.* **282**(1–2): 143–149 (2008).

63. K. E. Orwig and S. Schlatt, Cryopreservation and transplantation of spermatogonia and testicular tissue for preservation of male fertility, *J. Natl. Cancer Inst. Monogr.* **2005**(34): 51–56 (2005).

64. P. T. Ramirez, K. M. Schmeler, P. T. Soliman and M. Frumovitz, Fertility preservation in patients with early cervical cancer: Radical trachelectomy, *Gynecol. Oncol.* **110**(3 Suppl. 2): S25–S28 (2008).

65. Y. Sonoda, N. R. Abu-Rustum, M. L. Gemignani, D. S. Chi, C. L. Brown, E. A. Poynor *et al.*, A fertility-sparing alternative to radical hysterectomy: How many patients may be eligible? *Gynecol. Oncol.* **95**(3): 534–538 (2004).

66. M. Kyrgiou, G. Koliopoulos, P. Martin-Hirsch, M. Arbyn, W. Prendiville and E. Paraskevaidis, Obstetric outcomes after conservative treatment for intraepithelial or early invasive cervical lesions: Systematic review and meta-analysis, *Lancet* **367**(9509): 489–498 (2006).

67. T. Yahata, K. Fujita, Y. Aoki and K. Tanaka, Long-term conservative therapy for endometrial adenocarcinoma in young women, *Hum. Reprod.* **21**(4): 1070–1075 (2006).

68. L. Chiva, F. Lapuente, L. Gonzalez-Cortijo, N. Carballo, J. F. Garcia, A. Rojo *et al.*, Sparing fertility in young patients with endometrial cancer, *Gynecol. Oncol.* **111**(2 Suppl.): S101–S104 (2008).

69. P. Morice, Borderline tumours of the ovary and fertility, *Eur. J. Cancer* **42**(2): 149–158 (2006).

70. W. H. Wallace and A. B. Thomson, Preservation of fertility in children treated for cancer, *Arch. Dis. Child* **88**(6): 493–496 (2003).

30

Cancer and Thrombosis

Jerry Koutts

Abstract

The association between cancer and venous thromboembolism (VTE) has been known for over 150 years. Although the actual prevalence of cancer induced VTE is unclear, due largely to the frequent coexistence of cancer with other risk factors for VTE, including advanced age, immobilisation, surgery and chemotherapy. VTE is a common and life-threatening complication of and the second leading cause of morbidity and mortality amongst patients with cancer. Appropriate prophylactic practice for both surgical and non-surgical patients can significantly reduce this morbidity and mortality amongst patients with cancer.

Specific guidelines for the prevention and treatment of VTE in patients with cancer have been published by a number of expert groups and include the following recommendations:

(1) All hospitalised cancer patients should receive VTE prophylaxis with anticoagulant therapy in the absence of bleeding or other specific contraindications.
(2) Routine prophylaxis of ambulatory cancer patients with anticoagulants is not recommended, with the exception of patients receiving thalidomide or lenolidomide.
(3) Patients undergoing a surgical procedure of greater than 30 minutes anaesthetic time should be considered for pre-operative anticoagulant prophylaxis, which continues for

seven to ten days post-operatively or, for high risk patients, up to four weeks post-operatively.

(4) Specific prophylaxis to prevent VTE in patients with indwelling venous catheters is not recommended.

(5) Low molecular weight heparins (LMWH) are the preferred agent for both the initial and continuing treatment of cancer patients with established VTE. Recommended treatment duration for VTE is six months, or indefinite if active cancer or other risk factors persist.

(6) The impact of anticoagulants on cancer patient survival requires additional study and cannot be recommended at present.

Keywords: Deep vein thrombosis, pulmonary embolism, superficial thrombophlebitis, prophylaxis, anticoagulant therapy, heparins, vitamin K antagonists.

1. Introduction

Venous thromboembolic disease includes deep vein thrombosis (DVT) and pulmonary embolism (PE). Deep vein thrombosis includes upper extremity (brachial, axillary, subclavian and superior vena cava), lower extremity distal (calf veins), lower extremity proximal (popliteal and femoral) and central (iliac) and inferior vena cava. Catheter related DVT and superficial thrombophlebitis will also be considered separately.

The first reported association between cancer and VTE is generally attributed to Trousseau in 1865,[1] although the first cohort study which assessed the incidence of cancer in patients presenting with DVT was not published until 1982.[2] There is now extensive literature which documents the fact that VTE is a common and life-threatening complication of cancer, occurring in 4–20% of patients.[3-8] The risk of developing symptomatic VTE is six times higher in cancer patients, compared to non-cancer patients with a similar risk profile. The occurrence of VTE is reported to increase the likelihood of death for cancer patients by 2–8-fold. VTE has been documented as the most common cause of death in the month following surgery in patients with cancer.[6,9-14]

Active cancer accounts for at least 20% of all new VTE events in the community.[4] The increased risk of VTE in patients with cancer translates directly into increased morbidity and mortality, with approximately 10% of all hospital deaths attributed to PE.[15,16] The in-hospital fatality rate of VTE is estimated at 12% and the case-fatality rate at one year at 30%.[11,17]

High risk groups can be identified and stratified, but it is not possible to specifically predict which individual within a given risk group will develop clinically significant VTE. Massive PE occurs without warning in 70–80% of fatal cases and the diagnosis of VTE was not even considered prior to the event in most.[18–21]

Symptomatic DVT and PE are associated with significant acute and long term morbidity which consume substantial resources and adversely impact on patients' quality of life. Delayed discharge, re-admission (the majority of symptomatic VTE associated with hospitalisation occur after discharge), and complications of anticoagulant therapy represent the immediate consequences. The post-thrombotic syndrome of leg-swelling, discomfort and leg ulcers reduces patients' mobility, quality of life and economic well being.[22–24]

Although VTE is usually considered as a complication of surgery, the majority (60–80%) of symptomatic VTE events and fatalities from PE occur in non-surgical patients.[16,17,25–28] There have been numerous clinical trials which provide irrefutable evidence that primary prophylaxis reduces VTE, PE and fatalities.[29–33] Supporting these general trials is further strong evidence that prophylaxis with heparins effectively reduces the risk of VTE and fatal PE following cancer surgery.[29,34,35] It is important to recognise that cancer also represents an independent predictor of a poor response to prophylaxis. For patients with cancer, in general, a higher prophylactic dose is recommended for best outcomes.[36,37] The need to develop and promote specific guidelines to prevent VTE in cancer patients is underlined by the results of a recent survey of surgeons and oncologists, which reported that among hospitalised patients, VTE prophylaxis was used in 50% of surgical and 5% of the medical cancer patients.[38]

Patients with cancer and VTE fare significantly better if treated with low molecular weight heparin (LMWH), as compared to unfractionated heparin (UFH).[39,40] Five randomised controlled trials to evaluate the effects of LMWH on survival in cancer patients *without* thrombosis showed no consistent statistically significant benefit in cancer progression or overall survival.[41]

2. VTE as a Precursor of Cancer Diagnosis

Patients presenting with symptomatic VTE have an increased incidence of cancer, not known before the diagnosis of VTE. The incidence of detection of cancer at the time of VTE diagnosis is reported as 4–12% in large studies.[42] This incidence is 3–4-fold greater in patients with idiopathic VTE, as compared to VTE secondary to a known risk factor such as recent surgery or immobilisation.[42] In the general population approximately 50% of VTE are idiopathic and 50% are secondary. Approximately 50% of patients with cancer had metastatic disease at the time of VTE diagnosis, indicating that advanced disease represent a significant further risk factor.[43–45] In a three month follow-up study in which patients were treated initially with LMWH and then switched to oral vitamin K antagonist (VKA), the incidence of recurrence was increased 5-fold higher (11.4% versus 2.1%) in patients with cancer, compared to patients without cancer.[45] Although lung, prostate, colorectal and haematological malignancies were most commonly detected, virtually all sites are represented.

The incidence of cancer following VTE and the extent to which patients with VTE should be screened for occult cancer remains a subject of international debate. A recent meta-analysis of several cohort and population based studies calculated the incidence of newly diagnosed cancer in patients with idiopathic VTE to be 4–10% within 3 years of the VTE event.[42] The incidence of cancer is highest in the first few months after the VTE event, with the risk being approximately 2- to 5-fold in the first two to four months, compared to the expected incidence and becoming virtually equal after 12 months.[44] A recent large prospective study of over 17,000 patients with VTE reported that 16% of patients had cancer either before the VTE, or diagnosed within 15 days during their hospital admission. The incidence of cancer in the subsequent three months was only 1.2%.[45]

An ideal screening process should be safe and cost effective, with a high degree of sensitivity and specificity, and importantly, lead to improved outcomes for patients with VTE and cancer. Some experts recommend only a basic screening process, which includes a thorough history and physical examination, simple laboratory tests and a chest X-ray.[46] Others advocate a more extensive routine workup, which includes ultrasound and CT scanning and screening for cancer markers.[47] Six studies which have compared routine examination versus extensive screening suggest that on average the latter strategy resulted in a 1.8-fold higher detection of occult cancer. However all these studies have relatively low numbers and are subject to bias from non-detected additional confounding factors.[41] Both the one randomised trial[48] and the largest study[49] reported no additional significant value from extensive screening.

The finding of cancer subsequent to VTE is associated with a worse outcome.[43] At this stage however, benefit to the patient from early detection has not been established. A thorough history and physical examination, basic haematology and biochemistry screening and a chest X-ray at the time of VTE diagnosis represents an adequate and cost-effective strategy. Patients with recurrence may merit further investigation.[45] Further studies are required to settle this debate.

2.1   Risk assessment (Table 1)

Although cancer itself is associated with an increased risk of VTE, other risk factors, not exclusive to cancer, frequently coexist in this patient population (Table 1). Advancing age, particularly patients >60 years, hospitalisation and immobilisation, a history of previous VTE, and the presence of medical co-morbidities, are common in the cancer population. The risk of VTE increases with the number of risk factors present. For example, cancer patients hospitalised or confined to a nursing home have a 3-fold increased risk of VTE compared to non-institutionalised cancer patients.[7]

Cancer patients undergoing surgery, particularly major surgery (defined as a procedure lasting >30 minutes), have at least twice the risk of post-operative VTE and more than three times the risk of fatal PE compared to non-cancer patients undergoing similar procedures.[29,50]

Factor V (Leiden) and the prothrombin gene mutation (PGM) are the commonest inherited thrombophilic abnormalities, present in approximately 5% and 3% of the Caucasian population respectively.

Table 1. VTE risk factors.

Cancer-independent	Cancer-related	Treatment-related
Increasing age	Primary site	Central venous catheter
Previous VTE	Initial three to six months after diagnosis	Recent surgery
Co-morbid medical conditions (e.g. obesity, infection, cardiac)	Metastatic disease	Recent hospitalisation
Pregnancy/oral contraceptive	Myeloproliferative disorder	Chemotherapy
Familial or acquired thrombophilia		Hormonal therapy
Immobility		Anti-angiogenic therapy (thalidomide, lenolidomide)
Recent (< two months) surgery		Erythropoietic agents

Each is associated with a 3- to 8-fold increased risk of VTE in the general population[51] and an approximately 12-fold increased risk of VTE in patients with cancer.[52] Testing for FVL and PGM in cancer patients is not however recommended as a routine cost-effective strategy, since the results should not influence treatment decisions.[52]

Additional risk factors, exclusive to cancer patients or their treatment, can be identified. Pancreatic, lung, ovary and brain cancer and haematological malignancies have a strong, but not exclusive association with the development of VTE.[6,53–55] Patients with metastatic disease have been reported to have an odds ratio of up to 20 compared to localised disease.[8]

Chemotherapy and hormonal manipulation also affect the thrombosis risk. For example, in two large clinical studies of women with node negative breast cancer, the five-year incidence of VTE was 0.2% in the placebo group, 0.9% in the tamoxifen group and 4.2% in the tamoxifen plus chemotherapy group.[56,57] The risk of VTE declines rapidly once chemotherapy is completed.[58,59] Compared to patients without cancer, patients with cancer not receiving chemotherapy had a 4-fold increase in VTE and those receiving chemotherapy a 6.5-fold increase.[60] In breast cancer patients receiving tamoxifen the rate of VTE increases by 2- to 5-fold,[57,61] with the risk greatest in post-menopausal women.[62]

Anti-angiogenic agents (thalidomide, lenolidomide), particularly in association with Dexamethasone, have been associated with a high incidence of VTE: 17–26% for thalidomide[63,64] and 10–15% for lenolidomide.[65,66] Erythropoiesis stimulating agents have been reported on a meta-analysis to increase the relative risk of thrombosis 1.7-fold.[67] It is likely that, at least in part, this increased thrombotic risk is associated with attaining an Hb $> 130\,g/l$.[68]

The myeloproliferative disorders, particularly polycythemia rubra vera (PRV) and essential thrombocytosis (ET), are associated with a very significant increased risk of thrombosis, with prevalence at diagnosis of 34–39% for PRV[69,70] and 10–29% for ET.[71–73] The follow-up incidence of thrombosis are 8–19% for PRV and 8–31% for ET. Advanced aged, erythrocytosis, leukocytosis (but not thrombocytosis) and the presence of the JAK2 mutation are all independent predictors of thrombotic risk.

In all instances, 70% of thrombotic events in these myeloproliferative disorders were arterial (cerebrovascular, and coronary particularly) and 30% were venous.[74] Venous thrombotic disease in the myeloproliferative disorders includes catastrophic abdominal (i.e. portal and/or mesenteric) vein thrombosis at a reported incidence of 10% for PRV and 4–13% for ET[75] and is increased even in JAK2 positive patients without frank evidence of a myeloproliferative disorder.[76,77]

2.2   Thrombosis prophylaxis (Table 2)

2.2.1   Hospitalised and/or immobilised patients

Although formal risk assessment models have been published to allow individualised prophylaxis, this approach is cumbersome, and poorly validated. For this reason, published guidelines recommend group-specific prophylaxis routinely for all patients in the target group. The 2008 guidelines the American College of Chest Physicians (ACCP) and the 2007 American Society of Clinical

Table 2. Recommended prophylactic options.

Drug	Dosage
Unfractionated heparin	5000u S.C. every eight hours
* Dalteparin	5000u S.C. daily
* Enoxaparin	40 mgm S.C. daily
* Fondaparinux	2.5 mg S.C. daily

SC: Subcutaneous
Cautions:
* Low molecular weight heparin and fondaparinux should be used with caution in patients with:
    Creatine clearance < 30 ml/min
    Age > 75 years
    Weight < 50 kgm
* Platelet count should be checked every three days for first two weeks, and less frequently thereafter.

Oncology[33,84] strongly recommend pharmacological prophylaxis for hospitalised or bed-ridden patients with active cancer. These recommendations are based on clinical trials in which only a minority of patients had cancer, but the overall benefit for other medical patients and the low complication rates for prophylaxis justifies these recommendations.

2.2.2 Ambulatory patients

The data on whether the routine use of anticoagulants improves survival for cancer patients is inconclusive. A significant impact of Vitamin K antagonists seems unlikely.[85–87] Trials with unfractionated heparin (UFH) and LMWH are conflicting.[88,89] A recent analysis of 11 studies of anticoagulation in patients with cancer, but without VTE, found significantly improved overall survival, but an increased risk of bleeding. Most of these studies had significant methodological limitations and small numbers. Further study of this topic is warranted, but, based on the limitations of the available data, the use of anticoagulant prophylaxis in ambulatory cancer patients cannot be currently recommended.[90,91] The exceptions to this recommendation are the patients receiving thalidomide or lenolidomide, who should be prescribed low dose aspirin or Vitamin K antagonists,[84] and patients with PRV and ET who should be maintained on low dose aspirin.[92]

2.2.3 Surgery

Studies comparing UFH and LMWH on the rates of VTE in cancer patients suggest that both modalities are equally effective in reducing post-operative VTE.[33,36,93–95] A meta-analysis of 10 trials and over 900 patients with cancer demonstrated a reduction of DVT from 30.6% in the controlled group to 13.6% in the low dose UFH group.[95] The LMWH enoxaparin, dalteparin and tanzaparin all appear to be equally effective.[97] Cancer does however confer a relative resistance to standard prophylaxis measures and specific dosing schedules are required. Three times daily UFH is more effective than twice daily in gynaecology oncology patients,[37] and 5000 units dalteparin more effective than 2500 units (18.5% versus 14.9%) in general surgery patients.[36] The pantasaccharide Xa inhibitor, fondaparinux, has also been shown to be effective prophylaxis in a large group, the majority of whom had cancer.[98]

2.2.4 Prolonged prophylaxis

Two studies, each with Enoxaparin or dalteparin comparing one week versus four weeks of prophylaxis show a significant further reduction of VTE from 12% or 16% respectively for one week to 4.8% and 7.3% for four weeks therapy. Neither study demonstrated an increased risk of bleeding.[98–100]

2.2.5 Mechanical prophylaxis

Pneumatic calf compression is effective in reducing VTE rates by 50–66%, but it is less effective than anticoagulant prophylaxis, cumbersome to use and interferes with mobilisation. Their use is not recommended as the sole form of prophylaxis unless pharmacological therapy is contraindicated.[33,84,101]

2.2.6   Central venous catheter (CVC)

Initial reports suggested an incidence of catheter related deep vein thrombosis of approximately 25% in patients with cancer,[78,79] but recent well-designed studies have demonstrated a lower rate of 3–4%.[80,81] This may relate to the improvement in the quality of the catheter and better placement. Improved plastics, right-sided catheters, and catheters placed between the SVC and left atrium had lower risk of thrombosis, whereas repeated catheter insertions and catheter infections increased the risk of VTE.[82] A recent meta-analysis of trials with either low dose warfarin or LMWH did not demonstrate any significant reduction in the incidence of CVC-related DVT.[83]

2.3   Diagnosis of VTE in cancer patients

The diagnosis of VTE in cancer patients requires a high index of suspicion, particularly for hospitalised or immobilised patients where characteristic features such as leg swelling and pain may be absent. As a consequence, hospital-acquired DVT and PE are often clinically silent. On the other hand, the majority of VTE events occur outside the hospital setting. Pulmonary emboli frequently occur without warning. Approximately one-quarter to one-third of DVTs involve the proximal deep veins above the knee and these are much more likely to be symptomatic or cause PEs. Approximately 10–20% of calf (distal) thrombus will however extend to the proximal veins if untreated.[102,103]

Venous Doppler ultrasound is the preferred test for the diagnosis of lower limb DVT. This can have, in good hands, a sensitivity and specificity of 97% for the clinical significant proximal DVT, but about half this for distal, calf DVT.[104] This procedure is non-invasive and easily repeated if necessary. Ultrasonography does experience difficulties in visualising pelvic veins and the inferior vena cava. Reported sensitivity and specificity (80–100%) for upper limb vein thrombosis appear to be less than for proximal lower limbs thrombosis,[105,106] and contrast venography should be considered in equivocal cases.

A number of clinical pre-test probability scoring models, usually combined with a D-Dimer estimate, have been proposed to assist the decision to further image patients with DVTs.[107–109]

However, patients with active cancer and any suspicion of VTE automatically fall into the high risk group and are best immediately imaged appropriately. The D-Dimer assay methods show significant variability, with, in general, an inverse relationship between sensitivity and specificity; the latter is often less than 50%, or even lower for patients over the age of 60, and in patients with cancer.[110,111] These features compromise the test's utility in cancer patients. Alternate imaging modalities, particularly for the more proximal and central veins includes contrast enhanced CT venography and magnetic resonance venography.

2.3.1 *Superficial thrombophlebitis*

Superficial thrombophlebitis can be suspected on the basis of anatomically appropriate signs of tenderness, induration and erythema and can be confirmed by ultrasound.

2.3.2 *Pulmonary Embolism*

As for DVT, patients with active cancer and signs or symptoms suggestive of a PE should be investigated with appropriate imaging procedures. CT pulmonary angiography (CTPA) has replaced ventilation-perfusion scanning (V-Q scan) as the imaging modality of choice. A negative CTPA, in a setting of reasonable clinical suspicion should be followed by a compression ultrasound study (CUS) of the lower limbs. The combination of a negative CTPA and negative CUS has a high (> 99%) negative predictive value for the risk of subsequent VTE events.[112] Improved multi-detection scanners, which provide better definition at the segmental and sub-segmental pulmonary artery level provide a further improvement in diagnostic sensitivity and specificity.[113]

Ventilation-perfusion scanning may be appropriate for patients with renal insufficiency or contrast allergies. A normal V-Q scan essentially excludes a PE. Coexisting pulmonary or cardiac disease, more common in the elderly, can give abnormal V-Q scan results. Moreover, a high proportion of V-Q scan results fall into intermediate and low probability categories which lack diagnostic utility. Additional testing with ECG echocardiography and serum

Table 3. Recommended treatment options for established VTE.

S.C. dalteparin	100 u/kg S.C. every 12 hours for initial month or 200 u/kg S.C. daily then 150 u/kg S.C. daily
S.C. enoxaparin	1 mg/kg S.C. every 12 hours or 1.5 mg/kg S.C. daily
S.C. tinzaparin	175 u/kgm daily S.C
S.C. fondaparinux	> 50 kg 2.5 g S.C. daily 50–100 kg 5.0 g S.C. daily > 100 kg 7.5 g S.C. daily
IV Unfractionated heparin	80 u/kg initial bolus then 18 u/kg/hr, adjusted to APTT
Oral warfarin	5 mg P.O. daily, adjusted to INR

Cautions:

Heparins and fondaparinux should be used with caution with creatinine clearance < 60 ml/hr. Optimum dosage for patients < 50 kg and > 100 kg undefined.

Platelet count monitoring required every two to three days for first two weeks and then less frequent.

Heparin/warfarin overlap of at least four to five days and two therapeutic INRs required before stopping IV Heparin or LMWH.

Treatment duration of six months recommended or indefinite if active cancer persists.

troponin levels may provide an index of severity of right heart strain.[114]

2.4   *Treatment of VTE and PE (Table 3)*

Patients with VTE should be immediately commenced on heparin therapy.[115] The treatment approach for DVT and PE are similar. A meta-analysis of recent trials showed that subcutaneous LMWH and intravenous UFH are equally effective and safe. A statistically substantial mortality benefit in favour of LMWH was observed and this was essentially accounted for by patients with malignancy.[116] There was no significant difference between the different LMWHs. UFH has an unpredictable dose response and a narrow therapeutic range. UFH needs to be administered intravenously and requires regular monitoring, whereas LMWH can be safely administered at home without monitoring.[117–119] Administration of LMWH once daily is as effective as twice daily dosing, although subgroup analysis suggests that twice daily dosage may be more effective for patients with cancer.[119,120]

Whereas conventional treatment of VTE recommends switching to oral VKA after at least a five-day overlap, for cancer, most guidelines recommend continuing with LMWH.[84,114,115] Comparative studies show a significantly lower recurrence rate and a lower bleeding rate with LMWH (6–10%) as compared to VKA (16–20%) in patients with cancer.[121–123] Treatment with subcutaneous LMWH should be given for at least six months. Indefinite treatment is recommended for patients with active cancer, particularly patients with metastatic disease and those receiving chemotherapy since active cancer represents a strong continuing risk factor for recurrence.[84,115,121,122]

LMWH are predominantly excreted by the kidneys and caution needs to be exercised in patients with renal insufficiency. Downward adjustment of dosage in conjunction with anti-Xa monitoring in patients with creatinine clearance $< 50\,ml/min$, and alternative anticoagulants, should be considered with creatinine clearance $< 30\,ml/min$. Similarly, optimum dosages are unclear for obese patients (body mass index $> 40\,kg/m^2$), patients weighing $< 50kg$ and the elderly (> 70 yrs)[114–124] and anti-Xa monitoring should be considered. Clinicians needs to be alert to the risk of heparin-induced thrombocytopenia (HITS-defined as an unexplained fall in platelet count of $> 50\%$) in patients receiving heparins. Platelet monitoring (every two to three days for first two weeks and less frequently thereafter) is recommended.[125]

2.4.1 Thrombolytic therapy

There is little evidence to support the use of thrombolytic therapy in the majority of patients with VTE and it is associated with an increased bleeding risk. It is uncertain whether outcomes, particularly the post-phlebitic syndrome, are improved for patients with DVT. Once anticoagulant therapy is commenced in a patient with a DVT, the mortality for PE is $< 1\%$.[115,126]

2.4.2 Inferior vena cava (IVC) filters

The placement of IVC filters does not appear to improve early or late survival versus anticoagulation alone.[127,128] There are no studies on the effectiveness of such filters for patients with contra-indications to anticoagulation, which is the major group for whom filter placement is considered. IVC filter placement should be considered in patients with contraindication or major complication of anticoagulant therapy and in patients with recurrent embolic events despite adequate anticoagulation. However concurrent anticoagulant therapy should be instituted wherever possible. Appropriate clinical trials for the short term use of removable IVC filters may provide information in the future.

2.4.3 Catheter related thrombosis (CRT)

Treatment options for the management of CRT have few prospective studies to guide decision-making. Two important considerations are the significant risk of thrombus extension and embolism, versus the need to maintain adequate vascular access. The recommendation from the National Comprehensive Cancer Network (NCCN) is that, if the catheter is no longer required or if there is a contraindication to anticoagulant therapy, the catheter should be removed. Standard, therapeutic anticoagulant therapy is recommended if the catheter is left in place. Treatment should be continued for one to three months after removal. [82,114,129,130]

2.4.4 Superficial thrombophlebitis

The initial treatment of superficial thrombophlebitis should include compression, limb elevation and topical and oral anti-inflammatory agents. Intermediate dosages of LMWH or oral VKA therapy are recommended for symptomatic progression, for a duration of at least four weeks. [114,115,131]

2.5 Emerging anticoagulants

Current protocols for the prevention or treatment of VTE are based on UFH or LMWH, both of which need to be given parenterally, and/or oral VKAs, which have a narrow therapeutic range and require regular monitoring.

There are many newer anticoagulants presently undergoing clinical trials which have the potential to greatly improve the therapeutic options, safety and convenience of VTE prophylaxis and treatment.

2.5.1 *Factor Xa inhibitors*[114,125,132,133]

The Factor Xa inhibitor, fondaparinux has been extensively trialed and is of proven safety and efficiency in the prevention and treatment of VTE.[134,135] Like the LMWH, it needs to be given subcutaneously and is contraindicated in severe renal failure. At this stage there have been no specific studies on patients with cancer, although in a subgroup analysis of cancer patients within a large prophylactic study on patients undergoing abdominal surgery, fondaparinux was equal to dalteparin.

2.5.2 *Oral factor Xa inhibitors*

Several oral factor Xa inhibitors, of which rivoroxaban and apixaban are most advanced, are currently undergoing clinical trials for both the prophylaxis and treatment of VTE.

2.5.3 *Direct thrombin inhibitors*[132,133]

Lepirudin (recombinant hirudin), argatroban and bivalirudin are direct thrombin inhibitors, which are administered intravenously and which can be monitored by the APTT (partial thromboplastin time). All represent potential alternative therapy for patients with HITS. Lepirudin has a relatively narrow therapeutic window and is excreted predominantly by the kidneys. Argatroban is metabolised by the liver and is a useful alternative to the heparins in patients with severe renal impairment. Bivalirudin also has significant renal excretion and, at this stage, has been predominantly studied in association with cardiovascular procedures.

The oral direct thrombin inhibitor, ximelagatran, failed FDA approval in 2004 because of concerns with associated hepatic and coronary events. However its proven efficiency in both preventing and treating VTE provided 'proof of concept' for this class of agents. An alternative, dabigatran is currently undergoing clinical trials.

3.   Links Between Tumour Biology and Haemostasis

Activation of the coagulation system appears to promote the survival, growth and progression of cancer and leukaemic cells. Tissue factor (TF) is the best characterised cancer procoagulant. This transmembrane protein binds to Factor VII to activate the coagulation cascade, leading to thrombin generation and fibrin formation. Normally only expressed on resting stromal cells and fibroblasts of the vascular adventitia, TF is expressed constitutively on the surface of tumour cells.

The generation of thrombin, as well as leading to fibrin formation, initiates platelet, endothelial cell, and monocyte activation and the activation of inflammatory mediators. Activation of the coagulation cascade induces a complex process of expression of a multitude of cytokines and adhesive proteins including tumour necrosing factor (TNF), interleukins, cellular adhesion and permeability factor, vascular endothelial growth factors (VEGF) and basic fibroblast growth factor (bFGF) which influence tumour biology.[41]

The plasma level of TF is associated with clinical progression and a poor prognosis of cancers[136,137] and correlates with the malignant phenotype of various tumours, specifically with oncogenetic transformation due to K-ras mutation and p53 suppression.[138] Studies with TF knockout models demonstrate an inhibition of tumour growth and metastases,[139,140] and without TF there is no embryonic development.[141]

There is therefore a direct link between the clinical hypercoagulable state reflected in the incidence of VTE and disseminated intravascular coagulation (DIC) and tumour biology. The fibrin matrix formed around tumour cells protects against NK cell attack, and forms the scaffold for angiogenesis induced by the expression of VEGF and other angiogenic interleukins. The host immune response is suppressed and anti-apoptotic, cell adhesive and cell migration and permeability cytokines and receptors enhance growth and progression of the cancer.

At this stage, specific anticoagulant therapy, particularly LMWH, have been inconclusive in studies designed to demonstrate any benefit in cancer progression. Further studies, in patients with limited disease, are ongoing.

4.   Summary

Activation of the haemostatic pathways appears to be an integral part of malignant transformation of many, if not, to a greater or lesser degree, all malignant tumours. This activation appears to be a necessary prerequisite for the tumours' biological survival and advantage. A further understanding into these changes and their pharmacological manipulation is currently widely researched and is likely to provide clinical benefit at some stage in the future. In the meantime, clinicians need to appreciate the clinical consequences of the systemic effect of these changes induced by malignant tumours. The most obvious is the heightened risk of venous thromboembolic complications, which greatly adversely effect patient outcomes. Clinicians need to maintain a high index of suspicion and any symptom suggestive of a VTE or PE in a patient with a malignancy requires appropriate imaging investigation. The risk is greatest in the first six months after diagnosis and is greatest in patients with metastatic disease and those receiving chemotherapy. Patients hospitalised for surgical or medical reasons are at particular risk and all such patients should receive prophylactic anticoagulation.

References

1.   A. Trousseau, Phlegmasia alba dolens. In: *Clinique Medicanale de l'Hotel-Dieu de Paris*, 2nd ed., ed. A. Trousseau (Paris Bailliere J-B, 1865), Vol. 3, pp. 654–712.

2. J. M. Gore, J. S. Appelbaum, H. L. Greene *et al.*, Occult cancer in patients with pulmonary embolism, *Ann. Intern. Med.* **96**: 556–560 (1982).

3. A. A. Khorana, C. W. Francis, E. Culakova *et al.*, Thromboembolism is a leading cause of death in cancer patients receiving outpatient chemotherapy, *J. Thromb. Haemost* **5**: 632–634 (2007).

4. J. A. Heit, W. M. O'Fallon, T. M. Petterson *et al.*, Relative impact of risk factors for deep vein thrombosis and pulmonary embolism: A population based study, *Arch. Intern. Med.* **162**: 1245–1248 (2002).

5. H. K. Chew, T. Wun, D. Harvey *et al.*, Incidence of venous thromboembolism and its effects on survival amongst patients with common cancers, *Arch. Intern. Med.* **166**: 458–464 (2006).

6. N. Levitan, A. Dowlati, S. C. Remick *et al.*, Rates of initial and recurrent thromboembolic disease amongst patients with malignancy versus those without malignancy: Risk analysis using Medicare claims data, *Medicine (Baltimore)* **78**: 285–291 (1999).

7. J. A. Heit, D. N. Mohr, M. D. Silverstein, T. M. Petterson *et al.*, Predictors of recurrence after deep vein thrombosis and pulmonary embolism: A population based cohort study, *Arch. Intern. Med.* **160**: 761–768 (2000).

8. J. W. Blom, C. J. Doggen, S. Osanto *et al.*, Malignancies, prothrombotic mutations, and the risk of venous thrombosis, *J. Am. Med. Assoc.* **293**: 715–722 (2005).

9. P. Prandoni, A. Piccioli and A. Girolami, Cancer and venous thromboembolism: An overview, *Haematologica* **84**: 437–445 (1999).

10. P. Prandoni, A. Falanga and A. Piccioli, Cancer and venous thromboembolism, *Lancet Oncol.* **6**: 401–410 (2005).

11. J. A. Heit, M. D. Silverstein, D. N. Mohr *et al.*, Predictors of survival after deep vein thrombosis and pulmonary embolism: A population based cohort study, *Arch. Intern. Med.* **159**: 445–453 (1999).

12. H. T. Sorenson, L. Mellemkjaer, J. H. Olsen *et al.*, Prognosis of cancers associated with venous thromboembolism, *N. Engl. J. Med.* **343**: 1846–1850 (2000).

13. M. A. Martino, E. Williamson, S. Siegfreid *et al.*, Diagnosing pulmonary embolism: Experience with spiral CT pulmonary angiography in gynaecological oncology, *Gynecol. Oncol.* **98**: 289–293 (2005).

14. G. Agnelli, G. Bolis, L. Capussotti *et al.*, A clinical outcome based prospective study in venous thromboembolism after cancer surgery: The @RISTOS project, *Ann. Surg.* **243**: 89–95 (2006).

15. B. Lindblad, A. Eriksson and D. Bergqvist, Autopsy verified pulmonary embolism in a surgical department: Analysis of the period from 1951 to 1968, *Br. J. Surg.* **78**: 849–852 (1991).

16. D. A. Sandler and J. F. Martin, Autopsy proven pulmonary embolism in hospital patients: Are we detecting enough deep vein thrombosis? *J. R. Soc. Med.* **82**: 203–205 (1989).

17. F. A. Anderson, H. B. Wheeler, R. J. Goldberg *et al.*, A population based perspective of the hospital incidence and case fatality rates of deep vein thrombosis and pulmonary embolism: The Worcester DVT study, *Arch. Intern. Med.* **151**: 933–938 (1991).

18. P. D. Stein and J. W. Henry, Prevalence of acute pulmonary embolism amongst patients in a general hospital and at autopsy, *Chest* **108**: 978–981 (1995).

19. S. Z. Goldhaber, C. H. Hennekens, D. A. Evans *et al.*, Factors associated with correct antemotem diagnosis of major pulmonary embolism, *Am. J. Med.* **73**: 822–826 (1982).

20. B. Karwinski and E. Svendsen, Comparison of clinical and post mortem diagnosis of pulmonary embolism, *J. Clin. Pathol.* **42**: 135–139 (1989).

21. J. H. Ryu, E. J. Olsen and P. A. Pellikka, Clinical recognition of pulmonary embolism: Problems of unrecognized and asymptomatic cases, *Mayo Clin. Proc.* **73**: 873–879 (1998).

22. D. Bergqvist, S. Jendteg, L. Johansen *et al.*, Cost of long term complications of deep vein thrombosis of the lower extremities: An analysis of a defined patient population in Sweden, *Ann. Intern. Med.* **126**: 454–457 (1997).

23. J. A. Heit, T. W. Rooke, M. D. Silverstein *et al.*, Trends in the incidence of venous stasis syndrome and venous ulcers: A 25-year population based study, *J. Vasc. Surg.* **33**: 1022–1027 (2001).

24. S. R. Kahn, A. Hirsch and I. Shrier, Effects of post thrombotic syndrome on health related quality of life after deep vein thrombosis, *Arch. Intern. Med.* **162**: 1144–1148 (2002).

25. T. P. Baglin, K. White and A. Charles, Fatal pulmonary embolism in hospitalised medical patients, *J. Clin. Pathol.* **50**: 609–610 (1997).

26. J. Bouthier, The venous thrombotic risk in non-surgical patients, *Drugs* **52**(Suppl. 7): 16–29 (1996).

27. S. Z. Goldhaber, D. D. Savage, R. J. Garison *et al.*, Risk factors for pulmonary embolism: The Framingham study, *Am. J. Med.* **74**: 1023–1028 (1983).

28. B. Lindblad, N. H. Sternby and D. Bergqvist, Incidence of venous thromboembolism verified by necropsy over 30 years, *Br. Med. J.* **302**: 709–711 (1991).

29. International Multicentre Trial, Prevention of fatal pulmonary embolism by low doses of heparin, *Lancet* **2**: 45–51 (1975).

30. S. Sagar, J. Massey and J. M. Sanderson, Low dose heparin prophylaxis against fatal pulmonary embolism, *Br. Med. J.* **4**: 257–259 (1975).

31. H. Halkin, J. Goldberg, M. Modan *et al.*, Reduction in mortality in general medical in-patients by low dose heparin prophylaxis, *Ann. Intern. Med.* **96**: 561–565 (1982).

32. R. Collins, A. Scrimgeour, S. Yusuf *et al.*, Reduction in fatal pulmonary embolism and venous thrombosis by peri-operative administration of subcutaneous heparin: An overview of results of randomized trials in general, orthopaedic and urological surgery, *N. Engl. J. Med.* **318**: 1162–1173 (1988).

33. W. H. Geerts, D. Bergqvist, G. H. Pineo *et al.*, Prevention of venous thromboembolism. American College of Chest Physicians evidence based clinical practice guidelines (8th edition), *Chest* **126**: 381s–453s (2008).

34. P. Mismetti, S. Laporte, J. Y. Darmon *et al.*, Meta-analysis of low molecular weight heparin in the prevention of venous thromboembolism in general surgery, *Br. J. Surg.* **88**: 913–930 (2001).

35. Enoxacan Study Group, Efficiency and safety of enoxaparin versus unfractionated heparin for the prevention of deep vein thrombosis in elective cancer surgery: A double blind randomized multicentre trial with venographic assessment, *Br. J. Surg.* **84**: 1099–1103 (1997).

36. D. Bergqvist, U. S. Burmark, P. A. Flordal *et al.*, Low molecular weight heparin started before surgery as prophylaxis against deep vein thrombosis: 2500 versus 5000 XaI units in 2070 patients, *Br. J. Surg.* **82**: 496–501 (1995).

37. D. L. Clarke-Pearson, E. Delong, I. S. Synan *et al.*, Venous thromboembolism prophylaxis in gynaecological oncology: A prospective controlled trial of low dose heparin, *Am. J. Obstet. Gynaecol.* **145**: 606–613 (1983).

38. A. K. Kakkar, M. Levine, H. M. Pinedo *et al.*, Venous thrombosis in cancer patients: Insights from the FRONTLINE survey, *Oncologist* **8**: 381–388 (2003).

39. P. Prandoni, A. W. Lensing, H. R. Buller *et al.*, Comparison of subcutaneous low molecular weight heparin with intravenous standard

heparin in proximal deep vein thrombosis, *Lancet* **339**: 441–445 (1992).

40. R. J. Hettiarachi, S. M. Smorenburg, J. Ginsberg *et al.*, Do heparins do more than just treat thrombosis? The influence of heparins on cancer spread, *Thromb. Haemost.* **82**: 947–952 (1999).

41. H. R. Buller, F. F. Van Doormaal, G. L. Van Sluis *et al.*, Cancer and thrombosis: Form molecular mechanisms to clinical presentations, *J. Thromb. Haemost.* **5**(Suppl.): 246–254 (2007).

42. H. M. Otten and M. H. Prins, Venous thromboembolism and occult malignancy, *Thromb. Res.* **102**: 187–194 (2001).

43. H. T. Sorenson, L. Mellemkjaer, J. H. Olsen *et al.*, Prognosis of cancer associated with venous thromboembolism, *N. Engl. J. Med.* **343**: 1846–1850 (2000).

44. R. H. White, H. K. Chew, H. Zhou *et al.*, Incidence of thromboembolism in the year before the diagnosis of cancer in 528,693 adults, *Arch. Intern. Med.* **165**: 1782–1787 (2005).

45. J. Trujillo-Santos, P. Prandoni, K. Rivron-Guillot *et al.*, Clinical outcome in patients with venous thromboembolism and hidden cancer: Findings from the RIETE registry, *J. Thromb. Haemost.* **6**: 251–255 (2007).

46. A. Y. Lee, Screening for occult cancer in patients with idiopathic venous thromboembolism: No, *J. Thromb. Haemost.* **1**: 2273–2274 (2003).

47. A. Piciolli and P. Prandoni, Screening for occult cancer in patients with idiopathic venous thromboembolism: Yes, *J. Thromb. Haemost.* **1**: 2271–2272 (2003).

48. A. Piccioli, A. W. Lensing, M. H. Prins *et al.*, Extensive screening for occult malignant disease in idiopathic venous thromboembolism: A prospective randomized clinical trial, *J. Thromb. Haemost.* **2**: 884–889 (2004).

49. M. Monreal, A. W. Lensing, M. H. Prins *et al.*, Screening for occult cancer in patients with acute deep vein thrombosis or pulmonary embolism, *J. Thromb. Haemost.* **2**: 876–881 (2004).

50. G. P. Clagett and J. S. Reisch, Prevention of deep vein thrombosis in general surgical patients: Results of meta-analysis, *Ann. Surg.* **208**: 227–240 (1988).

51. U. Seligson and A. Lubetsky, Genetic susceptibility to venous thrombosis, *N. Engl. J. Med.* **344**: 1222–1231 (2001).

52. J. W. Blom, C. J. Doggen, S. Osanto *et al.*, Malignancies, prothrombotic mutations, and the risk of venous thrombosis, *J. Am. Med. Assoc.* **293**: 715–722 (2005).

53. P. D. Stein, A. Beemath, F. A. Meyers *et al.*, Incidence of venous thromboembolism in patients hospitalized with cancer, *Am. J. Med.* **119**: 60–68 (2006).

54. A. A. Khorana, C. W. Francis, E. Culakova *et al.*, Risk factors for chemotherapy associated venoous thromboembolism in a prospective observational study, *Cancer* **104**: 2822–2829 (2005).

55. S. Sallah, J. Y. Wan and N. P. Nguyen, Venous thrombosis in patients with solid tumours: Determination of frequency and characteristics, *Thromb. Haemost.* **87**: 575–579 (2002).

56. B. Fisher, J. Constantino, C. Redmond *et al.*, A randomized clinical trial evaluating Tamoxifen in the treatment of women with node-negative breast cancer who have estogen receptor positive tumours, *N. Engl. J. Med.* **320**: 479–484 (1997).

57. B. Fisher, J. Dignan, N. Woolmark *et al.*, Tamoxifen and chemotherapy for lymph node negative estrogen receptor positive breast cancer, *J. Natl. Cancer. Inst.* **89**: 1673–1682 (1997).

58. M. N. Levine, M. Gent, J. Hirsch *et al.*, The thrombogenic effect of anti-cancer drug therapy in women with stage II breast cancer, *N. Engl. J. Med.* **318**: 404–407 (1988).

59. T. Saphner, D. C. Tormey and R. Gray, Venous and arterial thrombosis in patients who receive adjuvant therapy for breast cancer, *J. Clin. Oncol.* **9**: 286–294 (1991).

60. J. A. Heit, M. D. Silverstein, D. N. Mohr *et al.*, Risk factors for deep vein thrombosis and pulmonary embolism: A population-based case control study, *Arch. Intern. Med.* **160**: 809–815 (2000).

61. A. Y. Y. Lee and M. N. Levine, Venous thromboembolism and cancer: Risks and outcomes, *Circulation* **107**: 117–121 (2003).

62. K. I. Pritchard, A. H. G. Paterson, N. A. Paul *et al.*, Increased thromboembolic complications with concurrent Tamoxifen and chemotherapy in a randomized trial of adjuvant therapy for women with metastatic breast cancer, *J. Clin. Oncol.* **14**: 2731–2737 (1996).

63. M. Cavo, E. Zamagni, C. Cellini *et al.*, Deep vein thrombosis in multiple myeloma receiving first-line thalidomide-dexamethasone therapy, *Blood* **100**: 2272–2273 (2002).

64. K. Osman, R. Comenzo and S. V. Rajkumar, Deep vein thrombosis and thalidomide therapy for multiple myeloma, *N. Engl. J. Med.* **344**: 1951–1952 (2001).

65. S. V. Rajkumar, Lenalidomide and venous thrombosis in multiple myeloma, *N. Engl. J. Med.* **354**: 2079–2080 (2006).

66. J. A. Zonder, B. Barlogie, B. G. Durie *et al.*, Thrombotic complications in patients with newly diagnosed multiple myeloma treated with lenalidamide and dexamethasone: Benefits of aspirin prophylaxis, *Blood* **108**: 403 (2006).

67. J. Bohlius, J. Wilson, J. Seidenfeld *et al.*, Recombinant human erythroeitins and cancer patients: Updated meta-analysis of 57 studies including 9,353 patients, *J. Natl. Cancer Inst.* **98**: 708–714 (2006).

68. H. Luksenberg, A. Weir and R. Wager, FDA briefing document. Oncologic Drugs Advisory Committee. Safety concerns associated with Aranesp (darbopoietin alpha) Amgen Inc., and Procrit (epopoietin alpha) Ortho Biotech, Lp, for the treatment of anaemia associated with cancer chemotherapy. Available at www.fda.gov/ ohrms/dockets/ac/04/briefing/4037B2_04_FDA-aranesp-procrit. htm. December 6, 2006.

69. Gruppo Italiano Studio Policitemia, Polycythaemia vera: The natural history of 1213 patients followed for 20 years, *Ann. Intern. Med.* **123**: 656–664 (1995).

70. R. Marchioli, G. Finazzi, R. Landolfi *et al.*, Vascular and neoplastic risk in a large cohort of patients with polycythemia vera, *J. Clin. Oncol.* **23**: 2224–2232 (2005).

71. A. P. Wolanskyj, S. M. Schwager, R. F. McClure *et al.*, Essential thrombocythemia beyond the first decade: Life expectancy, long term complication rates and prognostic factors, *Mayo Clin. Proc.* **81**: 159–166 (2006).

72. P. J. Campbell, L. M. Scot, G. Buck *et al.*, Definition of subtypes of essential thrombocythaemia and relation to polycythaemia vera based on JAK2 V614F mutation status: A prospective study, *Lancet* **366**: 1945–1953 (2005).

73. A. Carobbio, G. Finazzi, V. Guerini *et al.*, Leukocytosis is a risk factor for thrombosis in essential thrombocythemia: Interaction with treatment, standard risk factors and JAK2 mutation status, *Blood* **109**: 2310–2313 (2006).

74. V. De Stefano, T. Za, E. Rossi *et al.*, Recurrent thrombosis in patients with polycythemia vera or essential thrombocythemia: Efficacy of treatment in preventing re-thrombosis in different clinical settings, *Blood* **108**(11): 137 (abstract 119) (2006).

75. N. Gangat, A. P. Wolanskyj and A. Tefferi, Abdominal vein thrombosis in essential thrombocythemia: Prevalence, clinical correlates and prognostic implications, *Eur. J. Haematol.* **77**: 327–333 (2006).

76. D. Colaizzo, L. Amitrano, G. L. Tiscia *et al.*, The JAK2 V617F muta- tion frequently occurs in patients with portal and mesenteric vein thrombosis, *J. Thromb. Haemost.* **5**: 55–61 (2006).

77. M. Boissinot, E. lippert, F. Girodon *et al.*, Latent myeloproliferative disorder revealed by the JAK2 V617F mutation and endogenous megakaryocyte colonies in patients with splanchnic vein thrombosis, *Blood* **108**: 3223–3224 (2006).

78. R. D. Bona, Thrombotic complications of central venous catheters in cancer patients. *Semin. Thromb. Haemost.* **25**: 147–155 (1999).

79. M. M. Bern, J. J. Lokich, S. R. Wallach *et al.*, Very low doses of warfarin can prevent thrombosis in central venous catheters. A randomized prospective trial, *Ann. Intern. Med.* **112**: 423–428 (1990).

80. M. Verso, G. Agnelli, S. Bertoglio *et al.*, Enoxaparin for the prevention of venous thromboembolism associated with central vein catheter: A double blind placebo controlled, randomized study in cancer patients, *J. Clin. Oncol.* **23**: 4057–4062 (2005).

81. M. Karthaus, A. Kretzchmar, A. Kroning *et al.*, Dalteparin for the prevention of catheter-related complications in cancer patients with central venous catheters: Final results of a double-blind, placebo controlled phase III trial, *Ann. Oncol.* **17**: 289–296 (2006).

82. C. Freytes, Thromboembolic complications related to central venous access catheters in cancer patients, *Semin. Thromb. Haemost.* **33**: 389–396 (2007).

83. M. Carrier, J. Taty, D. Fergusson and S. Wells, Thromboprophylaxis for catheter related thrombosis in patients with cancer: A systematic review of the randomized controlled trials, *J. Thromb. Haemost.* **5**: 2552–2553 (2007).

84. G. H. Lyman, A. A. Khorana, A. Falanga *et al.*, American Society of Clinical Oncology Guideline: Recommendation for venous throm- boembolism prophylaxis and treatment in patients with cancer, *J. Clin. Oncol.* **25**: 5490–5505 (2007).

85. L. R. Zacharski, W. G. Henderson, F. R. Rickles *et al.*, Effect of war- farin anti coagulation on survival in carcinoma of the lung, colon and head and neck and prostate: Final report of VA Cooperative Study #75, *Cancer* **53**: 2046–2052 (1984).

86. A. P. Chahinian, K. J. Propert, J. H. Ware *et al.*, A randomized trial of anticoagulation with warfarin and of alternating chemotherapy in extensive small cell lung cancer by the Cancer and Leukemia Group B, *J. Clin. Oncol.* **7**: 993–1022 (1989).

87. L. H. Maurer, J. E. Herndon, D. R. Hollis *et al.*, Randomized trial of chemotherapy and radiation therapy with or without warfarin for limited stage small cell lung cancer: A Cancer and Leukemia Group B study, *J. Clin. Oncol.* **15**: 3378–3387 (1997).

88. A. K. Kakkar, M. N. Levine, Z. Kadziola *et al.*, Low molecular weight heparin, therapy with dalteparin, and survival in advanced cancer: The fragmin advanced malignancy outcome study (FAMOUS), *J. Clin. Oncol.* **22**: 1944–1948 (2004).

89. C. P. Klerk, S. M. Smorenburg, H. M. Otten *et al.*, The effect of low molecular weight heparin on survival in patients with advanced malignancy, *J. Clin. Oncol.* **23**: 2130–2135 (2005).

90. N. M. Kuderer, A. A. Khorana, G. H. Lyman *et al.*, A meta-analysis and systematic review of the efficacy and safety of anticoagulants as cancer treatment: Impact on survival and bleeding complications, *Cancer* **110**: 1149–1161 (2007).

91. A. Y. Y. Yee, Thrombosis and cancer: The role of screening for occult cancer and recognizing the underlying biological mechanisms, *Hematology* (Am Soc Hematol Educ Program) 438–443 (2006).

92. T. Barbui and G. Finazzi, Therapy for polycythemia vera and essential thrombocythemia is driven by the cardiovascular risk, *Semin. Thromb. Haemost.* **33**: 321–329 (2007).

93. The European Fraxiparin Study (EFS) Group, Comparison of low molecular weight heparin and unfractionated heparin for the prevention of deep vein thrombosis in patients undergoing abdominal surgery, *Br. J. Surg.* **75**: 1058–103 (1988).

94. Enoxacan Study Group, Efficacy and safety of enoxaparin versus unfractionated heparin for the prevention of deep vein thrombosis in elective cancer surgery: A double blind randomized multicentre trial with venographic assessment, *Br. J. Surg.* **84**: 1099–1103 (1997).

95. M. J. Leonardi, M. L. McGory and C. Y. Ko, A systematic review of deep vein thrombosis prophylaxis in cancer patients: Implications for improving quality, *Ann. Surg. Oncol.* **14**: 929–936 (2007).

96. G. P. Clagett and J. S. Reisch, Prevention of venous thromboembolism in general surgical patients. Results of meta-analysis, *Ann. Surg.* **208**: 227–240 (1988).

97. P. S. Wells, D. R. Anderson, M. A. Rodger *et al.*, A randomized trial comparing 2 low molecular weight heparins for the outpatient treatment of deep vein thrombosis and pulmonary embolism, *Arch. Intern. Med.* **165**: 733–738 (2005).

98. G. Agnelli, G. Bolis, L. Capussotti *et al.*, Clinical outcome based prospective study on venous thromboembolism after cancer surgery: The RISTOS project, *Ann. Surg.* **243**: 89–95 (2006).

99. D. Bergqvist, G. Agnelli, A. T. Cohen *et al.*, Duration of prophylaxis against venous thromboembolism with enoxaparin after surgery for cancer, *N. Engl. J. Med.* **346**: 975–980 (2002).

100. M. S. Rasmussen, L. N. Jorgensen, P. Wille-Jorgenson *et al.*, Prolonged prophylaxis with dalteparin to prevent late thromboembolic complications in patients undergoing major abdominal surgery: A multicentre randomizes open label study, *J. Thromb. Haemost.* **4**: 2384–2390 (2006).

101. A. Iorio and G. Agnelli, Low molecular and unfractionated heparin for prevention of venous thrombosis in neurosurgery: A meta-analysis, *Arch. Intern. Med.* **160**: 2327–2332 (2000).

102. V. V. Kakkar, C. T. Howe, C. Flanc *et al.*, Natural history of post operative deep vein thrombosis, *Lancet* **2**: 230–233 (1969).

103. C. Kearon, Natural history of venous thromboembolism, *Circulation* **107**: 122–130 (2003).

104. M. Pini, L. Marchini and A. Giordano, Diagnostic strategies in venous thromboembolism, *Haematologica* **84**: 535–540 (1999).

105. M. S. Sajid, N. Ahmed, M. Desai *et al.*, Upper limb deep vein thrombosis: A literature review to streamline the protocol for management, *Acta Haematol.* **118**(1): 8–10 (2007).

106. H. J. Baarslag, E. J. van Beek, M. M. Koopman *et al.*, Prospective study of colour duplex ultrasound compared with contrast venography in patients suspected of having deep vein thrombosis of the upper extremities, *Ann. Intern. Med.* **136**: 865–872 (2002).

107. P. A. Kyre and S. Eichinger, Deep vein thrombosis, *Lancet* **365**: 1163–1174 (2005).

108. P. S. Wells, C. Owen, S. Doucette *et al.*, Does this patient have deep vein thrombosis? *J. Am. Med. Assoc.* **295**: 199–207 (2006).

109. G. Le Gal, M. Righini, P. M. Roy *et al.*, Prediction of pulmonary embolism in emergency patients: The revised Geneva score, *Ann. Intern. Med.* **144**: 165–171 (2006).

110. A. Y. Y. Lee, J. A. Julian, M. N. Levine *et al.*, Clinical utility of a rapid whole blood d-dimer assay in patients with cancer who present with suspected acute deep vein thrombosis, *Ann. Intern. Med.* **131**: 417–423 (1999).

111. M. Di Nisio, A. Squizzato, A. W. S. Rutjes *et al.*, Diagnostic accuracy of d-dimer test for exclusion of venous thromboembolism: A systematic review, *J. Thromb. Haemost.* **5**: 296–304 (2007).

112. D. R. Anderson, M. J. Kovacs, C. Dennie *et al.*, Use of spiral computed tomography contrast angiography and ultrasonography to exclude the diagnosis of pulmonary embolism in the emergency department, *J. Emerg. Med.* **29**: 399–404 (2005).

113. Writing Group for the Christopher Study Investigators, Effectiveness of managing suspected pulmonary embolism using an algorithm combining clinical probability, d-dimer testing and computer tomography, *J. Am. Med. Assoc.* **295**: 172–179 (2006).

114. National Comprehensive Cancer Network, NCCN clinical guidelines in oncology: Venous thromboembolic disease. Available at www.ncca.org/professional/physician_gls/PDF/vte.pdf.

115. H. R. Buller, G. Agnelli, R. D. Hull *et al.*, Antithrombotic therapy for venous thromboembolic disease: The seventh ACCP conference on antithrombotic and thrombolytic therapy, *Chest* **126**: 401s–428s (2004).

116. L. R. Dolovich, J. S. Ginsberg, J. D. Douketis *et al.*, A meta-analysis comparing low molecular weight heparins with unfractionated heparin in the treatment of venous thromboembolism: Examining some unanswered questions regarding location of treatment, product type and dosing frequency, *Arch. Intern. Med.* **160**: 181–188 (2000).

117. M. Levine, M. Gent, J. Hirsh *et al.*, A comparison of low-molecular weight heparin administered primarily at home with unfractionated heparin administed in the hospital for proximal deep vein thrombosis, *N. Engl. J. Med.* **334**: 677–681 (1996).

118. M. M. Koopman, P. Prandoni, F. Piovella *et al.*, Treatment of venous thrombosis with intravenous unfractionated heparin administered in the hospital as compared with subcutaneous low-molecular weight heparin administered at home, *N. Engl. J. Med.* **334**: 682–687 (1996).

119. G. Merli, T. E. Spiron, C. G. Olsson *et al.*, Subcutaneous enoxaparin once or twice daily compared with intravenous unfractionated heparin for treatment of venous thromboembolic disease, *Ann. Intern. Med.* **134**: 191–202 (2002).

120. B. A. Charbonnier, J. N. Fiessinger, J. D. Banga *et al.*, Comparison of a once daily with a twice daily subcutaneous low molecular weight

heparin regimen in the treatment of deep vein thrombosis, *Thromb. Haemost.* **79**: 897–901 (1998).

121. A. Y. Y. Lee, M. N. Levine, R. I. Baker *et al.*, Low molecular weight heparin vesus a coumarin for the prevention of recurrent venous thromboembolism in patients with cancer, *N. Engl. J. Med.* **349**: 146–153 (2003).

122. G. Meyer, Z. Marjanovic, J. Valcke *et al.*, Comparison of low molecular weight heparin and warfarin for the secondary prevention of venous thromboembolism in patients with cancer: A randomized control study, *Arch. Intern. Med.* **162**: 1729–1735 (2002).

123. S. R. Detcher, C. M. Kessier, G. Merli *et al.*, Secondary prevention of venous thromboembolic events in patients with active cancer: Enoxparin alone versus initial enoxaparin followed by warfarin for a 180-day period, *Clin. Appl. Thromb. Hemost.* **12**: L389–396 (2006).

124. J. Hirsh and R. Raschke, Heparin and low molecular weight heparin: The seventh ACCP conference on antithrombotic and thrombolytic therapy, *Chest* **126**: 188s–203s (2004).

125. T. E. Warkentin and A. Greinacher, Heparin induced thrombocytopenia: Recognition, treatment and prevention: The seventh ACCP conference on antithrombotic and thrombolytic therapy, *Chest* **126**: 311s–337s (2004).

126. G. Agnelli, C. Becattini and T. Kirschstein, Thrombolysis vs. heparin in the treatment of pulmonary embolism: A clinical outcome-based meta-analysis, *Arch. Intern. Med.* **162**: 2537–2541 (2002).

127. H. Decousus, A. Leizorovicz, F. Parent *et al.*, A clinical trial of vena cava filters in the prevention of pulmonary embolism in patients with proximal deep vein thrombosis, *N. Engl. J. Med.* **338**: 409–415 (1998).

128. The PREPIC Study Group, Eight-year follow up of patients with permanent vena cava filters in the prevention of pulmonary embolism: The PREPIC randomized study, *Circulation* **112**: 416–422 (2005).

129. A. Y. Lee, M. N. Levine, G. Butler *et al.*, Incidence, risk factors and outcomes of catheter related thrombosis in adult patients with cancer, *J. Clin. Oncol.* **24**: 1404–1408 (2006).

130. M. J. Kovacs, S. R. Kahn, M. Rodger *et al.*, A pilot study of central venous catheter survival in cancer patients using low molecular weight heparin (dalteparin) and warfarin without catheter removal

for the treatment of upper extremity deep vein thrombosis (The Catheter Study), *J. Thromb. Haemost.* **5**: 1650–1653 (2007).

131. Superficial Thrombophlebitis Treated by Enoxaparin Study Group, A pilot randomized double blind comparison of a low molecular weight heparin, a non-steroidal anti-inflammatory agent and placebo in the treatment of superficial vein thrombosis, *Arch. Intern. Med.* **163**: 1657–1663 (2003).

132. J. I. Weitz, J. Hirsh and M. M. Samama, New anticoagulant drugs: The seventh ACCP conference on antithrombotic and thrombolytic therapy, *Chest* **126**: 265s–286 (2004).

133. S. M. Bates and J. I. Weitz, The status of new anticoagulants, *Br. J. Haematol.* **134**: 3–19 (2006).

134. H. R. Buller, B. L. Davidson, H. Decousus *et al.*, Fondaparinux or enoxaparin for the initial treatment of symptomatic deep vein thrombosis: A randomized trial, *Ann. Intern. Med.* **140**: 867–873 (2004).

135. The MATISSE Investigators, Subcutaneous fondaparinux versus intravenous unfractionated heparin in the initial treatment of pulmonary embolism, *N. Engl. J. Med.* **349**: 1695–1702 (2003).

Haematological Abnormalities in Cancer Patients

Philip J. Crispin and
Ian W. Prosser

Abstract

Haematological conditions frequently complicate cancer treatment, most commonly with reduced blood counts. Anaemia is common, and may respond to specific therapy with iron, or other haematinic therapy, immune suppression or erythropoietin, when there is an appropriate underlying cause. Whilst erythropoietin improves quality of life during chemotherapy, emerging evidence on the potential risks of erythropoietin in cancer patients needs to be weighed against the risks of transfusion support and where appropriate, non-pharmacological interventions should be considered.

Neutropenia is usually encountered as a complication of chemotherapy and increases the risk of sepsis. Granulocyte colony stimulating factor is widely available to assist in the prevention or management of neutropenia, but is not warranted in all cases. Cytokines directed at megakaryocytes have been used in chemotherapy-induced thrombocytopenia, but complications have limited their clinical development. Recent years have seen the emergence of promising thrombopoietin analogues, which may improve the management of thrombocytopenia into the future. At present, transfusion remains the mainstay of treatment for thrombocytopenia and coagulopathies, and should be given in accordance with evidence based guidelines.

Keywords: Malignancy, anaemia, erythropoietin, transfusion, neutropenia, granulocyte colony stimulating factor, thrombocytopenia.

1.   Introduction

Haematological abnormalities are commonly seen in cancer patients, and can be exacerbated by treatment. Peripheral blood cytopenias are most commonly encountered and may impair quality of life, increase the risk of complications during treatment, or delay the delivery of timely therapy. Coagulation disorders are also more common in malignancy, ranging from an increased risk of thrombosis, to more severe coagulopathies. This chapter will cover the aetiology and management of these disorders, with particular focus on cytopenias, which commonly contribute to symptoms and impact on treatment in cancer care. Deep vein thrombosis and the management of neutropenic sepsis will be dealt with in other chapters.

2.   Anaemia

2.1   *Incidence*

Anaemia, by definition, is a haemoglobin concentration lower than the reference range. While this condition is common in patients with malignancies, its exact incidence is difficult to define. Normal haemoglobin concentration is age and sex dependent; however, studies specifically examining the incidence of anaemia in cancer have used a variety of haemoglobin values to define it. The exact frequency of anaemia also depends on the study population and treatment administered.[1,2] Studies defining anaemia as a haemoglobin of less than 120g/L have shown incidence rates over 50%, whereas haemoglobin values below 100g/L (which may have greater clinical significance) were less common, occurring in fewer than 20% of patients during therapy.[3,4]

2.2　Impact of anaemia

Whilst there may be a lack of consensus regarding the exact incidence and severity of anaemia in cancer patients, there is general agreement that it commonly contributes to diminished quality of life.[1,5–8] Anaemia is recognised as a major contributor to cancer-related fatigue and it may also contribute to dyspnoea and decreased exercise tolerance, which have a measurable impact on quality of life. In patients with co-morbidities, impaired cerebral oxygenation may also contribute to confusion, and exacerbate cardio-respiratory disease, particularly in the elderly.

Anaemia is an adverse prognostic factor in many medical conditions, including renal failure and cardiac disease.[9,10] In the general population, older patients with anaemia have been shown to be at greater risk of death than comparable patients with normal haematocrits.[11,12] This may reflect a multitude of underlying co-morbidities, but appears to retain significance even when adjusted for confounding illnesses. It is unknown whether anaemia directly contributes to death, or whether it is simply an indicator of underlying disorders, but it is perhaps not surprising that anaemia is also an adverse prognostic factor in cancer. In a systematic review of the effect of anaemia on mortality, the risk was increased by an average of 65%, in all malignancies studied.[13] Anaemia is also recognised as a major prognostic factor in some malignancies, for example Hodgkin disease and multiple myeloma, where it has been used as a component of prognostic scoring systems.[14,15]

There are several potential reasons why anaemia can be associated with poorer outcomes. It may be an indicator of more advanced disease, such as bone marrow involvement. It may reflect underlying adverse biological features of cancers, which concurrently cause anaemia, possibly related to an adverse or exaggerated cytokine response. Additionally, anaemia may reflect co-morbidities that independently impact on survival or the ability to tolerate maximal therapy. Finally, it is possible that anaemia may decrease response to cancer therapy.

2.3　Aetiology

The causes of anaemia in cancer patients are diverse, although the most common pattern is consistent with anaemia of chronic disease.[1]

Reversible causes should first be considered, particularly bleeding and resultant iron deficiency, which may be more common in gastrointestinal and gynaecological malignancies. Other haematinic deficiencies, whilst not specific to malignancy, can also identify the need for specific and readily available therapies. Haemolytic anaemia is commonly seen in haematological malignancies, particularly B cell lymphocytic leukaemia and other lymphoproliferative disorders, and may occasionally be associated with medical therapy (e.g. methyldopa, fludarabine, or platinum agents).[16] A direct agglutination test and blood film should be part of the routine evaluation of normocytic anaemia. Myelosuppressive chemotherapy and radiotherapy encompassing haemopoietic bone marrow are amongst the iatrogenic causes for anaemia during cancer treatment. Direct marrow infiltration by malignancy can result in a myelopthisic anaemia, often associated with a leukoerythroblastic peripheral blood picture.

Production of cytokines by malignant cells, or the inflammatory response to malignant cells, can cause anaemia. Tumour necrosis factor-alpha and other cytokines directly impair erythropoiesis.[17] Indirectly, cytokines may impair erythropoietin production, or more commonly increase production of hepcidin. The latter leads to iron sequestration in marrow macrophages, decreased iron absorption, hypoferraemia and elevated ferritin, a mechanism common to the anaemia of chronic disorders. Interleukin 6 is a major mediator of increased hepcidin production in inflammatory and malignant disorders.[18]

Co-morbidities should always be considered when evaluating anaemia in the individual patient, particularly in the elderly, where anaemia is more common in the general population. Active inflammatory disease is commonly associated with anaemia. Renal impairment, which causes anaemia via decreased renal production of erythropoietin, may be an indicator for specific therapy. Bleeding and iron deficiency from causes other than cancer may also respond to specific therapy.

2.4   *Specific treatments for anaemia*

Although anaemia is an adverse prognostic factor, the optimal management of anaemia in cancer patients has yet to be determined.

2.4.1 *Iron administration*

The most common specifically correctable cause for anaemia is iron deficiency. Oral ferrous sulphate may be used, but responses may by slower in inflammatory states due to impaired absorption, and iron stores remain depleted during the initial weeks to months of oral iron treatment. The gastrointestinal side effects of constipation and nausea may also be significant in oncology patients and exacerbate the effects of other therapies.

Intravenous iron infusion is generally well tolerated and leads to a rapid increase in erythropoiesis in iron deficient patients. If bleeding has been arrested, a single dose can replace total body iron stores, so no repeat treatment is required. Timely intravenous iron may help to prevent red cell transfusion. While anaphylactoid reactions are uncommon, intravenous iron should be administered under close observation in an appropriate facility equipped to deal with any immediate complications. Intravenous iron may also be of benefit to improve the rate of response to erythropoietin.[6,19]

2.4.2 *Treatments for autoimmune haemolytic anaemia*

If autoimmune haemolytic anaemia (AIHA) is detected, immune suppression with corticosteroids is the treatment of choice. Further therapy may include specific treatment for underlying lymphoproliferative disease, or use of other immunosuppressive agents if response to steroids is suboptimal. Transfusion therapy for AIHA is complicated, and should not be undertaken without careful consideration of the risks and benefits. Autoantibodies will usually cross-react with all other red cells and in this circumstance it may be technically difficult to provide cross-matched blood. Transfusion may also have limited efficacy in AIHA due to the autoantibodies cross-reacting with transfused cells *in vivo*, resulting in rapid cell destruction.

A further complication of transfusion is the high rate of red cell alloantibody production in patients with AIHA. Alloantibodies are particularly difficult to identify in AIHA patients following recent transfusion, as the autoantibody may mask their presence, and an undetected alloantibody poses a risk of severe acute haemolytic transfusion reactions. Therefore, transfusion in AIHA should be reserved for those patients who have severe acute symptomatic anaemia or are at increased risk, due to co-morbidities such as critical vascular disease.

2.4.3 Red cell transfusions

There is no fixed threshold for blood transfusion based on haemoglobin concentration alone. Transfusion in chronic anaemia should be considered when underlying correctable causes for anaemia have been excluded or treated, or when there is clinical urgency to improve the anaemia. Transfusion is used primarily for symptomatic anaemia, although there may be specific circumstances where transfusion may be considered to improve outcome.

There are no specific symptoms of anaemia. While most people have significant symptoms warranting transfusion when haemoglobin concentrations fall below 70g/L, many will have dyspnoea at higher Hb concentrations, particularly on exertion, and the decision to transfuse is best made on symptoms when the haemoglobin is less than 100g/L. It is generally accepted that transfusion is seldom required when the haemoglobin concentration is above 100g/L.[20] Patients with significant cardio-respiratory impairment will be less tolerant of anaemia, and chronically anaemic patients will often have fewer symptoms than those with acute anaemia. Due to the lack of specific symptoms, it is important to assess the degree of improvement, if any, obtained by transfusing, especially if ongoing transfusional support is being considered.

The role of transfusion in altering prognosis is less clear. In critically ill patients a restrictive transfusion strategy, transfusing only when haemoglobin concentration is less than 70g/L, leads to similar outcomes as more liberal transfusion strategies, so a higher haemoglobin threshold for transfusion is not indicated simply because patients are anaemic and unwell.[21] There is debate about the ideal haemoglobin in patients with acute cardiac disease, with retrospective studies showing that transfusion may be appropriate at threshold haematocrits of 0.25 or 0.30.[22,23] The impact of concurrent cardiovascular disease should therefore be considered when deciding on whether to transfuse red cells.

Cytotoxic therapy requires adequate tissue perfusion. Tissue oxygenation is critical during radiotherapy in particular, which relies on oxygen-mediated, free radical-induced cell death. Necrotic or hypoxic tissue is less susceptible to radiotherapy. Anaemic patients have been shown to have less tumour reduction with radiotherapy and poorer outcomes than non-anaemic patients.[24-26] While there are potential confounding factors in anaemic patients which may contribute to poorer outcomes during radiotherapy, correction of anaemia by transfusion may obviate the adverse prognostic effect of anaemia. Local toxicity from radiotherapy is also reduced in anaemic patients, and is increased by transfusion.[26] These findings suggest a biologically plausible increase in the cytotoxicity of radiotherapy on normal and malignant tissues with improved haemoglobin concentrations due to improved tissue oxygenation. While the optimal haemoglobin concentration has not been defined, keeping the haemoglobin more than 120 g/L during radiotherapy may be of value.

The decision to transfuse needs to be weighed against the risk of potential complications. Increasingly, systematic attention has been given to blood safety, ensuring progressive decrease in transfusion associated risks. Viral infection, particularly with HIV, HBV and HCV has been reduced by donor vetting and serological screening. PCR testing for HIV and HBV has further reduced this risk. Bacterial contamination of blood products, acute haemolytic transfusion reactions and transfusion related acute lung injury, whilst rare, are now more common complications of transfusion than viral infections. Most blood services will monitor estimates of transfusion risk and make these available. In Australia, the estimated risks of infection with HIV or hepatitis viruses are less than one in a million.[27]

The immunological effects of transfusion may be particularly important in cancer patients. There is an increased risk of graft versus host disease in patients with impaired immunity, particularly Hodgkin disease or following purine analogues administration and they should receive irradiated cellular products if transfusion is required.[28,29] There have also been concerns about potential immune modulating effects of transfusion.[30] Increased risk of tumour recurrence has been noted in observational studies of transfused patients,[31] although this has not been confirmed in prospective randomised trials.[32-34] Whilst there is evidence of immune modulation secondary to blood transfusion, the magnitude and clinical relevance of this effect remains uncertain. It is probable that immune modulating effects are, at least in part, attributable to white cells in the transfused product and so may be reduced by leukodepletion.[30] It should therefore not be a reason to withhold transfusion when otherwise indicated.

Leukodepletion of blood products also reduces the risks of febrile non-haemolytic transfusion reactions and HLA antibody formation, which may cause platelet transfusion refractoriness. Therefore leukodepletion is recommended in all oncology patients, especially those who may require repeated transfusions.

2.5 Erythropoietin

Erythropoietin is produced by the kidney in response to tissue hypoxia. At physiological doses, the predominant effect of erythropoietin is to promote erythropoiesis. Erythropoietin receptors, once activated, bind to intracellular Jak-2 kinase, which dimerise STATs. The activated STATs translocate to the nucleus where they bind to DNA targets, promoting erythroid growth and preventing apoptosis.[35,36] Erythropoietin alpha, erythropoietin beta and darbopoietin all act on erythropoietin receptors to promote erythropoiesis, with the latter being a longer-acting analogue. Although each has different dosing regimens, the agents have similar therapeutic efficacy and complications.[5]

Erythropoietin production by the kidney is reduced in renal failure, and erythropoietin supplementation is standard therapy for anaemia of renal disease. Erythropoietin therapy may also increase the haematocrit in myelodysplasia,[37,38] anaemia due to platinum and non-platinum based chemotherapy, and in both haematological and non-haematological cancers.[39-44] In these settings, erythropoietin can improve fatigue scores and quality of life, concordant with the increase in haemoglobin concentration. It is not surprising that erythropoietin improves haemoglobin concentration and wellbeing in anaemic patients, as it is also known to increase haemoglobin concentration, maximal performance, endurance at submaximal performance, and general wellbeing in athletes with normal haemoglobin concentrations.[45] Erythropoietin also decreases transfusion requirements. Whilst this has been considered a worthy goal, direct comparisons between the risks and benefits of erythropoietin and transfusion with similar target haemoglobin values are lacking, and improvements in transfusion safety continue to alter the balance.

Whilst significant quality of life benefits with erythropoietin have been shown for haemoglobin concentrations of at least up to 140–150 g/L, recent studies have raised significant concerns regarding the safety of erythropoietin use in cancer patients. Earlier studies looked primarily at quality of life and transfusion end points. Most were of short duration and not powered to demonstrate changes in survival. On this basis erythropoietin was approved for use in cancer-associated anaemia. However, further studies have demonstrated safety concerns, particularly when erythropoietin is used to achieve higher haemoglobin levels (> 120 g/L), or when used for anaemia related to cancer in patients who are not undergoing radiotherapy or chemotherapy.[46] Specific outcomes include an increased risk of venous and arterial thrombosis,[47] hypertension, poorer local disease control during radiotherapy,[48,49] tumour progression,[50] and increased mortality.[50–52]

There are several potential mechanisms that may explain the poorer outcomes recently reported with erythropoietic agents. It has been postulated that erythropoietin may directly stimulate cell growth, as many tumour cells express erythropoietin receptors. This remains contentious, as erythropoietin receptor expression may be no higher in cancer cells than in corresponding normal tissues.[53–55] The effect may be indirectly mediated via the known increased risk of thrombosis. Erythropoietin also promotes angiogenesis during embryonic development, a role which appears to persist into adult life.[36] As angiogenesis is critical to tumour growth, and angiogenesis inhibitors are effective anti-tumour agents, it is feasible that erythropoietin analogues may promote tumour progression via enhanced angiogenesis.

Other non-erythropoietic functions of EPO have also been described. These include vascular repair and renal protection. High doses have been used in animal myocardial models and show decreased tissue infarction and preservation of myocardial function.[35,36]

Current recommendations support a limited role for erythropoietin in chemotherapy related anaemia, but not to increase haemoglobin concentrations beyond 120 g/L, as this may be associated with increased mortality. There is no role for erythropoietin at present in the treatment of anaemia of cancer in the absence of chemotherapy, and there remain uncertainties about the concurrent use of erythropoietin with radiotherapy. Due to current concerns about decreased survival, caution has been suggested when considering the role of erythropoietin in patients undergoing treatment with curative intent, and the European Medicines Agency has reiterated that blood transfusion remains the treatment of choice for symptomatic patients in this circumstance.[5,6,56] General recommendations for the use of erythropoietin are summarised in Table 1.

In view of the safety concerns regarding erythropoietin, it is important to consider the alternatives for managing anaemia in cancer patients. In the absence of correctable causes for anaemia, transfusion is the only other alternative to improve the haemoglobin concentration. For patients with borderline haemoglobin levels in whom the main aim of therapy is to improve fatigue, other treatments have proven value. Pharmacologic agents which have a modest effect on cancer-related fatigue include methylphenidate and corticosteroids, although the side effects may be limiting.[7] Non-pharmacological treatments may be preferable, with exercise in particular demonstrating improved fatigue and overall quality of life.[57] Given the prevalence of cancer-related fatigue in the cancer population, regular exercise should be advised. Whilst there may be benefit with erythropoietin in improving quality of life, this needs to be balanced with potential adverse effects. Transfusion is therefore best reserved for patients with symptomatic anaemia. There may also be a potential beneficial effect with transfusion during radiotherapy, but this requires further evaluation in prospective studies before it can be routinely recommended in clinical practice.

3.   Neutropenia

Neutropenia is a common complication of chemotherapy. Neutrophil counts below 1×10^9/L are associated with an increased risk of fever

Table 1. Recommendations for erythropoietin use in oncology.

Recommendation	ASH/ASCO Guidelines[5]	ESMO Guidelines[6]
Aim of treatment	Increase haemoglobin and decrease transfusions	Reduce transfusions
Eligible patients	Chemotherapy-related anaemia, Hb approaching or < 100g/L Hb 100–120 g/L with confounding factors for anaemia (e.g. angina, elderly with limited cardiopulmonary reserve) or with exceptionally reduced exercise capacity, energy or ability to carry out daily activities Exclude remedial causes prior to initiation	Chemotherapy-related anaemia (Hb 90–110 g/L)
Target haemoglobin concentration	< 120g/L	< 120g/L
Patients not receiving chemotherapy	Indicated in myelodysplasia Contraindicated in solid or non-myeloid haematological malignancies	Indicated in myelodysplasia Contraindicated in solid or non-myeloid haematological malignancies
Lack of response	Cease after six to eight weeks if no improvement in Hb by 10–20 g/L or reduction in transfusion requirements	No recommendation
Iron therapy	Periodic monitoring of iron status with iron repletion when appropriate	Concurrent parenteral iron recommended to increase the response to erythropoietin

and sepsis. The risk is further increased with more severe and longer duration of neutropenia. Neutropenic fever is considered a medical emergency, as the risks associated with untreated infection are high. The mortality rate for admission for febrile neutropenia was 9.5% in one study.[58] Age, significant co-morbidities and the type of organism were major factors that influenced the outcome. Strategies to reduce the risk of sepsis include antibiotic prophylaxis, reducing the duration of neutropenia by modification of the chemotherapy prescription, or the use of growth factors. An approach to the management of neutropenic sepsis is discussed elsewhere, so attention here will be focussed on the role of granulocyte growth factors during chemotherapy.

3.1   G-CSF and GM-CSF

There are two broad categories of granulocyte growth factors in common use. Granulocyte colony stimulating factor (G-CSF) is highly specific to neutrophil precursors with minimal effect on other lineages. Pharmacological preparations include filgrastim and lenograstim. The former has an N-terminal methionine differentiating it from endogenous G-CSF, whereas the latter is a glycosylated recombinant form of G-CSF. Both have short half lives and are used daily as subcutaneous doses following chemotherapy. Pegfilgrastim is a pegylated form of filgrastim, giving it a much longer half-life, and may be used as a single subcutaneous dose once per chemotherapy treatment cycle.[60]

Granulocyte-monocyte colony stimulating factor (GM-CSF) has broader haemopoietic effects than G-CSF, increasing granulocytes, monocytes and dendritic cells. There is also some effect on erythropoiesis, but GM-CSF knockout mice do not have haemopoietic deficiencies, so unlike G-CSF it does not appear essential for granulocyte development. Oedema, fatigue and diarrhoea are more common with GM-CSF, so it is less commonly used therapeutically. GM-CSF does shorten the duration of neutropenia, similar to G-CSF.[60]

Granulocyte colony stimulating factor may be used to prevent neutropenic sepsis and the adverse consequences associated with it. G-CSF may be used in several ways — as primary prophylaxis to prevent neutropenic sepsis, as secondary prophylaxis following an initial episode of sepsis, or to treat sepsis, in combination with antibiotics, in the neutropenic patient. In addition to preventing neutropenic sepsis, G-CSF may be used to support dose intensification, enabling shortened periods between chemotherapy cycles and assisting with stem cell harvesting for autologous stem cell transplantation.

3.1.1 Primary prophylaxis

Clinical trials have focused on the use of G-CSF as primary prophylaxis during treatments where the risk of febrile neutropenia is high. Seventeen randomised controlled trials in adults undergoing treatment for lymphoma and solid tumours were recently reviewed.[60] Most studies demonstrated a significant reduction in the risk of febrile neutropenia, with an overall relative risk of 0.54. In addition, the relative risks were significantly decreased in pooled analysis for infection related mortality (RR 0.55) and mortality during chemotherapy (RR 0.60). This reduced the absolute risk of death from infection from 2.8% to 1.5%. Current guidelines from several groups recommend the use of G-CSF after the first dose of chemotherapy as primary prevention for neutropenic sepsis when the risk is estimated at more than 20%.[61,62] Risk estimates for various chemotherapy regimens have been published, but clinicians may need to modify assessments based on individual patient risk factors for sepsis and subsequent adverse outcomes.[59,61]

3.1.2 Secondary prophylaxis

Secondary prophylaxis of neutropenic sepsis has been widely advocated following a first episode of neutropenic fever, and use of G-CSF in this setting has been approved by the Pharmaceutical Benefits Scheme in Australia. However, there are flaws in this approach, particularly in that febrile neutropenia may be more common with the first cycle of chemotherapy than with subsequent cycles, so a single episode may not predict recurrence. However, if the duration of neutropenia or neutropenic fever interferes with the ability to deliver the planned dose of chemotherapy on schedule, this may impact on outcome. Therefore, G-CSF support is recommended as secondary prophylaxis only when failure to maintain dosing schedule or intensity may adversely affect treatment outcome.[61,62]

3.1.3 Treatment of neutropenic sepsis

G-CSF has been used in conjunction with antibiotics for the treatment of neutropenic sepsis. A meta-analysis examining the role of G-CSF use compared with antibiotics alone in clinical trials showed a small benefit with the addition of G-CSF.[63] The mortality rate from sepsis in these studies was generally low, except in one study,[64] which showed a markedly increased mortality rate in the antibiotic alone group. Removing this study from the analysis negated the suggested mortality benefit from G-CSF. This may limit the generalisability of these findings. Although decreased duration of neutropenia and decreased hospitalisation time were noted, the authors of the meta-analysis did not recommend widespread use of G-CSF support in febrile neutropenia.[63] However, it is likely, based on these findings, that some patients may benefit, particularly those who are expected to have prolonged neutropenia, or those who fail to respond quickly to antibiotics. Decisions about whether to add G-CSF to antibiotics may need to be made giving consideration to the expected duration of neutropenia, based on the chemotherapy protocol, or previous response to chemotherapy, with the aim of limiting therapy to situations where neutrophil recovery is expected to be delayed. Current guidelines have supported the use of G-CSF in these circumstances.[61,62]

3.1.4 Increasing dose intensity

There is increasing evidence for the utility of dose dense chemotherapy. This is particularly the case for CHOP chemotherapy in elderly patients, where 14-rather than 21-day dosing increases survival, and many regard the 14-day cycle as the standard of care.[65] In order to maintain dose density, G-CSF support is required. Improved outcomes have also been reported in breast cancer and small cell lung cancer.[66,67] Clearly, where there is evidence of improved outcomes with G-CSF supported increased frequency regimens, this should be considered. In addition, increased dose intensity may be achieved by autologous stem cell transplantation. G-CSF is used to mobilise stem cells following chemotherapy, and to shorten the duration of neutropenia during transplantation procedures.[61,62]

3.1.5 *Adverse events from G-CSF*

The most significant immediate concern regarding G-CSF for most patients is bone pain, although other minor side effects do occur. More significant issues, including the potential for leukaemogenesis and increased anaemia in G-CSF treated patients, have been noted.[68,69] Although there have been suggestions that the rate of myelodysplasia and acute myeloid leukaemia (AML) may be increased in this population, there are multiple confounding factors. In a retrospective study patients who received G-CSF had done so due to increased haematological toxicity, which may reflect an increased effect of alkylating agents or topoisomerase inhibitors known to predispose to AML or MDS.[68] Firm conclusions cannot be drawn. As with erythropoietin, however, it would seem prudent to limit the use of G-CSF to those situations in which benefit has been clearly demonstrated.

4. Thrombocytopenia

Clinically significant thrombocytopenia is less common in cancer patients than anaemia or neutropenia. Causes include immune mediated thrombocytopenia, particularly in chronic lymphocytic leukaemia, B cell lymphoproliferative disorders or following fludarabine therapy. Marrow infiltration is a common cause of thrombocytopenia in haematological malignancies, but it may also be seen in metastatic solid tumours. Chemotherapy-induced thrombocytopenia is more common, but usually mild and transient. Thrombocytopenia may also be a feature of diffuse intravascular coagulation (DIC), heparin-induced thrombotic thrombocytopenia and thrombotic thrombocytopenic purpura.

4.1 *Platelet transfusion*

Although thrombocytopenia is usually mild, it may occasionally be severe following highly myelosuppressive chemotherapy, placing patients at risk of bleeding. Whilst surgical procedures may need careful consideration in patients with platelet counts less than $50 \times 10^9/L$, it is rare to have spontaneous bleeding with platelets more than $20 \times 10^9/L$. Spontaneous blood loss from the bowel increases when platelets are less than $5 \times 10^9/L$.[70] Studies in acute myeloid leukaemia have demonstrated equivalent safety of using a platelet transfusion threshold of $10 \times 10^9/L$ compared with $20 \times 10^9/L$.[71,72] This lower threshold has been widely adopted in clinical practice guidelines.[20,73] Lower prophylactic transfusion thresholds have been advocated, and some authors question the value of prophylactic transfusions at all.[74,75] Concurrent risk factors for haemorrhage, including age, known bleeding sites, intracerebral tumours and possibly fever, may be an indication to consider platelet transfusion at higher thresholds. For patients undergoing aggressive treatment with curative intent who develop severe thrombocytopenia, such as germ cell tumours, transfusion of platelets may be considered to support maintaining dose intensity, whereas for other patients, adjustment to the chemotherapy regimen is recommended.

In deciding whether to transfuse or not, special consideration needs to be given to the higher risks associated with platelet transfusion when compared with red cells. Platelets are inactivated by cold storage, so need to be kept on an agitator at room temperature (23°C). This makes an ideal environment for bacterial growth, so the risk of transfusion-associated bacterial sepsis is much higher with platelets than it is for red cells. Also due to the need for room temperature storage, platelets have a shelf life of only five days, and this severely limits the availability of this precious resource.

4.2   *Megakaryocyte stimulating agents*

Cancer therapy-related thrombocytopenia may also be amenable to treatment with cytokines. Megakaryopoiesis is complex, involving numerous cytokines including IL-1, IL-3, GM-CSF, IL-11 and thrombopoietin (TPO).[76] The latter is the most potent regulator of platelet production and is produced in relatively constant levels by the liver. TPO concentrations are therefore largely determined by its rate of metabolism, and increase as platelet production and numbers fall. Thrombopoietin analogues have been used clinically to treat chemotherapy related thrombocytopenia. Two agents, recombinant TPO and human megakaryocyte growth and development factor (MGDF) were used in clinical trials, with mixed results. In part, these may have related to the long lag time between administration and platelet response, as responses were sometimes seen with more rapidly increasing platelet counts after normal platelet recovery. Unfortunately, antibodies against MGDF developed, neutralising not only the effect of the drug, but also native thrombopoietin. This led to prolonged thrombocytopenia, and clinical development of both MGDF and TPO has now ceased.[76]

Interleukin 11 has been approved for use in the United States to prevent thrombocytopenia secondary to chemotherapy. It appears effective, but side effects including fluid retention and oedema, generalised myalgia and pleural effusions have been frequently noted.[76] Neutralising antibodies do not appear to be a major problem. The use of interleukin 1 and interleukin 3 has been studied, and whilst they appear effective, toxicity for both was unacceptable and this approach has also largely been abandoned.

Thrombopoietin receptor agonists theoretically may be suitable candidates for the treatment of chemotherapy induced thrombocytopenia. Romiplostim (formerly known as AMG 531), a peptide TPO receptor agonist, has recently been approved in the United States for treatment of immune thrombocytopenic purpura. Eltrombopag is a small molecule targeting the same receptor and has also been proven in clinical trials to have efficacy in ITP.[78] It has the advantage of good oral bioavailability. Both appear well tolerated, although concerns exist due to the development of increased marrow reticulum during romiplostim therapy. Whether these agents will be therapeutically useful in cancer therapy associated thrombocytopenia is as yet unknown.

5.   Disorders of Coagulation

5.1   *Diffuse intravascular coagulation (DIC)*

DIC has been defined by expert groups, but there is a clear spectrum of disordered coagulation with similar aetiology that does not fulfil diagnostic criteria.[79] Clinically, DIC may be identified as a consumptive coagulopathy syndrome, with evidence of clinical thrombosis, fibrinolysis (elevated cross-linked fibrin degradation products (XDP), and reduced platelets and coagulation factors. Laboratory screening tests usually show an elevated prothrombin time (PT), but activated partial thromboplastin time (APTT) may also be prolonged. Fibrinogen may be decreased, although as it is an acute phase reactant, increased production may mask some of the consumption. The platelet count is often reduced, and in severe cases the blood film may show evidence of red cell fragmentation. No one test is necessary, or sufficient for the diagnosis of DIC, which is a clinical diagnosis made on the basis of laboratory features in the appropriate clinical setting. Cancer is a risk factor for DIC, particularly in adenocarcinoma and with advanced stages.

The treatment of DIC is largely supportive. Effective treatment of the underlying cause is critical to resolution where this is possible.[80] Heparin is not recommended routinely, but may be indicated in patients with thromboses, and low dose heparin, or low molecular weight heparin is reasonable to consider in cancer patients with chronic DIC to prevent thrombosis. Transfusion may help to slow or stop bleeding, particularly with fresh frozen plasma to replace multiple coagulation factor deficiencies, combined with cryoprecipitate if fibrinogen levels are low.[20] Platelet transfusion may also be necessary. There is no specific therapy for DIC, but measures targeting the underlying contributing causes, such as sepsis, are mandatory.

5.2   *Thrombotic thrombocytopenic purpura (TTP)*

TTP is a clinical syndrome of thrombocytopenia, microangiopathic haemolytic anaemia, neurological symptoms, fever and renal impairment. Unlike DIC, coagulation studies are usually normal. It closely resembles haemolytic uraemic syndrome, although the pathogenesis differs. Idiopathic TTP is characterised by deficiency of ADAMTS13, a protease which cleaves von Willebrand factor, due to ADAMTS13 antibodies. Treatment of TTP with plasma exchange using fresh frozen or cryoprecipitate poor plasma is highly effective, as it removes the causative antibody and replaces depleted ADAMTS13.[81] Mortality rate with plasma exchange has been estimated at around 10%, compared with more than 90% without therapy.[82]

TTP occurs rarely in malignancy, but requires urgent assessment and treatment. TTP may be increased in solid tumours, but is also associated with mitomycin C therapy.[83] Although drug- and malignancy-associated TTP are less likely to respond to plasma exchange, the high mortality rates seen in this condition in patients who are untreated or fail to respond warrant consideration of plasma exchange in suitable patients.[82]

6.   Conclusion

Haematological complications are frequently encountered in cancer patients. Anaemia is common and should prompt a search for correctable causes. Correction of haematinic deficiency, particularly the use of intravenous iron, may lead to a rapid marrow response and avoid the need for transfusion. Red cell transfusion is safe and readily available, and should be considered for symptomatic anaemia. Whilst erythropoietin therapy may potentially decrease the need for transfusion and improve quality of life, recent data showing increased mortality in oncology settings suggest it should be used cautiously, particularly in patients not on active treatment. Renal impairment, where there is reduced erythropoietin production, remains an indication, but therapy should target a haemoglobin of not more than 120 g/L.

Cytokines are used in the management of chemotherapy-induced neutropenia to maintain the dose and intensity of chemotherapy where this is thought to improve the outcome. There are also specific circumstances where G-CSF is recommended to support dose intensification. Whilst cytokines have been trialled for thrombocytopenia, and thrombopoietin analogues are entering the market, transfusion with platelet concentrates or plasma products remains the primary therapy for thrombocytopenia and coagulopathy. Determining the cause underlying disorders of coagulation can also help to identify specific treatment options.

References

1. J. E. Groopman and L. M. Itri. Chemotherapy-induced anemia in adults: Incidence and treatment, *J. Natl. Cancer Inst.* **91**: 1616–1634 (1999).
2. J. Michon, Incidence of anaemia in pediatric cancer patients in Europe: Results of a large, international survey, *Med. Pediatr. Oncol.* **39**: 448–450 (2002).

3. H. Ludwig, S. Van Belle, P. Barrett-Lee, G. Birgegard, C. Bokemeyer, P. Gascon, P. Kosmidis, M. Krzakowski, J. Nortier, P. Olmi, M. Schneider and D. Schrijvers, The European Cancer Anaemia Survery (ECAS): A large, multinational, prospective survey defining the prevalence, incidence, and treatment of anaemia in cancer patients, *Eur. J. Cancer* **40**: 2293–2306 (2004).

4. T. Seshadri, H. M. Prince, D. R. Bell, P. B. Coughlin, P. P. James, G. E. Richardson, B. Chern, P. Briggs, J. Norman, I. N. Olver, C. Karapetis and J. Stewart, The Australian Cancer Anaemia Survey: A snapshot of anaemia in adult patients with cancer, *Med. J. Aust.* **182**: 453–457 (2005).

5. J. D. Rizzo, M. R. Somerfield, K. L. Hagerty, J. Seidenfeld, J. Bohlius, C. L. Bennett, D. F. Cella, B. Djulbegovic, M. J. Goode, A. A. Jakubowski, M. U. Rarick, D. H. Regan and A. Lichtin, Use of epoietin and darbopoietin in patients with cancer: 2007 American Society of Hematology/American Society of Clinical Oncology clinical practice guideline update, *Blood* **111**: 25–41 (2008).

6. R. Griel, R. Thödtman and F. Roila, Erythropoietins in cancer patients: ESMO recommendations for use, *Ann. Oncol.* **19**: ii 113–115 (2008).

7. O. Minton, P. Stone, A. Richardson, M. Sharpe and M. Hotopf, Drug therapy in the management of cancer related fatigue, *Cochrane Database Syst. Rev.* (**1**): CD006704 (2008).

8. M. Lind, C. Vernon, D. Cruickshank, P. Wilkinson, T. Littlewood, N. Stuart, C. Jenkinson, P. Grey-Amante, H. Doll and D. Wild, The level of haemoglobin in anaemic cancer patients correlates positively with quality of life, *Br. J. Cancer* **86**: 1243–1249 (2002).

9. S. M. Dunlay, S. A. Weston, M. M. Redfield. J. M. Killian and V. L. Roger, Anemia and heart failure: A community study, *Am. J. Med.* **121**: 726–732 (2008).

10. B. M. Robinson, M. M. Joffe, J. S. Berns, R. L. Pisoni, F. K. Port and H. I. Feldman, Anemia and mortality in hemodialysis patients: Accounting for morbidity and treatment variables updated over time, *Kidney Int.* **68**: 2323–2330 (2005).

11. N. A. Zakai, R. Katz, C. Hirsch, M. G. Shiplak, P. H. Chaves, A. B. Newman and M. Cushman, A prospective study of anemia status, haemoglobin concentration, and mortality in an elderly cohort: The Cardiovascular Health Study, *Arch. Intern. Med.* **165**: 2187–2189 (2005).

12. X. Dong, C. M. de Leon, A. Artz, Y. Tang, R. Shah and D. Evans, A population based study of haemoglobin, race, and mortality in elderly persons, *J. Gerontol. A Biol.* **63**: 873–878 (2008).

13. J. J. Caro, M. Salas, A. Ward and G. Goss, Anemia as an independent prognostic factor for survival in patients with cancer: A systemic qualitative review, *Cancer* **91**: 2214–2221 (2001).

14. D. Hasenclever and V. Diehl, A prognostic score for advanced Hodgkin's disease. Intenational Prognostic Factors Project on Advanced Hodgkin's Disease, *N. Engl. J. Med.* **339**: 1506–1514 (1998).

15. B. G. Durie and S. E. Salmon, A clinical staging system for multiple myeloma. Correlation of measured myeloma cell mass with presenting clinical features, response to treatment and survival, *Cancer* **36**: 842–854 (1975).

16. J. Desrame, H. Broustet, P. Darodes de Tailly, D. Girard and J. M. Saissy, Oxaliplatin-induced haemolytic anaemia, *Lancet* **354**: 1179 (1999).

17. M. T. Bertero and G. Caligaris-Cappio, Anemia of chronic disorders in systemic autoimmune diseases, *Haematologica* **82**: 375–381 (1997).

18. S. Sharma, E. Nemeth, Y. H. Chen, J. Goodnough, A. Huston, G. D. Roodman, T. Ganz and A. Lichtenstein, Involvement of hepcidin in the anemia of multiple myeloma, *Clin. Cancer Res.* **14**: 3262–3267 (2008).

19. Y. T. Kim, S. W. Kim, B. S. Yoon, H. J. Cho, E. J. Nahm, S. H. Kim, J. H. Kim and J. W. Kim, Effect of intravenously administered iron sucrose on the prevention of anemia in the cervical cancer patients treated with concurrent chemoradiotherapy, *Gynecol. Oncol.* **105**: 199–204 (2007).

20. National Health and Medical Research Council and Australian and New Zealand Society of Blood Transfusion, *Clinical Practice Guidelines on the Use of Blood Components*, Commonwealth of Australia (2001).

21. P. C. Hebert, G. Wells, M. A. Blajchman, J. Marshall, C. Martin, G. Pagliarello, M. Tweeddale, Schwitzer and E. Yetisir, A multicenter, randomized, controlled clinical trial of transfusion requirements in critical care. Transfusion requirements in Critical Care Investigators, Canadian Critical Care Trials Group, *N. Engl. J. Med.* **340**: 409–417 (1999).

22. S. V. Rao, J. G. Jollis, R. A. Harrington, C. B. Granger, L. K. Newby, P. W. Armstrong, D. J. Moliterno, L. Lindblad, K. Pieper, E. J. Topol,

J. S. Stamler and R. M. Califf, Relationship of blood transfusion and clinical outcomes in patients with acute coronary syndromes, *J. Am. Med. Assoc.* **292**: 1555–1562 (2004).

23. W. C. Wu, S. S. Rathore, Y. Wang, M. J. Radforf and H. M. Krumholz, Blood transfusion in elderly patients with acute myocardial infarction, *N. Engl. J. Med.* **345**: 1230–1236 (2001).

24. G. Thomas, The effect of haemoglobin level on radiotherapy outcomes: The Canadian experience, *Semin. Oncol.* **28**: 60–65 (2001).

25. K. L. Zhao, G. Liu, G. L. Jiang, Y. Wang, L. J. Zhong, Y. Wang, W. Q. Yao, X. M. Guo, G. D. Wu, L. X. Zhu and X. H. Shi, Association of haemoglobin level with morbidity and mortality of patients with locally advanced oesophageal carcinoma undergoing radiotherapy — A secondary analysis of three consecutive clinical phase III trials, *Clin. Oncol.* **18**: 621–627 (2006).

26. M. Grogan, G. M. Thomas, I. Melamed, F. L. W. Wong, R. G. Pearcey, P. K. Joseph, L. Portelance, J. Crook and K.D. Jones, The importance of haemoglobin levels during radiotherapy for carcinoma of the cervix, *Cancer* **86**: 1528–1536 (1999).

27. C. R. Seed, P. Kiely and A. J. Keller. Residual risk of transfusion transmitted human immunodeficiency virus, hepatitis B virus, hepatitis C virus and human T lymphotrophic virus, *Intern. Med. J.* **35**: 592–598 (2005).

28. L. M. Williamson, S. Love, E. M. Love, H. Cohen, K. Soldan, D. B. L, McClelland, P. Skacel and A. J. Barbara, Serious Hazards of Transfusion (SHOT) initiative: Analysis of the first two annual reports, *Br. Med. J.* **319**: 16–19 (1999).

29. N. Blumberg and J. M. Heal, Effects of transfusion on immune function, cancer recurrence and infection, *Arch. Pathol. Lab. Med.* **118**: 371–379 (1994).

30. E. C. Vamvakas and M. A. Blajchman, Universal WBC reduction: The case for and against, *Transfusion* **41**: 691–712 (2001).

31. E. Vamvakas, Perioperative blood transfusion and cancer recurrence: Meta-analysis for explanation, *Transfusion* **35**: 760–768 (1995).

32. M. N. Heiss, W. Mempel, C. Delanoff, K.W. Jauch, C. Gabka, M. Mempel, H. J. Dietrich, H. J. Eissner and F. W. Schildberg, Blood transfusion-modulated tumor recurrence: First results of a randomized study of autologous versus allogeneic blood transfusion in colorectal cancer surgery, *J. Clin. Oncol.* **12**: 1859–1867 (1994).

33. O. R. C. Busch, W. C. J. Hop, M. H. van Papendrecht, R. L. Marquet and J. Jeekel, Blood transfusion and prognosis in colorectal cancer, *N. Engl. J. Med.* **328**: 1372–1376 (1993).

34. L. M. G. van de Watering, A. Brand, J. G. A. Houbiers, W. M. Klien Kranenbarg, J. Hermans and C. van de Velde, Perioperative blood transfusions, with or without allogeneic leucocytes, relate to survival, not to cancer recurrence, *Br. J. Surg.* **88**: 267–272 (2002).

35. W. Jelkmann, Developments in the therapeutic use of erythropoiesis stimulating agents, *Br. J. Haematol.* **141**: 287–297 (2008).

36. D. Filser and H. Haller, Erythropoietin and treatment of non-anemic conditions — Cardiovascular protection, *Semin. Hematol.* **44**: 212–217 (2007).

37. M. Jadersten, L. Malcovati, I. Dybedal, M. G. Della Porta, R. Invernizzi, S. M. Montgomery, C. Pascutto, A. Porwit, M. Cazzola and E. Hellstrom-Lindberg, Erythropoietin and granulocyte-colony stimulating factor treatment associated with improved survival in myelodysplastic syndrome, *J. Clin. Oncol.* **26**: 3607–3613 (2008).

38. V. Moyo, P. Lefebvre, M. S. Duh, B. Yektashenas and S. Mundle, Erythropoiesis-stimulating agents in the treatment of anaemia in myelodysplastic syndromes: A meta-analysis, *Ann. Hematol.* **87**: 527–536 (2008).

39. R. Pirker, R. A. Ramlau, W. Schuette, P. Zatloukal, I. Ferreira, T. Lillie and J. F. Vansteenkiste, Safety and efficacy of darbopoietin alpha in previously untreated extensive-stage small-cell lung cancer treated with platinum plus etoposide, *J Clin. Oncol.* **26**: 2342–2349 (2008).

40. H. Ludwig, E. Sundal, M. Pechestorfer, C. Leitgeb, T. Bauernhofer, A. Beinhauer, H. Samonigg, A. W. Kappeler and E. Fritz, Recombinant human erythropoietin for the correction of cancer associated anemia with and without concomitant cytotoxic chemotherapy, *Cancer* **76**: 2319–2329 (1995).

41. P. J. Hesketh, F. Arena, D. Patel, M. Austin, P. D'Avirro, G. Rossi, A. Colowick and L. Schwartzberg, A randomized controlled trial of darbopoietin alfa administered as a fixed or weight-based dose using a front-loading schedule in patients with anaemia who have nonmyeloid malignancies, *Cancer* **100**: 859–868 (2004).

42. T. J. Littlewood, E. Bajetta, J. W. R. Nortier, E. Vercammen and B. Rapaport, Effects of epoietin alfa on hematologic parameters and quality of life in cancer patients receiving nonplatinum

chemotherapy: Results of a randomized, double-blind, placebo-controlled trial, *J. Clin. Oncol.* **19**: 2865–2874 (2001).

43. Y. Suzuki, Y. Tokuda, Y. Fujiwara, H. Minami, Y. Ohashi and N. Saijo, Weekly epoietin beta maintains haemoglobin levels and improves quality of life in patients with non-myeloid malignancies receiving chemotherapy, *Jpn. J. Clin. Oncol.* **38**: 214–221 (2008).

44. G. Thomas, S. Ali, F. J. Hoebers, K. M. Darcy, W. H. Rodgers, M. Patel, O. Abulafia, J. A. Lucci and A. C. Becc, Phase III trial to evaluate the efficacy of maintaining haemoglobin levels above 12.0g/dL with erythropoietin vs. above 10.0 g/dL without erythropoietin in anaemic patients receiving concurrent radiation and cisplastin for cervical cancer, *Gynecol. Oncol.* **108**: 317–325 (2007).

45. G. Ninot, P. Connes and C. Caillaud, Effects of recombinant human erythropoietin injections on physical self in endurance athletes, *J. Sports Sci.* **24**: 383–391 (2006).

46. R. E. Smith, M. S. Aapro, H. Ludwig, T. Pinter, M. Smakal, T. E. Ciuleanu, L. Chen, T. Lillie and J. A. Glaspy, Darbopoietin alpha for the treatment of anaemia in patients with active cancer not receiving chemotherapy or radiotherapy: Results of a phase III, multicenter, randomized, double-blind, placebo-controlled study, *J. Clin. Oncol.* **26**: 1040–1050 (2008).

47. C. L. Bennett, S. M. Silver, B. Djulbegovic, A. T. Samaras, C. A. Blau, K. J. Gleason, S. E. Barnato, K. M. Elverman, D. M. Courtney, J. M. McKoy, B. J. Edwards, C. C. Tigue, D. W. Raisch, P. R. Yarnold, D. A. Dorr, T. M. Kuzel, M. S. Tallman, S. M. Trifilio, D. P. West, S. Y. Lai and M. Henke, Venous thromboembolism and mortality associated with recombinant erythropoietin and darbopoietin administration for the treatment of cancer-associated anemia, *J. Am. Med. Assoc.* **299**: 914–924 (2008).

48. M. Henke, R. Laszig, C. Rube, U. Schafer, K. D. Haase, B. Schilcher, S. Mose, K. T. Beer, U. Burger, C. Dougherty and H. Fromhold, Erythropoietin to treat head and neck cancer patients with anaemia undergoing radiotherapy: Randomised, double-blind, placebo-controlled trial, *Lancet* **362**: 1255–1260 (2003).

49. M. Aapro, A. Scherhag and H. U. Burger, Effect of treatment with epoietin-β on survival, tumour progression and thromboembolic events in patients with cancer: An updated meta-analysis of 12 randomised controlled studies including 2301 patients, *Br. J. Cancer* **99**: 14–22 (2008).

50. B. Leyland-Jones, V. Semiglazov, M. Pawlicki, T. Pienkowski, S. Tjulandin, G. Manikhas, A. Makhson, A. Roth, D. Dodwell, J. Baselga, M. Biakhov, K. Valuckas, E. Voznyi, X. Liu and E. Vercammen, Maintaining normal haemoglobin levels with epoetin alfa in mainly nonanemic patients with metastatic breast cancer receiving first-line chemotherapy: A survival study, *J. Clin. Oncol.* **23**: 5960–5972 (2005).

51. M. Aapro, R. C. Leonard, A. Barnadas, M. Marangolo, M. Untch, N. Malamos, J. Mayordomo, D. Reichert, J. L. Pedrini, L. Ukarma, A. Scherhag and H. U. Burger, Effect of once-weekly epoetin beta on survival in patients with metastatic breast cancer receiving anthracycline-and/or taxane-based chemotherapy: Results of the Breast Cancer-Anemia and the Value of Erythropoietin (BRAVE) study, *J. Clin. Oncol.* **26**: 592–598 (2008).

52. J. R. Wright, Y. C. Ung, J. A. Julian, K. I. Pritchard, T. J. Whelan, C. Smith, B. Szechtman, W. Roa, L. Mulroy, L. Rudinskas, B. Gagnon, G. S. Okawara and M. N. Levine, Randomized, double-blind, placebo-controlled trial of erythropoietin in non-small-cell lung cancer with disease related anaemia, *J. Clin. Oncol.* **25**: 1027–1032 (2007).

53. M. Henke, D. Mattern, M. Pepe, C. Bezay, C. Weissenberger, M. Werner and F. Pajonik, Do erythropoietin receptors on cancer cells explain unexpected clinical findings?, *J. Clin. Oncol.* **24**: 4708–4713 (2006).

54. C. Lonnroth, M. Svensson, W. Wang, U. Korner, P. Daneryd, O. Nilsson and K. Lundholm, Survival and erythropoietin receptor protein in tumours from patients randomly treated with rhEPO for palliative care, *Med. Oncol.* **25**: 22–29 (2008).

55. A. M. Sinclair, N. Rogers, L. Busse, I. Archbeque, W. Brown, P. D. Kassner, J. E. V. Watson, G. E. Arnold, K. C. Q. Nguyen, S. Powers and S. Elliott, Erythropoietin receptor transcription is neither elevated nor predictive of surface expression in human tumour cells, *Br. J. Cancer* **98**: 1059–1067 (2008).

56. European Medicines Agency, *Questions and Answers on Epoetin and the Risk of Tumour Growth and Blood Clots in the Veins*, Press Release (June 2008).

57. F. Cramp and J. Daniel, Exercise for the management of cancer-related fatigue in adults, *Cochrane Database Syst. Rev.* (**2**): CD006145 (2008).

58. N. M. Kuderer, D. C. Dale, J. Crawford, L. E. Cosler and G. H. Lyman, Mortality, morbidity and cost associated with febrile neutropenia in adult cancer patients, *Cancer* **106**: 2258–2266 (2006).

59. M. Heuser, A. Ganser and C. Bokemeyer, Neutropenia: Review of current guidelines, *Semin. Hematol.* **44**: 148–156 (2007).

60. N. M. Kuderer, D. C. Dale, J. Crawford and G. Lyman, Impact of primary prophylaxis with granulocyte colony-stimulating factor on febrile neutropenia and mortality in adult cancer patients receiving chemotherapy: A systemic review, *J. Clin. Oncol.* **25**: 3158–3167.

61. M. S. Aapro, D. A. Cameron, R. Pettengell, J. Bohlius, J. Crawford, M. Ellis, N. Kearney, G. H. Lyman, V. C. Tjan-Heijnen, J. Walewski, D. C. Weber and C. Zielinski, EORTC guidelines for the use of granulocyte-colony stimulating factor to reduce the incidence of chemotherapy-induced febrile neutropenia in adult patients with lymphomas and solid tumors, *Eur. J. Cancer* **42**: 2433–2453 (2006).

62. T. J. Smith, J. Khatcheressian, G. H. Lyman, H. Ozer, J. O. Armitage, L. Balducci, C. L. Bennett, S. B. Cantor, J. Crawford, S. J. Cross, G. Demetri, C. E. Desch, P. A. Pizzo, C. A. Schiffer, L. Schwartzberg, M. R. Somerfield, G. Somlo, J. C. Wade, J. L. Wade, R. J. Winn, A. J. Wozniak and A.C. Wolff, 2006 update of recommendations for the use of white blood cell growth factors: An evidence based clinical practice guideline, *J. Clin. Oncol.* **24**: 3187–3205 (2006).

63. O. A. C. Clark, G. H. Lyman, A. A. Castro, L. G. O. Clark and B. Djulbegovic, Colony stimulating factors for chemotherapy induced febrile neutropenia: A meta-analysis of randomized controlled trials, *J. Clin. Oncol.* **23**: 4198–4214 (2005).

64. A. Aviles, R. Guzman, E. L. Garcia, A. Talavera and J. C. Diaz, Results of a randomized clinical trial of granulocyte colony-stimulating factor in patients with infection and severe granulocytopenia, *Anticancer Drugs* **7**: 392–397 (1996).

65. M. Pfreundshuh, L. Trumper, M. Kloess, R. Schmits, A. C. Feller, C. Rudolph, M. Reiser, D. K. Hossfeld, B. Metzner, D. Hasenclever, N. Schmitz, B. Glass, C. Rube and M. Loeffler, Two-weekly or 3-weekly CHOP chemotherapy with or without etoposide for the treatment of young patients with good-prognosis (normal LDH) aggressive lymphomas: Results of the NHL-B1 trial of the DSHNHL, *Blood* **104**: 626–633 (2004).

66. M. L. Citron, D. A. Berry, C. Cirricione, C. Hudis, E. P. Winer, W. J. Gradishar, N. E. Davidson, S. Martino, R. Liningston, J. N. Ingle,

E. A. Perez, J. Carpenter, D. Hurd, J. F. Holland, B. L. Smith, C. I. Sartor, E. H. Leung, J. Abrams, R. L. Schlisky, H. B. Muss and L. Norton, Randomized trial of dose-dense versus conventionally scheduled and sequential versus concurrent combination chemotherapy as post-operative adjuvant treatment of node-positive primary breast cancer: First report of Intergroup Trial C9741/Cancer and Leukemia Group B Trial 9741, *J. Clin. Oncol.* **21**: 1431–1439 (2003).

67. N. Thatcher, D. J. Girling, P. Hopwood, R. J. Sambrook, W. Qian and R. J. Stephens, Improving survival without reducing quality of life in small-cell lung cancer patients by increasing the dose-intensity of chemotherapy with granulocyte colony-stimulating factor support: Results of a British Medical Research Council multicenter randomized trial, *J. Clin. Oncol.* **18**: 395–404 (2000).

68. M. C. Le Deley, F. Suzan, B. Cutuli, S. Delaloge, A. Shamsaldin, C. Linassier, S. Clisant, F. De Vathaire, P. Fenaux and C. Hill, Anthracyclines, mitoxantrone, radiotherapy and granulocyte colony-stimulating factor: Risk factors for leukaemia and myelodysplastic syndrome after breast cancer, *J. Clin. Oncol.* **25**: 292–300 (2007).

69. P. Papaldo, F. Gianluigi, S. Di Cosimo, D. Giannarelli, P. Marolla, M. Lopez, E. Cortesi, M. Antimi, E. Terzoli, P. Carlini, P. Vici, C. Botti, L. Di Lauro, G. Naso, C. Nistico, M. Mottolese, F. Di Filippo, E. M. Ruggeri, A. Ceribelli and F. Cognetti, Does granulocyte colony-stimulating factor worsen anaemia in early breast cancer patients treated with epirubicin and cyclophosphamide?, *J. Clin. Oncol.* **24**: 3048–3055 (2006).

70. S. J. Slichter and L. A. Harker, Thrombocytopenia: Mechanisms and management of defects in platelet production, *Clin. Haematol.* **7**: 523–528 (1978).

71. P. Rebulla, G. Finazzi, F. Marangoni, G. Avvisati, L. Gugliotta, G. Tognoni, T. Barbui, F. Mandelli and G. Sirchia, The threshold for prophylactic platelet transfusions in adults with acute myeloid leukaemia, *N. Engl. J. Med.* **337**: 1870–1875 (1997).

72. K. D. Heckman, G. J. Weiner, C. S. Davis, R. G. Strauss, M. P. Jones and C. P. Burns, Randomized study of prophylactic platelet transfusion threshold during induction therapy for adult acute leukemia: 10,000/μL versus 20,000/μL, *J. Clin. Oncol.* **15**: 1143–1149 (1997).

73. C. A. Schiffer, K. C. Anderson, C. L. Bennett, S. Bernstein, L. S. Elting, M. Goldsmith, M. Goldstein, H. Hume, J. J. McCullough, R. E. McIntyre, B. L. Powell, J. M. Rainey, S. D. Rowley, P. Rebulla, M. B. Troner and

A. H. Wagnon, Platelet transfusion for patients with cancer: Clinical guidelines of the American Society of Clinical Oncology, *J. Clin. Oncol.* **19**: 1519–1538 (2001).

74. H. Wandt, K. Schaefer-Eckart, M. Frank, J. Birkmann and M. Wilhelm, A therapeutic platelet transfusion strategy is safe and feasible in patients after autologous peripheral blood stem cell transplantation, *Bone Marrow Transpl.* **37**: 387–392 (2006).

75. J. Gmür and A. Schaffner, Prophylactic platelet transfusion in acute leukaemia, *Lancet* **339**: 120–121 (1992).

76. S. O. Ciurea and R. Hoffman, Cytokines for the treatment of thrombocytopenia, *Semin. Hematol.* **44**: 166–192 (2007).

77. D. J. Kuter, J. B. Bussel, R. M. Lyons, V. Pullarkat, T. B. Gernsheimer, F. M. Senecal, L. M. Aledort, J. N. George, C. M. Kessler, M. A. Sanz, H. A. Leibman, F. T. Slovick, J. T. de Walt, E. Bourgeois, T. H. Guthrie, A. Newland, J. S. Wasser, S. I. Hamburg, C. Grande, F. Lefrere, A. E. Lichtin, M. D. Tarantino, H. R. Terebelo, J. F. Viallard, F. J. Cuevas, R. S. Go, D. H. Henry, R. L. Redner, L. Rice, M. R. Schipperus, D. M. Guo and J. L. Nichol, Efficacy of romiplostim in patients with chronic immune thrombocytopenic purpure: A double-blind randomised controlled trial, *Lancet* **371**: 395–403 (2008).

78. J. B. Bussel, G. Cheng, M. N. Saleh, B. Psaila, L. Kovaleva, B. Meddeb, J. Kloczko, H. Hassani, B. Mayer, N. L. Stone, M. Arning, D. Provan and J. M. Jenkins, Eltrombopag for the treatment of chronic idiopathic thrombocytopenic purpure, *N. Engl. J. Med.* **29**: 2237–2247 (2007).

79. S. Gando, T. Iba, Y. Eguchi, Y. Ohtomo, K. Okamoto, K. Koseki, T. Mayumi, A. Murata, T. Ikeda, H. Ishikura, M. Ueyama, H. Ogura, S. Kushimoto, D. Saitoh, S. Endo and S. Shimazaki, A multicenter, prospective validation of disseminated intravascular coagulation diagnostic criteria for critically ill patients: Comparing current criteria, *Crit. Care Med.* **34**: 899–900 (2006).

80. C. A. Labelle and C. S. Kitchens, Disseminated intravascular coagulation: Treat the cause, not the lab values, *Clevel. Clin. J. Med.* **72**: 377–378 (2005).

81. J. E. Sadler, Von Willebrand factor, ADAMTS13, and thrombotic thrombocytopenic purpura, *Blood* **112**: 11–18 (2008).

82. N. Bandarenko and M. E. Brecher, United States Thrombotic Thrombocytopenic Purpura Apheresis Study Group (US TTP ASG): Multicentre survey and retrospective analysis of current efficacy of therapeutic plasma exchange, *J. Clin. Apher.* **13**: 133–141 (1998).

83. S. Fontana H. E. Gerritsen, J. Kremer Hovinga, M. Furlan and
B. Lammle, Microangiopathic haemolytic anaemia in metastasizing
malignant tumours is not associated with a severe deficiency of the
von Willebrand factor-cleaving protease, *Br. J. Haematol.* **113**:
100–102 (2001).

Managing the Patient with Chronic Viral Hepatitis Receiving Chemotherapy

Venessa Pattullo and
Jacob George

Abstract

Immunosuppression associated with the use of chemotherapy for both solid tumours and haematological malignancies has been linked to the reactivation of hepatitis B in those with serological evidence of past or present hepatitis B infection. Reactivations may be unanticipated, unidentified or untreated, and can lead to fulminant liver failure and death. Hepatitis B flares may also interrupt chemotherapeutic regimens, thereby potentially increasing the risk of cancer-related morbidity and mortality.

Chronic hepatitis B is endemic worldwide, and in Australia its prevalence is rising, in part related to changing trends in migration. Clinicians caring for people with malignancy need to be aware of the potential for hepatitis B reactivation as a complication of chemotherapy in susceptible individuals. Thus, individuals at risk for chronic hepatitis B must be screened serologically for the virus before chemotherapy or immunosuppression is contemplated and prophylactic therapy with lamivudine or another nucleos(t)ide analogue, instituted. This chapter reviews hepatitis B prevalence, immunology, virology and the risk of reactivation in patients receiving chemotherapy. Recommendations regarding monitoring and prophylaxis are outlined. Other chronic hepatitis viral infections in the setting of chemotherapy are briefly discussed.

Keywords: Hepatitis B, reactivation, prophylaxis, lamivudine, chemotherapy.

1.   Epidemiology of Hepatitis-B Reactivation

It is estimated that two billion people worldwide have been infected with hepatitis B and approximately 350 million of these are chronically infected. Of those chronically infected, it is estimated that 75% reside in the Asia-Pacific region, where the disease is endemic.[1,2] This accounts for the higher prevalence of chronic hepatitis B (CHB) in certain at-risk groups, such as some migrant populations of Australia, in whom seroprevalence rates as high as 10% have been documented.[1-3] In the general population, only 0.4–2.1% have evidence of chronic hepatitis B infection (HBsAg positive), whilst 3.6–9.5% have serological evidence of previous exposure (HBsAg negative but anti-HBc positive).[3-5] Other at-risk groups for CHB in the population based on an Australian study are listed in Table 1.[3]

Chemotherapy (and immunosuppression) are associated with clinically significant reactivations of CHB in both cancer and non-cancer patients. The prevalence of CHB is not known amongst patients with non-malignant inflammatory, rheumatological or autoimmune diseases requiring immunosuppression, however, reactivation has been reported in patients receiving immunosuppression for Crohn's disease, rheumatoid arthritis and in those following liver and renal transplantation.[6-12]

Increasing numbers of clinically evident CHB reactivations following chemotherapy have been reported in the literature.[13-20] Amongst oncology patients, the prevalence of CHB has been reported to be as high as 26% in those with lymphoma and 12% of those with solid tumours.[21] Without antiviral prophylaxis, about 20% of CHB patients with malignancy will experience a reactivation.[21]

Table 1. Adjusted odds ratio for chronic hepatitis B in at risk groups within the Australian population.[3]

Chronic hepatitis B risk group	Adjusted odds ratio (95% confidence interval)
HIV infection	36.3 (6.93–180.06)
Born in Asia or the Pacific islands	12.4 (7.67–20.03)
Born in North Africa, the Middle East and the Mediterranean	6 (3.83–9.57)
Born abroad elsewhere in the world	2.7 (1.66–4.56)
Household contact with someone diagnosed with hepatitis between 1980 and 1990	3.9 (1.44–10.72)
Injected drugs between 1980 and 1990	4.4 (1.37–14.0)
Resident in a military establishment for > three months	2.3 (1.23–4.15)
Hospitalised for > three months	2.2 (1.04–4.58)
Received blood transfusion due to an accident and/or a haemorrhage	1.92 (1.10–3.44)
Never been vaccinated for hepatitis B	2.8 (1.67–4.79)
Male gender	1.59 (1.12–2.26)

In one study, 41% of breast cancer patients who were HBsAg positive and undergoing chemotherapy experienced CHB reactivation, as did 47% of lymphoma patients in another report.[15,21] The presence of CHB amongst haematology-oncology patients is therefore of great clinical relevance to patient outcomes.

2.   Hepatitis B Serology

To better understand the mechanisms and manifestations of hepatitis B reactivation in cancer patients, a basic overview of the immunology and clinical course of the infection is presented below.

Previous exposure to hepatitis B is signified by the presence of anti-HBc. In contrast, the presence of HBsAg for more than six months signifies the presence of chronic hepatitis B infection. Immunity to hepatitis B is characterised by the presence of anti-HBs. In the absence of anti-HBc, the presence of anti-HBs signifies successful immunisation. Table 2 summarises the interpretation of

Table 2. Interpretation of hepatitis B serology.

	Interpretation	Comments
Anti-HBc	Previous exposure to hepatitis B virus	
HBsAg	Chronic HBV infection if present for more than six months	May become negative in cases of viral clearance
Anti-HBs	Confers immunity	May be positive after past acute HBV infection with seroconversion OR after successful immunisation
HBeAg	In association with HBsAg indicates a high replicative state	
Anti-HBe	In association with HBsAg and normal ALT indicates a low replicative state	
HBV DNA	Indicates viraemia	HBV DNA may be negative in chronic hepatitis B in the 'immune tolerant' phase of the infection

ALT: Alanine aminotransferase, anti-HBc: hepatitis B core antibody, anti-HBe: hepatitis B e-antibody, anti-HBs: hepatitis B surface antibody, HBeAg: hepatitis B e-antigen, HBsAg: hepatitis B surface antigen, HBV: hepatitis B virus.

hepatitis B serology. Any individual with chronic infection (HBsAg positive) should be considered at risk of reactivation with chemotherapy.

In individuals with CHB, the immune system acts with varying levels of control on the virus, leading to the clinical, biochemical and serological manifestations that are observed over the course of the disease (Fig. 1).[22]

(1) The immune tolerant phase is characterised serologically by the presence of HBeAg, elevated levels of HBV DNA and a normal ALT. In this phase, in spite of elevations in HBV DNA, there is minimal hepatocyte damage.

(2) The immune clearance phase is characterised by a fall in HBV DNA, and may be associated with elevations in ALT, signifying

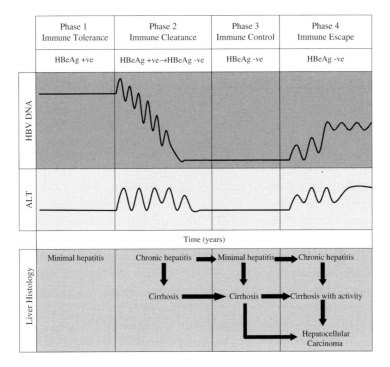

Phase 1 Immune Tolerance	Phase 2 Immune Clearance	Phase 3 Immune Control	Phase 4 Immune Escape
HBeAg +ve	HBeAg +ve→HBeAg -ve	HBeAg -ve	HBeAg -ve

Figure 1. The immune phases of chronic hepatitis B infection and corresponding serological, biochemical and clinical manifestations.

Adapted from Thomas (2007).[22]

bouts of hepatic necroinflammation. Repeated cycles of abortive immune clearance over many years result in chronic inflammation, hepatocyte damage and fibrosis seen in association with CHB.

(3) The immune control phase is characterised by the loss of HBeAg, and the development of anti-HBe. This is termed seroconversion. During this phase of variable duration (which may span decades), HBV DNA is suppressed and ALT is normal. This phase represents the switch of the hepatitis B virus to a low replicative state and is associated with reduced hepatocyte damage over the ensuing months to years. The onset of seroconversion cannot be predicted, and treatments aimed at achieving seroconversion are limited in their efficacy at this time.

(4) The immune escape phenomenon is characterised by a rise in HBV DNA and ALT, in association with chronic active hepatitis on liver histology in an individual who is HBeAg negative. During this phase, immune control of viral replication is lost and active hepatitis with progressive liver injury ensues. Over time, this hepatitis leads to hepatic fibrosis and eventually to cirrhosis. In some instances of viral reactivation, acute hepatitis with a rapid rise in HBV DNA, ALT, and symptoms of icteric liver failure may ensue.

The use of chemotherapy impacts on the ability of the host immune system to control hepatitis B replication. This therefore has the potential to result in rapid rises in HBV DNA during chemotherapy, causing direct hepatocyte necrosis. Alternatively, and more commonly, in the post-chemotherapy phase, massive immune reconstitution may cause severe immune mediated injury to infected hepatocytes. Both of these scenarios can result in asymptomatic biochemical hepatitis, or the more worrisome clinical presentation of acute symptomatic hepatitis that in severe cases can lead to liver failure and death.

In some circumstances patients with CHB reactivation may not have the usual pattern of serology described above.

2.1 *HBsAg negative patients*

Patients with previously documented CHB may spontaneously lose HBsAg at an annual rate of 0.5% and are said to have undergone 'spontaneous clearance'.[23] Such individuals however remain at risk of hepatitis B reactivation in the context of immunosuppression, owing to the persistence of HBV DNA within hepatocytes and other tissues that may or may not be detectable in serum.[24,25] Even in the presence of anti-HBs, this HBsAg negative state may represent 'occult' chronic hepatitis B infection and should always be considered in patients previously known to be carriers of hepatitis B, or who belong to a high risk group.

2.2 *Anti-HBc positive patients*

Documented cases of 'reverse seroconversion' (or sero-reversion) have been described in which an anti-HBc positive/anti-HBs positive individual undergoing immunosuppression re-develops hepatitis B surface antigenaemia, HBV DNA viraemia and/or clinically evident hepatitis, as a result of reactivation of 'occult' infection.[26]

2.3 'Undetectable' HBsAg

Mutation of the hepatitis B virus may also lead to the production of a 'mutant' form of HBsAg that is undetectable by routine assays. This is a rare occurrence with current laboratory assays, and occurs in persons who may have had either spontaneous mutations in the HBsAg-encoding region, or mutations secondary to previous antiviral treatment or HCV co-infection.[25] The diagnosis of hepatitis B reactivation in these individuals is made when HBV DNA is detectable by PCR. This phenomenon has been described in HBsAg negative patients experiencing hepatitis B reactivation with chemotherapy, organ transplant recipients developing chronic hepatitis B after receiving organs from HBsAg negative donors, and in chimpanzees developing hepatitis B after receiving HBsAg negative human blood transfusions.[25,27–29]

To summarise, anyone within a high risk group with past or present HBsAg positivity, or evidence of previous exposure (HB cAb positive) is at risk of hepatitis B reactivation with immunosuppression and should be considered for monitoring and/or antiviral prophylaxis prior to chemotherapy. Current recommendations for screening, monitoring and prophylaxis are outlined later.

3. Clinical Manifestations of Hepatitis B Reactivation

Reactivation of hepatitis B can be life-threatening and occurs when immune control of chronic infection is disrupted. Reactivation is defined as a 1 log (or ten-fold) rise in HBV DNA from baseline pre-chemotherapy levels.[30] Sero-reversion, i.e. the recurrence of HBsAg in a previously HBsAg negative/anti-HBc positive patient, also represents a form of hepatitis B reactivation.[31] HBV reactivation may occur with or without hepatitis (as defined by at least a 3-fold rise in serum ALT).[30] The manifestations of viral reactivation may range from an asymptomatic derangement of liver tests (transaminitis), to symptomatic acute hepatitis with jaundice, hepatomegaly and pain, to synthetic liver dysfunction with coagulopathy and hypoalbuminemia, to the extreme of fulminant liver failure with encephalopathy and death.

Two mechanisms underlie the liver damage that occurs as a result of a hepatitis B flare. Firstly, reactivation may occur during chemotherapy, due to loss of immune control of the virus leading to uncontrolled viral replication within hepatocytes and overwhelming cytolytic destruction of these cells. More commonly however, a flare may occur at a remote time (usually three to six weeks) after chemotherapy has ceased. The mechanism in this setting is immune reconstitution, which causes an exaggerated response against hepatocytes expressing viral proteins, again causing overwhelming necrosis of liver cells. The delayed flare may occur up to six months after cessation of chemotherapy.[30]

4.   Management of Hepatitis B Reactivation

HBV reactivation during chemotherapy, if detected, may be an indication to suspend or curtail chemotherapy. Interruption of chemotherapy may diminish the rate of HBV replication occurring during a reactivation. In a historic control cohort of 61 breast cancer patients with CHB, reactivation occurred in more than 40%, and chemotherapy had to be suspended in 46%, a significantly higher rate of chemotherapy interruption than for breast cancer patients given prophylactic lamivudine.[32] In lymphoma patients, chemotherapy was disrupted in 37% of a historic control cohort of 116 patients due to HBV reactivation.[33] Two-thirds of patients receiving chemotherapy for nasopharygeal carcinoma (common among Chinese, a population with a concomitant high prevalence of CHB) had treatment disrupted because of HBV reactivation.[17] The consequence of chemotherapy interruption is a higher rate of cancer related mortality.

The role of lamivudine treatment once HBV reactivation has occurred during chemotherapy has been examined in several studies. Lamivudine therapy started at the time of ALT elevation did not appear to change the natural course of chemotherapy-associated HBV reactivation in a prospectively followed cohort of patients treated for non Hodgkin's lymphoma.[30] Prophylactic lamivudine versus therapeutic lamivudine has been shown to reduce the incidence and severity of chemotherapy-related HBV reactivation in these patients.[30]

Thus, the key element in the management of hepatitis B reactivation in cancer patients receiving chemotherapy is prevention, rather than reactionary treatment, both to avoid chemotherapy interruption, and to reduce the rate and severity of HBV flares.

5.   Prevention of Hepatitis B Reactivation

As more reports of severe or fatal reactivations of CHB in the context of chemotherapy for solid tumours and haematological malignancies have appeared in the literature, awareness of this catastrophic complication has increased. The evidence for screening and management of patients with overt or occult CHB, which has accumulated over many years, is summarised below.

Two systematic reviews of studies examining the role of prophylaxis for hepatitis B reactivation in chemotherapy patients have been published.[34,35] Lamivudine prophylaxis in chemotherapy patients is associated with a relative risk of 0.0 to 0.21 for HBV reactivation and a relative risk of 0.0 to 0.2 for HBV-related death, when compared with no lamivudine prophylaxis.[34] No patient who received lamivudine prophylaxis in the studies included in this systematic review developed HBV-related liver failure.[34] These findings concur with a systematic review reporting that patients given lamivudine prophylaxis during chemotherapy showed an 87% decrease in HBV reactivation compared to patients not given prophylaxis. Most notably, the number needed to treat (NNT) to prevent one reactivation was just three patients.[35] Lamivudine prophylaxis also led to a 92% reduction in treatment delays and premature terminations of chemotherapy secondary to reactivation.[35]

The use of lamivudine prophylaxis has been demonstrated to be cost-effective, owing to the reduced number and severity of hepatitis B reactivations. In one study, the reduced numbers of cancer deaths in the prophylaxis group was presumably due to a reduced need for withholding chemotherapy in that group.[36]

6. Determining Risk Factors for Reactivation

Attempts have been made to determine risk factors for CHB reactivation amongst those receiving chemotherapy, in order to identify persons that should receive anti-viral prophylaxis. The serological risk factors associated with HBV reactivation include detectable HBsAg, HBV DNA, HBeAg and anti-HBc as described above.[22-26] Patient-specific risk factors associated with reactivation include younger age, male gender and treatment regimens that include corticosteroids or anthracyclines.[18,37] Pretreatment ALT and HBV DNA have been reported to be predictive for CHB reactivation, but cut-off levels are not available from existing studies. Interestingly, HBV reactivation appears to correlate with HBV genotypes C and B, prevalent in East Asia and the East Mediterranean.[38-40] However, whether this is a true finding or simply a reflection of the prevalent genotypes in these populations has been not been adequately addressed. Whilst these patient-specific and virus-specific associations have been made, there is insufficient evidence to support targeted lamivudine prophylaxis in these select groups. Thus, serological markers remain the main guide to monitoring and prophylaxis.

7. Timing and Duration of Lamivudine Prophylaxis

Existing trials of lamivudine prophylaxis are heterogeneous in methodology with regards to the timing of initiation of therapy. Lamivudine has been commenced most commonly from seven days prior to chemotherapy to day 1 of chemotherapy, with cessation occurring from one to 12 months after completion of chemotherapy.[34] In a randomized controlled prospective study of HBV infected non Hodgkin's lymphoma patients, the treatment group consisted of 26 subjects given lamivudine prophylaxis from day 1 of chemotherapy until two months after the cessation of chemotherapy. During chemotherapy, fewer patients in the prophylaxis group had HBV reactivation (11.5% versus 56%, $p = 0.001$) and HBV-related hepatitis (7.7% versus 48%, $p = 0.001$). No patient in the prophylaxis group had hepatitis B reactivation during the 12-month study period.[30] It is important to note that two patients died of HBV reactivation–related hepatitis, in spite of lamivudine prophylaxis, 173 and 182 days respectively after cessation of lamivudine.[30] One postulates that these delayed reactivations and deaths may have been prevented with more prolonged lamivudine therapy after the cessation of chemotherapy. However, whether this reactivation is part of the natural history of CHB (unrelated to cancer chemotherapy) or secondary to cancer-related immunosuppression is still unclear.

Delayed non-fatal reactivations of CHB have been reported after cessation of lamivudine prophylaxis, six weeks after chemotherapy completion. These patients were restarted on lamivudine with effective suppression of HBV DNA without adverse consequences.[41] Post-chemotherapy reactivation rates have not been reported in studies using lamivudine for 12 months after chemotherapy cessation. Thus, reactivation of hepatitis B can occur even in patients who have received lamivudine prophylaxis and the duration of ongoing prophylaxis after chemotherapy is debated. Therefore, continued monitoring of disease and viral replication is warranted in all cases.

Continuation of antiviral therapy may be necessary in patients who fulfill the criteria for the treatment of CHB outside of the chemotherapy setting. These include patients with elevated baseline ALT and DNA levels with evidence of chronic hepatitis on liver biopsy. Patients who have survived the underlying malignancy should be monitored long term by a hepatology service for the ongoing management of CHB, for example for the development of lamivudine resistance, and for any complications of chronic hepatitis B, including the progression to cirrhosis, portal hypertension, liver failure or hepatocellular cancer.

8.   Other Antiviral Agents

Other drugs in the available armamentarium for the current management of chronic hepatitis B include adefovir dipivoxil, entecavir, telbivudine and tenofovir disoproxil fumarate. None of these agents have been studied extensively to date in the context of hepatitis B reactivation for patients receiving immunosuppressive agents or chemotherapy. While no guidelines exist for their use in this setting, these drugs are likely to be equally efficacious in reducing the risk and severity of hepatitis B reactivation. With significantly less antiviral resistance than lamivudine, these newer agents are a more attractive choice as the first-line for HBV DNA suppression and prophylaxis, and are likely to be used by clinicians treating those receiving immunosuppressive agents.

9.   Recommendations

The American Association for the Study of Liver Disease (AASLD) recommends the following:[42]

9.1   *Screening*

HBsAg testing should be performed in persons who are at high risk for HBV infection (see Table 1), prior to the initiation of chemo- or immunosuppressive therapy. In addition, it is recommended that anti-HBc be tested in order to assess for previous exposure, which in some individuals may represent occult CHB.

9.2   *Prophylaxis of overt CHB*

Prophylactic antiviral therapy should be administered to those who are HBsAg positive at the onset of cancer chemotherapy.[42]

(1) Patients with baseline HBV DNA <2000 IU/ml should continue treatment for six months after completion of chemotherapy or immunosuppressive therapy.
(2) Patients with high baseline HBV DNA (>2000 IU/ml) level should continue treatment until they reach similar treatment end points as immunocompetent patients.

9.3   *Monitoring and prophylaxis of occult CHB*

Guidelines for the management of patients with occult HBV infection (HBsAg negative, anti-HBc positive) are unclear and further study is required. The AASLD does not give recommendations on how to manage these patients. Based on available experience, the

International Association for the Study of Liver Disease (IASLD) recommends that:[31]

(1) Oncology patients or those undergoing mild haematological therapies judged to be of low immunosuppressive potential, such as the ABVD [adriamycin (or doxorubicin), bleomycin, vinblastine, dacarbazine] or the CHOP [cyclophosphamide, doxorubicin (or adriamycin), vincristine (or oncovin) and prednisolone] 21-day scheme, HBsAg monitoring every one to three months is advised. Targeted prophylaxis or therapy should commence in the case of sero-reversion or hepatitis reactivation.
(2) Subjects receiving intense immunosuppression (chemotherapy with fludarabine, allogeneic transplantation, autologous myeloablative transplant, induction in acute leukaemia, use of monoclonal antibodies) should be considered for universal prophylaxis.

9.4 Monitoring after cessation of chemotherapy and cessation of lamivudine

There is no clear evidence on monitoring after the cessation of lamivudine therapy. Serum ALT measurements and HBV DNA measurements every one to two months for three to six months after cessation of lamivudine prophylaxis have been suggested,[34] but clinical experience would suggest that these patients should be monitored long term, particularly if there is a likelihood for the relapse of their underlying malignancy.

9.5 Hepatitis B and delta co-infection

There is currently no evidence-based guide for the management of hepatitis B and delta co-infection in the setting of immuno-suppression or cancer chemotherapy. The screening, prophylaxis and post-chemotherapy monitoring of these co-infected patients should therefore be the same as for CHB mono-infection, with the understanding that anti-viral therapy may prevent HBV reactivation, but may not influence the clinical course of delta virus co-infection.

10. Chemotherapy and Chronic Hepatitis C

Activation of chronic hepatitis C (CHC) is a far less common occurrence than reactivation of hepatitis B in the setting of malignancy and chemotherapy. In a cohort of patients who underwent allogeneic stem cell transplantation, the prevalence of chronic hepatitis B and C infections were 15.6% and 3.7% respectively. Whilst one patient had hepatitis B reactivation, none of these individuals had hepatitis C activation in the post-transplant phase.[43] Similarly, in a cohort of 98 patients with B-cell non Hodgkin's lymphoma treated with chemotherapy, the prevalence of HCV was 16% and whilst one of these patients developed hepatitis during chemotherapy, it was not attributed to the activation of hepatitis C.[44]

In contrast to the findings of these cohort studies, the development of acute symptomatic hepatitis C has been documented in patients who have undergone immunosuppression. One reported case of hepatitis C activation occurred in an individual one month after discontinuation of cyclosporin A, cyclophosphamide and cortisone given for immune thrombocytopenic purpura.[45] Similarly, a case of reactivation of hepatitis C has been reported in a patient receiving chemotherapy for colorectal cancer.[46]

On balance, the burden of hepatitis C reactivation appears to be far less than that of hepatitis B reactivation in the context of chemotherapy. This is likely due to differing immune control pathways that mediate chronic hepatitis B and C infection. Whilst we suggest that the HCV status of all patients undergoing chemotherapy should be checked at baseline (by testing for anti-HCV Ab), no specific therapy or prophylaxis for hepatitis C infection is recommended at this time.

11. Summary

Clinicians caring for people with a malignancy need to be aware of the potential for hepatitis B reactivation as a complication of chemotherapy in susceptible individuals. Those at risk for chronic hepatitis B must be screened serologically for the virus.

Prophylactic therapy with lamivudine or another nucleos(t)ide analogue should be commenced before the initiation of chemotherapy.

List of Abbreviations

ALT:	Alanine aminotransferase
Anti-HBc:	Hepatitis B core antibody
Anti-HBe:	Hepatitis B e-antibody
Anti-HBs:	Hepatitis B surface antibody
CHB:	Chronic hepatitis B
HBeAg:	Hepatitis B e-antigen
HBsAg:	Hepatitis B surface antigen
HBV:	Hepatitis B virus
ABVD:	Adriamycin (or doxorubicin), Bleomycin, Vinblastine, Dacarbazine
CHOP:	Cyclophosphamide, Doxorubicin (or adriamycin), Vincristine (or Oncovin) and Prednisolone.

References

1. J. Benson and W. Donohue, Hepatitis in refugees who settle in Australia, *Aust. Fam. Physician* **36**: 719–727 (2007).
2. R. Mohamed, P. Desmond, D. J. Suh, D. Amarapurkar, E. Gane, Y. Guangbi, J. L. Hou, W. Jafri, C. L. Lai, C. H. Lee, S. D. Lee, S. G. Lim, R. Guan, P. H. Phiet, T. Piratvisuth, J. Sollano and J. C. Wu, Practical difficulties in the management of hepatitis B in the Asia-Pacific region, *J. Gastroenterol. Hepatol.* **19**: 958–969 (2004).
3. H. M. Tawk, K. Vickery, L. Bisset, S. K. Lo, W. Selby and Y. E. Cossart, The current pattern of hepatitis B virus infection in Australia, *J. Viral Hepat.* **13**: 206–215 (2006).
4. P. Pavli, G. J. Bayliss, O. F. Dent and M. L. Lunzer, The prevalence of serological markers for hepatitis B virus infection in Australian Naval personnel, *Med. J. Aust.* **151**: 71, 74–75 (1989).
5. B. G. O'Sullivan, H. F. Gidding, M. Law, J. M. Kaldor, G. L. Gilbert and G. J. Dore, Estimates of chronic hepatitis B virus infection in Australia, 2000, *Aust. N. Z. J. Public Health* **28**: 212–216 (2004).
6. M. Esteve, C. Saro, F. Gonzalez-Huix, F. Suarez, M. Forne and J. M. Viver, Chronic hepatitis B reactivation following infliximab therapy

in Crohn's disease patients: Need for primary prophylaxis, *Gut* **53**: 1363–1365 (2004).

7. L. H. Calabrese, N. N. Zein and D. Vassilopoulos, Hepatitis B virus (HBV) reactivation with immunosuppressive therapy in rheumatic diseases: Assessment and preventive strategies, *Ann. Rheum. Dis.* **65**: 983–989 (2006).

8. V. G. Bain, Hepatitis B in transplantation, *Transpl. Infect. Dis.* **2**: 153–165 (2000).

9. A. Berger, W. Preiser, H. G. Kache, M. Sturmer and H. W. Doerr, HBV reactivation after kidney transplantation, *J. Clin. Virol.* **32**: 162–165 (2005).

10. G. Dusheiko, E. Song, S. Bowyer, M. Whitcutt, G. Maier, A. Meyers and M. C. Kew, Natural history of hepatitis B virus infection in renal transplant recipients — A fifteen-year follow-up, *Hepatology* **3**: 330–336 (1983).

11. E. Gane and H. Pilmore, Management of chronic viral hepatitis before and after renal transplantation, *Transplantation* **74**: 427–437 (2002).

12. J. Kletzmayr and B. Watschinger, Chronic hepatitis B virus infection in renal transplant recipients, *Semin. Nephrol.* **22**: 375–389 (2002).

13. M. G. Chheda, J. Drappatz, N. J. Greenberger, S. Kesari, S. E. Weiss, D. C. Gigas, L. M. Doherty and P. Y. Wen, Hepatitis B reactivation during glioblastoma treatment with temozolomide: A cautionary note, *Neurology* **68**: 955–956 (2007).

14. B. Coiffier, Hepatitis B virus reactivation in patients receiving chemotherapy for cancer treatment: Role of lamivudine prophylaxis, *Cancer Invest.* **24**: 548–552 (2006).

15. M. S. Dai, P. F. Wu, R. Y. Shyu, J. J. Lu and T. Y. Chao, Hepatitis B virus reactivation in breast cancer patients undergoing cytotoxic chemotherapy and the role of preemptive lamivudine administration, *Liver Int.* **24**: 540–546 (2004).

16. H. Higashiyama, T. Harabayashi, N. Shinohara, M. Chuma, S. Hige and K. Nonomura, Reactivation of hepatitis in a bladder cancer patient receiving chemotherapy, *Int. Urol. Nephrol.* **39**: 461–463 (2007).

17. W. Yeo, E. P. Hui, A. T. Chan, W. M. Ho, K. C. Lam, P. K. Chan, T. S. Mok, J. J. Lee, F. K. Mo and P. J. Johnson, Prevention of hepatitis B virus reactivation in patients with nasopharyngeal carcinoma with lamivudine, *Am. J. Clin. Oncol.* **28**: 379–384 (2005).

18. W. Yeo and P. J. Johnson, Diagnosis, prevention and management of hepatitis B virus reactivation during anticancer therapy, *Hepatology* **43**: 209–220 (2006).

19. W. Yeo, K. C. Lam, B. Zee, P. S. Chan, F. K. Mo, W. M. Ho, W. L. Wong, T. W. Leung, A. T. Chan, B. Ma, T. S. Mok and P. J. Johnson, Hepatitis B reactivation in patients with hepatocellular carcinoma undergoing systemic chemotherapy, *Ann. Oncol.* **15**: 1661–1666 (2004).

20. D. M. Nathan, P. W. Angus and P. R. Gibson, Hepatitis B and C virus infections and anti-tumor necrosis factor-alpha therapy: Guidelines for clinical approach, *J. Gastroenterol. Hepatol.* **21**: 1366–1371 (2006).

21. W. Yeo, P. K. Chan, S. Zhong, W. M. Ho, J. L. Steinberg, J. S. Tam, P. Hui, N. W. Leung, B. Zee and P. J. Johnson, Frequency of hepatitis B virus reactivation in cancer patients undergoing cytotoxic chemotherapy: A prospective study of 626 patients with identification of risk factors, *J. Med. Virol.* **62**: 299–307 (2000).

22. H. C. Thomas, Best practice in the treatment of chronic hepatitis B: A summary of the European Viral Hepatitis Educational Initiative (EVHEI), *J. Hepatol.* **47**: 588–597 (2007).

23. Y. F. Liaw, I. S. Sheen, T. J. Chen, C. M. Chu and C. C. Pao, Incidence, determinants and significance of delayed clearance of serum HBsAg in chronic hepatitis B virus infection: A prospective study, *Hepatology* **13**: 627–631 (1991).

24. C. Brechot, F. Degos, C. Lugassy, V. Thiers, S. Zafrani, D. Franco, H. Bismuth, C. Trepo, J. P. Benhamou, J. Wands *et al.*, Hepatitis B virus DNA in patients with chronic liver disease and negative tests for hepatitis B surface antigen, *N. Engl. J. Med.* **312**: 270–276 (1985).

25. I. Chemin, D. Jeantet, A. Kay and C. Trepo, Role of silent hepatitis B virus in chronic hepatitis B surface antigen(–) liver disease, *Antiviral Res.* **52**: 117–123 (2001).

26. J. R. Wands, C. M. Chura, F. J. Roll and W. C. Maddrey, Serial studies of hepatitis-associated antigen and antibody in patients receiving anti-tumor chemotherapy for myeloproliferative and lymphoproliferative disorders, *Gastroenterology* **68**: 105–112 (1975).

27. N. Schnepf, P. Sellier, M. Bendenoun, J. M. Zini, M. J. Sanson-le Pors and M. C. Mazeron, Reactivation of lamivudine-resistant occult hepatitis B in an HIV-infected patient undergoing cytotoxic chemotherapy, *J. Clin. Virol.* **39**: 48–50 (2007).

28. H. Marusawa, S. Imoto, Y. Ueda and T. Chiba, Reactivation of latently infected hepatitis B virus in a leukemia patient with antibodies to hepatitis B core antigen, *J. Gastroenterol.* **36**: 633–636 (2001).

29. J. K. Law, J. K. Ho, P. J. Hoskins, S. R. Erb, U. P. Steinbrecher and E. M. Yoshida, Fatal reactivation of hepatitis B post-chemotherapy for lymphoma in a hepatitis B surface antigen-negative, hepatitis B core antibody-positive patient: Potential implications for future prophylaxis recommendations, *Leuk. Lymphoma* **46**: 1085–1089 (2005).

30. C. Hsu, C. A. Hsiung, I. J. Su, W. S. Hwang, M. C. Wang, S. F. Lin, T. H. Lin, H. H. Hsiao, J. H. Young, M. C. Chang, Y. M. Liao, C. C. Li, H. B. Wu, H. F. Tien, T. Y. Chao, T. W. Liu, A. L. Cheng and P. J. Chen, A revisit of prophylactic lamivudine for chemotherapy-associated hepatitis B reactivation in non-Hodgkin's lymphoma: A randomized trial, *Hepatology* **47**: 844–853 (2008).

31. A. Marzano, E. Angelucci, P. Andreone, M. Brunetto, R. Bruno, P. Burra, P. Caraceni, B. Daniele, V. Di Marco, F. Fabrizi, S. Fagiuoli, P. Grossi, P. Lampertico, R. Meliconi, A. Mangia, M. Puoti, G. Raimondo and A. Smedile, Prophylaxis and treatment of hepatitis B in immunocompromised patients, *Dig. Liver Dis.* **39**: 397–408 (2007).

32. W. Yeo, W. M. Ho, P. Hui, P. K. Chan, K. C. Lam, J. J. Lee and P. J. Johnson, Use of lamivudine to prevent hepatitis B virus reactivation during chemotherapy in breast cancer patients, *Breast Cancer Res. Treat.* **88**: 209–215 (2004).

33. Y. H. Li, Y. F. He, W. Q. Jiang, F. H. Wang, X. B. Lin, L. Zhang, Z. J. Xia, X. F. Sun, H. Q. Huang, T. Y. Lin, Y. J. He and Z. Z. Guan, Lamivudine prophylaxis reduces the incidence and severity of hepatitis in hepatitis B virus carriers who receive chemotherapy for lymphoma, *Cancer* **106**: 1320–1325 (2006).

34. R. Loomba, A. Rowley, R. Wesley, T. J. Liang, J. H. Hoofnagle, F. Pucino and G. Csako, Systematic review: The effect of preventive lamivudine on hepatitis B reactivation during chemotherapy, *Ann. Intern. Med.* **148**: 519–528 (2008).

35. L. A. Martyak, E. Taqavi and S. Saab, Lamivudine prophylaxis is effective in reducing hepatitis B reactivation and reactivation-related mortality in chemotherapy patients: A meta-analysis, *Liver Int.* **28**: 28–38 (2008).

36. S. Saab, M. H. Dong, T. A. Joseph and M. J. Tong, Hepatitis B prophylaxis in patients undergoing chemotherapy for lymphoma: A decision analysis model, *Hepatology* **46**: 1049–1056 (2007).

37. G. Lalazar, D. Rund and D. Shouval, Screening, prevention and treatment of viral hepatitis B reactivation in patients with haematological malignancies, *Br. J. Haematol.* **136**: 699–712 (2007).

38. A. S. Lok and C. L. Lai, Acute exacerbations in Chinese patients with chronic hepatitis B virus (HBV) infection. Incidence, predisposing factors and etiology, *J. Hepatol.* **10**: 29–34 (1990).

39. A. S. Lok, R. H. Liang, E. K. Chiu, K. L. Wong, T. K. Chan and D. Todd, Reactivation of hepatitis B virus replication in patients receiving cytotoxic therapy. Report of a prospective study, *Gastroenterology* **100**: 182–188 (1991).

40. M. S. Jazayeri, A. A. Basuni, G. Cooksley, S. Locarnini and W. F. Carman, Hepatitis B virus genotypes, core gene variability and ethnicity in the Pacific region, *J. Hepatol.* **41**: 139–146 (2004).

41. G. K. Lau, H. H. Yiu, D. Y. Fong, H. C. Cheng, W. Y. Au, L. S. Lai, M. Cheung, H. Y. Zhang, A. Lie, R. Ngan and R. Liang, Early is superior to deferred preemptive lamivudine therapy for hepatitis B patients undergoing chemotherapy, *Gastroenterology* **125**: 1742–1749 (2003).

42. A. S. Lok and B. J. McMahon, Chronic hepatitis B, *Hepatology* **45**: 507–539 (2007).

43. D. Francisci, F. Aversa, V. Coricelli, A. Carotti, B. Canovari, F. Falcinelli, B. Belfiori, T. Aloisi, F. Baldelli, M. F. Martelli and G. Stagni, Prevalence, incidence and clinical outcome of hepatitis B virus and hepatitis C virus hepatitis in patients undergoing allogeneic hematopoietic stem cell transplantation between 2001 and 2004, *Haematologica* **91**: 980–982 (2006).

44. P. Faggioli, M. De Paschale, A. Tocci, M. Luoni, S. Fava, A. De Paoli, A. Tosi and E. Cassi, Acute hepatic toxicity during cyclic chemotherapy in non Hodgkin's lymphoma, *Haematologica* **82**: 38–42 (1997).

45. A. Gruber, L. G. Lundberg and M. Bjorkholm, Reactivation of chronic hepatitis C after withdrawal of immunosuppressive therapy, *J. Intern. Med.* **234**: 223–225 (1993).

46. M. E. Melisko, R. Fox and A. Venook, Reactivation of hepatitis C virus after chemotherapy for colon cancer, *Clin. Oncol. (R. Coll. Radiol.)* **16**: 204–205 (2004).

33

Management of Malignant Gastrointestinal Tract Obstruction

Eric Y. T. Lee, Vu Kwan and
Michael J. Bourke

Abstract

Malignant luminal obstruction is a potentially catastrophic occurrence in the management of patients with advanced gastrointestinal neoplasia. This chapter will deal with its presentation, assessment and treatment. Early recognition and effective treatment by minimally invasive means confers a rapid return to pre-obstruction functional status with prompt restitution of oral nutrition. In general, an endoscopic approach to palliation is the best option. Other alternatives will also be discussed.

Keywords: Gastroduodenal obstruction, colonic obstruction, oesophageal obstruction, stenting, malignant biliary obstruction.

1. Introduction

Malignant luminal obstruction is a frequent occurrence during the course of the management of patients with gastrointestinal malignancy. Early recognition and effective treatment by the least invasive means possible provides the best opportunity for patients to overcome this dramatic event, with its sudden impact on quality of life and potentially lethal consequences. This chapter will discuss each of the major anatomical sites of malignant luminal obstruction, their presentation, assessment and treatment.

1.1 General approach to the patient with gastrointestinal obstruction

The clinical presentation of gastrointestinal tract obstruction depends upon the site of mechanical obstruction. Dysphagia is the most common presentation of oesophageal obstruction, while gastroduodenal obstruction often presents with post-prandial nausea and vomitting and early satiety. Colonic obstruction typically presents with constipation or frequent small stools with a sense of incomplete evacuation, or abdominal pain and distension. Factors that increase the suspicion of a malignant process underlying the obstruction include a short but progressive history, advancing age of the patient, the presence of constitutional or alarm clinical manifestations such as weight loss, cachexia, and anorexia, a past history of malignancy, physical findings such as an abdominal mass, hepatomegaly or supraclavicular lymphadenopathy, and laboratory findings such as iron deficiency anaemia or obstructive liver biochemistry. These factors however are not sufficiently specific for confirmation of a malignant process. Other causes of 'obstructive' symptoms include the effects of oncological treatment such as radiotherapy-related fibrotic stricturing or neuropathy or medication such as narcotic-related constipation. A history of relentlessly progressive symptoms suggests a malignant process, whilst symptoms that are less consistent and fluctuating imply that the problem may be functional. Radiographic imaging with contrast studies and computed tomography may demonstrate the pattern of gastrointestinal tract obstruction, the primary tumour and metastatic neoplasia if present. However, histological confirmation of diagnosis remains essential and this is usually achieved with endoscopic assessment and biopsy. A multidisciplinary team approach enables early recognition, assessment and treatment of malignant gastrointestinal tract obstruction and its variants.

2.   Malignant Oesophageal Obstruction

2.1   *Presentation*

Primary oesophageal malignancy is the predominant cause of malignant oesophageal obstruction. Less commonly, extrinsic compression from mediastinal lymphadenopathy or lung cancer may also cause oesophageal obstruction. The most common and problematic presenting symptom is progressive, unrelenting dysphagia, which is almost invariably associated with progressive weight loss. Primary oesophageal malignancy presents late in its clinical course and, at the time of diagnosis, the disease is often advanced and either unresectable, or not amenable to surgical cure. The diagnosis is usually made in the elderly often with substantial co-morbidity and thus the poor functional status of the patient precludes surgery. The palliation of malignant dysphagia in patients with inoperable disease requires a multidisciplinary team approach. All patients require careful tumour staging, histological confirmation of the diagnosis and specialist surgical consultation before a palliative treatment plan is determined. The options include endoscopic therapies, chemo-radiotherapy, or nasogastric tube feeding. Surgical palliation (oesophageal bypass or oesophagectomy) is rarely attempted these days, given the significant morbidity (> 50%) and mortality (> 10%) associated with it and the availability of equally effective or superior minimally invasive options.[1,2] The selection of the most appropriate palliative treatment is individualised for each patient, and is discussed below.

2.2   *Endoscopic management*

Endoscopic palliation offers the most rapid path to safely restoring luminal patency, leading to symptom relief and prompt restitution of nutrition. Once the ability to swallow has been restored, further palliative treatment with chemo-radiotherapy can be considered if clinically appropriate. Endoscopic palliation of malignant dysphagia is undertaken in a number of clinical settings including:

- patients with significant dysphagia who require restoration of luminal patency and nutritional status prior to commencement of chemo-radiotherapy;

- recurrent malignant disease following previous treatment, including surgery or chemo-radiotherapy; and
- patients with inoperable disease and poor functional status precluding chemo-radiotherapy.

Established options for the endoscopic palliation of malignant dysphagia include:

- oesophageal stenting;
- tumour-ablative therapy (laser, argon plasma coagulation, photodynamic therapy) for tumour de-bulking; and
- endoscopic-guided nasogastric tube insertion.

The choice of endoscopic intervention depends on the stricture location and morphology, the presence of complicating features such as fistulising disease, the extent (stage) of disease, the patient's functional status, and importantly, the patient's preference. Where a tracheo-oesophageal or broncho-oesophageal fistula co-exists or is suspected, the first-line treatment is deployment of a covered oesophageal stent, with successful closure of fistula closure in 80–100% of cases.[3,4] When dealing with malignant obstruction of the upper oesophagus, bronchoscopic assessment with or without concurrent airway stenting may also be necessary if there is a clinical or radiologic suspicion of significant large airway (trachea or main bronchus) narrowing, given that a self-expandable oesophageal stent may compromise the airway lumen in this setting. Where the prognosis is poor and life expectancy is very limited, then if the patient and the family prefer, short-term enteral feeding can be established with a feeding tube inserted under combined endoscopic and fluoroscopic guidance, even if the stricture is endoscopically impassable.

Stricture morphology and site strongly influence the choice of endoscopic intervention. Assessment begins with a contrast swallow study, which complements the information obtained during endoscopy. Oesophageal stenting can be carried out for strictures throughout the oesophagus, although the upper margin of the tumour should be at least 2cm below the cricopharyngeus for the procedure to be safely performed. The endoscope does not have to traverse the stricture for stenting to be performed, as a guidewire can negotiate the vast majority of strictures under fluoroscopic guidance. In cases where the luminal diameter of the oesophageal stricture is still relatively large and permits the passage of the endoscope without resistance, oesophageal stenting may not be appropriate at that time, given the increased risk of distal stent migration. In this situation, tumour-ablative therapy should instead be considered if the patient is symptomatic.[5]

Endoscopic procedures are performed under conscious sedation using combinations of midazolam, fentanyl and propofol, and are often carried out on an out-patient basis, without the need for hospital admission. Following the endoscopic intervention, patients are commenced on a clear fluid diet on the same day, and this is gradually upgraded to a soft diet. In cases where the endoscopic treatment compromises the actions of the lower oesophageal sphincter (as it occurs with an oesophageal stent that traverses the gastro-oesophageal junction), anti-reflux measures (high-dose proton pump inhibition therapy and elevation of the head of the bed to 30 degrees) are imperative to minimise the impact of post-stenting gastro-oesophageal reflux. Severe reflux oesophagitis is a differential diagnosis for recurrent dysphagia following oesophageal stenting.

2.3   *Oesophageal stenting*

Oesophageal stents are self-expanding open mesh metallic tubes constrained on a narrow catheter, which can be placed across even very tight oesophageal strictures, with only minimal dilatation. Following deployment, the stent continues to expand against the tumour and adjacent normal tissue, thereby anchoring itself to the oesophagus. The portion of the oesophageal stent directly overlying the malignant tissue has a covering membrane which reduces the risk of tumour ingrowth, while the proximal and distal ends of the stent are uncovered, to help promote mucosal epithelialisation, and thereby reducing the risk of stent migration.

Palliative oesophageal stenting with self-expandable metal stents is highly effective in restoring oesophageal luminal patency in the setting of malignant obstruction, with technical and clinical success rates in excess of 90%.[6,7] Early complications include perforation (0.6%), bleeding (0.6%), and chest pain (12.2%). Delayed complications include stent obstruction due to tumour ingrowth/ overgrowth (11.3%) and stent migration (6.8%).[8] Almost a third of patients can expect to develop recurrent dysphagia due to tumour overgrowth at either end of the stent, stent migration or food bolus obstruction. Endoscopic reintervention involving additional stenting, ablative therapy or food bolus removal is effective in restoring luminal patency in the majority (> 90%) of patients.[9] Stents function best when their configuration is straight, and thus when the entire stent is within the oesophagus. However, the majority of oesophageal malignancy is adenocarcinoma complicating Barrett's oesophagus and thus stenting across the lower oesophageal sphincter with varying degrees of attendant angulation is the most common intervention. Migration is more frequent and dysfunction due to impaction on the gastric wall is also a possibility.

2.4 *Ablative therapy*

Options for ablative therapy include Nd-YAG laser, argon plasma coagulation and photodynamic therapy. These techniques can be costly, and generally require multiple treatment sessions. They can be utilised as a tumour-debulking strategy when the oesophageal stricture is deemed not narrow enough for successful stenting in symptomatic patients, or to treat tumour overgrowth after previous stenting.

2.5 *Summary*

Malignant oesophageal obstruction from primary oesophageal malignancy is frequently not resectable at presentation, due to the advanced stage of the disease, or the poor functional status of the patient. Endoscopic palliation, in particular oesophageal stenting, rapidly and safely enables patients to resume oral intake and be considered for further palliative treatment, such as chemo-radiotherapy.

3. Malignant Gastroduodenal Obstruction

3.1 *Presentation*

Gastric carcinoma and pancreatic carcinoma are the leading causes of gastroduodenal outlet obstruction. Cholangiocarcinoma or metastases from distant primary malignancies (such as colorectal carcinoma) are less common causes, through exerting extrinsic compression. Patients typically present with progressive, intractable nausea and vomitting. The clinical suspicion of gastroduodenal outlet obstruction can be confirmed radiologically or at endoscopy. Unfortunately the majority of patients are diagnosed with malignant gastroduodenal obstruction at an advanced stage, when curative surgery is no longer possible. Restoration of luminal patency with consequent resumption of adequate oral intake needs to be achieved prior to consideration of further palliative treatment, such as chemotherapy. Interventions available to achieve this include endoscopic enteral stenting or surgical gastroenterostomy.

3.2   *Endoscopic management*

Enteral stenting is now recognised as the most appropriate minimally invasive option for the palliation of incurable malignant gastroduodenal obstruction. This form of treatment is highly effective with a clinical success rate around 90%.[10,11] When compared to surgical gastroenterostomy, it has been shown to more rapidly restore oral intake and result in a shorter hospital stay.[12] A surgical gastroenterostomy should therefore only be considered as a first-line palliative treatment if the prognosis is good and survival is likely to exceed six months.

A significant proportion of palliative endoscopic stenting is performed on an out-patient basis, although a subset of patients with complete or near-complete gastroduodenal outlet obstruction are in-patients, due to their symptoms. The latter should remain nil by mouth or on a clear fluid only diet while awaiting endoscopy and a large bore nasogastric tube for pre-procedure gastric decompression should also be considered, to reduce the risk of aspiration of gastric contents while undergoing endoscopy.

Endoscopic enteral stenting is performed under conscious sedation, using combinations of intravenous midazolam, fentanyl and propofol. Enteral stents can be successfully deployed across malignant strictures at any level of the gastroduodenal tract, using a combination of fluoroscopic and endoscopic guidance. An endoscopically impassable stricture does not preclude gastroduodenal stenting, given that in these situations the stricture is traversed with a guidewire and the stricture morphology defined by contrast opacification. Enteral stents deployed across strictures below the level of the oesophagus are generally completely uncovered, due to the risk of stent migration with covered stents. On deployment, the stent expands against the malignant stricture as well as against normal tissue proximal and distal to the malignancy (Fig. 1). Subsequent pressure necrosis on both the tumour and surrounding tissue from the mesh of the self-expanding metal stent results in mucosal epithelisation around the struts of the stent, anchoring the stent to the desired site (Fig. 2).

Enteral stenting of the second part of the duodenum often involves covering the papilla of Vater. Most patients with duodenal obstruction will have newly diagnosed or previously treated biliary obstruction. The increased technical difficulties with endoscopic access of the biliary tree following enteral stenting covering the papilla and the higher morbidity of percutaneous transhepatic biliary drainage[13,14] compared to ERCP mean that assessment (with or without stenting) of the biliary tree prior to or at the time of enteral stenting is preferred if technically feasible.[15]

Following a technically successful procedure, a clear fluid diet is commenced on the same day and this is gradually upgraded to a soft diet, although leafy vegetables should be avoided, to reduce the risk of stent occlusion. A formal contrast study may be performed the following day to re-confirm stent position and patency. Endoscopic palliation of malignant gastroduodenal outlet obstruction is associated with technical and clinical success rates of 90% or higher.[10,11] In cases where patients do not improve clinically after

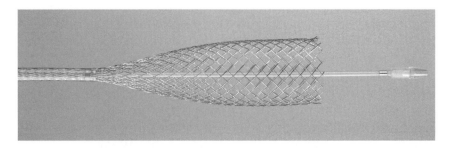

Figure 1. A partially deployed self-expandable metallic enteral stent.

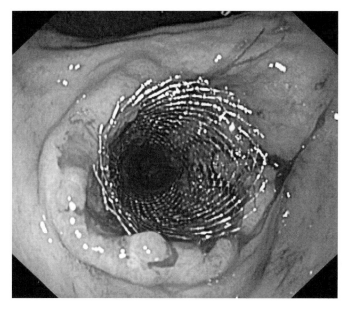

Figure 2. The endoscopic view following deployment of an enteral stent across a malignant stricture in the antrum.

technically successful enteral stenting, possible causes include the presence of additional sites of gastrointestinal obstruction distal to the stent unapparent prior to stenting, a motility dysfunction from malignant infiltration of the gastric or intestinal wall, early distal stent migration or food bolus obstruction of the stent.

Early complications of enteral stenting include sedation-related cardiorespiratory complications, such as aspiration of gastric contents, perforation, stent malposition, distal stent migration and bleeding. Late complications include stent obstruction and distal stent migration. Amongst long term survivors, re-intervention due to late-stent failure is necessary in more than 20% of patients.[16]

The predominant cause of late-stent failures is stent obstruction, which occurs due to of one or more factors including tumour ingrowth, tumour overgrowth, or mucosal hyperplasia. In the event of reintervention for stent obstruction, endoscopic procedures carried out include the deployment of one or more additional enteral stents across the pre-existing stent and stricture, local ablative therapy with argon plasma coagulation (APC) or laser, or balloon dilatation. Surgery is an option in the rare case where endoscopic reintervention is unsuccessful in restoring luminal patency, in a patient who continues to have excellent functional status.

The relationship between palliative chemo-radiotherapy and stent functional longevity remains uncertain. Chemotherapy has been associated with a prolongation of duration of stent patency and oral intake after palliative enteral stenting of malignant gastroduodenal obstruction.[11,17] While a response to chemotherapy may impede tumour ingrowth and overgrowth and therefore reduce the risk of stent obstruction, a reduction in tumour bulk may predispose to distal stent migration.[18] It is intuitively obvious however, that the benefits of palliative chemo-radiotherapy outweigh the risk of stent migration.

3.3   *Summary*

Malignancy complicated by gastroduodenal outlet obstruction is often advanced and inoperable. Endoscopic enteral stenting is a minimally invasive intervention which offers excellent palliation of malignant gastroduodenal obstruction with impressive technical and clinical outcomes. In the rare situation where endoscopic palliation fails (either as the primary intervention or re-intervention), palliative gastroenterostomy may be considered for patients with good functional status.

4.   Malignant Colorectal Obstruction

4.1   *Presentation*

Malignant colorectal obstruction is a frequently encountered clinical problem as more than 25% of patients with colorectal carcinoma present with a large bowel obstruction.[19] The rectosigmoid colon is the site of obstruction in the majority (75%) of cases, although more proximal sites of colonic obstruction are also seen. Primary colorectal carcinoma is the most common cause of malignant large bowel obstruction, while extrinsic compression of the rectosigmoid colon from another malignancy (such as ovarian tumours) arising in the pelvis is a less common cause.

Patients who present with a large bowel obstruction are often systemically unwell and urgent intervention to decompress the colon is imperative, as the risk of caecal perforation rises with an increasing caecal diameter (evident on imaging). Radiographic imaging (CT, gastrograffin enema) is a crucial part of the initial assessment of such patients, identifying the likely site of mechanical obstruction and excluding additional sites of obstruction more proximally. Patients should be kept nil by mouth and have a nasogastric tube inserted while awaiting the therapeutic intervention for colonic decompression. Options for colonic decompression include emergency surgery or endoscopic colonic stenting.

4.2 *Endoscopic management*

Emergency laparotomy for a temporary diverting colostomy in an unprepared bowel is associated with considerable morbidity (39%) and mortality (12%) as patients are often also systemically unwell, with active co-morbid medical problems.[20] Endoscopic colonic stenting is therefore an appealing minimally invasive intervention for the decompression of malignant colonic obstruction. Stenting of the colo-rectum can be performed as a bridge-to-surgery for systemically unwell patients, in whom curative resection will be considered at a later date, or as definitive palliation of an inoperable malignant large bowel obstruction. In the former setting, successful stenting of the colo-rectum allows colonic decompression, optimisation of co-morbid medical illnesses, staging of the extent of the malignancy, and planning for elective surgical resection which is associated with lower morbidity and mortality.

In most cases, bowel preparation is unnecessary, and in fact contraindicated in those with a complete mechanical bowel obstruction. Fortunately, the endoscopic view is usually adequate for the most commonly encountered scenario of a near-complete distal colorectal obstruction. Enemas should be considered for cases of incomplete colonic obstruction and more proximal lesions. In the rare case where bowel preparation is to be administered, this should be carried out cautiously (slowly) with close monitoring of the patient.

Endoscopic procedures are carried out under conscious sedation, although it is feasible to perform unsedated stenting of

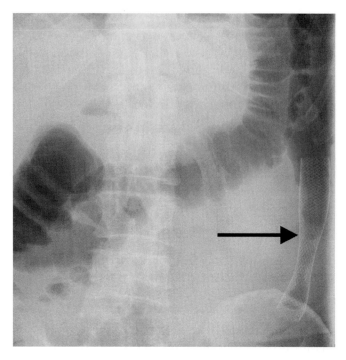

Figure 3. A colonic stent (→) deployed for decompression of a large bowel obstruction from a descending colon carcinoma.

the rectosigmoid colon in very frail patients. The self-expandable metallic colonic stents are similar in design to those used in the stomach and duodenum and they can be deployed across endo-scopically impassable malignant strictures (Fig. 3). Stenting of the colo-rectum can be undertaken successfully in the majority of cases, with median technical and clinical success rates of 94% and 91% respectively.[18] While most cases of colonic obstruction involve the rectosigmoid colon, colonic stenting can also be undertaken for proximal colonic lesions with comparable technical and clinical success rates.[21] A plain radiograph on the day following stenting confirms the position of the stent and successful colonic decom-pression. Patients are commenced on a clear fluid diet post-procedure, and this is gradually upgraded to a soft, low-fibre diet. Long-term stool softeners (Coloxyl) are advised, so as to reduce the risk of stool impaction of the stent.

Early complications include sedation-related cardiorespiratory complications, perforation, stent malposition, bleeding, and distal stent migration. In cases where technically successful stenting of the colo-rectum does not lead to clinical improvement, possible causes include the presence of additional sites of obstruction more proximally in the gastrointestinal tract, concurrent intestinal ileus in systemically unwell patients, or early stent migration. Post-procedure assessment can include a contrast enema to assess stent position and patency. Late-stent failures in long-term survivors are mainly related to stent obstruction, which occurs due to of one or more factors, including tumour ingrowth, tumour overgrowth, or mucosal hyperplasia. Endoscopic reintervention for stent obstruction is usually successful in restoring luminal patency. As with the upper gastrointestinal tract, a response to chemo-radiotherapy may delay stent obstruction from tumour ingrowth and overgrowth, but increase the risk of distal stent migration.[18]

4.3 Summary

Malignant large bowel obstruction is a serious clinical problem, which necessitates urgent intervention. The two viable treatment modalities to achieve colonic decompression in a timely manner are emergency surgical colostomy or endoscopic colonic stenting. Endoscopic colonic stenting is an effective minimally invasive intervention to decompress the colon, and can be therefore performed as a bridge-to-surgery for systemically unwell patients, or as definitive palliation of inoperable malignant large bowel obstruction.

5. Malignant Biliary Obstruction

5.1 Presentation and assessment of malignant biliary obstruction

Malignant biliary obstruction occurs most frequently as a result of adenocarcinoma of the head of the pancreas, but also occurs with cholangiocarcinoma, ampullary neoplasms and gallbladder carcinoma. Metastatic malignancy, particularly from sites such as the colo-rectum or breast, is also a relatively common cause, in which case the dominant mechanism is malignant lymphadenopathy at the porta hepatis, but may also be periampullary or at any site along the extrahepatic biliary tree. Less frequently, hepatocellular carcinoma can cause biliary obstruction.

Pancreatic adenocarcinoma is often locally advanced or metastatic at the time of presentation, with only 18% of patients being suitable for curative surgical resection.[22] Bile duct obstruction occurs in over 70%,[23] thus palliative biliary drainage is an important issue likely to be encountered in many new diagnoses of pancreatic cancer. Similarly, cholangiocarcinoma is unresectable in the majority of patients at presentation.[24]

Patients with malignant biliary obstruction usually present with painless jaundice. Significant neuropathic type pain generally indicates locally advanced disease. Pruritus, anorexia and weight loss are associated symptoms. As a direct result of biliary obstruction, other manifestations may be encountered, including coagulopathy, malabsorption and hepatocellular dysfunction.[23] In contrast to biliary obstruction due to gallstone disease, cholangitis is uncommon in the absence of prior biliary instrumentation. The aim of palliative drainage of the biliary tree is to allow bile to flow past the level of the stricture thereby minimising these features of biliary obstruction. Biliary drainage results in effective palliation by reducing symptoms of pruritus and biliary sepsis, and some data also exists to suggest improvement in other manifestations such as anorexia, fatigue, insomnia, cognition and overall quality of life.[25,26]

The initial assessment of patients with malignant biliary obstruction should aim to firstly determine the cause of the obstruction, and serve as a guide to the potential to surgically resect the lesion. Cross-sectional imaging with contrast enhanced computed tomography (MDCT) will confirm biliary dilatation and allow detection of mass lesions within the head of pancreas, but its sensitivity for detection of cholangiocarcinoma is low. CT scan provides an initial guide to the potential for surgical resection, which, if local vascular invasion or distant metastases are detected, is low. Endoscopic ultrasound (EUS) is an important diagnostic and staging tool, being of superior sensitivity to CT scan for the detection of mass lesions in the pancreas,[27] and hence should be considered as the next investigation when a patient presents with a clinical syndrome of malignant biliary obstruction, but with no mass seen on CT. EUS also allows for FNA to be performed, as well as accurate vascular staging. Magnetic resonance imaging and magnetic resonance cholangiopancreatography may have a role in the diagnosis and assessment of cholangiocarcinoma. Endoscopic retrograde cholangiopancreatography (ERCP) is the mainstay of assessment and management of malignant biliary strictures and is discussed in detail below.

5.2   *Endoscopic management*

Successful biliary drainage can be achieved by placement of a biliary stent at ERCP in more than 90% of cases, with low procedure-related morbidity and negligible mortality and in the majority of cases on a day only basis.[28,29]

Other options include percutaneous transhepatic cholangiography (PTC) or surgical bypass, however, these are more invasive, require inpatient admission and are attended by significantly greater morbidity and mortality.[30]

Furthermore, ERCP is more cost-effective and reduces length of stay compared with surgery.[31]

ERCP is performed under conscious sedation, with the procedure entailing the passage of a side viewing endoscope into the second part of the duodenum and cannulation of the bile duct via the ampulla of Vater. Contrast injected into the biliary tree allows delineation of the nature and location of the malignant stricture, and cytological brushings can also be performed. A biliary stent can then be placed to overcome the obstruction. There is a small risk of complications, such as post-ERCP pancreatitis and post-sphincterotomy bleeding; these occur in less than 2% of patients when the procedure is performed in a high volume centre by experienced endoscopists.[32–39]

5.3   *Biliary stents*

Two types of biliary stents exist, plastic and metal (Figs. 4–6). The optimal stent choice is dependent on multiple factors and varies from patient to patient. The main outcomes to consider in the context of the patient anticipated survival are stent efficacy and patency, need for reintervention and cost.

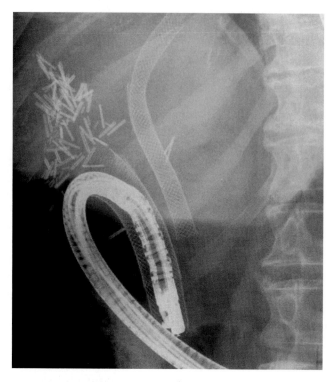

Figure 4. Palliation of malignant obstructive jaundice and duodenal obstruction by metal stenting in a patient with metastatic colorectal cancer. Two stents have been placed in both duodenal and biliary sites. Note the surgical clips from previous partial right hepatectomy for unilobar metastasis 18 months earlier.

The median patency of a plastic stent is three months.[40,41] The duration of patency is maximal with short strictures in the distal biliary tree (e.g. pancreatic cancer) and least at the hilum. The main disadvantage of plastic stents is occlusion from bacterial biofilm.[40] Stent occlusion usually presents with features of cholangitis, such as fever or jaundice[40–42] and stent change is indicated in the majority. If anticipated survival is significant (beyond three months), or the patient is found to have a hilar stricture at initial presentation, then generally a metal stent should be utilised.

Self-expandable metal stents (SEMS) were developed to overcome the problem of limited duration of patency of plastic stents. These stents expand after deployment to 10 mms diameter, in

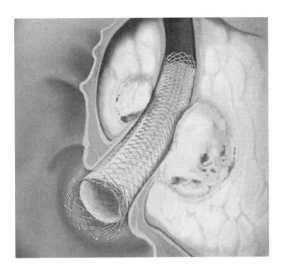

Figure 5. Covered biliary metal stent traversing a malignant stricture of the distal bile duct due to pancreatic cancer.

comparison to plastic stents in which the current maximal diameter is 3 mms. Most SEMS are made of stainless steel, or a nickel-titanium alloy (Nitinol) and are configured in an open mesh design (Figs. 4, 5).

Metallic stents are difficult to remove, so they are generally used only in patients with disease that is definitely unresectable. The larger lumen of these stents offers prolonged patency of up to four to ten months or more.[43–47] However, the cost per device is significantly higher than plastic stents (approximately AUD 2000 vs. AUD 100).

Metal stents can also occlude. Management usually entails mechanical clearance of biliary sludge, placement of a plastic stent within the metal stent, or placement of a second overlapping metal stent within the previous stent.

5.4   *Plastic versus metal stents*

There are no strict criteria for selecting one type of stent over another. Balancing life expectancy with stent patency to achieve optimal symptom-free survival in the most cost-effective fashion is the general aim. These decisions should be individualised and take into consideration patient factors. For example, a patient whose death appears imminent (i.e. within two months) will likely not live long enough to encounter the problems associated with obstruction of a plastic stent, hence this would be the most appropriate and cost-effective choice. However, a patient with a longer life expectancy, who is enjoying a relatively good quality of life would benefit from a metal stent, as the need for repeat procedures would be lessened. But even in patients with limited life expectancy, a metal stent may occasionally also be appropriate if, for example, they reside in a remote area, or are poorly compliant with follow-up.

In the presence of associated duodenal obstruction due to infiltrating pancreatic adenocarcinoma, or a primary or metastatic submucosal/mucosal duodenal lesion, early placement of a metal biliary stent prior to placement of a duodenal stent is optimal. Endoscopic access to the biliary tree will be limited after the ampulla of Vater is covered by the duodenal stent.

Once the stent is successfully placed, no major dietary restrictions exist. The patient should be instructed to present for medical attention in the case of recurrent jaundice or fever, as this could indicate stent occlusion. If a plastic stent has been placed, elective stent change at 3 months should be considered in those patients with good functional status.

5.5   *Other methods of biliary drainage*

Percutaneous transhepatic cholangiography (PTC) should be reserved for patients in whom ERCP performed by an experienced biliary endoscopist fails, or in those patients with duodenal obstruction that prevents passage of the endoscope. Randomised comparative studies have shown it to be less successful and associated with more complications than ERCP.[14] Quality of life is significantly impaired by the presence of a percutaneous drain and drainage bag and many patients develop complications, such as pain from transient biliary peritonitis or sepsis.

EUS guided drainage is a viable option in the rare event that endoscopic transpapillary access by ERCP fails. In experienced centres this should occur in less than 2% of cases.[33] EUS allows

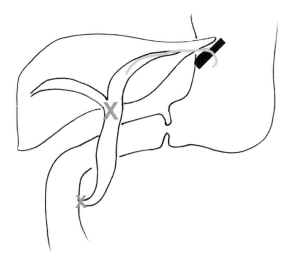

Figure 6. Schematic representation of EUS-guided transgastric puncture of intrahepatic ducts for hepaticogastrostomy formation.

real-time visualisation of extra-luminal structures, for example, the bile duct can be directly visualised and punctured with a needle and a guide wire placed, followed by the stent.[48–50] This can either be supra-papillary, or in cases of duodenal obstruction, where access to the papilla is not possible, a direct puncture into the left hepatic duct from the antrum of the stomach, creating an hepatico-gastrostomy (Fig. 6).[51] Compared to PTC, the EUS guided internal drainage achieves a better cosmetic result, without the encumbrance of an external drainage bag.

5.6   EUS-guided coeliac plexus blockade

The coeliac plexus, and even coeliac ganglia, can be directly visualised by EUS.[52,53] This allows the precise delivery of sclerosant or steroid agents to this region, providing effective relief of pancreatic pain.

Improved pain scores are achieved in almost 80% of patients at six months without major procedural-related complications.[54,55] EUS guided coeliac plexus blockade should be considered in patients with significant pancreatic cancer pain.

5.7 *Summary*

Patients with inoperable biliopancreatic malignancies are best palliated by endoscopic techniques. This approach provides rapid relief of symptoms in the majority with minimal morbidity. Quality of life is of the utmost importance in these patients, hence minimally invasive management techniques are preferable. Biliary stenting, with either plastic or metal stents, improves symptoms of biliary obstruction and reduces complications such as sepsis and coagulopathy.

6.   Conclusion

Malignant luminal obstruction is a common occurrence in the management of patients with advanced gastrointestinal malignancy. Early recognition is important to avoid a substantial and potentially irreversible decrement in the already inexorably declining quality of life amongst these patients. Endoscopic intervention provides prompt, minimally invasive, durable relief from the symptoms of gastrointestinal luminal obstruction in the majority. Radiologic and surgical techniques also have a role to play in a small proportion of patients.

References

1. A. Segalin, A. G. Little, A. Ruol *et al.*, Surgical and endoscopic palliation of esophageal carcinoma, *Ann. Thorac. Surg.* **48**(2): 267–271 (1989).
2. M. B. B. Orringer, Substernal gastric bypass of the excluded esophagus — Results of an ill-advised operation, *Surgery* **96**(3): 467–470 (1984).
3. I. Raijman, I. Siddique, J. Ajani and P. Lynch, Palliation of malignant dysphagia and fistulae with coated expandable metal stents: Experience with 101 patients, *Gastrointest. Endosc.* **48**(20): 172–179 (1998).
4. J. H. Shin, H. Y. Song, G. Y. Ko *et al.*, Esophagorespiratory fistula: Long term results of palliative treated with covered expandable metallic stents in 61 patients, *Radiology* **232**(1): 252–259 (2004).
5. M. J. Bourke, R. L. Hope, G. Chu *et al.*, Laser palliation of inoperable malignant dysphagia: Initial and at death, *Gastrointest. Endosc.* **43**: 29–32 (1996).

6. J. P. Ellul, A. Watkinson, R. J. Khan, A. Adam and R. C. Mason, Self-expanding metal stents for the palliation of dysphagia due to inoperable oesophageal carcinoma, *Br. J. Surg.* **83**(12): 1678–1681 (1995).

7. M. G. Cowling, H. Hale and A. Grundy, Management of malignant oesophageal obstruction with self-expanding metallic stents, *Br. J. Surg.* **85**(2): 264–266 (1998).

8. F. C. Ramirez, B. Dennert, S. T. Zierer and R. A. Sanowski, Esophageal self-expandable metallic stents — Indications, practice, techniques and complications: Results of a national survey, *Gastrointest. Endosc.* **45**(5): 360–364 (1997).

9. M. Y. Homs, E. W. Steyerberg, E. J. Kuipers *et al.*, Causes and treatment of recurrent dysphagia after self-expanding metal stent placement for palliation of esophageal carcinoma, *Endoscopy* **36**(10): 880–886 (2004).

10. A. J. Dorman, S. Meisner, N. Verin and A. W. Lang, Self-expanding metal stents for gastroduodenal malignancies: Systemic review of their clinical effectiveness, *Endoscopy* **36**: 543–550 (2004).

11. J. H. Kim, H. Y. Song, J. H. Shin *et al.*, Metallic stent placement in the palliative treatment of malignant gastro-duodenal obstructions: Prospective evaluation of results and factors influencing outcome in 213 patients, *Gastrointest. Endosc.* **66**: 256–264 (2007).

12. E. Fiori, A. Lamazza, P. Volpino *et al.*, Palliative management of malignant antro-pyloric strictures. Gastroenterostomy vs. endoscopic stenting. A randomized prospective trial, *Anticancer Res.* **24**(1): 269–271 (2004).

13. P. J. Pasricha, Stent or surgery for the palliation of malignant biliary obstructions: Is the choice clear now? *Gastroenterology* **109**: 1398–1400 (1995).

14. A. G. Speer, P. B. Cotton, R. C. Russell *et al.*, Randomized trial of endoscopic versus percutaneous stent insertion in malignant obstructive jaundice, *Lancet* **2**: 57–62 (2002).

15. M. Kaw, S. Singh and H. Gagneja, Clinical outcome of simultaneous self-expandable metal stents for palliation of malignant biliary and duodenal obstruction, *Surg. Endosc.* **17**: 457–461 (2003).

16. E. Y. T. Lee, A. Alrubaie, A. A. Bailey *et al.*, Predictors of re-intervention in palliative enteral stenting of malignant gastroduodenal or colonic obstruction, *Gastrointest. Endosc.* **63**(5): AB147 (2006).

17. J. J. Telford, D. L. Carr-Locke, T. H. Baron *et al.*, Palliation of patients with malignant gastric outlet obstruction with the enteral

wallstent: Outcomes from a multi-center study, *Gastrointest. Endosc.*
60: 916–920 (2004).

18. S. Sebastian, S. Johnston, T. Geoghegan, W. Torreggiani and M. Buckley, Pooled analysis of the efficacy and safety of self expanding metal stenting in malignant colorectal obstruction, *Am. J. Gastroenterol.* **99**: 2051–2057 (2004).

19. P. G. Carraro, M. Segala, B. M. Cessano and G. Tiberio, Obstructing colonic cancer: Failure and survival patterns over a ten year follow up after one stage curative surgery, *Dis. Colon Rectum* **44**(2): 243–250 (2001).

20. I. M. Leitman, J. D. Sullivan, D. Brams and J. J. DeCosse, Multivariate analysis of morbidity and mortality from the initial surgical management of obstructing carcinoma of the colon, *Surg. Gynecol. Obstet.* **174**(6): 513–518 (1991).

21. A. Repici, D. G. Adler, C. M. Gibbs *et al.*, Stenting of the proximal colon in patients with malignant large bowel obstruction: Techniques and outcomes, *Gastrointest. Endosc.* **66**: 940–944 (2007).

22. R. J. Geer and M. F. Brennan, Prognostic indicators for survival after resection of pancreatic adenocarcinoma, *Am. J. Surg.* **165**(1): 68–72, discussion 72–73 (1993).

23. M. J. Levy, T. H. Baron, C. J. Gostout, B. T. Petersen and M. B. Farnell, Palliation of malignant extrahepatic biliary obstruction with plastic versus expandable metal stents: An evidence-based approach, *Clin. Gastroenterol. Hepatol.* **2**(4): 273–285 (2004).

24. E. C. Burke, W. R. Jarnagin, S. N. Hochwald *et al.*, Hilar Cholangiocarcinoma: Patterns of spread, the importance of hepatic resection for curative operation, and a presurgical clinical staging system, *Ann. Surg.* **228**(3): 385–394 (1998).

25. W. A. Luman, A. Cull and K. R. Palmer, Quality of life in patients stented for malignant biliary obstructions, *Eur. J. Gastroenterol. Hepatol.* **9**(5): 481–484 (1997).

26. A. B. Ballinger, M. McHugh, S. M. Catnach, E. M. Alstead and M. L. Clark, Symptom relief and quality of life after stenting for malignant bile duct obstruction, *Gut* **35**(4): 467–470 (1994).

27. J. DeWitt, B. Devereaux, M. Chriswell *et al.*, Comparison of endoscopic ultrasonography and multidetector computed tomography for detecting and staging pancreatic cancer, *Ann. Intern. Med.* **141**(10): 753–763 (2004).

28. J. R. Anderson, S. M. Sorensen, A. Kruse, M. Rokkjaer and P. Matzen, Randomised trial of endoscopic endoprosthesis versus operative bypass in malignant obstructive jaundice, *Gut* **30**(8): 1132–1135 (1989).

29. H. A. Shepherd, G. Royle, A. P. Ross *et al.*, Endoscopic biliary endoprosthesis in the palliation of malignant obstruction of the distal common bile duct: A randomized trial, *Br. J. Surg.* **75**(12): 1166–1168 (1988).

30. A. C. Smith, J. F. Dowsett, R. C. Russell, A. R. Hatfield and P. B. Cotton, Randomised trial of endoscopic stenting versus surgical bypass in malignant low bile duct obstruction, *Lancet* **344**(8938): 1655–1660 (1994).

31. G. V. Raikar, M. M. Melin, A. Ress *et al.*, Cost effective analysis of surgical palliation versus endoscopic stenting in the management of unresectable pancreatic cancer, *Ann. Surg. Oncol.* **3**(5): 470–475 (1996).

32. A. J. Kaffes, M. J. Bourke, S. L. Ding *et al.*, A prospective randomised placebo controlled trial of transdermal glyceryl trinitrate in ERCP: Effects on technical success and post-ERCP pancreatitis, *Gastrointest. Endosc.* **64**: 351–357 (2006).

33. A. Bailey, M. J. Bourke, S. J. Williams *et al.*, A prospective randomised trial of cannulation technique in ERCP: Effects on technical success and post ERCP pancreatitis, *Endoscopy* **40**: 296–301 (2008).

34. R. P. Smilanich and G. H. Hafner, Complications of biliary stents in obstructive pancreatic malignancies — A case report and review, *Dig. Dis. Sci.* **39**(12): 2645–2649 (1994).

35. M. F. Gardiner, W. B. Long, Z. J. Haskal and G. R. Lichtenstein, Upper gastrointestinal hemorrhage secondary to erosion of a biliary wall stent in a woman with pancreatic cancer, *Endoscopy* **32**(8): 661–663 (2000).

36. D. J. Roebuck, P. Stanley, M. D. Katz, R. L. Parry and M. A. Haight, Gastrointestinal hemorrhage due to duodenal erosion by a biliary wallstent, *Cardiovasc. Intervent. Radiol.* **21**(1): 63–65 (1998).

37. B. J. Marano, Jr. and C. A. Bonanno, Metallic biliary endoprosthesis causing duodenal perforation and acute upper gastrointestinal bleeding, *Gastrointest. Endosc.* **40**(2 Pt. 1): 257–258 (1994).

38. P. Pescatore, H. J. Meier-Willersen and B. C. Manegold, A severe complication of the new self-expanding spiral nitinol biliary stent, *Endoscopy* **29**(5): 413–415 (1997).

39. C. C. Ainley, S. J. Williams, A. C. Smith *et al.*, Gallbladder sepsis after stent insertion for bile duct obstruction: Management by percutaneous cholecystostomy, *Br. J. Surg.* **78**(8): 961–963 (1991).

40. E. D. Libby and J. W. Leung, Prevention of biliary stent clogging: A clinical review, *Am. J. Gastroenterol.* **91**(7): 1301–1308 (1996).

41. M. Conio, J. F. Demarquay, L. De Luca, S. Marchi and R. Dumar, Endoscopic treatment of pancreatico-biliary malignancies, *Crit. Rev. Oncol. Hematol.* **37**(2): 127–135 (2001).

42. J. M. Smit, M. M. Out, A. K. Groen *et al.*, A placebo-controlled study on the efficacy of aspirin and doxycycline in preventing clogging of biliary endoprosthesis, *Gastrointest. Endosc.* **35**(6): 485–489 (1989).

43. P. H. Davids, A. K. Groen, E. A. Rauws, G. N. Tytgat and K. Huibregtse, Randomised trial of self expanding metal stents versus polyethylene stents for distal malignant biliary obstruction, *Lancet* **340**(8834–8835): 1488–1492 (1992).

44. K. Knyrim, H. J. Wagner, J. Pausch and N. Vakil, A prospective randomized controlled trial of metal stents for malignant obstruction of the common bile duct, *Endoscopy* **25**(3): 207–212 (1993).

45. F. Prat, O. Chapat, B. Ducot *et al.*, A randomized trial of endoscopic drainage methods for inoperable malignant strictures of the common bile duct, *Gastrointest. Endosc.* **47**(1): 1–7 (1998).

46. A. Schmassmann, E. Von Gunten, J. Knuchel *et al.*, Wall stents versus plastic stents in malignant biliary obstruction: Effects of stent patency of the first and second stent on patient compliance and survival, *Am. J. Gastroenterol.* **91**(4): 654–659 (1996).

47. M. Kaasis, J. Boyer, R. Dumas *et al.*, Plastic or metal stents for malignant stricture of the common bile duct? Results of a randomized prospective study, *Gastrointest. Endosc.* **57**(2): 178–182 (2003).

48. L. Bataille and P. Deprez, A new application for therapeutic EUS: Main pancreatic duct drainage with a "pancreatic rendezvous technique", *Gastrointest. Endosc.* **55**(6): 740–743 (2002).

49. E. Burmester, J. Niehaus, T. Leineweber and T. Huetteroth, EUS-cholangio-drainage of the bile duct: Report of 4 cases, *Gastrointest. Endosc.* **57**(2): 246–251 (2003).

50. S. Mallery, J. Matlock and M. L. Freeman, EUS-guided rendezvous drainage of obstructed biliary and pancreatic ducts: Report of 6 cases, *Gastrointest. Endosc.* **59**(1): 100–107 (2004).

51. E. Bories, C. Pesenti, F. Caillol, C. Lopes and M. Giovannini, Transgastric endoscopic ultrasonography-guided biliary drainage: Results of a pilot study, *Endoscopy* **39**(4): 287–291 (2007).

52. F. C. Gleeson, M. J. Levy, G. I. Papachristou *et al.*, Frequency of visualization of presumed celiac ganglia by endoscopic ultrasound, *Endoscopy* **39**(7): 620–624 (2007).

53. H. Gerke, R. G Silva Jr., D. Shamoun, C. J. Johnson and C. S. Jensen, EUS characteristics of celiac ganglia with cytologic and histologic confirmation, *Gastrointest. Endosc.* **64**(1): 35–39 (2006).

54. F. Gress, C. Schmitt, S. Sherman, S. Ikenberry and G. Lehman, A prospective randomized comparison of endoscopic ultrasound- and computed tomography-guided celiac plexus block for managing chronic pancreatitis pain, *Am. J. Gastroenterol.* **94**(4): 900–905 (1999).

55. N. T. Gunaratnam, A. V. Sarma, I. D. Norton and M. J. Wiersema, A prospective study of EUS-guided celiac plexus neurolysis for pancreatic cancer pain, *Gastrointest. Endosc.* **54**(3): 316–324 (2001).

34

Cancer and the Heart: The Good, the Bad and the Ugly

Liza Thomas and
David Richards

Abstract

Patients with cancer may present to the cardiologist with malignancy involving the heart, cardiac complications of cancer treatment, or with cardiac disease unrelated to cancer. In this chapter we address a variety of cardiac conditions (including primary and metastatic cardiac tumours, cardiac complications of chemotherapy and radiotherapy, and myocardial ischaemia) in cancer patients, and discuss diagnostic methods and management options.

Keywords: Cardiac tumours, mediastinal tumours, cardiotoxicity, ischaemic heart disease.

1. Masses Within the Pericardial Cavity: A 71-Year-Old Female with Lymphoma and Recurrent Pericardial Effusion

1.1 *History*

A 71-year-old female with diabetes mellitus and dyslipidaemia, presented with chest pain and dyspnoea. An ECG was normal and a moderate sized pericardial effusion was demonstrated on a transthoracic echocardiogram. The provisional diagnosis was viral pericarditis. Cytology and biochemistry on aspirated pericardial fluid were non-diagnostic.

Eighteen months after presentation, she underwent surgery for a presumed left inguinal hernia. There was a 2 cm necrotic mass in the inguinal region, but no hernia. Histopathology suggested chronic lymphadenitis. One month later she presented for cardiac consultation with symptoms of progressive dyspnoea, chest tightness, fever, lethargy and *"amaurosis fugax"*.

1.2 *Investigations*

A transthoracic echocardiogram suggested the presence of three masses. One mass appeared to be within the right ventricle (RV). A second mass appeared external to and compressing the right atrium (RA). The third mass, which appeared independently mobile, was attached to the left ventricular (LV) septum in the LV outflow tract. A subsequent transoesophageal echocardiogram (TOE) confirmed a mass external to the RA with extension into the RV cavity. Additionally, the RV mass appeared to have infiltrated the interventricular septum into the LV cavity (Figs. 1 and 2). The above findings were confirmed on a thoracic computed tomogram (CT). A left inguinal mass was seen on an abdominal CT scan. Histology of the left inguinal mass confirmed diffuse large B cell non-Hodgkin lymphoma. She received combination chemotherapy with rituximab and CHOP. Follow-up CT and echocardiography midway through chemotherapy demonstrated a significant reduction in tumour size.

The most commonly occurring cardiac tumour is myxoma. However in this instance, the extracardiac location and evidence of intracardiac infiltration was suggestive of a malignant tumour (including either an angiosarcoma or a lymphoma).

1.3 *Benign and malignant cardiac tumours*

Cardiac tumours, which are rare, range from benign to high grade malignant. Ninety percent of primary cardiac tumours are either myxomas or sarcomas.[1]

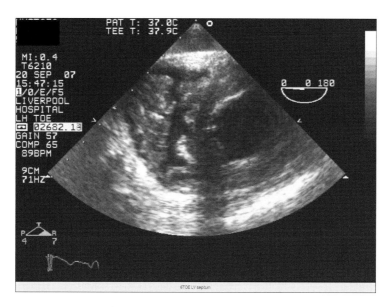

Figure 1. Transgastric echocardiographic image demonstrating a mass within the right ventricle (RV) with infiltration of the interventricular septum.

1.3.1 *Malignant cardiac tumours: Cardiac lymphomas*

Cardiac lymphomas are often part of disseminated disease. Approximately 20% of patients with non-Hodgkin lymphoma have evidence of cardiac involvement at autopsy. More recently primary cardiac lymphomas (PCL) have been described, especially in immunocompromised patients (HIV and allograft recipients). PCL is defined as an extranodal lymphoma involving only the heart or the pericardium, with an associated single asymptomatic extracardiac site.[2] These primary lymphomas account for ~1% of primary cardiac tumours[3] and arise primarily from the right heart chambers, most commonly the right atrium. PCL is commonly associated with pericardial effusions and in a series of 48 patients, 42% presented with a cardiac mass, 44% with a mass and pericardial effusion and 12% with an isolated pericardial effusion.[2] However cytology of pericardial fluid has demonstrated malignant cells in only 67% of cases.

Various imaging modalities can be used to evaluate these tumours. MRI appears to be superior in providing anatomical

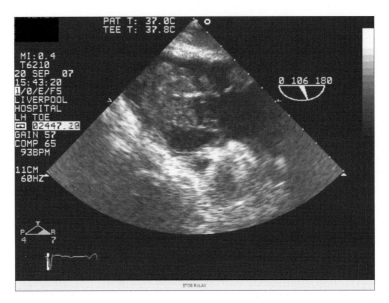

Figure 2. Transgastric echocardiographic image demonstrating a large mass within the right ventricle.

detail compared to echocardiography or CT.[2] Gallium scans are particularly useful in demonstrating accumulation in the heart without extracardiac uptake. PCL typically presents with obstructive symptoms (largely based on their location within the heart), chest pain and arrhythmias. Surgical excision is not the preferred treatment (since surgery is not curative), and chemotherapy with adjuvant radiotherapy is recommended. Surgical debulking may be performed, based on obstructive symptoms or if tumours are very large.

1.3.2 Malignant cardiac tumours: Angiosarcomas

Angiosarcomas, the most common malignant cardiac neoplasms, occur over a wide age range, peaking in the fourth decade.[1] Tumours most commonly occur in the RA and manifest with chest pain, right heart failure and arrhythmias. On echocardiography, these tumours are echogenic, nodular or lobulated, often with direct extension into the pericardium and surrounding mediastinal structures.[4] These tumours in general have a poor prognosis, with metastases to lung and liver.

1.3.3 Benign tumours: Cardiac myxomas

Myxomas typically occur in the left atrium (LA), are of uncertain histogenesis and are not seen in extracardiac locations. The mean age at presentation is ~50 years,[1,5] and almost 70% are reported in women.[6] Affected individuals may present with symptoms of obstruction (e.g. functional mitral valve stenosis for LA myxomas), or embolic phenomena[7] and constitutional symptoms are common.[7]

On echocardiography, myxomas are mobile pedunculated masses that demonstrate variable echocardiographic features with areas of hyperlucency representing haemorrhage or necrosis.[8] The thin stalk of myxomas may be difficult to identify on CT or magnetic resonance imaging (MRI).[9] Familial myxomas form an interesting subgroup and comprise about 5–7 % of all myxomas[10–12] and are associated with the "Carney complex".

Figures 3 and 4 are pre-operative transoesophageal echocardiographic images from a 32-year-old female with exertional dyspnoea with a secundum type atrial septal defect (ASD). The transoesophageal echocardiogram, performed prior to attempting

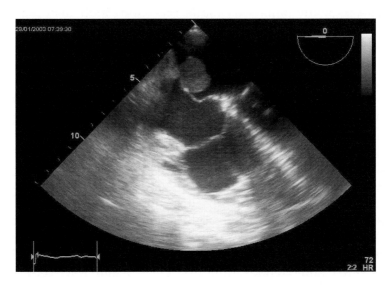

Figure 3. Transoesophageal echocardiographic image demonstrating a mass in the left atrium, arising from the interatrial septum.

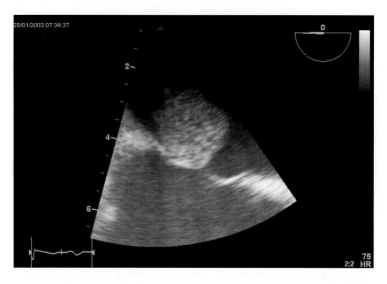

Figure 4. Magnified view of the left atrial mass with a possible pedicle arising from the interatrial septum.

percutaneous closure of the ASD, demonstrated additionally a mass in the LA arising from the interatrial septum and a clinical diagnosis of myxoma was made and confirmed histologically when the mass was excised and the ASD sewn over with a patch.

1.3.4 *Other benign cardiac tumours*

A variety of benign cardiac tumours have been reported and most of these lesions have no particular site predilection. Symptoms pertain to their position, size (in terms of obstructive symptoms) and several manifest as conduction abnormalities or arrhythmias.

Rhabdomyomas are common in childhood and are associated with the autosomal dominant disorder, tuberous sclerosis.[1] In patients with tuberous sclerosis, 40–86% have cardiac rhabdomyomas and although they can occur in any location, a ventricular origin is most common. On echocardiography, these are well circumscribed homogenous tumours. On CT and MRI they often have similar signal characteristics as normal myocardium and on occasion multiple tumours may be detected. In the subgroup with a familial form of tuberous sclerosis, at least 50% of patients have cardiac rhabdomyomas. Two genes have been identified in association with this familial form (TSC-1 at chromosome 9q34 and TSC-2 at chromosome 16p3.3).[1] Rhabdomyomas have a natural history of spontaneous regression and surgical excision is recommended for cases with obstructive or arrhythmic symptoms.

Fibromas, lipomas and hemangiomas are other benign cardiac tumours. All of these tumours present with symptoms based on their location within the cardiac chambers (e.g. obstruction, arrhythmia etc.) and occasionally based on local infiltration. Figure 5 is an echocardiographic image from a 34 weeks pregnant female who presented with significant dyspnoea on exertion. She declined any investigation or intervention until after an early induction and delivery of a healthy baby by caesarean section. She then proceeded to surgical excision of the right atrial mass. Histology demonstrated a lipoma.

1.3.5 Papillary fibroelastoma

Special mention is required of a tumour that occurs primarily on cardiac valves, the papillary fibroelastoma (Fig. 6). This lesion

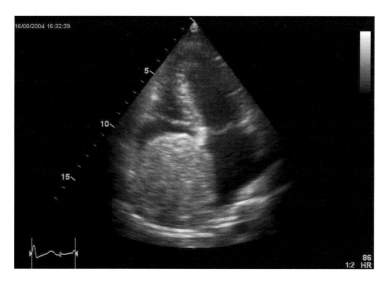

Figure 5. Transthoracic echocardiographic apical 4 chamber view, demonstrating an homogenous echogenic mass occupying almost the entire right atrium (RA).

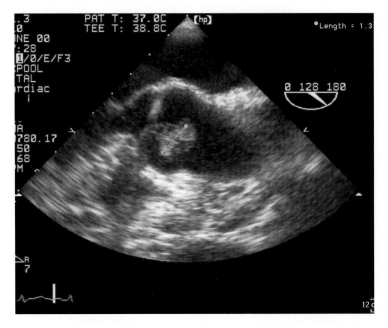

Figure 6. Transoesophageal echocardiographic image in a patient being evaluated for a cardiac source of embolus.

occurs only on endocardial surfaces, most commonly on valve leaflets and histologically is a collection of avascular fronds of dense connective tissue lined by endothelium.[13] There is a wide age range at presentation with no gender predominance.[14] The vast majority of patients are asymptomatic. However when symptoms are present, they are related to embolisation from fibrin clots that collect on tumours.[15,16] Fibroelastomas are slightly more common on left-sided valves (aortic 29%, mitral 25% , pulmonary 13% and tricuspid 17%).[16] Fibroelastomas are best visualised by echocardiography, especially transoesophageal echocardiography. CT and MRI are not as good at delineating these small mobile lesions attached to moving leaflets.[15] Excision is recommended, especially in patients who have had symptoms due to thromboembolism and in asymptomatic patients if the tumour is mobile.[13] If surgical resection is not possible, anticoagulation is recommended.

1.3.6 *Endocarditis*

Endocarditis should always be considered in patients with unexplained weight loss, or fever of unknown origin. A transthoracic echocardiogram is often sufficient to exclude valvular vegetation. A transoesophageal echocardiogram may be required if transthoracic acoustic access is poor (and no vegetation is seen), in an individual with likely endocarditis. Absence of visible vegetations on one occasion does not exclude endocarditis, and repeat echocardiograms may be required.

2. Masses Within the Mediastinum: A 56-Year-Old Male with Melanoma and a Mass in the Heart

2.1 *History*

A 56-year-old amateur cyclist presented with exertional dyspnoea for two weeks. He had had myelodysplasia eight years previously, and hypothyroidism for which he used replacement therapy. A melanoma (0.5 mm depth, Clark stage IV) had been excised from his left shoulder three years previously and an axillary lymph node clearance had been performed one year prior to the present illness.

Eight months prior to the present illness he was well. He reached 100% of his predicted maximum heart rate at 13 minutes of the Bruce Protocol without electrocardiographic changes to suggest myocardial ischaemia, and an echocardiogram was normal.

2.2 *Examination and investigations*

The blood pressure was 120/80 mmHg and the pulse was regular, at 65 per minute. Cardiovascular examination at rest was otherwise unremarkable. The electrocardiogram showed normal sinus rhythm. The echocardiogram (Fig. 7) now showed an irregular mass in the right atrium (RA), approximately 5 cm in diameter. There was no obstruction to blood flow within the heart.

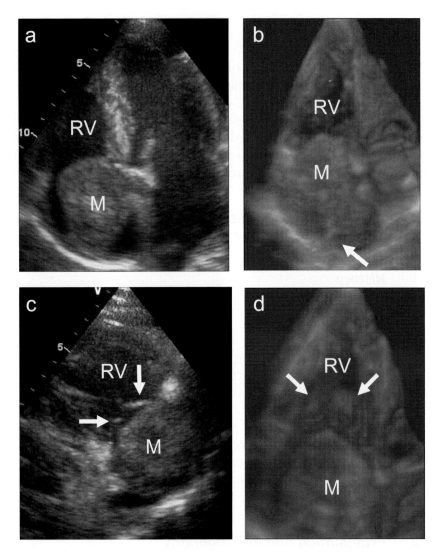

Figure 7. These are pre-operative echocardiographic images illustrating the mass in the right atrium. RV = Right ventricle, M = mass in right atrium (approximately 5 cm diameter, occupying most of the volume of the right atrium). **(a)** Apical long axis from 2D recording. **(b)** Apical long axis from 3D recording. Arrow indicates attachment of mass to the right atrial free wall. **(c)** 2D image showing tricuspid valve leaflets (indicated by arrows), clear of the mass. **(d)** 3D image showing tricuspid valve leaflets (indicated by arrows), clear of the mass.

A computed tomogram showed enlarged lymph nodes draining from the left shoulder, a mass in the right adrenal gland, and a mass in the RA.

The provisional diagnosis was disseminated melanoma with a large mass in the RA. Since this mass had grown rapidly in only a few months, it was considered likely that the atrial mass would continue to grow and would ultimately obstruct blood flow within the heart, or compromise function otherwise (due to haemopericardium, tamponade).

2.3 *Management*

The patient was reviewed promptly by the cardiologist, cardiothoracic surgeon and oncologists. The consensus was that there was a high risk for intracardiac obstruction and that with removal of the cardiac tumour followed by systemic chemotherapy, life expectancy would exceed one year. The patient was keen to proceed with surgery and chemotherapy. Since the adrenal mass was asymptomatic (and unlike the cardiac mass, did not threaten the circulation), it was decided that it would be treated by chemotherapy alone.

Three-dimensional transthoracic and two-dimensional transoesophageal images were obtained, confirming the original echocardiographic assessment. The tumour was attached to the right atrial free wall, clear of the tricuspid annulus. The patient proceeded to surgery two weeks following presentation and the mass was excised under cardiopulmonary bypass and the defect in the RA free wall (extending to the inferior vena cava) was repaired with bovine pericardium. Histologic examination of the excised tissue revealed malignant melanoma. Chemotherapy was commenced two months following surgery. He resumed exercise, but experienced dyspnoea on hills when carrying a backpack. Four months following surgery there was no echocardiographic evidence of tumour recurrence within the heart. Radiotherapy was applied to a lesion in the right lung. There was no echocardiographic evidence of tumour recurrence in the heart at seven months following surgery. There was gradual progression of extracardiac melanoma and the patient died under palliative care eighteen months following excision of the right atrial metastatic melanoma.

2.4   *Discussion*

A presentation with a large right atrial mass three years following excision of melanoma, suggested a diagnosis of disseminated malignant melanoma. Although the RA mass was not obviously obstructing blood flow within the heart, it was considered likely that as the mass grew there would be obstruction of flow within the heart.

The decision to offer surgery to reduce the risk of obstruction within the heart was made after determining that the intracardiac mass did not involve vital structures including valves, coronary arteries or the coronary sinus. The risk of major morbidity associated with surgery was considered to be less than 2%, and that there was a high chance that the mass could be completely excised, without threatening the structural integrity of the heart.

Prior to thoracotomy, there was no histologic confirmation of the nature of the cardiac mass. In our patient, it seemed most likely that the mass would be melanoma (rather than Grawitz or other tumour). The patient and involved clinicians elected to have the mass excised (irrespective of its aetiology), to reduce the risk of obstruction and there was no evidence of tumour recurrence in the heart until his death eighteen months after this presentation.

2.4.1   *Tumours metastasising to the heart*

Malignant melanoma has the highest rate of cardiac metastasis of any tumour.[17,18] Metastases can involve any cardiac structure, but most metastases occur in the myocardium and valvular involvement is rare.[19] In an autopsy series of 70 patients, all patients with cardiac involvement also had extensive metastatic disease at other sites.[17]

3. Cardiotoxicity of Chemotherapy: A 32-Year-Old Female with Left Ventricular Dysfunction after Chemotherapy

3.1 *History*

A 32-year-old female with no previous cardiac history and with no significant risk factors for cardiovascular disease, was diagnosed with multifocal infiltrating ductal breast cancer with lymph node and pulmonary metastases. She was treated with a left mastectomy and axillary node dissection in April 2005. She then underwent six cycles of 5-fluorouracil, doxorubicin (Adriamycin), and cyclophosphamide (FAC), to a total Adriamycin dose of $300\,mg/m^2$, followed by radiation therapy. In January 2006, she was commenced on adjuvant therapy with trastuzumab (Herceptin). Her left ventricular (LV) function prior to commencement of chemotherapy and prior to trastuzumab treatment was normal and gated heart pool scans (GHPS) demonstrated an LV ejection fraction (EF) of 55–58%. However, her GHPS in February 2007, after four cycles of trastuzumab and prior to being referred to a cardiologist was reduced at 41%. The specific question addressed by the cardiologist was regarding the safety of continuing trastuzumab therapy, in a patient whose breast cancer would likely benefit from this therapy.

At review, the patient denied any cardiac symptoms at rest or on exertion. Although there was no reported dyspnoea, she mentioned difficulty in performing her household chores. She denied any co-morbidities and was not on any medication. Physical examination was unremarkable; the jugular venous pressure was not elevated, there was no pedal oedema and there was no heart murmur. The ECG showed sinus bradycardia. She proceeded to have a resting and stress echocardiogram. The baseline echocardiogram showed normal LV size and mild to moderately impaired global systolic function. LVEF at baseline was estimated at 45%. She exercised to 95% of her predicted maximum heart rate at ten minutes of the Bruce protocol, without ischaemic ECG changes. Echocardiographic images immediately post-exercise demonstrated no segmental wall motion abnormality. However, no augmentation in overall LV function was noted, with an LVEF post exercise of 47%. The overall LV cavity size did not increase, but a lack of contractile reserve was demonstrated, with failure to increase her LVEF after a significant amount of exercise.

Thus the recommendation was made to cease her trastuzumab and a follow up stress echocardiogram was organized in three months' time. At follow-up, there was minimal global LV dysfunction, with the resting LVEF estimated at 54%. She exercised on a Bruce protocol to ten minutes, attaining a peak heart rate of 179 bpm. The ECG at peak exercise demonstrated no significant changes. Echocardiographic images obtained post-exercise demonstrated uniform augmentation of the LV with a decrease in LV cavity size and a post-exercise LVEF of 66%, demonstrating restoration of left ventricular contractile reserve with cessation of trastuzumab.

3.2   *Discussion*

This patient presented for cardiac evaluation following demonstrable cardiotoxicity with trastuzumab therapy. Chemotherapy-related cardiotoxicity is well described. Anthracyclines and trastuzumab are the most commonly implicated cardiotoxic agents. A recent editorial proposed a new classification for chemotherapy-related cardiotoxicity, namely Type I, caused by anthracyclines fluorouracil, doxorubicin (Adriamycin), and cyclophosphamide, with a greater tendency to cause cell death and result in irreversible changes, and Type II, caused by trastuzumab, that results in cell dysfunction and with a greater tendency to cause reversible cardiac dysfunction.[20] The ensuing discussion will focus essentially on anthracycline and trastuzumab cardiotoxicity and their diagnosis and management and a brief overview of cardiotoxicity related to 5 fluorouracil and cyclophosphamide.

3.2.1   *Anthracycline toxicity*

Anthracyclines are used in treatment of haematological and breast malignancies. Anthracyclines are thought to cause immediate damage to cardiac myocytes through the generation of free radicals, which may manifest as pericarditis, myocarditis, arrhythmias and LV dysfunction. The delayed effects include LV systolic dysfunction, with or without overt heart failure. Patients older than 70 years of age, who are female and have pre-existing hypertension and coronary artery disease are at an increased risk of developing anthracycline-induced cardiotoxicity.[21] Previous anthracycline exposure, as well as mediastinal or cardiac irradiation increase the risk for development of cardiotoxicity.[22,23]

Toxicity is dose-dependent and increases if the cumulative dose exceeds $500\,mg/m^2$.[24] There appears to be a reduction in toxicity with administration by infusion, rather than by bolus injection.[25,26] Toxicity varies with anthracycline type, with epirubicin being less cardiotoxic than doxorubicin.[24]

3.2.2 Trastuzumab toxicity

Trastuzumab is used as adjuvant treatment of breast cancers where human epidermal growth factor receptor 2 (HER-2)/*neu* is over-expressed or amplified.[27] The exact mechanism of cardiotoxicity is unclear.[28] The initial trials demonstrated a 2–4.7% incidence of cardiotoxicity, when used as monotherapy.[29,30] Concomitant treatment with doxorubicin is more likely to cause cardiotoxicity.[31] Varying degrees of cardiotoxicity have been reported from phase III trials of adjuvant trastuzumab therapy. The combined analysis of the North Central Cancer Treatment Group trial reported that 4.7% of patients developed symptomatic heart failure and 14.2% of patients had an asymptomatic decline in LVEF.[32] The Herceptin Adjuvant (HERA) Trial, where trastuzumab was administered thrice weekly for one to two years reported that development of severe congestive heart failure (CHF) was rare (0.5%); grade III and IV CHF occurred in 0.6%; grade II CHF in 1.5% and an asymptomatic decline in LVEF was noted in 3%.[33] The cardiotoxicity of trastuzumab is increased when administered after anthracyclines,[34] or when given concomitantly with paclitaxel.[34]

3.2.3 5-Fluorouracil cardiotoxicity

The antimetabolite 5-fluorouracil (5-FU) and its prodrug capecitabine, used in the palliative and adjuvant treatment of solid tumours are also cardiotoxic. The incidence of cardiotoxicity varies from 1–18%,[35–37] with the most common symptom being chest pain.[38] Arrhythmias, myocardial infarction, heart failure and even death have been reported.[38] The pathophysiological mechanisms of 5-FU-related cardiotoxicity are postulated to be due to vasospasm, coronary artery thrombosis, direct myocardial toxicity or an immunoallergic phenomenon. Several factors like age, pre-existing heart disease, high dose chemotherapy, 5-FU infusion, past or concomitant radiotherapy and impaired renal function increase the risk of developing cardiotoxicity.[38,39] Additionally, individuals who have experienced cardiac side effects are at an increased risk of developing cardiotoxic reactions. The recommended therapeutic options are adjustment of chemotherapy regimes with reduction of drug dosage, together with the administration of anti-anginal therapy (calcium channel blockers, beta blockers or long acting nitrates), although the efficacy of these treatments is somewhat uncertain.[38]

3.2.4 Alkylating agents: Cyclophosphamide

The cardiotoxicity consequent to cyclophosamide therapy is acute, occurring within ten days of its administration,[40,41] with no reported long term sequelae or late cardiotoxicity in those who survive the acute event. Thus far, there is no evidence of cumulative cyclophosphamide cardiotoxicity.[42] Cyclophosphamide-induced cardiotoxicity presents as a combination of signs and symptoms of myopericarditis (including heart failure, arrhythmias, pericardial effusions etc). The incidence of cyclophosphamide toxicity is dose-related and Goldberg *et al.* found that doses related to body surface area, rather than body weight, best correlated with and increased incidence of cardiotoxicity.[40] Thus, the incidence of symptomatic cardiotoxicity was 25%, with a 12% mortality in subjects who received a dose that exceeded $1.55\,mg/m^2$ as compared to a rate of symptomatic cardiotoxicity of 3% with no mortality in the group that received a dose below $1.55\,mg/m^2$.[40]

3.2.5 Monitoring cardiotoxicity

The aims of cardiac monitoring should be to (1) identify patients who are at an increased risk of developing cardiotoxicity, and (2) identify asymptomatic patients who have developed cardiotoxicity during or after chemotherapy. The estimation of LV function is predominantly done by echocardiography, or by radionuclide scanning. While the radionuclide scans are highly reproducible, they cannot provide additional information on ventricular or valvular status (which may contribute to heart failure). There is also the issue of cumulative radiation exposure that needs to be factored in, as repeated evaluation of LV function is necessary. Echocardiography is more widely available, is cheaper and is not associated with exposure to ionising radiation, but is more operator-dependent.

While estimation of resting LVEF is perhaps the most commonly used tool, evaluation of diastolic dysfunction[43,44] and stress echocardiography to evaluate contractile reserve[43] have also been employed. High risk patients should be identified by (1) an abnormal baseline LVEF of < 50–55%, (2) an absolute decline of ≥ 10% in baseline LVEF from a normal baseline to 50% or less, and (3) failure to augment LVEF by 5% with exercise (stress echocardiography).

In the case presented, the baseline LVEF was reduced and stress echocardiography demonstrated a lack of contractile reserve. Follow-up echocardiography after cessation of trastuzumab demonstrated the reversible nature of the associated cardiotoxicity.

3.2.6   Role of antifailure therapy

The current recommendations of the American College of Cardiology is the initiation of ACE inhibitors for patients with stage A heart failure (patients at a high risk of developing clinical heart failure (i.e. hypertension, diabetes, dyslipidaemia etc), but without detectable structural heart disease) and for the addition of β-blockers for patients with stage B heart failure (patients with detectable structural heart disease (i.e. LV hypertrophy, LV dysfunction), but no clinical signs or symptoms of heart failure). However, starting asymptomatic patients who have received cardiotoxic chemotherapy on these medications is not current practice.[45] Although data from randomised trials is lacking, there is a recent report that followed 114 patients treated with high dose chemotherapy, who had at least one elevated serum troponin-I level, when monitored over three days following chemotherapy. The group randomised to receive enalapril treatment had fewer cardiac events and no significant decline in LVEF on follow-up, compared with the group treated with a placebo.[46] Thus, it would seem reasonable to conduct a trial of standard anti-failure therapy, consisting of ACE inhibitors and β-blockers in patients with asymptomatic cardiac failure, as well as in those with symptomatic heart failure.

4. Cardiotoxicity of Radiotherapy: A 51-Year-Old Female with Breast Cancer and Angina

4.1 History

A 51-year-old ex-smoker awoke with central chest pain radiating to the neck and jaw. She had smoked ten cigarettes daily for approximately 15 years until the diagnosis of cancer in the left breast, 25 years prior to her current presentation with chest pain. She initially underwent lumpectomy and radiotherapy. Four years later she underwent right mastectomy and further radiotherapy, after the appearance of cancer in the contralateral breast. Another four years later there was recurrence of cancer in the left breast, for which she underwent mastectomy and further radiotherapy. Two years thereafter she underwent bilateral oophorectomy and chemotherapy. Her mother had died at 35 years of age from breast cancer. There was no known vascular disease in first degree relatives.

Her chest pain was relieved with sublingual nitrates in the emergency department. There was T wave inversion in leads V2 and V3 and the troponin-t was 0.34 ng/mL (reference range < 0.05 ng/mL). At selective coronary angiography (Fig. 8) there was a 90% narrowing at the junction of the middle and distal thirds of the left anterior descending artery (LAD). The narrowing was relieved by plain balloon angioplasty (1.5 mm × 12 mm at 14 atm). There was no further angina pectoris.

4.2 Management

At gated heart pool scan, the left ventricular ejection fraction was 59%, with mild hypokinesia in the anteroapical segment. Discharge

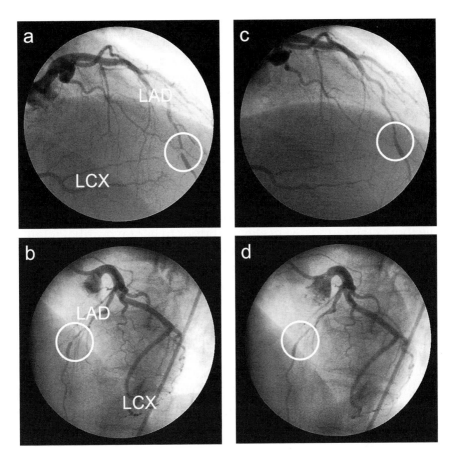

Figure 8. These are angiographic images before (Figs. 8a and 8b) and after (Figs. 8c and 8d) angioplasty to left anterior descending artery (LAD). The site of disease in the LAD is within the circle. The left circumflex artery (LCx) is visible as well. **(a)** Right anterior oblique (RAO) projection prior to percutaneous transluminal coronary angioplasty (PTCA). **(b)** Left anterior oblique (LAO) projection prior to PTCA. **(c)** RAO projection after PTCA. **(d)** LAO projection after PTCA.

medications included aspirin, clopidogrel, beta blocker, a statin and topical nitrate. Her serum lipids were elevated three months prior to presentation (total cholesterol 7.6 mmol/L, triglycerides 2.8 mmol/L). Her lipids gradually fell over the next few months (on simvastatin).

Four weeks following presentation (and angioplasty), she reached 95% of her predicted maximum heart rate at five minutes of the Bruce protocol, without chest pain and without electrocardiographic changes to suggest further myocardial ischaemia. Regular follow-ups with stress echocardiograms showed no demonstrable ischaemia in either the territory of the stented LAD or in other coronary artery territories.

4.3   *Discussion*

This patient presented with sub-endocardial infarction associated with localised narrowing in the distal left anterior descending artery, 25 years after the onset of cancer in the left breast. Over a period of 12 years she had received radiotherapy to both sides of the thorax. Her lipids were elevated prior to her myocardial infarction. In this case, narrowing of the distal left anterior descending coronary artery was probably due to atherosclerosis, in the context of previous smoking and hyperlipidaemia. The narrowing may have been aggravated by the chest wall irradiation. Narrowing in the artery was treated by angioplasty without stenting, because of the narrow diameter of the distal left anterior descending coronary artery and a high risk of restenosis within a bare metal stent (see below).

In this case, chemotherapy had not affected left ventricular contraction, since there was only localised hypokinesia at the site of sub-endocardial infarction, rather than global hypokinesia.

If the left anterior descending artery had been of larger calibre and if stenting had been required, then it would have been necessary to consider the risks and benefits of drug eluting stents versus bare metal stents. Bare metal stents become endothelialised within 1–2 months after stent deployment. If the endothelial growth is excessive, the arterial lumen may become narrowed, leading to ischaemia on exertion. Whereas in-stent restenosis may predispose to ischaemia under stress, it does not cause thrombosis within the stented segment.

Drug eluting stents (including sirolimus and paclitaxel) prevent endothelialisation within the stent for many months, and up to several years. This inhibition of endothelial proliferation prevents in-stent restenosis, but predisposes to acute thrombosis within the stent, particularly when clopidogrel or aspirin are withdrawn. Accordingly, it is important to determine prior to stent deployment if elective surgery would likely be required within the next year, or if any other co-morbidity exists that would preclude dual antiplatelet therapy. If elective surgery would be planned, then it would be safer to deploy a bare metal stent, particularly if the stented vessel would be > 2.5 mm in diameter. If the length of the lesion to be stented would be > 30 mm, or if the stented segment would be < 2.5 mm in diameter, and if elective surgery would not be likely within one year, it would be appropriate to consider the deployment of a drug eluting stent.

Even if localised coronary arterial narrowing was thought to be due to radiotherapy in the absence of atherosclerotic coronary arterial disease, risk factors for atherosclerosis should be addressed. Accordingly, advice should be given to avoid cigarette smoke (both active and passive smoking), to adopt a diet low in saturated fat, to adjust calorie intake to avoid being overweight, and to maintain a program of regular exercise. Pharmacotherapy should be offered if lipids or blood pressure remain elevated despite diet and exercise. In patients with atherosclerosis, high dose statin therapy (e.g. simvastatin 80 mg)[47,48] may reduce the risk of atherosclerotic plaque rupture (which may otherwise lead to intra-coronary thrombosis and myocardial infarction). Statin therapy to prevent atherosclerotic plaque rupture is of benefit even when the serum cholesterol is normal or low in those with pre-existing coronary artery disease.[49]

4.3.1 Cardiac effects of radiation

The acute cardiac problems consequent to radiation therapy are pericarditis, pericardial effusion and arrhythmias. The longer term complications relate to endothelial damage triggering inflammation and atherosclerosis, leading to myocardial ischaemia and fibrosis[50] (as was perhaps the case in our patient). Constrictive pericarditis is another well know complication of mediastinal irradiation,[51] with a median time to presentation of about 13 years post-radiation therapy. However, modern radiation protocols deliver less radiation to the heart, with techniques attempting to irradiate < 5% of the heart. Even so, more cardiac disease has been observed in patients who have undergone a left mastectomy with radiation to the left chest wall.[52] Radiation to the right breast does result in some cardiac exposure, especially if the internal mammary lymph nodes are irradiated. Finally, smoking has a synergistic effect on increasing the atherogenic potential of radiation.[53]

5.   When to Consult the Cardiologist?

It is important to consider cardiac pathology in patients with unexplained dyspnoea, chest pain, weight loss or fever, so early consultation is often warranted. In addition, sub-clinical left ventricular dysfunction should be actively excluded in patients receiving drugs which may be cardiotoxic. Cardiac pathology in cancer patients can often be treated effectively with simple medications or interventions. Cardiac surgery should be considered when the potential benefits of surgery exceed the risks. The possibility of cardiac pathology should be reviewed as necessary in patients with otherwise unexplained dyspnoea, chest pain, weight loss or fever.

References

1. A. Burke, J. Jeudy Jr. and R. Virmani, Cardiac tumours: An update, *Heart* **94**: 117–123 (2008).
2. G. L. Ceresoli, A. J. Ferreri, E. Bucci, C. Ripa, M. Ponzoni and E. Villa, Primary cardiac lymphoma in immunocompetent patients: Diagnostic and therapeutic management, *Cancer* **80**: 1497–1506 (1997).
3. R. M. Gowda and I. A. Khan, Clinical perspectives of primary cardiac lymphoma, *Angiology* **54**: 599–604 (2003).
4. P. A. Araoz, H. E. Eklund, T. J. Welch and J. F. Breen, CT and MR imaging of primary cardiac malignancies, *Radiographics* **19**: 1421–1434 (1999).
5. S. Bjessmo and T. Ivert, Cardiac myxoma: 40 years'experience in 63 patients. *Ann. Thorac. Surg.* **63**: 697–700 (1997).
6. D. H. Yoon and W. Roberts, Sex distribution in cardiac myxomas, *Am. J. Cardiol.* **90**: 563–565 (2002).
7. K. Reynen, Cardiac myxomas, *N. Engl. J. Med.* **333**: 1610–1617 (1995).
8. W. Thier, M. Schluter, H. J. Krebber, M. J. Polonius, G. Kloppel, K. Becker *et al.*, Cysts in left atrial myxomas identified by transesophageal cross-sectional echocardiography, *Am. J. Cardiol.* **51**: 1793–1795 (1983).

9. F. Tsuchiya, A. Kohno, R. Saitoh and A. Shigeta, CT findings of atrial myxoma, *Radiology* **151**: 139–143 (1984).

10. J. A. Carney, Carney complex: The complex of myxomas, spotty pigmentation, endocrine overactivity, and schwannomas, *Semin. Dermatol.* **14**: 90–98 (1995).

11. P. M. McCarthy, J. M. Piehler, H. V. Schaff, J. R. Pluth, T. A. Orszulak, H. J. Vidaillet Jr. *et al.*, The significance of multiple, recurrent, and "complex" cardiac myxomas, *J. Thorac. Cardiovasc. Surg.* **91**: 389–396 (1986).

12. M. L. Grebenc, M. L. Rosado-de-Christenson, C. E. Green, A. P. Burke and J. R. Galvin, Cardiac myxoma: Imaging features in 83 patients, *Radiographics* **22**: 673–689 (2002).

13. R. M. Gowda, I. A. Khan, C. K. Nair, N. J. Mehta, B. C. Vasavada and T. J. Sacchi, Cardiac papillary fibroelastoma: A comprehensive analysis of 725 cases, *Am. Heart J.* **146**: 404–410 (2003).

14. D. L. Ngaage, C. J. Mullany, R. C. Daly, J. A. Dearani, W. D. Edwards, H. D. Tazelaar *et al.*, Surgical treatment of cardiac papillary fibroelastoma: A single center experience with eighty-eight patients, *Ann. Thorac. Surg.* **80**: 1712–1718 (2005).

15. P. A. Araoz, S. L. Mulvagh, H. D. Tazelaar, P. R. Julsrud and J. F. Breen, CT and MR imaging of benign primary cardiac neoplasms with echocardiographic correlation, *Radiographics* **20**: 1303–1319 (2000).

16. J. M. Grinda, J. P. Couetil, S. Chauvaud, N. D'Attellis, A. Berrebi, J. N. Fabiani *et al.*, Cardiac valve papillary fibroelastoma: Surgical excision for revealed or potential embolization, *J. Thorac. Cardiovasc. Surg.* **117**: 106–110 (1999).

17. D. L. Glancy and W. C. Roberts, The heart in malignant melanoma. A study of 70 autopsy cases, *Am. J. Cardiol.* **21**: 555–571 (1968).

18. E. C. Klatt and D. R. Heitz, Cardiac metastases, *Cancer* **65**: 1456–1459 (1990).

19. P. Gibbs, J. S. Cebon, P. Calafiore and W. A. Robinson, Cardiac metastases from malignant melanoma, *Cancer* **85**: 78–84 (1999).

20. M. S. Ewer and S. M. Lippman, Type II chemotherapy-related cardiac dysfunction: Time to recognize a new entity, *J. Clin. Oncol.* **23**: 2900–2902 (2005).

21. D. D. Von Hoff, M. W. Layard, P. Basa, H. L. Davis Jr., A. L. Von Hoff, M. Rozencweig *et al.*, Risk factors for doxorubicin-induced congestive heart failure, *Ann. Intern. Med.* **91**: 710–717 (1979).

22. S. M. Swain, F. S. Whaley and M. S. Ewer, Congestive heart failure in patients treated with doxorubicin: A retrospective analysis of three trials, *Cancer* **97**: 2869–2879 (2003).

23. M. E. Billingham, M. R. Bristow, E. Glatstein, J. W. Mason, M. A. Masek and J. R. Daniels, Adriamycin cardiotoxicity: Endomyocardial biopsy evidence of enhancement by irradiation, *Am. J. Surg. Pathol.* **1**: 17–23 (1977).

24. B. R. Bird and S. M. Swain, Cardiac toxicity in breast cancer survivors: Review of potential cardiac problems, *Clin. Cancer Res.* **14**: 14–24 (2008).

25. G. N. Hortobagyi, D. Frye, A. U. Buzdar, M. S. Ewer, G. Fraschini, V. Hug *et al.*, Decreased cardiac toxicity of doxorubicin administered by continuous intravenous infusion in combination chemotherapy for metastatic breast carcinoma, *Cancer* **63**: 37–45 (1989).

26. M. S. Ewer, F. J. Martin, C. Henderson, C. L. Shapiro, R. S. Benjamin and A. A. Gabizon, Cardiac safety of liposomal anthracyclines, *Semin. Oncol.* **31**: 161–181 (2004).

27. M. L. Telli, S. A. Hunt, R. W. Carlson and A. E. Guardino, Trastuzumab-related cardiotoxicity: Calling into question the concept of reversibility, *J. Clin. Oncol.* **25**: 3525–3533 (2007).

28. T. Force, D. S. Krause and R. A. Van Etten, Molecular mechanisms of cardiotoxicity of tyrosine kinase inhibition, *Nat. Rev. Cancer* **7**: 332–344 (2007).

29. C. L. Vogel, M. A. Cobleigh, D. Tripathy, J. C. Gutheil, L. N. Harris, L. Fehrenbacher *et al.*, Efficacy and safety of trastuzumab as a single agent in first-line treatment of HER2-overexpressing metastatic breast cancer, *J. Clin. Oncol.* **20**: 719–726 (2002).

30. M. A. Cobleigh, C. L. Vogel, D. Tripathy, N. J. Robert, S. Scholl, L. Fehrenbacher *et al.*, Multinational study of the efficacy and safety of humanized anti-HER2 monoclonal antibody in women who have HER2-overexpressing metastatic breast cancer that has progressed after chemotherapy for metastatic disease, *J. Clin. Oncol.* **17**: 2639–2648 (1999).

31. D. J. Slamon, B. Leyland-Jones, S. Shak, H. Fuchs, V. Paton, A. Bajamonde *et al.*, Use of chemotherapy plus a monoclonal antibody against HER2 for metastatic breast cancer that overexpresses HER2, *N. Engl. J. Med.* **344**: 783–792 (2001).

32. E. H. Romond, E. A. Perez, J. Bryant, V. J. Suman, C. E. Geyer Jr., N. E. Davidson *et al.*, Trastuzumab plus adjuvant chemotherapy for

operable HER2-positive breast cancer, *N. Engl. J. Med.* **353**: 1673–1784 (2005).

33. M. J. Piccart-Gebhart, M. Procter, B. Leyland-Jones, A. Goldhirsch, M. Untch, I. Smith *et al.*, Trastuzumab after adjuvant chemotherapy in HER2-positive breast cancer, *N. Engl. J. Med.* **353**: 1659–1672 (2005).

34. E. Tan-Chiu, G. Yothers, E. Romond, C. E. Geyer Jr., M. Ewer, D. Keefe *et al.*, Assessment of cardiac dysfunction in a randomized trial comparing doxorubicin and cyclophosphamide followed by paclitaxel, with or without trastuzumab as adjuvant therapy in node-positive, human epidermal growth factor receptor 2-overexpressing breast cancer: NSABP B-31, *J. Clin. Oncol.* **23**: 7811–7819 (2005).

35. N. C. Robben, A. W. Pippas and J. O. Moore, The syndrome of 5-fluorouracil cardiotoxicity: An elusive cardiopathy, *Cancer* **71**: 493–509 (1993).

36. K. Becker, J. F. Erckenbrecht, D. Haussinger and T. Frieling, Cardiotoxicity of the antiproliferative compound fluorouracil, *Drugs* **57**: 475–484 (1999).

37. A. J. Anand, Fluorouracil cardiotoxicity, *Ann. Pharmacother.* **28**: 374–378 (1994).

38. S. A. Jensen and J. B. Sorensen, Risk factors and prevention of cardiotoxicity induced by 5-fluorouracil or capecitabine, *Cancer Chemother. Pharmacol.* **58**: 487–493 (2006).

39. K. J. Schimmel, D. J. Richel, R. B. van den Brink and H. J. Guchelaar, Cardiotoxicity of cytotoxic drugs, *Cancer Treat. Rev.* **30**: 181–191 (2004).

40. M. A. Goldberg, J. H. Antin, E. C. Guinan and J. M. Rappeport, Cyclophosphamide cardiotoxicity: An analysis of dosing as a risk factor, *Blood* **68**: 1114–1118 (1986).

41. J. S. Gottdiener, F. R. Appelbaum, V. J. Ferrans, A. Deisseroth and J. Ziegler, Cardiotoxicity associated with high-dose cyclophosphamide therapy, *Arch. Intern. Med.* **141**: 758–763 (1981).

42. M. I. Gharib and A. K. Burnett, Chemotherapy-induced cardiotoxicity: Current practice and prospects of prophylaxis, *Eur. J. Heart Fail.* **4**: 235–242 (2002).

43. M. Jarfelt, V. Kujacic, D. Holmgren, R. Bjarnason and B. Lannering, Exercise echocardiography reveals subclinical cardiac dysfunction in young adult survivors of childhood acute lymphoblastic leukemia, *Pediatr. Blood Cancer* **49**: 835–840 (2007).

44. B. Marchandise, E. Schroeder, A. Bosly, C. Doyen, P. Weynants, R. Kremer *et al.*, Early detection of doxorubicin cardiotoxicity: Interest

of Doppler echocardiographic analysis of left ventricular filling dynamics, *Am. Heart J.* **118**: 92–98 (1989).

45. S. A. Hunt, W. T. Abraham, M. H. Chin, A. M. Feldman, G. S. Francis, T. G. Ganiats *et al.*, ACC/AHA 2005 Guideline Update for the Diagnosis and Management of Chronic Heart Failure in the Adult: A report of the American College of Cardiology/American Heart Association Task Force on Practice Guidelines (Writing Committee to Update the 2001 Guidelines for the Evaluation and Management of Heart Failure): Developed in collaboration with the American College of Chest Physicians and the International Society for Heart and Lung Transplantation: Endorsed by the Heart Rhythm Society, *Circulation* **112**: e154–235 (2005).

46. D. Cardinale, A. Colombo, M. T. Sandri, G. Lamantia, N. Colombo, M. Civelli *et al.*, Prevention of high-dose chemotherapy-induced cardiotoxicity in high-risk patients by angiotensin-converting enzyme inhibition, *Circulation* **114**: 2474–2481 (2006).

47. C. P. Cannon, E. Braunwald, C. H. McCabe, D. J. Rader, J. L. Rouleau, R. Belder *et al.*, Intensive versus moderate lipid lowering with statins after acute coronary syndromes, *N. Engl. J. Med.* **350**: 1495–1504 (2004).

48. J. C. LaRosa, S. M. Grundy, D. D. Waters, C. Shear, P. Barter, J. C. Fruchart *et al.*, Intensive lipid lowering with atorvastatin in patients with stable coronary disease, *N. Engl. J. Med.* **352**: 1425–1435 (2005).

49. T. R. Pedersen, O. Faergeman, J. J. Kastelein, A. G. Olsson, M. J. Tikkanen, I. Holme *et al.*, High-dose atorvastatin vs usual-dose simvastatin for secondary prevention after myocardial infarction: The IDEAL study: A randomized controlled trial, *J. Am. Med. Assoc.* **294**: 2437–2445 (2005).

50. B. W. Corn, B. J. Trock and R. L. Goodman, Irradiation-related ischemic heart disease, *J. Clin. Oncol.* **8**: 741–750 (1990).

51. S. Schultz-Hector and K. R. Trott, Radiation-induced cardiovascular diseases: Is the epidemiologic evidence compatible with the radiobiologic data? *Int. J. Radiat. Oncol. Biol. Phys.* **67**: 10–18 (2007).

52. J. A. Violet and C. Harmer, Breast cancer: improving outcome following adjuvant radiotherapy, *Br. J. Radiol.* **77**: 811–820 (2004).

53. M. J. Hooning, A. Botma, B. M. Aleman, M. H. Baaijens, H. Bartelink, J. G. Klijn *et al.*, Long-term risk of cardiovascular disease in 10-year survivors of breast cancer, *J. Natl. Cancer Inst.* **99**: 365–375 (2007).

35

No-Man's Land: Between Paediatric and Adult Medical Oncology

Lisa M. Orme,
Susan Palmer and
David Thomas

Abstract

While dramatic improvements in cancer survival have been achieved over the past 30 years, the outcomes for adolescents and young adults (AYAs) are inferior to those of children for many cancer types. The reasons for this 'survival gap' which affects AYAs are complex, and relate to unique features of young people, the cancers that they are diagnosed with and the health care systems that care for them. Adolescence and young adulthood is a time of profound biological, psychological, and social change which powerfully affects the way they experience a cancer diagnosis and its treatment. AYA patients often are disengaged from the health care system and lack a usual place of care. The cancers that afflict AYA comprise a unique spectrum, including cancers of both children and older adults alongside a small range of tumours unique to this age range. Furthermore, paediatric and adult oncology specialities have evolved more or less independently, resulting in arbitrary differences in access to resources and expertise, and further dilution of caseloads.

Adult AYA health care in particular is widely dispersed across many institutions, exacerbating this situation. Finally, all of these factors and the relative rarity of cancer in this age group have resulted in a paucity of research on which to provide an evidence base for clinical care.

Keywords: Adolescent, young adult, cancer.

1. Introduction

When reflecting on the historic development of modern oncology, it is immediately apparent that paediatric and adult medical oncology arose largely independently. The division between the adult and paediatric cancer populations is not driven by biology, or by clinical care, or by any distinct difference in patient population. It is arguably shaped by nothing more than the age at which secondary schooling ends. Despite the blurry boundary between patient populations, there are very significant differences between the paediatric and adult cancer care systems, which are important to understand. Paediatric oncology services a very small part of the total community burden of cancer (<1%), because, thankfully, cancer in children is rare. This has led to the concentration of care in monolithic institutions, which has permitted remarkable efficiencies in clinical trials development and expertise in care. This fact, combined with the biological responsiveness of many paediatric cancers, has produced some of the major advances in outcomes in modern oncology.

By contrast, adult systems of care deal with an overwhelming burden of relatively un-responsive cancers of ageing. Treatment is dispersed at many institutions within each community, which has meant that clinical trials have focussed on very common cancer types, because the challenges of cross-institutional trials management have been balanced by the sheer number of cases for study. Additionally, adult and paediatric oncologists are trained completely independently of each other. Finally, the resources available per cancer case are remarkably different in any comparison between the paediatric and adult cancer systems. There is increasing recognition that those who are treated in *both* the paediatric and adult cancer systems have been systematically disadvantaged by the artificial separation of oncology into two disciplines. These are adolescents and young adults (AYA) with cancer. In this patient cohort, comparisons can be made between adult and paediatric oncology, and it is clear that the artificial boundaries have had potentially devastating consequences for AYA cancer patients, whose needs are poorly addressed in both domains. Moreover, the survival of AYA cancer patients is demonstrably worse than for children with many of the same cancers, and improvements in survival appear to have been slower in the AYA population than for either children or older adults with cancer.

2.   Definitions

Reflecting the enormous variation in the complex developmental timeline from childhood to adulthood, a variety of definitions of adolescence and young adulthood exist. The United Nations defines 'youth', as those persons between the ages of 15 and 24 years. This definition is used in combination with 'adolescence', defined by WHO as the period of time between 10 and 19 years, such that 'young people' or adolescents and young adults (AYA) are the combined cohort of 10 to 24 year olds.[1] It is important to recognise that the grouping of adolescence and young adulthood encompasses a diverse range of human development. Moreover, our conceptual frameworks for adolescence are much better defined than those for young adulthood, in part because adolescence is currently established within a paediatric model of care. The young adult age range is the most poorly defined, in part due to a gradual increase over the past 30 years in the age at which children have been leaving home, marrying and becoming parents — events which form natural hallmarks distinguishing young adulthood from mature adulthood.

Much of the impetus for change in how we care for AYA cancer patients is the poorer survival rates reported among AYA cancer patients, when compared to children. This 'survival gap' affects patients aged from 15 to 39 years.[2,3] From a medical perspective, there are distinct cancer types that afflict younger patients. Some of these represent the 'tail end' of cancers which are primarily occur in children, exemplified by rhabdomyosarcoma and acute lymphoblastic leukaemia. Others represent cancers which occur primarily in ageing populations, but which for various reasons may also be seen in young people. These may include breast and bowel cancer, particularly when associated with genetic predispositions. Finally, there is a small group of cancers which are relatively unique to the AYA range and are uncommon in children and older adults. These cancers include osteosarcoma, Ewing's sarcoma, Hodgkin's lymphoma and germ cell tumours.

3. The Adolescent and Young Adult Cancer Patient

Adolescence and young adulthood is a time of profound change during which the individual leaves behind a dependent self in a family-centred world and approaches autonomy amid the stresses and challenges of the adult world. Each individual travels their own complex developmental timeline that encompasses biological, cognitive, psychological, social, and existential realms. Under the best of circumstances, this journey is generally regarded as the most difficult transition of the lifespan. The diagnosis of a life-threatening illness can jeopardise this process and disrupt the young person's intended trajectory. However, normative development can occur if the care of young cancer patients is managed within a developmental context[4,5] that acknowledges how a cancer diagnosis and treatment may affect the personal identity, self-esteem, body image, life perspectives, future perspectives, distress levels, peer relationships, family dynamics and communication needs of an individual.[6]

3.1 *Physical development*

The physical transformation of adolescence and young adulthood, induced by powerful hormonal changes, includes puberty, the pubertal growth spurt, and accompanying maturational changes in other organ systems. This changing biological environment sets AYA cancer sufferers apart from both children and adults diagnosed with cancer, and exerts a profound effect on the young patient. It can influence their self-image; how other people respond to them; the nature and types of cancer to which they are susceptible; and how their body responds to treatment.

In AYA oncology, sexual differentiation is probably the single most underestimated biological change occurring during adolescence and young adulthood. The pubertal 'growth spurt' is manifested by significant increase in height, weight, size, and strength. For males, the age at which maximal growth commences is almost two years later than for females, and last until 18 years of age. Several cancers that arise in the AYA group appear to be correlated with rates of skeletal growth. For example, the incidence of osteosarcoma is higher in males than females, and outcomes for osteosarcoma appear to correlate with diagnosis at the time of maximal skeletal growth.[7] Recent recognition that some sarcomas are sensitive to agents which block signals associated normally with skeletal growth, reinforces the idea that physiologic processes of adolescence and young adulthood may directly bear on cancer biology.[8] In addition to effects on the skeleton, there are gender-related changes in body composition, with females having a higher ratio of fat to lean body mass, while males have a higher proportion of their lean body mass as muscle. Many drugs have differing lipid solubility and volumes of distribution, factors that are surprisingly poorly understood. Finally, both androgens and oestrogens not only act as oncogenic drivers in prostate and breast cancers, but they affect hepatic metabolism, which in turn may impact upon the efficacy and toxicities of treatment. These are issues that will be addressed in greater detail later.

These physical changes have direct implications for the clinical care of AYA patients, and add to the complexities of working with them. Body image is central to the world of the developing young person and the rapid transformations of puberty can induce feelings of awkwardness and body self-consciousness,[9,10] which may lead to delays in presentation to medical care. Such delays can have life-threatening consequences.[6] Following a diagnosis, the serious physical side effects that often accompany cancer treatment, such as alopecia, acne, weight loss or weight gain, major surgery to face or extremities, and stunted physical development can have an ongoing negative impact upon the body image of the young person and can influence the treatment choices made by the young patient. In addition while a young person may begin to *look* like an adult, there is also a danger that those working with AYA patients may relate to them like adults, and expect adult-like behaviours. In many instances these expectations are developmentally inappropriate — and can cause distress in a patient already under extreme pressure.

3.2 *Cognitive development*

It is during this period that young people expand their conceptual worlds, develop new cognitive capabilities, and begin to question and test the once unquestioned beliefs of their elders. For the first time the young person is able to think in abstract ways, to introspect and to examine their own thinking,[11,12] These increased powers require a considerable level of adjustment and have implications for a wide range of behaviours and attitudes.[11,12] However, although the majority of older adolescents and young adults are capable of formal operational thought, they are unlikely to be applying their new skills in a consistent way,[13] helping to explain the seemingly inconsistent thoughts and behaviours seen in this age group. Additionally, when these newly developed skills are placed under the stress of a cancer diagnosis, AYA patients may 'regress' to previously acquired skills which can impair a young person's capacity for insight or abstract thinking. These AYA characteristics may have implications for what the patient believes about prognosis and compliance with treatment. As a result, unlike working with younger patients (where decision making is more paternalistic) or older adult patients (where the focus is on patient–centred decision making), AYA patients need to be involved in decisions about their care, but treating teams need to be aware that their understanding and ability to think about the illness and treatment decisions may be incomplete or flawed.

3.3 *Psychological development*

Central to the process of becoming an independent human being is the formation of a personal identity, also known as 'self concept'.[14–17] Young people demonstrate this period by spending several years rehearsing alternative roles and ideologies. They consider various jobs and career possibilities, they enter into friendships and intimate relationships with different people, and they weigh the merits of divergent social, political, economic, and religious points of view. It is a time of newly developed needs for privacy, autonomy, independence, and peer interaction.[14–17]

Integral to the process of developing a sense of self is the opportunity to be as 'normal' as possible. For the young cancer patient, this includes the prospect of interacting with their peers, continuing with education and training, spending time away from parents, and exploring their sexuality. Without such opportunities, the 'sick role' can become central to the identity of the AYA patient and their newly developing sense of self can be altered or harmed.[18]

3.4   Social development

The development of advanced social skills and personal relationships are central to this life stage.[19] The role of the parent within the life of the AYA begins to diminish and the involvement of peers and the importance of intimate partners increase.[15] As a result of these changing relationships and support networks, negotiating the details of cancer care for the AYA patient is a complex process. It requires distinct communication skills and must acknowledge the potentially ambivalent role of the parent and family in decision making, all-the-while considering the inclusion of parents in discussions due to the potential loss of independence that can develop in the context of cancer treatment. Adding to the complexity of this negotiation is the presence of partners within the support dynamic of the AYA, the role of which is frequently underestimated in this age group.

Adolescence and young adulthood encompasses the full range of family situations, from complete dependence in a child-like role, to total independence, to full parental responsibility within a new family. It is therefore a stage during which assumptions about the social and familial context of the young person need to be carefully scrutinised.

3.5   Existential changes

It is during the AYA stage that young people begin to explore and struggle with the notions of isolation, morality, love, alienation, mortality, and taking responsibility for one's decisions.[20] Although not universal, this process can often involve religion and spirituality. These developing existential beliefs have a direct impact upon how the young person makes sense of their experience and further separate them from their childhood self. However, like the other changes occurring at this stage, these new skills are unstable at best and are often significantly challenged by a cancer diagnosis. If this is occurring in contrast with the existential beliefs of the parents and other family members, it can create a great deal of conflict for the family unit. Young people facing the prospect of their own death need opportunities to explore their feelings without fear of upsetting other members of their family.[21]

4. Epidemiology of Cancer in Adolescents and Young Adults

A cancer diagnosis between the ages of 15 and 30 years is 2.7 times more common than such a diagnosis during the first 15 years of life, yet it represents just 2% of all invasive cancers.[22] Cancer is diagnosed in over 350 adolescents and young adults each year in Victoria, and has increased by around 30% over the past 10 years.[23] Similar trends have been reported in the UK and USA.[24] The aetiology of AYA cancers has been relatively understudied, and most of the data are extrapolated from studies dominated by paediatric and older adult populations. It is likely that genetic factors play a larger role in AYA cancers than those seen in older populations, since early age of onset is a known marker for familial forms of cancer. Second cancers may occur in AYAs, partly due to genetic predisposition, and partly as a consequence of treatments used for a childhood cancers. Genetic factors are particularly important from a clinical perspective, because young adulthood is time for reproductive choices, and newer techniques enable antenatal diagnosis which may influence those decisions.

4.1 *Public health impact of cancer in adolescents and young adults*

The age, complexity and lethality of cancers affecting young adults suggests that the broader health economic and social impacts of cancer in this age group is disproportionate to its incidence. The disability-adjusted life year (DALY) is a measure for the overall burden of disease that is being used increasingly in the field of public health and health impact assessment.[25] It is designed to quantify the impact of premature death and disability on a population by combining them into a single, comparable measure. Using this measure, cancer in young people aged 15 to 30 accounted for 8785 disability adjusted life-years lost in 2003, which is a comparable to highly publicised health burdens of conditions such as asthma (10,762), cardiovascular disorders (7237), eating disorders (4994) and suicide (14,954).[26] Each year in Australia, a young person is diagnosed with cancer every six hours.

The long-term consequences for an AYA cancer survivor (such as quality of life, loss of productivity and fertility) represent an unquantified burden to the community. In 2003, the number of years lived with cancer-related disability in 15–30 year-old patients was 1622 years, which is comparable to diabetes mellitus (1611 years) and road trauma (1983).

4.2   *Types of cancer affecting AYA patients*

The cancer spectrum in AYA is uniquely diverse (Table 1) and changes across the age range, highlighting the need for a detailed and carefully targeted approach to both research and cancer management at the interface between paediatric and adult oncology. In describing United States Surveillance Epidemiology and End Results (SEER) data for cancer in 15–39 year-olds, Bleyer *et al.* conclude these AYA diagnoses to be a uniquely distinctive group that is beyond being a mere combination of those seen in the paediatric and adult settings.[27]. In fact the common developmental small blue round cell tumours of childhood are extremely rare in AYA, as are the typical aerodigestive and genitourinary carcinomas of older adulthood. In the 15–19 year-olds the most common diagnoses are lymphoma, leukaemia, sarcoma and brain tumours, while in the 20–29 year-olds this changes to lymphoma, melanoma, thyroid carcinoma and testicular cancer. Some tumours, such as Hodgkins lymphoma, testicular carcinoma, bone sarcomas and Kaposi sarcoma are at their incidence peak in the AYA years. Others (acute myeloid leukaemia, chronic myeloid leukaemia, non-Kaposi soft tissue sarcoma, and ovarian tumours) show an AYA peak prior to the main peak in later life, suggesting that perhaps there is a different age-dependent biology within the same histological diagnosis for these cancers.[27] Of note, in a number of diseases (such as testicular cancer,[28] breast[29] and colorectal carcinomas, thyroid carcinoma,[30] brain tumours,[31] leukaemia patients requiring stem cell transplant[32] and sarcoma),[33,34] there is evidence that caseload impacts outcome, with centres of excellence treating higher numbers of cases having superior survival data or surgical outcomes when compared to centres treating fewer. This heightens the vulnerability of this patient cohort with its diverse array of individually uncommon tumours scattered across adult and paediatric sites.

Melanoma is the most common cancer diagnosis among AYA cancer patients, accounting for 28% of cancer between 15 and 30 years of age.[35] Approximately 5% of melanoma occurs in the 15–30 age group. The majority of melanomas are presented at an early stage and curative therapy involves surgical excision with appropriate margins.

The five-year survival from testicular cancer for this age group is 94%, and these outcomes are comparable for all age groups. Treatment for testicular cancer requires a multidisciplinary approach that often combines surgery with chemotherapy or radiotherapy.

Hodgkin's disease accounts for approximately 32% of cancer in the 15–30 age range.[35] The five-year survival rate for Hodgkin's lymphoma is 92%. Treatment involves systemic chemotherapy, with or without radiotherapy, and is given over a three to four month period. The incidence of infertility following treatment for Hodgkin's lymphoma is low with first-line therapy, provided that reproductive organs are not exposed to radiotherapy. However, second-line treatment (bone marrow transplantation/use of alkylator agents/dose intensification) is associated with a high risk of infertility.[36,37]

Adult-type epithelial cancers (the majority comprising colorectal cancer and breast cancer) occur in older patients, with the 15–30 age group comprising less than 0.5% of all breast and colorectal cancer. In AYAs, the five-year survival rates are 74% and 68% for breast and colorectal cancer respectively. There is no evidence that AYA patients fare worse with these cancers, but there is substantial evidence that AYA patients with either breast or colorectal cancers have a ten-fold chance of having an inherited familial cancer risk. Treatment for both cancers is multidisciplinary, involving surgery, chemotherapy and radiotherapy.

The AYA cohort comprises 10% of all thyroid cancers. The crude five-year survival rate for AYA patients with thyroid cancers is 98%. Treatment for the great majority of thyroid cancers involves surgical resection. Systemic chemotherapy is rarely used for treating thyroid cancer, although radio-iodine treatment is effective in well-differentiated tumours, or those with nodal involvement or metastases. Infertility is not a significant clinical issue.

Brain tumours equate to 5% of all those diagnosed and account for 18% of cancer in the 15–30 age group.[35] The five-year survival rate from brain tumours in young people is 61%, and comparable to outcomes for children. The spectrum of brain tumours seen in AYA patients differs from that seen in children. Treatment in adult patients is primarily surgical, with adjuvant radiotherapy. While research into the treatment of brain tumours exists, AYA patients constitute a small subgroup of those studied. Chemotherapy is sometimes used, but is generally ineffective. Infertility may occur as a result of damage to the hypothalamic-pituitary-gonadal axis, secondary to direct tumour involvement, surgery or radiotherapy.

The majority of leukaemias *in children* are acute lymphoblastic leukaemia (ALL), whereas the main leukaemias affecting AYA patients include both acute myeloid and lymphoblastic leukaemias. The overall five-year survival rate for AYA patients with leukaemias is 46%, which contrasts with 76% in children. Treatment for acute lymphoblastic leukaemias involves intensive chemotherapy (up to two years in females and three years in males) with central nervous system chemoprophylaxis. Central nervous system and/or testicular radiotherapy are required in some circumstances. Acute myeloid leukaemia is treated with a shorter course of profoundly myelotoxic chemotherapy. Where leukaemias relapse, or in high-risk cases in first remission, allogeneic bone marrow transplantation is considered. While acknowledging that other factors have an impact, the evidence suggests that paediatric treatment protocols for ALL have better outcomes than adult-derived protocols.[38] There is also evidence that the biology of ALL becomes more aggressive in older patients — and the cytogenetic profile is also negatively affected by age (e.g. the incidence of Philadelphia chromosome positive disease increases with age, and this leads to adverse outcomes).

About half of sarcomas seen in AYA patients are osteosarcomas or Ewing's sarcomas, with the remainder being soft-tissue sarcomas, including rhabdomyosarcoma. Osteosarcoma, ewings and rhabdomyosarcoma represent 5%, 4% and 2% of cancer between 15 and 30 years respectively.[35] These cancers have extremely diverse pathologic profiles (with more than 70 subtypes, each with differing therapeutic and prognostic implications), and they require expert pathologic and molecular support. There are differences in sarcoma types seen in children compared to AYA patients; and AYA compared to older adults. The five-year survival rates for AYA patients with different cancers, compared to children with the same diagnoses are: 58% for osteosarcoma (68% in children); 50% for Ewing's sarcoma (63% in children); rhabdomyosarcoma 32% (65% in children); and other sarcomas 83% (75% in children). Treatment for osteosarcoma, Ewing's sarcoma and rhabdomyosarcoma is complex and multidisciplinary, requiring skilled surgical, medical oncology and radiation oncology expertise. Chemotherapy is both intense and prolonged (up to 12 months), and may cause significant long terms effects, which may also occur as a result of surgical intervention or radiation therapy. There is a substantial, but poorly quantified genetic component to these cancers. This is exemplified by the Li-Fraumeni syndrome (LFS), a cancer syndrome caused by inherited mutations in a major tumour suppressor gene, p53. Such individuals are at increased risk of a range of cancers, including sarcomas. Unlike BRCA1/2 mutation carriers, there is little evidence that intervention based on an awareness of carrier status will improve outcomes for an affected individual. This raises both ethical and scientific questions regarding the role of mutation testing.[39] Fertility is frequently affected in males, owing to the high doses of alkylator agents used to treat most sarcomas. The incidence of immediate premature ovarian failure is surprisingly low in females, although this is not well-studied. The incidence of premature ovarian failure (at 25 years of age) may be as high as 40% in young women who survive more than five years and who have regular menses at 21 years of age.[40] Pelvic irradiation is almost certainly sterilising.

These eight cancer types account for over 80% of cancers in the 15- to 30-year age group. The remaining 20% consist of a wide range of cancer types that are more commonly seen in older patients, including renal cancer, cervical cancer, lung cancer, liver cancer, and other very rare neoplasms. The spread of cancer types seen in the AYA group mean that any recommendations regarding referral lines or treatment location will depend on the disease-specific characteristics of each cancer.

4.3   *Mortality and survival*

Of all the young people diagnosed with cancer, over a quarter will eventually die from their disease. Cancer causes approximately 10% of deaths in young people aged 12 to 24, and it is the leading disease-related, and the third most common, cause of death in our community in this age group.[35]

Improvements in survival may be slower in the AYA group. Evidence from the surveillance, epidemiology and end results (SEER) program in the USA indicates that improvements in survival over the past 30 years seen in every other age group, have not occurred in adolescents and young adults.[2,3] The average annual improvement in survival in the US for both children under 15 years and for adults over 40 years is approximately 2%, while for older adolescents and young adults there has been no detectable improvement. There is robust data indicating that this group frequently has substantially worse outcomes than children with the same diseases.[38,41–43] Interestingly, the lack of improvement seen in the US over the past 30 years appears not to be duplicated in Australia, for reasons that may relate to access to universal health coverage in this country. In the US, the AYA group is the most likely to be under-insured.[44]

The reasons for the lack of improvements in survival, although poorly understood, are numerous and may include lack of participation in clinical trials,[23,45,46] the lack of concentration of clinical expertise in the cancers seen in this age group in adult cancer centres; poor adherence to complex, intense and prolonged treatments,[47] late presentation in advanced stages of disease; and unrecognised biological factors unique to this age group. The major conclusion by Boissel and colleagues was that in general the dose-intensity of adult protocols was lower than that used by paediatric trials.[38] In addition, the authors speculated somewhat provocatively on 'therapeutic nihilism' inherent in adult cancer care by virtue of the generally less curable nature of cancers seen in this age group.

However, the story is not so simple. A recent systematic review of outcomes in 14,371 Australian youths with cancer between 1982–2005, using Australian Institute of Health and Welfare data yielded interesting results (Table 1).[48] There were substantial differences in the spectrum of cancer types in AYA and children (e.g. an increasing proportion of cancers of epithelial origin with increasing age). While overall survival was 74.5% for AYA and 70.3% for children, on disease specific analysis, there were marked

Table 1. Cancer survival in Australian children and adolescents and young adults 1983–2005 by major subtypes.

		Age group	Numbers*	Five-year survival
Class I[†]	Acute lymphoblastic leukaemia	< 15	3112	79 ± 1
		15–30	790	45 ± 2
	Rhabdomyosarcoma	< 15	393	65 ± 2
		15–30	159	32 ± 4
	Ewings family tumours	< 15	270	63 ± 3
		15–30	302	50 ± 3
	Osteosarcoma	< 15	220	68 ± 3
		15–30	381	58 ± 3
	Hodgkins disease	< 15	433	95 ± 1
		15–30	2688	92 ± 1
Class II	Central nervous system tumours	< 15	1576	58 ± 1
		15–30	1460	61 ± 1
	Melanoma	< 15	52	90 ± 4
		15–30	2309	95 ± 1
	Sarcoma other	< 15	46	75 ± 7
		15–30	180	83 ± 3

*14,371 total cases: 6102 children under 15 years; 8269 adolescents and young adults 15–30 years. †Class I cancers comprise those in which AYA patients fare significantly worse than children; Class II cancers comprise those in which older patients fare better than in children.

age group differences in survival, with two broad groups of cancers identified. 'Class I' cancers, comprising acute lymphoblastic leukaemia, Ewing's family tumours, osteosarcoma, rhabdomyosarcoma and Hodgkin's lymphoma demonstrated a survival advantage in each case for children compared to AYA: these cancers represent important targets for research into causes for worse outcomes in AYA patients. 'Class II' tumours either showed no effect of age, or better outcomes for AYA than children.

A common thread in Class I cancers is chemosensitivity, and chemotherapy is critical to survival in rhabdomyosarcoma, ALL, Ewing's sarcoma, osteosarcoma, and Hodgkin's lymphoma. Although the absolute difference between survival for Hodgkin's lymphoma in AYA patients and children is only 3%, this represents a 60% greater chance of dying from this disease, and so is useful for this analysis. Notably, Class II tumours (melanoma, central nervous system tumours and otherwise unspecified sarcomas) are predominantly treated surgically in AYAs.

4.4   Gender effects

Gender has a very strong impact on survival for many cancer types that affect AYA. Overall, there is very little effect of gender on outcomes in children under 15 years, but AYA males have significantly higher death rates than females for Hodgkin's lymphoma, Ewing's sarcoma, osteosarcoma, and other sarcomas types. Notably, there is little gender effect for ALL and for rhabdomyosarcoma or CNS or colorectal cancers. Melanoma is unusual, in that females over 15 years have a striking reduction in risk, which may be related to stage at presentation. Importantly, almost the entire effect of age on adverse outcomes is limited to males with Ewing's sarcoma, osteosarcoma and Hodgkin's lymphoma, suggesting that gender-related factors are of critical importance in understanding and influencing survival in AYA patients with cancer.[48] Male survival disadvantage in AYA cancer has previously been reported in the literature for Hodgkins lymphoma and bone sarcomas.[49-51]

Remarkably, puberty and sexual differentiation have not been systematically analysed as variables that may impact upon survival differences between AYA and paediatric populations.

5. Adolescent and Young Adult Cancer and the Health Care System

Many of the major problems identified AYA cancer care arise from the dichotomisation of the paediatric and adult cancer systems. In essence, the arbitrary age limits applied to the paediatric and adult cancer systems have artificially divided the caseloads and clinical resources available to treat AYA cancer patients. This is significant, because gaining a critical mass of patients is central to achieving change in medical care, and because the feasibility of clinical trials, gathering of individual clinical expertise, and prioritising resources are all contingent on arguments based on numbers and case volume (usually on an institutional basis). There are significant differences between paediatric and adult cancer systems, which are important to consider. Paediatric and adult cancer training programmes have developed independently of each other with little or no regard for specific AYA training. As mentioned previously, paediatric and adult oncology systems operate with vastly differing resources and scales of disease burden. While childhood cancers are routinely referred to paediatric centres of excellence, the optimal lines of referral in adult oncology are far less defined. Differences in therapeutic philosophy may also impact AYA: some argue that in contrast to therapeutic optimism in paediatric oncology, the lack of responsiveness in adult cancer types has inculcated a form 'therapeutic nihilism' among adult oncologists.[36]

5.1 *Clinical trials*

Bleyer and colleagues have conclusively shown that AYA cancer patients in the US regardless of race, geography, gender or disease are the least likely of any age group (except those over 85) to be recruited into a clinical trial.[52] The age group over which this gap extends is from 15–40 years of age, and strongly correlates with the nadir in survival improvement. Mitchell and colleagues showed similar trends for clinical trial participation and survival in AYA sarcoma patients in Australia and demonstrated that treatment in specialised paediatric centres, where adherence to clinical trial regimens was more common, was associated with better outcomes.[23]

The problem with these analyses is that they are confounded by the effect of centralisation of care, and also by comparing cancer types whose biology is likely to have been fundamentally different. A second and under-estimated issue is that trials which are relevant to AYA-specific cancers are often biased towards older or younger populations of patients.

Purposefully accessing clinical trials relies on fully understanding the implications of a life-threatening cancer diagnosis, and the empowerment to make informed decisions about one's treatment pathway. Unlike younger and older patients, AYA patients are often disengaged from the health care system and lack a usual place of care. AYA health care is widely dispersed and haphazard. As such, young people may be less likely to trust the medical establishment and less likely to confidently navigate their way to centres of expertise where clinical trials may be offered. On a complex developmental timeline to adulthood, with a variable degree of family involvement and advocacy, young people are inexperienced decision makers, such that their understanding of information, empowerment to make decisions or obtain advice, may be lacking.

There are also barriers to clinical trials recruitment that operate at the point of decision making. It is speculated that AYA patients and families are more inclined to refuse participation in clinical trials. Perhaps they are having difficulty with the concept of being in an 'experiment' or feel that the question being asked is of no real or practical significance to them. Altruistic tendencies are not likely to predominate in this age group.

5.2   *Medico-legal implications for AYA cancer patients*

The AYA age span covers the transition from legal immaturity to full legal independence.[52] In Australia, the age of maturity is 18 years, and in general the responsibility for medical decision-making for patients under the age of 18 years falls to the legal guardian, usually the parent. However, there are circumstances where a young person under 16 years may be able to independently consent to treatment, provided s/he was deemed to possess sufficient understanding of what this involves (competency). Again, generally patients between 16 and 18 years of age are most likely to be able to give consent, while a young person between 14 and 16 years is reasonably likely to be able to give consent. Estimating competency may be difficult, because it is also dependent on the nature of the procedure in question. In addition, state-based laws vary with respect to the age at which a minor can be regarded as capable of consent to medical treatment. Whether competent young people can refuse consent is legally unclear in Australia, especially when a threat to the young person's health is involved. In these circumstances, inclusion of the parents in the decision-making process is very important, but not always possible. Where difficulties arise, legal opinion is useful, and resolution may require referral to the family court.

Confidentiality is of paramount importance in the care of young people. A competent young person, not yet 18 years of age, may deny parent's access to their medical record. In general, the Medical Practitioner's Board advises that "the most prudent course for the practitioner to take is not to reveal personal matters communicated in the course of the professional relationship to any other person, unless there is consent or it is essential to safeguard the wellbeing of the young person". The circumstances under which this is necessary include the usual criteria of personal or public risk, but specifically of interest is the issue of protection from physical, sexual or emotional abuse in AYA under 17 years of age. Regardless, it is good practice to discuss confidentiality (and its limits) with the young person.

6.   Summary

There are many aspects to care for the AYA cancer patient that are beyond the scope of this review, although they are of fundamental importance to practice in this area. Recognition of drug use and abuse, mental illness, risk behaviours, fertility and sexuality, the role of the family, privacy and confidentiality, communication, treatment and research, palliative care, survivorship and long term follow-up, have unique aspects extremely relevant to care of the AYA cancer patient. What is clear is that as we move forward in developing a coherent model of care for AYA cancer patients, it will be vital to bridge the paediatric and adult divide. In our view, this bridge will be created by recognising AYA oncology as a distinct discipline, which will draw its strengths from the best of paediatric and adult oncology.

References

1. http://www.un.org/esa/socdev/unyin/ganda.htm, http://www.who.int/topics/adolescent_health/en/
2. A. Bleyer, M. Montello, T. Budd and S. Saxman, National survival trends of young adults with sarcoma: Lack of progress is associated with lack of clinical trial participation, *Cancer* **103**: 1891–1897 (2005).
3. A. Bleyer, T. Budd and M. Montello, Adolescents and young adults with cancer: The scope of the problem and criticality of clinical trials, *Cancer* **107**(7 Suppl.): 1645-1655 (2006).
4. A. Mulhall, D. Kelly and S. Pearce, A qualitative evaluation of an adolescent cancer unit, *Eur. J. Cancer Care* **13**: 16–22 (2004).
5. J. Ellis, Coping with adolescent cancer: It's a matter of adaption, *J. Pediatr. Oncol. Nurs.* **8**(1): 10–17 (1991).
6. Report of the Adolescent and Young Adult Oncology Progress Review Group (AYAO-PRG), *Closing the Gap: Research and Care Imperatives for Adolescents and Young Adults with Cancer*, US Department of Health and Human Services (2006).
7. J. A. Lee *et al.*, Osteosarcoma developed in the period of maximal growth rate have inferior prognosis, *J. Pediatr. Hematol. Oncol.* **30**: 419–424 (2008).
8. J. A. Ludwig, Ewing sarcoma: Historical perspectives, current state-of-the-art, and opportunities for targeted therapy in the future, *Curr. Opin. Oncol.* **20**(4): 412–418 (2008).
9. K. Geldard and D. Geldard, *Counselling Adolescents: A Pro-active Approach* (SAGE Publications, London, 1999).
10. A. Ebata, A. Petersen and J. Conger, The development of psychopathology in adolescence. In: *Risk and Protective Factors in the Development of Psycho-Pathology*, eds. J. Rolf, A. Masten, D. Cicchetti, K. Nuechterlein and S. Weintraub (Cambridge University Press, New York, 1990).
11. J. Piaget, *The Construction of Reality in the Child* (Basic Books, New York, 1954).
12. J. Piaget, *The Moral Judgement of the Child* (Free Press, New York, 1965).
13. D. Elkind, *All Grown Up and No Place to Go: Teenagers in Crisis* (Addison-Wesley Publishing Co., California, 1984).

14. E. Erikson, *Childhood and Society* (Norton, New York, 1950).
15. E. Erikson, *Identity: Youth and Crisis* (Faber & Faber, London, 1968).
16. E. Erikson, *Identity and the Life Cycle* (Norton, New York, 1980).
17. J. Loevinger, *Ego Development* (Jossey-Blass, San Francisco, 1976).
18. R. Woodgate and S. McClement, Sense of self in children with cancer and childhood cancer survivors: A critical review. *J. Pediatr. Oncol. Nurs.* **14**(3): 137–155 (1997).
19. R. Havighurst, *Developmental Tasks and Education*, 3rd ed. (David McKay Co. Inc., New York, 1972).
20. G. Manaster, *Adolescent Development and the Life Tasks* (Allyn & Bacon Inc., Boston, 1977).
21. Joint Working Party on Palliative Care for Adolescents and Young Adults, *Palliative Care for Young People Aged 13–24* (Bristol, ACT, 2001).
22. A. Bleyer, A. Viner and R. Barr, Cancer in 15–29-year-olds by primary site, *Oncologist* **11**: 590–601 (2006).
23. A. E. Mitchell *et al.*, Cancer in adolescents and young adults: Treatment and outcome in Victoria, *Med. J. Aust.* **180**(2): 59–62 (2004).
24. J. M. Birch and A. Bleyer, Epidemiology and etiology of cancer. In: *Cancer in Adolescents and Young Adults*, eds. W. A. Bleyer and R. D. Barr (Springer Verlag, Berlin Heidelberg, 2007), p. 50.
25. World Health Organization, Global Burden of Disease (GBD). Available at www.who.int/healthinfo/global-burden-disease/en/index.html (21 April 2009).
26. S. Begg, T. Vos, B. Barker, C. Stevenson, L. Stanley and A. Lopez, *The Burden of Disease and Injury in Australia 2003* (PHE 82, Australian Institute of Health and Welfare, 2007). Available at www.aihw.gov.au/publications/index.cfm/title/10317.
27. A. Bleyer *et al.*, The distinctive biology of cancer in adolescents and young adults, *Nat. Rev. Cancer* **8**: 288–298 (2008).
28. E. J. Feuer, C. M. Frey, O. W. Brawley, S. G. Nayfield, J. B. Cunningham, N. L. Geller, G. J. Bosl and B. S. Kramer, After a treatment breakthrough: A comparison of trial and population-based data for advanced testicular cancer, *J. Clin. Oncol.* **12**: 368–377 (1994).
29. R. Sainsbury, B. Haward, L. Rider, C. Johnston and C. Round, Influence of clinician workload and patterns of treatment on survival from breast cancer, *Lancet* **345**(8960): 1265–1270 (1995).
30. J. A. Sosa, H. M. Bowman, J. M. Tielsch, N. R. Powe, T. A. Gordon and R. Udelsman, The importance of surgeon experience for clinical and economic outcomes from thyroidectomy, *Ann. Surg.* **228**(3): 320–330 (1998).

31. F. G. Barker II, T. C. William Jr., and B. S. Carter, Surgery for primary supratentorial brain tumors in the United States, 1988 to 2000: The effect of provider caseload and centralization of care, *Neuro. Oncol.* **7**(1): 49–63 (2005).

32. M. M. Horowitz, D. Przepiorka, R. E. Champlin *et al.*, Should HLA-identical sibling bone marrow transplants for leukemia be restricted to large centers?, *Blood* **79**: 2771–2774 (1992).

33. G. Bacci *et al.*, Role of surgery in local treatment of Ewing's sarcoma of the extremities in patients undergoing adjuvant and neoadjuvant chemotherapy, *Oncol. Rep.* **11**: 111–120 (2004).

34. J. C. Gutierrez, Improved outcome in patients with soft tissue sarcoma treated at high-volume centers. *Nature Clin. Pract. Oncol.* **4**: 504–505 (2007).

35. Australian Institute of Health and Welfare, *Young Australians: Their Health and Wellbeing* (PHE 87, Australian Institute of Health and Welfare, Canberra, 2007). Available at www.aihw.gov.au/publications/index.cfm/title/10451.

36. J. F. Seymour, Ovarian tissue cryopreservation for cancer patients: Who is appropriate? *Reprod. Fertil. Dev.* **13**: 81–89 (2001).

37. C. J. Stern and J. F. Seymour, Defining the cost of cure: Infertility among female survivors of lymphoma, *Leuk. Lymphoma* **47**(4): 574–575 (2006).

38. N. Boissel, M. Auclerc, V. Lheritier *et al.*, Should adolescents with acute lymphoblastic leukemia be treated as old children or young adults? Comparison of the French FRALLE-93 and LALA-94 trials, *J. Clin. Oncol.* **21**(5): 774–780 (2003).

39. M. Tischkowitz and E. Rosser, Inherited cancer in children: Practical/ethical problems and challenges, *Eur. J. Cancer* **40**: 2459–2470 (2004).

40. J. Byrne *et al.*, Early menopause in long-term survivors of cancer during adolescence, *Am. J. Obstet. Gynecol.* **166**: 788–793 (1992).

41. H. E. Grier *et al.*, Addition of ifosfamide and etoposide to standard chemotherapy for Ewing's sarcoma and primitive neuroectodermal tumor of bone, *N. Engl. J. Med.* **348**: 694–701 (2003).

42. R. B. Womer, D. C. West, M. D. Krailo, P. S. Dickman and B. Pawel. Chemotherapy intensification by interval compression in localized Ewing sarcoma family of tumors (ESFT), Abstract & 855, *Proc. 13th Annu. Meet. Connective Tissue Oncol. Soc.*, 31 October–3 November 2008, Seattle, Washington, USA.

43. A. Ferrari *et al.*, Rhabdomyosarcoma in adults. A retrospective analysis of 171 patients treated in a single institution. *Cancer* **98**: 571–580 (2003).

44. A. Ziv, J. R. Boulet and G. B. Slap, Utilization of physician offices by adolescents in the United States, *Pediatrics* **104** (1.1): 35–42 (1999).

45. K. Albritton and W. A. Bleyer, The management of cancer in the older adolescent, *Eur. J. Cancer* **39**: 2584–2599 (2003).

46. A Bleyer, Older adolescents with cancer in North America deficits in outcome and research, *Pediatr. Clin. North Am.* **49**: 1027–1042 (2002).

47. A. Bleyer, The adolescent and young adult gap in cancer care and outcome, *Curr. Probl. Pediatr. Adolesc. Health Care* **35**: 182–217 (2005).

48. K. K. Khamly, V. J. Thursfield, J. Desai, M. Fay, G. C. Toner, P. F. M. Choong, S. Y. K. Ngan, G. J. Powell and D. M. Thomas, Gender and survival for adolescents and young adults with cancer in Australia, *Int. J. Cancer* **125**: 426–431 (2009).

49. B. Klimm *et al.*, Role of hematotoxicity and sex in patients with Hodgkin's lymphoma: An analysis from the German Hodgkin Study Group, *J. Clin. Oncol.* **23**: 8003–8011 (2005).

50. G. Bacci *et al.*, Prognostic factors in non-metastatic Ewing's sarcoma tumor of bone: An analysis of 579 patients treated at a single institution with adjuvant or neoadjuvant chemotherapy between 1972 and 1998, *Acta Oncol.* **45**: 469–475 (2006).

51. G. Bacci *et al.*, Prognostic factors for osteosarcoma of the extremity treated with neoadjuvant chemotherapy: 15-year experience in 789 patients treated at a single institution. *Cancer* **106**: 1154–1161 (2006).

52. Medical Practitioners Board of Victoria, Consent for Treatment and Confidentiality in Young People, September 2004 … provided s/he is deemed to possess sufficient understanding of what this involves (competency).

36

Cancer and the Geriatrician — Managing Cancer in Older People

Robert J. Prowse

Abstract

More cancers occur in people older than 65 than in younger individuals. Demographic changes will result in increasing numbers of cancer diagnoses into the mid-21st century. Despite this, older patients with cancer are treated less often than younger patients and, when they are treated, are treated less intensively. Older patients have more concurrent illnesses than younger ones, requiring management in parallel with treatment of the cancer and influencing outcome of the latter. The complexity of the management of older patients is being increasing recognised by oncologists and a number of approaches are being used to increase the skills available to them. These include direct involvement of geriatricians, but also the use of instruments to identify concurrent problems, and may be used to stratify patients, in order to make effective use of limited resources.

Keywords: Oncogeriatrics, comprehensive geriatric assessment, co-morbidities, polypharmacy, frailty.

1.   Introduction

The twentieth century saw the new demographic phenomenon of increasing survival of humans into later life, so that both the proportions and, more importantly for service provision, the absolute numbers, of people over the age of 65 are greater than at any previous time. This began in countries with developed economies, notably in Western Europe, but now also involves the developing world. Demographic projections have this phenomenon continuing until the middle of the twenty-first century.

Cancer is the third most common cause of death in people over 65, after heart disease and stroke. Fifty per cent of cancers occur in this age group. Incidence of cancer increased in adults of all ages between 1950 and 1990, but this increase was greater in people over 65 years. However, in younger adults there was a reduction in mortality over that period, whereas the mortality in people over 65 increased.[1]

The combination of an ageing population and the increased incidence and prevalence of cancer in later life leads to the great increase in the importance of cancer in older people. In Australia in 2005, 57% of new diagnoses of cancer and 73% of the deaths occurred in people older than 65.[2] Projections of cancer incidence in Australia estimate that 23,000 extra new cases of cancer will occur in young older adults (65–74) from 2005–2015 over the 25,000 cases which occurred in 2004.

The most frequent cancers in older people include carcinomata of prostate, colon and rectum, lung and breast. These are all common cancers and are thus non-oncologists are likely to have some basic knowledge of them. The other common group of malignancies in older people is of cancers presenting as a metastasis from an unknown primary site; often called "Cancer of Unknown Primary". This group has particular issues in older people, involving the fitness of the patient and overall relevance of a search for the primary site.

Older people with cancer are less likely than younger patients to receive standard cancer therapy.[3]

Geriatric Medicine and Oncology are relatively young subspecialities in medicine, both developing in the second half of the twentieth century. They share concern for holistic management of the patient, for achieving as good a functional outcome from treatment as possible and for focussing on quality of life ahead of its length. These similarities of approach to patient care should promote close cooperation in patient care. Yet, the subspecialities have developed in isolation from each other.

2. Geriatricians with Patients with Cancer

Despite being the acknowledged experts in management of patients over 65, geriatricians rarely see new patients whose primary reason for referral is cancer. Primary care doctors refer to other specialities for diagnosis of possible cancer; commonly to surgeons and organ specific physicians. Geriatricians are likely to encounter new or recurrent cancers in those under their care for other illnesses. They will, often appropriately, make decisions about the need for treatment of cancer based on their knowledge of the effect of co-morbidities on the quality of life of the patient. However, there will be situations in which palliative, or even curative, treatment of the cancer would be available. Geriatricians will not know of the appropriateness of the intervention without consultation with an oncologist. Subspecialties which have developed with mutual respect, but essentially in isolation from each other, are likely to contain highly relevant expertise which is mutually opaque. Some oncologists recommend referral of all patients with newly diagnosed cancer, whether from geriatricians or others, for at least a single opinion on specific treatment. Departments of Oncology may need increased resources to deal with the increased workload this recommendation would require.

3. Older Patients in Departments of Cancer Care

Most older patients with newly diagnosed cancer arrive in departments of oncology following diagnosis, and oncologists are increasingly realising the range of fitness in these patients, which extends from extremely healthy, apart from the cancer, through having one or many co-morbid conditions, to frail and impaired. Geriatricians could bring to the care of this group of patients their expertise in management of complex co-morbidities, frailty, polypharmacy and cognitive impairment. They could also share their insights and experience in working in multidisciplinary teams.

This has led to the recommendations to incorporate standard geriatric practice into cancer clinics.[4] The concept of Comprehensive Geriatric Assessment (CGA) aims to encompass all aspects of an individual which are relevant to decision making and provision for his or her care. These are more extensive than are considered in a standard medical consultation, including in oncology. The domains of a CGA are shown in Table 1.

Oncologists traditionally assess the functional status of their patients, using scales such as Karnofsky performance status (KPS) and Eastern Co-operative Oncology Group (ECOG) performance status. These tools are limited to physical function, do not cover the range of deficits experiences in older people and have not been evaluated in that group. Comprehensive Geriatric Assessment has been shown to provide additional information about function over ECOG status.[5]

Terret *et al.*[6] identified four questions needing particular consideration in older cancer patients:

(1) Is the patient going to die with or of cancer?
(2) Is the patient going to live long enough to suffer from cancer?
(3) Is the patient going to tolerate treatment of cancer?
(4) How will treatment impact quality of life, given other co-existing illnesses and geriatric issues?

Table 1.   Components of comprehensive geriatric assessment.

- Co-morbidities
- Medications
- Cognition
- Functional ability
  - Personal activities of daily living
  - Instrumental activities of daily living
- Nutrition
- Frailty
- Social support
- Psychological support

Answering these questions adequately will require information about the patient which will be captured by CGA. Ideally, each case should be discussed by a multidisciplinary team, with representatives from both geriatrics and oncology.

A pioneer program of geriatric oncology is that of Balducci and Extermann at the H. Lee Mofitt Cancer Center in Florida.[7] Similar programs have been introduced at centres in France, Italy and the United States of America.[8] The assessment at the H. Mofitt Lee Centre is performed at the patient's first visit, and takes on average two and a half hours. While this may be appropriate in some major centres, it will, clearly, not be available universally, either because of limited geriatrician time, or indeed, no available geriatrics service at all.

The recognition of the need for a more comprehensive assessment of older people with cancer, coupled with the unavailability of geriatrician to many services, has led to the development of assessment questionnaires, which can be completed by the patient, alone or with help of others, prior to initial oncology clinic appointment.[8,9] This can then be used to guide referrals to supportive services or for further assessment. In services in which a geriatrician is part of the team, the responses to the questionnaire will be a guide to those who most need specialised assessment, rationalising the use of a usually limited resource.

The approach chosen will depend on local circumstances and will include the nature of the centre, whether geriatric services are available to assist, or whether oncologists are working alone, but adopting principles of geriatrics in their assessments. Whichever approach is used in the assessment of older patients, one aim is to allocate patients into streams: fit, vulnerable or frail. Fit patients could be planned for standard oncology therapy, with adjustments if treatment is less well tolerated than expected; frail patients should be offered palliative therapy, while the vulnerable patients (the middle group), are likely to be the most numerous, who will need further assessment in at least one area of function and are likely to require supportive therapy to complete oncological treatment. This may need to be modified, at least in the initial course of therapy, to ensure tolerability of treatment. As oncogeriatric services develop, assessment instruments will be modified and evaluated for local use.

While such approaches have been shown to more fully identify the range of problems interacting with cancer management in the older population, the expected benefits, which may include: improved outcomes for treated patients, increased delivery of therapeutic doses of chemotherapy to older patients, reduced toxicity, less treatment of frail patients and reduction of cost, have yet to be shown to result from this integrated approach to management.

3.1 *Specific management issues*

One of the specific issues in the oncological management of older people concerns the requirement to modify therapy, in this case chemotherapy, in the light of ageing changes in drug metabolism and excretion. This especially involves drugs excreted by the kidney because the majority of older individuals, even those apparently in good health, have reduced renal function. This is not apparent on standard biochemical testing because the reduction in muscle mass in older people, resulting in reduced serum creatinine estimations, balances the reduced renal function, resulting in a 'normal' serum creatinine. Numerous methods are available to determine the actual renal function as accurately as possible.[10] No existing test is ideal, however, more important than determining the perfect test is the use of one of them to guide drug dosing.

One of the maxims of pharmacological therapy in geriatric medicine is 'Start low and go slow'. This advocates caution in initial dose and rate of escalation, so as to provide time to evaluate effects of therapy, in light of altered pharmacokinetics and pharmacodynamics. However, its injudicious application may result in patients never reaching an adequate therapeutic dose. Examples of this include sub-optimal doses of antidepressants or of beta-blockers for cardiac failure. In oncological treatment of older people, while doses reduction in the first cycle may be appropriate in more frail individuals to assess tolerability, as near to full dose should be given once it has been established treatment will continue. Sub-therapeutic doses are likely to be ineffective at tumour control, but to have most, if not all, the side effects of a full dose.

4. Consent in Relation to Cognitive Impairment

A particular problem in providing care to older individuals with any medical illness is the frequency of the co-morbidity of cognitive impairment. The incidence of Alzheimer's disease increases from 0.1% in people between 60 and 64, to 1% over 65 years and greater than 2% over 80 years. The prevalence of dementia is 20% over the age of 80. There are further older individuals with mild cognitive impairment, many of which will progress to clinical Alzheimer's disease. In many patients with dementia, the diagnosis has not been made at the time they are seen by the health system for other reasons and they may seem superficially to have normal cognition.

These patients are a potential cause of difficulty in oncology, particularly because they may not understand the complexities of the treatment choices being offered them and the consequences of undertaking, or omitting, particular courses of action. Additionally, chemotherapy and the stresses imposed by its administration may worsen the cognitive function of patients at risk because of underlying impairment, especially if not recognised.

Screening for cognitive problems is thus an important part of oncogeriatric assessment. Patients found by screening to have possible dementia need referral to a geriatrician, or other expert in cognitive assessment, whether a member of the oncogeriatric team or part of a separate service.

Some older adults will have planned for possible mental incapacity in the future by appointing a Medical Agent or expressing their wishes in an Advanced Directive. Such future planning is a helpful guide to decision making by the treating oncologist, if the patient proves to be cognitively impaired. Most older people, however, have not made such provisions, which can result in close family members being left to consent to treatment courses as substitute decision makers. The complex interaction of close relatives' own views of cancer and their emotional involvement with the patient can make this one of the most difficult aspects of management of older cancer patients.

Older patients may also have a different view of the place of their treating doctors in decision making, expecting their oncologist to be more than the expert providing them with treatment choices. "What do you think, Doctor?" can be seen as maintaining outdated paternalism, but some argue that, given the complexity of the decisions to be made and, especially, of the possible treatments offered, this response has a continued place in management and should not be automatically dismissed.

5.   Older Patients in Cancer Research Trials

Historically, older people were not included as subjects in clinical trials, even when the disease under study primarily affected them. Treatment of older people was empirical, at best extrapolated from the results of trials in younger individuals. Over time, the upper age limit for inclusion in trials was progressively raised, so that older subjects were included. In recent years, trials of therapy have been specifically conducted in older people. The results of these trials may challenge widely held beliefs. For example, the recent HYVET study of hypertension, of patients over the age of 80, in which the mean age of the patients was 83.5 and the oldest was 105, showed benefit in reducing death from stroke, but also from mortality from any cause. This contradicted the belief that anti-hypertensive therapy in this population increases the risk of death.[11]

Trials in cancer in older people follow a similar pattern to those in other areas. Many trials have specifically excluded older patients and those with older subjects have often selected particularly fit individuals, who are not representative of the usual patient with cancer.[12] Trials which include older patients are now being conducted. However, trials which specifically study older patients, including those with co-morbidities and the other common problems of ageing, are required. End points may not simply be increased survival, but improved quality of life, effective palliation of symptoms or cost-effective care.

6.   Conclusion

Cancer will be an increasing problem in older adults in first half of the 21st Century. Geriatricians can work with oncologists to improve outcomes for older cancer patients. Collaboration between these specialties should lead to improved care of cancer patients in all settings. Research should focus on whether this approach improves outcomes for older people with cancer. Specific clinical trials with appropriate end points in all older adults, including those at risk from the co-morbidities common in ageing, will be required.

References

1. G. Lyman, Cancer care in the elderly: Cost and quality of life considerations, *Cancer Control* **5**: 347–354 (1998).
2. Australian Institute of Health and Welfare (AIHW), Australian Cancer Incidence and Mortality (ACIM) Books (2007).
3. T. Mahoney, K. Yen-Hong, A. Topilow *et al.*, Stage III colon cancers: Why adjuvant chemotherapy is not offered to elderly patients, *Arch. Surg.* **135**: 182–185 (2000).
4. M. Extermann, M. Aapro, R. Bernabei *et al.*, Use of comprehensive geriatric assessment in older cancer patients: Recommendations from the task force on CGA of the International Society of Geriatric Oncology, *Crit. Rev. Oncol. Haematol.* **55**: 241–252 (2005).
5. L. Repetto, L. Fratino, R. A. Audisio *et al.*, Comprehensive geriatric assessment adds information to Eastern Cooperative Oncology Group Performance Status in elderly cancer patients: An Italian group for geriatric oncology study, *J. Clin. Oncol.* **20**: 494–502 (2002).
6. C Terret, G. B. Zulian, A. Naiem *et al.*, Multidisciplinary approach to the geriatric oncology patient, *J. Clin. Oncol.* **25**(14): 1876–1881 (2007).
7. L. Balducci and J. Yates, General guidelines for the management of older patients with cancer, *Oncology* **14**: 221–227 (2000).
8. C. Terret, *Clinical Assessment in Geriatric Oncology*, Vol. 6 (American Society of Clinical Oncology Educational Book, 2006), pp. 297–299.
9. A. Hurria, S. M. Lichtman, J. Gardes *et al.*, Identifying vulnerable older adults with cancer: Integrating geriatric assessment into oncology practice, *J. Am. Geriatr. Soc.* **55**: 1604–1608 (2007).
10. C. Steer, Renal function in the elderly, *Cancer Forum* **32**: 11–16 (2008).
11. N. S. Beckett, R. Peters, A. E. Fletcher *et al.*, Treatment of hypertension in patients 80 years of age or older, *N. Engl. J. Med.* **358**: 1887–1898 (2008).
12. L. F. Hutchins, J. M. Unger, J. J. Crowley *et al.*, Underrepresentation of patients 65 years of age or older in cancer-treatment trials, *N. Engl. J. Med.* **341**: 2061–2067 (1999).

37

Cancer and the General Practitioner. The Role of the GP in Cancer Diagnosis and Treatment

Moyez Jiwa

Abstract

The experience of people with advanced or life threatening cancers speaks volumes for the health care system of their home country. The overall prognosis of many cancers reflects the effectiveness of screening services, because screening allows the detection of treatable malignancies. The prognosis also reflects timely access to appropriate and competent health care and the extent of team-work and collaboration across the primary, secondary and tertiary health care sectors. The theme of this chapter is that primary care, more than any other sector in health, can reduce the burden of morbidity and mortality from cancer. Because the majority of contact with cancer patients in primary care is in the period following diagnosis and treatment, some people believe that primary care has a relatively minor role in cancer care, yet nothing could be further from the truth. In many countries, policy makers are promoting a move away from the biomedical practice model to a community-based, primary care practice model, acknowledging that it will deliver 'better' health outcomes for a lower cost than a health system that focuses on hospital-based medical practice. Nowhere are the potential gains greater than in the improvements that could be made to patients with cancer by rethinking our approach. People with a cancer diagnosis increasingly want to have a say in their treatment and how they live their life during and after treatment. This chapter explores the role of the general practitioner and of primary care in cancer management, currently and in the future.

Keywords: Cancer, general practice, primary care, challenges, opportunities.

1. Cancer and Primary Care: Opportunities and Challenges

One in three men and one in four women in Australia will be diagnosed with cancer in the first 75 years of life, meaning that cancer is overtaking heart disease as the biggest cause of death in some parts of the country.[1] Overall five-year cancer survival is 58.4% for males and 64.1% for females, but to the general public, cancer remains the most feared disease.[2,3] However the term 'cancer' encompasses a great variety of conditions with a very indolent course, such as most skin cancers, but also those that have a very poor prognosis, including pancreatic cancer.

Cancer has both environmental and genetic causes, and so a diagnosis of cancer in one member of a family could provide the opportunity to work with the family and wider community around quantifying cancer risk. This might see encouragement of some forms of screening, support for smokers to quit smoking or advice around healthy lifestyle, as a means of reducing risk for developing cancer and improving mental and physical wellbeing. It is noteworthy that a significant number of patients presenting to general practitioners in Australia are at risk of developing cancer, but only a small proportion have a preventive intervention initiated by their GP.[4] While GPs generally see their role in prevention as important, the role of general practice in future cancer prevention is scarcely encouraged by national health policies in most countries. In Australia for example, a growing concern is that the Medicare system only pays GPs for services delivered if and when the patient visits their practice, and does not foster better prevention, early intervention and management of chronic illnesses, including cancer. There are major lessons to be learned from the United Kingdom, where despite an investment of 43 billion pounds sterling in the National Health Service since 2002, people have not benefitted from greater efficiency in health care, because of a lack of commitment to public health objectives, such as tackling obesity, smoking, physical activity and diet.[5]

While 'cancer' per se is a relatively rare presentation in primary care, symptoms that may be suggestive of cancer are very common. .The proportion of both males and females who report consulting a GP in a two-week period increases with age. For males this proportion ranges from one in six people aged 24–34 years, to over 40% of those aged 75 years and older. The proportion for women ranges from a fifth of women aged 16–24 years, to over 40% of those 75 years and older. Females report a greater frequency of GP consultation in every age group, even as people get older.[6] The proportion of people presenting with symptoms that cannot be attributed to a specific diagnosis is relatively high. For example, it is reported that 2.1 of every 100 encounters in general practice is for the investigation of abdominal pain, a rate which varies with age. In more than two-thirds of cases the general practitioner does not prescribe, supply or advise any medication, but 40% of patients with abdominal pain will be offered some sort of investigation or test, and in 25% of cases, the practitioner won't be able to make any definitive diagnosis.[7] On the other hand, gastrointestinal malignancies present at a rate of 0.2 per 100 encounters and the most common reason for contact with these patients is a request for a prescription.[8] In Australia the average practitioner will encounter about four new cancer diagnoses in their patients each year and have about 16 patients at any one time with a diagnosed cancer under their care.[9]

The evidence consistently shows that collaboration between care providers in different sectors, coordination of care and patient involvement all contribute to better quality healthcare.[10] In Australia as elsewhere, there is a move away from the biomedical practice model to a community-based, primary care practice model.[11] Nowhere would the benefits be felt more acutely than in the care provided for cancer patients.

2. The Role of Primary Care in Cancer Diagnosis

Screening asymptomatic people for treatable cancers is touted as the most promising strategy for timely diagnosis of some cancers. I would also argue that in primary care prompt referral of symptomatic people is also important. However in general practice patients present with undifferentiated illness, often with a host of other needs. Symptoms may originate in the physical, psychological and/or social domains. It is up to the practitioner to selectively refer those most likely to benefit from diagnostic tests, often in close consultation with the patient and taking on-board the patient's ideas, concerns and expectations. Unfortunately in many countries access to such expensive tests is rationed to those with so-called recognised 'red flag' symptoms. In these circumstances, general practitioners are often forced to err on the side of caution, for fear of litigation or complaint, and the sensitivity of a GP referral is often very poor.[12]

It is sometimes said that many life limiting cancers, depending on the histology and site, present at a late stage with few, if any, symptoms and that the doctors can do little to aid survival once people have developed symptoms.[13] However, there is evidence that many treatable cancers are not completely asymptomatic and there is potential to ensure a good prognosis by more effective case finding.[14] It is plausible that the group of patients with a short symptom-to-diagnosis interval is comprised of a mixture of patients with more aggressive tumours, but also patients with less biologically active tumours, who seek care sooner. Conversely, those diagnosed a long time after the onset of symptoms may include patients with relatively benign tumours, as well as patients with more aggressive disease, who delay seeking care.[15] Therefore it is incumbent on the general practitioner to identify and refer people who are at high risk of malignant disease. The possibility of advanced disease once symptoms appear cannot be interpreted as an invitation to diagnostic and treatment nihilism. Failure to diagnose malignant disease in primary care is frequently a cause for litigation and complaint in general practice.[16] Diagnosis requires practitioners to notice deviations from normal. While in countries with largely privatised primary care arrangements, the model of fee-for-service offers choice but it does not encourage people to consult a limited number of practitioners, thereby reducing the scope for significant new symptoms to be fully appreciated. Organisational and financial structures underpin high quality care.

Effective tools to alert general practitioners to the possibility of cancer among the symptomatic patients are needed. In time, it may be that genetic markers for cancers may be identified and patients will be selected for urgent referral in the presence of significant genetic profiles.[17] However, at present this seems a long way off and there may be potential benefits in widening the 'dragnet of case finding' to effectively and efficiently incorporate a larger host of primary care providers. For example, pharmacists have been estimated to have as many as 75 million contacts with Australian consumers annually.[18] The ongoing patient-practitioner relationship enjoyed by many community pharmacists and their clients has been undervalued and its impact across the spectrum of the cancer care in most health care systems remains ill-defined and unquantified. The decision to consult a medical practitioner is based on perceived benefit and offset against the monetary and other costs, as well as the inconvenience of scheduling a medical appointment.[19] Many patients seek over-the-counter remedies for symptoms, and the opportunity for pharmacists to identify high risk patients and refer them to a doctor at a time when the condition is amenable to treatment is well recognised, despite their impact on case detection being under-explored.[20] The public is also becoming increasingly better informed through the Internet and other media. In the coming years it may be possible that many patients will seek independent information to confirm advice from their general practitioner, when worried about a possible cancer diagnosis, or making choices about when to have investigations. Instruments such as the patient consultation questionnaire depend on history alone and could be used to aid communication with specialists. In conjunction with the weighted numerical score, which removes operator bias, it can be used as an accurate system for prediction of symptomatic colorectal cancer.[21]

It is important to offer patients advice and information that is consistent with current research evidence and for all health providers to have access to that information. The British experience suggests that published guidelines as the basis of a strategy to stream referrals to appropriate specialists has failed to benefit patients.[22] Effective case finding warrants appropriate and timely referral of people with 'red flag' cancer symptoms. While there is growing literature on the positive predictive value of some red flag cancer symptoms, there are few recognised effective strategies to implement this evidence.[23] Information technology (IT) offers the best prospect of enabling practitioners to make referrals, share data and refer to the latest evidence on an interactive basis. However, such innovations will only succeed if they are designed for and with the consultation of general practitioners, to allow the users to address patients' multiple needs, without feeling burdened by the technology. Such developments may significantly improve compliance to guidelines, such as those published by peak bodies, such as the Royal Australian College of General Practitioners.[24]

2.1 *The role of primary care during cancer treatment*

The acute phase of cancer treatment will continue to be managed by specialists, given the need to apply costly, technologically intensive and scarce treatment modalities. However, of growing importance is the involvement of primary care providers during 'active' treatment, as oral chemotherapeutic and biological agents are becoming more common in cancer treatment and in-patient stays for surgery shorten.[25] GPs have a role in identifying and managing acute toxicities during treatment, or perhaps administering chemotherapy in close consultation with the specialist team. A recent Australian paper suggests that information about chemotherapy (CT) faxed to GPs is a simple and inexpensive intervention that increases the primary care practitioners' confidence in managing chemotherapy adverse effects and enhances patients' satisfaction with shared care. This intervention could have widespread application.[26] In Australia, shared care arrangements, particularly those emphasising 'informational continuity of care', (so that primary care professionals are kept abreast of how their patients are being managed by a multidisciplinary team), offer prospects for improved patient care.[27] **Schemes that hold particular promise are those** where practitioners in different sectors have access to the same data on patients managed between them, either through patient-held records, or shared access to computer databases.[28] The notion that the 'physician knows best what's appropriate for the patient' has also been questioned, even in cases where therapy may prolong life. It seems that most patients with colorectal cancer would trade as much as a third of their life expectancy to avoid various forms of treatment. Researchers from Sydney interviewed 103 colorectal cancer patients to determine their preference and views on five treatment options, including abdomino-perineal resection, pre- and post-operative radiotherapy, chemotherapy and chemoradiotherapy. Patient preferences were measured on their willingness to trade remaining life expectancy for the treatment. More than 60% of patients would relinquish an average of 34% of their life expectancy to avoid having a colostomy. Also, 50% of patients indicated they would forgo almost 25% of their life expectancy to avoid chemoradiotherapy.[29] Therefore, primary care may have a substantial role as an independent advocate for the patient. This is especially the case when advising patients who wish to challenge the assumptions made about their need to accept radical and 'life prolonging' therapies. Patients today have relatively little contact with their primary care provider in the active treatment phase of cancer. I and others have argued that this is counter-productive, as greater involvement of professionals in the community, functioning within a care hub could offer better practical and psycho-social support for patients.[30]

2.2 The role of primary care in cancer survivorship and support

People with serious illnesses have consistently expressed the need for continuity of care from a care provider who is available, is genuinely interested in them, provides emotional support and takes the time to understand and communicate with them and important others.[31,32] Modern medicine should not fail in this regard. It remains a challenge to guide patients who may be desperate because of a bleak prognosis to accept evidence-based approaches, rather than seek miracle cures. Information and care are largely delivered in specialist centres, which are seldom in attuned to the large range of cultural, familial or social backgrounds of their patients. Arguably, the coordination of care could be better managed by a primary care provider with an understanding of the person's social context.

Following diagnosis and treatment a person may be cured, or experience troublesome sequelae, a recurrence or face death. Therefore 'surviving' cancer does not guarantee an acceptable quality of life for either the patient or their family. How an individual copes depends not only on the biological characteristics of the cancer and available treatments, but also on their social supports, reserves for dealing with uncertainty and ability to participate in decisions around treatment options, as well as the treatment itself. Most people experience some physical, social, economic and psychological sequelae, leading the World Health Organization to include cancer in its list of chronic conditions.[33,34] Recognition is overdue that providers of primary care extend beyond medical practitioners to a wider spectrum of practitioners in the community, including patients themselves and their families.[11] To this end, it is essential that those aspects that assist the person cope with their cancer are recognised, acknowledged and supported. Financing arrangements in many countries do not enable direct access to health professionals, other than medical practitioners, even when other health care providers may be better placed to address many aspects of cancer care.

Landmark qualitative research on living with a chronic condition highlights three aspects that the patient must manage: the disease/symptoms, the emotional consequences, and the impact on daily function/life roles.[35] With acute care symptoms focussed on the former, even when clinical guidelines recommend otherwise, systems of care do not ensure coordination or continuity. For example, while evidence-based interventions for fatigue are available, they rarely form part of usual care. Likewise, emotional concerns are recognised, but rarely approached systematically or comprehensively.

Occupational therapists, physiotherapists, community nurses, psychologists, counsellors, social workers and nutritionists also have a valued role to play in assisting patients to manage symptoms, emotional consequences and impact on daily life roles. Examples include rehabilitation to better maintain or regain independence in self care, modifications to homes, self-management programmes for common cancer symptoms (e.g. fatigue, psychosocial distress and anxiety), pain management techniques; lymphoedema care; graded exercise programs; carer education; and nutritional advice. While these interventions are included in algorithms for best practice (such as the NCCN Practice Guidelines in Oncology: Cancer-Related Fatigue), the mechanisms to ensure patients' access to such services do not yet exist in all countries, nor do mechanisms to allow multiple professionals to communicate with each other or the patient.[36]

Partners of patients with cancer experience similar levels of psychological stress to the patient, with some studies revealing higher levels of distress in the partner.[37,38] Many couples confront cancer as a team and adjustment to cancer by one partner affects the other.[39] However, spouses receive minimal support from the medical team.[40] It is well documented that partners deserve greater focus as recipients of support and care. Recent work has focused on family and friends of cancer patients, as well as the patients themselves. Results from targeted educational programs show high levels of participant satisfaction and positive changes in measures such as illness perceptions and emotional functioning. In many cases, the pattern of change was different for people with cancer, compared to family and friends. Such programs may be useful for helping people with cancer cope with the disease, with some distinct benefits for family and friends.[41] Children of older patients with cancer are also a particularly vulnerable group and often at a loss to know how to respect their parent's privacy, but yet be involved in the treatment plan and gain an understanding of the nature of the illness for their own and their parent's psychological health. Often there are supportive friends who would also like to be involved by providing assistance in day-to-day care. All too often, the role of significant others and the wider impact of the diagnosis on them represent unmet needs.

Finally, there is a need to adapt programs to ensure they also meet the needs of minority and vulnerable groups. It remains an indictment of our health care system that in many parts of the world indigenous people experience later cancer diagnosis, lower five-year survival, higher mortality rates than non-indigenous people and lower participation in screening programs.[42-44] While there has been a 30% reduction in cancer mortality rates in countries such as Australia over the last two decades, there has been little change in indigenous cancer mortality and such a situation illustrates a need for reconsideration of how all aspects of cancer control are managed for this group.[45] Surprisingly, little is understood about the experience of Culturally and Linguistically Diverse (CALD) groups with cancer. Culture is known to exert a profound influence on lifestyle and behaviour and often determines when and where the patient will present with symptoms to a medical practitioner. CALD groups are often excluded from mainstream research studies and their needs seldom documented. Minority groups also include those with non-traditional sexual behaviours, which can also increase risk for some cancers.[46] It has been documented that women who categorise themselves as homosexual may have equal numbers of male and female sexual partners over a lifetime and are therefore at equal risk of cervical cancer as women who are heterosexual. However homosexual women seldom present for contraceptive advice and therefore may not be offered Pap smears as often as other women.[47]

3.   Conclusions

Cancer is a leading cause of death in the Western world, although more people will survive cancer in the coming decades. The diagnosis of cancer is relatively uncommon among the people who present to a general practitioner with cancer symptoms. Therefore new algorithms will have to be developed to help the GP decide which symptomatic people should be referred for invasive, risky and expensive tests. It is also possible that other health care professionals in primary care will also be involved in the diagnosis of cancer and making referrals of patients to GPs.

In the future GPs will also advise, advocate for and perhaps be involved in the treatment of patients immediately following the diagnosis of cancer. This role will greatly enhance the potential for providing timely support and empowering people to make appropriate choices. Patients' ability to cope with the sequelae of cancer and its impact on significant others will depend on a re-organisation of healthcare, with a greater emphasis on practical and psychological support throughout the cancer journey. The extent to which all people will benefit from this reform will depend on our determination to ensure that no groups are disadvantaged by virtue of their culture or other differences.

References

1. Australian Bureau of Statistics, *Causes of Death*, Australia, 2006. Available at abs.gov.au/Ausstats/abs@.nsf/e8ae5488b598839cca256 82000131612/2093da6935db138fca2568a9001393c9!OpenDocument (accessed April 2008).
2. R. Borland, N. Donaghue and D. Hill, Illnesses that Australians most feared in 1986 and 1993, *Aust. J. Public Health* **18**: 366–369 (1994).
3. Australia's Health, 2008. Available at www.aihw.gov.au/publications/ index.cfm/title/10585 (accessed July 2008).
4. A. Heywood, R. Sanson-Fisher, I. Ring and P. Mudge, Risk prevalence and screening for cancer by general practitioners, *Prev. Med.* **23**(2): 152–159 (1994).
5. Commonwealth Government Health Budget Bulletin, June 2008. Available at www.macroeconomics.com.au/pdfs/commonwealth-healthbudgetbulletin-june2008-abridged.pdf (accessed July 2008).
6. New South Wales Government, Visited a general practitioner in the last 2 weeks, available from http://www.nursesreg.health.nsw.gov. au/PublicHealth/surveys/hsa/07/i_genprac1/i_genprac1_bar.asp (accessed May 2009).
7. BEACH Program, AIHW General Practice Statistics and Classification Unit, Presentations of abdominal pain in Australian general practice, *Aust. Fam. Physician* **33**: 968–969 (2004).
8. J. Charles, G. Miller and A. Ng, GI malignancies in Australian general practice, *Aust. Fam. Physician* **35**: 186–187 (2006).
9. B. McAvoy, M. Elwood and M. Staples, Cancer in Australia — An update for GPs, *Aust. Fam. Physician* **34**: 41–45 (2005).
10. Canadian Health Services Research Foundation, *Interdisciplinary Teams in Primary Healthcare can Effectively Manage Chronic Illnesses*, Evidence Boost for Quality, 2005. Available at www.chsrf.ca/ mythbusters/pdf/boost3_e.pdf (accessed January 21, 2008).
11. J. Doggett, *A New Approach to Primary Care for Australia*, Centre for Policy Development, Occ paper 1 (2007).
12. M. Jiwa and C. Saunders, Fast track referral for cancer, *Br. Med. J.* **335**: 267–268 (2007).

13. M. Porta, E. Fernandez, J. Belloc, N. Malats, M. Gallén and J. Alonso, Emergency admission for cancer: A matter of survival? *Br. J. Cancer* **77**: 477–484 (1998).

14. J. Corner, J. Hopkinson, D. Fitzsimmons *et al.*, Is late diagnosis of lung cancer inevitable? Interview study of patients' recollections of symptoms before diagnosis, *Thorax* **60**(4): 314–319 (2005).

15. E. Fernandez, M. Porta, N. Malats, J. Belloc and M. Gallén, Symptom-to-diagnosis interval and survival in cancers of the digestive tract, *Dig. Dis. Sci.* **47**: 2434–2440 (2002).

16. S. Bird, Failure to diagnose breast cancer, *Aust. Fam. Physician* **31**: 623–625 (2002).

17. A. V. Ryan, S. Wilson, M. J. Wakelam, S. A. Warmington, J. A. Dunn, R. F. Hobbs, A. Martin and T. Ismail, A prospective study to assess the value of MMP-9 in improving the appropriateness of urgent referrals for colorectal cancer, *Br. Med. J. Cancer* **6**: 251 (2006).

18. H. Howarth, G. Peterson, S. Jackson *et al.*, *Report of Health Promotion and Screening Activities by Community Pharmacists*, 2005. Community Pharmacy Research Support Centre. Available at www.guild.org.au/research/project_display.asp?id=259 (accessed June 2007).

19. A. Tversky and D. Kahneman, The framing of decision and the psychology of choice, *Science* **211**: 453–458 (1981).

20. D. Connelly, Community pharmacists can play a key role raising awareness of bowel cancer, *Pharm. J.* **278**: 580 (2007).

21. S. N. Selvachandran, R. J. Hodder, M. S. Ballal, P. Jones and D. Cade, Prediction of colorectal cancer by a patient consultation questionnaire and scoring system: A prospective study, *Lancet* **360**: 278–283 (2002).

22. M. F. Harris and N. A. Zwar, Care of patients with chronic disease: The challenge for general practice, *Med. J. Aust.* **187**: 104–107 (2007).

23. W. Hamilton, T. J. Peters, A. Round and D. Sharp, What are the clinical features of lung cancer before the diagnosis is made? A population based case-control study, *Thorax* **60**: 1059–1065 (2005).

24. The RACGP, *Guidelines for Preventive Activities in General Practice (The Red Book)*, 6th ed., 2005. Available at www.racgp.org.au/guidelines/redbook (accessed September 2007).

25. M. D. DeMario and M. J. Ratain, Oral chemotherapy: Rationale and future directions, *J. Clin. Oncol.* **16**: 2557–2567 (1998).

26. M. Jefford, C. Baravelli, P. Dudgeon, A. Dabscheck, M. Evans, M. Moloney and P. Schofield, Tailored chemotherapy information faxed to general practitioners improves confidence in managing adverse

effects and satisfaction with shared care: Results from a randomized controlled trial, *J. Clin. Oncol.* **26**: 2272–2277 (2008).

27. J. L. Haggerty, R. J. Reid, G. K. Freeman *et al.*, Continuity of care: A multidisciplinary review, *Br. Med. J.* **327**:1219–1221 (2003).

28. M. Hickman, N. Drummond and J. Grimshaw, A taxonomy of shared care for chronic disease, *J. Public Health Med.* **16**: 447–454 (1994).

29. J. M. Young, M. J. Solomon, J. D. Harrison, G. Salkeld and P. Butow, Measuring patient preference and surgeon choice, *Surgery* **143**: 582–588 (2008).

30. M. Jiwa, C. M. Saunders, S. C. Thompson, L. K. Rosenwax, S. Sargant, E. L. Khong, G. K. Halkett, G. Sutherland, H. C. Ee, T. L. Packer, G. Merriman and H. R. Arnet, Timely cancer diagnosis and management as a chronic condition: Opportunities for primary care, *Med. J. Aust.* **189**: 78–82 (2008).

31. Australian Institute of Health and Welfare (AIHW) and Australasian Association of Cancer Registries (AACR) 2004, *Cancer in Australia 2001*, AIHW Cat. No. CAN 23 (AIHW: Canberra Cancer Series No. 28).

32. J. R. Curtis, M. D. Wenrich, J. D. Carline, S. E. Shannon, D. M. Ambrozy and P. G. Ramsey, Patients' perspectives on physician skill in end-of-life care: Differences between patients with COPD, cancer, and AIDS, *Chest* **122**: 356–362 (2002).

33. No authors listed, Cancer survivors: Living longer, and now, better, *Lancet* **364**: 2153–2154 (2004).

34. 58th World Health Assembly Resolution on Cancer Prevention and Control. Available at www.who.int/cancer/eb1143/en/index.html (accessed 27 November 2007).

35. NCCN Practice Guidelines in Oncology: Cancer-Related Fatigue. Available at www.nccn.org/professionals/physician_gls/PDF/fatigue.pdf (accessed November 2007).

36. J. Corbin and A. Strauss, Managing chronic illness at home: Three lines of work, *Qual. Sociol.* **8**(3): 224–247 (1985).

37. L. Baider, U. Koch, R. Esacson and A. K. De-Nour, Prospective study of cancer patients and their spouses: The weakness of marital strength, *Psychooncology* **7**: 49–56 (1998).

38. J. Harden, A. Schafenacker, L. Northouse, D. Mood, D. Smith, K. Pienta, M. Hussain and K. Baranowski, Couples' experiences with prostate cancer: Focus group research, *Oncol. Nurs. Forum* **29**: 701–709 (2002).

39. L. Northouse, T. Templin and D. Mood, Couples' adjustment to breast disease during the first year following diagnosis, *J. Behav. Med.* **24**: 115–136 (2001).

40. J. Harrison, P. Haddad and P. Maguire, The impact of cancer on key relatives: A comparison of relative and patient concerns, *Eur. J. Cancer* **31A**: 1736–1740 (1995).

41. G. Sutherland, L. H. Dpsych, V. White, M. Jefford and S. Hegarty, How does a cancer education program impact on people with cancer and their family and friends?, *J. Cancer Educ.* **23**: 126–132 (2008).

42. J. R. Condon, C. Cunningham, T. Barnes *et al.*, Cancer diagnosis and treatment in the Northern Territory: Assessing health service performances for indigenous Australians, *Intern. Med. J.* **36**: 498–505 (2006).

43. Australian Institute of Health and Welfare, *Cervical screening in Australia 2001–2002*, Cancer Series No. 27 (AIHW: Canberra, 2004).

44. Australian Institute of Health and Welfare, *Breast Screen Australia Monitoring Report 2001–2002*, Cancer Series No. 29 (AIHW: Canberra, 2005).

45. R. M. Lowenthal, P. B. Grogan and E. T. Kerrins, Reducing the impact of cancer in indigenous communities: Ways forward, *Med. J. Aust.* **182**(3): 105–106 (2005).

46. J. S. Anderson, C. Vajdic and A. E. Grulich, Is screening for anal cancer warranted in homosexual men?, *Sex Health* **1**(3): 137–140 (2004).

47. A. K. Matthews, D. L. Brandenburg, T. P. Johnson and T. L. Hughes, Correlates of underutilization if gynaecological cancer screening among lesbian and heterosexual women, *Prev. Med.* **38**(1): 105–113 (2004).

38

Genetic Testing for Cancer Susceptibility: How and When?*

Judy Kirk

Abstract

There is now an improved ability to detect people at high risk of cancer through analysis of their family history and genetic testing. Advances in cancer screening, cancer surveillance and cancer prevention have accompanied this. It is important to identify individuals at high cancer risk so that these advances can be applied in their management. Equally important is the identification of those not at high risk, so that they are spared unnecessary cancer screening and concern. Risk assessment and genetic testing is available through familial cancer services. This article introduces the common syndromes requiring referral to such a service and the general principles of cancer genetic testing.

Keywords: Genetic testing, genetic susceptibility, germline mutation, BRCA1 mutation, BRCA2 mutation, Multiple Endocrine Neoplasia (Types 1 and 2), retinoblastoma, Familial Adenomatous Polyposis (FAP) and Von-Hippel Lindau syndrome, Peutz-Jeghers syndrome, Li–Fraumeni syndrome, PARP inhibitors.

* This article was first published in *Cancer Forum: Clinical Cancer Genetics*, Vol. 31, No. 3, November 2007 (by Cancer Council Australia). Reproduced with permission from the authors and publishers.

1. Cancer is a Genetic Disease

Cancer is a genetic disease, associated with alterations (mutations) in genes that normally act to control cell growth, proliferation and DNA repair. These genetic mutations usually occur in somatic (tissue) cells over the course of a lifetime. In this way, cancer is usually due to a series of acquired mutations ('hits') in genes that control cell growth, eventually allowing cells with these faults to grow in an uncontrolled fashion. Up to 95% of all cancers are caused by these somatic mutations in cancer-associated genes. Because they occur in somatic cells, these genetic mutations are not inherited.

However, some rare families have an inherited mutation in one of these same genes. In these families, the 'first hit' is usually inherited either in the egg or the sperm (this is known as a germline mutation). It affects all cells of the body. People who inherit a germline mutation in a cancer-associated gene are at increased risk of developing cancer. The pattern of cancer seen in such a family will depend on the specific gene involved and sometimes on the type and location of mutation in that gene. There are tools available with which to assess the probability of a genetic susceptibility to cancer, e.g. CancerGene http://www4.utsouthwestern.edu/breasthealth/cagene/.

There have been considerable advances in the area of cancer genetics over the last 15 years, with the identification and characterisation of genes in which germline mutations predispose to a high risk of cancer. These scientific advances in understanding genetic susceptibility have been translated into clinical practice as genetic testing for families with cancer predisposition has become available. This has been achieved by the development of familial cancer services in most major centres throughout the developed world, often within public-sector comprehensive cancer centres. Such services are staffed by clinical geneticists and/or oncologists with expertise in cancer genetics, supported by trained genetic counsellors and a molecular genetics laboratory. The role of the familial cancer service is to identify individuals at high genetic risk of cancer so that appropriate intervention strategies can be implemented for early detection or prevention, with the ultimate aim being to reduce the impact of cancer for the individual and their family.

2.   Genetic Predisposition to Cancer

Family history has long been recognised as an important risk factor for cancer. The taking of a good family history is more important than ever.[1] Published guidelines[2,3] and computer programs (e.g. http://www4.utsouthwestern.edu/breasthealth/cagene/) can assist health professionals in estimating the risk of cancer based on family history and to determine whether referral to a familial cancer service might be appropriate. In general, family histories of cancer that suggest genetic susceptibility include those with:

- either three or more relatives on the same side of the family with the same (or related) cancer; or
- two affected individuals with the same (or related) cancer where there is an additional 'high risk feature', such as:
  - earlier than average age at diagnosis; or
  - the presence of more than one primary cancer in a family member.

3.   The Role of the Familial Cancer Service

A familial cancer service can be expected to construct a full three-generation pedigree on both sides of the family. Importantly, family history is often poorly reported and verification of the described family history is necessary. Gynaecological malignancy is commonly misreported and confirmation that the family account of ovarian cancer was actually a cervical intra-epithelial neoplasia, or that a reported breast cancer was simply a fibroadenoma, can dramatically change the assessment of familial risk. Verification of family history is time-consuming and involves the genetic counsellor obtaining consent from family members to enable access to pathology reports and medical records. Seemingly diverse cancer types can be present in certain 'inherited cancer predisposition syndromes', and recognition of such patterns is important. For example, both breast and ovarian cancers occur in families with a BRCA1 or BRCA2 mutation, colorectal cancers in association with gynaecological cancers may point to a defect in the mismatch repair genes, and the combination of medullary carcinoma of the thyroid and phaeochromocytoma occurs in families with Multiple Endocrine

Neoplasia due to a heritable mutation in the RET proto-oncogene. Occasionally the finding of phenotypic clues, such as peri-oral freckling in Peutz–Jeghers syndrome or skin tricholemmomas in Cowden syndrome, will assist with making a cancer genetic diagnosis.

While an assessment of cancer risk may be made on the basis of family history, this is generally a broad categorisation, placing an individual at "average risk", "moderate risk" or "potentially high risk", based on the verified family history. For those at potentially high risk, due to a stronger family history, genetic testing (discussed below in further detail) can assist in further clarifying risk within some families. An offer of genetic testing can only be made if there are known genes in which heritable mutations cause an increased risk of cancer.

The well-known cancer susceptibility syndromes are reviewed in Nagy[4] and Garber[5] for general reference and further information is available through websites such as Genetests (http://www.genetests.org/). It should be recognised that the offer of genetic counselling and testing should now be an integral part of the clinical management of Multiple Endocrine Neoplasia (Types 1 and 2), retinoblastoma, Familial Adenomatous Polyposis (FAP) and Von-Hippel Lindau syndrome, where the genes tested are MEN1, RET, Rb, APC and VHL, respectively. In these conditions there is a clear role for screening and prevention in reducing the impact of cancer for those at proven high risk.

For families with a strong family history of breast and ovarian cancer, clinical testing usually involves the genes BRCA1 and BRCA2.[6] Certain specific founder mutations in BRCA1 and BRCA2 are more common in individuals of Ashkenazi Jewish descent. Breast and thyroid malignancies with intestinal hamartomas (consistent with Cowden syndrome) may be investigated by testing the PTEN gene. A family history of bowel cancer, especially early onset (aged < 50 years) and other cancers, including uterus, ovary, stomach, small bowel, renal pelvis or ureter, suggests the involvement of the mismatch repair genes in the syndrome of Hereditary Non-Polyposis Colon Cancer (HNPCC), also called Lynch syndrome.[7] Genetic testing for other polyposis syndromes, including Juvenile Polyposis and Peutz–Jeghers syndrome is now possible. On the other hand, genetic testing for familial melanoma is usually only available when a family CDKN2A mutation has already been identified as a result of participation in a research study. Furthermore, despite intensive research, no genes have yet been firmly identified in which mutations cause a hereditary tendency to prostate cancer. Finally, for some syndromes, such as the Li–Fraumeni syndrome, where there is a high risk of varied cancers (including paediatric sarcoma, haematological malignancy, early onset breast cancer, adrenal cancer, brain tumour and lung cancer), genetic testing for p53 may identify a causative mutation. However, for individuals with the Li–Fraumeni syndrome, there is currently little to offer in the way of proven screening or prevention, and so genetic testing needs to be considered with care.

Families with a significant family history of cancer can be enrolled in studies involved in genetic research. Population and family-based research efforts, such as the Modifiers and Genetics in Cancer (MAGIC), Epidemiological study of BRCA1 and BRCA2 mutation carriers (EMBRACE), Genetic Modifiers of cancer risk in BRCA1/2 mutation carriers (GEMO), the Kathleen Cuningham Consortium for Research on Familial Breast Cancer (http://www.kconfab.org) and the National Cancer Institute Breast and Colon Cancer Family Registries (http://epi.grants.cancer.gov/CFR/) will continue to make significant contributions to understanding the familial aspects of cancer.

4. Genetic Testing for Cancer Susceptibility

In 2003, the American Society of Clinical Oncology (ASCO) published an updated policy statement concerning genetic testing for cancer susceptibility: "ASCO recommends that genetic testing be offered when:

1) the individual has personal or family history features suggestive of a genetic cancer susceptibility condition;
2) the test can be adequately interpreted; and
3) the results will aid in diagnosis or influence the medical or surgical management of the patient or family members at hereditary risk of cancer. ASCO recommends that genetic testing only be done in the setting of pre- and post-test counselling, which should include discussion of possible risks and benefits of cancer early detection and prevention modalities."[8]

It is recommended that prior to consideration of cancer genetic testing, key components of the consultation should include medical and family history, cancer risk assessment and discussion of the limitations, as well as possible risks (e.g. impact on future applications for life/disability insurance) and benefits of molecular genetic testing for the person and their family members. Informed consent must be obtained.[9]

Genetic testing is now available through familial cancer services for some of the common hereditary cancer syndromes outlined above. Whatever the gene(s) to be tested, the general principles remain the same. The first step in genetic testing is usually to take blood from one of the family members affected by the condition, although sometimes an unaffected obligate carrier may be tested instead. This must be done with fully-informed consent. Counselling before testing must cover the potential harms, benefits and limitations of such testing. The laboratory then searches the relevant gene(s) to determine whether a causative gene mutation can be found.

This first phase, the 'mutation search', may take some months in some centres. A causative gene mutation cannot be found in every family, as mutations may be missed, or mutations may be present in other genes that are not yet identified. Importantly, this means that if the family history is strong and the genetic test (mutation search) fails to identify a gene mutation in an affected family member (with a significant family history), that test result should be considered 'inconclusive' and all relatives remain at potentially high risk. However, if a causative mutation is identified in the relevant gene, e.g. in BRCA1 or BRCA2 for a breast cancer family, or in a mismatch repair gene for an HNPCC (also called Lynch syndrome) family, then other at-risk family members (males and females) can be offered 'predictive' genetic testing. Predictive tests are relatively cheap and quick, with results generally available in four to six weeks. Once the family gene mutation has been identified in the mutation search phase, using a predictive test, others in the family can simply be tested for the presence or absence of that same gene fault.

The risk of cancer associated with the gene mutation and the approach to that risk requires discussion before testing. Those who are found not to carry the family mutation (at predictive testing) should be considered to be at average risk of cancer. They and their offspring can be spared unnecessary cancer screening and concern.

Predictive genetic testing for cancer risk is usually restricted to adults unless there is a case for medical intervention in childhood, such as in families with Familial Adenomatous Polyposis, where screening starts in the teenage years. Pre-natal testing and pre-implantation genetic diagnosis is feasible once the family mutation is identified, but is not often considered in cancer families.

5.   Conclusion

Genetic susceptibility to cancer is rare. It can generally be identi-fied by taking a good family history. If genetic testing identifies a causative gene mutation, then predictive testing can identify those family members who do not carry the mutation and are 'not at risk'. It also identifies those who are 'at high risk'. The latter can take the opportunity to have intensive cancer screening, including newer modalities such as breast magnetic resonance imaging. They may wish to consider risk-reducing surgery, particularly in circumstances where this has a proven role. Restorative procto-colectomy is the standard care for preventing bowel cancer in FAP, as the risk of cancer without such intervention is 100%. In carriers of a BRCA1 or BRCA2 gene mutation, bilateral mastectomy reduces the risk of breast cancer.[10] For these women, risk-reducing salpingo-oophorectomy not only dramatically reduces the risk of ovarian cancer, but if done before menopause, halves the risk of breast cancer.[11] For children with an inherited RET gene mutation, prophylactic thyroidectomy prevents medullary thyroid cancer.[12] In some cases chemoprevention can be used to reduce the risk of cancer. Tamoxifen may be considered as a risk-reducing option for high-risk women,[13] although there are side effects and evidence is not yet available regarding the impact of preventative tamoxifen on mortality from breast cancer.

Finally, for those at high genetic risk who do develop cancer, targeted therapies are being designed for tumours, depending on their molecular basis.[14] As an example, BRCA1/2 deficient breast/ovarian cancers seem to rely on poly (ADP-ribose) polymerase (PARP) in response to DNA damage and specific inhibition. The use of PARP inhibitors is now being studied in a phase II trial of recurrent breast/ovarian cancers in BRCA1/2 carriers. Such devel-opments will no doubt continue.

The improved ability to detect people at high-risk (through analysis of their family history and genetic testing) has been accompanied by advances in cancer screening, cancer surveillance and cancer prevention. It is important to identify these individuals so that these advances can be applied in their management, offering hope of making an impact on the international goals of cancer control.

References

1. A. E. Guttmacher, F. S. Collins and R. H. Carmona, The family history — more important than ever, *N. Engl. J. Med.* **351**(22): 2333–2336 (2004).
2. National Breast Cancer Centre, Advice about familial aspects of breast cancer and epithelial ovarian cancer [monograph on the Internet], available from: http://www.nbocc.org.au/resources/resource.php?code=BOG [accessed August 2007].
3. The Australian Cancer Network, Familial aspects of bowel cancer: A guide for health professionals [monograph on the Internet], available from: http://www.cancer.org.au/File/HealthProfessionals/Familial BowelCancerCardfinal.pdf [accessed March 2008].
4. R. Nagy, K. Sweet and C. Eng, Highly penetrant hereditary cancer syndromes, *Oncogene* **23**(38): 6445–6470 (2004).
5. J. E. Garber and K. Offit, Hereditary cancer predisposition syndromes, *J. Clin. Oncol.* **23**(2): 276–292 (2005).
6. A. Antoniou, P. Pharoah, S. Narod, H. Risch, J. Eyfjord, J. Hopper *et al.*, Average risks of breast and ovarian cancer associated with BRCA1 and BRCA2 mutations detected in case series unselected for family history: A combined analysis of 22 studies, *Am. J. Hum. Genet.* **72**: 1117–1130 (2003).
7. H. T. Lynch and A. de la Chapelle, genomic medicine: Hereditary colorectal cancer, *N. Engl. J. Med.* **348**: 919–932 (2003).
8. American Society of Clinical Oncology (ASCO), American Society of Clinical Oncology policy statement update: Genetic testing for cancer susceptibility, *J. Clin. Oncol.* **21**: 1–10 (2003).
9. A. Trepanier, M. Ahrens, W. McKinnon, J. Peters, J. Stopfer, S. C. Grumet *et al.*, National Society of Genetic Counselors. Genetic cancer risk assessment and counseling: Recommendations of the national society of genetic counsellors, *J. Genet. Couns.* **13**(2): 83–114 (2004).

10. T. Rebbeck, T. Friebel, H. Lynch *et al.*, Bilateral prophylactic mastectomy reduces breast cancer risk in BRCA1 and BRCA2 mutation carriers: The PROSE Study Group, *J. Clin. Oncol.* **22**: 1055–1062 (2004).

11. S. M. Domchek, T. M. Friebel, S. L. Neuhausen *et al.*, Mortality after bilateral salpingo-oophorectomy in BRCA1 and BRCA2 mutation carriers: A prospective cohort study, *Lancet Oncol.* **7**(3): 223–229 (2006).

12. M. L. Brandi, R. F. Gagel, A. Angeli *et al.*, Guideline for diagnosis and therapy of MEN type 1 and MEN type 2, *J. Clin. Endocrinol. Metab.* **86**: 5658–5671 (2001).

13. IBIS Investigators, First results from the International Breast Cancer Intervention Study (IBIS 1): A randomised prevention trial, *Lancet* **360**: 817–824 (2002).

14. W. Rubinstein, Hereditary breast cancer: Pathobiology, clinical translation, and potential for targeted cancer therapeutics, *Fam. Cancer* **7**(1): 83–89 (2008).

39

Management of Women at High Familial Risk of Breast and Ovarian Cancer*

Kathryn M. Field and
Kelly-Anne Phillips

Abstract

Women with a strong family history of breast and/or ovarian cancer have a greatly increased risk for the development of these diseases. The key question for these women is what they can do to ameliorate their cancer risk. Fortunately, there are now several interventions which clearly reduce breast and ovarian cancer risk in high-risk women. These include risk-reducing bilateral mastectomy, salpingo-oophorectomy and chemoprevention with tamoxifen or raloxifene. For those women who do not undergo risk-reducing bilateral mastectomy, screening is generally recommended in order to try and detect breast cancers at an early stage. Breast magnetic resonance imaging has an emerging role in such screening programs. Cancer screening does not reduce cancer risk and its impact on reduction of mortality in this group is uncertain. Women at high risk should be fully informed of their surgical,

* This article was first published in *Cancer Forum: Clinical Cancer Genetics*, Vol. 31, No. 3, November 2007 (by Cancer Council Australia). Reproduced with permission from the authors and publishers.

chemopreventive and screening options. A risk management plan should be tailored to each woman, particularly taking into account the level of her short-term (rather than lifetime) risk, her lifestyle plans (such as child-bearing), competing risks (particularly in women with a prior cancer) and her personal preferences. The risk management plan should be reviewed regularly and altered as the individual's short-term risk level and circumstances change, and as the evidence base for various interventions builds. Participation in appropriate clinical trials should be offered.

Keywords: Family history, risk-reducing mastectomy, risk-reducing salpingo-oophorectomy, chemoprevention, tamoxifen.

1. Who is at High Risk for Breast/Ovarian Cancer?

Breast cancer and ovarian cancer are diagnosed in about 12,000 and 1100 Australian women per year respectively.[1] Between 1% and 5% of all breast cancer cases and around 10% of invasive epithelial ovarian cancer cases are due to the inheritance of mutations in known cancer predisposition genes.[2,3]

In less than 1% of the population, the number of blood relatives affected with cancer, their ages at diagnosis and the types of cancers suggest a high likelihood of a dominantly-inherited mutation in a breast cancer and/or ovarian cancer-predisposition gene (see Table 1).

Referral of such women to a family cancer centre for formal risk assessment, consideration of genetic testing and discussion of management options is considered by many to be a standard of care.

BRCA1 and BRCA2 are the genes most commonly associated with breast and ovarian cancer predisposition. Carriers of mutations in these genes have a significantly elevated lifetime risk of breast cancer or ovarian cancer.[4,5] Several other genes are also associated with an increased risk of breast and/or ovarian malignancy (see Table 2).

Families meeting high risk criteria (see Table 1), but in whom a mutation cannot be found, are still considered at high risk because genetic testing is not 100% sensitive, and because there may be a mutation in an as yet unidentified cancer predisposition gene.

Table 1. Risk of breast or ovarian cancer based on family history alone.[113,114]

Cancer type	Features	Lifetime risk	% of population
Breast cancer	Two 1st or 2nd degree relatives (same side of family) with breast or ovarian cancer. PLUS one or more of the following conditions:	25–50%[†]	< 1%
	• additional relative(s) with breast or ovarian cancer; • onset of breast cancer before the age of 40; • bilateral breast cancer; • breast and ovarian cancer in the same woman; • Ashkenazi Jewish ancestry; • breast cancer in a male relative.		
	Or One 1st or 2nd degree relative diagnosed with breast cancer ≤ 45yo, plus another 1st or 2nd degree relative (same side of family) with sarcoma (bone or soft tissue) ≤ 45yo.		
Ovarian cancer	One 1st degree relative diagnosed with epithelial ovarian cancer in a family of Ashkenazi Jewish ancestry.	3–30%[†]	< 1%
	Two 1st or 2nd degree relatives (same side of the family) diagnosed with ovarian cancer, especially if ≥ 1 of the following:		
	• additional relative(s) with breast or ovarian cancer; • onset of breast cancer before the age of 40; • bilateral breast cancer; • breast and ovarian cancer in the same woman; or • breast cancer in a male relative.		

(*Continued*)

Table 1.   (Continued)

Cancer type	Features	Lifetime risk	% of population
	Three or more 1st or 2nd degree relatives on the same side of the family diagnosed with any cancers associated with HNPCC*:		
	• colorectal cancer (especially if < 50y);		
	• endometrial cancer;		
	• ovarian cancer;		
	• gastric cancer; or		
	• cancers involving the renal tract.		

* HNPCC = Hereditary non-polyposis colorectal cancer.

† Higher if woman documented to carry a mutation in a breast and ovarian cancer predisposition gene.

2.   What are the Risk Management Options for High-Risk Women?

Management of women with a strong family history and/or a documented gene mutation is complex and dynamic. Optimal risk management is likely to be in the context of a multidisciplinary team. Multidisciplinary risk management clinics have been set up at several family cancer centres within Australia.[6] Figures 1 and 2 outline the options with respect to risk management strategies currently available.

3.   Risk-Reducing Surgery

An individual's level of risk should be fully clarified prior to undertaking risk-reducing surgery. If possible, genetic testing of a family member with cancer should occur. If a mutation is found, the woman contemplating surgery should be tested for that mutation. In that way, unnecessary surgery in women who have not inherited the cancer-causing family mutation can be avoided.

Table 2. High risk genes, frequency and increased risks of breast and ovarian cancer.[115,116]

Gene	Syndrome	Breast cancer risk by age 70	Ovarian cancer risk by age 70	Associated cancers
BRCA1	Hereditary breast/ovarian cancer	39–87%	20–40%	Pancreas
BRCA2	Hereditary breast/ovarian cancer	26–91%	10–20%	Prostate Pancreas
p53	Li–Fraumeni syndrome	> 90%	n/a	Soft tissue sarcoma Osteosarcoma Brain tumours Adrenocortical carcinoma Leukaemia Colon
PTEN	Cowden syndrome	25–50%	~1%	Thyroid Endometrial Genitourinary
STK11/LKB1	Peutz–Jeghers syndrome	45–54%	(Usually sex cord tumors rather than epithelial ovarian cancer)	Small intestine Colorectal Uterine Testicular
CDH1	Hereditary diffuse gastric carcinoma	39% (lobular)	n/a	Diffuse gastric cancer
MLH1, MSH2 MSH6, PMS1, PMS2 (mismatch repair)	Hereditary non-polyposis colorectal cancer/Lynch syndrome	n/a	10%	Small intestine Colorectal Stomach Uterus Ureter/renal pelvis

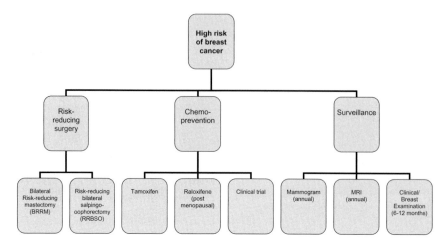

Figure 1. Breast cancer: Risk reduction and surveillance strategies.

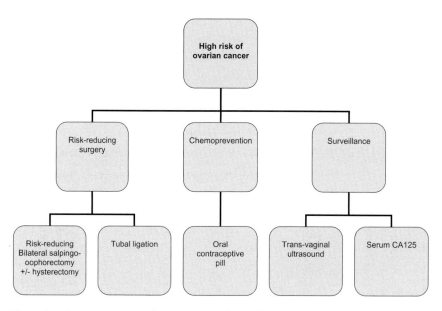

Figure 2. Ovarian cancer: Risk reduction and surveillance strategies.

3.1   *Bilateral risk-reducing mastectomy*

Bilateral risk-reducing mastectomy (BRRM) is the most effective method of breast cancer prevention, reducing risk by about 90%.[7–10]

It is usually done in conjunction with immediate reconstruction. Total mastectomy is likely to reduce risk more than subcutaneous mastectomy, however the latter is a reasonable option for women wishing to retain the native nipple and areola complex,[11] provided they are informed that the benefits may be slightly less. BRRM carries the risk of surgical complications;[12] additionally, cosmetic complications following reconstruction may occur.[13]

In descriptive studies women who have undergone BRRM report lessened concern about cancer[14,15] and decreased perceived cancer risk,[16] but also dissatisfaction with reconstruction,[17] feelings of femininity and sexual relationships.[14,18] Because BRRM can have adverse psychological and body image consequences, it should not be performed without prior counselling.

In Australia, uptake rates for BRRM have been relatively low by international standards.[19] In high-risk women attending family cancer clinics (90% of whom were not known mutation carriers), the uptake rate over a three-year follow-up period was 4.4%. Those who underwent the procedure were more likely to have more first-degree relatives with breast cancer than those who did not.[16] In another study of mutation carriers in the kConFab research cohort,[20] the uptake rate of BRRM was 11%, three years after learning their mutation result.[21]

3.2 Risk-reducing bilateral salpingo-oophorectomy

Risk-reducing bilateral salpingo-oophorectomy (RRBSO) reduces ovarian and fallopian tube cancer risk by about 90% and, for pre-menopausal women, it also reduces breast cancer risk by about 50% in BRCA1 and BRCA2 mutation carriers.[22–27] RRBSO has recently been shown to reduce overall and cancer-specific mortality.[22] It is an appropriate option for women who carry a BRCA1 or BRCA2 mutation, or who have a family history of breast and epithelial ovarian cancer (but is not generally recommended for women with a breast cancer-only family history). In Australia, uptake rates for RRBSO have been higher than for BRRM, with approximately 30% of mutation carriers undergoing RRBSO within three years of learning of their mutation result.[21]

RRBSO includes removal of the fallopian tube because of the increased risk of fallopian tube cancer in these women. Concurrent hysterectomy increases the complexity of the surgery, but is sometimes advocated to avoid the risk of endometrial cancer if progesterone-containing HRT or tamoxifen is planned for subsequent use. Primary peritoneal carcinoma may occur despite RRBSO,[28] with the rates of such malignancies varying from 2–11%.[29]

For pre-menopausal women, RRBSO causes abrupt menopause. Observational studies suggest that the use of hormone replacement therapy (HRT), after RRBSO in BRCA1/2 mutation carriers, does not offset the breast cancer risk reduction conferred by the procedure.[30] Results from the US-based Women's Health Initiative Study suggest caution in advising prolonged post-menopausal HRT in women.[31,32]

Optimal timing of RRBSO is controversial and needs to be individualised. Clearly it should not be undertaken until childbearing is completed. Ovarian cancer risk does not generally start to increase above that of the general population until about age 40 (BRCA1 carriers) or 50 (BRCA2 carriers). Thus, if ovarian cancer risk reduction is the major objective (e.g. the patient is using other strategies to decrease breast cancer risk), surgery can be delayed until ages 35–40 in BRCA1 carriers and ages 45–50 in BRCA2 carriers. However, if reduction in breast cancer risk is also an objective, earlier RRBSO may be appropriate.

3.3   Tubal ligation

Tubal ligation has been associated with decreased risk for ovarian cancer in observational studies.[33–35] One case-control study showed that tubal ligation reduced ovarian cancer risk by about 60% in BRCA1 carriers. A protective effect was not seen in BRCA2 carriers, however was not excluded as this subgroup was small.[36] In BRCA1/2 mutation carriers, who have completed childbearing but who choose not to undergo pre-menopausal RRBSO, tubal ligation should be considered as an effective contraceptive means which may also decrease ovarian cancer risk.

4.   Chemoprevention

4.1   Breast cancer chemoprevention

Chemoprevention, with the selective oestrogen receptor modulators (SERMs) tamoxifen or raloxifene, reduces breast cancer risk by about 40%.[37–42] Tamoxifen is the only evidence-based option for pre-menopausal women; for post-menopausal women raloxifene is also an option. These two agents have been compared in a randomised trial[43] and are equally efficacious in preventing oestrogen receptor positive invasive breast cancers, with tamoxifen superior for prevention of non-invasive cancers. Raloxifene is associated with fewer gynaecological side effects, thromboembolic events and cataracts than tamoxifen. These agents probably should not be used in women with previous history of deep venous thrombosis, smokers, or those with other uncontrolled cardiovascular risk factors.

SERMs have not been shown to reduce risk for oestrogen receptor negative breast cancer and this has been used as an argument against using them in BRCA1 carriers, who usually develop ER negative tumours.[44,45] Indeed, a sub-analysis of mutation carriers in the largest prevention trial suggested that the benefit of tamoxifen might be limited to BRCA2 carriers; however, the study was under-powered and included fewer than 10 BRCA1 carriers.[46] Although BRCA1-associated breast cancers are usually oestrogen receptor negative, initiation of these tumours may well involve the oestrogen pathway,[47,48] which is consistent with the observation that interventions reducing oestrogen exposure in these women (e.g. pre-menopausal oophorectomy) appear to reduce risk. For this reason, tamoxifen chemoprevention may be considered a reasonable option, although enrolment in trials of novel chemoprevention agents such as retinoids should be considered.[49]

Aromatase inhibitors show promise as chemopreventive agents based on their ability to reduce contralateral breast cancer risk in the adjuvant disease setting.[50] A clinical trial of anastrozole as chemoprevention (IBIS II) is underway. Participation should be discussed with high risk women, particularly those with a contraindication to SERMs.

4.2 *Ovarian cancer chemoprevention*

While there are no randomised trials, observational studies demonstrate a reduced risk of ovarian cancer in the general population and in high risk individuals who take the oral contraceptive pill.[33,51–54] Most studies suggest up to a 50% reduction in the risk of ovarian cancer in BRCA1/2 carriers.[53,55,56] Oral contraceptive pill use in this setting has been tempered by concern about the effect on breast cancer risk (discussed below in Section 6.3). However, as ovarian cancer carries a higher mortality rate than breast cancer, in pre-menopausal women who choose not to undergo RRSO, the oral contraceptive pill is a reasonable strategy to reduce risk while being mindful of the uncertainty regarding impact on breast cancer risk. For women who have undergone BRRM, but wish to postpone RRSO until later, it is potentially a useful strategy as there is no concern about the possible impact on breast cancer risk.

5. Surveillance Strategies

Surveillance strategies do not reduce cancer risk, but are aimed at detecting malignancy at an early stage when it may be amenable to curative treatment. Evidence on the efficacy of intensive surveillance in high risk women is limited.

5.1 *Breast cancer screening/surveillance*

5.1.1 *Mammography*

In the general population, mammographic screening has been demonstrated to reduce breast cancer mortality in women older than 50 years by 20–25%.[57,58] The efficacy of mammographic screening in younger, high risk women remains controversial.[59] Anecdotal reports document both the success and failure of mammography to detect breast cancer in carriers of BRCA1 mutations,[60] and the sensitivity of mammographic screening in high-risk women over a variety of studies ranges from 50–91%.[61]

Some have suggested that annual mammography may not be frequent enough in BRCA1 mutation carriers because these cancers are usually high grade and may develop between screens.[9,62–64] However, enthusiasm for more frequent mammographic screening is limited, partly by the question of whether ionising radiation may induce cancers in mutation carriers, because these individuals may have difficulty repairing DNA damage caused by radiation.[65] Studies have had conflicting results. Two studies of BRCA1/2 carriers found no increased risk of breast cancer associated with mammography.[66,67] However, a recent retrospective cohort study of 1601 BRCA1/2 carriers demonstrated an increased risk of breast cancer (HR1.54, $p = 0.007$) with any reported exposure to chest x-rays, especially in younger women.[68]

Currently, women at high risk are recommended to undergo annual mammography, either from the age of 40 or five years earlier than the age at diagnosis of the youngest breast cancer case in the family, whichever is earlier. For women with proven gene mutations mammographic screening is often considered in the 30s.

5.1.2 Magnetic resonance imaging

Magnetic resonance imaging (MRI) is an emerging screening modality for high risk women because of its high sensitivity.[69–75,76] The American Cancer Society supports annual MRI screening for individuals with a known BRCA mutation, individuals untested but with a first-degree relative with a BRCA mutation and individuals with an estimated lifetime breast cancer risk > 20–25%.[76] The European National Institute for Health and Clinical Excellence (NICE) guidelines recommend annual MRI in similar circumstances and in those with TP53 mutations; a ten-year risk of > 8% (30–39 years of age); or a ten-year risk > 12% with dense breasts on mammography (40–49 years of age).[77]

The high sensitivity of MRI screening is offset to some extent by its low specificity. This results in high false-positive rates, which may result in anxiety and unnecessary biopsy. There is no data on mortality benefits and lead-time bias may be a factor. While further research is needed, many Australian clinicians have begun to adopt the practice of MRI surveillance in high-risk women.

5.1.3 Breast clinical and self-examination

Clinical breast examination (CBE) may be an important adjunct in breast cancer screening in young, high risk women, as it may detect mammographically silent cancers, or may detect interval cancers between mammographic screenings. In addition, CBE is a potentially useful modality when women are pregnant or breast-feeding and other screening modalities are contraindicated. It is generally recommended that CBE be carried out every six to 12 months in high risk women. While there is no evidence of survival benefits from breast self-examinations, women should be encouraged to be aware of how their breasts look and feel, and report any changes promptly.

5.2 *Ovarian cancer screening/surveillance*

Despite mounting evidence from observational studies that it is of no benefit, ovarian screening is sometimes considered for high risk women who have not undergone RRBSO.[78] Screening tests usually consist of trans-vaginal ultrasonography with serum CA125 levels.[78–81] Women who choose ovarian screening rather than RRBSO should be fully informed of the lack of evidence for any benefit.

6. Lifestyle Factors

Lifestyle and environmental factors may modify breast cancer risk, although the effects are modest compared with surgery or chemo-prevention. Current evidence is limited for several reasons. Most studies of modifiers of cancer risk in high risk women have been retrospective, prevalent case-control designs, which have a high likelihood of systematic biases, including recall and survivorship bias. The few prospective studies are small or cobbled together from multiple institutions, using non-systematic and non-uniform follow-up strategies. Non-random loss to follow-up is a major potential source of bias in these studies. Additionally, most studies have focused on mutation carriers rather than the much larger pop-ulation of women who have a strong family history but lack an identified gene mutation.

6.1 *Parity*

Increasing parity and early age at first childbirth are protective in the general population against breast cancer development. While several studies have investigated the effect of parity and age at first birth on breast cancer risk in BRCA1 and BRCA2 mutation carriers, results have been inconsistent.[82–87] However, the advantage of early childbearing for mutation carriers is that it allows earlier use of other effective risk management strategies such as risk-reducing surgery and chemoprevention.

6.2 Breastfeeding

In the general population, a woman's breast cancer risk reduces by about 4% for every 12 months of breastfeeding.[88] Several studies of mutation carriers have shown a reduction in breast cancer risk associated with breastfeeding.[85,86,89] The single study which did not show any risk reduction was inadequately powered to exclude benefit.[84] Women who are at high risk should breastfeed for as long as practical and preferably beyond one year.

6.3 Oral contraceptive use

Use of the combined oral contraceptive pill reduces ovarian cancer risk in the general population and in BRCA1 and BRCA2 mutation carriers. Whether oral contraceptive pill use affects breast cancer in high risk individuals remains controversial. A meta-analysis of 54 studies showed that current oral contraceptive pill use is associated with a 24% increase in breast cancer risk, but the risks were similar for those with and without a family history of breast cancer.[90] Two other studies have not demonstrated a significant effect of oral contraceptive pill use on breast cancer risk in women with a family history.[91,92] Conversely, one study showed a three-fold increase in breast cancer risk among women who used the oral contraceptive pill and had a first-degree relative with breast cancer.[93]

In BRCA mutation carriers, two studies have shown no increase in risk in BRCA1 carriers who used oral contraceptive pills for at least one year[94,95] and one showed an increased risk of about 20% in continual users of the oral contraceptive pill.[96] Of these three studies, two showed no effect of oral contraceptive pills on breast cancer risk in BRCA2 mutations, however one showed an increased risk for BRCA2 carriers after at least five years of use. Thus, at this stage, there is no consistent evidence to suggest that the oral contraceptive pill is either safe or contraindicated in women at high risk for breast cancer.

6.4 Obesity

There is clear evidence in the general population that obesity is associated with significantly increased breast cancer risk.[97,98] Data on the effect of weight control on breast cancer risk in mutation carriers is very limited, however the published data does suggest that this may be an important area of risk management.[99,100]

6.5 Alcohol consumption

Alcohol is clearly associated with breast cancer risk in the general population, with the risk increasing by about 9% per daily standard drink.[101–104] Few studies have addressed the influence of alcohol in high risk women. One study found a 2.4-fold increase in breast cancer risk in daily drinkers with a strong family history of breast cancer.[105] Conversely, the only published study in mutation carriers showed no increased risk of breast cancer associated with alcohol consumption in carriers aged less than 50.[106] Given the other adverse health effects of excessive alcohol, it may be prudent to recommend that high risk women drink no more than one standard drink per day.

7. What about Risk Management in High-Risk Women with Cancer?

Women with a personal diagnosis of breast cancer may be identified as belonging to a high risk family. Risk management for such women should consider the risk for a subsequent breast cancer or ovarian cancer and the competing risk of dying from their prior cancer which would attenuate the prevention benefits. Referral to a family cancer centre for urgent genetic testing may be appropriate in planning both loco-regional and systemic management. For women who carry a mutation in BRCA1 or BRCA2, the risk of a second breast cancer is around 40%[107,108] and ovarian cancer risk is also increased.[109]

The most effective preventative strategy against development of a new breast cancer, in BRCA1/2 positive individuals with a prior history of breast cancer, is complete mastectomy (if the previous operation on the affected breast was less than a mastectomy) with contralateral mastectomy, which reduces the risk of contralateral breast cancer by 90%.[110] In mutation carriers with a low risk of systemic recurrence of their prior breast cancer, this operation should be considered prior to adjuvant breast irradiation, as the latter can limit the reconstructive options. Similarly, RRSO should be considered if the prognosis from the breast cancer is reasonably good; additionally, the subsequent oestrogen deprivation may be an effective adjuvant therapy in pre-menopausal hormone receptor positive women.[111]

Conversely, in women who are at high risk for systemic recurrence, it may be pertinent to wait two to five years before proceeding with risk-reducing surgery, which will be of no benefit if her previous cancer recurs systemically. However, these decisions are complex and should involve the input of experts in breast cancer genetics, the treating oncologist and the woman herself.

If risk-reducing mastectomy is not performed, secondary chemoprevention may be considered. Tamoxifen appears to reduce contralateral breast cancer risk by about 50% in mutation carriers, including BRCA1 carriers (who usually do not receive adjuvant tamoxifen for treatment of their hormone receptor negative breast cancers).[112]

Management of subsequent breast cancer risk in women with prior ovarian cancer will be highly influenced by the stage and prognosis of the ovarian cancer. For women with advanced ovarian cancer, where the five-year survival rates are low (even taking into account the possible better survival from ovarian cancer in BRCA mutation carriers), management of breast cancer risk with screening and/or chemoprevention may be preferable to BRRM, whereas BRRM may be appropriate for women with early stage ovarian cancer.

8.   Conclusion

The management of women at high risk of breast and ovarian cancer is complex and requires individualisation based on a woman's age, childbearing potential, personal risk and wishes. The great promise of predictive genetic testing for cancer predisposition in improving public health will only be realised with widespread implementation of evidence-based risk reduction strategies by the oncology and genetics community.

Acknowledgements

We would like to thank Dr Prue Francis for her critical review of the section of this article pertaining to management of high risk women with prior cancer.

References

1. Australian Institute of Health and Welfare, *Cancer in Australia: An Overview*, available from http://www.aihw.gov.au/publications/can/ca08/ca08.pdf (2008).
2. M. Reedy, H. Gallion, J. M. Fowler, R. Kryscio and S. A. Smith, Contribution of BRCA1 and BRCA2 to familial ovarian cancer: A gynecologic oncology group study, *Gynecol. Oncol.* **85**(2): 255–259 (2002).
3. T. Pal, J. Permuth-Wey, J. A. Betts, J. P. Krischer, J. Fiorica, H. Arango *et al.*, BRCA1 and BRCA2 mutations account for a large proportion of ovarian carcinoma cases, *Cancer* **104**(12): 2807–2816 (2005).
4. A. Antoniou, P. D. Pharoah, S. Narod, H. A. Risch, J. E. Eyfjord, J. L. Hopper *et al.*, Average risks of breast and ovarian cancer associated with BRCA1 or BRCA2 mutations detected in case series unselected for family history: A combined analysis of 22 studies, *Am. J. Hum. Genet.* **72**(5): 1117–1130 (2003).
5. H. A. Risch, J. R. McLaughlin, D. E. Cole, B. Rosen, L. Bradley, E. Kwan *et al.*, Prevalence and penetrance of germline BRCA1 and BRCA2 mutations in a population series of 649 women with ovarian cancer, *Am. J. Hum. Genet.* **68**(3): 700–710 (2001).
6. Y. Antill, M. Shanahan and K.-A. Phillips, The integrated, multidisciplinary clinic: A new model for the ongoing management of women at high genetic risk for breast and ovarian cancer, *Cancer Forum* **29**(2): 107–110 (2005).
7. L. C. Hartmann, T. A. Sellers, D. J. Schaid, T. S. Frank, C. L. Soderberg, D. L. Sitta *et al.*, Efficacy of bilateral prophylactic mastectomy in BRCA1 and BRCA2 gene mutation carriers, *J. Natl. Cancer Inst.* **93**(21): 1633–1637 (2001).

8. L. C. Hartmann, D. J. Schaid, J. E. Woods, T. P. Crotty, J. L. Myers, P. G. Arnold *et al.*, Efficacy of bilateral prophylactic mastectomy in women with a family history of breast cancer, *N. Engl. J. Med.* **340**(2): 77–84 (1999).

9. H. Meijers-Heijboer, B. van Geel, W. L. van Putten, S. C. Henzen-Logmans, C. Seynaeve, M. B. Menke-Pluymers *et al.*, Breast cancer after prophylactic bilateral mastectomy in women with a BRCA1 or BRCA2 mutation, *N. Engl. J. Med.* **345**(3): 159–164 (2001).

10. T. R. Rebbeck, T. Friebel, H. T. Lynch, S. L. Neuhausen, L. van 't Veer, J. E. Garber *et al.*, Bilateral prophylactic mastectomy reduces breast cancer risk in BRCA1 and BRCA2 mutation carriers: the PROSE Study Group, *J. Clin. Oncol.* **22**(6): 1055–1062 (2004).

11. K. A. Metcalfe, J. L. Semple and S. A. Narod, Time to reconsider subcutaneous mastectomy for breast-cancer prevention? *Lancet Oncol.* **6**(6): 431–434 (2005).

12. M. B. Barton, C. N. West, I. L. Liu, E. L. Harris, S. J. Rolnick, J. G. Elmore *et al.*, Complications following bilateral prophylactic mastectomy, *J. Natl. Cancer Inst. Monogr.* **35**: 61–66 (2005).

13. B. A. Heemskerk-Gerritsen, C. T. Brekelmans, M. B. Menke-Pluymers, A. N. van Geel, M. M. Tilanus-Linthorst, C. C. Bartels *et al.*, Prophylactic mastectomy in BRCA1/2 mutation carriers and women at risk of hereditary breast cancer: Long-term experiences at the Rotterdam Family Cancer Clinic, *Ann. Surg. Oncol.* **14**: 3335–3344 (2007).

14. M. H. Frost, D. J. Schaid, T. A. Sellers, J. M. Slezak, P. G. Arnold, J. E. Woods *et al.*, Long-term satisfaction and psychological and social function following bilateral prophylactic mastectomy, *J. Am. Med. Assoc.* **284**(3): 319–324 (2000).

15. M. B. Hatcher, L. Fallowfield and R. A'Hern, The psychosocial impact of bilateral prophylactic mastectomy: Prospective study using questionnaires and semistructured interviews, *Br. Med. J.* **322**(7278): 76 (2001).

16. Y. Antill, J. Reynolds, M. A. Young, J. Kirk, K. Tucker, T. Bogtstra *et al.*, Risk-reducing surgery in women with familial susceptibility for breast and/or ovarian cancer, *Eur. J. Cancer* **42**(5): 621–628 (2006).

17. M. E. Stefanek, K. J. Helzlsouer, P. M. Wilcox and F. Houn, Predictors of and satisfaction with bilateral prophylactic mastectomy, *Prev. Med.* **24**(4): 412–419 (1995).

18. D. K. Payne, C. Biggs, K. N. Tran, P. I. Borgen and M. J. Massie, Women's regrets after bilateral prophylactic mastectomy, *Ann. Surg. Oncol.* **7**(2): 150–154 (2000).

19. S. Wainberg and J. Husted, Utilization of screening and preventive surgery among unaffected carriers of a BRCA1 or BRCA2 gene mutation, *Cancer Epidemiol. Biomarkers Prev.* **13**(12): 1989–1995 (2004).

20. G. J. Mann, H. Thorne, R. L. Balleine, P. N. Butow, C. L. Clarke, E. Edkins *et al.*, Analysis of cancer risk and BRCA1 and BRCA2 mutation prevalence in the kConFab familial breast cancer resource, *Breast Cancer Res.* **8**(1): R12 (2006).

21. K. A. Phillips, M. A. Jenkins, G. J. Lindeman, S. A. McLachlan, J. M. McKinley, P. C. Weideman *et al.*, Risk-reducing surgery, screening and chemoprevention practices of BRCA1 and BRCA2 mutation carriers: a prospective cohort study, *Clin. Genet.* **70**(3): 198–206 (2006).

22. S. M. Domchek, T. M. Friebel, S. L. Neuhausen, T. Wagner, G. Evans, C. Isaacs *et al.*, Mortality after bilateral salpingo-oophorectomy in BRCA1 and BRCA2 mutation carriers: A prospective cohort study, *Lancet Oncol.* **7**(3): 223–229 (2006).

23. J. P. Struewing, P. Watson, D. F. Easton, B. A. Ponder, H. T. Lynch and M. A. Tucker, Prophylactic oophorectomy in inherited breast/ovarian cancer families, *J. Natl. Cancer Inst. Monogr.* **17**: 33–35 (1995).

24. T. R. Rebbeck, H. T. Lynch, S. L. Neuhausen, S. A. Narod, L. Van't Veer, J. E. Garber *et al.*, Prophylactic oophorectomy in carriers of BRCA1 or BRCA2 mutations, *N. Engl. J. Med.* **346**(21): 1616–1622 (2002).

25. J. L. Kramer, I. A. Velazquez, B. E. Chen, P. S. Rosenberg, J. P. Struewing and M. H. Greene, Prophylactic oophorectomy reduces breast cancer penetrance during prospective, long-term follow-up of BRCA1 mutation carriers, *J. Clin. Oncol.* **23**(34): 8629–8635 (2005).

26. A. Eisen, J. Lubinski, J. Klijn, P. Moller, H. T. Lynch, K. Offit *et al.*, Breast cancer risk following bilateral oophorectomy in BRCA1 and BRCA2 mutation carriers: An international case-control study, *J. Clin. Oncol.* **23**(30): 7491–7496 (2005).

27. N. D. Kauff, J. M. Satagopan, M. E. Robson, L. Scheuer, M. Hensley, C. A. Hudis *et al.*, Risk-reducing salpingo-oophorectomy in women with a BRCA1 or BRCA2 mutation, *N. Engl. J. Med.* **346**(21): 1609–1615 (2002).

28. J. K. Tobacman, M. H. Greene, M. A. Tucker, J. Costa, R. Kase and J. F. Fraumeni, Jr., Intra-abdominal carcinomatosis after prophylactic

oophorectomy in ovarian-cancer-prone families, *Lancet* **2**(8302): 795–797 (1982).

29. H. N. Nguyen, H. E. Averette and M. Janicek, Ovarian carcinoma. A review of the significance of familial risk factors and the role of prophylactic oophorectomy in cancer prevention, *Cancer* **74**(2): 545–555 (1994).

30. T. R. Rebbeck, T. Friebel, T. Wagner, H. T. Lynch, J. E. Garber, M. B. Daly *et al.*, Effect of short-term hormone replacement therapy on breast cancer risk reduction after bilateral prophylactic oophorectomy in BRCA1 and BRCA2 mutation carriers: The PROSE Study Group, *J. Clin. Oncol.* **23**(31): 7804–7810 (2005).

31. J. E. Rossouw, G. L. Anderson, R. L. Prentice, A. Z. LaCroix, C. Kooperberg, M. L. Stefanick *et al.*, Risks and benefits of estrogen plus progestin in healthy postmenopausal women: Principal results from the Women's Health Initiative randomized controlled trial, *J. Am. Med. Assoc.* **288**(3): 321–333 (2002).

32. R. T. Chlebowski, S. L. Hendrix, R. D. Langer, M. L. Stefanick, M. Gass, D. Lane *et al.*, Influence of estrogen plus progestin on breast cancer and mammography in healthy postmenopausal women: The Women's Health Initiative Randomized Trial, *J. Am. Med. Assoc.* **289**(24): 3243–3253 (2003).

33. A. S. Whittemore, R. Harris and J. Itnyre, Characteristics relating to ovarian cancer risk: Collaborative analysis of 12 US case-control studies. II. Invasive epithelial ovarian cancers in white women. Collaborative Ovarian Cancer Group, *Am. J. Epidemiol.* **136**(10): 1184–1203 (1992).

34. S. E. Hankinson, D. J. Hunter, G. A. Colditz, W. C. Willett, M. J. Stampfer, B. Rosner *et al.*, Tubal ligation, hysterectomy, and risk of ovarian cancer. A prospective study, *J. Am. Med. Assoc.* **270**(23): 2813–2818 (1993).

35. K. A. Rosenblatt and D. B. Thomas, Reduced risk of ovarian cancer in women with a tubal ligation or hysterectomy. The World Health Organization Collaborative Study of Neoplasia and Steroid Contraceptives, *Cancer Epidemiol. Biomarkers Prev.* **5**(11): 933–935 (1996).

36. S. A. Narod, P. Sun, P. Ghadirian, H. Lynch, C. Isaacs, J. Garber *et al.*, Tubal ligation and risk of ovarian cancer in carriers of BRCA1 or BRCA2 mutations: A case-control study, *Lancet* **357**(9267): 1467–1470 (2001).

37. J. Cuzick, J. Forbes, R. Edwards, M. Baum, S. Cawthorn, A. Coates *et al.*, First results from the International Breast Cancer Intervention Study (IBIS-I): A randomised prevention trial, *Lancet* **360**(9336): 817–824 (2002).

38. B. Fisher, J. P. Costantino, D. L. Wickerham, C. K. Redmond, M. Kavanah, W. M. Cronin *et al.*, Tamoxifen for prevention of breast cancer: Report of the National Surgical Adjuvant Breast and Bowel Project P-1 Study, *J. Natl. Cancer Inst.* **90**(18): 1371–1388 (1998).

39. T. Powles, R. Eeles, S. Ashley, D. Easton, J. Chang, M. Dowsett *et al.*, Interim analysis of the incidence of breast cancer in the Royal Marsden Hospital tamoxifen randomised chemoprevention trial, *Lancet* **352**(9122): 98–101 (1998).

40. U. Veronesi, P. Maisonneuve, A. Costa, V. Sacchini, C. Maltoni, C. Robertson *et al.*, Prevention of breast cancer with tamoxifen: Preliminary findings from the Italian randomised trial among hysterectomised women. Italian Tamoxifen Prevention Study, *Lancet* **352**(9122): 93–97 (1998).

41. J. Cuzick, T. Powles, U. Veronesi, J. Forbes, R. Edwards, S. Ashley *et al.*, Overview of the main outcomes in breast-cancer prevention trials, *Lancet* **361**(9354): 296–300 (2003).

42. P. A. Ganz, S. R. Land, D. L. Wickerham, M. Lee, M. Ritter, V. Vogel *et al.*, The study of tamoxifen and raloxifene (STAR): First report of patient-reported outomes from the NSABP P-2 breast cancer prevention study, *J. Clin. Oncol.* **24**(18S): LBA561 (2006).

43. V. G. Vogel, J. P. Costantino, D. L. Wickerham, W. M. Cronin, R. S. Cecchini, J. N. Atkins *et al.*, Effects of tamoxifen vs raloxifene on the risk of developing invasive breast cancer and other disease outcomes: The NSABP Study of Tamoxifen and Raloxifene (STAR) P-2 trial, *J. Am. Med. Assoc.* **295**(23): 2727–2741 (2006).

44. K. A. Phillips, Breast carcinoma in carriers of BRCA1 or BRCA2 mutations: Implications of proposed distinct histologic phenotypes, *Cancer* **83**(11): 2251–2254 (1998).

45. K. A. Phillips, K. Nichol, H. Ozcelik, J. Knight, S. J. Done, P. J. Goodwin *et al.*, Frequency of p53 mutations in breast carcinomas from Ashkenazi Jewish carriers of BRCA1 mutations, *J. Natl. Cancer Inst.* **91**(5): 469–473 (1999).

46. M. C. King, S. Wieand, K. Hale, M. Lee, T. Walsh, K. Owens *et al.*, Tamoxifen and breast cancer incidence among women with inherited mutations in BRCA1 and BRCA2: National Surgical Adjuvant

Breast and Bowel Project (NSABP-P1) Breast Cancer Prevention Trial, *J. Am. Med. Assoc.* **286**(18): 2251–2256 (2001).

47. W. Li, C. Xiao, B. K. Vonderhaar and C. X. Deng, A role of estrogen/ERalpha signaling in BRCA1-associated tissue-specific tumor formation, *Oncogene* **26**(51): 7204–7212 (2007).

48. L. Hilakivi-Clarke, Estrogens, BRCA1, and breast cancer, *Cancer Res.* **60**(18): 4993–5001 (2000).

49. A. Decensi, D. Serrano, B. Bonanni, M. Cazzaniga and A. Guerrieri-Gonzaga, Breast cancer prevention trials using retinoids, *J. Mammary Gland Biol.* **8**(1): 19–30 (2003).

50. J. Cuzick, Aromatase inhibitors for breast cancer prevention, *J. Clin. Oncol.* **23**(8): 1636–1643 (2005).

51. M. L. Gwinn, N. C. Lee, P. H. Rhodes, P. M. Layde and G. L. Rubin, Pregnancy, breast feeding, and oral contraceptives and the risk of epithelial ovarian cancer, *J. Clin. Epidemiol.* **43**(6): 559–568 (1990).

52. S. Franceschi, F. Parazzini, E. Negri, M. Booth, C. La Vecchia, V. Beral *et al.*, Pooled analysis of 3 European case-control studies of epithelial ovarian cancer: III. Oral contraceptive use, *Int. J. Cancer* **49**(1): 61–65 (1991).

53. S. A. Narod, H. Risch, R. Moslehi, A. Dorum, S. Neuhausen, H. Olsson *et al.*, Oral contraceptives and the risk of hereditary ovarian cancer. Hereditary Ovarian Cancer Clinical Study Group, *N. Engl. J. Med.* **339**(7): 424–428 (1998).

54. V. McGuire, A. Felberg, M. Mills, K. L. Ostrow, R. DiCioccio, E. M. John *et al.*, Relation of contraceptive and reproductive history to ovarian cancer risk in carriers and noncarriers of BRCA1 gene mutations, *Am. J. Epidemiol.* **160**(7): 613–618 (2004).

55. B. Modan, P. Hartge, G. Hirsh-Yechezkel, A. Chetrit, F. Lubin, U. Beller *et al.*, Parity, oral contraceptives, and the risk of ovarian cancer among carriers and noncarriers of a BRCA1 or BRCA2 mutation, *N. Engl. J. Med.* **345**(4): 235–240 (2001).

56. A. S. Whittemore, R. R. Balise, P. D. Pharoah, R. A. Dicioccio, I. Oakley-Girvan, S. J. Ramus *et al.*, Oral contraceptive use and ovarian cancer risk among carriers of BRCA1 or BRCA2 mutations, *Br. J. Cancer* **91**(11): 1911–1915 (2004).

57. R. A. Smith, S. W. Duffy, R. Gabe, L. Tabar, A. M. Yen and T. H. Chen, The randomized trials of breast cancer screening: what have we learned? *Radiol. Clin. North. Am.* **42**(5): 793–806 (2004).

58. L. Nystrom, I. Andersson, N. Bjurstam, J. Frisell, B. Nordenskjold and L. E. Rutqvist, Long-term effects of mammography screening: Updated overview of the Swedish randomised trials, *Lancet* **359**(9310): 909–919 (2002).

59. K. Kerlikowske, D. Grady, J. Barclay, E. A. Sickles, A. Eaton and V. Ernster, Positive predictive value of screening mammography by age and family history of breast cancer, *J. Am. Med. Assoc.* **270**(20): 2444–2450 (1993).

60. D. G. Evans, G. Ribiero, D. Warrell and D. Donnai, Ovarian cancer family and prophylactic choices, *J. Med. Genet.* **29**(6): 416–418 (1992).

61. M. Kriege and J. G. Klijn, Efficacy of MRI and mammography for breast cancer screening in women with genetic predisposition. In: *Educational Book of the American Society of Clinical Oncology Annual Meeting*, Chicago, USA (2007), pp. 135–141.

62. I. K. Komenaka, B. A. Ditkoff, K. A. Joseph, D. Russo, P. Gorroochurn, M. Ward *et al.*, The development of interval breast malignancies in patients with BRCA mutations, *Cancer* **100**(10): 2079–2083 (2004).

63. L. Scheuer, N. Kauff, M. Robson, B. Kelly, R. Barakat, J. Satagopan *et al.*, Outcome of preventive surgery and screening for breast and ovarian cancer in BRCA mutation carriers, *J. Clin. Oncol.* **20**(5): 1260–1268 (2002).

64. K. A. Phillips, Re: biologic characteristics of interval and screen-detected breast cancers, *J. Natl. Cancer Inst.* **93**: 151–152 (2001).

65. M. Jasin, Homologous repair of DNA damage and tumorigenesis: The BRCA connection, *Oncogene* **21**(58): 8981–8993 (2002).

66. S. A. Narod, J. Lubinski, P. Ghadirian, H. T. Lynch, P. Moller, W. D. Foulkes *et al.*, Screening mammography and risk of breast cancer in BRCA1 and BRCA2 mutation carriers: A case-control study, *Lancet Oncol.* **7**(5): 402–406 (2006).

67. D. Goldfrank, S. Chuai, J. L. Bernstein, Y. C. T. Ramon, J. B. Lee, M. C. Alonso *et al.*, Effect of mammography on breast cancer risk in women with mutations in BRCA1 or BRCA2, *Cancer Epidemiol. Biomarkers Prev.* **15**(11): 2311–2313 (2006).

68. N. Andrieu, D. F. Easton, J. Chang-Claude, M. A. Rookus, R. Brohet, E. Cardis *et al.*, Effect of chest X-rays on the risk of breast cancer among BRCA1/2 mutation carriers in the international BRCA1/2 carrier cohort study: A report from the EMBRACE, GENEPSO, GEO-HEBON, and IBCCS Collaborators' Group, *J. Clin. Oncol.* **24**(21): 3361–3366 (2006).

69. E. A. Morris, L. Liberman, D. J. Ballon, M. Robson, A. F. Abramson, A. Heerdt *et al.*, MRI of occult breast carcinoma in a high-risk population, *Am. J. Roentgenol.* **181**(3): 619–626 (2003).

70. A. R. Hartman, B. L. Daniel, A. W. Kurian, M. A. Mills, K. W. Nowels, F. M. Dirbas *et al.*, Breast magnetic resonance image screening and ductal lavage in women at high genetic risk for breast carcinoma, *Cancer* **100**(3): 479–489 (2004).

71. M. Kriege, C. T. Brekelmans, C. Boetes, P. E. Besnard, H. M. Zonderland and I. M. Obdeijn *et al.*, Efficacy of MRI and mammography for breast-cancer screening in women with a familial or genetic predisposition, *N. Engl. J. Med.* **351**(5): 427–437 (2004).

72. E. Warner, D. B. Plewes, K. A. Hill, P. A. Causer, J. T. Zubovits, R. A. Jong *et al.*, Surveillance of BRCA1 and BRCA2 mutation carriers with magnetic resonance imaging, ultrasound, mammography, and clinical breast examination, *J. Am. Med. Assoc.* **292**(11): 1317–1325 (2004).

73. C. D. Lehman, J. D. Blume, P. Weatherall, D. Thickman, N. Hylton, E. Warner *et al.*, Screening women at high risk for breast cancer with mammography and magnetic resonance imaging, *Cancer* **103**(9): 1898–1905 (2005).

74. M. O. Leach, C. R. Boggis, A. K. Dixon, D. F. Easton, R. A. Eeles, D. G. Evans *et al.*, Screening with magnetic resonance imaging and mammography of a UK population at high familial risk of breast cancer: A prospective multicentre cohort study (MARIBS), *Lancet* **365**(9473): 1769–1778 (2005).

75. C. K. Kuhl, S. Schrading, C. C. Leutner, N. Morakkabati-Spitz, E. Wardelmann, R. Fimmers *et al.*, Mammography, breast ultrasound, and magnetic resonance imaging for surveillance of women at high familial risk for breast cancer, *J. Clin. Oncol.* **23**(33): 8469–8476 (2005).

76. D. Saslow, C. Boetes, W. Burke, S. Harms, M. O. Leach, C. D. Lehman *et al.*, American Cancer Society guidelines for breast screening with MRI as an adjunct to mammography, *CA Cancer J. Clin.* **57**(2): 75–89 (2007).

77. Familial breast cancer: The classification and care of women at risk of familial breast cancer in primary, secondary and tertiary care. *Partial Update of NICE Clinical Guideline 41*, National Institute for Health and Clinical Excellence (October 2006).

78. R. Hogg and M. Friedlander, Biology of epithelial ovarian cancer: Implications for screening women at high genetic risk, *J. Clin. Oncol.* **22**(7): 1315–1327 (2004).

79. NIH consensus conference, ovarian cancer. Screening, treatment, and follow-up. NIH Consensus Development Panel on Ovarian Cancer, *J. Am. Med. Assoc.* **273**(6): 491–497 (1995).

80. W. Burke, M. Daly, J. Garber, J. Botkin, M. J. Kahn, P. Lynch *et al.*, Recommendations for follow-up care of individuals with an inherited predisposition to cancer. II. BRCA1 and BRCA2. Cancer Genetics Studies Consortium, *J. Am. Med. Assoc.* **277**(12): 997–1003 (1997).

81. Y. Antill and K. A. Phillips, Ovarian cancer screening for high risk women. In: *Gynecologic Cancer: Controversies in Management*, eds. D. M. W. Gershenson, M. Gore, M. A. Quinn and G. Thomas (Elsevier, Philadelphia, 2004), pp. 341–354.

82. A. C. Antoniou, A. Shenton, E. R. Maher, E. Watson, E. Woodward, F. Lalloo *et al.*, Parity and breast cancer risk among BRCA1 and BRCA2 mutation carriers, *Breast Cancer Res.* **8**(6): R72 (2006).

83. J. Kotsopoulos, J. Lubinski, H. T. Lynch, J. Klijn, P. Ghadirian, S. L. Neuhausen *et al.*, Age at first birth and the risk of breast cancer in BRCA1 and BRCA2 mutation carriers, *Breast Cancer Res. Treat.* **105**(2): 221–228 (2007).

84. N. Andrieu, D. E. Goldgar, D. F. Easton, M. Rookus, R. Brohet, A. C. Antoniou *et al.*, Pregnancies, breast-feeding, and breast cancer risk in the International BRCA1/2 Carrier Cohort Study (IBCCS), *J. Natl. Cancer Inst.* **98**(8): 535–544 (2006).

85. J. Gronwald, T. Byrski, T. Huzarski, C. Cybulski, P. Sun, A. Tulman *et al.*, Influence of selected lifestyle factors on breast and ovarian cancer risk in BRCA1 mutation carriers from Poland, *Breast Cancer Res. Treat.* **95**(2): 105–109 (2006).

86. L. Tryggvadottir, E. J. Olafsdottir, S. Gudlaugsdottir, S. Thorlacius, J. G. Jonasson, H. Tulinius *et al.*, BRCA2 mutation carriers, reproductive factors and breast cancer risk, *Breast Cancer Res.* **5**(5): R121–R128 (2003).

87. C. A. Cullinane, J. Lubinski, S. L. Neuhausen, P. Ghadirian, H. T. Lynch, C. Isaacs *et al.*, Effect of pregnancy as a risk factor for breast cancer in BRCA1/BRCA2 mutation carriers, *Int. J. Cancer* **117**(6): 988–991 (2005).

88. Collaborative Group on Hormonal Factors in Breast Cancer, Breast cancer and breastfeeding: Collaborative reanalysis of individual data from 47 epidemiological studies in 30 countries, including 50302 women with breast cancer and 96973 women without the disease, *Lancet* **360**(9328): 187–195 (2002).

89. H. Jernstrom, J. Lubinski, H. T. Lynch, P. Ghadirian, S. Neuhausen, C. Isaacs *et al.*, Breast-feeding and the risk of breast cancer in BRCA1 and BRCA2 mutation carriers, *J. Natl. Cancer Inst.* **96**(14): 1094–1098 (2004).

90. Collaborative Group on Hormonal Factors in Breast Cancer, Breast cancer and hormonal contraceptives: Collaborative reanalysis of individual data on 53297 women with breast cancer and 100239 women without breast cancer from 54 epidemiological studies, *Lancet* **347**(9017): 1713–1727 (1996).

91. S. A. Silvera, A. B. Miller and T. E. Rohan, Oral contraceptive use and risk of breast cancer among women with a family history of breast cancer: A prospective cohort study, *Cancer Causes Control* **16**(9): 1059–1063 (2005).

92. G. A. Colditz, B. A. Rosner and F. E. Speizer, Risk factors for breast cancer according to family history of breast cancer. For the Nurses' Health Study Research Group, *J. Natl. Cancer Inst.* **88**(6): 365–371 (1996).

93. D. M. Grabrick, L. C. Hartmann, J. R. Cerhan, R. A. Vierkant, T. M. Therneau, C. M. Vachon *et al.*, Risk of breast cancer with oral contraceptive use in women with a family history of breast cancer, *J. Am. Med. Assoc.* **284**(14): 1791–1798 (2000).

94. R. L. Milne, J. A. Knight, E. M. John, G. S. Dite, R. Balbuena, A. Ziogas *et al.*, Oral contraceptive use and risk of early-onset breast cancer in carriers and noncarriers of BRCA1 and BRCA2 mutations, *Cancer Epidemiol. Biomarkers Prev.* **14**(2): 350–356 (2005).

95. R. W. Haile, D. C. Thomas, V. McGuire, A. Felberg, E. M. John, R. L. Milne *et al.*, BRCA1 and BRCA2 mutation carriers, oral contraceptive use, and breast cancer before age 50, *Cancer Epidemiol. Biomarkers Prev.* **15**(10): 1863–1870 (2006).

96. S. A. Narod, M. P. Dube, J. Klijn, J. Lubinski, H. T. Lynch, P. Ghadirian *et al.*, Oral contraceptives and the risk of breast cancer in BRCA1 and BRCA2 mutation carriers, *J. Natl. Cancer Inst.* **94**(23): 1773–1779 (2002).

97. C. M. Friedenreich, Review of anthropometric factors and breast cancer risk, *Eur. J. Cancer Prev.* **10**(1): 15–32 (2001).

98. S. Loi, R. L. Milne, M. L. Friedlander, M. R. McCredie, G. G. Giles, J. L. Hopper *et al.*, Obesity and outcomes in premenopausal and postmenopausal breast cancer. *Cancer Epidemiol. Biomarkers Prev.* **14**(7): 1686–1691 (2005).

99. J. Kotsopoulos, O. I. Olopado, P. Ghadirian, J. Lubinski, H. T. Lynch, C. Isaacs *et al.*, Changes in body weight and the risk of breast cancer in BRCA1 and BRCA2 mutation carriers, *Breast Cancer Res.* **7**(5): R833–R843 (2005).

100. A. Nkondjock, A. Robidoux, Y. Paredes, S. A. Narod and P. Ghadirian, Diet, lifestyle and BRCA-related breast cancer risk among French-Canadians, *Breast Cancer Res. Treat.* **98**(3): 285–294 (2006).

101. S. A. Smith-Warner, D. Spiegelman, S. S. Yaun, P. A. van den Brandt, A. R. Folsom, R. A. Goldbohm *et al.*, Alcohol and breast cancer in women: A pooled analysis of cohort studies, *J. Am. Med. Assoc.* **279**(7): 535–540 (1998).

102. A. Schatzkin and M. P. Longnecker, Alcohol and breast cancer. Where are we now and where do we go from here? *Cancer* **74** (Suppl. 3): 1101–1110 (1994).

103. M. P. Longnecker, Alcoholic beverage consumption in relation to risk of breast cancer: Meta-analysis and review, *Cancer Causes Control* **5**(1): 73–82 (1994).

104. R. C. Ellison, Y. Zhang, C. E. McLennan and K. J. Rothman, Exploring the relation of alcohol consumption to risk of breast cancer, *Am. J. Epidemiol.* **154**(8): 740–747 (2001).

105. C. M. Vachon, J. R. Cerhan, R. A. Vierkant and T. A. Seller, Investigation of an interaction of alcohol intake and family history on breast cancer risk in the Minnesota Breast Cancer Family Study, *Cancer* **92**(2): 240–248 (2001).

106. V. McGuire, E. M. John, A. Felberg, R. W. Haile, N. F. Boyd, D. C. Thomas *et al.*, No increased risk of breast cancer associated with alcohol consumption among carriers of BRCA1 and BRCA2 mutations ages < 50 years, *Cancer Epidemiol. Biomarkers Prev.* **15**(8): 1565–1567 (2006).

107. K. Metcalfe, H. T. Lynch, P. Ghadirian, N. Tung, I. Olivotto, E. Warner *et al.*, Contralateral breast cancer in BRCA1 and BRCA2 mutation carriers, *J. Clin. Oncol.* **22**(12): 2328–2335 (2004).

108. Y. M. Kirova, D. Stoppa-Lyonnet, A. Savignoni, B. Sigal-Zafrani, N. Fabre and A. Fourquet, Risk of breast cancer recurrence and contralateral breast cancer in relation to BRCA1 and BRCA2 mutation status following breast-conserving surgery and radiotherapy, *Eur. J. Cancer* **41**(15): 2304–2311 (2005).

109. D. Ford, D. F. Easton, D. T. Bishop, S. A. Narod and D. E. Goldgar, Risks of cancer in BRCA1-mutation carriers. Breast Cancer Linkage Consortium, *Lancet* **343**(8899): 692–695 (1994).

110. T. C. van Sprundel, M. K. Schmidt, M. A. Rookus, R. Brohet, C. J. van Asperen, E. J. Rutgers *et al.*, Risk reduction of contralateral breast cancer and survival after contralateral prophylactic mastectomy in BRCA1 or BRCA2 mutation carriers, *Br. J. Cancer* **93**(3): 287–292 (2005).

111. B. Wirk, The role of ovarian ablation in the management of breast cancer, *Breast J.* **11**(6): 416–424 (2005).

112. J. Gronwald, N. Tung, W. D. Foulkes, K. Offit, R. Gershoni, M. Daly *et al.*, Tamoxifen and contralateral breast cancer in BRCA1 and BRCA2 carriers: An update, *Int. J. Cancer* **118**(9): 2281–2284 (2006).

113. Genetic risk assessment and BRCA mutation testing for breast and ovarian cancer susceptibility: Recommendation statement, *Ann. Intern. Med.* **143**(5): 355–361 (2005).

114. *Clinical Practice Guidelines for the Management of Women with Epithelial Ovarian Cancer*, National Breast Cancer Centre, Camperdown, NSW (2004).

115. M. Robson and K. Offit, Clinical practice. Management of an inherited predisposition to breast cancer, *N. Engl. J. Med.* **357**(2): 154–162 (2007).

116. L. Kasprzak, W. D. Foulkes and A. N. Shelling, Fortnightly review: Hereditary ovarian carcinoma, *Br. Med. J.* **318**(7186): 786–789 (1999).

40

Management of High Genetic Risk Bowel Cancer*

Barbara Leggett

Abstract

The identification and appropriate genetic counselling of individuals at high genetic risk of bowel cancer is an excellent example of how improved understanding of the genetic basis of disease can lead to reduction in morbidity and mortality. The key to good management is to make as accurate a diagnosis of the family syndrome as possible, since different syndromes require different surveillance regimens. Diagnosis requires not only verification of cancer diagnoses in the family, but also consideration of the number and types of polyps detected at colonoscopy and in colectomy specimens. In addition, assays to detect microsatellite instability in cancer specimens aid in the diagnosis of Lynch syndrome. Since so much can be done to prevent cancer developing in at risk individuals, a major challenge in the future is how best to disseminate knowledge within a family and how to encourage compliance with appropriate surveillance.

Keywords: Colorectal cancer, polyposis, Lynch syndrome, HNPCC.

* This article was first published in *Cancer Forum: Clinical Cancer Genetics*, Vol. 31, No. 3, November 2007 (by Cancer Council Australia). Reproduced with permission from the authors and publishers.

1.   Introduction

Bowel cancer offers an opportunity for prevention available for virtually no other solid tumours. Not only can mortality be reduced by early detection of cancer, but in many cases the very occurrence of cancer can be greatly reduced without major surgery. This is because the disease develops in pre-malignant polyps which can be removed during surveillance colonoscopy, upper endoscopy and enteroscopy. Even in cases where the polyps are too numerous to safely control endoscopically, they can be identified in the pre-malignant phase and appropriate surgery planned electively.

However endoscopic procedures are relatively invasive and carry some risk of morbidity and mortality. To use them appropriately in individuals at high genetic risk requires understanding of the natural history of the various genetic syndromes. Most polyps are adenomas and occur predominantly in the colon and rectum. They generally take between 5 and 15 years to evolve into invasive cancer. Thus for individuals with a moderately increased risk of bowel cancer without the features of the specific genetic syndromes discussed below, colonoscopy every 5 years is appropriate to interrupt the natural history and greatly reduce the risk of cancer. If polyps are identified, increased frequency of colonoscopy may be appropriate according to published guidelines.[1] For all the specific inherited susceptibility syndromes discussed below, the natural history of the polyps differs significantly from the above. Thus the first and most important step in recommending appropriate surveillance is to make the most accurate diagnosis possible based on the verified clinical history of as many family members as possible, and include consideration not only of cancers but also the numbers, location and histological characteristics of polyps. This may be confirmed by finding a causative germline mutation in an affected family member, but if the family has convincing clinical features of a genetic syndrome, a negative mutation search in a definitely affected family member should be regarded as "inconclusive" rather than negative, and the family should be managed according to the clinical diagnosis with periodic attempts to clarify the mutation status as technology and knowledge advances.

2. Familial Adenomatous Polyposis (FAP)

In classical FAP, individuals develop over 100 and often thousands of adenomatous polyps in the second and third decade of life.[2] Although each individual polyp is no more likely than any other adenoma to progress to cancer, the sheer numbers of adenomas and the early onset mean that colorectal cancer is virtually inevitable, with an average age of onset of 39 years. Adenomas also occur in the duodenum and periampullary adenocarcinoma is the most common threat to life in patients who have undergone colectomy.[3] Patients are also at risk of other extracolonic tumours, including intra-abdominal fibromatosis (desmoid tumours), papillary carcinoma of the thyroid and hepatoblastoma, but the lifetime risk of these is relatively low and there is no evidence to support screening.

FAP is due to mutation in the *APC* tumour suppressor gene and is inherited as an autosomal dominant trait with very high penetrance. About 30% of cases are due to *de novo* mutations.[4] Mutation searching is successful in over 85% of families. There is some genotype-phenotype correlation in classical FAP but there is heterogeneity in clinical course even between family members with the same mutation and thus identification of the exact mutation is of limited value in planning management.

The recommended surveillance protocol for at risk individuals is flexible sigmoidoscopy annually or biennially from age 12–15 years to at least age 30–35 years.[5] Once polyps are identified prophylactic colectomy is planned. Appropriate surgical options are either total colectomy and ileorectal anastomosis or restorative proctocolectomy with pouch formation. Lifetime surveillance of the rectum or pouch is needed because of the ongoing risk of cancer. If the causative mutation has been identified in the family, predictive testing is usually offered at the age at which flexible sigmoidoscopy screening would commence. Mutation positive individuals should then undergo annual sigmoidoscopy and surgery is not planned until there is pathological confirmation of the development of adenomas. Regular upper endoscopy to identify duodenal adenomas is advised after age 25.[5] Management of duodenal polyposis is very challenging, as it is technically difficult to remove the polyps endoscopically and duodenectomy may be associated with high morbidity and mortality. Management of such patients should be in a tertiary centre.

It is now recognised that certain *APC* mutations result in an attenuated phenotype, where individuals develop less than 100 adenomas, onset is at a later age and adenomas tend to be flat and may only be present in the proximal colon.[2] The lifetime risk of colorectal cancer is very high. Surveillance needs to be with colonoscopy, rather than flexible sigmoidoscopy, since significant adenomas may be present in the proximal colon when none have developed distally. Because of the later age of onset surveillance does not usually need to commence until age 18. In some cases prophylactic surgery can be avoided if polyp numbers remain low enough for the colonoscopist to be confident that all adenomas can be removed at each colonoscopy but this decision needs to be individualised. Patients are also at risk of duodenal adenomas.

3.   MYH-Associated Polyposis

The phenotype of this autosomal recessive condition mimics attenuated FAP. This is not surprising, since the molecular defect is biallelic inactivating germline mutations in the base excision repair gene *MYH*, which normally produces a protein which repairs G to T transversions in the *APC* gene.[2] Thus individuals with this genetic defect frequently inactivate APC in colonocytes and develop large numbers of adenomas at a young age. Affected or at risk individuals need to be managed as described above for attenuated FAP. Generally genetic testing is only offered for the common mutations but more extensive mutation searching is worthwhile especially in individuals with a typical clinical picture and who are heterozygous for a common mutation.

3.1 *Hereditary nonpolyposis colorectal cancer (HNPCC)/Lynch syndrome*

The natural history of colorectal carcinogenesis is fundamentally different in HNPCC, as compared to that described above in moderate risk families, FAP and MYH-associated polyposis.[6] Despite its name, cancer does develop in polyps in this syndrome but rather than there being a vast excess of adenomas, individual adenomas in individuals with HNPCC have a much greater risk of rapidly developing into invasive cancer. The estimated risk of colorectal cancer in affected individuals is approximately 70% by age 70 years and about two-thirds of cancers are in the proximal colon, unlike sporadic colorectal cancers which are more common distally.[7] Development of multiple primary cancers is common. The estimated life time risk for affected women developing endometrial cancer is 40–60%.[7] There is also an increased risk of cancers of the small intestine, ovary, hepatobiliary system, kidney and ureter.

HNPCC is an autosomal dominant condition, due to germline mutation in one of the family of DNA mismatch repair genes. Most families have mutations in *MLH1* or *MSH2*, but a significant minority have mutations in *MSH6* or *PMS2*. Unlike FAP *de novo* mutations are very rare and there is nearly always a family history of the disease if the family history is truly known. Mutation of *MSH6* is associated with a somewhat lower risk of colorectal cancer with a later age of onset but the risks of endometrial cancer are at least as high as for the other genetic defects.[7] Dysfunction of the mismatch repair system leads to defective repair of mutations occurring during normal cell division and thus in susceptible tissues, such as colonic polyps, somatic mutations occur in important cancer related genes and cancer rapidly develops.

In cancers that develop due to defective DNA mismatch repair, repetitive DNA sequences known as microsatellites are especially prone to accumulate mutations and microsatellite instability (MSI) can be assayed in cancer tissue as a biomarker of HNPCC. Interpretation of MSI results needs to include an understanding that 10% of sporadic colorectal cancers exhibit MSI due to somatic inactivation of *MLH1*. Interestingly both HNPCC and sporadic colorectal cancers which display a high level of MSI have distinctive histological features, including mucinous histology, poor differentiation and tumour infiltrating lymphocytes.[8] Deficiency in mismatch repair in cancer tissue can also be assayed by performing immunohistochemistry for MLH1, MSH2, MSH6 and PMS2 proteins. Absence of one of these proteins indicates mismatch repair deficiency. Since these proteins act as heterodimers and loss of one partner destabilises the other protein, loss of MLH1 is accompanied by secondary loss of PMS2 and loss of MSH2 by secondary loss of MSH6. The results of MSI testing correlate very closely with immunohistochemistry although occasionally a protein may be detectable on staining despite being dysfunctional.[9]

The ability to test cancer tissue for MSI is very useful in diagnosing HNPCC, since the phenotype of an individual patient is much less distinctive than in any of the polyposis syndromes. Before the genetic defect was understood, the Amsterdam criteria, which specify a very strong family history of colorectal cancer with early age of onset and autosomal dominant inheritance, were used as a diagnostic tool.[7] However many HNPCC families do not meet these criteria, especially if the family size is small, and some families with other, as yet not understood genetic predispositions do meet them. It is now recommended that MSI and/or immunohistochemistry be performed on the cancers of a much broader range of individuals who have some indication of possible HNPCC.[5,7,10,11] These criteria have been formalised into the Bethesda criteria as outlined in Fig. 1.[11] In 2006 the Royal College of Pathologists of Australasia issued a position statement recommending there be no requirement for additional consent or genetic counselling prior to performing MSI or immunohistochemistry for mismatch repair proteins. If this testing indicates HNPCC is likely in an individual meeting the Bethesda criteria, they should then be offered genetic counselling

Bethesda Guidelines

1. CRC under 50 years.
2. Synchronous or metachronous CRC (or other HNPCC-associated cancer) regardless of age.
3. CRC with MSI-H histology under age 60.
4. CRC with one first degree relative with CRC or other HNPCC-associated cancer with one of the cancers being diagnosed under 50 years.
5. CRC with two or more first or second degree relatives with CRC or other HNPCC-associated cancers regardless of age.

Figure 1. Guidelines for patients whose cancers should be tested for MSI to identify possible HNPCC (Lynch Syndrome).

and further investigation to confirm the diagnosis for other high risk families. If a family is referred directly to a genetic service with a history suggestive of HNPCC, archival cancer material on affected family members will be retrospectively tested to help confirm the diagnosis before a mutation search is undertaken. Immunohistochemistry is especially helpful in this regard since it indicates which gene is likely to be mutated.

Once a family has been diagnosed as transmitting HNPCC, all affected individuals and those at risk of the disease should be offered surveillance. If the germline mutation has been identified those at risk can be offered predictive testing so that only those carrying the mutation need continue with surveillance. Surveillance should be by colonoscopy to the caecum annually or at least once every two years beginning at age 25 or five years younger than the youngest affected family member (whichever is the earliest).[5,7] This frequent screening is essential to prevent interval cancers, which would otherwise occur due to the different mechanism of carcinogenesis in HNPCC. Individuals with HNPCC often develop cancer in very small recently formed adenomas. There is no evidence that CT colography ('virtual colonoscopy') is a safe alternative, as it is known to have poor sensitivity for small polyps. The efficacy of screening for extracolonic cancers has not been demonstrated, but it is generally recommended that patients be offered the following tests annually:

— transvaginal ultrasound from age 30 to 35 with endometrial sampling if there is endometrial thickening;
— CA–125 measurement (after the menopause); and
— consideration of upper endoscopy in families where upper GI tract cancers have occurred.

If an individual with HNPCC presents with a colorectal cancer, consideration should be given to total colectomy and ileorectal anastomosis, because of the high risk of metachronous cancer. In addition, if the patient is female and past childbearing years prophylactic hysterectomy and oophorectomy should be discussed. However these decisions need to be individualised according to co-morbidities and patient preference.

4.   Juvenile Polyposis

This is a rare condition characterised by the histologically distinctive juvenile polyp with cystically dilated tubules embedded in abundant lamina propria. The epithelium lining the tubules and covering the surface of the polyp is normal, but when the polyps are numerous and longstanding there is a significant risk of malignancy. All the malignancies associated with the condition occur in the gastrointestinal tract but are not confined to the colon.[12] It is inherited as an autosomal dominant condition with variable penetrance and is genetically heterogeneous. The two genetic causes defined so far are mutations in *SMAD4* and *BMPR1A* and interestingly both these genetic defects would be expected to disrupt the TGF beta signalling pathway. A closely related but distinct disorder is Cowden syndrome, due to mutations in *PTEN.* Although some of the polyps in Cowden syndrome may have the histology of juvenile polyps, the majority of polyps do not. There is essentially no risk of GI malignancy in Cowden's syndrome which is instead associated with breast and thyroid cancer.

It is recommended that patients at risk of juvenile polyposis start having colonoscopy from age 15 or earlier if symptomatic.[12] Upper endoscopy and even capsule endoscopy should be considered, especially if there is a family history of gastric or small bowel cancer.[13] If possible all polyps should be removed and if they are too numerous, surgery should be considered especially if polyps start to show dysplasia.

5.   Peutz–Jeghers Syndrome

This rare syndrome is also characterised by a particular histological type of polyp, in which there is prominent hypertrophy of the smooth muscle layer, which extends and branches up towards the epithelium which does not usually show dysplasia. Polyps are most common in the small intestine and in addition to conferring a risk of malignancy, they are associated with acute bowel obstruction. There are extraintestinal manifestations, including mucocutaneous pigmentation on the lips and an increased risk of breast, pancreatic, ovarian and testicular cancers.[14] It is an autosomal dominant condition and in many families is due to mutation in *STK11* (*LKB1*). *De novo* mutations are common, so there may be no family history. Surveillance with regular colonoscopy and endoscopy should commence in the late teens or earlier if there are symptoms. A most important aspect of management is surveillance for small intestinal polyps beyond the reach of the endoscope and capsule endoscopy followed by push enteroscopy has made a major contribution to better management of these patients.

6.   Hyperplastic Polyposis

This increasingly recognised syndrome is characterised by multiple (> 20), large (> 1cm) and proximal hyperplastic polyps.[15] It is now recognised that this syndrome confers a high risk of colorectal cancer and this has prompted a review of the pathological classification of hyperplastic polyps which were previously thought to have no malignant potential. It is now recognised that the polyps occurring in this syndrome are in fact a particular form of serrated polyp, named a sessile serrated adenoma.[16] This syndrome is associated with a marked tendency to hypermethylation of the CpG islands in the promoters of key cancer-associated genes. Many of the cancers have silenced *MLH1* by hypermethylation of its promoter and are thus show a high level of MSI. However this condition is distinct from HNPCC (Lynch syndrome) and screening for a germline mutation in *MLH1* is not productive.[5]

In many cases of hyperplastic polyposis, there is no family history of polyposis or even of colorectal cancer and the genetic aetiology of the condition is unclear. No predictive genetic testing can be offered at present. It seems likely that the polyps precede development of cancer by several years and thus it is recommended that first degree relatives be offered screening as for moderate risk families (five-yearly colonoscopy from ten years younger than the youngest affected subject in the family).[5] Management of affected individuals is complex and clear guidelines are only recently emerging. It is recommended that sessile serrated adenomas be completely removed endoscopically and that colonoscopy be repeated every one to two years if the subject meets the definition of hyperplastic polyposis (> 20 polyps).[5,16] The risk of cancer increases if the polyps show dysplasia and in these subjects and those in whom polyps are too numerous to be safely removed during colonoscopy, colectomy and ileo-rectal anastomosis should be considered.

7.   Conclusion

Bowel cancer offers great opportunities for cancer prevention, as pre-malignant polyps can be removed, or risk reducing elective surgery planned before malignant transformation occurs. While for individuals at moderately increased risk of colorectal cancer, five-yearly colonoscopy is an appropriate surveillance strategy; in specific inherited susceptibility syndromes, considerations of appropriate surveillance should include a thorough clinical history of as many family members as possible and consideration of the numbers, location and histological characteristics of polyps. If the family has convincing clinical features of a genetic syndrome, a negative mutation search in a definitely affected family member should be regarded as 'inconclusive,' rather than negative and periodic attempts to clarify the mutation status need to be made, in line with advancements in technology and scientific knowledge.

References

1. S. J. Winawer, A. G. Zauber, R. H. Fletcher, J. S. Stillman, M. J. O'Brien, B. Levin *et al*. Guidelines for colonoscopy sureveillance after polypectomy: A consensus update by the US Multi-Society Task Force on Colorectal Cancer and the American Cancer Society, *Gastroenterology* **130**: 1872–1875 (2006).
2. J. R. Jass, What's new in hereditary colorectal cancer? *Arch. Pathol. Lab. Med.* **129**: 1380–1384 (2005).
3. M. L. Aravantid, D. G. Jagelman, A. Romania, V. W. Fazio, I. C. Lavery and E. McGannon, Mortality in patients with familial adenomatous polyposis. *Dis. Colon Rectum* **33**: 639–642 (1990).
4. P. Rozen and F. Macrae, Familial adenomatous polyposis: the practical applications of clinical and molecular screening, *Familial Cancer* **5**: 227–235 (2006).
5. Australian Cancer Network Colorectal Cancer Guidelines Revision Committee, *Guidelines for the Prevention, Early Detection and Management of Colorectal Cancer*, The Cancer Council Australia and Australian Cancer Network, Sydney (2005).

6. K. W. Kinzler and B. Vogelstein, Lessons from hereditary colorectal cancer, *Cell* **87**: 159–170 (1996).

7. N. M. Lindor, G. M. Petersen, D. W. Hadley, A. Y. Kinney, S. Miesfeldt, K. H. Lu *et al.*, Recommendations for the care of individuals with an inherited predisposition to Lynch syndrome, *J. Am. Med. Assoc.* **296**: 1507–1517 (2006).

8. J. R. Jass, K.-A. Do, L. A. Simms, H. Iino, C. Wynter, S. P. Pillay *et al.*, Morphology of sporadic colorectal cancer with DNA replication errors, *Gut* **42**: 673–679 (1998).

9. N. M. Lindor, L. J. Burgart, O. Leontovich, R. M. Goldberg, J. M. Cunningham, D. J. Sargent *et al.*, Immunohistochemistry versus microsatellite instability testing in phenotyping colorectal tumours, *J. Clin. Oncol.* **20**: 1043–1048 (2002).

10. M. C. Southey, M. A. Jenkins, L. Mead, J. Whitty, M. Trivett, A. A. Tesoriero *et al.*, Use of molecular tumor characteristics to prioritize mismatch repair gene testing in early-onset colorectal cancer, *J. Clin. Oncol.* **23**: 1–9 (2005).

11. A. Umar, C. R. Boland, J. P. Terdiman, S. Syngal, A. de la Chapelle, J. Ruschoff *et al.* Revised Bethesda guidelines for hereditary nonpoly-posis colorectal cancer (Lynch syndrome) and microsatellite instability, *J. Natl. Cancer Inst.* **96**: 261–268 (2004).

12. E. Chow and F. Macrae, Review of juvenile polyposis syndrome, *J. Gastroenterol. Hepatol.* **20**: 1634–1640 (2005).

13. B. A. Leggett, L. R. Thomas, N. Knight, S. Healey, G. Chenevix-Trench and J. Searle, Hereditary juvenile polyposis is not due to a defect in the APC or MCC genes, *Gastroenterology* **105**: 1313–1316 (1993).

14. B. A. Leggett, J. P. Young and M. Barker, Peutz-Jeghers syndrome: Genetic screening, *Expert Rev. Anticancer Ther.* **3**: 518–524 (2003).

15. E. Chow, L. Lipton, E. Lynch, R. D'Souza, C. Aragona, L. Hodgkin *et al.*, Hyperplastic polyposis syndrome: Phenotypic presentations and the role of *MBD4* and *MYH*, *Gastroenterology* **131**: 30–39 (2006).

16. D. C. Snover, J. R. Jass, C. Fenoglio-Preiser and K. P. Batts, Serrated polyps of the large intestine, *Am. J. Clin. Pathol.* **124**: 380–391 (2005).

41

Hereditary Mutations and Cancer Management

Alison H. Trainer and
Robyn Ward

Abstract

Over the last decade, our capacity to dissect out and identify different tissue-specific tumour subtypes has greatly expanded. The ability to classify tumours on their molecular and biochemical characteristics has already delivered improved prognostic models for some common tumours like breast cancers. The development of sophisticated tumour classification systems is a first step towards developing treatments which are tailored at the patient-specific level — so-called personalised medicine.

In addition, our ability to identify the small population of tumours that have arisen due to a familial genetic predisposition has fundamentally altered our approach to the identification and management of these cases. In the future, it is anticipated that germline testing for cancer pre-disposition mutations will be routinely performed in some individuals at the time of their initial diagnosis in order to estimate their risk of tumour recurrence and predict their response to therapy. In this scenario, germline genetic testing would move from the domain of a family cancer clinic to the routine clinical setting.

Keywords: Tumour testing, BRCA, mismatch repair, colorectal cancer, breast cancer.

1. Tumour Evolution as an Indicator of a Germline Cancer Susceptibility Mutation

In the clinical setting, individuals who develop cancer are divided into two groups: those who have a family history of a similar or associated cancer, and those who do not. The distinction between these two groups forms the basis of the current familial cancer service, by helping to identify families and individuals at increased risk of developing tissue-specific cancers.

Over the last decade an increasing body of evidence has shown that tumours arising due to a familial predisposition have distinctive molecular and biochemical characteristics. An individual with a tumour displaying these specific attributes warrants referral to a familial cancer service for consideration of germline mutation testing, regardless of his or her family history. It is also recognised that this tumour specific information may carry prognostic information and also determine the sensitivity of the tumour to various treatments.

Tumour cells display an aberrant cellular genome indicative of current or previous genomic instability. This instability can arise at different levels: abnormal chromosome number or structure, loss or amplification of chromosomal regions and nucleotide sequence variations, deletions or insertions. These DNA sequence changes are often accompanied by gross perturbations in the epigenetic state of the genome. These epigenetic changes are often associated with alterations in the pattern of DNA methylation, specifically inappropriate hypermethylation of gene promoters, accompanied by widespread genomic demethylation. Abnormal DNA methylation, together with changes in chromatin packaging, can adversely affect the regulation of gene expression without an underlying change in the DNA sequence. Since these changes functionally mimic genomic alterations, they are often called 'epimutations'.

The fundamental importance of DNA repair pathways in ensuring genomic stability and thus protecting against malignant transformation is evidenced by the high cancer susceptibility seen in those individuals with a germline mutation in genes associated with the recognition (ATM[1]) or repair (BRCA1,[2] BRCA2,[3] and the mismatch repair genes[4]) of DNA damage.

Through the accumulation of these genetic and epigenetic alterations, tumour cells slowly evolve, often through a pre-malignant stage, until they develop six major characteristics which allow them to grow independent of normal tissue and cellular restraints.[5] The sequence or mechanisms by which these end-points are achieved vary within and across tissue-specific tumour types.

The pathways involved in the evolution of a specific tumour can be surmised by analysing the resultant cancer at five inter-locking levels:

1) chromosome number and structure;
2) DNA sequence and chromatin context;
3) gene expression profile;
4) protein levels; and
5) functional pathway readouts.

Access to the technology required to undertake these analyses varies greatly between the research setting and routine clinical diagnostic service provision.

Based on the results from these molecular and biochemical approaches, tumours of similar histopathological classification can be separated and grouped into subtypes depending on their under-lying evolutionary pattern. The important clinical significance of this approach lies in our increasing ability to recognise evolutio-nary tumour patterns that are associated with germline mutations in cancer predisposition genes. Increasingly, the information gleaned though this approach is used to identify new therapeutic targets, or treatments which are applicable not only to the rare indi-viduals who have developed cancer as a result of a germline mutation in cancer predisposition genes, but also to the larger pop-ulation of individuals whose cancers, although not due to familial predisposition, have evolved through similar evolutionary path-ways at the somatic level.

This information could fundamentally change the way that familial cancer service provision is offered. In the future it may be placed at the heart not only of familial risk assessment strate-gies, but also as an arbiter of treatment options for the affected individual.

2. Identification of Individuals with Germline Cancer Predisposition Mutations

Classically, familial cancer services identify families with an increased predisposition to cancer by merit of the number of affected individuals within multigenerational families, and the early age of onset of their cancers. This approach is biased towards large families with good communication skills, and against small families, non paternity or adoption, and newly arisen mutations or low penetrant alleles. More importantly, it is fundamentally a retrospective diagnosis, only possible once multiple members of the family have already developed cancer. It is also limited by numerous administrative hurdles, including access to clinical records for tumour verification, consent and confidentiality issues. Once a family has been identified, germline testing is only possible if there is a living affected individual who wishes to pursue this option. Additional problems include the presence of individuals with sporadic tumours within a family with a genetic predisposition and non-guaranteed access to the most appropriate person for mutation screening. Taken together this means that expensive genetic testing services are often used sub-optimally.

Interestingly, and indeed worryingly for the family history-dependent model of familial cancer service provision, in population series of breast cancer patients, 30–50% of women with an identified BRCA mutation had either no significant family history of the condition, or the family history was not known to the patient at the time of her diagnosis.[6-8]

From a clinical prospective, a functional, reliable and cost-effective screen for individuals with a heterozygous cancer susceptibility gene mutation would be invaluable, but to date, no non-cancerous heterozygote phenotype has been identified.[9,10] However, in keeping with Knudson's two hit hypothesis,[11] the majority of tumours within this population arise through loss of the wildtype allele in the tumour. Assays to detect loss of gene function within the tumour are more robust and easily translated into the clinical setting.

This model of targeting germline genetic tests to individuals on the basis of their tumour phenotype has many clinical advantages. Firstly and most importantly, it means only one individual need develop cancer for a familial genetic diagnosis to be possible. Secondly, it avoids undertaking expensive germline mutation screening in individuals whose tumours have arisen sporadically even within the context of a strong family history, whilst still allowing testing to be offered to individuals independent of their family history. Finally, it allows novel, lower penetrance mechanisms in cancer predisposition to be identified which may not be associated with the strong family history.

The means and significance of identifying familial tumours will be discussed in the next sections.

3. Colorectal Cancer and Mismatch Repair Pathway

Colorectal cancer can be divided into two main sub-groups on the basis of the major form of genetic instability observed within the tumour. The two types comprise chromosomal instability (CIN), which encompasses about ~85% of all colorectal cancer, and microsatellite instability (MIN), present in the remaining 15%. Although the mechanism for the chromosome instability displayed by the majority of colorectal tumours is unknown, our understanding regarding the evolution of MIN tumours is more advanced. In particular, the recognition that 14% of MIN-type tumours arise through germline mutations within the mismatch repair pathway (Lynch syndrome) has greatly increased our knowledge of the genetic predisposition to autosomal dominant, highly penetrant forms of familial colorectal cancer.[4,12]

3.1 *MIN colorectal cancer high risk features*

The mismatch repair (MMR) pathway comprises a network of interdependent proteins. Germline heterozygous mutations in one of the four major gene loci (*MSH2, MLH1, PMS2, MSH6*) are associated with an increased predisposition to colorectal, small bowel, endometrial, gastric, transitional cell, brain and ovarian cancers.[13,14]

The original genetic testing criteria based on family history alone required the confirmation of three affected individuals within a family over at least two generations, with one being affected under the age of 50.[15] As the function of the mismatch repair pathway has been further elucidated and more clinical reagents become available, testing for an aberrant mismatch repair pathway is becoming established at part of routine clinical evaluation of all colorectal tumours.

3.1.1 Microsatellite instability and immunohistochemistry

An accepted part of routine colorectal cancer assessment includes testing for the presence of the four main mismatch repair genes, *MLH1, MSH2, PMS1* and *MSH6* by immunohistochemistry. Immunohistochemistry is a well established technique used throughout clinical pathology departments. The surgical requirement for a clear, tumour-free margin also provides a good internal positive control for this test, as the surrounding normal tissue should express the protein of interest, which is lacking in the tumour cells. However, although robust, this technique is technically limited as the presence of a protein does not guarantee that it is functional.

An alternative method to characterise MIN tumours is to identify the unrepaired DNA damage which accumulates in the absence of a functional mismatch repair pathway. DNA replication is an error-prone process which relies heavy on post-replication repair pathways to restore DNA fidelity.

Microsatellites are short repetitive DNA sequences, which are prone to errors during DNA replication. In cells with defective mismatch repair, aberrant microsatellite regions accumulate. These abnormalities often occur in dinucleotide and mononucleotide repeat sequences and indicate microsatellite instability. Microsatellite Instability (MSI) can be detected in tumour DNA in a diagnostic molecular laboratory as part of routine pathological reporting.

3.1.2 Somatic versus germline loss of mismatch repair gene expression

Of the 15–20% of colorectal cancers associated with MSI, 5% of individuals have lost MMR due to a predisposing germline MMR mutation, whilst most of the remaining 10–15% of tumours have lost a functional MMR pathway through bi-allelic somatic methylation of *MLH1*.[16] Thus, the absence of *MLH1* staining on immunohistochemistry does not have the same predictive value of a germline mutation as that indicated by the absence of the *MSH2* or *MSH6*. Loss of either of these two proteins on immunohisto-chemistry, in the presence of MSI, leads directly to a search for a germline mutation and places first degree relatives of the affected patient at high risk of developing colorectal and other cancers. Thus, they would be offered high risk cancer reduction surveillance. In addition, this result highlights a high risk of synchronous and metachronous tumours to the patient themself.

Interestingly, it has been known for over 20 years that the RAS-RAF-MEK-MAP kinase network, which is involved in cellular responses to growth signals, is often inappropriately activated in many solid tumours.[17] Somatic point mutations within the *K-RAS* gene are found in 50% of colorectal cancers, often at an early stage of tumorigenesis.[18] Recent studies have identified that in a further 12% of colorectal cancers, activation of this pathway is associated with activating point mutations in one member of the RAF group of genes, *BRAF*,[19] the most common point mutation being BRAF-V600E. No colorectal tumour has been found to contain both a *K-RAS* mutation and the BRAF-V600E mutation, which suggests that these mutations activate a similar pathway and are functionally redundant.[20] The presence of a BRAF-V600E in a MSI colorectal cancer has been found to strongly correlate with somatic methylation of the *MLH1* gene.[21,22]

Thus, from a clinical perspective, independent of age or family history, the absence of *MLH1* staining on IHC in the context of wildtype BRAF is highly indicative that this tumour has arisen due to a germline mutation within the *MLH1* gene locus. This result again alerts the familial cancer service that first-degree relatives of the patient are at a high risk of developing colorectal cancer.

3.2 *Novel cancer predisposition due to germline epimutations*

An additional strength of a tumour-focused approach is in identifying novel mechanisms of cancer predisposition, independent of family history. Gene expression is regulated both at the DNA and chromatin levels. Although methylation of the *MLH1* gene locus within a MSI colorectal cancer is normally limited to tumours cells, recent work has revealed that in a rare number of individuals, germline methylation of the *MLH1* locus can occur as a cancer predisposing phenomenon, a germline epimutation.[23–27]

Although these mutations occur in individuals who do not have a strong family history of cancer, there is evidence that the epimutation, or a predisposition to the epimutation can be transmitted from parent to offspring[28] and therefore the implementation of surveillance regimes to other close family members is recommended. Although the extent of the familial risk is not clear, the presence of a germline epimutation confers a high risk of synchronous or metachronous tumour formation to the individuals themselves.

3.3 *Prognostic indicator*

Colorectal tumours with high frequency MSI tend to be more proximally placed in the colon, poorly differentiated, mucinous, have marked lymphocytic infiltration and retain a diploid chromosomal karyotype.[29]

Population studies[30,31] as well as a meta-analysis[32] have shown that the presence of a MSI phenotype is associated with a 15–33% relative survival advantage when compared to microsatellite stable tumours. The basis of this increased survival is not clear, but may relate to a relatively low somatic mutation rate in the K-RAS locus during MSI tumour development.[33] Alternatively, the presence of a high lymphocytic infiltrate within MSI tumours may reflect the positive influence of an active anti-tumour immunogenic response. The use of MSI as a prognostic indicator in colorectal cancer has not as yet been adopted as part of the most recent 2006 American Society of Clinical Oncologist (ASCO).[34]

Although this meta-analysis[32] was corrected for tumour stage, there is independent evidence that MSI tumours are less likely to develop metastases, both locally and distantly, compared to CIN tumours.[30,35] Again, this difference may be attributable to differences in somatic mutation patterns in MSI compared to CIN tumours.[35]

Whether this survival advantage is also manifest in the smaller subgroup of MSI positive tumours associated with Lynch syndrome due to a germline defect in the mismatch repair pathway, rather than somatic methylation, is still unclear.[36–38]

3.4   *Treatment response and tailored therapy*

Until recently, the majority of chemotherapeutic treatment options were based on data obtained from empiric studies correlating histopathology of the tumours and response to treatment. As our knowledge of tissue-specific tumorigenesis has expanded, certain biological markers are becoming established as either surrogate biomarkers for response to already established chemotherapeutic agents, or as targets for the production of novel agents.

Since 1999, *in vitro* data has suggested that MSI colorectal cell lines were less sensitive to 5-Fluorouracil treatments.[39,40] Although early studies investigating the clinical relevance of these *in vitro* results were unclear,[41] there is now gathering evidence that MSI tumours respond less well to the standard fluoropyrimidine therapy given as an adjuvant therapy in early-stage disease compared to MSS tumours.[42,43] Indeed, the results suggest that treatment with 5-FU in these cases may indeed reduce the survival benefit inherent to a MSI phenotype.[42]

4.   Breast Cancer and BRCA Mutations

Our understanding of the underlying causes of a genetic predisposition to breast and ovarian cancer has become much clearer over the last decade. It is evident that mutations within the *BRCA1* and *BRCA2* gene loci account for the major autosomal dominant high risk genetic predisposition, whilst the remaining familial predisposition relates to multiple low and moderate risk alleles.[44] The clinical utility of testing for the presence of these lower penetrant alleles is still unclear,[45] whilst BRCA mutation searches are typically limited to those families with a strong, young-onset multigenerational family history of breast and/or ovarian cancer.

4.1   *BRCA and high risk breast cancer features*

A role for both *BRCA1* and *BRCA2* in the repair of DNA double strand breaks by homologous recombination (HR), and in the Fanconi network is now well established.[46]

Interestingly, mutations in other gene loci implicated in these processes are also associated with a moderately increased familial risk of breast cancer.[47,48] However, unlike the situation with the mismatch repair proteins, the ability to identify tumours with aberrant homologous recombination due to the presence of pathognomic DNA lesions is not currently possible, although recent evidence suggests that the mutation spectrum found in *BRCA1*-related tumours does differ from that present in sporadic breast tumours and may directly relate to loss of HR.[49]

4.1.1 *Triple negative breast tumours*

For many years, invasive breast carcinomas were classified according to histological type, grade, presence of hormone receptors and more recently, HER2 expression.

With the advent of gene expression profiling studies, breast cancer can be systematically stratified into five main subgroups, two of which are oestrogen receptor positive (ER+): Luminal type A and type B, whilst three are oestrogen receptor negative (ER–): normal breast, basal-like and HER2 positive.[50,51]

The basal-like carcinomas express the gene transcript profile found in the epithelial basal myoepithelial, rather than luminal cells, including the high molecular weight cytokeratins (CK) 5/6, CK14 and CK17.[51] Basal-like tumours account for about 15% of all breast tumours, often affect young women and are associated with aberrant P53 expression. They are usually of high histological grade. Moreover, they often have metaplastic elements and medullary or atypical medullary features. Basal-like breast tumours have a more aggressive course, distinct metastatic pattern targeting brain and lungs, rather than lymph nodes and bones, and poorer prognosis.[52]

The basal-like phenotype includes many breast tumours which are found to be negative for oestrogen, progesterone and HER2 receptor staining (triple negative) on immunohistochemistry, although whether triple negative tumours can be directly correlated with basal-like tumours is still contenious.[53–55]

Previous work had suggested that *BRCA1*-related tumours had a seven-fold higher incidence of atypical medullary breast cancer features, namely high mitotic index, continuous pushing margins and lymphocyte infiltration, compared to the sporadic breast tumour population,[56,57] whilst more recently gene expression profiling indicates an overlap between medullary and basal-like breast cancer subtypes.[58]

Recent reviews of BRCA1-, but not BRCA2-related breast cancers indicate that the prevalence of triple negative, CK5/6 positive breast cancers are enriched for in this population.[59–61] Indeed, it has been predicted that by focusing on triple negative, CK5/6 positive breast tumours, a BRCA1 mutation detection rate of 10% may be achieved independent of family history,[59] although direct, prospective evidence for this approach is still awaited.

4.2   BRCA and high risk ovarian cancer features

The most common ovarian tumours are epithelial ovarian malignancies, which can be stratified on histopathology into different subtypes: papillary serous, cystadenocarcinomas, endometrioid, serous, mucinous and clear cell carcinomas. BRCA mutation screening on an unselected population of women with ovarian cancer detected a germline mutation in 3–15% of cases.[7,62–64] This wide variation in detection rate is dependent on the prevalence of women with other high risk features, such as a strong family history or a high risk ethnic ancestry. In these studies, the two main features associated with germline BRCA1 mutations, other than that of a strong family history, were early age of onset and serous ovarian histopathology. Although some population studies indicate that 10% women who develop a serous ovarian cancer harbour a predisposing heterozygous BRCA1 mutation independent of family history,[7,62,63] these results appear to be population-dependent, as neither serous histology nor early age of onset were consistent features in all studies.[7,62,64,65] However, although other epithelial ovarian subtypes are seen in BRCA mutation carriers, no mucinous ovarian carcinomas have been identified in any studies, suggesting that BRCA testing of individuals with this subtype of ovarian cancer may have no clinical utility, even within the context of a high risk family history.

At present, there are no molecular or biochemical markers which can further refine the BRCA-related subgroup of ovarian cancers.

4.3 Prognostic indicator

To date, surveillance regimes for BRCA-related ovarian cancers have been ineffective in detecting early stage disease.[66,67] However, BRCA ovarian tumours may have a better prognosis than their sporadic counterparts.[68] Studies which adjusted for other confounding prognostic factors showed disease-free survival[69] and overall survival was improved in *BRCA1* and *BRCA2* mutation carriers, compared to the non hereditary group.[69–72] Whether this observation extends to those tumours with somatic loss of *BRCA1* is undetermined.[73,74]

4.4 Treatment response and tailored therapy for BRCA-related breast and ovarian cancer

The current clinical trials aimed at tumours that arise in the context of a BRCA germline mutation highlight the possibility of tailoring well-established chemotherapeutic agents to specific tumours and also of designing new targeted agents.

Both *BRCA1* and *BRCA2* proteins have been implicated in the repair of both endogenously and exogenously produced double strand breaks through homologous recombination (HR).[46] Tumours arising from a germline mutation in either of these genes show aberrant HR repair pathways.

The Fanconi pathway is intimately involved in the repair of DNA cross-linking agents. Indeed, increased sensitivity to these agents forms the diagnostic clinical test for patients with Fanconi syndrome. With the recognition that mutations within the *BRCA2* locus were responsible for Fanconi syndrome D1[75] came the suggestion that *BRCA1*- and *BRCA2*-related tumours would be more sensitive to chemotherapeutic agents known to increase the incidence of DNA cross-links.[76,77] Clinical trials are now in progress, targeting already well established therapeutic agents such as Cisplatinum, specifically to BRCA-related tumours.

Poly (ADP-ribose) polymerase (PARP) is involved in the cell signalling of single strand DNA breaks (SSBs) and the recruitment of DNA repair networks. Inhibition of PARP results in the accumulation of SSBs, which are converted during DNA replication to double strand breaks (DSB). PARP inhibitors have been shown to increase the sensitivity of tumours cells to irradiation induced DSBs.[78,79] Cells lacking either *BRCA1* or *BRCA2* homologous repair pathways are more sensitive *in vitro* to PARP inhibitors than wild-type cells.[77,80] This has led to the first clinical phase II trials using PARP inhibitors and Cisplatinum aimed at BRCA-related tumours, based on targeting and harnessing their aberrant DNA repair function as part of their treatment.

Evolution is a constantly changing and adaptive process, and it is not unexpected that cancer therapies targeted to specific molecular pathways will ultimately select for chemoresistant tumour cells. In *BRCA2*-related tumours, resistance to both PARP inhibitors and Cisplatinum correlates with re-expression of a truncated form of *BRCA2* due to the acquisition of a second 'rescue' mutation.[81] The future challenge will be to understand, and tailor treatment to circumvent these adaptive changes.

5. PTEN Associated Hamartomatous Syndromes and the PI3K/Akt/mTor Pathway

Unlike the previous examples, the rare patients with heterozygous germline mutations at the PTEN locus manifest a set of distinct clinical features, which allow a diagnosis to be made often before a tumour develops.[82] PTEN hamartomatous tumour syndrome (PHTS) includes Cowdens syndrome (CS), Bannayan–Riley–Ruvalcaba syndrome (BRRS) and Lhermitte–Duclos syndrome (LDS). These syndromes are also associated with the overgrowth disorder, Proteus and Proteus-like syndrome,[83] although this connection is not well established. Most patients with PTEN germline mutations develop hamartomas, whilst patients with Cowdens and BRRS also develop thyroid and breast cancer at an earlier age and greater incidence than the general population.[84,85] PTEN encodes both a protein and lipid phosphatase which suppresses the PI3K/Akt/mTOR kinase signalling pathway. Loss of PTEN function within a tumour cell results in constitutional activation of this pathway, and increased phosphorylation of many proteins integral to processes such as cell cycle progression, apoptosis, transcription and translation.

As activation of the PI3K/Akt/mTOR pathway correlates with increased tumour susceptibility in these patients, agents which inhibit this pathway could be used to treat tumours and possibly prevent the cancers which arise in these overgrowth syndromes.

Although heterozygous germline PTEN mutations were identified in patients with Cowden syndrome through classical linkage analysis,[86-88] somatic mutations within the PTEN locus have been identified in breast, brain and prostate tumours[89] and are now known to be somatically altered by mutation or epigenetic gene silencing in most tumour types. Thus, chemotherapeutic agents that target a constitutionally active PI3k/Akt/mTOR pathway have a broad clinical application in the treatment of tumours arising not only from an inherited predisposition, but also from somatic activation of this pathway.

5.1 *Akt/PI3K/mTOR inhibitors*

Although *in vitro* models have suggested that many inhibitors of this pathway are effective in suppressing this pathway and thereby reducing the proliferative capacity of tumour cells, toxicity in the clinical setting has limited their use.[90]

To date the most well studied inhibitors of Akt activation are Perifosine and Triciribine. Although these agents have shown limited efficacy as monotherapy,[91-93] they are showing promise as radiation sensitisers,[94,95] and as therapy when used in combination with other chemotherapeutic agents.[96,97] These drugs are however associated with gastrointestinal toxicity, hyperglycaemia and hypertriglyceridemia.

Inhibitors of the downstream effectors in this pathway, the mTOR complexes, include Rapamycin, Rad001/Everolimus and CCI-779/temsirolimus. These drugs have produced objective responses and disease stabilisation as single agents, although unexpected toxicity has limited their efficacy when used in combination therapy. In particular, Temsirolimus has been shown to be effective in the treatment of advanced renal cancer[96] in which PTEN mutations are associated with advanced stage, aggressive disease.[98]

The optimal use of these agents may be in those tumours which have arisen through a genetic predisposition to a constitutively active mTOR pathway, or those tumours which on immunohistochemistry show increased phosphorylation of mTOR associated proteins.[99,100]

Interestingly, suggestive of functional redundancy between signalling networks, mTOR inhibitors also appear to augment
the actions of other tyrosine kinase (TK) inhibitors, such as the
EGFR TK inhibitor (gefitinab)[101,102] and non-EGFR TK inhibitors
(Imatinib) as well as overcoming resistance to these other TK
inhibitors.

6.   VHL and VEGF Targeted Therapy

Von Hippel Lindau (VHL) syndrome is a genetic disorder associated with vascular anomalies and an increased predisposition to
the development of renal clear cell tumours. Although individuals with VHL syndrome are rare in the population, they have
greatly informed our understanding of the pathogenesis of this
renal cell cancer. The cloning of the VHL gene in 1993 in families
with VHL,[103] and the recognition of its fundamental role in
the regulation of angiogenesis-associated growth factors was
pivotal to the design of novel anti-angiogenesis targeted therapeutic drugs.

Mutations within the VHL locus have been detected in 40–50%
of sporadic clear cell renal cell carcinomas, with methylation of the
locus present in a further 10–20% of tumours.[104] VHL regulates the
action of hypoxia-induced transcription factors, including HIF-α.
Loss of VHL function within a tumour simulates a hypoxic environment and the aberrant expression of hypoxia-associated genes,
vascular endothelial growth factor (VEGF), transforming growth
factor (TGF)-α and Met in a HIF-α dependent fashion.[105,106] Since
over 50% of clear cell renal carcinomas over-express HIF1/2α associated genes, including VEGF, there is a strong rationale for
targeting this pathway.[107]

Trials treating such patients with the functionally inactivating
recombinant human monoclonal α-VEGF receptor antibody,
bevacizumab, have shown an increased progression-free survival
time.[108–110] An additive or alternative approach using small-
molecule inhibitors of VEGF function, such as sorafenib or sunitinib,
have also been found to produce objective treatment responses.[111–113]
These inhibitors are less specific than the monoclonal antibody
and alter the function of other kinase-related pathways. HIF levels
are also increased by activation of the mTOR pathway, leading

to the biological rational for the use of mTOR inhibitors in the treatment of advanced renal carcinoma.[114,115]

7. Conclusions

Our increasingly sophisticated understanding of the mechanisms by which tumours evolve is radically changing our approach to both their treatment and in assessing future cancer risk in both the affected patient and their relatives. This approach will help rationalise current resources and target them at those pre-selected patients in whom they will have most benefit. Currently, germline testing of cancer predisposition genes is becoming part of the acute management plan in some patients, dissolving the boundaries between medical oncology and familial cancer services. This joint approach in cancer management will only increase in the future, as inherited germline susceptibilities to treatment response,[116] and other aspects of tumour physiology are slowly identified.

References

1. A. M. Taylor, Ataxia telangiectasia genes and predisposition to leukaemia, lymphoma and breast cancer, *Br. J. Cancer* **66**: 5–9 (1992).
2. Y. Miki *et al.*, A strong candidate for the breast and ovarian cancer susceptibility gene BRCA1, *Science* **266**: 66–71 (1994).
3. R. Wooster *et al.*, Localization of a breast cancer susceptibility gene, BRCA2, to chromosome 13q12–13, *Science* **265**: 2088–2090 (1994).
4. R. Fishel *et al.*, The human mutator gene homolog MSH2 and its association with hereditary nonpolyposis colon cancer, *Cell* **75**: 1027–1038 (1993).
5. D. Hanahan and R. A. Weinberg, The hallmarks of cancer, *Cell* **100**: 57–70 (2000).
6. S. de Sanjose *et al.*, Prevalence of BRCA1 and BRCA2 germline mutations in young breast cancer patients: A population-based study, *Int. J. Cancer* **106**: 588–593 (2003).
7. T. Pal *et al.*, BRCA1 and BRCA2 mutations account for a large proportion of ovarian carcinoma cases, *Cancer* **104**: 2807–2816 (2005).
8. P. Moller *et al.*, Genetic epidemiology of BRCA mutations — Family history detects less than 50% of the mutation carriers, *Eur. J. Cancer* **43**: 1713–1717 (2007).

9. I. Locke *et al.*, Loss of heterozygosity at the BRCA1 and BRCA2 loci detected in ductal lavage fluid from BRCA gene mutation carriers and controls, *Cancer Epidemiol. Biomarkers Prev.* **15**: 1399–1402 (2006).

10. Z. Kote-Jarai *et al.*, Accurate prediction of BRCA1 and BRCA2 heterozygous genotype using expression profiling after induced DNA damage, *Clin. Cancer Res.* **12**: 3896–3901 (2006).

11. A. G. Knudson, Jr., Mutation and cancer: Statistical study of retinoblastoma, *Proc. Natl. Acad. Sci. USA* **68**: 820–823 (1971).

12. A. de la Chapelle, Genetic predisposition to colorectal cancer, *Nat. Rev. Cancer* **4**: 769–780 (2004).

13. P. Watson and B. Riley, The tumor spectrum in the Lynch syndrome, *Fam. Cancer* **4**: 245–248 (2005).

14. D. C. Chung and A. K. Rustgi, The hereditary nonpolyposis colorectal cancer syndrome: Genetics and clinical implications, *Ann. Intern. Med.* **138**: 560–570 (2003).

15. J. G. Park *et al.*, Suspected hereditary nonpolyposis colorectal cancer: International Collaborative Group on Hereditary Non-Polyposis Colorectal Cancer (ICG-HNPCC) criteria and results of genetic diagnosis, *Dis. Colon Rectum* **42**: 710–715; discussion 715–716 (1999).

16. J. M. Cunningham *et al.*, Hypermethylation of the hMLH1 promoter in colon cancer with microsatellite instability, *Cancer Res.* **58**: 3455–3460 (1998).

17. J. L. Bos, Ras oncogenes in human cancer: A review, *Cancer Res.* **49**: 4682–4689 (1989).

18. B. Vogelstein *et al.*, Genetic alterations during colorectal-tumor development, *N. Engl. J. Med.* **319**: 525–532 (1988).

19. H. Davies *et al.*, Mutations of the BRAF gene in human cancer, *Nature* **417**: 949–954 (2002).

20. H. Rajagopalan *et al.*, Tumorigenesis: RAF/RAS oncogenes and mismatch-repair status, *Nature* **418**: 934 (2002).

21. G. Deng *et al.*, BRAF mutation is frequently present in sporadic colorectal cancer with methylated hMLH1, but not in hereditary nonpolyposis colorectal cancer, *Clin. Cancer Res.* **10**: 191–195 (2004).

22. K. Koinuma *et al.*, Mutations of BRAF are associated with extensive hMLH1 promoter methylation in sporadic colorectal carcinomas, *Int. J. Cancer* **108**: 237–242 (2004).

23. C. M. Suter, D. I. Martin and R. L. Ward, Germline epimutation of MLH1 in individuals with multiple cancers, *Nat. Genet* **36**: 497–501 (2004).

24. L. Valle *et al.*, MLH1 germline epimutations in selected patients with early-onset non-polyposis colorectal cancer, *Clin. Genet.* **71**: 232–237 (2007).

25. M. Hitchins *et al.*, MLH1 germline epimutations as a factor in hereditary nonpolyposis colorectal cancer, *Gastroenterology* **129**: 1392–1399 (2005).

26. I. Gazzoli, M. Loda, J. Garber, S. Syngal and R. D. Kolodner, A hereditary nonpolyposis colorectal carcinoma case associated with hypermethylation of the MLH1 gene in normal tissue and loss of heterozygosity of the unmethylated allele in the resulting microsatellite instability-high tumor, *Cancer Res.* **62**: 3925–3928 (2002).

27. Y. Miyakura *et al.*, Extensive but hemiallelic methylation of the hMLH1 promoter region in early-onset sporadic colon cancers with microsatellite instability, *Clin. Gastroenterol. Hepatol.* **2**: 147–156 (2004).

28. M. P. Hitchins *et al.*, Inheritance of a cancer-associated MLH1 germline epimutation, *N. Engl. J. Med.* **356**: 697–705 (2007).

29. H. T. Lynch *et al.*, Genetics, natural history, tumor spectrum, and pathology of hereditary nonpolyposis colorectal cancer: An updated review, *Gastroenterology* **104**: 1535–1549 (1993).

30. R. Gryfe *et al.*, Tumor microsatellite instability and clinical outcome in young patients with colorectal cancer, *N. Engl. J. Med.* **342**: 69–77 (2000).

31. W. S. Samowitz *et al.*, Microsatellite instability in sporadic colon cancer is associated with an improved prognosis at the population level, *Cancer Epidemiol Biomarkers Prev.* **10**: 917–923 (2001).

32. S. Popat, R. Hubner, and R. S. Houlston, Systematic review of microsatellite instability and colorectal cancer prognosis, *J. Clin. Oncol.* **23**: 609–618 (2005).

33. H. J. Andreyev, A. R. Norman, D. Cunningham, J. R. Oates, and P. A. Clarke, Kirsten ras mutations in patients with colorectal cancer: The multicenter "RASCAL" study, *J. Natl. Cancer Inst.* **90**: 675–684 (1998).

34. G. Y. Locker *et al.*, ASCO 2006 update of recommendations for the use of tumor markers in gastrointestinal cancer, *J. Clin. Oncol.* **24**: 5313–5327 (2006).

35. A. Malesci *et al.*, Reduced likelihood of metastases in patients with microsatellite-unstable colorectal cancer, *Clin. Cancer Res.* **13**: 3831–3839 (2007).

36. R. A. Barnetson *et al.*, Identification and survival of carriers of mutations in DNA mismatch-repair genes in colon cancer, *N. Engl. J. Med.* **354**: 2751–2763 (2006).

37. R. Sankila, L. A. Aaltonen, H. J. Jarvinen and J. P. Mecklin, Better survival rates in patients with MLH1-associated hereditary colorectal cancer, *Gastroenterology* **110**: 682–687 (1996).

38. P. Watson *et al.*, Colorectal carcinoma survival among hereditary nonpolyposis colorectal carcinoma family members, *Cancer* **83**: 259–266 (1998).

39. J. M. Carethers *et al.*, Mismatch repair proficiency and *in vitro* response to 5-fluorouracil, *Gastroenterology* **117**: 123–131 (1999).

40. M. Meyers, M. W. Wagner, H. S. Hwang, T. J. Kinsella and D. A. Boothman, Role of the hMLH1 DNA mismatch repair protein in fluoropyrimidine-mediated cell death and cell cycle responses, *Cancer Res.* **61**: 5193–5201 (2001).

41. P. L. Barratt *et al.*, DNA markers predicting benefit from adjuvant fluorouracil in patients with colon cancer: A molecular study, *Lancet* **360**: 1381–1391 (2002).

42. C. M. Ribic *et al.*, Tumor microsatellite-instability status as a predictor of benefit from fluorouracil-based adjuvant chemotherapy for colon cancer, *N. Engl. J. Med.* **349**: 247–257 (2003).

43. J. M. Carethers *et al.*, Use of 5-fluorouracil and survival in patients with microsatellite-unstable colorectal cancer, *Gastroenterology* **126**: 394–401 (2004).

44. C. Turnbull and N. Rahman, Genetic predisposition to breast cancer: Past, present, and future, *Annu. Rev. Genomics Hum. Genet.* **9**: 321–345 (2008).

45. G. B. Byrnes, M. C. Southey and J. L. Hopper, Are the so-called low penetrance breast cancer genes, ATM, BRIP1, PALB2 and CHEK2, high risk for women with strong family histories? *Breast Cancer Res.* **10**: 208 (2008).

46. W. Wang, Emergence of a DNA-damage response network consisting of Fanconi anaemia and BRCA proteins, *Nat. Rev. Genet.* **8**: 735–748 (2007).

47. N. Rahman *et al.*, PALB2, which encodes a BRCA2-interacting protein, is a breast cancer susceptibility gene, *Nat. Genet.* **39**: 165–167 (2007).

48. S. Seal *et al.*, Truncating mutations in the Fanconi anemia J gene BRIP1 are low-penetrance breast cancer susceptibility alleles, *Nat. Genet.* **38**: 1239–1241 (2006).

49. L. H. Saal *et al.*, Recurrent gross mutations of the PTEN tumor suppressor gene in breast cancers with deficient DSB repair, *Nat. Genet.* **40**: 102–107 (2008).

50. C. M. Perou *et al.*, Molecular portraits of human breast tumours, *Nature* **406**: 747–752 (2000).
51. T. Sorlie *et al.*, Gene expression patterns of breast carcinomas distinguish tumor subclasses with clinical implications, *Proc. Natl. Acad. Sci. USA* **98**: 10869–10874 (2001).
52. J. S. Reis-Filho and A. N. Tutt, Triple negative tumours: A critical review, *Histopathology* **52**: 108–118 (2008).
53. E. Rakha, I. Ellis and J. Reis-Filho, Are triple-negative and basal-like breast cancer synonymous? *Clin. Cancer Res.* **14**: 618; author reply 618–619 (2008).
54. E. A. Rakha *et al.*, Are triple-negative tumours and basal-like breast cancer synonymous? *Breast Cancer Res.* **9**: 404; author reply 405 (2007).
55. B. Kreike *et al.*, Gene expression profiling and histopathological characterization of triple-negative/basal-like breast carcinomas, *Breast Cancer Res.* **9**: R65 (2007).
56. S. R. Lakhani *et al.*, Multifactorial analysis of differences between sporadic breast cancers and cancers involving BRCA1 and BRCA2 mutations, *J. Natl. Cancer Inst.* **90**: 1138–1145 (1998).
57. Breast Cancer Linkage Consortium, Pathology of familial breast cancer: Differences between breast cancers in carriers of BRCA1 or BRCA2 mutations and sporadic cases, *Lancet* **349**: 1505–1510 (1997).
58. F. Bertucci *et al.*, Gene expression profiling shows medullary breast cancer is a subgroup of basal breast cancers, *Cancer Res.* **66**: 4636–4644 (2006).
59. S. R. Lakhani *et al.*, Prediction of BRCA1 status in patients with breast cancer using estrogen receptor and basal phenotype, *Clin. Cancer Res.* **11**: 5175–5180 (2005).
60. W. D. Foulkes *et al.*, Germline BRCA1 mutations and a basal epithelial phenotype in breast cancer, *J. Natl. Cancer Inst.* **95**: 1482–1485 (2003).
61. N. Turner, A. Tutt and A. Ashworth, Hallmarks of 'BRCAness' in sporadic cancers, *Nat. Rev. Cancer* **4**: 814–819 (2004).
62. H. A. Risch *et al.*, Prevalence and penetrance of germline BRCA1 and BRCA2 mutations in a population series of 649 women with ovarian cancer, *Am. J. Hum. Genet.* **68**: 700–710 (2001).
63. L. Sarantaus, A. Auranen and H. Nevanlinna, BRCA1 and BRCA2 mutations among Finnish ovarian carcinoma families, *Int. J. Oncol.* **18**: 831–835 (2001).

64. M. Soegaard *et al.*, BRCA1 and BRCA2 mutation prevalence and clinical characteristics of a population-based series of ovarian cancer cases from Denmark, *Clin. Cancer Res.* **14**: 3761–3767 (2008).

65. S. R. Lakhani *et al.*, Pathology of ovarian cancers in BRCA1 and BRCA2 carriers, *Clin. Cancer Res.* **10**: 2473–2481 (2004).

66. K. N. Gaarenstroom *et al.*, Efficacy of screening women at high risk of hereditary ovarian cancer: Results of an 11-year cohort study, *Int. J. Gynecol. Cancer* **16** (Suppl. 1): 54–59 (2006).

67. E. R. Woodward *et al.*, Annual surveillance by CA125 and trans-vaginal ultrasound for ovarian cancer in both high-risk and population risk women is ineffective, *Br. J. Obstet. Gynaecol.* **114**: 1500–1509 (2007).

68. S. C. Rubin *et al.*, Clinical and pathological features of ovarian cancer in women with germ-line mutations of BRCA1, *N. Engl. J. Med.* **335**: 1413–1416 (1996).

69. J. Boyd *et al.*, Clinicopathologic features of BRCA-linked and sporadic ovarian cancer, *J. Am. Med. Assoc.* **283**: 2260–2265 (2000).

70. Y. Ben David *et al.*, Effect of BRCA mutations on the length of survival in epithelial ovarian tumors, *J. Clin. Oncol.* **20**: 463–466 (2002).

71. T. Pal, J. Permuth-Wey, R. Kapoor, A. Cantor and R. Sutphen, Improved survival in BRCA2 carriers with ovarian cancer, *Fam. Cancer* **6**: 113–119 (2007).

72. A. Chetrit *et al.*, Effect of BRCA1/2 mutations on long-term survival of patients with invasive ovarian cancer: The national Israeli study of ovarian cancer, *J. Clin. Oncol.* **26**: 20–25 (2008).

73. R. L. Baldwin *et al.*, BRCA1 promoter region hypermethylation in ovarian carcinoma: A population-based study, *Cancer Res.* **60**: 5329–5333 (2000).

74. J. P. Geisler, M. A. Hatterman-Zogg, J. A. Rathe and R. E. Buller, Frequency of BRCA1 dysfunction in ovarian cancer, *J. Natl. Cancer Inst.* **94**: 61–67 (2002).

75. N. G. Howlett *et al.*, Biallelic inactivation of BRCA2 in Fanconi anemia, *Science* **297**: 606-609 (2002).

76. A. Bhattacharyya, U. S. Ear, B. H. Koller, R. R. Weichselbaum and D. K. Bishop, The breast cancer susceptibility gene BRCA1 is required for subnuclear assembly of Rad51 and survival following treatment with the DNA cross-linking agent cisplatin, *J. Biol. Chem.* **275**: 23899–23903 (2000).

77. B. Evers *et al.*, Selective inhibition of BRCA2-deficient mammary tumor cell growth by AZD2281 and cisplatin, *Clin. Cancer Res.* **14**: 3916–3925 (2008).

78. A. Chalmers, P. Johnston, M. Woodcock, M. Joiner and B. Marples, PARP-1, PARP-2, and the cellular response to low doses of ionizing radiation, *Int. J. Radiat. Oncol. Biol. Phys.* **58**: 410–419 (2004).

79. W. A. Brock *et al.*, Radiosensitization of human and rodent cell lines by INO-1001, a novel inhibitor of poly(ADP-ribose) polymerase, *Cancer Lett.* **205**: 155–160 (2004).

80. H. Farmer *et al.*, Targeting the DNA repair defect in BRCA mutant cells as a therapeutic strategy, *Nature* **434**: 917–921 (2005).

81. S. L. Edwards *et al.*, Resistance to therapy caused by intragenic deletion in BRCA2, *Nature* **451**: 1111–1115 (2008).

82. C. Eng, Will the real Cowden syndrome please stand up: Revised diagnostic criteria, *J. Med. Genet.* **37**: 828–830 (2000).

83. X. Zhou *et al.*, Association of germline mutation in the PTEN tumour suppressor gene and Proteus and Proteus-like syndromes, *Lancet* **358**: 210–211 (2001).

84. T. M. Starink *et al.*, The Cowden syndrome: A clinical and genetic study in 21 patients, *Clin. Genet.* **29**: 222–233 (1986).

85. C. A. Schrager, D. Schneider, A. C. Gruener, H. C. Tsou and M. Peacocke, Clinical and pathological features of breast disease in Cowden's syndrome: An underrecognized syndrome with an increased risk of breast cancer, *Hum. Pathol.* **29**: 47–53 (1998).

86. W. Marsh Rde *et al.*, A phase II trial of perifosine in locally advanced, unresectable, or metastatic pancreatic adenocarcinoma, *Am. J. Clin. Oncol.* **30**: 26–31 (2007).

87. N. B. Leighl *et al.*, A Phase 2 study of perifosine in advanced or metastatic breast cancer, *Breast Cancer Res. Treat.* **108**: 87–92 (2008).

88. K. Hoffman *et al.*, Phase I-II study: Triciribine (tricyclic nucleoside phosphate) for metastatic breast cancer, *Cancer Chemother. Pharmacol.* **37**: 254–258 (1996).

89. S. R. Vink *et al.*, Phase I and pharmacokinetic study of combined treatment with perifosine and radiation in patients with advanced solid tumours, *Radiother Oncol.* **80**: 207–213 (2006).

90. S. Weiss, M. Diaz-Lacayo, R. Birch *et al.*, Online Collaborative Oncology Group, a phase I study of daily oral perifosine and weekly gemcitabine, *J. Clin. Oncol. ASCO Annu. Meet. Proc.* **24**(Suppl. 18): 13117 (2006).

91. S. M. Chang *et al.*, Phase II study of CCI-779 in patients with recurrent glioblastoma multiforme, *Invest. New Drugs* **23**: 357–361 (2005).

92. M. B. Atkins *et al.*, Randomized phase II study of multiple dose levels of CCI-779, a novel mammalian target of rapamycin kinase inhibitor, in patients with advanced refractory renal cell carcinoma, *J. Clin. Oncol.* **22**: 909–918 (2004).

93. K. W. Yee *et al.*, Phase I/II study of the mammalian target of rapamycin inhibitor everolimus (RAD001) in patients with relapsed or refractory hematologic malignancies, *Clin. Cancer Res.* **12**: 5165–5173 (2006).

94. C. J. Punt, J. Boni, U. Bruntsch, M. Peters and C. Thielert, Phase I and pharmacokinetic study of CCI-779, a novel cytostatic cell-cycle inhibitor, in combination with 5-fluorouracil and leucovorin in patients with advanced solid tumors, *Ann. Oncol.* **14**: 931–937 (2003).

95. S. Pacey, N. Steven, C. Brock *et al.*, Results of a phase I clinical trial investigting a combination of the oral mOTR-inhibotor everolimus (ERAD001) and gemcitabine (GEM) in patients (pts) with advanced cancers, *J. Clin. Oncol. ASCO Annu. Meet. Proc.* **22** (Suppl. 14): 3120 (2004).

96. G. Hudes *et al.*, Temsirolimus, interferon alfa, or both for advanced renal-cell carcinoma, *N. Engl. J. Med.* **356**: 2271–2281 (2007).

97. T. F. Goggins, T. F. Shiffman, R. Birch *et al.*, Online Collaborative Oncology Group, a phase I study of daily oral perifosine with every 3-week paclitaxel, *J. Clin. Oncol. ASCO Annu. Meet. Proc.* **24** (Suppl. 18): 13117 (2006).

98. K. Kondo *et al.*, PTEN/MMAC1/TEP1 mutations in human primary renal-cell carcinomas and renal carcinoma cell lines, *Int. J. Cancer* **91**: 219–224 (2001).

99. I. Duran *et al.*, A phase II clinical and pharmacodynamic study of temsirolimus in advanced neuroendocrine carcinomas, *Br. J. Cancer* **95**: 1148–1154 (2006).

100. E. Galanis *et al.*, Phase II trial of temsirolimus (CCI-779) in recurrent glioblastoma multiforme: A North Central Cancer Treatment Group Study, *J. Clin. Oncol.* **23**: 5294–5304 (2005).

101. D. A. Reardon *et al.*, Phase 1 trial of gefitinib plus sirolimus in adults with recurrent malignant glioma, *Clin. Cancer Res.* **12**: 860–868 (2006).

102. D. T. Milton *et al.*, Phase 1 trial of everolimus and gefitinib in patients with advanced nonsmall-cell lung cancer, *Cancer* **110**: 599–605 (2007).

103. F. Latif *et al.*, Identification of the von Hippel-Lindau disease tumor suppressor gene, *Science* **260**: 1317–1320 (1993).

104. M. Yao *et al.*, VHL tumor suppressor gene alterations associated with good prognosis in sporadic clear-cell renal carcinoma, *J. Natl. Cancer Inst.* **94**: 1569–1575 (2002).

105. O. Iliopoulos, A. P. Levy, C. Jiang, W. G. Kaelin, Jr. and M. A. Goldberg, Negative regulation of hypoxia-inducible genes by the von Hippel-Lindau protein, *Proc. Natl. Acad. Sci. USA* **93**: 10595–10599 (1996).

106. D. Mukhopadhyay, B. Knebelmann, H. T. Cohen, S. Ananth and V. P. Sukhatme, The von Hippel-Lindau tumor suppressor gene product interacts with Sp1 to repress vascular endothelial growth factor promoter activity, *Mol. Cell Biol.* **17**: 5629–5639 (1997).

107. B. I. Rini and E. J. Small, Biology and clinical development of vascular endothelial growth factor-targeted therapy in renal cell carcinoma, *J. Clin. Oncol.* **23**: 1028–1043 (2005).

108. J. C. Yang *et al.*, A randomized trial of bevacizumab, an anti-vascular endothelial growth factor antibody, for metastatic renal cancer, *N. Engl. J. Med.* **349**: 427–434 (2003).

109. R. M. Bukowski *et al.*, Randomized phase II study of erlotinib combined with bevacizumab compared with bevacizumab alone in metastatic renal cell cancer, *J. Clin. Oncol.* **25**: 4536–4541 (2007).

110. B. Melichar *et al.*, First-line bevacizumab combined with reduced dose interferon-{alpha}2a is active in patients with metastatic renal cell carcinoma, *Ann. Oncol.* **19**(8): 1470–1476 (2008).

111. D. Strumberg *et al.*, Safety, pharmacokinetics, and preliminary anti-tumor activity of sorafenib: a review of four phase I trials in patients with advanced refractory solid tumors, *Oncologist* **12**: 426–437 (2007).

112. M. J. Ratain *et al.*, Phase II placebo-controlled randomized discontinuation trial of sorafenib in patients with metastatic renal cell carcinoma, *J. Clin. Oncol.* **24**: 2505–2512 (2006).

113. R. J. Motzer *et al.*, Sunitinib versus interferon alfa in metastatic renal-cell carcinoma, *N. Engl. J. Med.* **356**: 115–124 (2007).

114. S. Radulovic and S. K. Bjelogrlic, Sunitinib, sorafenib and mTOR inhibitors in renal cancer, *J. BUON.* **12**(Suppl. 1): S151–162 (2007).

115. R. J. Motzer *et al.*, Efficacy of everolimus in advanced renal cell carcinoma: A double-blind, randomised, placebo-controlled phase III trial, *Lancet* **372**(9637): 449–456 (2008).

116. R. Fagerholm *et al.*, NAD(P)H: quinone oxidoreductase 1 NQO1*2 genotype (P187S) is a strong prognostic and predictive factor in breast cancer, *Nat. Genet.* **40**: 844–853 (2008).

42

Cancer and the Psycho-Oncologist. Psychosocial Well-Being of Cancer Survivors

Jane Turner,
Katharine Hodgkinson and
Allison Boyes

Abstract

Adjusting to the diagnosis and treatment of cancer is a complex process which evolves over time, and individuals, their family members and health professionals may have diverse opinions about what constitutes the status of survivor. Whilst significant psychiatric disorder is not the norm, many of those diagnosed with cancer experience a degree of psychological distress and changes in their attitudes, beliefs and worldview as they negotiate a new and different life compared with before cancer.

This chapter describes the process of adjustment, factors which affect adjustment, and provides practical suggestions for health professionals to assist them in exploring the specific concerns of their patients. Information is provided about simple interventions which can be delivered in routine clinical care by non-specialist providers, as well as details about risk factors for the development of psychiatric disorder. Practical suggestions about facilitating referral for specialist psychosocial treatment are also provided.

Keywords: Psychosocial well-being, cancer survivors, adjustment, psychological distress, psychiatric disorder.

1. Introduction

Improved survival has resulted in increased attention to the longer-term psychosocial wellbeing of survivors, including the impact on partners and family members, and occupational and social functioning. Traditionally a five-year interval from diagnosis conferred "survivor" status, although current definitions employed by medical professionals, researchers and consumers vary widely. Terms such as short term and long term survival are used with little consistency and may have disparate meaning for different cancer types. A person may define themselves as a survivor at any time point along the continuum from diagnosis and active treatment to completion of treatment; furthermore the person may or may not have active disease. For example a woman with advanced breast cancer may define herself as a survivor, asserting that she is indeed surviving until she dies from the disease. Thus *"the word 'survival' can mean different things to those who have cancer, those who care for them, and those who treat their illness"* (pp. 501).[1]

Health professionals should seek to understand how each patient defines themselves in terms of survival.

2. The Process of Adjustment

High rates of psychiatric morbidity have been reported in patients diagnosed and treated for cancer, resulting in calls for distress to be considered the "sixth vital sign" of wellbeing in cancer populations.[2] Whilst distress often declines over time, it cannot be assumed that pre-morbid levels of adjustment are invariably achieved. The process of adjustment is a dynamic process occurring over time, and whilst there may be obvious milestones (such as completion of active treatment), other less obvious factors such as social support and attitudes can also affect adjustment and so merit exploration as described below.

2.1   Cessation of active treatment

While many patients anticipate completion of active treatment with enthusiasm, the reality may be that they feel highly ambivalent for a number of reasons. There is no longer such regular contact with health professionals who have acted as a "safety net" monitoring response to treatment, and providing support. Furthermore there is no longer a sense of being an active participant in dealing with the cancer, now being replaced by waiting to see what happens: *"As treatments finished and visits to specialists decreased, I began to feel uneasy — I felt that things could go wrong again and I wasn't being monitored. This feeling of being 'left alone' after treatment finishes is a difficult one."*[3]

2.2   The opportunity for reflection

Demands of active treatment are often considerable, and the person who is exhausted may have little time to reflect on what has happened, instead just "getting on with it". Many people find that it is only when they have completed active treatment that they actually contemplate what has happened, and how this changes their life, relationships and world view. Long-standing problems may be brought into sharp focus, and the person may be more or less tolerant of adversity. *"It was a pivotal event. It made me focus on my mortality, what was important in life, how I wanted to live, and to take on my weaknesses, indulgences etc. But it took away my blissful ignorance."*[3]

2.3   Residual symptoms and disability

Physical morbidity causing problems with speech, or bladder or bowel symptoms may lead to cascading losses and undermine some of the social relationships which provide support and balance. Anxiety about recurrence often makes it difficult to cope with residual symptoms which are a constant reminder of the cancer diagnosis. Even with good prognosis, few people will be "as good as new": *"Surviving the disease is the initial challenge. Surviving the aftermath of the disease is the next major step"* (pp. 1478).[4]

2.4 *Burden of gratitude and positive thinking*

Despite the absence of confirmatory evidence, it is commonly believed that a positive attitude will favourably influence outcome. Pressure to be positive negates the enormity of the experience and inhibits the ability of the person to express their feelings, fears and concerns, all necessary steps in adjustment to a life after diagnosis and treatment of cancer. Overt pressure to "move forward" and resume "normal" function compounds the common concern that to express distress represents a lack of gratitude.[5] *"It is very hard to find people with the time or inclination to have any understanding of the impact cancer has had on life."*[3]

3. Adjustment Problems in Cancer Survivors

Approximately one-quarter to one-third of cancer survivors experience significant problems such as anxiety or depression within the first few years.[6–8] It is important to recognise however that research has tended to focus on the diagnosis of disorder, and that absence of disorder does not necessarily mean absence of distress.

3.1 *Who is at risk?*

Some subgroups of survivors are more likely than others to experience difficulty adapting to life after cancer.[9–11] Responses are mediated by several variables: biological vulnerability (history of depression or anxiety, drug or alcohol abuse); concurrent life stressors and caring roles; social circumstances (access to health care and social support, financial strain); sociodemographic factors (younger or older age, being female) and residual disease and treatment characteristics, in particular pain and fatigue.[12] The process of adjustment is not linear, and risk factors may exert more or less effect over time, as may medical and disease-related factors.[13]

3.2 *Common concerns*

Patients may experience concerns in a number of domains, with diverse modes of presentation. Table 1 summarises some of the

Table 1. Common psychosocial concerns of cancer survivors.

Patient's concern	Things to explore
Physical	
Physical limitations e.g. fatigue, lymphoedema	Weight gain, apparent difficulty resuming former roles.
Pain	Poor sleep, impaired capacity to resume former social and occupational roles.
Fertility	Depressed mood. Even if the person has children the sense of further choice being taken away can be a source of sadness.
Cognitive functioning	Complaints of poor memory, disorganisation, frustration about being 'in a fog'.
Psychological	
Depression/anxiety	Impaired capacity to make decisions, reduced optimism, lack of initiative, feeling 'stuck', panic, poor sleep, needing reassurance.
Fear of recurrence	Preoccupation with physical symptoms, frequent presentations, reduced sense of control, vulnerability and uncertainty, hypervigilance, inability to make plans.
Sexuality/body image	Reduced intimacy and sexual activity, difficulty re-establishing sexual relationships, anxiety about establishing new relationships.
Social	
Relationships	Loneliness, perceived lack of support, social withdrawal, attempts to be positive to avoid distressing others, difficulty relating to others, concerns about familial cancer risk.
Socioeconomic	Financial strain, job insecurity/discrimination, insurance matters.
Spiritual/existential	
Existential/grief	Feeling burdened, sad or having lost optimism; managing the expectations of self and others; survivor guilt. Sometimes feeling liberated because of letting go of previous burdens, redefining priorities and challenging or reaffirming of spiritual beliefs.

common concerns, and identifies specific issues the health professional can explore further with the patient.

3.3 *How to elicit concerns*

Reflecting on personal and professional beliefs about survival and appreciating the diversity of perspectives on survival is a very helpful step for those caring for people with cancer. An analogy might be that of staff at a maternity hospital who see delivery of a baby as a defining event, their job effectively completed when the mother and baby are discharged; yet for the parents, the birth is just the beginning of a long journey. Likewise, health professionals who may have considered their major role as focusing on diagnosing, initiating and monitoring cancer treatment may need to reconsider this view, as for patients the cancer diagnosis and subsequent treatment represent the beginning of a new and different life. Discussion about the tasks facing patients and their priorities can be initiated as follows: *"Although treatment is now finished, that doesn't mean that everything is back to normal, and many aspects of life are different now. Can you tell me how things are going?"* Or: *"How would you say the experience of cancer has affected you? We know that not everything is as it seems, and I am keen to hear what you personally feel about it all, good and bad."* The following summarises some of the specific concerns commonly experienced by cancer survivors, and outlines approaches to assessment.

3.3.1 *Exploration of psychosocial issues*

Cancer survivors experience psychosocial concerns and worries across the cancer continuum, with transitions from one phase of care to another being particularly stressful. Nearly all individuals experience some psychosocial impairment at diagnosis and during treatment which usually abates over time. However a range of issues such as fatigue, sexual difficulties, fear of recurrence and uncertainty about the future may not necessarily recede with time. Other issues such as difficulties in decision-making and social isolation may emerge months or years after treatment has finished. Personality style, flexibility, social support and past experiences will all influence the individual's appraisal of the cancer experience, and the person who appears to have recovered well may in fact be angry or fearful. The key issue is to not make assumptions about psychosocial concerns. Because the burden posed by the cancer experience and how an individual copes fluctuates over time, it is important to continue to assess adjustment, rather than assuming that over time the person has achieved their optimal adjustment.

> **The survivorship experience is dynamic and changes over time. Psychosocial needs should be identified, systematically followed up, and re-evaluated over time.**

3.3.2 Attention to physical concerns

At diagnosis and during treatment, priority is given to major morbidities especially life-threatening complications. However 'medically minor' residual symptoms can erode functional capacity, adversely impacting on occupational and social functioning, this in turn leading to isolation, lack of support and financial strain, all risk factors for the development of psychosocial distress. Recognition that the patient's agenda may differ from the health professional's agenda in this regard can be addressed using open-ended questions: *"How would you say things are going for you physically? I know that during treatment we often focused on what we called 'serious' problems, but even more mild symptoms are important, especially if they persist."*

3.3.3 Fear of recurrence

Fears of disease recurrence are commonly reported across the survivorship continuum and have been consistently identified as the highest unmet supportive care need expressed in survivorship groups even up to 11 years after diagnosis.[14,15] *"I used to think that once I got to the five-year mark it would be over, but I'm starting to realise it will never be over… there is always this nagging fear — will it come back?"* Whilst health professionals appraise risk in terms of statistics and evidence, the individual may appraise their risk based on family experience, popular reading, information gleaned from Internet sources, or "gut feelings" which are not inherently logical. These concerns may not be volunteered unless directly explored, especially if they are at odds with the social expectations of being a brave cancer survivor. Awareness of the factors shaping appraisal is important: *"We have talked about the cancer and I have said that it is highly likely that you have been cured. But I know that feelings aren't always logical, and I wonder if you could tell me what you really think in your heart about how things might go for you in the future?"*

3.3.4 *Roles and relationships*

It is not uncommon for individuals to feel disappointed about the response of family and friends to the diagnosis of cancer. Friends sometimes withdraw, perhaps because of uncertainty about how to respond. Family members may be reluctant to acknowledge the enormity of the diagnosis because to do so would be distressing, but this avoidance can lead to resentment as the patient feels misunderstood and isolated. Even subtle changes in roles and relationships which are not immediately apparent to observers can exert a major influence on adjustment. Feelings of disappointment or resentment may contaminate relationships long after the initial diagnosis.

3.3.5 *Assessment of distress*

The Distress Thermometer and associated Problem List were designed as a non-stigmatising tool for cancer patients to record their distress and delineate specific concerns to guide further enquiry and interventions.[16,17] The patient rates their level of distress on a scale ranging from zero representing "No distress" to ten which represents "Extreme distress". In addition, the person indicates the specific source of their distress, for example practical problems (such as childcare, finances), family problems, emotional problems (such as sadness, worry), spiritual or religious concerns, and physical problems (including fatigue and body image concerns). The tool is quick to administer and has been demonstrated to be sensitive to change over time. A score of four or more has been demonstrated to have greatest sensitivity and specificity compared with other validated measures.[18,19] Open questions exploring mood and adjustment are described in relevant guidelines.[12] Standardised, self-administered questionnaires such as Quality of Life in Adult Cancer Survivors[20] or Impact of Cancer[21] can also be used to capture the individual's perspective across multiple areas of wellbeing.

Patients' unmet supportive care needs can be assessed across the disease continuum using the Supportive Care Needs Survey (SCNS)[22] or the shorter 34 item version.[23] Persistent or new unmet care needs arising post treatment can be identified using questionnaires specifically designed to assess the unique needs of cancer survivors (Cancer Survivors Unmet Needs measure, CaSUN)[24] and their partners (Cancer Survivors' Partners Unmet Needs measure, CaPSUN)[25] and/or caregivers (Supportive Care Needs Survey — Partners and Caregivers Measure — SCNS — P & Cs).[26] Needs may change over time and cannot be assumed to be identical within couples.[27] Such measures assist the tailoring of individualised interventions as well as the evaluation of supportive care services and generation of service delivery recommendations.

Survivors should be routinely assessed about distress, particularly at times of vulnerability such as the end of treatment, remission, recurrence. Their partners' and caregivers' needs should also be considered.

4.   Promoting Adjustment

The majority of cancer survivors will not require specialist psychosocial interventions, and specialist treatment should be reserved for those at particular risk or those whose distress is affecting their functioning and relationships.[28] However there is evidence that a range of interventions can promote adjustment and quality of life for all patients, even in the absence of significant adjustment problems. Moreover, many of these strategies are simple and can be effectively delivered by non-specialist health professionals during routine clinical care, as described below.

4.1 Information and support

All patients are likely to benefit from the provision of appropriate information and empathic support from their health professional.[12] For example it may be helpful for cancer survivors to hear that many people report positive outcomes following treatment for cancer. This can include an enhanced appreciation of life, strengthened relationships, enhancement of self-concept, living a fuller and more meaningful life, and existential gains,[29-31] as typified by this statement: *"I know cancer has had a very positive side effect and has taught me many lessons. I have grown in understanding and actually feel better about life than I used to. I am more assertive and spiritual."* An acknowledgement that the experience of cancer can undermine optimism and self-confidence can be very valuable for the person who feels pressured by family or friends to 'move forward'.

4.2 Physical activity

There is evidence about strategies to enhance adjustment, and these can be discussed with all patients, not only those who are distressed. Exercise has been demonstrated to improve physical and psychosocial outcomes in patients treated for cancer,[32] in particular regarding mood, body image, quality of life and fatigue. Emerging evidence also links active lifestyle with lower risk of cancer recurrence.[33] Health professionals should explore patients' attitudes to physical activity and encourage gentle exercise, as advice to be more active despite illness is counterintuitive for many patients. It is important to explore the personal beliefs the individual may have about any potential deleterious impact of activity especially if they have residual physical symptoms.

4.3 Lifestyle changes

Many cancer survivors spontaneously adopt lifestyle changes (e.g. dietary changes) and use of complementary therapies (e.g.

meditation, relaxation, food supplements) in the hope of achieving improved health. There is insufficient evidence specific to cancer survivors to make recommendations regarding diet and healthy weight. However cancer survivors can be advised of the existing recommendations for cancer prevention. These can be summarised as: maintain a healthy body weight; be physically active every day; limit intake of energy-dense foods, red meat, alcohol, salt; eat mostly foods of plant origin; meet nutritional needs through diet rather than supplements.[34]

In parallel with the expanding evidence-base, complementary therapies are increasingly being integrated into conventional cancer care. For example, acupuncture is effective in reducing nausea, vomiting and pain, and relaxation therapy is effective in reducing anxiety and pain.[35] Given the potential harm (e.g. abandonment of conventional treatment, adverse drug interactions) associated with the use of complementary medicines, it is important that open discussions take place between survivors and health care providers. Health professionals should explore their patients' behaviour changes, including use of complementary therapies, and promote lifestyle changes that may improve the length and quality of life. The National Breast and Ovarian Cancer Centre's evidence-based Communication Skills Module *Effectively discussing complementary therapies in a conventional oncology setting* (CAM) provides an overview of the significant issues and the basis for discussion.[36]

4.4   *Psychosocial interventions*

Whilst there are few evaluations of psychosocial interventions to promote well-being, a cognitive approach encouraging women to define their concerns, actively seek information, and develop strategies for responding has been highly acceptable to women after treatment for breast cancer.[37] Although this intervention drew on a cognitive behavioural framework, many health professionals who have not received specific training in this area could offer some assistance with a similar problem-solving approach. Details of the process are provided in Table 2.

Table 2. A structured approach to problem-solving.

Step 1:	Discuss the common feeling of being overwhelmed when facing a number of problems, leading to difficulty making decisions (commonly expressed as: *"I don't know which way to turn"*).
Step 2:	Ask the person to write a complete list of all of their concerns, even if they seem trivial. Be as specific as possible, for example, having to carry groceries upstairs after shopping being limited by lymphoedema.
Step 3:	Rank the problems in order of the stress they pose, highest stress being number 1. If the person says "everything" is stressful, use prompts such as: *"OK, what if I could magically fix just one thing on the list, what would it be?"*.
Step 4:	Select the most pressing problem. Generate ideas about how to approach the problem, including even "out of left field" options. Brainstorm all possibilities and outline how these could be enacted. This may necessitate obtaining further information, checking on potential external sources of support, etc. (For example if the problem is concerns about sexuality, options may include exploration of menopausal status, obtaining a medical review, considering the use of lubricants, possible hormonal options, couple counselling, etc.)
Step 5:	Choose a response and follow-through. Evaluate its effectiveness, and modify the priority for that stressor, or move down the list of possible options to 'value add' in dealing with the problem.

Further examples of practical approaches can be found in a text edited by Hodginson and Gilchrist (2008).[38]

5. Rehabilitation

All health professionals involved in the care of patients with cancer need access to a variety of skilled professionals such as physiotherapists, occupational therapists and social workers, along with psychologists and sometimes psychiatrists. A patient with residual shoulder and chest pain after treatment for breast cancer may gradually relinquish previous activities, and over time become less fit, deskilled and socially isolated. Comprehensive assessment and active rehabilitation may limit this decline and reduce the risk of adverse psychological impact. Whilst chronic conditions can be challenging for health professionals who strive to cure, many patients are more flexible in their expectations: *"I don't really expect it to be fixed. But if I could just move my arm enough to be able to drive safely again that would make all the difference to my quality of life."* For patients struggling to adjust to ongoing physical limitations, psychological interventions can be helpful in reducing distress (such as through relaxation therapy or guided imagery) and promoting adaptation.

6. Identification and Treatment of Psychiatric Disorder

Persistent or severe levels of distress should raise concern that the person has a significant psychiatric disorder such as Major Depression or Anxiety. Differentiating between an understandable response to adversity and a disorder can be difficult, and the desire to avoid medicalising emotional responses must be balanced against the benefits of identifying and treating a significant disorder. Features suggestive of Major Depression are feelings of guilt, worthlessness, helplessness and lack of hope for the future. Depression is also strongly implicated if the person's functional ability is affected by their mood (for example due to lack of motivation), or if there is an adverse impact on relationships or on occupational functioning. Effective treatments are available and described in *Clinical Practice Guidelines for the Psychosocial Care of Adults with Cancer*,[12] which also provides prompts which health professionals can use to explore mood.

Despite this, there remain barriers to initiation of treatment, including lack of access to specialist service providers and patient reluctance to accept referral.[11] Some health professionals may feel ambivalent about referral or even feel that they should be the one who helps their patient. In the same way that a surgeon does not administer radiotherapy treatment or an oncologist does not administer anaesthetics, it is not reasonable for an untrained health professional to expect that they can provide specialist treatment of disorders such as Major Depression. The development of a solid referral network of social workers, psychologists and psychiatrists represents an investment in patient care and is likely to reduce the professional stress inherent in trying to address problems outside of one's area of expertise. Strategies to facilitate acceptance of referral include using physical analogies (*"If you had a broken leg you would accept the need to see a specialist for treatment"*); stating the evidence-base (*"There has been extensive research into depression and cancer, and we now have very effective treatments"*) and citing clinical experience (*"I have had several patients who were struggling with depression, and treatment really helped them get back into living again"*). It is important to note that the impact of disorder extends beyond the individual, powerfully affecting family relationships.

7.   Summary

In contrast with the traditional conceptualisations of cancer treatment, for most patients and their families, definitive cancer treatment is not the 'end point', but rather the beginning of a process of adjustment, at times involving uncertainty, frustration, grief and loss, and also possible benefit-finding. All health professionals involved in the care of patients who have been diagnosed and treated for cancer need to appreciate the differing perspectives brought by individuals to their experience. Moving beyond an emphasis on disorder or a focus on only potentially life-threatening complications is necessary to appreciate the complex interplay of apparently 'minor' problems which impact on adjustment and so is preparedness to listen to the individual and explore their views. Challenging the notion that it is possible to provide a 'one stop shop' is fundamental, and liaison with a variety of health professionals from different disciplines is essential for quality care of cancer survivors.

References

1. M. Little, E. J. Sayers, K. Paul and C. F. C. Jordens, On surviving cancer, *J. R. Soc. Med.* **93**: 501–503 (2000).
2. B. D. Bultz and L. E. Carlson, Emotional distress: The sixth vital sign in cancer care, *J. Clin. Oncol.* **23**: 6440–6441 (2005).
3. A. Boyes, V. Hansen and A. Girgis, A qualitative study of the supportive care needs of recent cancer survivors (abstract), *Asia Pac. J. Clin. Oncol.* **3**(Suppl. 2): A73 (2007).
4. S. Leigh, Myths, monsters, and magic: Personal perspectives and professional challenges of survival, *Oncol. Nurs. Forum* **19**: 1475–1480 (1992).

5. P. Maguire, Improving communication with cancer patients, *Eur. J. Cancer* **35**: 2058–2065 (1999).

6. D. Polsky, J. A. Doshi, S. Marcus, D. Oslin, A. Rothbard, N. Thomas and C. L. Thompson, Long-term risk for depressive symptoms after a medical diagnosis, *Arch. Int. Med.* **165**: 1260–1266 (2005).

7. M. J. Massie, Prevalence of depression in patients with cancer, *J. Natl. Cancer Inst.* **32**: 57–71 (2004).

8. S. Broers, A. A. Kaptein, S. Le Cessie, W. Fibbe and M. W. Hengeveld, Psychological functioning and quality of life following bone marrow transplantation: A 3-year follow-up study, *J. Psychosom. Res.* **48**: 11–21 (2000).

9. G. T. Deimling, K. F. Bowman, S. Sterns, L. J. Wagner and B. Kahana, Cancer-related health worries and psychological distress among older adult, long-term cancer survivors, *Psycho-Oncology* **15**: 306–320 (2006).

10. P. A. Parker, W. F. Baile, C. de Moor and L. Cohen, Psychosocial and demographic predictors of quality of life in a large sample of cancer patients, *Psycho-Oncology* **12**: 183–193 (2003).

11. Y. M. Chan, H. Y. S. Ngan, P. S. F. Yip, B. Y. G. Li, O. W. K. Lau and G. W. K. Tang, Psychosocial adjustment in gynecologic cancer survivors: A longitudinal study on risk factors for maladjustment, *Gynecol. Oncol.* **80**: 387–394 (2001).

12. National Breast Cancer Centre (NBCC) and National Cancer Control Initiative (NCCI), *Clinical Practice Guidelines for the Psychosocial Care of Adults with Cancer* (NBCC, Camperdown, 2003).

13. V. S. Helgeson, P. Snyder and H. Seltman, Psychological and physical adjustment to breast cancer over 4 years: Identifying distinct trajectories of change, *Health Psychol.* **23**: 3–15 (2004).

14. K. Hodgkinson, P. Butow, G. E. Hunt, A. Fuchs, A. Stenlake, K. Hobbs *et al.*, Long term survival from gynecologic cancer: Psychosocial outcomes, supportive care needs and positive outcomes, *Gynecol. Oncol.* **104**: 381–389 (2007a).

15. K. Hodgkinson, P. Butow, G. Hunt, S. Pendlebury, K. Hobbs and G. Wain, Breast cancer survivors' supportive care needs 2–10 years after diagnosis, *Support. Care Cancer* **15**: 515–523 (2007b).

16. A. J. Roth, A. B. Kornblith, L. Batel-Copel, E. Peabody, H. I. Scher and J. C. Holland, Rapid screening for psychologic distress in men with prostate carcinoma: A pilot study, *Cancer* **82**: 1904–1908 (1998).

17. National Comprehensive Cancer Network, Distress management clinical practice guidelines, *J. Natl. Compreh. Cancer Netw.* **1**: 344–374 (2003).

18. P. B. Jacobsen, K. A. Donovan, P. C. Trask, S. B. Fleishman, J. Zabora, F. Baker F *et al.*, Screening for psychological distress in ambulatory cancer patients, *Cancer* **103**: 1494–1502 (2005).

19. A. J. Mitchell, Pooled results from 38 analyses of the accuracy of distress thermometer and other ultra-short methods for detecting cancer-related mood disorders, *J. Clin. Oncol.* **25**: 4670–4681 (2007).

20. N. E. Avis, K. W. Smith, S. McGraw, R. G. Smith, V. M. Petronis and C. S. Carver, Assessing Quality of Life in Adult Cancer Survivors (QLACS), *Qual. Life Res.* **14**: 1007–1023 (2005).

21. B. J. Zebrack, P. A. Ganz, C. A. Bernaards, L. Petersen and L. Abraham, Assessing the impact of cancer: Development of a new instrument for long term survivors, *Psycho-Oncology* **15**: 407–421 (2006).

22. B. Bonevski, R. Sanson-Fisher, A. Girgis, L. Burton, P. Cook and A. Boyes, The Supportive Care Review Group, Evaluation of an instrument to assess the needs of patients with cancer, *Cancer* **88**: 217–225 (2000).

23. A. Boyes, A. Girgis and C. Lecathelinais, Brief assessment of adult cancer patients perceived needs: Development and validation of the 34-item Supportive Care Needs Survey (SCNS-SF34), *J. Eval. Clin. Pract.*, in press (accepted May 2008).

24. K. Hodgkinson, P. Butow, G. E. Hunt, S. Pendlebury, K. M. Hobbs, S. K. Lo and G. Wain, The development and evaluation of a measure to assess cancer survivors' unmet supportive care needs: The CaSUN (Cancer Survivors' Unmet Needs measure), *Psycho-Oncology* **16**: 796–804 (2007).

25. K. Hodgkinson, P. Butow, K. M. Hobbs, G. E. Hunt, S. K. Lo and G. Wain. Assessing unmet supportive care needs in partners of cancer survivors: The development and evaluation of the Cancer Survivors' Partners Unmet Needs measure (CaSPUN), *Psycho-Oncology* **16**: 805–813 (2007).

26. Supportive Care Needs Survey — Partners and Caregivers, Centre for Health Research and Psycho-Oncology, Newcastle (2005).

27. K. Hodgkinson, P. Butow, G. E. Hunt, R. Wyse, K. M. Hobbs and G. Wain, Life after cancer: Couples' and partners' psychological adjustment and supportive care needs, *Support. Care Cancer* **15**: 405–415 (2007).

28. S. D. Hutchison, S. K. Steginga and J. Dunn, The tiered model of psychosocial intervention in cancer: A community-based approach, *Psycho-Oncology* **15**: 541–546 (2006).

29. K. Hodgkinson, P. Butow, K. M. Hobbs and G. Wain, After cancer: The unmet supportive care needs of survivors and their partners, *J. Psychosoc. Oncol.* **24**: 89–104 (2007c).

30. J. Dunn, B. Lynch, M. Rinaldis, K. Pakenham, L. McPherson, N. Owen *et al.*, Dimensions of quality of life and psychosocial variables most salient to colorectal cancer patients, *Psycho-Oncology* **15**: 20–30 (2006).

31. U. Schulz and N. E. Mohamed, Turning the tide: Benefit finding after cancer surgery, *Soc. Sci. Med.* **59**: 653–662 (2004).

32. K. S. Courneya, Exercise in cancer survivors: An overview of research, *Med. Sci. Sport Exer.* **35**: 1846–1852 (2003).

33. C. N. Holick, P. A. Newcomb, A. Trentham-Dietz, L. Titus-Ernstoff, A. J. Bersch, M. J. Stampfer *et al.*, Physical activity and survival after diagnosis of invasive breast cancer, *Cancer Epidemiol. Biomarkers Prev.* **17**: 379–386 (2008).

34. World Cancer Research Fund and American Institute for Cancer Research, *Food, Nutrition, Physical Activity, and the Prevention of Cancer: A Global Perspective* (AICR, Washington DC, 2007).

35. E. Ernst and B. Cassileth, How useful are unconventional cancer treatments?, *Eur. J. Cancer* **35**: 1608–1613 (1999).

36. National Breast and Ovarian Cancer Centre (NBOCC), http://www.nbcc.org.au/bestpractice/commskills/modules.html

37. B. Cimprich, N. K. Janz, L. Northouse, P. A. Wren and B. Given CW, Taking CHARGE: A self-management program for women following breast cancer treatment, *Psycho-Oncology* **14**: 704–717 (2005).

38. K. Hodgkinson and J. Gilchrist (eds.), *Psychosocial Care of Cancer Patients* (Ausmed Publications, Melbourne, 2008).

43

Understanding and Managing Changes in Survivor Identity and Relationships

Paul Y. Cheung and
Ian H. Kerridge

Abstract

Cancer and its treatment are associated with profound changes to a person's identity and relationships. Some of these changes result in distress, while others contribute to flourishing. Understanding what these changes are and how they can be managed constitute important elements in contemporary post-treatment care. This chapter examines the evidence of the psychosocial impact of cancer and its treatment not only on survivors, but also on their significant others. Changes to survivor identity and intimate relationships, especially those within the first five years post-treatment, are discussed by drawing on and comparing a wide range of research findings. A number of practice implications are noted for counsellors, psychologists, psychiatrists, social workers and others caring for cancer survivors in professional roles.

Keywords: Distress, intimacy, treatment outcomes, quality of life, recurrence, response shift, self-concept, sexuality, survivorship, wellbeing.

1. Surviving and Thriving?

In introducing a special issue of the journal *Psycho-Oncology* in 2002, the editor posed a rhetorical question — "Surviving and thriving?"[1] The goal of flourishing after treatment of cancer is not only an aspiration held by those faced with the sequelae of disease and therapy, but one to which healthcare professionals increasingly strive to contribute. In academic research, as well as professional practice, the notion of flourishing after a cancer diagnosis has broadened considerably to include not only the physical sequelae of treatment, but also the psychological and the interpersonal. The latter sequelae are often considered to be inextricably interconnected and are usually designated as the psychosocial impact of treatment. Accordingly, research and practice have expanded to cover not only the psychosocial impact on the patient as an individual, but as a person living in relation to partners, children, parents, some of whom act as care-givers, and also colleagues and members of various communities. In turn, survival and thriving are increasingly considered in terms of how well patients and those around them play these common but life-defining roles following cancer and its treatment.

The profound and predominantly adverse changes to identity and relationship are a common theme in the research literature, although what these changes are precisely and how they can be best managed have not been jointly examined. This chapter begins by outlining the impact of adult cancer and its treatment on identity and relationships. This impact is examined with reference to research conducted with patients, including those who have completed primary treatment for cancer, their intimate partners and care-givers. The second part of the chapter highlights the issues connected with particular identities stemming from these roles, especially those of a sexual being and a provider of care. The last part of the chapter considers the practice implications of research into these and related issues for those counsellors, psychologists, psychiatrists and social workers.

2. Who are Cancer Survivors?

2.1 *Healthy but not quite healthy?*

Cancer patients, particularly those who have completed primary treatment, are commonly referred to as *survivors*. This is an important, but often taken-for-granted change in identity as a direct result of cancer treatment. In the research literature, the identity label 'survivor' is important for a number of reasons. First, it signals a significant disruption in the lives of those affected by cancer and implies a discount to their quality of life. Second, it highlights the overcoming of a potentially life-threatening condition, although not necessarily the lingering fear of recurrence. Third, it is also a compact reference to the cessation of active treatment for cancer and as such, dissociates the 'former' patient from terminal illness and chronic illness. Survivors are viewed almost in a class of their own.

Not quite patients, terminally ill or chronically ill, survivors are in some sense in a liminal state, or a state between two defined categories. The question of the wellbeing of survivors, then, becomes one of discontinuity, both with life prior to cancer and with life as reflected in the broader, non-cancerous population. Despite the implied distinctions between 'survivors', 'patients' and healthy adults', some researchers acknowledge the partial continuity of life over the course of treatment and across health states in the population at large. Research has shown that survivors do not always fare worse than the rest of the population in every respect, even when comparisons are made with healthy adults. By the same token, pre-diagnosis issues such as identity confusion or relationship tensions may persist and account for the level of psychosocial wellbeing post-treatment. As one would expect of the general population, the wellbeing of survivors is far from uniform. Identity as well as relationship issues are diverse among survivors. To the extent that survivors in all their varieties can be distinguished from the general population by the sequelae of cancer diagnosis and cancer treatment, the characteristics of living as survivors are encapsulated by the term 'cancer survivorship'. Much of the survivorship research literature is therefore concerned with distinguishing survivors from their pre-diagnosis selves or from the rest of the population. Such distinctions are far from straightforward, as shown in the review below.

2.2   *Capturing the identity of survivors*

Apart from the conferment of survivor identity, and the range of possibilities of survivorship associated with it, researchers have sought to operationalise the construct 'identity' in order to examine in detail the impact of cancer diagnosis and of its treatment. Early attempts at studying the identity of cancer patients, which had a strong influence on research into cancer survivors, centered on the related construct of self-concept, defined as the totality of the regard towards oneself. Some authors conceived of regard in *affective* terms, as feelings about the self,[2] or in *cognitive* terms, as representations of the self by the self.[3] Self-concept has also been unpacked into constituent components, namely the body, interpersonal, achievement and identification 'compartments' in one meta-analytical account.[2] The 'body compartment' is further divided into the 'functional self' and 'body image' while the 'interpersonal compartment' is further divided into the 'psychosocial self' and the 'sexual self'. The 'achievement' and 'identification' compartments pertain to employment and religious/ethical orientation respectively. In a later meta-analytical account,[3] self-concept is not as rigidly structured but includes 'domains' salient to the self that are subject to different degrees of impairment based on lived experiences including cancer and its completed treatment. One patient's or survivor's self-concept may therefore include the domains of 'athlete', 'sexual partner', 'parent', 'worker' and 'religious participant', whereas for another survivor, the self domains 'athlete' and 'worker' may not be relevant. In this account, variability in the impact of cancer and its treatment is held to be the result of differences in domain salience, diagnosis, stage of disease, prognosis, treatment and care givers on the one hand, and personality, lifestyle and demographics on the other. Moreover, some domains are held to revert to pre-diagnosis, minor levels of impairment.

These early attempts to unpack cancer patient and survivor identity intersected with those aimed at quantifying quality of life using self-report questionnaires and coincided with the rise of quality of life measurement as a health-related outcome assessment practice. Some of the abovementioned components of self-concept can be found in the scales and sub-scales of the most commonly used instruments such as the FACT-G (Functional Assessment of Cancer Treatment), the EORTC QLQ-C30 (European Organisation for Research and Treatment of Cancer) and the SF-36 (Short Form of the Medical Outcomes Survey).[4-6] FACT-G and EORTC QLQ-C30 in particular were developed to assess the impact of cancer treatment without a specific focus on survivorship issues while the SF-36 is a generic health-related quality of life instrument. While the functionally and interpersonally oriented elements of self-concept are well represented in these quality of life measures, intrapersonal elements pertaining to body image, achievements and spirituality are not. In other words, the less tangible, visible and external aspects of self-regard are not included in the bulk of quality of life assessments of cancer survivors in empirical studies.

There have been recent attempts to incorporate the less tangible qualities of self-regard into the measurement of quality of life. The Quality of Life — Cancer Survivors (QOL-CS) tool adds a spiritual wellbeing scale to the physical, psychological and social but has only been applied in a small number of studies of cancer survivors.[7] The Quality of Life in Adult Cancer Survivors (QLACS) instrument includes sub-scales relating to financial problems,[8] benefits of cancer, distress to family, appearance and distress to self due to the fear of recurrence. The QLACS is a relatively new instrument whose psychometric properties have only been recently investigated.[9] The Impact of Cancer (IOC) instrument is designed for survivors who have completed treatment for five or more years.[10] The sub-scales of the IOC instrument cover the physical, psychological, existential, social domains of quality of life as well the 'meaning of cancer' and 'health worry'. The psychometric properties of the IOC instrument are still under investigation and the instrument does not appear to have been employed in a study of survivor quality of life as yet.[11]

The call for refinements in survivor-specific quality of life measures notwithstanding,[11] a number of points are noteworthy when interpreting the results of research seeking to quantify the quality of life of cancer survivors. First, quality of life data provide a valid picture of survivor identity to the extent that identity-related domains comprehensively represent survivors. Data collected using instruments designed for cancer patients are more prevalent and it is not yet clear whether additional information will be gained from cancer survivor-specific instruments. Most questionnaire data relates largely to the relatively tangible, visible and external aspects of self-regard. The relatively intangible, invisible and internal aspects of self-regard among survivors have been investigated using qualitative and mixed methods.

Second, the validity of quality of life data in picturing survivor identity is somewhat reduced by pre-determining domains on the assumption of their unchanging levels of high salience to all survivors. As has been argued in the meta-analysis of self-concept among cancer patients and survivors,[3] not all domains are equally valued by survivors due to different life experiences including those of cancer. Restricting responses to fixed domains may also result in the failure to capture the often nuanced identity changes evident in professional practice.

Third, where quality of life data show that survivors' sense of identity becomes more or less like the healthy adults in the population, either over time or by comparing groups who have completed treatment at different times, there is no way of avoiding the confounding effects of adjustment on scores. For instance, higher-than-normal levels of quality of life enjoyed by younger Norwegian survivors of testicular cancer in an identity-related area such as sexual satisfaction could be explained both by altered personal evaluation of what constitutes satisfaction and increased intimacy with partners through the sharing of the experience of facing and coping with cancer treatment.[12] The lower expectations of sexual performance and strengthened bonds through adversity are very different kinds of impact of treatment on self-regard and call for different responses by professionals offering care. As the self undergoes changes over time, the changes in valuation or response shifts draw attention to the need to supplement the understanding of identity based on quality of life data.[13] Given the very real possibility of response shift, it can be said that new domains of importance will arise even over the course of the same survivor's life, bringing on new identities that may be a matter either of distress or flourishing.

2.3   *How survivors see themselves over time*

While quantitative self-report instruments offer 'still images' of the functional aspects of survivor identity, qualitative and mixed-methods studies have produced somewhat less static images of identity in formation. Below, we examine the findings of select qualitative and mixed-methods studies and where relevant, compare them with those of quantitative studies to produce more detailed pictures of identity changes following cancer treatment.

In recently reported interviews conducted with 39 US women who had previously completed primary treatment for breast cancer for between three to 18 months,[14] a range of meanings attached to the conferred survivor identity was found. Being regarded as a survivor meant anything from being permanently free of disease, to having marginally escaped death, or being a member of an exclusive, courageous elite. The survivor identity was adopted by 19 of the women, while the remaining 20 women had difficulty in seeing themselves as survivors. In a qualitative study of Australian survivors of breast cancer,[15] there was limited evidence of the adoption of the chronically ill identity. When asked what they learned about themselves and their lives as a result of having cancer, the women reported altered qualities such as increased compassion, spontaneity, decisiveness, broadened perspective and decreased selfishness. Further, these survivors portrayed themselves as actual or potential beneficiaries of continued health care services and monitoring, suggesting a self-regard imbued with health concerns. In another qualitative study of 47 US women within 18 months of breast cancer treatment completion,[16] a number of women expressed difficulty with the notion that being a survivor primarily means being disease-free. Cancer was described metaphorically by the women as an integral part of their new identity, which they describe as the burden of being mentally strong and being normal once more. In another study, data from telephone interviews with 18 Australian women breast cancer survivors suggests that those who were pre-menopausal at diagnosis, or those with younger children were more likely than others to distance themselves from the identity of the chronically ill,[17] instead identifying themselves as pursuers of careers and selectors of lifestyles. Accordingly, they also presented themselves as beneficiaries or consumers of non-hospital based services to support informed choices in diet and physical exercises.

Interviews conducted with breast cancer survivors up to two years following treatment show a general demand for care which is not always dependent on the identification with the survivor identity or that of the chronically ill. The major concern is of recurrence of cancer, regardless of whether one identifies oneself as a survivor or as chronically ill. Very few survivors identify themselves as being depressed or anxious,[17] a finding which is of interest as elevated levels of depression and anxiety are commonly expected of cancer patients at the completion of treatment. In a survey of 94 breast cancer survivors, 30% ($n = 28$) scored 16 or above on the Center for Epidemiological Studies-Depression scale (CES-D) on the last day of radiotherapy. A score above 15 is normally interpreted as a marker of clinical depression. By the second measurement two weeks later, the group average had returned to the non-clinically significant level of 10 and no further elevation was found in three subsequent measurements during the next six months. Similarly, no clinically significant levels of depression were found in the baseline survey of the Moving Beyond Cancer study of 558 women breast cancer survivors, conducted within four weeks of the completion of treatment.[18] Based on more global measures of wellbeing such as FACT, researchers have reported improved quality of life in breast cancer survivors over the first six months post-treatment,[17–19] peaking between two to five years, but declining from that point onwards. Whether identity as measured in quality of life assessment changes further beyond two or five years awaits confirmation in future research. Importantly, there is some evidence suggesting that at five years post-diagnosis, breast cancer survivors share a very similar SF-36 subscale score profile as female population controls, and are more clearly distinguishable only in terms of psychological variables not normally within the scope of quality of life measurement such as locus of control.[20] Independently of any possible effects of time since treatment, treatment modality has been shown to be correlated with quality of life scores among breast cancer survivors.[18] Moreover, different quality of life score profiles have been identified among survivors of other cancers, such as ovarian cancer and among recipients of a particular treatment modality, such as haematopoietic stem cell transplantation.[21,22] Irrespective of the type of diagnosis and mode of treatment however, a high level of demand for and acceptance of professional care is consistently found in studies, for example among another sample of survivors of early ovarian cancer five years after completion of treatment.[23] Even though survivors may not proactively seek professional care post-treatment, they are very likely to expect it. They are also likely to accept care when offered in ways perceived to be consistent with the varying regard they have of themselves.

2.4 *How survivors work on their identity*

A number of qualitative and mixed method studies of survivors have shed light on the dynamics of identity changes occasioned by a cancer diagnosis and treatment. These studies demonstrate the often delicate and difficult work performed on identity by survivors within themselves and in interaction with partners, children, parents, care-givers, colleagues and community members. It is clear from these studies that the identities of cancer survivors are not determined rigidly and exclusively by diagnosis, stage of disease, prognosis and treatment. Rather, as survivors relate their experiences to interviewers in the research setting, they are constantly engaged with the question of their identity and confronted with the disruptions to life brought about by cancer and its treatment. There is indirect evidence to show that the greater the experience of life disruption, the more complicated the accounts would be.[24] Accordingly, the offering of a structurally complicated account of the experience of cancer treatment, as opposed to a relatively straightforward chronology hints strongly at identity in formation or transformation. The twists and turns in the accounts provided by cancer survivors are closely tied to the experiences of discontinuity with one's former self, separation from other people, especially those deemed to be leading a normal, cancer-free life, and from one's future now that possibilities seem so drastically narrowed down.[25] Responses to these threats of identity vary between and within individuals and include 'alienation' (the sense of being targeted, isolated and socially dislocated by cancer); 'reconstruction' (or the attempt to be the same person as before cancer); 'incorporation' (the creation of a new, often superior identity based on the experience of cancer); and 'meaning-making' (the attribution of significance to past events including cancer). Over time, the same survivors may respond in a combination of these ways, re-evaluating their priorities in life in the process. The majority of survivors strive towards reconstruction,[26] although this appears to be dependent on the amount of time since treatment and any signs of recurrence.

The orientation towards identity reconstruction is corroborated by analyses of metaphors used by cancer survivors to describe their experiences.[27] Although elaborate new metaphors and analogies are created by cancer survivors, the majority are based on taken-for-granted experiences of being healthy and the ordinary self-body relations these imply. There are other sources of metaphors, including popular conceptions and representation of cancer in terms of victorious armed conflict.[28] These metaphors may be indicative of the desire for incorporation and often cast survivors as heroic in their respective battles against cancer. A recent study of survivors of stroke has provided preliminary evidence for links between the usage of antagonistic metaphors and lower levels of functioning, as well as higher levels of depression.[29] While it is not clear what metaphors are favoured by survivors who focus on meaning-making and those who feel alienated, these studies of survivor accounts and metaphor usage demonstrate that survivors are active to various degrees in identity work.

What precipitates reorientation in identity work and how orientations correlate with well-being are questions awaiting clarification in further research. Fear of recurrence is a potential explanation of reorientation. There is preliminary evidence of survivors recently diagnosed with metastases reviewing and changing their priorities in life over a period of six months,[30] confirming the idiosyncrasies of domain salience, a point previously noted in the study of self-concept.[3] Relinquishing positively-rated domains of importance or priorities was linked to increases in quality of life as measured by FACT-G over this period; conversely, retaining negatively-rated domains was conversely linked to decreases in FACT-G scores.

3.   Cancer Survivors and Intimate Relationships

Depending on the orientation towards their pre-cancer identity and towards meaning-making, survivors may identify with the roles of the 'outcast', the 'cured', the 'hero' or 'heroine', the 'advocate', or the 'philosopher'. The research reviewed above suggests that these roles are not always adopted independently by survivors, but in the course of their interaction with others. The negotiation of roles is not unique to survivorship but the encounter with death makes it somewhat hazardous. A relevant scenario is where the survivor, over time, comes to a profound sense of their own vulnerability to death, whether through recurrence or not. In contrast, their partner, who is also the care-giver during and after treatment, also shares a heightened awareness of death, although only in a more general sense.[31] Consequently, the partner opts for reconstruction and seeks affirmation of a continued sense of identity from the survivor while the survivor tries to grapple with this strong sense of death. The partner often wishes for the relationship to return to normal along with other aspects of their pre-cancer life while the survivor often has difficulty with feeling 'cured', leading the survivor to feel somewhat isolated.

This scenario of growing dissatisfaction and distance in intimate relationships, which has been constructed on the basis of qualitative interviews, matches closely with that generated in a prospective, longitudinal quantitative study of 76 US survivors of haematopoietic stem cell transplantation (HSCT) for chronic myelogenous leukaemia, acute leukaemias, myelodysplasias, lymphomas, breast cancer and multiple myeloma and of their partner-care-givers.[32] While scores on the marital satisfaction sub-scale of the Dyadic Adjustment Scale were comparable between survivors and their partners pre-transplant, those of partners followed a statistically-significant downward trend at six and 12 months post-transplantation. Survivor marital satisfaction, in contrast, remained at pre-transplant levels at these two points in time. Over the one-year period following transplantation, changes in marital satisfaction among partners were significantly associated only with gender, with female partners accounting almost entirely for the downward trend. Survivor quality of life as measured by SF-36 did not predict changes in partner marital satisfaction. This study also found evidence of elevated depression among partners pre-transplant and at six months post-transplantation while survivors remained on par with a group of adult controls at both points. Although the design of the study did not allow the gender effect on marital satisfaction among partners or their depressive tendencies to be explained, the findings are a clear indication of the psychosocial impact on treatment on the survivor's partner across a range of cancer diagnoses.

It is unsurprising that the wellbeing of partners, like that of survivors, and of the general population, will be influenced by a large range of factors. Whether partners' experiences follow a particular trajectory over time remains to be shown. Across a number of studies, it had been found that distress in one member of the dyad predicts distress in the other member during cancer treatment and post-treatment for at least 12 months.[33] This co-existence of distress is not as consistently found at the point of diagnosis and at the completion of treatment, suggesting different psychosocial responses among partners compared to survivors that lead to distress over time. In the light of this, the growing distance between dyads in terms of marital satisfaction for at least 12 months post-HSCT is due not only to intrapersonal but also interpersonal factors.[32] An important set of interpersonal factors stems from the intimate relationships shared by survivors and their sexual partners, who are often, but not always their care-givers. While sexual function and intimate relationships are generally accepted to be adversely impacted upon by cancer and its treatment, the nature, extent and duration of this impact are not well understood, especially from the perspective of partners.

3.1   *The roles of the sexual partner and care-giver*

Cancer diagnosis, treatment and survival can alter identity and social roles in ways that may transform intimate relationships. Becoming a patient and later, a survivor, can be such a disruptive experience that one's identity as a sexual being is overshadowed. Given the well-known impact of cancer treatment on fertility, some people regard the sexual being as important only insofar as the procreator identity is concerned. The role of sexual partner may be regarded as a lower priority, even by the survivor himself or herself. In addition, pre-diagnosis living arrangements, such as domestic duties may have been disrupted, so that for example, a female partner takes on additional responsibilities aside from providing care to the cancer survivor. Especially where good health prevailed pre-cancer, the role of the care-giver may be a relatively new one for the partner. Or perhaps a male partner receives assistance from family members such as the survivor's parents with domestic duties while being the primary care-giver.[32,34] The partner may consequently focus less on sexual relations and more on caring for the survivor. The survivor is thereby conferred the identity of 'care-recipient' rather than 'lover' or 'sexual partner'. The ensuing reduction in sexual activity or in sexual satisfaction may not only be the result of the focus on survival; it may be part of well-meaning, if often unannounced, attempts to consider the other's need before one's own.[35] Whether this is done by engaging in sexual activity when the desire is not strong, or disengaging from it in spite of desire, communication of intent is often absent. Such reciprocal and tacit accommodation in sexual relations may lead to distress both for the survivor and the partner, compounding the effects of identity changes arising from intrapersonal aspects of cancer survivorship reviewed above. Doubts concerning the self and the body, and guilt over providing inadequate sexual satisfaction are commonly reported by partners and survivors in the context of research.

3.2   *Studies of survivors and their partners*

Research into the impact of cancer on sexual relations between survivors and their partners has focused on capturing survivor perceptions and attitudes. Few studies have investigated couples, and where they have, only heterosexual couples have been studied. Most studies are cross-sectional in design and typically conducted around five years post-diagnosis or post-treatment. To-date, no study of couples has included suitable comparison groups from the general population, making it difficult to evaluate the degree of cancer-related distress in sexual relations reported. Self-report instruments are often administered in these studies, but the many measures of sexual functioning and satisfaction used have not all been cross-validated or standardised.

Although potentially relevant indicators such as quality of life measures (e.g. SF-36 and FACT) are included in some studies, their scores have not been found to discriminate between people facing different kinds and levels of distress in sexual relations. For these reasons we still lack a clear and reliable picture of cancer-related changes in sexual relations in the first two years post-treatment. In an early study of US survivors of testicular cancer ($n = 34$), Hodgkin's Disease ($n = 24$) and their female marriage partners three to four years post-treatment, it was found that couples reached greater agreement over items concerned with sexual functioning of the survivor (for example in terms of erectile response) than those concerned with the frequency of sexual intercourse, physical attractiveness and sexual satisfaction.[36] For example, 32.8% of survivors reported decreases in sexual satisfaction, while only 12% of partners did so. While approximately half of survivors and partners reported no change in sexual satisfaction, over 80% of respondents claimed that cancer had brought them closer to their partner. The level of concordance of responses on the impact of illness on relationship was relatively high, suggesting great agreement over global qualities of the relationship than on specific aspects such as sexual satisfaction. That there was disagreement over a seemingly objective matter, such as the frequency of sexual intercourse is another indication of the disparity of survivor and partner perceptions. Further, decreases in sexual satisfaction appeared to be associated with increased distance in relationship to a greater degree from the perspective of survivors of Hodgkin's disease, while the same applied to partners of survivors of testicular cancer. This and other findings strongly suggest different adjustments towards challenges to sexual relations among survivors compared to their partners, adjustments that are influenced by the sequelae of different treatment regimes, such as unilateral orchidectomy plus radiotherapy, or chemotherapy versus splenectomy plus combination therapy.

Focus group interviews with ten heterosexual dyads surviving prostate cancer in the US[37] provide insights into possible reasons for the disparity of perceptions between survivors and their partners. Female partners reported switching of relationship roles with survivors, for example in becoming protectors of their male partners' ego. At the same time, the lack of sexual response, such as erection, cast doubts over the female partners' sense of attractiveness even though they were not the ones receiving cancer treatment. They thought their male partners refrained from showing physical intimacy by touching in fear of it leading to sexual intercourse in which normal erectile performance is expected. In contrast, the survivors themselves did not describe the processes of sexual relations in quite such detail, but did report increased difficulty and decreased romance. Both groups expressed a desire for more information on the management of intimate relationships, but survivors preferred such information in the form of reading materials while their partners were interested in support groups. Survivors and their partners also showed interest in seeking help from healthcare professionals.

In a study of 26 women with invasive cervical cancer and their male partners,[38] divergence in the level of concern in different disease, treatment and psychosocial domains was found to be significantly associated with lower marital satisfaction, as rated separately by both groups. In the cross-section of dyads at different stages pre- and post-treatment, the mean rating of concern for sexuality was three out of six while male partners at earlier stages were more concerned with a mean rating of five. Male partners of women at later stages were less concerned with a mean rating of lower than three but higher than two. It may be the case, therefore, that concerns dissipate somewhat among male partners over time, while survivors remain worried about sexuality. The intensity of concern reported by male partners early in the cancer journey in this study is corroborated by the findings of another study, this time in the UK of partners of women six to eight months post-diagnosis of gynaecological cancer.[34] In this study, one male was distressed by the evident, but unexplained loss of interest in sexual activity on the part of his post-treatment partner. At the same time, and unbeknownst to the make partner, the survivor described her fear that intercourse would be painful. Another male described how whereas he used to be the initiator of sexual intercourse pre-diagnosis, he now left the initiation of intercourse to his partner. As she never initiated intercourse he gradually lost interest in sexual relations altogether. These findings suggest that over time, lack of interest in sexual intercourse may lead to lessening of concern and potentially to distress.

On the other hand, studies of long term survivors suggest the possibility of long term recovery in sexual relations. For example, at four to five years post-diagnosis, a number of US studies have found survivors of breast and gynaecological cancers to be just as satisfied with their sexual relationships as female members of the general population.[39,40] Norwegian survivors of testicular cancer under 40 years of age who had completed treatment for at least four years even reported a higher level of sexual satisfaction than age-matched counterparts in the general population.[12] A reasonable interpretation of these findings is that these survivors had adapted their thinking and behaviour to allow them to remain sexual beings, albeit with different expectations and practices.

Not all survivors exhibit the same adaptations over the long term. Considerable distress in sexual relations has been reported in other studies such as those of long term early-stage ovarian cancer survivors in the US.[22,23] In one qualitative study of long-term ethnic Chinese survivors of gynaecological cancers in Hong Kong, some participants remained married to their male partners, despite the partners' involvement in extra-marital affairs since diagnosis.[41] Little is known about the long term impact on partners or variety of adjustments they make in sexual relations, as the majority of studies of care-givers continue to focus on care-giver burden and their overall quality of life.

3.3   *Predictors of outcomes in sexual relations*

Given the tremendous variety in sexual relations post-cancer treatment and the differential impact on partners as opposed to survivors, there is some interest among researchers in identifying outcome predictors. In one such line of inquiry, which is based on the construct of sexual self-concept or sexual self-schema, studies have focused on grouping personality dispositions predictive of sexual behaviour, such as frequency of intercourse, or other intimate acts, and of sexual response, such as desire, and evaluating personal identification with these dispositions. One list of adjectives had been developed for females (50 items) and one for males (45 items) for self rating along a 7-point scale from 'Not descriptive at all" to 'Very descriptive'.[42,43] The two self sexual schema (SSS) scales reflect the putatively different domain salience in self-regard as sexual beings among women and men. According to this view, it is argued that women and men are disposed to different degrees to passionate-romantic emotions and behavioural openness. In addition, women are disposed to different degrees also to embarrassment-conservatism and men to being powerful and aggressive. Using the SSS, researchers have categorised women into those with positive and negative self-regard and men into those with very positive (schematic) and positive (aschematic) self-regard. In one study of 40 largely post-menopausal women over 18 months post-treatment for gynaecological cancer,[44,45] women with positive self-regard were more likely to be sexually responsive and engaged in sexual behaviour. SSS scores from these and 59 women sharing a similar demographic profile but with a higher level of quality of life as measured by SF-36, by themselves, accounted for an additional 28% of variance in sexual responsiveness and 6% of that of sexual behaviour. As a further indication of the potential utility of the SSS as a measure of sexual identity predictive of outcomes in sexual relations, scores from cancer survivors and female controls were comparable overall.

Categorising survivors on the basis of sexual self-regard may be useful in elucidating the poorly understood interactions between cancer treatment, time since treatment, sexual relations, depression and quality of life. In one recent cross-sectional study of 175 women who had completed treatment for gynaecological cancer for a period between two to ten years,[39] SSS scores were found to be significantly correlated with depression (as measured by CES-D) and quality of life (as measured by FACT). Where sexual satisfaction was lower, women with positive self-regard were less likely to be classified as clinically depressed than those with negative self-regard. Likewise, negative self-regard was associated with lower quality of life even where sexual satisfaction was higher. The conceptual and methodological difficulties of this line of inquiry notwithstanding, these findings highlight the interaction between intrapersonal and interpersonal factors in producing or mitigating distress following cancer treatment.

4.   Practice Implications

The question "surviving and thriving?" is still pertinent today, despite the more sophisticated understanding we now have of survivorship today than previously. Distress arising from identity work and the negotiation of roles in sexual relations is real, whatever its duration. But so is the possibility of resolution, at least among some survivors. And while some survivors are able to maintain or initiate stable and functional relationships, psychosocial deterioration and the recurrence of distress are also prospects for long-term survivors.

Given this, what can counsellors, psychologists, psychiatrists, social workers and others in professional roles do to mitigate distress and contribute to the flourishing of survivors and their intimate partners? The review of evidence in this chapter suggests a number of implications for professional practice. First, and perhaps the most crucial, is the recognition of the diversity of survivorship experiences, not only across individuals, but across the span of an individual survivor's cancer journey. This requires skillful and tactful assessment of any changes (which are often subtle and unannounced), in preferences, desires, perceptions and attitudes. Survivors will be more likely to turn to those practitioners who show an understanding of how they regard themselves for the help they feel they need in the manner they believe to be suitable. The relationship between the professional and the client needs to be adjusted as necessary to take into account the process and hazards of identity work performed by the survivor. The lack of clear, consistent and lasting impact of intervention programs on the psychosocial wellbeing of survivors or their intimate relationships underscores the importance of developing and nurturing the professional-client relationship over time,[40,46–49] and being able to provide care appropriate to survivors' changing needs, roles and circumstances rather than as part of a standard intervention bundle. The practitioner's personal and personalising touch may be the single most important element in this relationship, which serves as a safe environment for the often difficult and unavoidable task of identity formation and transformation. Within this environment, clients may, without the threat of judgment or misunderstanding, explore the regard they have of themselves, along with changes they themselves or other people have perceived, either coincidentally or otherwise. The professional's facilitation of this process is not restricted to empathic affirmation of the client and may include the offering-up of alternative identities and roles for the client's consideration. For example, if a survivor showed increasing reliance on a 'heroic' identity, the professional may extend the exploration to cover other possible identities, possibly through the use of less antagonistic metaphors. In the consulting room, the professional's flexibility in modeling roles commensurate with these alternatives is important in making these explorations concrete and true-to-life for the client. It would not be consistent for example to given an extended hero's welcome to the long term heroic client who has been struggling to cope.

Discussions of modes of post-treatment care have highlighted the way that survivors may form therapeutic or otherwise helpful relationships with a variety of people other than in formal health care delivery settings.[50-52] Some survivors may prefer to seek support not from professionals, but from others such as fellow survivors affiliated with support organisations. But even here, health professionals can contribute training and advice to those coordinating these services and to volunteers working with survivors.

Few issues in cancer care are as neglected as discussions of intimacy. In this regard, sensitive and timely discussions regarding intimate relationships are of particular importance to cancer patients, cancer survivors and their partners. The involvement of the partner in these discussions would be a matter of mutual agreement and continual negotiation. Whether the partner is directly involved in these discussions, communication within and about the intimate relationship itself is to be encouraged. Areas where communication is needed include the initiation of sexual activity, its frequency, its form and its evaluation. Fertility and child bearing are often closely related topics also requiring communication. With appropriate advice and facilitation, some couples have discovered anew that intimacy can be achieved and communicated by means other than sexual intercourse, that touching, for instance, can be of great comfort to both persons without leading to unwanted penetration. This requires clarification of expectations and intent in a manner that is sensitive to both persons' perceptions and self-regard. The survivor and the partner need to be informed of the range of sexual activities that may be appropriate given the diagnosis, mode of treatment and its long term effects. Assurance needs to be given where appropriate that sexual activity is safe for the survivor and their partner and not linked to cancer.

While the research on psychological profiling is yet to reach the stage of application in psycho-oncology and related settings, it does highlight the need to offer care in a targeted manner. Managing clients by manipulating psychological variables such as locus of control, sexual self schema and hope may contribute to flourishing but not necessarily for all survivors at all stages of their cancer journey.

References

1. J. R. Bloom, Surviving and thriving?, *Psycho-Oncology* **11**: 89–92 (2002).
2. A. T. Foltz, The influence of cancer on self-concept and life quality, *Sem. Oncol. Nurs.* **3**: 303–312 (1987).
3. B. Curbrow, M. Somerfield, M. Legro and J. Sonnega, Self-concept and cancer in adults: Theoretical and methodological issues, *Soc. Sci. Med.* **31**: 115–128 (1990).
4. N. K. Aaronson *et al.*, The European Organization for Research and Treatment of Cancer QLQ-C30: A quality-of-life instrument for use in international clinical trials in oncology, *J. Natl. Cancer Inst.* **85**: 365–376 (1993).
5. D. F. Cella *et al.*, The Functional Assessment of Cancer Therapy scale: Development and validation of the general measure, *J. Clin. Oncol.* **11**: 570–579 (1993).
6. A. L. Stewart and J. E. Ware Jr, (eds.). *Measuring Functioning and Well-Being: The Medical Outcomes Study Approach* (Duke University Press, Durham, NC, 1992).
7. B. R. Ferrell, K. Hassey Dow and M. Grant, Measurement of the quality of life in cancer survivors, *Qual. Life Res.* **4**: 523–531 (1995).
8. N. E. Avis *et al.*, Assessing Quality of Life in Adult Cancer Survivors (QLACS), *Qual. Life Res.* **14**: 1007–1023 (2005).
9. N. Avis, E. Ip and K. Foley, Evaluation of the Quality of Life in Adult Cancer Survivors (QLACS) scale for long-term cancer survivors in a sample of breast cancer survivors, *Health Qual. Life Outcomes* **4**: 92 (2006).
10. B. J. Zebrack, P. A. Ganz, C. A. Bernaards, L. Petersen and L. Abraham, Assessing the impact of cancer: Development of a new instrument for long-term survivors, *Psycho-Oncology* **15**: 407–421 (2006).
11. N. J. M. Pearce, R. Sanson-Fisher and H. S. Campbell, Measuring quality of life in cancer survivors: A methodological review of existing scales, *Psycho-Oncology* **17**: 629–640 (2008).
12. A. A. Dahl *et al.*, Is the sexual function compromised in long-term testicular cancer survivors?, *Eur. Urol.* **52**(5): 1438–1447 (2007).
13. I. S. Breetvelt and F. S. van Dam, Underreporting by cancer patients: The case of response-shift, *Soc. Sci. Med.* **32**: 981–987 (1991).
14. K. Kaiser, The meaning of the survivor identity for women with breast cancer, *Soc. Sci. Med.* **67**(1): 79–87 (2008).

15. M. Oxlad, T. D. Wade, L. Hallsworth and B. Koczwara, 'I'm living with a chronic illness, not ... dying with cancer': A qualitative study of Australian women's self-identified concerns and needs following primary treatment for breast cancer. *Eur. J. Cancer. Care. (Engl.)* **17**: 157–166 (2008).

16. J. D. Allen, S. Savadatti and A. G. Levy, The transition from breast cancer 'patient' to 'survivor', *Psycho-Oncology* **18**(1): 71–78 (2008).

17. B. Thewes, P. Butow, A. Girgis and S. Pendlebury, The psychosocial needs of breast cancer survivors: A qualitative study of the shared and unique needs of younger versus older survivors, *Psycho-Oncology* **13**: 177–189 (2004).

18. P. A. Ganz *et al.*, Quality of life at the end of primary treatment of breast cancer: First results from the moving beyond cancer randomized trial, *J. Natl. Cancer Inst.* **96**: 376–387 (2004).

19. B. Holzner *et al.*, Quality of life in breast cancer patients — not enough attention for long-term survivors? *Psychosomatics* **42**: 117–123 (2001).

20. P. L. Tomich and V. S. Helgeson, Five years later: A cross-sectional comparison of breast cancer survivors with healthy women, *Psycho-Oncology* **11**: 154–169 (2002).

21. U. Gruber, M. Fegg, M. Buchman and H.-J. Kolb, The long-term psychosocial effects of haematopoetic stem cell transplantation, *Eur. J. Cancer Care* **12**: 249–256 (2003).

22. U. A. Matulonis *et al.*, Long-term adjustment of early-stage ovarian cancer survivors, *Int. J. Gynecol. Cancer* **18**(6): 1183–1193 (2008).

23. L. B. Wenzel *et al.*, Resilience, reflection, and residual stress in ovarian cancer survivorship: A gynecologic oncology group study, *Psycho-Oncology* **11**: 142–153 (2002).

24. C. F. C. Jordens, M. Little, K. Paul and E.-J. Sayers, Life disruption and generic complexity: A social linguistic analysis of narratives of cancer illness, *Soc. Sci. Med.* **53**: 1227–1236 (2001).

25. M. Little, K. Paul, C. F. C. Jordens and E.-J. Sayers, Survivorship and the discourse of identity, *Psycho-Oncology* **11**: 170–178 (2002).

26. M. Little and E.-J. Sayers, While there's life ... hope and the experience of cancer, *Soc. Sci. Med.* **59**: 1329–1337 (2004).

27. R. W. Gibbs and H. Franks, Embodied metaphor in women's narratives about their experiences with cancer, *Health Commun.* **14**: 139–165 (2002).

28. C. Skott, Expressive metaphors in cancer narratives, *Cancer Nurs.* **25**: 230–235 (2002).

29. C. Boylstein, M. Rittman and R. Hinojosa, Metaphor shifts in stroke recovery, *Health Commun.* **21**: 279–287 (2007).

30. L. Sharpe, P. Butow, C. Smith, D. McConnell and S. Clarke, Changes in quality of life in patients with advanced cancer: Evidence of response shift and response restriction, *J. Psychosom. Res.* **58**: 497–504 (2005).

31. M. Little and E.-J. Sayers, The skull beneath the skin: Cancer survival and awareness of death, *Psycho-Oncology* **13**: 193–198 (2004).

32. S. Langer, J. Abrams and K. Syrjala, Caregiver and patient marital satisfaction and affect following hematopoietic stem cell transplantation: A prospective, longitudinal investigation, *Psycho-Oncology* **12**: 239–253 (2003).

33. L. J. Hodges, G. M. Humphris and G. Macfarlane, A meta-analytic investigation of the relationship between the psychological distress of cancer patients and their carers, *Soc. Sci. Med.* **60**: 1–12 (2005).

34. K. Maughan, B. Heyman and M. Matthews, In the shadow of risk: How men cope with a partner's gynaecological cancer, *Int. J. Nurs. Stud.* **39**: 27–34 (2002).

35. B. M. Atwell, Sex and the cancer patient: An unspoken concern, *Patient Educ. Couns.* **5**: 123–126 (1984).

36. M. T. Hannah *et al.*, Changes in marital and sexual functioning in long-term survivors and their spouses: Testicular cancer versus Hodgkin's disease, *Psycho-Oncology* **1**: 89–103 (1992).

37. S. Sanders, L. W. Pedro, E. O. C. Bantum and M. E. Galbraith, Couples surviving prostate cancer: Long-term intimacy needs and concerns following treatment, *Clin. J. Oncol. Nurs.* **10**: 503–508 (2006).

38. J. M. D. Groot *et al.*, The psychosocial impact of cervical cancer among affected women and their partners, *Int. J. Gynecol. Cancer* **15**: 918–925 (2005).

39. K. M. Carpenter, B. L. Andersen, J. M. Fowler and G. L. Maxwell, Sexual self schema as a moderator of sexual and psychological outcomes for gynecologic cancer survivors, *Arch. Sex Behav.* (2008).

40. V. S. Helgeson and P. L. Tomich, Surviving cancer: a comparison of 5-year disease-free breast cancer survivors with healthy women, *Psycho-Oncology* **14**: 307–317 (2005).

41. A. Molassiotis, C. W. H. Chan, B. M. C. Yam, E. S. J. Chan and C. S. W. Lam, Life after cancer: Adaptation issues faced by Chinese gynaecological cancer survivors in Hong Kong, *Psycho-Oncology* **11**: 114–123 (2002).

42. B. L. Andersen and J. M. Cyranowski, Women's sexual self-schema, *J. Pers. Soc. Psychol.* **67**: 1079–1100 (1994).

43. B. L. Andersen, J. M. Cyranowski and D. Espindle, Men's Sexual self-schema, *J. Pers. Soc. Psychol.* **76**: 645–661 (1999).

44. B. L. Andersen, Surviving cancer: The importance of sexual self-concept, *Med. Pedia. Oncol.* **33**: 15–23 (1999).

45. B. L. Andersen, X. A. Woods and L. J. Copeland, Sexual self-schema and sexual morbidity among gynecologic cancer survivors, *J. Consult. Clin. Psychol.* **65**: 221–229 (1997).

46. B. L. Andersen, R. A. Shelby and D. M. Golden-Kreutz, RCT of a psychological intervention for patients with cancer: I. Mechanisms of change, *J. Consult. Clin. Psychol.* **75**: 927–938 (2007).

47. F. M. Lewis *et al.*, Helping Her Heal: A pilot study of an educational counseling intervention for spouses of women with breast cancer, *Psycho-Oncology* **17**(2): 131–137 (2007).

48. A. L. Stanton *et al.*, Outcomes from the moving beyond cancer psychoeducational, randomized, controlled trial with breast cancer patients, *J. Clin. Oncol.* **23**: 6009–6018 (2005).

49. P. C. Trask, D. Jones and A. G. Paterson, Minimal contact intervention with autologous BMT patients: Impact on QOL and emotional distress, *J. Clin. Psychol. Med. S.* **10**: 109–117 (2003).

50. P. N. Butow *et al.*, What is the ideal support group? Views of Australian people with cancer and their carers, *Psycho-Oncology* **17**(3): 209–218 (2007).

51. E. Grunfeld *et al.*, Randomized trial of long-term follow-up for early-stage breast cancer: A comparison of family physician versus specialist care, *J. Clin. Oncol.* **24**: 848–855 (2006).

52. M. Hewitt, S. Greenfield and E. Stovall (eds.), *From Cancer Patient to Cancer Survivor: Lost in Transition* (National Academies Press, Washington, D.C., 2006).

44

Survivors of Childhood Cancer: Issues and Challenges

Carmen L. Wilson,
Richard J. Cohn and
Lesley J. Ashton

Abstract

Over 600 children under the age of 14 years are diagnosed with a childhood cancer each year in Australia and more than 80% survive their therapy each year and move into adulthood. For the majority of children the battle against cancer is won, but cure is often accompanied by a range of adverse health events, some of which may manifest many years after ceasing therapy. Changes in therapeutic approaches and increased survival command the need for ongoing research that focuses on the long term health outcomes of childhood cancer survivors. In this chapter we examine common health problems that can manifest in survivors of childhood cancer and discuss some of the challenges for long term care in this area.

Keywords: Childhood, cancer, survivor, late effects, paediatric.

1. Introduction

On average, one in every 5000 children living in Australia develops cancer each year (Fig. 1).[1] Although cancer is the leading cause

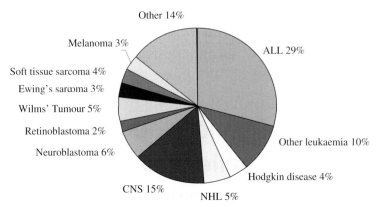

Figure 1. Percentage distribution of childhood cancers in New South Wales, Australia.[162]

of non-accidental death among children ≤14 years of age,[2] improvements in diagnosis, multimodal therapy and supportive care over the past several decades have resulted in substantial reductions in mortality rates for childhood cancer in Australia. Almost 80% of individuals diagnosed with cancer during childhood are now expected to survive for at least five years after their initial diagnosis, with 1 in every 900 individuals currently aged between 16 and 44 years estimated to be a cancer survivor.[3] Despite improvements in therapy, survival rates across all types of cancer remain variable, differing by diagnosis and age of diagnosis (see Table 1).

As survival rates for paediatric cancers have increased over time, so too have concerns for the long term complications that may occur as a direct result of cancer-related therapies received during childhood. Long term complications resulting from therapy for cancer during childhood are often referred to as 'late effects' or 'therapy-related sequelae'. Late effects may either arise during treatment, or shortly thereafter and persist as chronic conditions, or be absent at the end of therapy only to manifest later in life as a consequence of growth, development, or ageing. Hence, it is often difficult to determine the effects of anti-cancer therapies on specific tissue or organ function until survivors have grown into adulthood.

Previous studies have suggested that between 60% and 75% of survivors of childhood cancer will develop at least one medical

Table 1. Age-specific relative 5-year survival rates for brain cancer and leukaemia by age group and period of diagnosis.[2]

	1982–86		1992–97	
Age at diagnosis	Rate[a] (%)	95% CI[b]	Rate[a] (%)	95% CI[b]
Leukaemia				
0–4	67.5	63.0–71.6	73.9	70.1–77.7
5–9	71.4	64.7–77.1	72.0	66.5–77.5
10–14	46.2	38.4–53.5	60.8	53.1–68.5
0–14	62.4	59.0–65.7	69.7	66.5–72.7
Brain cancer				
0–4	57.3	49.7–64.1	53.0	46.7–59.2
5–9	57.7	49.6–64.9	62.3	55.1–69.5
10–14	67.1	58.2–74.5	76.3	70.8–82.6
0–14	60.1	55.5–64.5	61.9	57.9–65.6

[a] Age-standardised to the 2001 Australian population.
[b] Confidence interval.

disability as a direct result of their cancer therapy, with approximately 25% to 36% of survivors expected to develop a serious or life-threatening physical health condition.[4–7] The late effects of cancer treatment observed in survivors of childhood cancer are diverse in nature, with survivors at risk of developing a range of health conditions including neurocognitive deficits, skeletal problems, renal and hepatic damage, as well as endocrine and cardiopulmonary dysfunction. As individual treatment is largely determined by the type of cancer diagnosed, a strong relationship can often be observed between an individual's childhood cancer diagnosis, the treatment they receive, and the nature of the late effects they develop. For instance, as mediastinal irradiation is associated with cardiac and pulmonary sequelae, conditions such as atherosclerotic heart disease, cardiomyopathy and lung fibrosis are predominantly reported in survivors of Hodgkin disease or Wilms' tumour who receive irradiation to the chest or abdomen.[8–11] Survivors at highest risk of late effects are survivors of Hodgkin disease, bone tumours and central nervous system malignancies.[7]

2. Common Late Effects of Childhood Cancer

Numerous studies have examined the most frequently occurring late effects of childhood cancer treatment and several reviews have been published on the topic.[12-17] The most common late effects of treatment are listed in Table 2 and are the subject of further review in this chapter.

2.1 *Mortality*

Previous studies have shown survivors of childhood cancer to be at an increased risk of early death relative to age- and sex-specific rates observed in the general population, with estimates of relative mortality ranging between 8- and 17-fold.[18-21] In general, rates of mortality among survivors are highest five to nine years after a diagnosis of a childhood cancer and decline over time. The leading cause of death among long term survivors of childhood cancer is relapse of the primary childhood malignancy, accounting for approximately 57–75% of deaths.[18] However, survivors are also at increased risk of excess mortality from second cancers, cardiac and pulmonary conditions, a consequence of therapies received during childhood.[19] Among those surviving childhood cancer, mortality rates are generally highest in those diagnosed with central nervous system (CNS) malignancies, while survivors of non-Hodgkin's lymphoma, neuroblastoma and kidney tumour exhibit the lowest rates.[19]

2.2 *Second malignant neoplasms*

The cumulative incidence of second malignancies following treatment for childhood cancer has been reported to range between 2.5% and 4.2% at 25 years, which is 3- to 6-fold higher than that observed in the general population.[22-26] The type of second cancer diagnosed in survivors is often associated with the therapy received in childhood, with solid tumours being more prevalent in patients treated with radiation, while secondary leukaemia and myelodysplasia syndromes are more frequently observed in those treated with chemotherapy.[22,27-30]

The most common second malignant neoplasms arising after treatment with radiotherapy include soft tissue sarcoma,

Table 2. Long-term health outcomes in childhood cancer survivors.

Health condition	Cumulative incidence	Risk factors
Second malignant neoplasms[22–24,39,42]	2.5–4.2% at 25 years	— HD, soft tissue sarcoma, hereditary retinoblastoma — Younger age at diagnosis — Radiation therapy — Exposure to alkylating agents, or topoisomerase II inhibitors
Congestive heart failure[55,58–60,155,156]	0–16% at five years	— Higher cumulative dose of anthracyclines — Female sex — Younger age at diagnosis — Presence of trisomy 21 — Radiation therapy involving the heart — Exposure to cyclophosphamide, ifosfamide or amsacrine
Myocardial infarction[11,64–66]	21% at 20–25 years following HD	— Radiation therapy to the mediastinum — Dose > 30Gy — Increased time since irradiation — Younger age at irradiation — Hypertension, high blood cholesterol levels, smoking, obesity

(Continued)

Table 2. (*Continued*)

Health condition	Cumulative incidence	Risk factors
Ischaemic stroke [67–69]	12% at 15 years in patients treated with irradiation for head and neck cancers	— Radiation therapy to head or neck — Younger age at irradiation — Hypertension, high blood cholesterol levels, smoking
Hypothyroidism [70,71,157]	40–90% at seven years in patients treated with >15Gy of irradiation for HD, NHL, or head/neck malignancies	— Radiation therapy involving the neck — Female sex
Osteoporosis [114,117,158–160]	Not determined	— High cumulative doses of methotrexate — Corticosteroids — Growth hormone deficiency (cranial irradiation) — Gonadotropin deficiency/ovarian failure or Leydig cell dysfunction — Nutritional deficiencies and reduced activity levels
Neurocognitive deficits [141,142,161]	40–100% of brain tumour survivors at five years* 20–30% of ALL survivors at five years*	— Intrathecal or high dose methotrexate — Corticosteroids — Radiotherapy involving the CNS system — Surgical resection involving the CNS system

* Prevalence; ALL, acute lymphoblastic leukaemia; CNS, central nervous system; Gy, Gray; HD, Hodgkin disease; NHL, Non-Hodgkin lymphoma.

osteosarcoma, brain, thyroid, and breast cancer.[22,28,31-38] Radiation-associated second cancers typically develop within the field of radiation, are more common with higher radiation dose and are characterised by long latency periods following treatment during childhood.[22,28,31-39] The risk of second cancers is highest among survivors of hereditary retinoblastoma, Hodgkin disease and soft tissue sarcoma.[22,40] Female survivors previously treated with mediastinal irradiation for Hodgkin disease have a particularly high risk for developing breast cancer,[22,32,34-37] with the cumulative incidence of developing a secondary breast cancer as a function of age reported to be around 20% at 45 years of age.[35]

The incidence of secondary leukaemia following childhood cancer is approximately 0.5% to 3.8% at five to six years post-diagnosis,[30,41] and has been associated with exposure to alkylating agents and epipodophyllotoxins.[42] Unlike secondary solid tumours, which continue to appear many years after therapy, secondary leukaemias tend to arise early; one to three years after treatment with epipodophyllotoxins and five to ten years after treatment with alkylating agents, and then plateau.[15] The risk of alkylator-induced secondary leukaemia increases with cumulative dosing.[43] However, no apparent dose effect over time has been observed for epipodophyllotoxin-induced leukaemias,[44] rather the intensity of the dosing schedule appears to be more carcinogenic.[41]

Although the occurrence of second cancers in survivors of childhood cancer is largely thought to be a direct consequence of the anti-cancer therapies received during childhood, the aetiology of second cancers may also be influenced by a individual's underlying genetic predisposition for cancer.[24] Previous studies have described several clinical syndromes for which the evidence for an excess cancer risk in children is persuasive, such as familial retinoblastoma, Li-Fraumeni syndrome, Bloom's syndrome and neurofibromatosis.[45-48] While most of the polymorphisms (variants) in cancer susceptibility genes discovered to date are highly penetrant and confer a high level of cancer risk in affected families, these gene variants are relatively rare in the general population and account for less than 5% of all cases of cancer among children. However, genetic studies examining polymorphisms in genes encoding drug metabolising enzymes and DNA repair enzymes have suggested inter-individual genetic susceptibility to treatment-related health outcomes.[49–53] Further studies are required to provide information on how gene polymorphisms interact with environmental exposures, such as pesticide use in the home and workplace, diet and viral exposures.

2.3   *Cardiovascular late effects*

In individuals treated for childhood cancer, both radiotherapy to the mediastinum and chemotherapy, especially anthracyclines, have been associated with the development of cardiotoxicity. Cardiotoxicity can manifest as an acute response during the administration of treatment, or occur after completion of treatment, sometimes manifesting many years after therapy. The most frequently observed late cardiac sequelae in survivors of childhood cancer and their associated risk factors are summarised in Table 2.

2.3.1   *Congestive heart failure*

While anthracyclines have been shown to display anti-neoplastic activity against a wide variety of tumour types, their usefulness in the clinical setting is limited by the life-threatening cardiotoxicity that can result from their administration.[54] Cardiomyopathy and congestive heart failure are long term cardiac sequelae that can develop as a consequence of exposure to doxorubicin and daunorubicin in childhood. Anthracycline-induced cardiotoxicity is usually due to changes in the cardiac muscle that result in inappropriate thinning of the left ventricular wall and diminished left ventricular contractility, which over time can lead to cardiomyopathy and congestive heart failure.[54]

The incidence of anthracycline-induced congestive heart failure among patients receiving cumulative doses of anthracyclines of approximately $300\,mg/m^2$ is 5% at 15 years from therapy.[55] However, anthracycline-induced cardiotoxicity is a dose-dependent phenomenon, with the incidence of congestive heart failure increasing to approximately 18% at doses of $700\,mg/m^2$.[55,56] As cumulative anthracycline dose is a major factor influencing the risk of congestive heart failure, most paediatric protocols limit exposure to cumulative doses below $400\,mg/m^2$. Additional factors which can also increase the risk of cardiomyopathy and congestive heart failure include younger age at diagnosis (age < five years), increasing length of follow-up, and female sex.[57–61]

2.3.2 Ischaemic heart disease and myocardial infarction

Long term survivors of childhood cancer treated with mantle irradiation have been shown to be at an increased risk of ischemic heart disease and myocardial infarction. The cumulative incidence of ischemic heart disease among children and adults treated for Hodgkin disease has been reported to be 21.3% at 20 years.[11] Mediastinal irradiation at doses in excess of 30Gy has been shown to increase the risk of subsequent death from myocardial infarction.[11,62–64] The risk of myocardial infarction increases with minimal protective cardiac blocking, younger age at irradiation and increasing duration of follow-up.[64–66]

2.3.3 Ischaemic stroke

Radiation fields involving the head and neck may lead to carotid stenosis and ischemic stroke, particularly among survivors of Hodgkin disease, CNS tumours and leukaemia.[67,68] The risk of stroke following irradiation to the head and neck region increases in a dose-dependent fashion at >30 Gy.[68] Among patients receiving cranial irradiation for head and neck squamous cell carcinoma the incidence of stroke is 12% at 15 years.[69] While the underlying mechanisms leading to ischemic stroke in cancer survivors are not fully understood, acceleration of the atherosclerotic process through irradiation-induced endothelial cell damage and fibrosis of the arterial wall may play a role in the development of ischemic disease.[67]

2.4 Thyroid

As the thyroid gland is one of the most radiation sensitive organs in the human body, thyroid abnormalities are commonly observed in survivors treated with craniospinal or mantle radiation, or in patients who have received total body irradiation in preparation for haemopoietic stem cell transplantation.[17] Abnormalities in thyroid gland structure and function following treatment with radiotherapy may be due to direct damage to the thyroid gland itself, or may be secondary to damage to the hypothalamic-pituitary axis. Estimates of the prevalence of thyroid abnormalities among survivors are variable, owing to differences in study design, small sample sizes, variation in the types of cancers considered, or limited clinical observation. One of the most frequently reported thyroid abnormalities among survivors is hypothyroidism,[70,71] which is associated with increasing radiation dose, older age at diagnosis and female sex.[72] Additional thyroid abnormalities such as hyperthyroidism, nodules, goitres, and carcinomas are also frequently observed among survivors of childhood cancer.[71,72]

2.5   Fertility

2.5.1   Chemotherapy

The effect of chemotherapy on testicular and ovarian function depends on the age and sex of the individual receiving therapy and the nature and dosage of the drugs given.[14] Alkylating agents such as cyclophosphamide, melphalan, busulfan, and procarbazine can cause irreparable damage to the gonads.[17] The exact doses known to cause infertility are unclear for most agents, except for cyclophosphamide, where cumulative doses $>7.5\,g/m^2$ are known to affect fertility.[73] Most children and adolescents treated on current protocols will maintain or recover fertility following chemotherapy, except for male survivors of Hodgkin disease treated with multiple courses of alkylating agent-based chemotherapy.[74–78] Although young females may not become amenorrheic following treatment with alkylating agents, the risk of premature menopause is increased.[79,80]

2.5.2   Radiotherapy

Germ cells (sperm producing cells) are very sensitive to the effects of radiotherapy and most males who receive 3–6Gy of testicular irradiation will become infertile.[81] In contrast, Leydig cell (testosterone producing cells) failure and androgen insufficiency are comparatively less common following treatment with radiotherapy.[82] While most pre-pubertal boys who receive >20Gy will require androgen-replacement to proceed to puberty, >30Gy is needed to induce Leydig cell failure in adolescent males and young adults.[83,84]

Ovarian damage following abdominal, pelvic or total body irradiation is dependent on dose, fractionation schedule and age. In general, the ovaries of younger females are considered to be more resistant to radiation injury,[85–87] with doses in excess of 20Gy required to induce permanent ovarian damage in pre-pubertal girls.[88] Radiation fields involving the uterus may also increase the risk of early pregnancy loss, premature labour, and delivery of low birth-weight infants.[89–91] Although the mechanism underlying these findings is yet to be determined, uterine changes such as reduced muscle elasticity and blood vessel damage have been suggested.[92–94]

2.6   *Growth and body composition*

Poor linear growth and short adult stature are well-recognised late complications that can occur as a consequence of cranial irradiation received in childhood. Severe growth retardation, which is defined as a standing height below the 5th percentile, has been observed in 30–35% of children treated with irradiation for brain tumours, and 10–15% of patients treated for acute lymphoblastic leukaemia (ALL) in an era when prophylactic cranial irradiation was widely used.[95–97] While endocrine dysfunction such as growth hormone deficiency and gonadal dysfunction may contribute to reduced growth, poor growth rates and reduced stature may also result from the direct effects of irradiation on the spinal column.[98]

Cranial irradiation can influence linear growth through its effect on growth hormone production.[99] In children, growth hormone deficiency is characterised by reduced growth velocity, delayed physical maturation and bone age, as well as stature below that expected from family data.[100] Over 80% of brain tumour survivors who receive doses >30Gy have been reported to exhibit impaired growth hormone activity within one to five years of treatment, while 35% of patients who receive doses <30Gy demonstrate normal growth hormone responses during testing two to five years after radiotherapy.[101] Children who have received whole brain irradiation for ALL or 10Gy of total body irradiation as a single fraction have also been shown to be at an increased risk of growth hormone insufficiency.[102–104]

Linear growth in survivors of childhood cancer can also be influenced by the effect of cranial irradiation on additional pituitary hormones.[99,105] Moderate doses of irradiation may result in the premature activation of the hormonal axis leading to early or precocious puberty.[106,107] Precocious puberty can further shorten the final height of survivors, by accelerating skeletal maturation and premature closure of the growth plates.[108] It is generally thought that the younger the child at the time of therapy, the earlier the onset of puberty.

Irradiation of the spinal column can impair final height through direct inhibition of vertebral growth.[98] This complication is most frequently observed in brain tumour survivors who may receive more than 35Gy of radiation to the entire spinal column. In severe cases, spinal irradiation may also result in disproportion, with sufferers exhibiting disproportionately short torsos, but normal limb length.[109]

In addition to reduced adult stature, survivors of childhood cancer are also at increased risk of obesity.[12] This phenomenon is most frequently reported in survivors of ALL.[110,111] Cranial irradiation, particularly >18Gy, female sex and younger age at diagnosis (< four years) have been associated with increased risk of obesity.[110] Concurrent medical conditions, such as growth hormone deficiency and hypothyroidism, may also contribute to weight management issues.

2.7 Bone health

Survivors of childhood cancer are at risk of osteoporosis as a result of disturbances in normal bone metabolism during childhood or adolescence that may lead to reductions in bone mineral density (BMD).[112,113] As shown in Table 2, these disturbances may develop as a direct or indirect consequence of risk factors such as nutritional deficiencies and reduced exercise capacity,[114,115] hormonal deficits following cranial irradiation,[116–119] or from therapy with corticosteroids and chemotherapeutic agents, which can influence normal bone mineral accretion and skeletal development.[115,120–122] The effects of cancer therapy on BMD may be far-reaching, with some studies reporting evidence of reduced BMD and asymptomatic vertebral fractures in adults more than ten years after treatment for childhood cancer.[123,124] Accordingly, reductions in BMD may place long term survivors of childhood cancer at an increased risk for osteoporosis and fractures in later life.[125]

2.8   Neurocognitive and psychosocial late effects

The use of cranial irradiation and intrathecal methotrexate has been previously shown to be associated with the occurrence of neurological and sensory sequelae in long term survivors of childhood cancer.[126] Neurocognitive late effects are among the most prevalent neurological sequelae observed in survivors of childhood cancer and manifest as deficits in overall global function, as measured by Intelligence Quotient (IQ) tests, or more commonly, as diminished capacity in specific areas, such as attention and concentration,[127,128] memory,[129,130] non-verbal abilities,[127,131] visual-spatial and perceptual motor skills.[132] Accordingly, long term survivors may experience difficulties with language, reading and mathematics, as well as diminished academic performance.[132–135] Declines in IQ observed among survivors of childhood cancer are most likely to result from the inability of survivors to learn at an age appropriate rate, rather than from a loss of previous knowledge.[136] In general, neurocognitive function is observed to decline following the cessation of treatment,[137,138] stabilising approximately three to five years from diagnosis.[139,140] Previous studies have reported the prevalence of neurocognitive late effects as assessed by various psychometric tests to range from between 40 and 100% among survivors of brain tumours,[141] while the reported prevalence of neurocognitive impairment is lower among survivors of ALL treated with cranial irradiation, ranging from between 20 and 30%.[142]

The incidence of neurocognitive deficits is related to the volume of brain irradiated,[143,144] total dose received,[145] and the age at which the cranial irradiation is received. While children younger than six years who receive radiation doses of between 18 and 24Gy as prophylactic cranial irradiation for leukaemia may experience difficulties learning basic skills, equivalent treatments given to older children may not result in impaired learning capacity, except for acquisition of complex skills, such as learning a new language or high-level mathematics.[15] Anti-cancer drugs such as glucocorticoids and intrathecal or high-dose methotrexate have also been found to influence the development of neurocognitive deficits in survivors of childhood cancer.[142,146–149]

Difficulties securing and maintaining employment are often reported among survivors of brain tumours and leukaemia, and are generally attributed to neurocognitive deficits that can result as a consequence of CNS directed therapy.[150,151] However, physical and functional late sequelae resulting from intensive multimodality therapy, for example, following treatment for bone and soft tissue sarcoma, may place restrictions on activity that can impact on employment opportunities.[152,153] In instances where survivors experience difficulties securing gainful employment, the burden of care may be transferred to the families of survivors and the community.

3. Challenges for Future Research and Care

Although research examining the long term effects of childhood cancers has been ongoing over the last two decades or more, changes in anti-cancer therapies and the growing number of adolescents and adult survivors of childhood cancer highlights the continuing need to assess the health issues faced by survivors and develop strategies to minimise the long term health burden associated with a childhood cancer diagnosis and its treatment. The characterisation of late effects and associated risk factors is also necessary to direct appropriate clinical care for patients and assist in the development of new treatment regimens to minimise long term morbidity in survivors. Moreover, identification of those at increased risk provides opportunities to develop preventive strategies to minimise the long term risk of adverse health outcomes.

To date, much of the research on childhood cancer survivors has focused on events occurring in the first decade following diagnosis and treatment. However, the diversity and risk of late effects is likely to increase over time, as underlying cancer susceptibility, lifestyle factors and the natural ageing process modify the impact of previous cancer treatment on general health. Therapies targeting childhood cancers will also continue to change with the introduction of new chemotherapeutic protocols, radiation oncology techniques, and surgical procedures. Thus, there will be an ongoing need to systematically follow survivors of childhood cancer produced by these new treatment strategies, to identify changes in the pattern of late effects, and to detect the emergence of previously unrecognised long term complications of anti-cancer therapies.[154] Because survivors are a heterogeneous population, it is difficult for health care providers in the community to be very knowledgeable about these risks and what they imply. Approaches to the follow-up and long term health care required will vary depending on the needs of the survivor, and are likely to change with time. Moving forward, the development of standardised, evidence-based follow-up programs relevant to the specific needs of survivors of childhood cancer will be essential to evaluate, manage and optimise the care of common health problems faced by childhood cancer survivors.

References

1. Australian Paediatric Cancer Registry Report, Part I & II, *Department of Paediatrics and Child, Royal Children's Hospital* (2000).
2. AIHW, A picture of Australia's children, *Cat. No. PHE 58* (Australian Institute of Health and Welfare, Canberra, 2005).
3. J. A. Heath, Monitoring after childhood cancer — an update for GPs. *Aust. Fam. Physician* **34**(9): 761–767 (2005).
4. K. C. Oeffinger, D. A. Eshelman, G. E. Tomlinson, G. R. Buchanan and B. M. Foster, Grading of late effects in young adult survivors of childhood cancer followed in an ambulatory adult setting, *Cancer* **88**(7): 1687–1695 (2000).
5. D. B. Crom, D. K. Chathaway, E. A. Tolley, R. K. Mulhern and M. M. Hudson, Health status and health-related quality of life in long-term adult survivors of pediatric solid tumors, *Int. J. Cancer Suppl.* **12**: 25–31 (1999).
6. M. M. Geenen, M. C. Cardous-Ubbink, L. C. Kremer, C. van den Bos, H. J. van der Pal, R. C. Heinen *et al.*, Medical assessment of adverse health outcomes in long-term survivors of childhood cancer, *J. Am. Med. Assoc.* **297**(24): 2705–2715 (2007).
7. K. C. Oeffinger, A. C. Mertens, C. A. Sklar, T. Kawashima, M. M. Hudson, A. T. Meadows *et al.*, Chronic health conditions in adult

survivors of childhood cancer, *N. Engl. J. Med.* **355**(15): 1572–1582 (2006).

8. F. Villani, S. Viviani, V. Bonfante, P. De Maria, F. Soncini and A. Laffranchi, Late pulmonary effects in favorable stage I and IIA Hodgkin's disease treated with radiotherapy alone, *Am. J. Clin. Oncol.* **23**(1): 18–21 (2000).

9. M. E. Wohl, N. T. Griscom, D. G. Traggis and N. Jaffe, Effects of therapeutic irradiation delivered in early childhood upon subsequent lung function, *Pediatrics* **55**(4): 507–516 (1975).

10. D. M. Green, Y. A. Grigoriev, B. Nan, J. R. Takashima, P. A. Norkool, G. J. D'Angio *et al.*, Congestive heart failure after treatment for Wilms' tumor: A report from the National Wilms' Tumor Study group, *J. Clin. Oncol.* **19**(7): 1926–1934 (2001).

11. J. G. Reinders, B. J. Heijmen, M. J. Olofsen-van Acht, W. L. van Putten and P. C. Levendag, Ischemic heart disease after mantlefield irradiation for Hodgkin's disease in long-term follow-up, *Radiother. Oncol.* **51**(1): 35–42 (1999).

12. P. C. Rogers, L. R. Meacham, K. C. Oeffinger, D. W. Henry and B. J. Lange, Obesity in pediatric oncology, *Pediatr. Blood Cancer* **45**(7): 881–891 (2005).

13. R. Nandagopal, C. Laverdiere, D. Mulrooney, M. M. Hudson and L. Meacham, Endocrine late effects of childhood cancer therapy: A report from the Children's Oncology Group, *Horm. Res.* **69**(2): 65–74 (2008).

14. W. H. Wallace, A. Blacklay, C. Eiser, H. Davies, M. Hawkins, G. A. Levitt *et al.*, Developing strategies for long term follow up of survivors of childhood cancer, *Br. Med. J.* **323**(7307): 271–274 (2001).

15. C. L. Schwartz, Long-term survivors of childhood cancer: The late effects of therapy, *Oncologist* **4**(1): 45–54 (1999).

16. J. D. Dickerman, The late effects of childhood cancer therapy, *Pediatrics* **119**(3): 554–568 (2007).

17. H. K. Gleeson, K. Darzy and S. M. Shalet, Late endocrine, metabolic and skeletal sequelae following treatment of childhood cancer, *Best. Pract. Res. Clin. Endocrinol. Metab.* **16**(2): 335–348 (2002).

18. A. C. Mertens, Cause of mortality in 5-year survivors of childhood cancer, *Pediatr. Blood Cancer* **48**(7): 723–726 (2007).

19. A. C. Mertens, Y. Yasui, J. P. Neglia, J. D. Potter, M. E. Nesbit, Jr., K. Ruccione *et al.*, Late mortality experience in five-year survivors

of childhood and adolescent cancer: The Childhood Cancer Survivor Study, *J. Clin. Oncol.* **19**(13): 3163–3172 (2001).

20. M. C. Cardous-Ubbink, R. C. Heinen, N. E. Langeveld, P. J. Bakker, P. A. Voute, H. N. Caron *et al.*, Long-term cause-specific mortality among five-year survivors of childhood cancer, *Pediatr. Blood Cancer* **42**(7): 563–573 (2004).

21. T. R. Moller, S. Garwicz, L. Barlow, J. Falck Winther, E. Glattre, G. Olafsdottir *et al.*, Decreasing late mortality among five-year survivors of cancer in childhood and adolescence: A population-based study in the Nordic countries, *J. Clin. Oncol.* **19**(13): 3173–3181 (2001).

22. J. P. Neglia, D. L. Friedman, Y. Yasui, A. C. Mertens, S. Hammond, M. Stovall *et al.*, Second malignant neoplasms in five-year survivors of childhood cancer: Childhood cancer survivor study, *J. Natl. Cancer Inst.* **93**(8): 618–629 (2001).

23. J. H. Olsen, S. Garwicz, H. Hertz, G. Jonmundsson, F. Langmark, M. Lanning *et al.*, Second malignant neoplasms after cancer in childhood or adolescence. Nordic Society of Paediatric Haematology and Oncology Association of the Nordic Cancer Registries. *Br. Med. J.* **307**(6911): 1030–1036 (1993).

24. H. C. Jenkinson, M. M. Hawkins, C. A. Stiller, D. L. Winter, H. B. Marsden and M. C. Stevens, Long-term population-based risks of second malignant neoplasms after childhood cancer in Britain, *Br. J. Cancer* **91**(11): 1905–1910 (2004).

25. M. C. Cardous-Ubbink, R. C. Heinen, P. J. Bakker, H. van den Berg, F. Oldenburger, H. N. Caron *et al.*, Risk of second malignancies in long-term survivors of childhood cancer, *Eur. J. Cancer* **43**(2): 351–362 (2007).

26. A. C. MacArthur, J. J. Spinelli, P. C. Rogers, K. J. Goddard, N. Phillips and M. L. McBride, Risk of a second malignant neoplasm among 5-year survivors of cancer in childhood and adolescence in British Columbia, Canada, *Pediatr. Blood Cancer* **48**(4): 453–459 (2007).

27. J. P. Neglia, A. T. Meadows, L. L. Robison, T. H. Kim, W. A. Newton, F. B. Ruymann *et al.*, Second neoplasms after acute lymphoblastic leukemia in childhood, *N. Engl. J. Med.* **325**(19): 1330–1336 (1991).

28. S. Bhatia, H. N. Sather, O. B. Pabustan, M. E. Trigg, P. S. Gaynon and L. L. Robison, Low incidence of second neoplasms among children diagnosed with acute lymphoblastic leukemia after 1983, *Blood* **99**(12): 4257–4264 (2002).

29. M. C. Le Deley, T. Leblanc, A. Shamsaldin, M. A. Raquin, B. Lacour, D. Sommelet *et al.*, Risk of secondary leukemia after a solid tumor in childhood according to the dose of epipodophyllotoxins and anthracyclines: A case-control study by the Societe Francaise d'Oncologie Pediatrique, *J. Clin. Oncol.* **21**(6): 1074–1081 (2003).

30. M. M. Hawkins, L. M. Wilson, M. A. Stovall, H. B. Marsden, M. H. Potok, J. E. Kingston *et al.*, Epipodophyllotoxins, alkylating agents, and radiation and risk of secondary leukaemia after childhood cancer, *Br. Med. J.* **304**(6832): 951–958 (1992).

31. B. Le Vu, F. de Vathaire, A. Shamsaldin, M. M. Hawkins, E. Grimaud, C. Hardiman *et al.*, Radiation dose, chemotherapy and risk of osteosarcoma after solid tumours during childhood, *Int. J. Cancer* **77**(3): 370–377 (1998).

32. S. Bhatia, L. L. Robison, O. Oberlin, M. Greenberg, G. Bunin, F. Fossati-Bellani *et al.*, Breast cancer and other second neoplasms after childhood Hodgkin's disease, *N. Engl. J. Med.* **334**(12): 745–751 (1996).

33. D. G. Gold, J. P. Neglia and K. E. Dusenbery, Second neoplasms after megavoltage radiation for pediatric tumors, *Cancer* **97**(10): 2588–2596 (2003).

34. C. Metayer, C. F. Lynch, E. A. Clarke, B. Glimelius, H. Storm, E. Pukkala *et al.*, Second cancers among long-term survivors of Hodgkin's disease diagnosed in childhood and adolescence, *J. Clin. Oncol.* **18**(12): 2435–2443 (2000).

35. S. Bhatia, Y. Yasui, L. L. Robison, J. M. Birch, M. K. Bogue, L. Diller *et al.*, High risk of subsequent neoplasms continues with extended follow-up of childhood Hodgkin's disease: Report from the Late Effects Study Group, *J. Clin. Oncol.* **21**(23): 4386–4394 (2003).

36. L. B. Kenney, Y. Yasui, P. D. Inskip, S. Hammond, J. P. Neglia, A. C. Mertens *et al.*, Breast cancer after childhood cancer: A report from the Childhood Cancer Survivor Study, *Ann. Intern. Med.* **141**(8): 590–597 (2004).

37. D. M. Green, A. Hyland, M. P. Barcos, J. A. Reynolds, R. J. Lee, B. C. Hall *et al.*, Second malignant neoplasms after treatment for Hodgkin's disease in childhood or adolescence, *J. Clin. Oncol.* **18**(7): 1492–1499 (2000).

38. M. P. Little, F. de Vathaire, A. Shamsaldin, O. Oberlin, S. Campbell, E. Grimaud *et al.*, Risks of brain tumour following treatment for cancer in childhood: Modification by genetic factors, radiotherapy and chemotherapy, *Int. J. Cancer* **78**(3): 269–275 (1998).

39. S. Bhatia and C. Sklar, Second cancers in survivors of childhood cancer, *Nat. Rev. Cancer* **2**(2): 124–132 (2002).

40. F. L. Wong, J. D. Boice, Jr., D. H. Abramson, R. E. Tarone, R. A. Kleinerman, M. Stovall *et al.*, Cancer incidence after retinoblastoma. Radiation dose and sarcoma risk, *J. Am. Med. Soc.* **278**(15): 1262–1267 (1997).

41. C. H. Pui, R. C. Ribeiro, M. L. Hancock, G. K. Rivera, W. E. Evans, S. C. Raimondi *et al.*, Acute myeloid leukemia in children treated with epipodophyllotoxins for acute lymphoblastic leukemia, *N. Engl. J. Med.* **325**(24): 1682–1687 (1991).

42. J. P. Perentesis, Genetic predisposition and treatment-related leukemia, *Med. Pediatr. Oncol.* **36**(5): 541–548 (2001).

43. D. Grimwade, H. Walker, F. Oliver, K. Wheatley, C. Harrison, G. Harrison *et al.*, The importance of diagnostic cytogenetics on outcome in AML: Analysis of 1,612 patients entered into the MRC AML 10 trial. The Medical Research Council Adult and Children's Leukaemia Working Parties, *Blood* **92**(7): 2322–2333 (1998).

44. M. A. Smith, L. Rubinstein, J. R. Anderson, D. Arthur, P. J. Catalano, B. Freidlin *et al.*, Secondary leukemia or myelodysplastic syndrome after treatment with epipodophyllotoxins, *J. Clin. Oncol.* **17**(2): 569–577 (1999).

45. M. Tischkowitz and E. Rosser, Inherited cancer in children: Practical/ethical problems and challenges, *Eur. J. Cancer* **40**(16): 2459–2470 (2004).

46. C. A. Stiller, Epidemiology and genetics of childhood cancer, *Oncogene* **23**(38): 6429–6444 (2004).

47. R. Nagy, K. Sweet and C. Eng, Highly penetrant hereditary cancer syndromes, *Oncogene* **23**(38): 6445–6470 (2004).

48. R. S. Houlston and J. Peto, The future of association studies of common cancers, *Hum. Genet.* **112**(4): 434–435 (2003).

49. M. Stanulla, C. Dynybil, D. B. Bartels, M. Dordelmann, L. Loning, A. Claviez *et al.*, The NQO1 C609T polymorphism is associated with risk of secondary malignant neoplasms after treatment for childhood acute lymphoblastic leukemia: A matched-pair analysis from the ALL-BFM study group, *Haematologica* **92**(11): 1581–1582 (2007).

50. M. V. Relling, J. E. Rubnitz, G. K. Rivera, J. M. Boyett, M. L. Hancock, C. A. Felix *et al.*, High incidence of secondary brain tumours after radiotherapy and antimetabolites, *Lancet* **354**(9172): 34–39 (1999).

51. J. M. Allan, C. P. Wild, S. Rollinson, E. V. Willett, A. V. Moorman, G. J. Dovey *et al.*, Polymorphism in glutathione S-transferase P1 is associated with susceptibility to chemotherapy-induced leukemia, *Proc. Natl. Acad. Sci. USA* **98**(20): 11592–11597 (2001).

52. M. V. Relling, W. Yang, S. Das, E. H. Cook, G. L. Rosner, M. Neel *et al.*, Pharmacogenetic risk factors for osteonecrosis of the hip among children with leukemia, *J. Clin. Oncol.* **22**(19): 3930–3936 (2004).

53. R. Aplenc, W. Glatfelter, P. Han, E. Rappaport, M. La, A. Cnaan *et al.*, CYP3A genotypes and treatment response in paediatric acute lymphoblastic leukaemia, *Br. J. Haematol.* **122**(2): 240–244 (2003).

54. M. A. Grenier and S. E. Lipshultz, Epidemiology of anthracycline cardiotoxicity in children and adults, *Semin. Oncol.* **25**(4 Suppl. 10): 72–85 (1998).

55. L. C. Kremer, E. C. van Dalen, M. Offringa, J. Ottenkamp and P. A. Voute, Anthracycline-induced clinical heart failure in a cohort of 607 children: Long-term follow-up study, *J. Clin. Oncol.* **19**(1): 191–196 (2001).

56. D. D. Von Hoff, M. W. Layard, P. Basa, H. L. Davis, Jr., A. L. Von Hoff, M. Rozencweig *et al.*, Risk factors for doxorubicin-induced congestive heart failure, *Ann. Intern. Med.* **91**(5): 710–717 (1979).

57. C. B. Pratt, J. L. Ransom and W. E. Evans, Age-related adriamycin cardiotoxicity in children, *Cancer Treat. Rep.* **62**(9): 1381–1385 (1978).

58. S. E. Lipshultz, S. D. Colan, R. D. Gelber, A. R. Perez-Atayde, S. E. Sallan and S. P. Sanders, Late cardiac effects of doxorubicin therapy for acute lymphoblastic leukemia in childhood, *N. Engl. J. Med.* **324**(12): 808–815 (1991).

59. S. E. Lipshultz, S. R. Lipsitz, S. M. Mone, A. M. Goorin, S. E. Sallan, S. P. Sanders *et al.*, Female sex and drug dose as risk factors for late cardiotoxic effects of doxorubicin therapy for childhood cancer, *N. Engl. J. Med.* **332**(26): 1738–1743 (1995).

60. J. P. Krischer, S. Epstein, D. D. Cuthbertson, A. M. Goorin, M. L. Epstein and S. E. Lipshultz, Clinical cardiotoxicity following anthracycline treatment for childhood cancer: The Pediatric Oncology Group experience, *J. Clin. Oncol.* **15**(4): 1544–1552 (1997).

61. J. H. Silber, R. I. Jakacki, R. L. Larsen, J. W. Goldwein and G. Barber, Increased risk of cardiac dysfunction after anthracyclines in girls, *Med. Pediatr. Oncol.* **21**(7): 477–479 (1993).

62. F. Eriksson, G. Gagliardi, A. Liedberg, I. Lax, C. Lee, S. Levitt *et al.*, Long-term cardiac mortality following radiation therapy for

Hodgkin's disease: Analysis with the relative seriality model, *Radiother. Oncol.* **55**(2): 153–162 (2000).

63. S. L. Hancock, M. A. Tucker and R. T. Hoppe, Factors affecting late mortality from heart disease after treatment of Hodgkin's disease, *J. Am. Med. Soc.* **270**(16): 1949–1955 (1993).

64. S. L. Hancock, S. S. Donaldson and R. T. Hoppe, Cardiac disease following treatment of Hodgkin's disease in children and adolescents, *J. Clin. Oncol.* **11**(7): 1208–1215 (1993).

65. C. Glanzmann, P. Kaufmann, R. Jenni, O. M. Hess and P. Huguenin, Cardiac risk after mediastinal irradiation for Hodgkin's disease, *Radiother. Oncol.* **46**(1): 51–62 (1998).

66. J. F. Boivin, G. B. Hutchison, J. H. Lubin and P. Mauch, Coronary artery disease mortality in patients treated for Hodgkin's disease, *Cancer* **69**(5): 1241–1247 (1992).

67. D. C. Bowers, D. E. McNeil, Y. Liu, Y. Yasui, M. Stovall, J. G. Gurney *et al.*, Stroke as a late treatment effect of Hodgkin's Disease: A report from the Childhood Cancer Survivor Study, *J. Clin. Oncol.* **23**(27): 6508–6515 (2005).

68. D. C. Bowers, Y. Liu, W. Leisenring, E. McNeil, M. Stovall, J. G. Gurney *et al.*, Late-occurring stroke among long-term survivors of childhood leukemia and brain tumors: A report from the Childhood Cancer Survivor Study, *J. Clin. Oncol.* **24**(33): 5277–5282 (2006).

69. L. D. Dorresteijn, A. C. Kappelle, W. Boogerd, W. J. Klokman, A. J. Balm, R. B. Keus *et al.*, Increased risk of ischemic stroke after radiotherapy on the neck in patients younger than 60 years, *J. Clin. Oncol.* **20**(1): 282–288 (2002).

70. M. B. Rosenthal and I. D. Goldfine, Primary and secondary hypothyroidism in nasopharyngeal carcinoma, *J. Am. Med. Assoc.* **236**(14): 1591–1593 (1976).

71. S. L. Hancock, R. S. Cox and I. R. McDougall, Thyroid diseases after treatment of Hodgkin's disease, *N. Engl. J. Med.* **325**(9): 599–05 (1991).

72. C. Sklar, J. Whitton, A. Mertens, M. Stovall, D. Green, N. Marina *et al.*, Abnormalities of the thyroid in survivors of Hodgkin's disease: Data from the Childhood Cancer Survivor Study, *J. Clin. Endocrinol. Metab.* **85**(9): 3227–3232 (2000).

73. L. B. Kenney, M. R. Laufer, F. D. Grant, H. Grier and L. Diller, High risk of infertility and long term gonadal damage in males treated with high dose cyclophosphamide for sarcoma during childhood, *Cancer* **91**(3): 613–621 (2001).

74. E. J. Mackie, M. Radford and S. M. Shalet, Gonadal function following chemotherapy for childhood Hodgkin's disease, *Med. Pediatr. Oncol.* **27**(2): 74–78 (1996).

75. J. H. Bramswig, U. Heimes, E. Heiermann, W. Schlegel, E. Nieschlag and G. Schellong, The effects of different cumulative doses of chemotherapy on testicular function. Results in 75 patients treated for Hodgkin's disease during childhood or adolescence, *Cancer* **65**(6): 1298–1302 (1990).

76. E. A. Livesey and C. G. Brook, Gonadal dysfunction after treatment of intracranial tumours, *Arch. Dis. Child.* **63**(5): 495–500 (1988).

77. L. E. Bath, R. A. Anderson, H. O. Critchley, C. J. Kelnar and W. H. Wallace, Hypothalamic-pituitary-ovarian dysfunction after prepubertal chemotherapy and cranial irradiation for acute leukaemia, *Hum. Reprod.* **16**(9): 1838–1844 (2001).

78. W. H. Wallace, S. M. Shalet, L. J. Tetlow and P. H. Morris-Jones, Ovarian function following the treatment of childhood acute lymphoblastic leukaemia, *Med. Pediatr. Oncol.* **21**(5): 333–339 (1993).

79. C. A. Sklar, A. C. Mertens, P. Mitby, J. Whitton, M. Stovall, C. Kasper *et al.*, Premature menopause in survivors of childhood cancer: A report from the childhood cancer survivor study, *J. Natl. Cancer. Inst.* **98**(13): 890–896 (2006).

80. W. Chemaitilly, A. C. Mertens, P. Mitby, J. Whitton, M. Stovall, Y. Yasui *et al.*, Acute ovarian failure in the childhood cancer survivor study, *J. Clin. Endocrinol. Metab.* **91**(5): 1723–1728 (2006).

81. S. J. Howell and S. M. Shalet, Spermatogenesis after cancer treatment: Damage and recovery, *J. Natl. Cancer. Inst.* **34**: 12–17 (2005).

82. C. A. Sklar, Growth and neuroendocrine dysfunction following therapy for childhood cancer, *Pediatr. Clin. North. Am.* **44**(2): 489–503 (1997).

83. S. M. Shalet, A. Horner, S. R. Ahmed and P. H. Morris-Jones, Leydig cell damage after testicular irradiation for lymphoblastic leukaemia, *Med. Pediatr. Oncol.* **13**(2): 65–68 (1985).

84. R. Brauner, P. Caltabiano, R. Rappaport, G. Leverger and G. Schaison, Leydig cell insufficiency after testicular irradiation for acute lymphoblastic leukemia, *Horm. Res.* **30**(2–3): 111–114 (1988).

85. S. Howell and S. Shalet, Gonadal damage from chemotherapy and radiotherapy, *Endocrinol. Metab. Clin. North. Am.* **27**(4): 927–943 (1998).

86. W. H. Wallace, S. M. Shalet, E. C. Crowne, P. H. Morris-Jones and H. R. Gattamaneni, Ovarian failure following abdominal irradiation

in childhood: Natural history and prognosis, *Clin. Oncol. (R. Coll. Radiol.)* **1**(2): 75–79 (1989).

87. C. C. Lushbaugh and G. W. Casarett, The effects of gonadal irradiation in clinical radiation therapy: A review. *Cancer* **37**(Suppl. 2): 1111–1125 (1976).

88. R. J. Stillman, J. S. Schinfeld, I. Schiff, R. D. Gelber, J. Greenberger, M. Larson *et al.*, Ovarian failure in long-term survivors of childhood malignancy, *Am. J. Obstet. Gynecol.* **139**(1): 62–66 (1981).

89. W. H. Wallace, S. M. Shalet, J. H. Hendry, P. H. Morris-Jones and H. R. Gattamaneni, Ovarian failure following abdominal irradiation in childhood: The radiosensitivity of the human oocyte, *Br. J. Radiol.* **62**(743): 995–998 (1989).

90. J. E. Sanders, J. Hawley, W. Levy, T. Gooley, C. D. Buckner, H. J. Deeg *et al.*, Pregnancies following high-dose cyclophosphamide with or without high-dose busulfan or total-body irradiation and bone marrow transplantation, *Blood* **87**(7): 3045–3052 (1996).

91. D. M. Green, B. Hall and M. A. Zevon, Pregnancy outcome after treatment for acute lymphoblastic leukemia during childhood or adolescence, *Cancer* **64**(11): 2335–2339 (1989).

92. H. O. Critchley, W. H. Wallace, S. M. Shalet, H. Mamtora, J. Higginson and D. C. Anderson, Abdominal irradiation in childhood; the potential for pregnancy. *Br. J. Obstet. Gynaecol.* **99**(5): 392–394 (1992).

93. H. O. Critchley, C. H. Buckley and D. C. Anderson, Experience with a 'physiological' steroid replacement regimen for the establishment of a receptive endometrium in women with premature ovarian failure, *Br. J. Obstet. Gynaecol.* **97**(9): 804–810 (1990).

94. K. Holm, K. Nysom, V. Brocks, H. Hertz, N. Jacobsen and J. Muller, Ultrasound B-mode changes in the uterus and ovaries and Doppler changes in the uterus after total body irradiation and allogeneic bone marrow transplantation in childhood, *Bone Marrow Transplant.* **23**(3): 259–263 (1999).

95. S. E. Oberfield, J. C. Allen, J. Pollack, M. I. New and L. S. Levine, Long-term endocrine sequelae after treatment of medulloblastoma: Prospective study of growth and thyroid function, *J. Pediatr.* **108**(2): 219–223 (1986).

96. L. L. Robison, M. E. Nesbit, Jr., H. N. Sather, A. T. Meadows, J. A. Ortega and G. D. Hammond, Height of children successfully treated for acute lymphoblastic leukemia: A report from the Late Effects Study

Committee of Childrens Cancer Study Group, *Med. Pediatr. Oncol.* **13**(1): 14–21 (1985).

97. C. Sklar, A. Mertens, A. Walter, D. Mitchell, M. Nesbit, M. O'Leary *et al.*, Final height after treatment for childhood acute lymphoblastic leukemia: Comparison of no cranial irradiation with 1800 and 2400 centigrays of cranial irradiation, *J. Pediatr.* **123**(1): 59–64 (1993).

98. J. H. Silber, P. S. Littman and A. T. Meadows, Stature loss following skeletal irradiation for childhood cancer, *J. Clin. Oncol.* **8**(2): 304–312 (1990).

99. B. M. Brennan, A. Rahim, E. M. Mackie, O. B. Eden and S. M. Shalet, Growth hormone status in adults treated for acute lymphoblastic leukaemia in childhood, *Clin. Endocrinol.* **48**(6): 777–783 (1998).

100. A. L. Carrel and D. B. Allen, Effects of growth hormone on body composition and bone metabolism, *Endocrine* **12**(2): 163–172 (2000).

101. P. E. Clayton and S. M. Shalet, Dose dependency of time of onset of radiation-induced growth hormone deficiency, *J. Pediatr.* **118**(2): 226–228 (1991).

102. S. M. Shalet, C. G. Beardwell, P. Morris-Jones, F. N. Bamford, G. G. Ribeiro and D. Pearson, Growth hormone deficiency in children with brain tumors, *Cancer* **37**(Suppl. 2): 1144–1148 (1976).

103. J. A. Kirk, P. Raghupathy, M. M. Stevens, C. T. Cowell, M. A. Menser, M. Bergin *et al.*, Growth failure and growth-hormone deficiency after treatment for acute lymphoblastic leukaemia, *Lancet* **1**(8526): 190–193 (1987).

104. A. L. Ogilvy-Stuart, D. J. Clark, W. H. Wallace, B. E. Gibson, R. F. Stevens, S. M. Shalet *et al.*, Endocrine deficit after fractionated total body irradiation, *Arch. Dis. Child.* **67**(9): 1107–1110 (1992).

105. L. S. Constine, P. D. Woolf, D. Cann, G. Mick, K. McCormick, R. F. Raubertas *et al.*, Hypothalamic-pituitary dysfunction after radiation for brain tumors, *N. Engl. J. Med.* **328**(2): 87–94 (1993).

106. A. D. Leiper, R. Stanhope, P. Kitching and J. M. Chessells, Precocious and premature puberty associated with treatment of acute lymphoblastic leukaemia, *Arch. Dis. Child.* **62**(11): 1107–1112 (1987).

107. B. Lannering, C. Jansson, S. Rosberg and K. Albertsson-Wikland, Increased LH and FSH secretion after cranial irradiation in boys, *Med. Pediatr. Oncol.* **29**(4): 280–287 (1997).

108. L. R. Meacham, T. T. Ghim, I. R. Crocker, M. S. O'Brien, J. Petronio, P. Davis *et al.*, Systematic approach for detection of endocrine

disorders in children treated for brain tumors, *Med. Pediatr. Oncol.* **29**(2): 86–91 (1997).

109. H. A. Davies, E. Didcock, M. Didi, A. Ogilvy-Stuart, J. K. Wales and S. M. Shalet, Disproportionate short stature after cranial irradiation and combination chemotherapy for leukaemia, *Arch. Dis. Child.* **70**(6): 472–475 (1994).

110. K. C. Oeffinger, A. C. Mertens, C. A. Sklar, Y. Yasui, T. Fears, M. Stovall *et al.*, Obesity in adult survivors of childhood acute lymphoblastic leukemia: A report from the Childhood Cancer Survivor Study, *J. Clin. Oncol.* **21**(7): 1359–1365 (2003).

111. H. A. Davies, E. Didcock, M. Didi, Ogilvy-A. Stuart, J. K. Wales and S. M. Shalet, Growth, puberty and obesity after treatment for leukaemia, *Acta. Paediatr. Suppl.* **411**: 45–50; discussion 51 (1995).

112. K. Nysom, K. Holm, K. F. Michaelsen, H. Hertz, J. Muller and C. Molgaard, Bone mass after treatment for acute lymphoblastic leukemia in childhood, *J. Clin. Oncol.* **16**(12): 3752–3760 (1998).

113. P. Arikoski, J. Komulainen, P. Riikonen, M. Parviainen, J. S. Jurvelin, R. Voutilainen *et al.*, Impaired development of bone mineral density during chemotherapy: A prospective analysis of 46 children newly diagnosed with cancer, *J. Bone Miner. Res.* **14**(12): 2002–2009 (1999).

114. S. A. Atkinson, J. M. Halton, C. Bradley, B. Wu and R. D. Barr, Bone and mineral abnormalities in childhood acute lymphoblastic leukemia: Influence of disease, drugs and nutrition, *Int. J. Cancer Suppl.* **11**: 35–9 (1998).

115. J. T. Warner, W. D. Evans, D. K. Webb, W. Bell and J. W. Gregory, Relative osteopenia after treatment for acute lymphoblastic leukemia, *Pediatr. Res.* **45**(4 Pt 1): 544–551 (1999).

116. R. C. Henderson, C. D. Madsen, C. Davis and S. H. Gold, Bone density in survivors of childhood malignancies, *J. Pediatr. Hematol. Oncol.* **18**(4): 367–371 (1996).

117. A. M. Boot, M. M. van den Heuvel-Eibrink, K. Hahlen, E. P. Krenning and S. M. de Muinck Keizer-Schrama, Bone mineral density in children with acute lymphoblastic leukaemia, *Eur. J. Cancer* **35**(12): 1693–1697 (1999).

118. S. S. Nussey, S. L. Hyer, M. Brada, A. D. Leiper and M. Pazianas, Bone mineralization after treatment of growth hormone deficiency in survivors of childhood malignancy, *Acta. Paediatr. Suppl.* **399**: 9–14; discussion 15 (1994).

119. R. D. Barr, T. Simpson, C. E. Webber, G. J. Gill, J. Hay, M. Eves *et al.*, Osteopenia in children surviving brain tumours, *Eur. J. Cancer* **34**(6): 873–877 (1998).

120. B. Meister, I. Gassner, W. Streif, K. Dengg and F. M. Fink, Methotrexate osteopathy in infants with tumors of the central nervous system, *Med. Pediatr. Oncol.* **23**(6): 493–496 (1994).

121. S. Gnudi, L. Butturini, C. Ripamonti, M. Avella and G. Bacci, The effects of methotrexate (MTX) on bone. A densitometric study conducted on 59 patients with MTX administered at different doses. *Ital. J. Orthop. Traumatol.* **14**(2): 227–231 (1988).

122. E. C. Abramson, J. Chang, M. Mayer, L. J. Kukla, D. H. Shevrin, T. E. Lad *et al.*, Effects of cisplatin on parathyroid hormone- and human lung tumor-induced bone resorption, *J. Bone Miner. Res.* **3**(5): 541–546 (1988).

123. J. Aisenberg, K. Hsieh, G. Kalaitzoglou, E. Whittam, G. Heller, R. Schneider *et al.*, Bone mineral density in young adult survivors of childhood cancer, *J. Pediatr. Hematol. Oncol.* **20**(3): 241–245 (1998).

124. B. M. Brennan, A. Rahim, J. A. Adams, O. B. Eden and S. M. Shalet, Reduced bone mineral density in young adults following cure of acute lymphoblastic leukaemia in childhood, *Br. J. Cancer* **79**(11–12): 1859–1863 (1999).

125. S. C. Kaste, R. W. Chesney, M. M. Hudson, R. H. Lustig, S. R. Rose and L. D. Carbone, Bone mineral status during and after therapy of childhood cancer: An increasing population with multiple risk factors for impaired bone health, *J. Bone Miner. Res.* **14**(12): 2010–2014 (1999).

126. R. K. Mulhern and R. W. Butler, Neurocognitive sequelae of childhood cancers and their treatment, *Pediatr. Rehabil.* **7**(1): 1–14; discussion 15–16 (2004).

127. M. Moleski, Neuropsychological, neuroanatomical, and neurophysiological consequences of CNS chemotherapy for acute lymphoblastic leukemia, *Arch. Clin. Neuropsychol.* **15**(7): 603–630 (2000).

128. C. B. Reeves, S. L. Palmer, W. E. Reddick, T. E. Merchant, G. M. Buchanan, A. Gajjar *et al.*, Attention and memory functioning among pediatric patients with medulloblastoma, *J. Pediatr. Psychol.* **31**(3): 272–280 (2006).

129. D. D. Roman and P. W. Sperduto, Neuropsychological effects of cranial radiation: Current knowledge and future directions, *Int. J. Radiat. Oncol. Biol. Phys.* **31**(4): 983–998 (1995).

130. M. D. Ris and R. B. Noll, Long-term neurobehavioral outcome in pediatric brain-tumor patients: Review and methodological critique, *J. Clin. Exp. Neuropsychol.* **16**(1): 21–42 (1994).

131. R. T. Brown, A. Madan-Swain, G. A. Walco, I. Cherrick, C. E. Ievers, P. M. Conte *et al.*, Cognitive and academic late effects among children previously treated for acute lymphocytic leukemia receiving chemotherapy as CNS prophylaxis. *J. Pediatr. Psychol.* **23**(5): 333–340 (1998).

132. K. A. Espy, I. M. Moore, P. M. Kaufmann, J. H. Kramer, K. Matthay and J. J. Hutter, Chemotherapeutic CNS prophylaxis and neuropsychologic change in children with acute lymphoblastic leukemia: A prospective study. *J. Pediatr. Psychol.* **26**(1): 1–9 (2001).

133. R. T. Brown, M. B. Sawyer, G. Antoniou, I. Toogood, M. Rice, N. Thompson *et al.*, A 3-year follow-up of the intellectual and academic functioning of children receiving central nervous system prophylactic chemotherapy for leukemia, *J. Dev. Behav. Pediatr.* **17**(6): 392–398 (1996).

134. K. L. Kaemingk, M. E. Carey, I. M. Moore, M. Herzer and J. J. Hutter, Math weaknesses in survivors of acute lymphoblastic leukemia compared to healthy children, *Child Neuropsychol.* **10**(1): 14–23 (2004).

135. I. M. Moore, K. A. Espy, P. Kaufmann, J. Kramer, K. Kaemingk, P. Miketova *et al.*, Cognitive consequences and central nervous system injury following treatment for childhood leukemia, *Semin. Oncol. Nurs.* **16**(4): 279–90; discussion 291–299 (2000).

136. R. K. Mulhern, S. L. Palmer, T. E. Merchant, D. Wallace, M. Kocak, P. Brouwers *et al.*, Neurocognitive consequences of risk-adapted therapy for childhood medulloblastoma, *J. Clin. Oncol.* **23**(24): 5511–5519 (2005).

137. C. L. Rubenstein, J. W. Varni and E. R. Katz, Cognitive functioning in long-term survivors of childhood leukemia: A prospective analysis, *J. Dev. Behav. Pediatr.* **11**(6): 301–305 (1990).

138. R. K. Mulhern, D. Fairclough and J. Ochs, A prospective comparison of neuropsychologic performance of children surviving leukemia who received 18-Gy, 24-Gy, or no cranial irradiation, *J. Clin. Oncol.* **9**(8): 1348–1356 (1991).

139. E. Hoppe-Hirsch, D. Renier, A. Lellouch-Tubiana, C. Sainte-Rose, A. Pierre-Kahn and J. F. Hirsch, Medulloblastoma in childhood: Progressive intellectual deterioration, *Child's Nerv. Syst.* **6**(2): 60–65 (1990).

140. I. M. Moore, J. H. Kramer, W. Wara, F. Halberg and A. R. Ablin, Cognitive function in children with leukemia. Effect of radiation dose and time since irradiation, *Cancer* **68**(9): 1913–1917 (1991).

141. T. A. Glauser and R. J. Packer, Cognitive deficits in long-term survivors of childhood brain tumors, *Child's Nerv. Syst.* **7**(1): 2–12 (1991).

142. P. D. Cole and B. A. Kamen, Delayed neurotoxicity associated with therapy for children with acute lymphoblastic leukemia, *Ment. Retard. Dev. Disabil. Res. Rev.* **12**(3): 174–183 (2006).

143. J. Grill, V. K. Renaux, C. Bulteau, D. Viguier, C. Levy-Piebois, C. Sainte-Rose *et al.*, Long-term intellectual outcome in children with posterior fossa tumors according to radiation doses and volumes, *Int. J. Radiat. Oncol. Biol. Phys.* **45**(1): 137–145 (1999).

144. B. Lannering, I. Marky, A. Lundberg and E. Olsson, Long-term sequelae after pediatric brain tumors: Their effect on disability and quality of life, *Med. Pediatr. Oncol.* **18**(4): 304–310 (1990).

145. M. Deutsch, P. R. Thomas, J. Krischer, J. M. Boyett, L. Albright, P. Aronin *et al.*, Results of a prospective randomized trial comparing standard dose neuraxis irradiation (3,600 cGy/20) with reduced neuraxis irradiation (2,340 cGy/13) in patients with low-stage medulloblastoma. A Combined Children's Cancer Group-Pediatric Oncology Group Study, *Pediatr. Neurosurg.* **24**(4): 167–176; discussion 176–177 (1996).

146. D. P. Waber, S. C. Carpentieri, N. Klar, L. B. Silverman, M. Schwenn, C. A. Hurwitz *et al.*, Cognitive sequelae in children treated for acute lymphoblastic leukemia with dexamethasone or prednisone, *J. Pediatr. Hematol. Oncol.* **22**(3): 206–213 (2000).

147. J. Ochs, R. Mulhern, D. Fairclough, L. Parvey, J. Whitaker, L. Ch'ien *et al.*, Comparison of neuropsychologic functioning and clinical indicators of neurotoxicity in long-term survivors of childhood leukemia given cranial radiation or parenteral methotrexate: A prospective study, *J. Clin. Oncol.* **9**(1): 145–151 (1991).

148. R. T. Brown, A. Madan-Swain, R. Pais, R. G. Lambert, K. Baldwin, R. Casey *et al.*, Cognitive status of children treated with central nervous system prophylactic chemotherapy for acute lymphocytic leukemia, *Arch. Clin. Neuropsychol.* **7**(6): 481–497 (1992).

149. D. E. Hill, K. T. Ciesielski, L. Sethre-Hofstad, M. H. Duncan and M. Lorenzi, Visual and verbal short-term memory deficits in childhood leukemia survivors after intrathecal chemotherapy, *J. Pediatr. Psychol.* **22**(6): 861–870 (1997).

150. J. W. Pang, D. L. Friedman, J. A. Whitton, M. Stovall, A. C. Mertens, L. L. Robison *et al.*, Employment status among adult survivors in the Childhood Cancer Survivor Study, *Pediatr. Blood Cancer* **50**(1): 104–110 (2008).

151. C. H. Pui, C. Cheng, W. Leung, S. N. Rai, G. K. Rivera, J. T. Sandlund *et al.*, Extended follow-up of long-term survivors of childhood acute lymphoblastic leukemia, *N. Engl. J. Med.* **349**(7): 640–649 (2003).

152. R. Nagarajan, J. P. Neglia, D. R. Clohisy, Y. Yasui, M. Greenberg, M. Hudson *et al.*, Education, employment, insurance, and marital status among 694 survivors of pediatric lower extremity bone tumors: A report from the childhood cancer survivor study, *Cancer* **97**(10): 2554–2564 (2003).

153. J. A. Punyko, J. G. Gurney, K. Scott, Baker, R. J. Hayashi, M. M. Hudson, Y. Liu *et al.*, Physical impairment and social adaptation in adult survivors of childhood and adolescent rhabdomyosarcoma: A report from the Childhood Cancer Survivors Study, *Psycho-Oncology* **16**(1): 26–37 (2007).

154. L. L. Robison, D. M. Green, M. Hudson, A. T. Meadows, A. C. Mertens, R. J. Packer *et al.*, Long-term outcomes of adult survivors of childhood cancer, *Cancer* **104**(S11): 2557–2564 (2005).

155. F. Pein, O. Sakiroglu, M. Dahan, J. Lebidois, P. Merlet, A. Shamsaldin *et al.*, Cardiac abnormalities 15 years and more after adriamycin therapy in 229 childhood survivors of a solid tumour at the Institut Gustave Roussy, *Br. J. Cancer* **91**(1): 37–44 (2004).

156. E. C. van Dalen, H. J. van der Pal, W. E. Kok, H. N. Caron and L. C. Kremer, Clinical heart failure in a cohort of children treated with anthracyclines: A long-term follow-up study, *Eur. J. Cancer* **42**(18): 3191–3198 (2006).

157. L. L. Robison and S. Bhatia, Late-effects among survivors of leukaemia and lymphoma during childhood and adolescence, *Br. J. Haematol.* **122**(3): 345–359 (2003).

158. B. L. van Leeuwen, W. A. Kamps, H. W. Jansen, H. J. Hoekstra, The effect of chemotherapy on the growing skeleton, *Cancer Treat. Rev.* **26**(5): 363–376 (2000).

159. S. C. Kaste, Bone-mineral density deficits from childhood cancer and its therapy. A review of at-risk patient cohorts and available imaging methods, *Pediatr. Radiol.* **34**(5):373–378; quiz 443–444 (2004).

160. A. J. Strauss, J. T. Su, V. M. Dalton, R. D. Gelber, S. E. Sallan and L. B. Silverman, Bony morbidity in children treated for acute lymphoblastic leukemia, *J. Clin. Oncol.* **19**(12): 3066–3072 (2001).
161. R. W. Butler and R. K. Mulhern, Neurocognitive interventions for children and adolescents surviving cancer, *J. Pediatr. Psychol.* **30**(1): 65–78 (2005).
162. E. B. Tracey, D. Chen, W. Stavrou and E. Bishop, *Cancer in New South Wales: Incidence, Mortality and Prevention* (Cancer Institute NSW, Sydney, 2005).

45

The Benefits of Nutrition and Physical Activity for Cancer Survivors

Kathy Chapman,
Erica L. James,
Jane Read and
Judy Bauer

Abstract

Cancer survivors may benefit from lifestyle interventions which can mitigate their increased risk of other health problems after a diagnosis of cancer, including heart disease, diabetes and functional impairment.

There is emerging evidence that weight management and physical activity will positively impact on key outcomes measures for cancer survivors; including quality of life, cancer recurrence and survival rates. Although dietary supplement use is very common among cancer survivors, there are very few studies documenting the effect nutritional supplements have on cancer recurrence and survival.

Overall, lifestyle interventions have the potential to improve the health and wellbeing of cancer survivors, in particular for women with breast cancer. Key recommendations for cancer survivors include:

- maintaining a healthy body weight;
- being physically active;
- eating more vegetables and fruit; and
- limiting or avoiding alcohol consumption.

These recommendations are consistent with evidence-based advice on reducing the risk of cancer and with national dietary recommendations to promote general health and need to be considered in the context of a cancer survivor's individual health and social circumstances. Further research is required to determine the efficacy and effectiveness of specific lifestyle interventions designed for breast cancer survivors, as well as for survivors of other forms of cancer.

Keywords: Nutrition, physical activity, diet supplements, overweight, obesity, fruit, vegetables, alcohol, soy, phytoestrogens.

1. Background

The role of lifestyle factors, such as nutrition, physical activity and a healthy weight in improving survival rates for people with cancer is an emerging, albeit challenging area of research. Differences in the health status of cancer survivors at different stages of illness, the various types of cancers involved and the effect of the cancer treatments used can significantly impact the overall outcomes and complicate outcome measurements. Reviews of the evidence linking obesity to breast cancer recurrence is of good quality, while the evidence linking obesity to adverse prognosis in other cancers is also beginning to accumulate.[1] Physical activity may be important for reducing the risk of recurrence and in extending survival for cancer survivors.[1]

Although survivorship should be celebrated, it is important to acknowledge that the impact of cancer is significant and associated with several long term health and psychosocial sequelae.[2] Cancer survivors may be at an increased risk of weight gain, functional impairment, fatigue, other chronic diseases (particularly cardiovascular disease, diabetes and osteoporosis), secondary cancers, and death from non-cancer causes and it is noteworthy that some of these effects may be amenable to lifestyle interventions. There is evidence that cancer patients die of non-cancer causes at a higher rate than people in the general population.[3-6] Increased weight is of particular concern, because of the adverse effects of some chemotherapy agents on the cardiovascular system and because of an observed association between weight gain and cancer mortality.[7] As an example, in the American Cancer Society Cancer Prevention Study II (a longitudinal cohort study), obesity was strongly associated with an increased risk of dying of breast cancer. The risk of dying from cancer in people with a BMI > 40 was 52% higher for men and 62% higher for women, compared to people of normal weight.[7] While moderate increases in mortality with obesity (RR ≤ 2) occurred for colon cancer and post-menopausal breast cancer in women, significantly higher relative risks were identified for uterine and kidney cancer in women and for cancer of the pancreas in both genders.[7]

Similarly, in an analysis of obesity on breast cancer survival in premenopausal women, Daling and colleagues reported that women younger than 45 years of age who had invasive breast cancer and a BMI > 25 kg/m^2 were 2.5 times more likely to die of their disease within five years of diagnosis, compared with women with a BMI < 21 kg/m^2.[8] These findings remain significant even after adjustment for stage at diagnosis and the adequacy of treatment, but the very broad weight ranges in the highest quartiles (BMI ranging from 25.9 to 52.6 kg/m^2), the relatively small sample size of the group (< 300 cases) and the fact that the study only examined ductal breast carcinomas may limit the generalisability of these findings to all breast cancers.

2. Lifestyle Habits of Cancer Survivors

Early research suggested that the practice of healthful behaviours was higher among cancer survivors than in the population at large, but many of these studies relied on modest-sized convenience samples, had limited follow-up and enrolled patients with many different cancer types.[2,9] More recent reports using much larger data sets and assessing behaviours in longer-term cancer survivors indicate that few lifestyle differences exist between individuals diagnosed with cancer and the general population — a population marked by inactivity; overweight and obesity, and suboptimal fruit and vegetable consumption.[10,11] This marks a paradigm shift and the realisation that although some cancer patients make healthful lifestyle changes after diagnosis, these changes may not generalise to all populations of cancer survivors or may be temporary.

3. Body Weight Issues and Outcomes in Cancer Survivors

Being overweight or obese has been associated with an increased risk for dying of cancer.[7] A large cohort study in the USA estimated that the current patterns of overweight and obesity could account for 14% of cancer deaths in men and 20% in women.[7]

Increased body mass index or body weight has been found to be a significant risk factor for breast cancer recurrence and decreased survival.[12] Studies have found that the risk of death was up to five times greater (30–54%) in heavier women with breast cancer, compared to women in the healthy weight range.[12] Epidemiological studies have also shown that weight gain after a cancer diagnosis is associated with an increased risk for recurrence and death, compared with maintaining normal weight after diagnosis.[13] This is especially worrisome given the fact that especially among women treated for breast cancer, a majority of them gain a significant amount of weight in the year following breast cancer diagnosis, and that return to pre-diagnosis weight is rare.[14] Results from the Nurses Health Study showed that large weight gains after a breast cancer diagnosis were associated with a 64% greater risk of recurrence, compared with those women who maintained their weight.[13] Smaller weight gains were associated with smaller increases in risk.[13]

Being overweight or obese has also been associated with an increased likelihood of recurrence of colorectal cancer.[15,16]

Results from the Women's Intervention Nutrition Study (WINS) study, a randomised controlled trial involving over 2400 women (aged 48–79 years) with early stage breast cancer, have further highlighted the importance of weight management for cancer survivors. In this randomised controlled trial, the intervention group received nutrition counselling to decrease their fat intake. After five years of follow up, the dietary fat intake of the intervention group was significantly lower ($p < 0.001$), corresponding with a significantly lower ($p = 0.005$) mean body weight in intervention participants.[17] The risk of recurrence was decreased by 24% in the intervention group compared to the control group, which was a statistically significant result ($p = 0.034$).[17] The low-fat diet was most beneficial in women with oestrogen- or progesterone-receptor negative tumours.[17] Further analysis is required to determine whether the beneficial results could be attributable to decreased in fat intake, a changed fatty acid profile, an increase in fibre intake or to the weight loss and to determine if the results can be generalisable to all breast cancers, or whether they are specific to oestrogen- or progesterone-receptor negative tumours.

Another randomised controlled trial, the Women's Healthy Eating and Living (WHEL) study including over 3000 women, evaluated the effects of a reduced-fat diet and increased intake of fruits and high-fibre vegetables among both pre- and postmenopausal women with early-stage breast cancer.[18] The intervention in the WHEL study was delivered by telephone, whereas the WINS intervention was delivered by face-to-face counselling. In contrast to the WINS trial, the WHEL trial did not show an improvement in survival. After seven years of follow up, there was no difference in breast cancer recurrence, new breast cancer, or all cause mortality between the intervention and control groups.[19] Unlike the WINS study, in the WHEL study women in both the intervention and control groups experienced small increases in weight, and this may be a factor in explaining the different results.

4. Exercise and Physical Activity

The benefits of exercise and physical activity for cancer survivors are becoming more apparent, especially the evidence that physical activity can help to alleviate fatigue and improve quality of life.[20–22] Other proven benefits of exercise for cancer survivors include improved cardiovascular fitness, muscle strength, body composition, anxiety, depression, self-esteem, and several components of quality of life (physical, functional and emotional).[21]

4.1 *Effect of physical activity on psychosocial outcomes and cardiovascular fitness*

Recent systematic reviews and meta-analyses have reported clear benefits of physical activity for cardiovascular fitness among cancer survivors, but more modest outcomes with respect to reducing fatigue or improving mood or quality of life.[1,21] A breast cancer-specific meta-analysis found exercise to be associated with small but statistically significant improvements in quality of life, physical functioning, and fatigue.[21] In one of the largest studies to date, Courneya and colleagues examined the effects of aerobic exercise alone, resistance exercise alone, or usual care, on fitness, muscular strength, body composition, and quality of life in 242 breast cancer survivors initiating chemotherapy.[23] There were significant favourable effects of both aerobic and resistance exercise on multiple outcomes including self-esteem, fitness, and body composition, as well as increased chemotherapy completion rates compared with usual care.[23] Furthermore, no significant adverse events were reported; in particular, lymphoedema did not increase and was not exacerbated by aerobic or resistance exercise.[23]

In the recent World Cancer Research Fund (WCRF) systematic review, twenty-three physical activity randomised controlled trials met the criteria for inclusion.[24] Interventions ranged from simple advice to increase physical activity, to enrolment in supervised exercise programs. These were mostly small trials and of short duration. In half of the studies, compliance levels were unclear, and the majority failed to record physical activity levels in the control group, which severely limits their value. Of the 20 physical activity trials that investigated quality of life, 18 reported a benefit from the intervention on at least one of the outcome measures reported in the study.[24] None of the trials reported harmful effects of the physical activity interventions on any of the outcomes studied.[24]

4.2 *Effect of physical activity on cancer specific survival and overall survival*

Only three of the physical activity intervention trials included in the WCRF review reported on mortality or cancer recurrence,[25–27] and none of these studies reported significant effects. Whilst there is insufficient evidence from RCTs to suggest increased disease-free survival for those who are more physically active, there is observational data that points in this direction. The Nurses Health Study was one of the first studies to show that physical activity improved breast cancer survival rate and not just quality of life, and showed that the greatest survival benefit occurred in women who performed moderate activity, such as the equivalent of walking three to five hours per week at an average pace, compared with those women who were sedentary.[28] There was a 26 to 40% improvement in survival outcomes (including death, breast cancer death, and breast cancer recurrence) for the more active women, compared to the least active women.[28] Other large observational studies have recently been published demonstrating that participation in moderate-intensity recreational physical activity after diagnosis is associated with improved survival in women who develop breast cancer.[28–30] These studies demonstrated a 24–67% reduction in the risk of total deaths and a 50–53% reduction in the risk of breast cancer deaths in women who are physically active after breast cancer diagnosis, compared with women reporting no recreational physical activity after diagnosis.

Taken together, the WCRF concluded that there is some evidence for the benefit of physical activity on post-treatment quality of life in cancer survivors.[24] The general consensus appears to be that physical activity is beneficial both from a physical and mental well-being perspective.

It is currently not know what exercise prescription is the most beneficial for which types of cancer, or at which stage of disease or treatment.[31] There are no specific fitness or physical activity guidelines that are effective for maintaining a threshold of optimal health for this population. However, a combination of aerobic and resistance training is potentially most beneficial and case reports describing exercise capacity of cancer survivors throughout various treatment regimes are emerging.[32] Two large observational studies demonstrated that participation in three hr/wk of moderate intensity recreational physical activity after diagnosis is associated with a 39–59% reduction in the risk of colon cancer death and a 50–63% reduction in the risk of total deaths in men and women who are physically active after a colon cancer diagnosis, compared with inactive men and women.[33,34] The inverse relations between post-diagnosis physical activity and colon cancer mortality remained largely unchanged across strata of sex, BMI, age, disease stage, or year of diagnosis. These observational findings of post-diagnosis physical activity and improved survival suggest that exercise may confer additional improvements in breast cancer survival beyond surgery, radiation and chemotherapy.

The simplest evidence based recommendation at present would be to undertake 30 minutes of moderate intensity recreational physical activity, such as brisk walking, five times per week. Since a majority of cancer survivors are not currently participating in recommended levels of physical activity, resulting in greater disease risk and health care costs, this targeted therapy has the potential to benefit a large number of cancer survivors.

4.3   *Sedentary behaviour*

A related, but separate behaviour to physical activity, sedentary behaviour (prolonged periods of inactivity and absence of whole body movement), is distinctly related to the risk of chronic disease independent of physical activity.[35] This accumulating evidence base has led for calls for public health recommendations regarding limiting total sedentary time, and breaking up bouts of sedentary time.[36]

> **Further reading on exercise prescription for cancer survivors:** C. Schneider, C. Dennehy and S. Carter, Exercise and cancer recovery. In: *Human Kinetics* (Champaign, IL, 2003).

5.   Dietary Factors

Many epidemiology studies demonstrate an association of diet with cancer incidence. Other than smoking cessation, a healthy diet is perhaps the most important lifestyle change a person can make to help prevent cancer, as well as cardiovascular disease, diabetes, and other chronic conditions. On the other hand, special dietary regimens have had very few trials among patients after a cancer diagnosis. One of two studies among patients with breast cancer reported an increased risk of recurrence with more servings of butter, margarine, lard, and beer,[37] and the other study reported reduced risk of death with more protein, vegetables, fibre, and omega-3 fatty acids.[38]

Evidence that dietary intakes of vegetables, fruit or related nutrients (e.g. beta carotene, vitamin C) affect cancer recurrence or survival is somewhat supportive but not conclusive.[12] The effect on risk is likely to only be modest. In a review of eight studies that examined the effect of fruit and vegetable intake on breast cancer outcomes, three studies found a significant association between increased intake of fruit and vegetables with a decreased risk of death in breast cancer cohorts, with the risk ratios ranging from 0.1–0.8.[12] One study found a trend for risk reduction that was not significant, and another study found a significant inverse association only in women with node-negative disease.[12]

For oral cancers, the consumption of vegetables, citrus fruit and orange juice has been associated with a better prognosis.[39] Fruit and vegetables are recommended for their important role as a low energy density source of nutrients (vitamins, minerals, phytochemicals and fibre) and for their contribution to weight management, as well as for their probable cancer protective effect.

5.1　*Role of dietary supplements*

Among the most common complementary therapies used by cancer survivors are dietary treatments, such as special diets, herbal remedies, and dietary supplements, including megavitamins and/or antioxidants. There is some controversy and debate about the use of dietary supplements, primarily due to the substantial gap between cancer survivors' beliefs about and use of these treatments and the lack of scientific evidence about their safety and effectiveness.

Dietary supplements are usually available in pill or powder form, and may include herbs, amino acids, vitamins, minerals and different bioactive substances found in plants (e.g. antioxidants), either singly or in combination. Micronutrients include both vitamins (e.g. folate, beta-carotene, Vitamin C and E) and minerals (e.g. selenium, calcium). Some bioactive substances or phytochemicals (e.g. phytoestrogens, lycopenes) have been investigated for cancer protective properties. Antioxidants exist naturally in many foods such as fruits, vegetables, grains and nuts, and as oxidative damage may be important in the development of cancer, it has been proposed that antioxidants may be useful chemopreventive agents.

However, the use of some antioxidants has been associated with an increased cancer incidence and/or mortality (for example, the use of beta-carotene to prevent lung cancer in smokers led to a 27% increase in mortality in smokers who developed lung cancer in the CARET study, which enrolled > 18,000 participants[40,41]). It remains unclear at present whether antioxidants may be beneficial in preventing or treating cancer or not.

A systematic review of trials of antioxidant supplements, which included 68 randomised trials with 232,606 participants found no significant effect on mortality (RR = 1.02; 95% CI, 0.98–1.06).[42] Interestingly when the meta-analysis was restricted to high quality trials (47 trials with 180,938 participants), there was an increased risk of mortality from antioxidant supplements (RR = 1.05; 95% CI, 1.02–1.08). The authors concluded that treatment with beta carotene, vitamin A, and vitamin E may increase mortality. Vitamin C and selenium had no significant effect on mortality and require further study.[42] A double-blind placebo controlled study examining the use of vitamin E and beta-carotene supplements in over 500 people being treated for head and neck cancers also suggested that long-term supplementation with high-dose antioxidant vitamins could lead to increased mortality.[43]

Across studies, the use of dietary supplements is reported by 25 to 80% of cancer survivors,[44–47] and at higher levels in cancer survivors compared with the general population or controls who have not been diagnosed with cancer.[46] The types of dietary supplements taken vary across different cancer sites — for example, the use of cranberry extract is more common among patients with bladder cancer, folic acid supplementation among patients with colorectal and uterine cancer, soy and oestrogen supplementation among women with breast cancer, and vitamin A supplementation among women diagnosed with ovarian cancer, as well as both men and women who have been diagnosed with melanoma.[46,48]

The purported benefits of the supplements are usually supported by preclinical studies. Although some supplements have been evaluated in clinical trials, the small numbers of participants, design problems, and mixed outcomes have limited the validity of their findings. The concurrent use of supplements, especially high-dose antioxidants or complex botanical agents during chemotherapy or radiation therapy can be problematic, due to drug-supplement interaction.[49,50] Some botanicals, based on their chemical structure, may have adverse effects when used perioperatively. They may have antiplatelet activity, or they may adversely interact with corticosteroids, opioid analgesics and central nervous system depressant drugs or they may produce gastrointestinal effects, hepatotoxicity, and nephrotoxicity.[51]

5.2   *Dietary supplements versus whole foods*

Although dietary supplement use is very common among cancer survivors, there are very few studies assessing the effect of nutritional supplements on cancer recurrence and survival.

Foods, like vegetables and fruits, are complex and contain many different types of nutrients and phytochemicals, which cannot always be replicated in a supplement form. Research cannot definitively identify which specific component of foods, in particular in vegetables and fruit, provide a cancer protective effect — whole foods appear to be most beneficial.[24] Studies suggest that people who eat more vegetables and fruits, which are rich sources of antioxidants (including vitamin C, vitamin E, carotenoids, and many other antioxidant phytochemicals), may have a lower risk for some types of cancer.[24]

Most of the water soluble vitamins are thought to be harmless at pharmacological doses, but there are some concerns about the safety of certain vitamins. Other nutrients, including fat soluble vitamins and minerals, are known to be toxic at pharmacological doses. The results from clinical trials using vitamin supplements (e.g. beta-carotene) to prevent cancer in particular high-risk groups have been disappointing.[40] Much of the evidence for dietary supplements is mostly derived from experimental studies and not properly conducted clinical trials. However the results from the large-scale randomised controlled trials on the efficacy of dietary supplements to reduce the risk of cancer have raised serious safety concerns.[41–43]

5.3   *Advice for cancer survivors*

The WCRF in their major review of the evidence linking food and nutrition to the prevention of cancer, concluded that there is convincing evidence that beta-carotene supplements increase the risk of lung cancer.[24] In contrast to the results for beta-carotene, the WCRF concluded that there was probable evidence that calcium protects against bowel cancer and selenium protects against prostate cancer.[24]

The WCRF concluded that the evidence does not support the use of high dose micronutrient supplements as a means of improving outcomes in people with a diagnosis of cancer, and that high dose supplements may be harmful.[24]

It is still prudent to encourage cancer survivors to obtain the potentially beneficial compounds from food. Nutritional supplements are rarely a replacement for a diet rich in vegetables and fruit and their complex mixture of phytochemicals. In Australia, the Dietary Guidelines[52] recommend two servings of fruit a day and five servings of vegetables a day, which provide optimal vital vitamins and minerals in the diet. Table 1

Table 1. Food sources and recommended dietary intakes for nutrients.

Nutrient and food sources	RDI — men	RDI — women	Upper intake limit
Selenium found in cereals, meat and fish	65 μg/day	55 μg/day	400 μg/day
Calcium found in dairy foods	1000 mg/day	1000 mg/day	2500 mg/day
Vitamin A Beta-carotene is found in orange coloured vegetables and fruits, such as carrots, sweet potato, apricots, peaches and rockmelon	900 μg/day	700 μg/day	3000 μg/day
Vitamin C found in fruits and vegetables, particularly citrus fruits	45 mg/day	45 mg/day	Not possible to set
Vitamin E found in whole grains, seeds, nuts and vegetable oils	10 mg/day	7 mg/day	300 mg/day

RDI = Recommended dietary intake.

describes food sources and the National Health and Medical Research Council (NHMRC) recommended dietary intakes[53] for some of the common anti-oxidant nutrients used by cancer survivors.

There are however some indications for lower dose nutrient supplementation (at levels at or below the recommended dietary intake) by cancer patients and survivors. These include the following:[1]

- biochemically confirmed nutrient deficiency (e.g. low plasma vitamin D levels, Vitamin B12 deficiency), where dietary approaches have been inadequate;
- nutrient intakes persistently below recommended intake levels (e.g. due to poor appetite or persistent nausea and vomiting, swallowing difficulties, etc.);
- to meet public health recommended levels of intake (i.e. calcium or vitamin D supplementation for bone health, folate among women of child-bearing age planning pregnancy) if not contraindicated due to cancer therapy; and
- known health sequelae related to cancer therapy (i.e. bone loss requiring calcium and/or vitamin D supplementation) or other comorbidites, such as osteoporosis.

A daily multivitamin supplement in amounts equivalent to 100% of the recommended dietary intakes is a good choice for those cancer survivors who are not able to eat a healthy diet. As high doses of dietary supplements may be associated with toxicity, the use of vitamin and mineral supplements in higher doses should be assessed and discussed on an individual basis.

Discussion between patients and health care providers should occur regarding dietary supplementation, to assure there is no contraindication in relation to the prescribed cancer therapy or for longer term health effects. In turn, health care providers should make an effort not only to provide time to review dietary supplement decisions with patients, but also to stay abreast of current research in this area, particularly related to potential drug interactions.

In order for cancer survivors to be better informed about complementary and alternative therapies, including dietary

Table 2. Checklist for assessing dietary supplements.

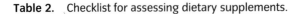

☐ Is the dietary supplement suitable for treating the condition? Is there any scientific evidence for its use?

☐ Does the dietary supplement have the potential to prevent, alleviate and/or cure symptoms or in other ways contribute to improved health and well-being?

☐ Is the dietary or herbal supplement provided by a qualified (preferably registered and certified) practitioner with adequate training background, good skills and knowledge?

☐ Are the products or materials of assured quality and what are the contraindications and precautions?

☐ Are the dietary or herbal supplements available at a competitive price?

supplements, the checklist in Table 2 may assist them to assess the benefits and harms of taking a particular dietary supplement.[54]

5.4   *Soy and phytoestrogens*

Soy and phytoestrogen supplements are commonly taken by women with breast cancer, due to their possible health benefits for a number of conditions, including cardiovascular disease, menopausal symptoms, osteoporosis and cancer. Phytoestrogens are bioactive substances that occur in plant foods with naturally occurring oestrogenic activity. Particularly high concentrations of phytoestrogens are found in soy beans and other foods containing soy.

Phytoestrogens achieved notoriety in the 1940s in Western Australia, when sheep fed large quantities of clover fodder developed a reproductive abnormality known as clover disease, which resulted in fertility problems and loss of productivity. The phytoestrogens in the clover were subsequently identified as the bioactive substance responsible for the reproductive abnormality.[55]

The lower breast and prostate cancer incidence in Asian countries and the potential anti-oestrogenic effects of phytoestrogens have led to speculations that soy foods may reduce cancer risk. Soy phytoestrogens (isoflavones) comprise mainly genistein and daidzein.[56] Genistein and daidzein have a similar structure to oestradiol, and are able to bind to oestrogen receptors, albeit with a lower affinity than oestradiol.[57]

5.4.1 Issues for women with a breast cancer diagnosis

As phytoestrogens are strikingly similar in chemical structure to oestradiol, a potential mechanism of action for phytoestrogens is their ability to bind to oestrogen receptors.

Most of the actions of phytoestrogens occur only at pharmacologic concentrations (30–185μM) in experimental studies, rather than at the lower concentrations achievable from a dietary intake. However at concentrations within the range achievable from dietary soy exposures (< 4μM in the blood), genistein (a type of phytoestrogen) exhibits oestrogenic properties, some of which could theoretically enhance breast cancer risk.[58]

In contrast, daidzein, the other key phytoestrogen in soy, has been shown to enhance tamoxifen efficacy at physiologic levels in a rat model.[59]

It is not clear whether it is safe for women with existing breast cancer to consume soy supplements, or even large quantities of soy-based foods. The results of scientific studies are contradictory, with cell culture studies reporting both the oestrogenic stimulation of oestrogen receptor positive breast cancer cell lines and the antagonism of tamoxifen activity at physiological phytoestrogen concentrations.[60,61]

Thus phytoestrogens (genistein and daidzein) may stimulate existing tumour growth and antagonise the effects of tamoxifen.[60,62] Women with current or a history of breast cancer should be aware of the risks of potential tumour growth when taking soy products.

There are no clinical trials available to definitively answer this question. While they may have a protective effect, there is also some evidence that phytoestrogens might stimulate the growth of existing hormone dependent cancers.

5.4.2 Recommendations

Although the evidence is not conclusive for soy foods to protect against cancer risk or cancer recurrence, soy foods can be encouraged as part of a varied and nutritious diet. This is consistent with national dietary guidelines to eat a diet rich in plant foods.

As the results of some experimental studies suggest adverse effects from phytoestrogens, high dose phytoestrogen supplementation is not recommended at this stage, especially for women with existing breast cancer.

5.5 *Alcohol*

No studies have found a significant association between post-diagnosis alcohol intake and cancer survival, despite the convincing evidence for alcohol being associated with the incidence of some types of cancer.[12,24] However in view of the consistency of the evidence suggesting alcohol is a modifiable risk factor for some types of cancer, and its contribution to other health problems, it is prudent to recommend alcohol be drunk in moderation by cancer survivors.

6. Recommendations

Recommendations for Cancer Survivors:

- Maintain a healthy body weight with a body mass index between 18.5 and 25
- Be physically active — aim for at least 30 minutes of moderate activity daily
- Eat more fruit and vegetables — aim for two servings of fruit and five servings of vegetables a day
- Limit or avoid alcohol — no more than two standard drinks a day for men and no more than one standard drink a day for women.

Most of these recommendations are consistent with advice to reduce the risk of cancer and promote general health and well being, and should be considered within the context of the individual survivor's overall health and social circumstances. Further research is required to determine the efficacy and effectiveness of specific lifestyle interventions designed for all cancer survivors.

References

1. C. Doyle, L. H. Kushi, T. Byers, K. S. Courneya, W. Demark-Wahnefried, B. Grant *et al.*, Nutrition and physical activity during and after cancer treatment: An American Cancer Society guide for informed choices, *CA Cancer J. Clin.* **56**(6): 323–353 (2006).
2. V. B. Stull, D. C. Snyder and W. Demark-Wahnefried, Lifestyle interventions in cancer survivors: Designing programs that meet the needs of this vulnerable and growing population, *J. Nutr.* **137**(Suppl. 1): 243S–248S (2007).
3. B. W. Brown, C. Brauner and M. C. Minnotte, Noncancer deaths in white adult cancer patients, *J. Natl. Cancer Inst.* **85**(12): 979–987 (1993).
4. S. Chang, S. R. Long, L. Kutikova, L. Bowman, D. Finley, W. H. Crown *et al.*, Estimating the cost of cancer: Results on the basis of claims data analyses for cancer patients diagnosed with seven types of cancer during 1999 to 2000, *J. Clin. Oncol.* **22**(17): 3524–3530 (2004).
5. P. A. Wingo, L. A. Ries, S. L. Parker and C. W. Heath, Jr. Long-term cancer patient survival in the United States, *Cancer Epidemiol. Biomarkers Prev.* **7**(4): 271–282 (1998).
6. K. R. Yabroff, W. F. Lawrence, S. Clauser, W. W. Davis and M. L. Brown, Burden of illness in cancer survivors: Findings from a population-based national sample, *J. Natl. Cancer Inst.* **96**(17): 1322–1330 (2004).
7. E. E. Calle, C. Rodriguez, K. Walker-Thurmond and M. J. Thun, Overweight, obesity, and mortality from cancer in a prospectively studied cohort of U.S. adults, *N. Engl. J. Med.* **348**(17): 1625–1638 (2003).
8. J. R. Daling, K. E. Malone, D. R. Doody, L. G. Johnson, J. R. Gralow and P. L. Porter, Relation of body mass index to tumor markers and

survival among young women with invasive ductal breast carcinoma, *Cancer* **92**(4): 720–729 (2001).

9. W. Demark-Wahnefried, N. M. Aziz, J. H. Rowland and B. M. Pinto, Riding the crest of the teachable moment: Promoting long-term health after the diagnosis of cancer, *J. Clin. Oncol.* **23**(24): 5814–5830 (2005).

10. K. M. Bellizzi, J. H. Rowland, D. D. Jeffery and T. McNeel, Health behaviors of cancer survivors: Examining opportunities for cancer control intervention, *J. Clin. Oncol.* **23**(34): 8884–8893 (2005).

11. E. J. Coups and J. S. Ostroff, A population-based estimate of the prevalence of behavioral risk factors among adult cancer survivors and noncancer controls, *Prev. Med.* **40**(6): 702–711 (2005).

12. C. L. Rock and W. Demark-Wahnefried, Nutrition and survival after the diagnosis of breast cancer: A review of the evidence, *J. Clin. Oncol.* **20**(15): 3302–3316 (2002).

13. C. H. Kroenke, W. Y. Chen, B. Rosner and M. D. Holmes, Weight, weight gain, and survival after breast cancer diagnosis, *J. Clin. Oncol.* **23**(7): 1370–1378 (2005).

14. M. L. Irwin, A. McTiernan, R. N. Baumgartner, K. B. Baumgartner, L. Bernstein, F. D. Gilliland *et al.*, Changes in body fat and weight after a breast cancer diagnosis: Influence of demographic, prognostic, and lifestyle factors, *J. Clin. Oncol.* **23**(4): 774–782 (2005).

15. P. I. Tartter, G. Slater, A. E. Papatestas and A. H. Aufses, Jr., Cholesterol, weight, height, Quetelet's index, and colon cancer recurrence, *J. Surg. Oncol.* **27**(4): 232–235 (1984).

16. M. L. Slattery, K. Anderson, W. Samowitz, S. L. Edwards, K. Curtin, B. Caan *et al.*, Hormone replacement therapy and improved survival among postmenopausal women diagnosed with colon cancer (USA), *Cancer Causes Control* **10**(5): 467–473 (1999).

17. R. Chlebowski, Lifestyle change including dietary fat reduction and breast cancer outcome, *J. Nutr.* **137**(Suppl. 1): 233S–235S (2007).

18. V. A. Newman, C. A. Thomson, C. L. Rock, S. W. Flatt, S. Kealey, W. A. Bardwell *et al.*, Achieving substantial changes in eating behavior among women previously treated for breast cancer — an overview of the intervention, *J. Am. Diet. Assoc.* **105**(3): 382–391 (2005).

19. J. P. Pierce, L. Natarajan, B. J. Caan, B. A. Parker, E. R. Greenberg, S. W. Flatt *et al.*, Influence of a diet very high in vegetables, fruit, and fiber and low in fat on prognosis following treatment for breast cancer: the Women's Healthy Eating and Living (WHEL) randomized trial, *J. Am. Med. Assoc.* **298**(3): 289–298 (2007).

20. K. Ahlberg, T. Ekman, F. Gaston-Johansson and V. Mock, Assessment and management of cancer-related fatigue in adults, *Lancet* **362**(9384): 640–650 (2003).

21. K. S. Courneya and C. M. Friedenreich, Physical exercise and quality of life following cancer diagnosis: A literature review, *Ann. Behav. Med.* **21**(2): 171–179 (1999).

22. D. A. Galvao and R. U. Newton, Review of exercise intervention studies in cancer patients, *J. Clin. Oncol.* **23**(4): 899–909 (2005).

23. K. S. Courneya, R. J. Segal, J. R. Mackey, K. Gelmon, R. D. Reid, C. M. Friedenreich *et al.*, Effects of aerobic and resistance exercise in breast cancer patients receiving adjuvant chemotherapy: A multi-center randomized controlled trial, *J. Clin. Oncol.* **25**(28): 4396–4404 (2007).

24. The World Cancer Research Fund and American Institute for Cancer Research, *Food, Nutrition, Physical Activity and the Prevention of Cancer: A Global Perspective* (AICR, Washington DC, 2007).

25. G. Berglund, C. Bolund, U. L. Gustafsson and P. O. Sjoden, One-year follow-up of the 'Starting Again' group rehabilitation programme for cancer patients, *Eur. J. Cancer* **30A**(12): 1744–1751 (1994).

26. B. A. Cunningham, G. Morris, C. L. Cheney, N. Buergel, S. N. Aker and P. Lenssen, Effects of resistive exercise on skeletal muscle in marrow transplant recipients receiving total parenteral nutrition, *JPEN J. Parenter. Enteral. Nutr.* **10**(6): 558–563 (1986).

27. D. C. Nieman, V. D. Cook, D. A. Henson, J. Suttles, W. J. Rejeski, P. M. Ribisl *et al.*, Moderate exercise training and natural killer cell cytotoxic activity in breast cancer patients, *Int. J. Sports Med.* **16**(5): 334–337 (1995).

28. M. D. Holmes, W. Y. Chen, D. Feskanich, C. H. Kroenke and G. A. Colditz, Physical activity and survival after breast cancer diagnosis, *J. Am. Med. Assoc.* **293**(20): 2479–2486 (2005).

29. C. N. Holick, P. A. Newcomb, A. Trentham-Dietz, L. Titus-Ernstoff, A. J. Bersch, M. J. Stampfer *et al.*, Physical activity and survival after diagnosis of invasive breast cancer, *Cancer Epidemiol. Biomarkers Prev.* **17**(2): 379–386 (2008).

30. M. L. Irwin, A. W. Smith, A. McTiernan, R. Ballard-Barbash, K. Cronin, F. D. Gilliland *et al.*, Influence of pre- and postdiagnosis physical activity on mortality in breast cancer survivors: the health, eating, activity, and lifestyle study, *J. Clin. Oncol.* **26**(24): 3958–3964 (2008).

31. N. Humpel and D. C. Iverson, Review and critique of the quality of exercise recommendations for cancer patients and survivors, *Support Care Cancer* **13**(7): 493–502 (2005).

32. J. Riggs, K. Callahan and K. Golik, Exercise capacity of a breast cancer survivor: A case study, *Med. Sci. Sports Exer.* **40**(10): 1711–1716 (2008).

33. J. A. Meyerhardt, D. Heseltine, D. Niedzwiecki, D. Hollis, L. B. Saltz, R. J. Mayer *et al.*, Impact of physical activity on cancer recurrence and survival in patients with stage III colon cancer: Findings from CALGB 89803, *J. Clin. Oncol.* **24**(22): 3535–3541 (2006).

34. J. A. Meyerhardt, E. L. Giovannucci, M. D. Holmes, A. T. Chan, J. A. Chan, G. A. Colditz *et al.*, Physical activity and survival after colorectal cancer diagnosis, *J. Clin. Oncol.* **24**(22): 3527–3534 (2006).

35. M. T. Hamilton, D. G. Hamilton and T. W. Zderic, Role of low energy expenditure and sitting in obesity, metabolic syndrome, type 2 diabetes, and cardiovascular disease, *Diabetes* **56**(11): 2655–2667 (2007).

36. G. N. Healy, D. W. Dunstan, J. Salmon, E. Cerin, J. E. Shaw, P. Z. Zimmet *et al.*, Breaks in sedentary time: Beneficial associations with metabolic risk, *Diabetes Care* **31**(4): 661–666 (2008).

37. J. Hebert, T. Hurley and Y. Ma, The effect of dietary exposures on recurrence and mortality in early stage breast cancer, *Breast Cancer Res. Treat.* **51**: 17–28 (1998).

38. M. D. Holmes, M. J. Stampfer, G. A. Colditz, B. Rosner, D. J. Hunter and W. C. Willett, Dietary factors and the survival of women with breast carcinoma, *Cancer* **86**(5): 826–835 (1999).

39. P. Crosignani, A. Russo, G. Tagliabue and F. Berrino, Tobacco and diet as determinants of survival in male laryngeal cancer patients, *Int. J. Cancer* **65**(3): 308–313 (1996).

40. A. J. Gescher, R. A. Sharma and W. P. Steward, Cancer chemoprevention by dietary constituents: A tale of failure and promise, *Lancet Oncol.* **2**(6): 371–379 (2001).

41. K. Smigel, Beta carotene fails to prevent cancer in two major studies; CARET intervention stopped, *J. Natl. Cancer Inst.* **88**(3–4): 145 (1996).

42. G. Bjelakovic, D. Nikolova, L. L. Gluud, R. G. Simonetti and C. Gluud, Mortality in randomized trials of antioxidant supplements for primary and secondary prevention: Systematic review and meta-analysis, *J. Am. Med. Assoc.* **297**(8): 842–857 (2007).

43. I. Bairati, F. Meyer, E. Jobin, M. Gelinas, A. Fortin, A. Nabid *et al.*, Antioxidant vitamins supplementation and mortality: A randomized

trial in head and neck cancer patients, *Int. J. Cancer* **119**(9): 2221–2224 (2006).

44. D. M. Eisenberg, R. B. Davis, S. L. Ettner, S. Appel, S. Wilkey, R. M. Van *et al.*, Trends in alternative medicine use in the United States, 1990–1997: Results of a follow-up national survey, *J. Am. Med. Assoc.* **280**(18): 1569–1575 (1998).

45. K. McDavid, R. A. Breslow and K. Radimer, Vitamin/mineral supplementation among cancer survivors: 1987 and 1992 National Health Interview Surveys, *Nutr. Cancer* **41**(1–2): 29–32 (2001).

46. C. L. Rock, V. A. Newman, M. L. Neuhouser, J. Major and M. J. Barnett, Antioxidant supplement use in cancer survivors and the general population, *J. Nutr.* **134**(11): 3194S–3195S (2004).

47. E. Ernst and B. R. Cassileth, The prevalence of complementary/alternative medicine in cancer: A systematic review, *Cancer* **83**(4): 777–782 (1998).

48. H. Greenlee, E. White, R. E. Patterson and A. R. Kristal, Supplement use among cancer survivors in the Vitamins and Lifestyle (VITAL) study cohort, *J. Altern. Complement. Med.* **10**(4): 660–666 (2004).

49. D. Labriola and R. Livingston, Possible interactions between dietary antioxidants and chemotherapy, *Oncology (Williston Park)* **13**(7): 1003–1008 (1999).

50. H. E. Seifried, S. S. McDonald, D. E. Anderson, P. Greenwald and J. A. Milner, The antioxidant conundrum in cancer, *Cancer Res.* **63**(15): 4295–4298 (2003).

51. N. B. Kumar, K. Allen and H. Bell, Perioperative herbal supplement use in cancer patients: Potential implications and recommendations for presurgical screening, *Cancer Control* **12**(3): 149–157 (2005).

52. National Health and Medical Research Council, *Dietary Guidelines for Australian Adults* (NHMRC, Canberra, 2003).

53. National Health and Medical Research Council, *Nutrient Reference Values for Australia and New Zealand Including Recommended Dietary Intakes* (Commonwealth Department of Health and Ageing, Canberra, Australia, 2006).

54. World Health Organization, *WHO Guidelines on Developing Information on Proper Use of Traditional, Complementary and Alternative Medicine* (World Health Organization, Geneva, 2004).

55. D. A. Shutt, R. H. Weston and J. P. Hogan, Quantitative aspects of phytoestrogen metabolism in sheep fed on Subterranean Clover (*Trifolium subterraneum cultivar Clare*) or Red Clover (*Trifolium pratense*), *Aust. J. Agric. Res.* **21**: 713–722 (1970).

56. A. C. Eldridge and W. F. Kwolek, Soybean isoflavones: Effect of environment and variety on composition, *J. Agric. Food Chem.* **31**(2): 394–396 (1983).

57. A. C. Eldridge and W. F. Kwolek, Soybean isoflavones: Effect of environment and variety on composition, *J. Agric. Food Chem.* **31**(2): 394–396 (1983).

58. M. J. Messina and C. L. Loprinzi, Soy for breast cancer survivors: A critical review of the literature, *J. Nutr.* **131**(Suppl. 11): 3095S–3108S (2001).

59. A. I. Constantinou, B. E. White, D. Tonetti, Y. Yang, W. Liang, W. Li *et al.*, The soy isoflavone daidzein improves the capacity of tamoxifen to prevent mammary tumours, *Eur. J. Cancer* **41**(4): 647–654 (2005).

60. M. L. de Lemos, Effects of soy phytoestrogens genistein and daidzein on breast cancer growth, *Ann. Pharmacother.* **35**(9): 1118–1121 (2001).

61. J. L. Limer and V. Speirs, Phyto-oestrogens and breast cancer chemo-prevention. *Breast Cancer Res.* **6**(3): 119–127 (2004).

62. C. Duffy and M. Cyr, Phytoestrogens: Potential benefits and implications for breast cancer survivors, *J. Womens Health (Larchmt)* **12**(7): 617–631 (2003).

46

Palliative and Supportive Care

Geoffrey Mitchell
and David C. Currow

Abstract

Supportive and palliative care services are integral to the provision of comprehensive cancer care (and no cancer service should call itself 'comprehensive' without a comprehensive supportive and palliative care team). All people diagnosed with cancer should have access to supportive care and the one in two people who will have their lives shortened as a result of cancer need to be able to access palliative care. The skill base, competencies and clinical evidence base for these disciplines is shared.

Properly resourced and integrated supportive and palliative care services have been shown to deliver *improved health outcomes* without compromising life expectancy to:

- people with cancer,
- their caregivers (while in the role and subsequently), and
- health services that are prepared to adequately invest in these services, with more efficient use of resources.

In order to achieve these improved health outcomes, early identification of people who have more complex needs becomes a responsibility of each member of the clinical cancer care team. Systematic assessment of current and likely future needs is imperative to improve the patient-defined outcomes that are necessary to live well with cancer or to ensure that life goals are met if premature death will occur because of cancer.

Keywords: Palliative care, supportive care, terminal care, service planning, needs assessment.

1.   Introduction

This chapter examines the delivery of palliative care in Australia. It describes both those who are provided with care, and those who miss out on accessing it. The nature of the interaction between care providers is examined and the chapter also outlines the potential benefits of access to palliative care.

The care of people in the latter stages of their life, when the objective is to maximise symptom management rather than seek a cure, is often termed palliative care. Palliative care has been defined by the World Health Organisation (WHO) as:

> ..."an approach that improves the quality of life of patients and their families facing the problems associated with life-threatening illness, through the prevention and relief of suffering by means of early identification and impeccable assessment and treatment of pain and other problems, physical, psychosocial and spiritual".[1]

Further, palliative care ideally:

- provides relief from pain and other distressing symptoms;
- affirms life and regards dying as a normal process;
- intends neither to hasten, nor to postpone death;
- integrates the psychological and spiritual aspects of patient care;
- offers a support system to help patients live as actively as possible until death;
- offers a support system to help the family cope during the patient's illness and in their own bereavement;
- uses a team approach to address the needs of patients and their families, including bereavement counselling, if indicated;
- will enhance quality of life, and may also positively influence the course of the illness; and
- is applicable early in the course of illness, in conjunction with other therapies that are intended to prolong life, such as chemotherapy or radiation therapy, and includes those

investigations needed to better understand and manage distressing clinical complications.[1]

To further define these issues, this chapter uses the following definitions for different types of care:

Supportive care is provided to optimise symptom control and functional status, irrespective of the outcomes from cancer (cure, living with cancer in the long term or premature death because of cancer) for a person and occurs throughout the cancer trajectory. Such care includes symptom control, psychosocial support and rehabilitation.

Palliative care is a subset of supportive care where the cancer is likely to be responsible for the death of this person. Continuing disease modifying therapy where appropriate is an option, in parallel with receiving good palliative care. Most importantly, this definition is not limited by prognosis, nor by a diagnosis that is limiting a person's life expectancy. It explicitly does not limit palliative care to the terminal stages of an illness. Further, the definition outlines the ability to simultaneously provide disease modifying treatment, while providing excellent palliative care and does not support a model where palliative care is only (sequentially) involved in care when all disease modifying treatments have been exhausted.

Terminal care is a subset of palliative care where the person is in the last few days or hours of life. It is characterised by increasing fatigue, rapid weight loss and anorexia as systemic manifestations of uncontrolled cancer, irrespective of the primary or secondary sites of cancer. Goals of care here are entirely directed to comfort for the person as they die, as the course of the illness at this time cannot be altered.

The threshold for referral for palliative or supportive care is defined by a systematic needs assessment done as often as necessary throughout the course of the life-limiting illness. Such a model also acknowledges that many people do not need to access specialist services — the care provided by family and health professionals is meeting their needs. Unmet needs for the patient, their family caregivers or the health professionals providing care for them, can all trigger referral for further assessment and treatment by a specialist supportive and palliative care team.

Key issues facing someone with cancer are also issues that many people expect health professionals to raise because they are uncomfortable raising the topics themselves. These include issues around finances, self-identity, sexuality and relationships.[2] Ensuring that these issues can be adequately addressed is a key responsibility for all health professionals in cancer care. Counter-intuitively, the longer the relationship between health professional and patient, the more likely it is that these issues may not be addressed.

The skill base for supportive and palliative care is identical, with each drawing upon similar research and practice literature.

Palliative and supportive care is provided by a wide range of health practitioners and services, apart from palliative care specialists. These include generalist practitioners (GPs), and nurses in community services and acute hospital settings; specialist medical practitioners, and different services (oncology, radiation therapy, surgery, and medical subspecialties, like respiratory medicine, and psychiatry). In addition, allied health practitioners frequently provide advice and treatment. Psychologists, counsellors and pastoral care workers all have important skills to contribute.

This multiplicity of professionals that can be involved in the care of people with advanced cancer should ideally work as a coordinated team. In reality, often this does not happen, with the patient being in receipt of independent and sometimes conflicting advice and care from a range of health professionals.

1.1   *Goals of care*

In parallel with therapies designed to cure, improve survival or better palliate symptoms through modifying the course of the cancer, is the process of optimising a person's level of functioning and comfort. Wherever people are in their disease trajectory, there is a need to address their symptoms and their functional status. Within this context it should be noted that extremely poor five-year survival persists for many cancers, including cancers of the lung, mesothelioma, pancreas, liver and unknown primary, and expectant assessment by a palliative care service may be justified even at the time of diagnosis for any of these cancers.

Supportive and palliative clinical care therefore also provides for the direct effects of the cancer and the effects of its treatment. The physical, psychological and spiritual effects of cancer and its treatment sit directly within the remit of comprehensive cancer care. Even for people whose cancer will not further compromise their physical health, there is still often a reappraisal and reprioritisation of life goals, and the need for physical rehabilitation as a minimum.

In-depth interviews and population-based surveys identified common issues among people facing an expected death, which include: excellent symptom control, avoiding unnecessary or futile treatments, not being a burden to others, reconciling relationships and putting one's affairs in order.[3,4] The ability to be cared for in their environment of choice is surprisingly less an issue for patients than it is for their caregivers.[4]

There is a sense that health-related quality of life is what is sought in this setting and in order to focus on patient-valued outcomes in a more concrete way, the aim of care is to optimise function and comfort in all domains that define personhood: the physical, social, sexual (including changes in body image as the result of the cancer or its treatment), financial, existential, cultural and emotional aspects of a person's life. In such a model, the focus is on better addressing unmet needs following a comprehensive assessment.

1.2 What are the demonstrated benefits of appropriate involvement of specialist palliative care?

Net benefits arising from supportive and palliative care need to measure many aspects of the service provided and no single measure is able to capture the breadth of such involvement. Outcomes must be measured for the person with cancer[5] and their caregivers, while in the role and after they have relinquished it. Caregiver outcomes include their health status, survival, health service utilisation, mental health and physical functioning. The third level of outcomes examines the impact of supportive and palliative care on the entire health system.

Evidence of the net benefit of supportive and palliative care can be measured at community and individual levels. As a community, quality end-of-life care is consistently valued.[6] Such care requires resources, a trained workforce and use of best evidence to inform practice.[7]

Overall, there are benefits identified in systematic reviews.[8–11] Measurable associations with improved outcomes for patients who access palliative care services include:

- pain assessment and management,[12,13]
- symptom management,[14]
- better maintained dignity,[15]
- perception that needs were better met,[16]
- potentially increasing the likelihood that the place of care and place of death is that of the patient's choosing,[15,17]
- the "quality of dying" and comfort in the last two weeks of life,[18,19] and
- satisfaction with care.[20–22]

The associations between the use of palliative care services and domains important to caregivers while in the role include:

- reduced anxiety,[22]
- better meeting spiritual and emotional needs,[15,23]
- improved communication,[15,24]
- improved satisfaction with care,[16,21,23] and
- fewer identified unmet needs.[25,26]

Having completed their caring, caregivers who have accessed palliative care services are more likely to:

- adjust to their new circumstances,[25] and
- have better intermediate term survival themselves.[27]

The health and social systems may also derive measurable benefit from the adequate use of specialised palliative care services *without compromising survival*.[28 29] Such benefits may include:

- reduced inpatient bed days,[20,30]
- reduced number of hospital admissions,[31] and
- decreased costs.[20,24,32,33]

Despite widely differing health systems and referral patterns, benefits have been described at a population level in several countries.[8,34–39]

Comprehensive cancer care requires quality care for all people seen in a cancer centre and must include adequate provision of supportive and palliative services. Cancer care is much more than simply trying to influence the course of cancer.

There are still cancer services that fail to invest in supportive and palliative care services, despite the evidence of benefit at all levels of evaluation. It could be argued that the title 'Comprehensive Cancer Centre' cannot be used without an adequately resourced and integrated specialist supportive and palliative care team. Given that approximately one-half of all people diagnosed with cancer will die as a result of their disease, such care is not an elective service in comprehensive care. In service planning, as the workload for oncologists increase, it is inevitable that the workload for the palliative and supportive care team will also increase.

1.3 *Who gets care for what and where?*

It is often assumed that everyone gets adequate palliative care. In order to determine if this is the case, it is useful to define the numbers of patients who should be seen with certain problems, what symptoms they have and what care they should be receiving. For example, Higginson used national cancer death figures to estimate that the incidence of death from cancer would be expected to be 28 deaths from advanced cancer in a typical general practice list of 10,000 patients each year.[40] Extrapolating the symptoms these patients would have experienced from bereaved caregiver reports,[41] it can be estimated that of these, 24 would experience pain, 13 breathlessness, 14 vomiting or nausea, and 20 a loss of appetite.[42] Seven to 18 of these will require specialist community support, and between four and seven would require in-patient hospice care.[40] If non-malignant diseases with a palliative phase are included in the count, these numbers would triple.[42]

Attempts have been made to quantify the levels of service provision required to provide adequate palliative care. Franks *et al.*,[43] examining usage in the United Kingdom and therefore relevant to their health service delivery, in a systematic review of palliative care needs, calculated that the following palliative care services should be provided:

(1) pain control for 2800 patients per million population (p/M) dying from cancer each year and 3400 p/M for people dying of non-cancer terminal illnesses;
(2) palliative home nursing for 700–1800 p/M with cancer and 350–1400 p/M with non-cancer terminal illness; and
(3) 400–700 cancer p/M and 200–700 non-cancer p/M requiring inpatient terminal care.

Franks *et al.* identified published literature which showed that these needs were being serviced (in 1999) by palliative care services providing 40–50 palliative care beds/million population. In the Australian setting, it is estimated that a minimum of 67 palliative care beds per million population is required to service the patients who will require an average of seven days per annum as in-patients in dedicated in-patient palliative care units.[44]

Specialist palliative care services see cancer patients far more commonly than other life-limiting illnesses. In Australia, a population study indicated that 61% of cancer patients accessed specialist palliative care services, compared with 34% of non-cancer patients. Palliative care services indicate that cancer patients comprise around 80 to 85% of patients.[45] However, cancer is not the only cause of predictable death. Lynn describes three trajectories of dying:

- slow decline with a rapid terminal phase (most cancer fits this trajectory);
- slow decline with periodic relapses and remissions (for example, organ failure); and
- generalised poor functioning and slow decline to death (for example, dementia).[46]

In the UK, the first trajectory is estimated to account for 25% of deaths per annum, the second (relapsing and remitting course) comprises 30% and deaths in the context of generalised poor function comprise 35%; sudden and accidental deaths comprise

10%.[47] Research questions are developing around the needs of patients with non-malignant disease and their access to palliative care, and the sort of palliative care they need, compared to that provided within a model of palliative care that has developed around the needs of people with advanced cancers.

1.4   *Access to services*

Both the number of people who are diagnosed with cancer and the number of people who die from cancer are known. The challenge is to identify the sub-group of people who will benefit most from the involvement of palliative and supportive service specialist teams. The outcomes generated by timely involvement of palliative and supportive services need to be measured in order for social and health systems to adequately invest in these services.

Some of these outcomes include:

- Overall, how effectively do people access specialist palliative care services in Australia, and are the people who most need a service being seen at the right time?
- Are the people with more complex needs being seen in the current processes? This is an important question for a service that relies on the selective referral of a subset of the whole population who may or may not benefit from service involvement.

Modelling derived from whole-of-population and whole-of-health-system data in Western Australia suggests that the current level of service provision is probably providing care for approximately the right number of people, given that many people will have excellent care from their general practitioner, community nurse and family or friends.[48] Work done in South Australia using a randomised whole-of-population approach suggests that for people with cancer, the people who most identify a need for services are indeed the people seen by those services.[19] However, a small percentage of caregivers identified that their needs would have been better met with improved access to palliative care services. Whether these results can be extrapolated to all jurisdictions remains to be seen, although both areas of research reflect very similar overall findings.

People with demonstrably lower uptake of specialist palliative care services include people from lower socioeconomic communities and people whose country of birth was not Australia. Lack of uptake does not, however, necessarily equate with greater unmet need.[19] In studies from the United Kingdom, the other group in the community who were less likely to access services were the very elderly.

Gaps in services, beyond whole groups in the community who are systematically under-represented in referrals, are otherwise sporadic. The investment in palliative care service provision varies widely between jurisdictions and within jurisdictions. Few services are funded at the levels set out in the Guidelines from Palliative Care Australia, although there are now examples where adequate resources are being made available, mostly in the jurisdictions with smaller populations.[49]

Some people with cancer have more complex needs, and when such care needs are identified, health care professionals whose substantive work is in supportive and palliative care should be included in care. Such specialist palliative care will help to:

- meet the complex needs of the person with advanced cancer
- ensure that quality research is informing practice (clinical, health service and basic science research) and
- provide education for other health professionals (existing practitioners and those in training) and the community more broadly.

A smaller number of people will need high levels of expertise. Not surprisingly, confidence in dealing with palliative care patients is predicted by practitioner experience.[50] What is not as well known is to what extent a lack of exposure may deter practitioners from commencing involvement in palliative care. A recent Australian study of GPs showed that the 25% of the surveyed sample who did *not* provide palliative care were younger, had less general practice experience, worked fewer hours, were employees rather than practice owners and had their medical education overseas.[51] Moreover, non-involvement in palliative care predicted a lack of confidence in a wide range of skills required to provide palliative care. While lifestyle issues may impact on whether some GPs would elect to offer palliative care or not, it is also likely that the longer involvement in palliative care is deferred, the less likely it is for it to ever eventuate. The changing nature of general practice means that there are more female and more part time practitioners in the general practice workforce,[52] and more GPs are making a choice not to provide such care. There is a possibility that, in the near future, the proportion of involved practitioners will fall, at a time when the number of patients needing palliative care will rise as the population ages.

The degree of matching between the needs of people who have advancing cancer with appropriate and timely referral to palliative care services, together with identification of more objective measures of the need for continuing service involvement has been reviewed systematically.[53] The review suggested measures to optimise the matching of needs and risk factors with referral to a range of health professionals including (but not limited to) specialist palliative care services. Currently, at the national level, referrals are largely limited to people experiencing uncontrolled (or the threat of uncontrolled) physical symptoms, regardless of the breadth of needs that may initiate a referral.[54]

2. Developing a Competent Workforce: Training for Palliative Care Service Delivery

Palliative care requires skills in clinical practice, in communicating with distressed patients and their caregivers, and the ability to identify and marshall community resources to meet these needs. Palliative care is an area of health care, where multidisciplinary team-based care is essential.

Not all health professionals will need or want to provide palliative care. However, all health practitioners require an understanding of the principles that underpin supportive and palliative care. This is because the underlying assumptions about care differ in this setting. In acute care settings, the focus is often on the disease process and the objective is to remove the disease, or at least to control its manifestations. The objective of palliative care is to maximise patients' quality of life and allow them and their families to function as effectively as possible during their final illness. This is unfamiliar territory for many clinicians, and an approach that has to be deliberately adopted in the right setting. This level of training should be offered at undergraduate vocational training levels, as part of broader learning of all health disciplines. In Australia, a generic palliative care undergraduate level course has been developed, with the objective of developing competence in several domains: to show empathy and compassion; to respect each individual's personal and social circumstances, preferences and choices; to optimise an individual's sense of control and personal resources; to provide holistic, person-centered care; to provide an interdisciplinary approach to meeting a person's needs; and to ensure excellence in care, being accountable to individuals and the community.[55] These materials are available at http://www.caresearch.com.au/caresearch/ PCC4UHome.

Ongoing surveys of palliative care teaching in the UK indicate a considerable expansion, with the most recent survey indicating that all medical schools had at least some palliative care teaching in their curricula.[56] Such a palliative approach is necessary because of the range and complexity of needs that people experience as death approaches.

Considerable effort needs to be made to encourage participation in palliative care. Most GPs state they would like further training in palliative care. However, palliative care suffers from being one of many skills a GP is required to maintain. While patient numbers are very small, the skills required are broad. Considerable funding is being expended to give primary care practitioners including GPs' experience in palliative care through supported short term placements — the Program of Experience in the Palliative Approach (PEPA).[57] This will encourage participation in palliative care and development of personal links with local palliative care programs.

Practitioners who have a high level of professional commitment to palliative care should have access to university level qualifications, or professional qualifications overseen by learned bodies, like medical colleges. Many western countries have specialist qualifications for palliative care, as well as Masters level higher degree qualifications.

3. Populations that Illustrate Specific Issues in Supportive and Palliative Care

Children are not supposed to die before their parents, so in those rare events, the situation poses unique challenges for everyone concerned. Most cancers are now curable, with only a small proportion leading to death. Thus most expected deaths in children occur in non-malignant conditions.[58] Many are genetically determined, which adds to the awful burden of parents, fearing that other siblings may well be affected too. For the child, there are several issues. In addition to the symptoms that the child will suffer, the child may have an incomplete understanding of their own illness and dying. Additionally, siblings of affected children are affected by the relatively large degree of attention paid to the ill child. The distress of the parents and siblings is another factor not present to the same extent in dying adults. Finally, there are issues of consent to treatment, given that children are usually not competent to make decisions for themselves. Paediatric palliative care expertise can be of real help in this setting.

Most of these life-limiting conditions have a relapsing, remitting course, where most patients will respond to initial treatment. The problem is that it is impossible to predict which relapse will be the terminal event — each relapse is probably treatable, but response lessens with the number of recurrences. Additionally, the physiological characteristics of children and the treatment regimes utilised are different to adults, so specialist medical, nursing and allied health professionals are almost inevitably involved in the care. Children with life-limiting conditions are frequently cared for by a range of sub-specialists including neurologists, pulmonologists and clinical geneticists. Palliative care services for children are scarce and the interface between them and the treating team can be strained by perceived differences in treatment objectives. Adult palliative care services may struggle with the unique problems paediatric patients bring. If the paediatric specialist and the palliative care team can work together, the patient has the benefit of both worlds, where the patient is treated by a team that hopes for the best, but prepares for the worst.[58]

Certainly in cancer there has been a concerted effort to incorporate palliative care experts at an earlier stage, both at a service level,[59] and through education and service planning.[60] Improvements have been achieved, for example in one US tertiary centre,[61] where the topics of palliation and the possibility of the child's dying were discussed earlier, and death occurred less often in intensive care after the introduction of a palliative care team. Parents reported feeling more prepared for the child's death, and were less distressed by it.

4. The Elderly in Nursing Homes — Terminal Care, Rather than Palliative Care

Another set of problems arises where patients have a terminal illness, such as disseminated cancer, and live in a residential aged care facility. While the medical needs are considerable and equal those of the elderly living at home, they may also have significant physical frailty, or dementia, or both.

In Australia, and elsewhere,[46] the care of people in residential aged care facilities is complicated by funding constraints, staffing levels, and the level of training across the workforce. Finally, there are issues around access to timely medical care from the patient's GP, due to variable after-hours accessibility and differing policies on visiting people at the facility.[62] Considerable work has been undertaken to develop evidence-based assessment and treatment for these patients.[62] Central to this care is the idea of advance care planning. Legally this involves a mentally competent person expressing in writing what they wish for in terms of medical care, in particular or what treatments they would and would not accept if they were competent to make those decisions when they become severely ill. They can appoint a person to make decisions on their behalf. Clearly these plans have to be made while the person is still competent. Once dementia is established, the person is usually not capable of formulating an advance health directive. Should these provisions not be made while the person is competent, the patient's legal and financial affairs become the responsibility of the state authorities.

Care planning in this situation also means anticipating potential medical problems, and putting plans to deal with them in place.

Finally, clear instructions for the provision of after hours medical care is a matter of priority for these patients.

5.   A Person with an Acute Haematological Malignancy

The conflict here is between attempts at curative treatment that are highly technical and palliative care which utilises technology only to improve patient comfort. Difficult decisions have to be made when the patient relapses in spite of chemotherapeutic and radio-therapeutic interventions, up to and including bone marrow transplantation. Conversations about curative and palliative interventions should occur in parallel. A "cost-benefit analysis" is required to ensure that the cost of second and third line treatment regimes is worth the effort in terms of physical effort, time, cost and morbidity. Who makes this decision? At what point is it made? Australian research shows that variability in referral patterns relates to the approach different haematologists take to referral to palliative care services. These range from refractory attitudes to referral, through to the integration of palliative care from the time of diagnosis, with roles defined for palliative care services in pain and symptom control and psychosocial support.[63] Clearly the latter approach is preferable, and contingent upon individual patient circumstances. In spite of inherent difficulties in determining the clinical course of haematological malignancies, there are clear signs that a malignancy *may not* respond to disease modifying therapy.[64] These include the number of treatments already undertaken, if and how often the patient had relapsed, how long the patient remained in remission, signs of increasing symptoms and indications of the refractory nature of the disease to treatment protocols.[64] These should be acknowledged and possibly used as the triggers to a referral to palliative care, if these services are not already in place.

6.   How are Supportive and Palliative Care Services Actually Delivered in Australia?

Supportive and palliative care services have developed largely at a local level in Australia. Most services have evolved from the interest of a small number of clinicians. This is despite a National Palliative Care Plan endorsed by all health ministers in 2000, and specific payments for these services in the last four Commonwealth State/Territory health care agreements, over the last 20 years. Ultimately, such an evolution has meant that some major hospitals and health services have invested few or no resources in funding such services, while others have robust resourcing, service provision and strategic directions.

The models of care also vary widely across the country, typified by various formal and informal relationships between inpatient, outpatient and community services. The referral base to services from cancer and other services varies widely and is often dictated by local clinical relationships, rather than needs-based planning. Given that the majority of all palliative care is delivered in the community, relationships between general practitioners, practice nurses, community health nurses and specialist palliative care services will continue to dictate the care that most people with advancing cancer receive as their illness progresses.

7. Conclusions

There is a strong evidence base for the benefits derived from timely access to an adequately resourced palliative care services. Such an investment delivers measurable benefits for the person with advancing cancer, their caregivers and the health system in which that care is delivered.

Much needs to be done to improve timely access to specialist supportive and palliative care at every level of the health system, from university teaching hospitals (which should all have acute inpatient symptom assessment units) to community-based care. Without such an investment, key benefits valued by patients and their caregivers will be foregone, causing ongoing needless suffering.

References

1. World Health Organization, *WHO Definition of Palliative Care*. Available at www.who.int/cancer/palliative/definition/en/ (accessed October 2004).
2. P. Maguire, Barriers to psychological care of the dying, *Br. Med. J.* **291**: 1711–1713 (1985).

3. P. A. Singer, D. K. Martin and M. Kelner, Quality end-of-life care: Patients' perspectives. *J. Am. Med. Assoc.* **281**: 163–168 (1999).
4. K. E. Steinhauser, N. A. Christakis, E. C. Clipp, M. McNeilly, L. McIntyre and J. A. Tulsky, Factors considered important at the end of life by patients, family, physicians, and other care providers, *J. Am. Med. Assoc.* **284**(19): 2476–2482 (2000).
5. J. Hearn and I. J. Higginson, Outcome measures in palliative care for advanced cancer patients, *J. Public Health Med.* **19**(2): 193–199 (1997).
6. T. Bodenheimer, The Oregon Health Plan — Lessons for the nation, first of two parts, *N. Engl. J. Med.* **337**(9): 651–656 (1997).
7. Anon, ASCO Policy Statement, Cancer care during the last phase of life, *J. Clin. Oncol.* **16**(5): 1986–1996 (1998).
8. I. G. Finlay, D. M. Higginson, A. M. Goodwin *et al.*, Palliative care in hospital, hospice, at home: Results from a systematic review, *Ann. Oncol.* **13**(Suppl. 4): 257–264 (2002).
9. D. M. Goodwin, I. J. Higginson, A. G. K. Edwards, I. G. Finlay, A. M. Cook, K. Hood, H. Douglas and C. E. Normand, An evaluation of systematic reviews of palliative care services, *J. Palliat. Care* **18**(2): 77–83 (2002).
10. I. J. Higginson, I. Finlay, D. M. Goodwin, A. M. Cook, K. Hood, A. G. K. Edwards, H. Douglas and C. E. Norman, Do hospital-based palliative care teams improve care for patients of families at the end of life?, *J. Pain Symptom Manage.* **23**(2): 96–106 (2002).
11. R. Harding and I. J. Higginson, What is the best way to help caregivers in cancer and palliative care? A systematic literature review of interventions and their effectiveness, *Palliat. Med.* **17**(1): 63–74 (2003).
12. S. C. Miller, V. Mor and J. Teno, Hospice enrolment and pain assessment and management in nursing homes, *J. Pain Symptom Manage.* **26**(3): 791–799 (2003).
13. I. J. Higginson, I. G. Finlay, D. M. Goodwin, K. Hood, A. G. K. Edwards, A. Cook, H. R. Douglas and C. E. Normand, Is there evidence that palliative care teams alter end-of-life experiences of patients and their caregivers?, *J. Pain Symptom Manage.* **25**(2): 150–168 (2003).
14. J. B. Hillier, A. Williams and J. Oldham, Hospital based palliative care teams improve the symptoms of cancer patients, *Palliat. Med.* **17**(6): 498–502 (2003).
15. D. Casarett, A. Pickard, F. A. Bailey, C. Ritchie, C. Furman, K. Rosenfeld, S. Shreve, Z. Chen and J. A. Shea, Do palliative consultations improve patient outcomes?, *J. Am. Geriatr. Soc.* **56**(4): 595–599 (2008).

16. J. M. Teno, B. R. Clarridge, V. Casey *et al.*, Family perspectives on end-of-life care at the last setting of care, *J. Am. Med. Assoc.* **291**(1): 88–93 (2004).

17. M. Ahlner-Elmqvist, M. S. Jordhøy, M. Jannert, P. Fayers and S. Kaasa, Place of death: Hospital-based advanced home care versus conventional care. A prospective study in palliative cancer care, *Palliat. Med.* **18**(7): 585–593 (2004).

18. K. A. Wallston, C. Burger, R. A. Smith *et al.*, Comparing the quality of death for hospice and non-hospice cancer patients, *Med. Care* **26**(2): 177–182 (1988).

19. D. C. Currow, M. Agar, C. Sanderson and A. Abernethy, Populations who die without specialist palliative care: Does lower uptake equate with unmet need? *Palliat. Med.* **22**(1): 43–50 (2008).

20. R. D. Brumley, S. Euguidanos and D. A. Cherin, Effectiveness of a home-based palliative care program for end-of-life, *J. Palliat. Med.* **6**(5): 715–724 (2003).

21. S. L. Hughes, J. Cummings, F. Weaver *et al.*, A randomized trial of the cost effectiveness of VA hospital-based home care for the terminally ill, *Health Serv. Res.* **26**(6): 801–817 (1992).

22. R. L. Kane, L. Bernstein, J. Wales *et al.*, A randomized controlled trial of hospice care, *Lancet* **323**(8382): 890–894 (1984).

23. L. P. Gelfman, D. E. Meier and R. S. Morrison, Does palliative care improve quality? A survey of bereaved family members, *J. Pain Symptom Manage.* **36**(1): 22–28 (2008).

24. G. Gade, I. Venohr, D. Conner, K. McGrady, J. Beane, R. H. Richardson, M. P. Williams, M. Liberson, M. Blum and R. Della Penna, Impact of an inpatient palliative care team: A randomized control trial, *J. Palliat. Med.* **11**(2): 180–190 (2008).

25. A. P. Abernethy, D. C. Currow, B. S. Fazekas *et al.*, Palliative care services make a difference to short- and long-term caregiver outcomes, *J. Support Care Cancer* **16**(6): 585–597 (2008).

26. S. Aoun, L. Kristjanson, D. C. Currow *et al.*, The experience of supporting a dying relative: Reflections of caregivers, *Prog. Palliat. Care* **13**(6): 317–325 (2005).

27. N. A. Christakis and T. J. Iwashyna, The health impact of health care on families: A matched cohort study of hospice use by decedents and mortality outcomes in surviving, widowed spouses, *Soc. Sci. Med.* **57**(3): 465–475 (2003).

28. B. Pyenson, S. Connor, K. Fitch and B. Kinzbrunner, Medicare in cost matched hospice and non-hospice cohorts, *J. Pain Symptom Manage.* **28**: 200–210 (2004).

29. S. R. Connor, B. Pyenson, K. Fitch, C. Spence and K. Iwasaki, Comparing hospice and non-hospice patient survival among patients who die within a three-year window, *J. Pain Symptom Manage.* **33**(3): 238–246 (2007).

30. M. Constantini, I. J. Higginson, L. Bon, M. A. Orengo, E. Garrone, F. Henriquet and P. Bruzzi, Effect of palliative home care team on hospital admissions among patients with advanced cancer, *Palliat. Med.* **17**(4): 315–321 (2003).

31. T. M. Shelby-James, D. C. Currow, P. A. Phillips *et al.*, Promoting patient-centred palliative care through case conferencing, *Aust. Fam. Phys.* **36**(11): 961–964 (2007).

32. D. H. Taylor Jr., J. Ostermann, C. H. Van Houtven, J. A. Tulsky and K. Steinhauser, What length of hospice use maximizes reduction in medical expenditures near death in the US Medicare program? *Soc. Sci. Med.* **65**(7): 1466–1478 (2007).

33. J. Hearn and I. J. Higginson, Do specialist palliative care teams improve outcomes for cancer patients? A systematic literature review, *Palliat. Med.* **12**: 317–332 (1998).

34. N. A. Christakis, T. J. Iwashyna and J. X. Zhang, Care after the onset of serious illness: A novel claims-based dataset exploiting substantial cross-set linkages to study end-of-life care, *J. Palliat. Med.* **5**(4): 515–529 (2002).

35. D. C. Currow, A. P. Abernethy and B. S. Fazekas, Specialist palliative care needs of whole populations: A feasibility study using a novel approach, *Palliat. Med.* **18**(3): 239–247 (2004).

36. B. McNamara, L. Rosenwax and C. Holman, A method for defining and estimating the palliative care population, *J. Pain Symptom Manage.* **32**: 5–12 (2006).

37. S. R. Connor, F. Elwert, C. Spence and N. A. Christakis, Geographic variation in hospice use in the United States in 2002, *J. Pain Symptom Manage.* **34**(3): 277–285 (2007).

38. T. J. Iwashyna, J. X. Zhang and N. A. Christakis, Disease-specific patterns of hospice and related healthcare use in an incidence cohort of seriously ill elderly patients, *J. Palliat. Med.* **5**(4): 531–538 (2002).

39. E. B. Lamont and N. A. Christakis, Physician factors in the timing of cancer patient referral to hospice palliative care, *Cancer* **94**(10): 2733–2737 (2002).

40. I. Higginson, Health needs assessment: Palliative and terminal care. In: *Health Care Needs Assessment*, eds. A. Stevents and J. Raftery (Radcliffe Medical Press, Oxford, 1997), pp. 183–260.

41. A. Cartwright, Changes in life and care in the year before death 1969–1987, *J. Public. Health Med.* **13**(2): 81–87 (1991).

42. J. Koffman, R. Harding and I. Higginson, Palliative care: The magnitude of the problem. In: *Palliative Care: A Patient-centered Approach*, ed. G. Mitchell (Radcliffe, Abdingdon, UK, 2007), pp. 7–77.

43. P. J. Franks, C. Salisbury, N. Bosanquet, E. K. Wilkinson, S. Kite, A. Naysmith *et al.*, The level of need for palliative care: A systematic review of the literature, *Palliat. Med.* **14**: 93–104 (2000).

44. Palliative Care Australia, *Palliative Care Service Provision in Australia: A Planning Guide* (Palliative Care Australia, Canberra, 2003).

45. N. A. Christakis and J. J. Escarce, Survival of Medicare patients after enrolment in hospice programs, *N. Engl. J. Med.* **335**(3): 172–178 (1996).

46. J. Lynn, Perspectives on care at the close of life. Serving patients who may die soon and their families: The role of hospice and other services, *J. Am. Med. Assoc.* **285**(7): 925-932 (2001).

47. E. Davies and I. Higginson, *The Solid Facts: Palliative Care* (World Health Organization, Copenhagen, 2004).

48. L. K. Rosenwax, B. McNamara, A. M. Blackmore and C. D. Holman, Estimating the size of a potential palliative care population, *Palliat. Med.* **19**: 556–562 (2005).

49. D. C. Currow and E. Nightingale, Palliative service provision in Australia — Planning resources, *Med. J. Aust.* **179**: S23–S25 (2003).

50. A. Lopez de Maturana, V. Morago, E. San Emeterio, J. Gorostiza and A. O. Arrate, Attitudes of general practitioners in Bizkaia, Spain, towards the terminally ill patient, *Palliat. Med.* **7**(1): 39–45 (1993).

51. J. J. Rhee, N. Zwar, S. Vagholkar, S. Dennis, A. M. Broadbent and G. Mitchell, Attitudes and barriers to involvement in palliative care by Australian urban general practitioners, *J. Palliat. Med.* **11**(7): 980–985 (2008).

52. J. Harding, The supply and distribution of general practitioners. In: *General Practice in Australia* (Commonwealth Department of Health and Aged Care, Canberra, 2007), pp. 41–74.

53. A. Girgis, C. Johnson, D. C. Currow, A. Walker, L. Kristjanson, G. Mitchell, P. Yates, A. Neil, B. Kelly, M. Tattersall and D. Bowman, *Palliative Care Needs Assessment Guidelines* (The Centre for Health Research and Psycho-oncology, Newcastle, NSW, 2006).

54. C. E. Johnson, A. Girgis, C. L. Paul and D. C. Currow, Cancer specialists' palliative care referral practices and perceptions: Results of a national survey, *Palliat. Med.* **22**(1): 51–57 (2008).

55. P. Yates, R. Nash, G. Mitchell, D. Canning, D. C. Currow, M. Hegarty *et al.*, *Principles for Including Palliative Care in Undergraduate Curricula* (Department of Health and Ageing, Canberra, 2005).

56. D. Field and B. Wee, Preparation for palliative care: Teaching about death, dying and bereavement in UK medical schools 2000–2001, *Med. Educ.* **36**(6): 561–567 (2002).

57. Department of Health and Ageing, *Program of Experience in the Palliative Approach (PEPA): A Clinical Placement Program* (Department of Health and Ageing, Canberra, 2005).

58. J. L. Hynson, J. Gillis, J. J. Collins, H. Irving and S. J. Trethewie, The dying child: How is care different? *Med. J. Aust.* **179**(6 Suppl.): S20–S22 (2003).

59. F. J. Meyers, J. Linder, L. Beckett, S. Christensen, J. Blais and D. R. Gandara, Simultaneous care: A model approach to the perceived conflict between investigational therapy and palliative care, *J. Pain Symptom Manage.* **28**(6): 548–556 (2004).

60. A. M. Sullivan, M. D. Lakoma, J. A. Billings, A. S. Peters and S. D. Block, Creating enduring change: Demonstrating the long-term impact of a faculty development program in palliative care, *J. Gen. Intern. Med.* **21**(9): 907–914 (2006).

61. J. Wolfe, J. F. Hammel, K. E. Edwards, J. Duncan, M. Comeau, J. Breyer *et al.*, Easing of suffering in children with cancer at the end of life: Is care changing? *J. Clin. Oncol.* **26**(10): 1717–1723 (2008).

62. L. J. Kristjanson, *Guidelines for a Palliative Approach in Residential Aged Care* (Australian Government Department of Health and Ageing, Canberra, 2006).

63. D. Joske and P. McGrath, Palliative care in haematology, *Intern. Med. J.* **37**(9): 589–590 (2007).

64. P. McGrath and H. Holewa, Special considerations for haematology patients in relation to end-of-life care: Australian findings, *Eur. J. Cancer Care* **16**(2): 164–171 (2007).

47

Cancer Care and General Practice Palliative Care

Paul Mercer

Abstract

With around 90% of people dying with cancer preferring to die at home, palliative care is an important aspect of General Practice work as GPs care for 5–8 patients dying of cancer each year on average. This chapter seeks to explore the experience of GP palliative care from three perspectives.

(1) Palliative care as a paradigm of excellence for the generalist. The specific nature of palliative care allows GPs to showcase the strength of a generalist approach. This 'excellence' manifests as a creative tension between evidence-based biomedical care, a patient-centred approach and the more traditional role of 'healer'. GPs think and reflect around patient stories, rather than the abstraction of data to achieve best practice care. Teamwork is an emerging aspect of such care.
(2) Palliative care can be a catalyst for maturity for General Practitioners. One quarter of GPs choose not to become involved in palliative services. For the majority who do so, they embark on a journey towards maturity as a practitioner. In this section the issues explored include maturity and suffering, educational challenges, communication and relational skills, self-awareness including cultural and spiritual awareness and the strength of becoming a 'wounded healer'.

(3) Palliative care and the challenge of self-care. GPs do not have a strong tradition of self-care activities. The experience of palliative care has the potential to cause stress and burn out. GPs need to pay attention to self-care and there is emerging evidence to help in this area. The 'experience of dying' again has specific challenges which need both thoughtful care and self-care. This can extend into the 'aftermath' period when managing one's grief and supporting the wider family take precedence.

Keywords: General practice, palliative care, patient-centred best practice, mature practice, teamwork, self-care.

My doctor's bag is a gift from a family I had got to know well in a palliative context. Together we had cared for a man who died at home with bowel cancer. Another patient dying with leukaemia, refused to see me if I came to his home with my Doctor's bag.

There is a fine line between good and bad outcomes in palliative cancer care in General Practice. With this awareness, I want to explore both the 'Story' and the evidence available around palliative care in this primary care context.

It is recognised that general practitioners care for 5–8 patients dying of cancer each year[1] and around 1.6% of all general practice consultations deal with cancer care.[2] In this chapter, I want to discuss the proposition that:

(1) palliative care is a paradigm of excellence for the generalist;
(2) palliative care can be a catalyst for maturity for general practitioners; and
(3) palliative care calls out a challenge to self-care for general practitioners.

1. Palliative Care as a Paradigm of Excellence for the Generalist

Modern general practice is a complex, challenging and evolving discipline. Palliative care is a window into the way general practice delivers excellence in care. This excellence manifests as a creative tension between evidence-based biomedical care, a patient-centred approach and the more traditional role of 'healer.' In general practice and especially care for dying human beings, there are times we need to set aside the evidence and "walk hand in hand with the patient through the territory."[3]

McWhinney is a champion for the patient-centred approach in primary care.[3] This approach develops from the challenge to both understand the patient and their disease. The approach then is the reconciling of the doctor's agenda to achieve biomedical diagnoses with the patient's agenda, which will include expectations, feelings and fears. The integration of these two agendas is the patient-centred approach. While symptoms and signs will be categorised into potential diagnoses or issues requiring investigations by a GP, the expectations, feelings and fears will be specific for each patient.

Research has shown that 90% of people, given the choice, prefer to die at home.[4] As McWhinney observes, GPs often know their patients before they develop a terminal illness. This 'knowing' will involve the development of trust through multiple brief episodes of care, supporting wider family challenges, facilitating episodes of mental health care and developing preventive partnerships.

Parker has published a review of his experience with 95 end-of-life case stories.[5] He observes that "relationships among the patient, physician and family built over time usually allow a 'good death' and almost always prevent unwarranted resuscitation, futile interventions, and unnecessary suffering."

1.1   *Best practice care*

Best practice guidelines and care pathways are a way the evidence around clinical issues is synthesized for practitioners. Uptake by GPs has been reserved. The patient-centred approach has implied a resistance by GPs to 'recipe style' care. Mature practice requires a reconciliation of the evidence-based approach with patient-centred care.[5] Guidelines are helpful for teaching, difficult clinical contexts, audits of care and benchmarking.

Balaban outlined a four-step guideline to conducting end-of-life discussions with patients and their families:

(1) initializing discussion;
(2) clarifying prognosis;

(3) identifying end-of-life goals; and

(4) developing a treatment plan.[6]

The paper confirms that following these steps leads to improved outcomes.

A paper around attitudes of rural GPs in Western Australia identifies six themes in terms of best practice[7]:

(1) Maintaining patients' quality of life;

(2) Providing continuity of care;

(3) Experiencing emotional issues;

(4) Collaborating with a multidisciplinary team;

(5) Acknowledging the need for education and training; and

(6) Dealing with the wider context (locally).

1.2   *Teamwork*

With the establishment of Divisions of General Practice throughout Australia in the early 1990s, there has been a steady trend towards primary care teams in General Practice, with 5% of GP patient encounters now involving a practice nurse.[8] For palliative care, the role of teams broadens to include family carers, community nurses, oncology departments, community-based palliative care services, domiciliary nursing care services and pastoral care workers. The introduction of Care Planning and Case Conferencing items for GPs has strengthened the potential formation of palliative care teams.

The implication of team care can be significant in terms of better outcomes and some research has also shown a reduction of GP patient contact time by around 50% per episode of palliative care.[9]

GP availability to conduct home visits[10] is seen as a "very important aspect of care for people with palliative care needs.[10,11] BEACH data shows a decline in home visit numbers (from 1.9% per 100 encounters in 1988–1989, down to 0.9% in 2006–2007), as well as the percentage of GPs conducting home visits.[8] The development of GP-Nurse teams may reverse this trend. Grande and colleagues also established that accessible team care is critical for lay carers to support loved ones in the end of life context.[11] A Dutch study identified that co-operation in teams is "most prevalent in younger patients, patients with cancer as the underlying disease and if psychosocial care is important."[12]

A study by Goldschmidt *et al.* confirms a growing trend in palliative care service where GPs and district nurses form a team with a palliative home-care team service.[13] The key ingredient here is good communication. Such communication often fails or is delayed at the hospital-GP interface.

Whilst case conferencing can facilitate coordination of care, the literature suggests that GPs are not so keen to put time into organising case conferences; and there is some ambivalence about the use of time (average duration is 39 minutes)[14] when there is no clear agenda, or the GP is involved by teleconference.[15] However, if well planned and with a clear agenda, case conferencing can be invaluable in defining roles and responsibilities, creating open lines of communication for the patient and their family and developing a plan which everyone 'owns'. Personal experience suggests a case conference at the family home is the best context.

Mitchell *et al.* looked at the value of case conferences for the specialist-GP interface and found that "there are improvements in patient adherence to follow-up and in physicians' clinical behaviour, and there are marginal improvements in patient health outcome which could be long-term."[16]

A literature review by the National Palliative Care Program makes a number of observations about GPs and a team approach.[17] I quote a number of points:

(1) GPs are rated by carers as not performing palliative care as effectively as specialist teams. According to carers, GPs who perform best are those who work closely with specialist teams, and GPs who rated as performing worst are those who work alone.[18]
(2) Whilst GPs have questioned the extent that they should defer to the specialist team.[19]
(3) Their participation in palliative care teams has been shown to result in improved diagnostic accuracy,[20] application of evidence-based treatments, identification of systematic problems in the delivery of care,[21] and improved ability to facilitate death at home.[22]

Teamwork transcends the palliative care context for GP's. In an editorial surveying the current literature on teamwork, Wagner noted patients value both team care and continuity of care.[23] Citing the evidence he concluded: "Continuity is associated with better health outcomes, cost of care and patient satisfaction." The editorial finished with an important recommendation for general practice, that: "more concentrated attention needs to be given to testing ways that we can make teams function as a 'coherent whole' that is visible to and appreciated by patients."

2. Palliative Care and the General Practitioner — A Catalyst for Maturity

It has been observed that "the only difference between standard general practice and palliative care is the intense nature of the problem and a short time frame."[24] In making this call, the author also notes that 25% of GPs do not become involved in palliative care and that a deliberate choice needs to be made by junior GPs on what is a steep learning curve. There are a number of pathways to mature practice. Involvement in palliative care is undoubtedly one of these paths and this section of the chapter expands this proposition.

2.1 *Maturity and suffering*

Biomedical education does not necessarily prepare us to face suffering. Suffering fits more readily into a patient-centred approach. Arthur Frank (1991) writes that "caring has nothing to do with categories, it shows the person that her life is valued because it recognises what makes her experience particular," and "care being when difference is recognised." There is no 'right thing' to say to a cancer patient, because the 'cancer patient' as a generic entity does not exist.[25] In palliative care, evidence suggests 40% of patients have moderate to high levels of unmet needs relating to fears about their prognosis, coping abilities and emotional response.[26]

Patients' most common needs can be grouped into the following categories:

- psychosocial (spiritual);
- health systems and information;
- physical and daily living;

- patient care and support; and
- services and resources.[27]

Suffering can emerge in the context of any of these needs. Researchers report 20–40% incidence of depression in early stages of cancer[28] and 12–15% levels of anxiety.[29] About 30% of people facing end of life challenges have moderate to high needs in managing pain and nausea.[30] Florian Strasser notes the association between unrelieved pain and anxiety, depressive symptoms and general distress[31]: "The phenomenon of psychospiritual pain and amplification may become a powerful trigger for a vicious cycle of increased pain expression, anxiety, escalation of opioid and benzodiazepine use and impaired cognition."

2.2   Communication skills

A 2001 study[32] in Sydney highlighted the threat poor communication poses to good patient outcomes, both to GPs and to a palliative care service.[32] GPs need accessibility and after hours support to maintain their role and the paper warns that communication failure leads to unnecessary hospitalisation. The role of assessment tools to facilitate communication has not impacted GP practice to date.[33]

A Belgian study demonstrated the need for a comprehensive communication guideline from the perspective of caregivers.[34] They identified four major communication themes

(1) truth telling;
(2) exploration of the patient's wishes regarding the end of life;
(3) dealing with disproportionate interventions; and
(4) dealing with requests for euthanasia in the terminal phase of life.

Such a guideline envisaged the combining of evidence, patient values and professional experience.

2.3   Time management

The current context of general practice in Australia is of workforce shortage. Time pressure is significant and palliative care needs time and patient-centred energy. While GPs will adopt a range of strategies, providing home visits before surgery sessions, at lunchtime or after work, this may not be sustainable if there is a heavy workload. Involving a practice nurse, palliative care service and telephone accessibility will reduce GP time involvement, but it is not always clear that reduced GP contact is effective. Hence, decisions need to be made on a case by case basis and by determining whether the patient has high needs.

2.4　*Self-awareness*

Others have noted that palliative patients and their carers value GP care and can feel betrayed when their GP does not 'deliver' when the need is greatest. Some families will change their GPs as a result of the perceived poor care their loved one received. Paradoxically, anger unrelated to care can still be directed toward a GP before or after death. Kissane *et al.* found that 9% of patients, 13% of spouses and 26% of children experienced anger in the palliative context.[35] Knowing oneself and setting professionally defensible limits to work activity is critical to sustainable palliative care. Practising in an environment of hostility and anger can readily lead to burnout.

Under the many pressures of palliative care, a GP needs to exercise a well developed sense of 'moral deliberation' or ethics. Ethical challenges are wide, ranging from communication of bad news, confidentiality in the context of team care and carer involvement, resource allocation, co-modification of health services, cultural and spiritual awareness and respect, and so on.

A Dutch study published in 2004 concluded that "striving for the highest quality of life at the end of life is best facilitated by a shared process of decision making."[36] The research around this issue suggested GPs were less likely to propose an extensive technological approach to issues. The GP needs to factor in the emotional aspects of care and the capacity of a family to endure a given situation. Home visits provide an overview not available to hospital specialists. Nurses felt that it was easier to care for patients if they had been present when the doctor had communicated about problems and management options. A patient-centred approach will mean ethical decisions will need modest guidelines. For the authors the only argument against implementing moral deliberation was the potential time this may take.

2.5 Develop cultural and spiritual awareness

Existential distress is a widespread phenomenon in the palliative context. Kissane cites a Japanese study which found meaninglessness (37%), hopelessness (37%), role loss (29%), dependency (39%) and concern about being a burden (34%) in a group of hospice patients.[37] The challenges of death itself, meaning, grief, aloneness, freedom and dignity in the palliative context all contribute to distress.

2.6 A wounded healer?

This chapter has developed the concept that dying patients need understanding and care as much as they need palliative medical skill. The words of Dame Cecily Saunders ring true here: "they need the friendship of the heart more than the skills of the mind."[38] Palliative care provides the opportunity to mature from doctor to healer. Our own wounds and suffering can be the impetus for this. Our own stories of illness or failure may have a strong resonance with the experience of dying patients. As McWhinney observes: "to be a healer one must recognize and respond to all forms of suffering; at least by listening and comforting and, if not possessing the necessary experience ourselves, calling on others who have."[39]

3. Palliative Care and the Challenge of Self-Care

As French GP philosopher Paul Tournier states: "Suffering knows no frontiers." This is true for our patients, but also is a warning not to miss. There is no tradition of pastoral care or supervision in general practice, despite the often intense demands and transference issues at play. With the increasing demands of chronic disease care, patient load and palliative care at a community level, attention to the health of doctors is emerging. Confidential doctors' health services provide backup for distressed or ill doctors. Professional bodies now encourage all doctors to have their own GP. There are regular discussions in the medical field about work life balance. The RACGP has published a resource to support GP well-being[40] and Divisions offer 'a doctor for doctors training' programme to up-skill GPs to care for colleagues. There is a growing emphasis on the value of participating in a peer support group for important care areas such as palliative care.

3.1   *What do we know about self-care in the palliative context?*

A study among nursing staff in 2004 found that for both stressed and unstressed nurses the major source of support was family and friends at home, rather than colleagues at work.[41] Only one-third practised relaxation skills and most felt there was little opportunity to genuinely debrief with colleagues. My own experience would confirm this. Attempts to set up support networks among GPs are patchy and unsustainable, but given the right circumstances, peer support can be very helpful.

Accessing timely training is a way many GPs respond to stress. In a recent survey of a post-graduate training course in the UK, 100% of respondents felt they needed more training with half indicating no previous specific palliative care training at all.[42] An Irish study revealed over 40% of GP trainees had no confidence in using a syringe driver, managing stoma problems, bereavement in children and euthanasia issues; and 57% of these trainees identified the need for further palliative care training as a priority for themselves.[43]

Palliative care is a developing discipline and timely education opportunities are valuable for the confidence of GPs who are active in this area. One study concluded that "to maintain GPs' feeling of being at ease with palliative care requires helping them to acquire the appropriate balance between technical and organisational interventions and a compassionate orientation to their terminally ill patients."[44] It is therefore not surprising that the length of time spent in general practice has been shown to be the best predictor of GP comfort in palliative care management.[45]

3.2   *The experience of dying*

Communication with the dying patient needs to balance honesty with the maintenance of hope. Ramsey *et al*. identified six areas which are of central importance in such communication[46]:

(1) talking with patients in an honest and straightforward way;
(2) being willing to talk about dying;
(3) giving bad news in a sensitive way;
(4) listening to patients;
(5) encouraging questions from patients; and
(6) being sensitive when patients are ready to talk about death.

Three issues have been reported in relation to the "experience of dying"[47]:

(1) Privacy and autonomy, principally in regard to families. As people become more frail, they struggle with their loss of control and it can be challenging for GPs to respect confidentiality in relation to the expectations of family members.
(2) A perception of lack of information about the physical changes and medication use as death approaches may be best addressed by a team approach, with reference to websites and consumer medication information.
(3) The desire to shorten life, expressed by patients, may range from fleeting thoughts that life was not worth living, or had gone on long enough, through to the expressed wish that they were dead to an outright plan for suicide; relatives may hold a different view on this.

One of my patients has been a young mother with disseminated breast cancer. She was reaching the end stage of her life as Christmas approached, and expressed a wish to die. I tried to reframe her wish by suggesting she may be able to attend a very special party if she made it to heaven before Christmas day. I also wondered with her if her family would struggle with Christmas in years to come. At my next visit she grinned and told me I had been very mischievous to talk as I had. She now had decided to live and almost miraculously she did so for the next four months. She got up from the bed and started to socialise again. Her husband was totally confused and eventually told his wife he might divorce her if she went into complete remission. Within two weeks she was dead. No one encourages suffering, but it is often very difficult to assess what is the 'real suffering' for our patients.

Advanced health directives have become a popular document to help individuals express their wishes about a palliative death. Death and dying is part of the package deal of life. Parker reports that in the context of a good doctor-patient relationship, a discussion of this nature is not usually time consuming.[5] He says: "although physicians are exhorted to discuss end-of-life issues with healthy patients, I find I can address the issue more naturally when the patient is significantly ill and more likely to be thinking of dying." He goes on "I favour directives as a stimulus for patients and families to clarify their feelings." A Finnish study confirms this by concluding that "many problems could be avoided if physicians and patients conducted progressive discussions about living wills."[48]

3.3   *The aftermath of death*

The last gasps of Cheyne-Stokes breathing herald in the finality of death, but many members of a palliative team continue to support a family by attending a funeral. The act of 'paying respect' can also help a GP finish the business of the episode of care and honour personal feelings of grief. It may act as a type of debriefing. Attending a funeral also creates openness to ongoing solidarity with carers. It has been established that bereaved carers are at a high risk of morbidity and indeed have a higher mortality in the 12 months after a spousal death. As Mitchell observes, "someone has to care for those left behind — who, if not the GP?"[1] Other research[49] shows that "for 10–20% of people, the experience of grief can become complicated and significantly impact on their ability to function." Accepting some responsibility to monitor spouses/family wellbeing can be a value added service and, because it is a shared experience, may help GPs deal with their own feelings of grief. Risk factors for complicated grief include: adversities in childhood,[50] a dependent type of relationship with the deceased,[51] and having an insecure attachment style.[52]

4.   Conclusion

I have attempted to capture the 'natural' but challenging nature of palliative care for people with cancer in the Australian general practice context. I have demonstrated that palliative care rides the creative tension for all general practice work, of evidence-based care and a patient-centred approach. GPs work with guidelines and evidence and listen to patients' stories. We try to "form a picture of what life is like for these people, of their own understanding of the illness, of their hopes and fears, of the disruptions to their social world, and of the strengths and resources they bring to bear in their struggle to die well."[53]

A recent major review of palliative care services acknowledges "GPs independently provide most of the palliative medical care required by patients who die in the community and this trend is likely to continue in to the future."[17] Advances in the techniques of palliation, the evolution of palliative teams and training to improve the skills associated with caring will help GPs fulfil their role.

Dr. Paul Mercer
General Practitioner
Manly, Queensland

References

1. M. A. Wakefield, J. Beilby and M. A. Ashby, General practitioners and palliative care, *Palliat. Med.* **7**: 117–126 (1993).
2. H. Britt, G. C. Miller, J. Charles, C. Bayram, Y. Pan, J. Henderson, L. Valenti *et al.*, *General Practice Activity in Australia 2006–07*, (Australian Institute of Health and Welfare, Canberra, 2008).
3. I. R. McWhinney, *A Textbook of Family Medicine*, 2nd ed. (Oxford University Press, Oxford, 1997), pp. 79.
4. S. T. Tang, When death is imminent: Where terminally ill patients with cancer prefer to die and why, *Cancer Nurs.* **26**: 245–251 (2003).
5. R. A. Parker, Caring for patients at the end of life: Reflections after 12 years of practice, *Ann. Intern. Med.* **136**: 175 (2002).
6. R. B. Balaban, A physician's guide to talking about end of life care, *J. Gen. Intern. Med.* **15**: 195–200 (2000).

7. M. O'Connor and R. Lee-Steere, General practitioners' attitudes to palliative care: A Western Australia rural perspective, *Palliat. Med.* **9**: 1271–1281 (2006).

8. J. Charles, Practice nurses working with GPs, *GPreview* **May**: 15 (2005).

9. P. Hall, L. Weaver, D. Gravelle and H. Thibault, Developing collaborative person-centred practice: A pilot project on a palliative care unit, *J. Interprof. Care* **21**: 69–81 (2007).

10. K. J. Yuen, M. M. Behrndt, C. Jacklyn and G. K. Mitchell, Palliative care at home: General practitioners working with palliative care teams, *Med. J. Aust.* **179**: S38–40 (2003).

11. G. E. Grande, M. C. Farquahar, S. I. Barclay and C. J. Todd, Valued aspects of primary care: content analysis of bereaved carers' descriptions, *Br. J. Gen. Pract.* **54**: 772–778 (2004).

12. S. D. Borgsteed, I. Deliens, G. van der Wal, A. L. Francke, W. A. Stalman and J. T. van Eijk, Interdisciplinary cooperation of GP's in palliative care at home: A nationwide survey in The Netherlands, *Scand. J. Prim. Health Care* **25**: 226–231 (2007).

13. D. Goldschmidt, M. Groenvold, A. T. Johnsen, A. S. Stromgren, A. Krasnik and L. Scmidt, Cooperating with a palliative home-care team: Expectations and evaluations of GP's and district nurses, *Palliat. Med.* **19**: 241–250 (2005).

14. T. M. Shelby-James, D. C. Currow, P. A. Phillips, H. Williams and A. P. Abernethy, Promoting patient centred palliative care through case conferencing, *Aust. Fam. Phys.* **37**: 1–2 (2007).

15. G. K. Mitchell, I. C. de Jong, C. B. Del Mar, A. M. Clavarino and R. Kennedy, General practitioner attitudes to case conferences: How can we increase participation and effectiveness?, *Med. J. Aust.* **177**: 95–97 (2002).

16. G. Mitchell, M. Cherry, R. Kennedy, K. Weeden, L. Burridge, A. Clavarino *et al.*, General practitioner, specialist providers case conferences in palliative care: Lessons learned from 56 case conferences, *Aust. Fam. Phys.* **34**: 389–392 (2005).

17. The National Palliative Care Program, Prepared for the Australian Government Department of Health and Ageing by Mount Olivet Community Services Ltd, *Research Study into the Educational, Training and Support Needs of General Practitioners in Palliative Care*, Final Report, 2003.

18. N. Sykes, Quality of care of the terminally ill: The carer's perspective, *Palliat. Med.* **6**: 227–236 (1992).

19. D. Field, Special not different: General practitioners' accounts of their care for dying people, *Soc. Sci. Med.* **46**: 111–120 (1998).

20. G. E. Grande, S. Barclay and C. J. Todd, Difficulty of symptom control and general practitioners' knowledge of patients' symptoms, *Palliat. Med.* **11**: 399–406 (1997).

21. L. Robinson and R. Stacy, Palliative care guidelines in the community: Setting practice guidelines for primary care teams, *Br. J. Gen. Pract.* **44**: 461–464 (1994).

22. M. Costantini, E. Camoirano, L. Madeddu, P. Bruzzi, E. Verganelli and F. Henriquet, Palliative home care and place of death among cancer patients: A population based study, *Palliat. Med.* **7**: 323–331 (1993).

23. E. H. Wagner and R. J. Reid, Are continuity of care and teamwork compatible?, *Med. Care* **45**(1): 6–7 (2007).

24. G. K. Mitchell, How well do general practitioners deliver palliative care? A systematic review, *Palliat. Med.* **16**: 457–464 (2002).

25. I. R. McWhinney, *A Textbook of Family Medicine*, 2nd ed. (Oxford University Press, Oxford, 1997), pp. 94.

26. B. Bonevski, R. Sanson-Fisher, A. Girgis, L. Burton, P. Cook and A. Boyes, Evaluation of an instrument to assess the needs of patients with cancer, *Cancer* **88**: 217–225 (2000).

27. N. Hiramanek and B. R. McAvoy, Meeting the needs of patients with cancer: A GP guide to support services, *Aust. Fam. Phys.* **34**: 365–367 (2005).

28. J. Zabora, K. Brintzenhofeszoc, B. Curbow, C. Hooker and S. Piantadosi, The prevalence of psychological distress by cancer site, *Psychooncology* **12**: 19–28 (2001).

29. S. Moorey, S. Greer, M. Watson, C. Gorman, L. Rowden, R. Tunmore *et al.*, The factor structure and factor stability of the Hospital Anxiety and Depression Scale in patients with cancer, *Br. J. Psychiatry* **158**: 255–259 (1991).

30. J. Harrison, P. Maguire, T. Ibbotson, R. MacLeod and P. Hopwood, Concerns, confiding and psychiatric disorder in newly diagnosed cancer patients: A descriptive study, *Psychooncology* **3**: 179 (1994).

31. F. Strasser, Palliative pain management: When both pain and suffering hurt, *J Palliat. Care* **21**: 69–79 (2005).

32. J. A. Low, R. K. Liu and R. Chye, Specialist community palliative care services — A survey of general practitioners' experience in Eastern Sydney, *Support. Care Cancer* **9**: 474–476 (2001).

33. B. H. Osse, K. J. Vernooij-Dassen, E. Schade and R. P. Grol, A practical instrument to explore patients' needs in palliative care: The problems and needs in palliative care questionnaire short version, *Palliat. Med.* **21**: 391–399 (2007).

34. R. Deschepper, R. Vander Stichele, J. L. Bernheim, E. De Keyser, G. Van der Kelen, F. Mortier *et al.*, Communication on end-of-life decisions with patients wishing to die at home: The making of a guideline for GPs in Flanders, *Br. J. Gen. Pract.* **56**: 14–19 (2006).

35. D. Kissane, S. Bloch, W. I. Burns, D. McKenzie and M. Posterino, Psychological morbidity in the families of patients with cancer, *Psychooncology* **3**: 47–56 (1994).

36. M. Hermsen and H. ten Have, Decision-making in palliative care practice and the need for moral deliberation: A qualitative study, *Patient Educ. Couns.* **56**: 268–275 (2005).

37. D. Kissane, Existential distress in palliative care, *Aust. Doc.* 27 September 2007.

38. C. Saunders and N. Sykes, *The Management of Terminal Malignant Disease* (Edward Arnold, London, 1993).

39. I. R. McWhinney, *A Textbook of Family Medicine*, 2nd ed. (Oxford University Press, Oxford, 1997), pp.101.

40. D. Clode and J. Bolden, *Keeping the Doctor Alive: A Self-Care Guidebook for Medical Practitioners* (RACGP Publication, 2006).

41. K. de Vries, Enhancing creativity to improve palliative care: The role of an experienced self-care workshop, *Int. J. Palliat. Nurs.* **7**: 505–511 (2001).

42. M. M. Groot, M. J. F. Vernooij-Dassen, B. J. P. Crul and R. P. T. Grol, General practitioners (GPs) and palliative care: Perceived tasks and barriers in daily practice, *Palliat. Med.* **19**: 111–118 (2005).

43. S. Dowling, A. Leary and D. Broomfield, Education in palliative care: A questionnaire survey of Irish general practitioner trainees, *Educ. Prim. Care* **16**: 42–50 (2005).

44. A. Lopez de Maturana, V. Morago, E. San Emeterio, J. Gorostiza and A. Olaskoaga Arrate, Attitudes of general practitioners in Bizkaia, Spain, towards the terminally ill patient, *Palliat. Med.* **7**: 39–45 (1993).

45. E. Wilson and K. Cox, Community palliative care development: Evaluating the role and impact of a general practitioner with a special interest in palliative medicine, *Palliat. Med.* **21**: 527–535 (2007).

46. M. D. Wenrich, J. R. Curtis, S. E. Shannon, J. D. Carline, D. M. Ambrozy and P. G. Ramsey, Communicating with dying patients within the spectrum of medical care from clinical diagnosis to death, *Arch. Intern. Med.* **161**: 868–874 (2001).

47. W. Terry, L. G. Olson, L. Wilss and G. Boulton-Lewis, Experience of dying: Concerns of dying patients and of carers, *Intern. Med. J.* **36**: 338–346 (2006).

48. H. M. Hilden, P. Louhiala and J. Palo, End of life decisions: Attitudes of Finnish physicians, *J. Med. Ethics* **30**: 362–365 (2004).

49. G. K. Silverman, J. G. Johnson and H. G. Prigerson, Preliminary explorations of the effects of prior trauma and loss on risk for psychiatric disorders in recently widowed people, *Isr. J. Psychiatry Relat. Sci.* **38**: 2002–2015 (2001).

50. G. A. Bonanno, C. B. Wortman, D. R. Lehmann *et al.*, Resilience to loss and chronic grief: A prospective study from pre-loss to 18 months post-loss, *J. Pers. Soc. Psychol.* **83**: 1150–1164 (2002).

51. C. van Doom, S. Kasl, L. C. Beery, S. Jacobs and H. G. Prigerson, The influence of marital quality and attachment styles on traumatic grief and depressive symptoms, *J. Nerv. Mental Dis.* **186**: 566–573 (1998).

52. I. R. McWhinney, *A Textbook of Family Medicine*, 2nd ed. (Oxford University Press, Oxford, 1997), pp. 94.

53. I. R. McWhinney, *A Textbook of Family Medicine*, 2nd ed. (Oxford University Press, Oxford, 1997), pp. 78.

48

Spiritual and Existential Issues at the End of Life

Bruce Rumbold

Abstract

Spiritual and existential issues are significant concerns for many people nearing the end of life. While the healthcare literature continues to debate definitions of spirituality, a reasonable consensus is emerging that the core themes addressed and affirmed in spiritual discourse are identity, community, purpose and coherence. Evidence indicates that spiritual wellbeing is correlated with an increased capacity to handle symptom load, higher quality of life and life satisfaction, and reduced anxiety.

It is argued here that it is important for these issues of spiritual significance to be explored, even if the term 'spirituality' is not used explicitly in the conversation. While debate continues about the level of engagement that healthcare practitioners should have in spiritual care, the evidence available suggests that the core competencies underpinning spiritual care are substantially the same as those required for good personal care: relational capacity and communication skills.

This chapter suggests that spirituality should be acknowledged by clinicians in ways that are appropriate to each person in their care, so that it is clear to that person that their caregivers see spirituality as important. Spiritual needs should be addressed in a care plan at least at the level of 'doing no harm' — respecting understandings, beliefs, practices and relationships important to the person. However, more active spiritual interventions should not be undertaken, unless it is the person's explicit wish that spiritual care of this sort be provided by the clinical team. If this is the case, the team can decide upon the degree to which they accede to this request or involve, perhaps by referral, other appropriately qualified practitioners. In a hospital context this may be achieved by including pastoral care practitioners in the caring team; in a community context such a request is more likely to require referral.

Keywords: Existential issues, spirituality, wellbeing, quality of life, end-of-life.

1. Introduction

Living with life-threatening illness, let alone entering a palliative care program for end-of-life care, can raise existential issues — questions about the meaning and purpose of life. Whether these existential issues should be classified as spiritual concerns is a moot point, although the trend over the past decade has been to do precisely that.[1] Assuming significant correspondence between religious beliefs and practices, spiritual needs, and existential issues is even more problematic. Evidence accumulated since the time spiritual need became a category of interest to some health-care researchers indicates that attention to spiritual concerns can ameliorate symptoms and improve quality of life, but whether clinicians should be the providers of the spiritual care that produces these outcomes continues to be debated.[2-4] Opinions expressed range from assertions that healthcare practitioners should be actively involved in providing spiritual care,[4] to counter-assertions that spiritual issues are beyond the scope and competence of health care providers and ought be dealt with by referral should they happen to arise in clinical conversation.[5]

These diverging opinions arise from, and continue to contribute to, differing ideas about spirituality. They also reflect differing ideas about the nature and scope of clinical relationships. This chapter will review the principal debates and the evidence that is available, and suggest some strategic responses.

2. Existential, Spiritual, Religious

Existential issues — issues concerning the ultimate meaning and purpose of life — arise when we as humans are confronted with our mortality. This can take place in a variety of ways; having ambitions thwarted or relationships crumble can cause us to question the meaning and purpose of our lives, for example. Similarly the death of someone we love can make us aware of our own mortality, as does the disruption of life-threatening illness in our own lives or the life of another close to us. Usually existential issues arise as we find ourselves forced to live with uncertainty, which in turn calls into question the assumptions we make about life or the beliefs by which we have been attempting to live. Changing and uncertain circumstances bring about a heightened awareness of the brevity and vulnerability of life, and the threat that death may negate everything for which we have striven.

Our responses to existential awareness are typically anxiety or dread, but these in turn can elicit courage that enables us to continue to live constructively and find meaning in the face of death.[6,7] The meaning we find will be our personal commitment made in the face of uncertainty and finitude; it will not remove uncertainty or incompleteness so much as give us a way of living constructively with these conditions.

The language of existentialism is less prevalent today, in part because existential philosophy has been replaced by other philosophical approaches. A few clinicians prefer to retain existentialist language, presumably because it is more obviously secular, and because it links with a strand of psychotherapeutic practice that draws attention to human becoming in the face of death.[8,9]

In recent years, however, the word 'spiritual' has been used increasingly to denote issues that might previously have been labelled 'existential'. This usage has become possible as spirituality has, for western cultures at least, become distanced from specific religious connotations,[10] and this social shift in the understanding of spirituality has been reflected in the healthcare literature.[11] It is encapsulated in the oft-quoted phrase: "I'm spiritual, but I'm not religious" (although this is by no means a universal distinction, particularly among older adults[12]).The spirituality referred to may vary from a vague sense that there might be 'something more' than the observable material world to a well-developed belief system based in alternative realities. The common ground appears to be a perception of one's spirit as the vitalising or animating force of the self.

A major reason for preferring the term 'spiritual' to 'existential' is that the former concept is broader in scope. Spirituality encompasses real-world practices and relationships, as well as beliefs, while existentialism focuses upon individualised inner meaning.[13] An over-emphasis on the meaning or beliefs aspects of spirituality, as existential approaches encourage, can focus on intellectual functioning and ignore people's practices and associations. A consequence can be the neglect of the spirituality and spiritual needs of cognitively-affected people in particular.

The backdrop to both mid-twentieth century existentialism and the new spiritualities of the late-twentieth century is provided by religious traditions. For existentialism the context is Christianity, while the new spiritualities tend to draw eclectically from individualist western consumerism and on the religious traditions of both the East and West.[14,15] Religions have traditionally provided frameworks that gave answers to existential questions and provided spiritual practices through which people's daily lives might be conformed to their beliefs. Interestingly, existential confrontation was a standard spiritual exercise in many of these religious traditions: reflection upon death and its imminence was prescribed as a daily exercise allowing people to live 'in the moment' as well as prepare themselves for a life after death.[16]

Religious belief systems usually include propositions concerning an afterlife, although the degree to which religiously-committed people adhere to these formal theories varies.[17] Perhaps ironically, theorising about afterlife is stronger in many of the new spiritualities, as even a cursory investigation of media and information sites like Amazon.com will show.

This chapter will use spirituality in the general sense in which it is employed in the healthcare literature; as an umbrella term that includes religious affiliation and existential encounter as aspects of a web of relationships that provides a sense of belonging and security. The content of spirituality understood in this way is personal in its detail, but it usually encompasses issues of identity, community, and purpose, while the search for operational answers to the underlying questions (Who am I? Who are we? What are we doing here?) provides some sense of coherence to the person's experience.[18,19] This consensus on a multidimensional understanding of spirituality seems to be emerging more strongly in Europe and Australia than North America. Some US studies, presumably reflecting the continuing role of religion in US society, present spirituality as more akin to religious participation and belief. Thus Breitbart, for example, defines spirituality as a construct involving 'faith' and meaning', a construct that is easily individualised and assimilated to propositional religion on the one hand or psychology on the other.[20]

Three further general comments should be made. First, in conceptualising spirituality as a construct involving identity, community and purpose it is clear that the spiritual domain is not a separate entity alongside physical, psychological and social domains, but rather a meta-narrative that constructs and maintains meaning based upon experiences in these other domains.

Second, it follows that spirituality can be an asset, or a liability, supporting resilience or fostering resistance and denial.[21] It appears that spirituality, including its religious forms, is at its best when it is intrinsic to a person, integrated into his or her practice and perception. Conversely, it is least helpful when used to avoid personal realities by means such as uncritically adopting other people's answers to avoid the risk of working out one's own.

Third, alongside discussions of the meaning of spirituality, it is important to consider its social significance: that is, what is being attempted or achieved by introducing spirituality into healthcare conversations. Understanding this has important implications for responding to spiritual issues in clinical practice contexts. An overview of the literature suggests that practitioners and patients have rather different — albeit potentially complementary — interests.[22] For healthcare practitioners and theorists, discussions of spirituality are used to:

- challenge biomedical hegemony (hence nursing and allied health interest in particular); and/or

- introduce questions of values and meaning into clinical practice.

For patients, spirituality is used to:

- regain expertise concerning one's own life: a sense of agency and identity;
- challenge the dominance of medical interpretations of their experience; and/or
- legitimise a personal quest for meaning in the treatment of their illness, including exploration of alternative healing strategies (Complementary and Alternative Medicine or CAM).

A key implication is that, if the term spirituality is to be used by either clinician or patient, the practical outcomes of the concept must be explored. The inter-subjective nature of spirituality has been used to suggest that the term might best be dispensed with.[23] This critique has some value if 'spirituality' is to be used as an objective clinical measure. It has little relevance if spirituality is seen (as it is in this chapter) as the ground upon which people's experience of illness and treatment intersects their personal history and destiny. Adopting this latter perspective, this chapter suggests that spirituality is to be taken into account in relationships and communication in healthcare settings, as an aspect of the culture in which both clinician and patient participate.

3.   Evidence for Spiritual Need and the Effects of Spiritual Care

The discussion above alerts us to one of the core issues in assembling evidence, the lack of an agreed definition of terms. As a consequence, much of the material published is descriptive, and comparisons between the quantitative studies that are available are not always straightforward. Nevertheless, consensus is emerging around a number of key points. This section draws upon systematic reviews to identify consensus. Anyone who wishes to explore the original studies in detail can do so by searching the references provided in the reviews.

3.1 Evidence for spiritual need

The principal repositories of evidence to date include two linked reviews on palliative and supportive care undertaken by the National Institute for Clinical Excellence, London[24,25] and the Palliative Care Guidelines commissioned by the National Palliative Care Program, Australia.[26] At least two relevant Cochrane reviews are in process, and no doubt others will follow. Key findings from these reviews include:

- spiritual and/or religious beliefs are important to the majority of patients with advanced cancer;
- spiritual wellbeing increases patients' capacity to handle symptom load;
- higher spiritual wellbeing correlates with higher quality of life (QoL) and life satisfaction, as well as reduced anxiety; and
- existential concerns are often as prevalent as psychological and physical symptoms in people with advanced cancer.

The evidence here comes from people consciously nearing the end-of-life; but it's important to remember that issues of meaning and purpose are engaged with at other times in the life course, and that existential crises may be precipitated by diagnosis and treatment, not just at the point where treatment options are exhausted. Survivors of cancer also demonstrate existential/spiritual need.[27] That is, an encounter with life-threatening illness may cause us to revisit earlier understandings and commitments in the light of our mortality, of which we are forcibly reminded by our current situation, even if we don't die of this particular illness. Recognising that spiritual and existential issues may occur at any point of the illness trajectory contrasts however with guidelines that assign spiritual care a role only when death is imminent.[28]

It is important to recognise that the presence of existential issues does not necessarily equate with existential distress.[29] That is, spiritual need may be identified by others, but may not necessarily be experienced by the individual as any kind of distress or lack.

It is also important to note that spiritual need usually presents as an aspect of a general need for supportive care, as quality of life may be impaired by emotional, social, spiritual and communication needs.[30] Spiritual wellbeing is thus a core domain in the assessment of quality of life in cancer,[31] although these authors also remark that the clinical utility of spiritual assessment is unclear, a point to which we will return.

3.2 *Religion, spirituality and pain*

The hospice movement introduced the concept of spiritual pain as part of a construct of 'total pain'.[32] Cecily Saunders, founder of the movement, reflecting on the years of practice in which she developed and refined hospice philosophy, explained it thus[33]:

> It soon became clear that each death was as individual as the life that preceded it and that the whole experience of that life was reflected in a patient's dying. This led to the concept of "total pain", which was presented as a complex of physical, emotional, social and spiritual elements. The whole experience for a patient includes anxiety and depression, and fear; concern for the family who will become bereaved; and often a need to find some meaning in the situation, some deeper reality in which to trust.

Chibnall *et al.*[34] correlate death distress (death anxiety, death depression) with living alone, greater physical symptom severity, more severe depressive symptoms, lower spiritual well-being, and less physician communication as perceived by the patient. They note that death distress so understood both includes, and has elements distinct from, depression. McClain, Rosenfeld and Breitbart[35] similarly equate spiritual pain with end-of-life despair, expressed in a desire for hastened death, hopelessness, suicidal ideation, loss of meaning, loss of dignity, or demoralisation, and find that spiritual well-being (as measured by the functional assessment of chronic illness therapy — spiritual well-being scale [FACIT-SWB][36]) offers some protection against this despair.[35,37]

Others[38,39] see spiritual pain or distress as caused by the loss of relationships with others, with loss of autonomy, and loss of the future. They thus locate spiritual pain in the life of the person, adding weight to Johnson's suggestion that spiritual pain might more usefully, or more comprehensively, be framed as biographical pain.[40] This approach is more consistent with Saunders' total pain concept that attends to the interaction of multiple dimensions, rather than attempting to isolate and treat a spiritual component. Whether spiritual pain becomes in fact the suffering that Breitbart, Chibnall and others describe is again a function of biography and the context, supportive or otherwise, in which people find themselves at the end of their lives.

3.2.1   Pain and suffering

Cassell notes that people in pain frequently report suffering from pain when they feel out of control, when the pain is overwhelming, when the source of the pain is unknown, when the meaning of the pain is dire, when others will not validate the pain, or when the pain is apparently without end. Conversely, suffering can often be relieved in the presence of continuing pain, by making the source of the pain known, changing its meaning, and demonstrating that it can be controlled and an end is in sight.[41] It is not surprising, then, that the experiences described as spiritual pain are amenable to interventions that range from good physical pain control through supportive presence, life review, and seeking reconciliation, to developing or renewing religious or spiritual practice.[42,43]

Wall makes a similar point when, in his dual role of career pain expert and current cancer sufferer, he states that[44]:

> There is no chance of coping if attention is monopolised by fear, anxiety and depression. There is no chance of coping while passively awaiting death or the invention of a cure. Coping is an active process directed at everything other than the pain itself. It needs inspiration and inspired help to live with pain.

3.3   Religion, spirituality and decision-making

The impact of spirituality on decision-making at the end of life is under-researched, as indeed is the general participation of patients with advanced cancer in their own treatment.[45] It is logical to think that a person's values will affect decisions about treatment, while recognising that effects are not always what we might assume. For example, there is some evidence that religious commitment correlates with aggressive treatment aimed at extending life rather than limitation or cessation of treatment.[46] Other studies have found that spiritual involvement could be linked with decisions to forgo conventional treatment in order to explore complementary or alternative treatments.[47] These studies did not explore reasons for such correlations, but one plausible hypothesis would be that, to retain a sense of hope, patients have needed either to conform to their practitioner's curative hopes or look outside the clinical relationship altogether. Gaston and Mitchell, in reviewing information giving and decision making in advanced cancer, conclude[48]:

> Better information giving and opportunity for participation in decision-making both require a shift in attitude of the doctor, given the long history of the more paternalistic model of medical care. This will involve training in consultation skills in more specialities, together with discussion of shared decision-making in all clinical situations, including that of advanced cancer.
>
> Passing in a poor prognosis, or ceasing active treatment will not affect patients adversely by destroying hope. Rather, sensitive informing and involving of the patient will involve resetting of goals and establishing an atmosphere of openness, trust and cooperation between the patient and carers.

The growth of programs in Advanced Care Planning should begin to generate more insight here by providing a framework for explicit discussion of end-of-life care — although most of these programs, it must be said, focus more upon clinicians' interests than those that might be central to patients. That considerable work has to be done in this area is evident from, for example, the recent study of Desharnais et al.,[49] which found that physicians' awareness of their patients' preferences concerning pain management, place of death, and the impact of religious/spiritual or financial concerns upon patients' treatment decisions correlated poorly with their patients' reports on these matters.

3.4   Spirituality and hope

Interestingly, increased discussion of spirituality in recent years seems to have led to fewer discussions of hope, perhaps because hope is assumed to be included in the broader concept of spirituality, or perhaps because too often hope in common parlance is limited to hope for cure, a return to the known rather than a journey into the unknown.

Hope should be understood less as specific ideas about the future and more as a capacity that enables us to engage with the present in order to move with some degree of confidence into an unknown future. Hope is the capacity to perceive possibility in each situation and to engage with that situation despite uncertainty. It is a multi-dimensional process, with experiential, spiritual, rational, relational and social elements.[50] Hope is strongly dependent upon the resources people bring from their past, the support of their communities, and clarity about their present circumstances. That is, as Gaston and Mitchell imply, hope is not something retained as long as adverse possibilities are withheld.[48] Hope must emerge from a realistic appraisal of the situation, which among other things requires clear communication of prognosis and treatment options. It should of course also be stated that clear communication concerning a person's medical condition is not guaranteed to lead to hope — simply to make it possible.[51]

Hope may be expressed in a search or quest for some sense of agency and purpose in the present circumstances,[52] perhaps one reason that complementary and alternative measures are so frequently explored by cancer sufferers: these modalities offer some sense of control and participation in treatment which conventional therapies often fail to do.[53,54] Hope can thus be seen as an aspect of spirituality: it manifests a person's spirit.

3.5   Religion, spirituality and the clinical relationship

It has already been stated that understandings of the clinical relationship will affect whether or not spiritual issues are engaged within it. Many people, while expressing a wish that their doctor would address spiritual issues in some way, are reluctant to raise these themselves because they are unsure as to whether they have the right to do so, or how their doctor will respond.[55] On the clinicians' side, different understandings of the boundaries of clinical relationships will affect whether a doctor is prepared to raise spiritual issues explicitly, or indicate awareness of their possible relevance, or acknowledge them only if they are introduced by the patient. As discussed below, the issue is not whether there should be a single best practice approach, but the pragmatic one of how to deal with different explanatory models on both sides of the clinical encounter.

4. Key Issues in Providing Spiritual Care

Those who believe that clinicians should not enter the territory of spiritual care argue that it is not in the competence of clinically-trained practitioners to offer spiritual care, and thus spiritual discussion should not be initiated by the practitioner.[5] Those arguing for clinicians' involvement in spiritual issues point to evidence that spiritual beliefs and practices can influence clinical concerns such as pain control, patient compliance, and capacity to tolerate symptoms.[56] They argue that, because spiritual issues intersect with clinical concerns, attention should be paid to spiritual factors. Others would argue more broadly that anything that enables clinicians to understand their patients better is relevant to clinical practice, and thus spiritual beliefs and practices are legitimately included in taking a clinical history. This in turn raises the matter of training in spiritual care, and has led to curricula developed in a number of medical, nursing and allied health programs, particularly in North America.[57]

The evidence that spiritual care is needed is matched with evidence that there is a role for clinicians in the provision of care.[58,59] There is however no evidence that identifies standard strategies by which care might be delivered. That is, evidence indicates that practitioners' awareness and validation of spiritual need is important to a majority of patients, but that no particular response can be identified as 'best-practice', apart that is from a person-centred approach that allows exploration of a particular person's possibilities and needs. NICE guidelines[25] conclude that core spiritual care strategies encompass:

- listening to the person's experience and questions that may arise;

- affirming the person's humanity;
- protecting the person's dignity, self-worth and identity; and
- ensuring that spiritual care is offered as an integral part of an holistic approach to health, within the framework of the person's beliefs or philosophy of life.

As noted above, the practice issue is not what clinicians think about spirituality, so much as how patients use the word and what content they ascribe to it. Introducing spirituality into the clinical conversation can be a way of ensuring that care incorporates possibilities, in addition to addressing problems.

4.1 Provision of spiritual care

4.1.1 Assessment

There is a wide range of assessment tools available.[60,61] Most have been developed for research purposes, and have little utility for clinical practice. They tend to focus upon the researcher's interests rather than the patient's concerns, and in this way undermine the social role of spirituality in current health discourse. If spirituality is about patients preserving a sense of identity and agency in the face of the strange and uncertain world of medical treatment, then having that world attempt to capture spirituality through a set of assessment tools is surely counterproductive.[62]

This is not however to suggest that spirituality cannot be constructively introduced into clinical conversation. Puchalski's spiritual history is an approach that introduces faith or belief explicitly as an aspect of clinical process, and is referenced frequently. The brief interview schedule follows the acronym FICA, for Faith or beliefs, Importance and influence, Community, and Address.[63,64]

F   What is your faith or belief?

Do you consider yourself spiritual or religious?
What things do you believe that give meaning to your life?

I   Is your faith or belief important in your life?

What influence does it have on how you take care of yourself?

How have your beliefs influenced your behaviour during this illness?

What role do your beliefs play in regaining your health?

C   Are you part of a spiritual or religious community?

Is this of support to you, and how?

Is there a person or group of people you really love or who are really important to you?

A   How would you like me as your healthcare provider to address these issues in your healthcare?

Clearly this approach signals both the clinician's recognition of the potential significance of spiritual issues and a willingness to engage them, whilst also respecting the patient's wishes about whether, and how, to incorporate them in a treatment plan.

4.1.2   *Who should provide spiritual care?*

Because spiritual need may appear in any or all domains of human experience, all practitioners can expect to encounter it as an integral aspect of treatment in some patients. However, while spiritual issues emerge within healthcare contexts, the implications range well beyond the scope of healthcare disciplines. It seems reasonable then to suggest that medical personnel are responsible in the recognition of spiritual need but not necessarily in the attempt to meet it themselves. It also seems reasonable to warn against attempting to confine spiritual issues to clinical areas of expertise, by treating them as a further complication of the symptoms and experiences from which they arise.

In so far as spirituality is grounded in human and humanising relationships, spiritual care begins with good care, respect, openness, and willingness to engage with the other as a person. Spiritual care thus has the potential to take practitioners beyond the realm of their expertise into the human experience they share in common with patients.

4.2   *Strategies for spiritual care*

As already reported, competencies for spiritual care are more about relational capacity and communication skills than about specific knowledge or specialist skills in spirituality per se. An excellent evidence-informed practical guide to communication around end-of-life issues is provided in *Clinical Practice Guidelines for Communicating Prognosis and End-of-life Issues with Adults in the Advanced Stages of a Life-limiting Illness, and their Caregivers*,[65] although admittedly the guidelines are sparse when it comes to explicit discussion of spiritual issues.

As with other aspects of supportive care, spiritual care can also be structured in a tiered approach.[66,67] In such models it becomes the responsibility of each practitioner to decide the levels at which he or she is competent to operate, and to organise referral for levels of practice beyond his or her competence or capacity. Some will choose to refer almost immediately when spiritual issues are raised; others will accompany their patients for a considerable part of the journey.

In practice, the multiple ways in which the word spirituality may be used suggests it may not be appropriate to introduce it into a conversation until it becomes obvious that spirituality is a term with which a patient feels comfortable. As spiritual and existential issues are strongly linked with meaning, one avenue into discussion is to explore the 'explanatory framework'[68] or model through which patients understand their illness. Kleinman suggests a series of questions to do this[69]:

- What do you think has caused your problem?
- Why do you think it started when it did?
- What do you think your sickness does to you?
- How does it work?
- How severe is your sickness?
- What kind of treatment do you think you should receive?

Discussing the explanatory models through which patients approach their illness not only gives an opportunity for beliefs and values to be introduced, using spiritual language if a patient so desires; but also provides the opportunity to clarify with patients the different explanatory model with which the clinician operates.

Finally, the main categories of spiritual care strategy can usefully be described as attention to settings, to stories, and to systems of belief.[70]

Settings are the contexts of self-care and informal care in which all professional interventions are embedded. It is important to remember that the actual time patients spend in professional care (be it institutional care or office appointments) is usually a small fraction of the time spent living with life-threatening illness. Hence encouragement of self-care strategies, support of informal carers, and referral to community resources, is vital. Spiritual care is not provided principally by clinicians, but by communities of family, friends, colleagues, local community groups and associations in which people live their lives. Clinicians can encourage patients to use these resources and explore further options, but cannot substitute for them. In this respect spiritual care, as with end-of-life care in general, is a public health issue[71-73] and clinical organisations would do well to seek community partnerships that support self-care and informal carers in the community.

Stories are the vehicle through which people process present experience and link it with their own past experiences and other stories — personal, cultural, religious — that transcend their own limited perspective.[74] The narratives that support identity and purpose are disrupted by serious illness[75, 52] and must be revised in order to accommodate a changed sense of self, a different community, and a revised purpose. Listening to stories, assisting people to recover damaged or forgotten strands of their story and to achieve a new coherence, is something to which clinicians can contribute. Through careful listening,[76,64] by encouraging patients to mobilise all the resources at their disposal, and not tacitly permitting them to reduce their story to that of a patient in treatment,[52,77] practitioners can elicit and enrich storytelling. Stories can provide the integration of experience that is at the heart of spirituality.

Systems of belief are best dealt with by referral. This is not to say that clinicians should not enquire about them, but that issues clearly related to religious or spiritual institutions are best dealt with by practitioners authorised by those institutions. Often this will involve a referral into the community, perhaps via a pastoral care, or chaplaincy department if care is being provided in a hospital context.

5.   Conclusion

It is clear, then, that spiritual care should take a cooperative, multi-disciplinary, competency-based approach. This in turn requires that clinicians increase their capacity to refer for supportive issues, in particular spiritual issues, as well as symptom control.[78,79] Nevertheless, the foundational capacities for spiritual care tend to be those of good care-giving in general: flexibility, openness, and the ability to communicate. Spiritual care begins with encouraging patients to create the space in their lives for reflective engagement with existential-spiritual issues. It may or may not lead to active intervention on the clinician's part. If it does, it should be because the patient has requested this. Involvement in spiritual care beyond the affirmation and encouragement outlined above is not a professional obligation, but an offering made from recognising and responding from our common humanity.

References

1. P. Speck, The meaning of spirituality in illness. In: *The Spiritual Challenge of Health Care*, eds. M. Cobb and V. Robshaw (Churchill Livingstone, London, 1998), pp. 21–33.
2. R. Sloan, E. Bagiella and T. Powell, Religion, spirituality and medicine, *Lancet* **353**: 664–667 (1999).
3. H. Peach, Religion, spirituality and health: How should Australia's medical professionals respond? *Med. J. Aust.* **178**: 86–88 (2003).
4. H. Koenig, Religion, spirituality and health: An American physician's response, *Med. J. Aust.* **178**: 51–52 (2003).
5. L. Vandercreek, Should physicians discuss spiritual concerns with patients? *J. Relig. Health* **38**: 193–201 (1999).
6. W. Kaufman, ed. *Existentialism from Dostoevsky to Sartre* (Meridian, New York, 1956).
7. S. Wein, Is courage the counterpoint of demoralization? *J. Palliat. Care* **23**: 40–43 (2007).
8. I. Yalom, *Existential Psychotherapy* (Basic Books, New York, 1980).
9. M. Lavoie, D. Blondeau and T. De Koninck, The dying person: An existential being until the end of life, *Nurs. Philos.* **9**: 89–97 (2008).
10. P. Heelas and K. Woodward with B. Seel, B. Szerszynski and K. Tusting, *The Spiritual Revolution: Why Religion is Giving Way to Spirituality* (Blackwell, Oxford, 2005).
11. M. Stefanek, P. McDonald and S. Hess, Religion, spirituality and cancer: Current status and methodological challenges, *Psychooncology* **14**: 450–463 (2005).

12. M. Schlehofer, A. M. Omoto and J. R. Adelman, How do 'religion' and 'spirituality' differ? Lay definitions among older adults, *J. Sci. Study Relig.* **47**: 411–425 (2008).

13. M. Cobb, *The Dying Soul: Spiritual Care at the End of Life* (Open University Press, Buckingham, 2001).

14. P. Heelas, *The New Age Movement: The Celebration of the Self and the Sacralization of Modernity* (Blackwell, Oxford, 1996).

15. P. Heelas, *Spiritualities of Life: New Age Romanticism and Consumptive Capitalism* (Blackwell, Oxford, 1998).

16. W. Law, *A Serious Call to a Devout and Holy Life* (Fontana, London, 1965 [1728]).

17. T. Walter, *The Eclipse of Eternity: A Sociology of the Afterlife* (Macmillan, London, 1996).

18. B. Rumbold, Guidelines concerning spirituality and spiritual care in palliative care. In: *Spirituality and Palliative Care: Social and Pastoral Perspectives,* ed. B. Rumbold (Oxford University Press, Melbourne, 2002), pp. 221–228.

19. M. Wright, Good for the soul? The spiritual dimension of hospice and palliative care. In: *Palliative Care Nursing: Principles and Evidence for Practice,* eds. S. Payne, J. Seymour and C. Ingleton (Open University Press, Maidenhead, 2004), pp. 218–240.

20. W. Breitbart, Spirituality and meaning in cancer, *Rev. Francoph. Psycho-Oncol.* **4**: 237–240 (2005).

21. B. Rumbold, Spiritual dimensions in palliative care. In: *The Creative Option of Palliative Care: A Manual for Health Professionals,* eds. P. Hodder and A. Turley (Melbourne City Mission, Melbourne, 1989), pp. 110–127.

22. B. Rumbold, Caring for the spirit: Lessons from working with the dying, *Med. J. Aust.* **179**: S11–S13 (2002).

23. J. Paley, Spirituality and nursing: A reductionist approach, *Nurs. Philos.* **9**: 3–18 (2008).

24. M. Gysels and I. Higginson with M. Rajasekaran, E. Davies and R. Harding, *Improving Supportive and Palliative Care for Adults with Cancer: Research Evidence Manual* (King's College, London, 2004).

25. National Institute of Clinical Excellence (NICE), *Guidance on Cancer Services: Improving Supportive and Palliative Care for Adults with Cancer* (NICE, London, 2004).

26. A. Girgis, C. Johnson, D. Currow, A. Waller, L. Kristjanson, G. Mitchell, P. Yates, A. Neil, B. Kelly, M. Tattersall and D. Bowman,

Palliative Care Needs Assessment Guidelines (The Centre for Health Research and Psycho-oncology, Newcastle, NSW, 2006).

27. M. Little, K. Paul, C. Jordens C and E. Sayers, Survivorship and discourses of identity, *Psychooncology* **11**: 170–178 (2002).

28. National Breast Cancer Centre and National Cancer Control Initiative, *Clinical Practice Guidelines for the Psychosocial Care of Adults with Cancer* (National Breast Cancer Centre, Camperdown, NSW, 2003).

29. C. Blinderman and N. Cherny, Existential issues do not necessarily result in existential suffering: Lessons from cancer patients in Israel, *Palliat. Med.* **19**: 371–380 (2005).

30. I. Higginson and M. Constantini, Dying with cancer, living well with advanced cancer, *Eur. J. Cancer* **44**: 1414–1424 (2008).

31. H. Whitford, I. N. Olver and M. J. Peterson, Spirituality as a core domain in the assessment of quality of life in oncology, *Psychooncology* **17**: 1121–1128 (2008).

32. C. Saunders, The philosophy of terminal care. In: *The Management of Terminal Disease,* ed. C. Saunders (Edward Arnold, London, 1978), pp. 193–202.

33. C. Saunders, Into the valley of the shadow of death: A personal therapeutic journey, *Br. Med. J.* **313**: 1599–1601 (1996).

34. J. T. Chibnall, S. Videen, P. Duckro and D. K. Miller, Psychosocial-spiritual correlates of death distress in patients with life-threatening medical conditions, *Palliat. Med.* **16**: 331–338 (2002).

35. C. S. McClain, B. Rosenfeld and W. Breitbart, Effect of spiritual wellbeing on end-of-life despair in terminally-ill cancer patients, *Lancet* **361**: 1603–1607 (2003).

36. M. Brady, A. Peterman, G. Fitchett, M. Mo and D. Cella, A case for including spirituality in quality of life measurement in oncology, *Psychooncology* **8**: 417–428 (1999).

37. H. Chochinov and B. Cann, Interventions to enhance the spiritual aspects of dying, *J. Palliat. Med.* **8**: S103–S115 (2005).

38. P. McGrath, Spiritual pain: A comparison of findings from survivors and hospice patients, *Am. J. Hosp. Palliat. Care* **20**: 23–33 (2003).

39. H. Murata and T. Morita, Conceptualization of psycho-existential suffering by a Japanese task force: The first step of a nationwide project, *Palliat. Support. Care* **4**: 279–285 (2006).

40. T. Walter, Spirituality in palliative care: Opportunity or burden? *Palliat. Med.* **16**: 133–139 (2002).

41. E. Cassell, *The Nature of Suffering and the Goals of Medicine,* 2nd ed. (Oxford University Press, New York, 2004), pp. 361.

42. P. Rousseau, Spirituality and the dying patient, *J. Clin. Oncol.* **18**: 2000–2002 (2000).

43. W. Breitbart, Spirituality and meaning in supportive care: Spirituality- and meaning-centered group psychotherapy interventions in advanced cancer, *Support. Care Cancer* **10**: 272–278 (2002).

44. P. Wall, *Pain: The Science of Suffering* (Weidenfeld & Nicholson, London, 1999), pp. 161.

45. C. Gaston and G. Mitchell, Information giving and decision-making in patients with advanced cancer: A systematic review, *Soc. Sci. Med.* **61**: 2252–2264 (2005).

46. T. Balboni, L. Vanderwerker, S. Block, M. E. Paulk, C. Lathan, J. R. Peteet and H. G. Prigerson, Religiousness and spiritual support among advanced cancer patients and associations with end-of-life treatment preferences and quality of life, *J. Clin. Oncol.* **25**: 555–560 (2007).

47. M. White and M. Verhoef, Cancer as part of the journey: The role of spirituality in the decision to decline conventional prostate cancer treatment and to use complementary and alternative medicine, *Integr. Cancer Ther.* **5**: 117–122 (2006).

48. C. Gaston and G. Mitchell, Information giving and decision-making in patients with advanced cancer: A systematic review, *Soc. Sci. Med.* **61**: 2252–2264, p. 2261 (2005).

49. S. Desharnais, R. Carter, W. Hennessy, J. Kurent and C. Carter, Lack of concordance between physician and patient: Reports on end-of-life care discussions, *J. Palliat. Med.* **10**: 728–740 (2007).

50. C. Farren, C. Wilken and J. Popovich, Clinical assessment of hope, *Issues Ment. Health* **13**: 129–138 (1992).

51. B. Rumbold, *Helplessness and Hope: Pastoral Care in Terminal Illness* (SCM Press, London, 1986).

52. A. Frank, *The Wounded Storyteller: Body, Illness and Ethics* (University of Chicago Press, Chicago, 1995).

53. A. Furnham, The psychology of complementary and alternative medicine, *Evid. Based Integr. Med.* **1**: 57–64 (2003).

54. F. Bishop and L. Yardley, Constructing agency in treatment decisions: Negotiating responsibility in cancer, *Health* **8**: 465–482 (2004).

55. E. Grant, S. Murray, M. Kendall, K. Boyd, S. Tilley and D. Ryan, Spiritual issues and needs: Perspectives from patients with advanced

cancer and non-malignant disease. A qualitative study, *Palliat. Support. Care* **2**: 371–378 (2004).

56. P. Mueller, D. Plevak and T. Rummans, Religious involvement, spirituality and medicine: Implications for clinical practice, *Mayo Clin. Proc.* **76**: 1225–1235 (2001).

57. C. Puchalski and D. Larson, Developing curricula in spirituality and medicine, *Acad. Med.* **73**: 970–974 (1998).

58. R. D'Souza, The importance of spirituality in medicine and its application to clinical practice, *Med. J. Aust.* **186**: S57–S59 (2007).

59. W. Larimore, M. Parker and M. Crowther, Should clinicians incorporate positive spirituality into their practices? What does the evidence say? *Ann. Behav. Med.* **24**: 69–73 (2002).

60. Fetzer Institute, *Multidimensional Measurement of Religiousness/Spirituality for Use in Health Research: A Report of the Fetzer Institute/National Institute on Aging Working Group* (Fetzer Institute Kalamazoo, Michigan, 1999).

61. E. Idler, M. Musick, C. Ellison *et al.*, Measuring multiple dimensions of religion and spirituality for health research, *Res. Aging* **25**: 327–365 (2003).

62. B. Rumbold, A review of spiritual assessment in health care practice, *Med. J. Aust.* **186**: S60–S62 (2007).

63. C. M. Puchalski and A. Romer, Taking a spiritual history allows clinicians to understand patients more fully, *J. Palliat. Med.* **3**: 129–137 (2000).

64. C. M. Puchalski, Spirituality and the care of patients at the end-of-life: An essential component of care, *Omega* **56**: 33–46 (2008).

65 J. Clayton, K. Hancock, P. Butow, M. Tattersall and D. Currow, Clinical practice guidelines for communicating prognosis and end-of-life issues with adults in the advanced stages of a life-limiting illness, and their caregivers, *Med. J. Aust.* **186**: S77–S108 (2007).

66. M. Fitch, Supportive care for cancer patients, *Hosp. Quart.* **3**: 39–46 (2000).

67. T. Gordon and D. Mitchell, A competency model for the assessment and delivery of spiritual care, *Palliat. Med.* **18**: 646–651 (2004).

68. S. Dein, *Culture and Cancer Care: Anthropological Insights in Oncology* (Open University Press, Maidenhead, 2006), pp. 24–27.

69. A. Kleinman, *The Illness Narratives: Suffering, Healing and the Human Condition* (Basic Books, New York, 1986), pp. 227–251.

70. A. Kellehear, Spirituality and palliative care: A model of needs, *Palliat. Med.* **14**: 149–155 (2000).

71. A. Kellehear, *Compassionate Cities: Public Health and End of Life Care* (Routledge, London, 2005).

72. J. Rao, L. Anderson and S. Smith, End of life is a public health issue, *Am. J. Prev. Med.* **23**: 215–220 (2002).

73. J. Rao, J. Alongi, L. Anderson, L. Jenkins, G. Stokes and M. Kane, Development of public health priorities for end-of-life initiatives, *Am. J. Prev. Med.* **29**: 453–460 (2005).

74. A. McIntyre, *After Virtue: A Study in Moral Theory* (Duckworth, London, 1986).

75. M. Bury, Illness narratives: Fact or fiction?, *Soc. Health Illness* **23**: 263–285 (2001).

76. R. Choron, *Narrative Medicine: Honouring the Stories of Illness* (Oxford University Press, New York, 2006).

77. B. Hurwitz, T. Greenhalgh and V. Skultans, eds., *Narrative Research in Health and Illness* (Blackwell, Oxford, 2004).

78. C. Johnson, A. Girgis, C. Paul and D. Currow, Cancer specialists' palliative care referral practices and perceptions: Results of a national survey, *Palliat. Med.* **22**: 51–57 (2008).

79. C. Willard and K. Luker, Supportive care in the cancer setting: Rhetoric or reality? *Palliat. Med.* **19**: 328–333 (2005).

Index

ablation   507, 510, 526
acute and late effects   179
acute compartment syndrome
   569, 570, 593
adolescent   885, 887, 888, 890,
   892, 897, 898, 900
alcohol   1078, 1092
amputation   570, 582, 585, 592,
   595, 596
anaemia   783–793, 797, 800,
   801
anticoagulant therapy   753, 755,
   765, 766, 768, 769
appendicitis   422, 428, 432

biliary obstruction   422, 429, 430,
   431
body mass index (BMI)   52–54,
   68
bowel
      function   465, 466, 468–473,
         478

obstruction   422, 425, 426,
   428
perforation   421–424
BRCA (breast cancer)   984,
989–993
   BRCA1 mutation   933–937
   BRCA2 mutation   933, 935
breast cancer   111, 113, 114,
   118–121, 124, 125, 984, 989,
   990, 991, 996

cancer   33, 34, 40–43, 161–170,
   172–175, 231–235, 239–246,
   248–252, 256, 317–319,
   322–333, 885–902, 917–926,
   1047–1056, 1058–1061
   aetiology   80
   cluster   132, 133, 151, 152,
      153
   oncology   647, 657, 663, 664
   survivor   1005, 1008–1010,
      1012–1015, 1018

cardiac tumour 859–862, 864, 865, 869
cardiotoxicity 871–876
cerebral metastases 345, 347, 352, 354
cervical cancer 550–554
challenge 918, 923
chemoprevention 941, 946, 948, 949, 952, 953, 955
chemotherapy 161, 162, 165, 167–175, 231–234, 236–238, 243–246, 250, 251, 253–256, 507, 510, 516, 518, 520–522, 525, 527–529, 813–827
childhood 1047–1051, 1053–1061
Chinese herbs 290–304
cholangiocarcinoma 519
cholecystitis 422, 428, 429, 430
colonic obstruction 834, 842–844
colorectal cancer 971–975, 977, 978, 985–988
colorectal liver metastases 520–522, 526
communication 317, 318, 320, 322, 325–327, 328, 330, 333
co-morbidity 909, 910, 913–915
complications 627, 628, 630, 637–639, 642
comprehensive geriatric assessment 910
consumer product 132, 133, 149, 151
cryopreservation 729, 737, 739–743, 746

debulking surgery 561
deep vein thrombosis 352, 353, 754, 762

diagnosis 367–372, 627, 628, 630, 631, 637
diet 49–51, 58, 62, 68
dietary
    counseling 268
    intake 267, 271, 274, 275, 278, 279
    supplement 1077, 1078, 1085–1087, 1089, 1090
    vitamin D 85, 86, 90, 96, 99, 102, 103
distress 1023, 1027, 1028, 1034, 1035, 1037–1040
drug-herb interaction 287, 288, 290, 294, 295, 297

early and differential diagnosis 604, 606
embryo 729, 735–737, 739–742, 746
end of life 1139, 1140, 1145–1148, 1153, 1154
endometrial cancer 111, 112, 115, 121, 125
ENT surgeon 673, 678, 679, 684, 691, 693, 695–698
enteral nutrition 439, 443, 449–455, 457–459
environmental
    carcinogen 147, 150
    tobacco smoke 6, 9, 10, 11
erectile dysfunction 628, 638, 640
erythropoietin 783, 786, 787, 790–793, 797, 801
existential issues 1139–1141, 1145, 1153

Familial Adenomatous Polyposis (FAP)   934, 937

family history   941, 943, 944, 947, 952–954

fast track surgery   439–441

febrile neutropenia   212, 213, 215–220, 227

fertility preservation   730, 731, 737, 746

flap   650–662, 664–668

foetus   231–240, 242, 245, 249, 250, 252, 253, 256

fruit   1078, 1079, 1081, 1085, 1087, 1088, 1092

gastroduodenal obstruction   834, 838, 839, 842

gastrointestinal
   bleeding   422, 431
   dysmotility   487, 488, 493, 494
   malignancies   439, 440

general practice   918–920, 1121–1124, 1126, 1127, 1129, 1130, 1133

genetic susceptibility   932, 933, 937

genetic testing   931, 932, 934–938

germline mutation   932

granulocyte colony stimulating factor   783, 794

head and neck cancer   674–677, 679, 681, 683–685, 691–698

health information   317, 319, 320, 322–327

health seeking behaviour   319–326, 333

help lines   33

heparin   754, 755, 760, 764, 765, 767

hepatitis B   813–827

hepatocellular carcinoma   507–510, 518

hereditary nonpolyposis colorectal cancer (HNPCC)   972–975, 977

hormone replacement therapy (HRT)   111–113, 116–125

hyponatraemia   201, 204–206, 209

hysterectomy   548, 551, 553, 554, 559

impending fracture   574–577

incontinence   627, 628, 639, 640, 642

infection   570, 571, 585, 587, 589, 590, 593

Internet   317–319, 322–327, 331

intimacy   1028, 1036, 1041

ischaemic heart disease   871

lamivudine   813, 820–825, 827

late effects   1048–1050, 1054, 1059–1061

Li-Fraumeni syndrome   935

lung cancer   368–370, 372, 380–384

lymphoedema   603–622

Lynch syndrome   969, 972, 974, 977

malabsorption   487–489, 495

malignancy   784, 786, 800, 801

malignant biliary obstruction   845, 846

malignant bowel obstruction 225, 226

malnutrition 267, 269–273, 279, 443, 445–449, 455, 459

massive haemoptysis 222, 223

mature practice 1123, 1126

mediastinal tumour 862, 873, 879

medical oncology 286–288, 302, 304

microsurgery 648, 656

mismatch repair 982, 985, 986, 988, 990

multidisciplinary team 673, 696–698

Multiple Endocrine Neoplasia (Types 1 and 2) 934

needs assessment 1101

neuro-cognitive outcome 354

neuroendocrine liver metastases 508, 528, 529

neurosurgery 350

neutropenia 783, 792–797, 801

neutropenic enterocolitis 422, 427–429

normal tissues 179, 180, 182, 183

nutrition 51, 268–275, 278, 279, 1077, 1078, 1080, 1087

nutritional
  management 495–498
  risk assessment 271, 439, 447

obesity 1078–1080

occupational cancer 131, 133–135, 137, 139, 140, 395, 396, 397, 399–401, 404, 414, 415

oesophageal obstruction 834, 835, 838

oestrogen 111–113, 117–125

oncogeriatric 911, 913

oocyte 729, 732, 734, 736–742

oophorectomy 548

opportunity 918, 921

oral contraceptive 111–116, 122, 124, 125

orthopedic oncologic emergency 569, 570

outcome expectation 604, 607, 610, 612, 616, 619, 622

ovarian cancer 111, 112, 114, 115, 120, 121, 125, 548, 559–563

overweight 1079, 1080

paediatric 1054

palliative care 1099–1114, 1121, 1122, 1124–1130, 1133

pancreatectomy 488, 489, 491, 492, 495, 497

pancreatic cancer 488

pancreatic insufficiency 489, 496

paraneoplastic syndrome 161, 163, 164, 172

parenteral nutrition 439, 449, 450, 452–455, 457–459

pathologic fracture 569–571, 573–586, 595, 596

patient-centred best practice 1121–1123, 1126, 1128, 1133

pericardial effusion 223–225

peri-operative care 440, 441

Peutz-Jeghers syndrome 934

pharmacotherapy 33, 35, 42, 43

physical activity 49–51, 54, 65–68, 1077, 1078, 1081–1084

phytoestrogen   1085, 1090, 1091
plastic surgery   655, 668
pollution   131, 133, 141–143, 145, 146, 148, 149
poly (ADP-ribose) polymerase PARP inhibitor   937
polypharmacy   910
polyposis   971, 972, 974, 976, 977
pregnancy   231–246, 248–256
premature ovarian failure   733, 738
primary care   917–924, 926
progestogen   111–114, 117–121, 125
prognosis   703, 704, 706, 707, 715
prognostic nutritional index   447
prophylaxis   753–755, 759–761, 767, 769, 814, 819, 821–826
prostate cancer   628, 632, 633, 635, 636
psychiatric disorder   1005, 1006, 1017
psychological
    consequences   465, 478
    distress   1005
psycho-social adjustment   1005, 1006, 1008, 1011–1014, 1018
psychosocial well-being   1005
pulmonary embolism   352–354, 754, 763

quality of life   487, 488, 490, 498, 1025–1028, 1030, 1032, 1033, 1035, 1038, 1039, 1139, 1140, 1145, 1146

radiation therapy   179
radical hysterectomy   548, 551, 553, 554, 627–634, 637–642

radioactive iodine   703, 704, 707–710, 714, 717, 718
raised intracranial pressure   208, 209
reactivation   814–816, 818–826
reconstruction   647–668
    graft   649–652, 657, 658, 660–662
rectal cancer   465–470, 472–475, 478
recurrence   627–637, 1025, 1027, 1029, 1031–1033, 1039
response shift   1028
restoration   729, 743
retinoblastoma   934
risk-reducing
    mastectomy   946, 955
    salpingo-oophorectomy 946, 947

sarcoma   520, 529
self-care   1122, 1129, 1130
self-concept   1026–1028, 1032, 1038
service planning   1105, 1112
sex hormone   736, 745
sexual dysfunction   465, 474, 478
sexuality   1037
shared decision making   318, 328
side effects   161–163, 167–169, 174
smoking cessation   33–37, 39–43
soy   1086, 1090, 1091
spermatogenesis   734, 736, 743
spinal cord compression 210–212, 226, 569–571, 585
spinal metastases   356, 358
spirituality   1139–1144, 1146, 1147, 1149, 1151–1154

staging   367, 369, 370, 372–378, 380, 381, 395, 396, 399, 401, 402, 406, 408

stenting   836–845, 848, 852

stoma   465–467, 471, 472, 474, 478

sun exposure   79, 81, 83, 84, 87–95, 98, 99, 101–105

superficial thrombophlebitis   754, 763, 766

superior vena caval (SVC) obstruction   221, 222

supportive care   1099–1102, 1105

surgery   367–369, 371, 378, 380–383, 395, 396, 402–404, 407–413, 415, 507, 508, 518–529

survival   396, 402, 404–407, 412, 414

survivor   1047–1061

survivorship   1025, 1027, 1032, 1035, 1039, 1040

tamoxifen   941, 946, 948, 949, 955

teachable moment   2, 12, 16

teamwork   1121, 1124, 1125

terminal care   1101, 1106, 1112

thrombocytopenia   783, 784, 797–801

thyroglobulin   703, 704, 706, 708, 712, 713, 716, 718, 719

thyroid
  hormone   703, 704, 707, 709, 711–713
  neoplasm   704–706, 720

tobacco   1–15, 17–20, 22, 23

transfusion   783–793, 797, 798, 800, 801

treatment   703, 704, 707, 709–711, 713, 715–720
  effect   18
  option   604
  outcome   1026, 1038, 1039

tumour lysis syndrome   206

tumour testing   981, 982, 984–986, 989, 991, 996

UV radiation   80

vegetables   1078, 1081, 1084, 1085, 1087, 1088, 1092

vitamin D levels   82, 83, 86, 90, 91, 99, 101–103, 105

vitamin K antagonist   756, 760, 761

Von-Hippel Lindau syndrome   934

vulvar cancer   548, 554–559

vulvectomy   555–558

well-being   1025, 1027, 1033, 1040, 1139, 1145, 1146

young adult   887, 888, 900